DEDICATION

The twelfth edition of Healthy Healing is dedicated to the profound role that the higher spirit of the universe plays in our everyday health and happiness. Our hearts instinctively reach toward a higher force beyond ouselves. We may turn from it when we reach the limits of our understanding. Our scientific successes may seem to obscure the real force behind all science. Yet it is always there—unmoving, eternal energy—expressed to each of us in every wonder of our lives. Sometimes we can see it more clearly if we think of angels as the part of this marvelous, universal force that can touch us and that we can recognize with our own highest selves.

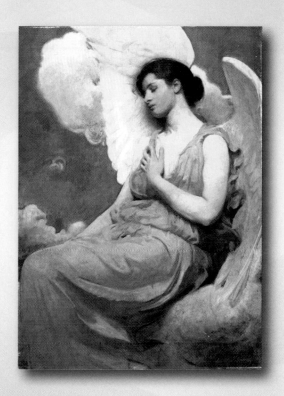

Look throughout this book for sayings of the spirit that might speak to you. I've collected sayings that mean something to me all my life. I use them in my life (and in all my books when I have a little extra room), as an easy way to inspire the spirit of healing. A simple technique of focusing on a saying that fits a situation while you breathe deeply really works to recenter your mind and spirit, and open channels for healing. In many healing circles, this technique is believed to open the crown chakra, allowing healing spirit energy to flow more smoothly through the body.

Even one miracle cure can show the value of a therapy with the body's own healing powers. When the evidence is good enough to affect the behavior of researchers, why pretend it is too preliminary for consumers? If a therapy is natural, non-invasive and does no harm, consumers should be able to act upon it as a valid choice.

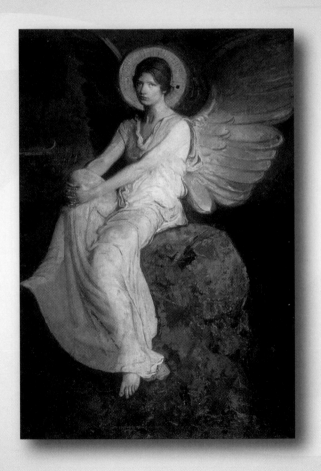

The highest calling of the healer

is to rally the mind and body against the disease.

After a forest fire in Yellowstone National Park, forest rangers began their trek up a mountain to assess the inferno's damage. One ranger found a bird literally petrified in ashes, perched statuesquely on the ground at the base of a tree. Somewhat sickened by the eerie sight, he knocked over the bird with a stick. When he gently struck it, three tiny chicks scurried from under their dead mother's wings. The loving mother, keenly aware of impending disaster, had carried her offspring to the base of the tree and had gathered them under her wings, instinctively knowing that the toxic smoke would rise. She could have flown to safety but had refused to abandon her babies. When the blaze had arrived and the heat had scorched her small body, the mother had remained steadfast. Because she had been willing to die, those under the cover of her wings would live. Being loved this much makes a huge difference in your life… and then you become different because of it.

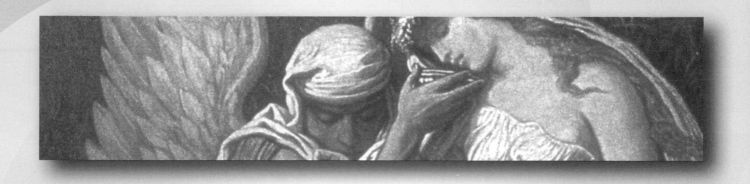

Healing comes in many ways… even a hug can rescue a life. A newspaper article recently detailed the first week of life of a set of twins. Each were in their respective incubators, but one was not expected to live. A hospital nurse fought against the hospital rules that separated the babies and moved them to the same incubator for comfort. When they were placed in the same incubator, the healthier of the two threw an arm over her sister in an endearing embrace. The smaller baby's heart rate stabilized and her temperature rose to normal. She got a new chance for life.

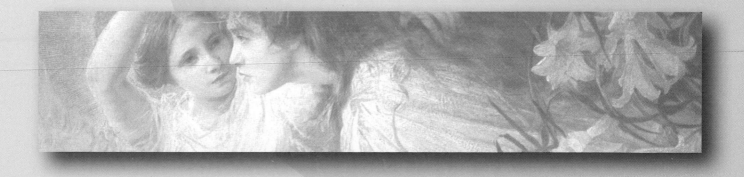

Linda Page, N.D., Ph.D.

Long before natural foods and herbal formulas became a "chic," widely accepted method for healing, Linda Page was sharing her extensive knowledge with those who dared to listen.

Through what some would call an accident of fate but she calls a blessing, she was compelled to research alternative avenues of healing. Sequestered in a hospital with a life-threatening illness, watching her 5-foot frame wither to 69 pounds, her hair drop out, and her skin peel off, doctors told her they had no cure. With only a cursory knowledge of herbs, she began a frantic research process of testing herbal formulas and healing food combinations on herself. She read voraciously about herbal healing. Good friends shopped for herbs and she began to formulate the many compounds, which would eventually save her life, revitalize her health and restore beautiful new hair and skin. It was that incident that led her to seek her degrees in Naturopathy and Nutrition from Clayton College of Natural Health in Birmingham, Alabama, where she is now adjunct professor.

Linda's rewarding career as a leader in natural health and healing spans almost three decades. She is a prolific author and educator. Her best-selling book, *Healthy Healing™– A Guide To Self-Healing For Everyone*, is used as a textbook at many higher educational institutions teaching natural health courses. She has also written other books including: *Cooking For Healthy Healing, How To Be Your Own Herbal Pharmacist, Party Lights, Detoxification* and a popular series of library books which address specific healing therapies for topics like menopause, weight loss, sexuality, colds and flu and cancer.

A master classical herbalist, she founded the herbal nutrition company, Crystal Star® in 1978 and she has formulated over 250 whole herb combinations. She received some of the first United States Patents for herbal formulations for her women's hormone balancing formulas.

Linda is in demand by the media and she has appeared weekly on CBS television with a report on natural healing; she is a principle speaker at national health symposiums and conventions; she is featured regularly in national magazines and newspapers; she appears on hundreds of radio and television programs and she regularly contributes to WebMD and other health websites. Currently, she is featured on the television program, "The World of Healthy Healing" airing on PBS television and she leads educational tours to destinations as China, Southwest USA and Kauai, Hawaii.

Today, Linda delights in having come full circle. "I am so grateful that knowledge of healing through herbal formulas and good foods is becoming so widespread. I see it as an opportunity for people to seize the power to heal themselves. Knowledge is power. Whether one chooses conventional medicine, alternative healing avenues, or combines them both in a complementary process, the real prescription for healing is knowledge."

Linda has spoken before Congressional and Senate Committees on behalf of DSHEA and she continues to be a staunch advocate for the freedom of all to choose natural health protocols and products. She is a member of The American Naturopathic Medical Association, The California Naturopathic Association, The American Herbalist Guild, The American Botanical Council and The Herb Research Foundation.

About the Cover

The new "Self Healing for Everyone" cover design for the twelfth edition reminds us
that natural healing is eternal, universal and all around us.
The many colors of the cover recalls the wonderful
rainbow of our world.
The energy swirl surrounding a bright point of light speaks
to the spiritual quality that is always part
of real healing.

Natural healing helps us grow in maturity.
In order to use it we must take a measure of responsibility for our health.
In order to help the world's great rainbow of peoples
we must keep adding to our wisdom.
It brings us together because it helps us care for each other.

Natural healing represents timeless knowledge.
It is for everyone.

Neither drugs nor herbs nor vitamins are a cure for anything.
The body heals itself.
The human body is incredibly intelligent.
It usually responds to intelligent therapies.
The healing professional can help this process
by offering intelligent therapies.

My thanks to:
the design talent of Michael Kohler for the cover and inspiring "angel pages;"
the enormous coordination and promotional effort of Leah Thomson;
and the tireless dedication of talented research associate Sarah Abernathy.

This reference is to be used for educational information.
It is not a claim for cure or mitigation of disease, but rather an adjunctive approach,
supplying individual nutritional needs
that otherwise might be lacking
in today's lifestyle.

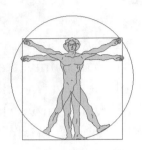

FIRST EDITION, JUNE 1985. COPYRIGHT NOV. 1985.
SECOND EDITION, JANUARY 1986.
THIRD EDITION, REVISED, SEPTEMBER 1986.
FOURTH EDITION, REVISED/UPDATED, MAY 1987.
FIFTH EDITION, NOVEMBER 1987.
SIXTH EDITION, REVISED/UPDATED, JUNE 1988.
SEVENTH EDITION, REVISED/UPDATE, JAN. 1989, SEPT. 1989, MARCH 1990.
EIGHTH EDITION, REVISED/UPDATED/EXPANDED, JULY, 1990.
NINTH EDITION, REVISED/UPDATED/EXPANDED, SEPT., 1992 AND 1994.
TENTH EDITION, REVISED/UPDATED/EXPANDED, 1997 AND 1998.
ELEVENTH EDITION, REVISED/UPDATED, MARCH 2000.
TWELFTH EDITION, REVISED/UPDATED/EXPANDED, SEPTEMBER 2004.
TWELFTH EDITION, REVISED/UPDATED, AUGUST 2006.

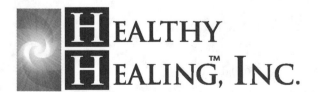

Copyright © August 2006 by Linda Page.
Published by Healthy Healing, Inc.
Internet Address: healthyhealing.com

Publisher's Cataloging-in-Publication
(Provided by Quality Books, Inc.)

Rector-Page, Linda G.
    [Healthy healing]
    Linda Page's healthy healing : a guide to
self-healing for everyone / by Linda Page. -- 12th ed.,
Expanded & updated.
    p. cm.
    Includes bibliographical references and index.
    ISBN 1-884334-92-X
    ISBN 1-884334-93-8 (Spiral bound)

    1. Holistic medicine. 2. Alternative medicine.
3. Diet therapy.   I. Title.

R733.R43 2004   615.5
                                 QBI04-563

Books by Dr. Linda Page

Healthy Healing - *Twelfth Edition, A Guide to Self Healing for Everyone*

Diets for Healthy Healing - *Natural Solutions to America's 10 Biggest Health Problems*

How To Be Your Own Herbal Pharmacist - *Herbal Traditions, Expert Formulations*

Detoxification - *All You Need to Know to Recharge, Renew and Rejuvenate Your Body, Mind and Spirit!*

Cooking For Healthy Healing - Book One: The Healing Diets - *Food Is Your Pharmacy*

Cooking For Healthy Healing - Book Two: The Healing Recipes

The Healthy Healing Library Series
- Revealing The Secrets Of Anti-aging
- Colds, Flu & You - Building Optimum Immunity
- Boosting Immunity With Power Plants
- Renewing Male Health & Energy

Expanded Library Series
- Fatigue Syndromes
- Renewing Female Health
- Menopause & Osteoporosis
- Cancer
- Sexuality
- Weight Loss & Cellulite Control
- Stress & Energy

with Sarah Abernathy

Do You Want to Have a Baby? - *Natural Fertility Solutions and Pregnancy Care*

with Doug Vanderberg

Party Lights - *Healthy Party Foods & Earthwise Entertaining*

Video:
"Unleashing The Healing Power of Herbs"

VISIT www.HealthyHealing.com

Your Complete Online Natural Healing & Wellness Resource.

The official website for Dr. Linda Page, Healthy Healing Publications and Crystal Star products.

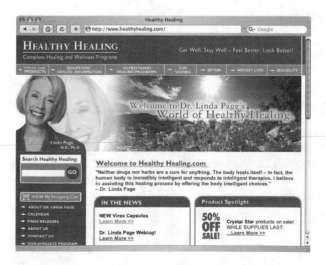

- Extensive Crystal Star Product Information
- Books by Dr. Linda Page
- Dr. Linda Page Weblog
- Free Recipes, Self Tests, Therapy Plans and Articles
- Download Catalogs, Audio Interviews
- Store Locator
- Special Announcement Email Subscription
- Natural Health Tips

Table of Contents

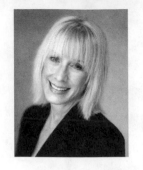

How to use this book....
an old friend with a new look

This book is the 12th Edition of HEALTHY HEALING: A Guide To Self-Healing For Everyone. Whether this is your first look at HEALTHY HEALING or you're an old hand at playing a major role in your health care, this book is a completely new version with a brand new look. Over a million copies have been sold since this book first went into publication in 1985, and many of you have made good suggestions and comments that I have tried to incorporate into each new edition. HEALTHY HEALING 12 now has the larger type and tighter format you've requested, along with updated and expanded information about each ailment. The sideways "Ailments pages" of previous editions are now "pink pages," so they're easier to find and reference right away.

Regardless of its new look and format, HEALTHY HEALING remains a complete, detailed reference for people who are interested in a more personal kind of health care… health care they can practice at home with every confidence that the recommended remedies have been used and found to be effective by hundreds, if not thousands of people. I develop and work with the healing programs over many years; they are constantly updated with new information, often from people who have had success in dealing with the problem themselves. I always believe that the most significant information I can offer is the evidence of people who have used the natural healing methods for themselves, experienced real improvement in their health, and wish to share their success with others. *Check out the "highly recommended" notations for this type of information.*

Every page in HEALTHY HEALING 12 is new, offering you the latest knowledge from a wide network of natural healing professionals - nutritional consultants, holistic practitioners, naturopaths, nurses, world health studies and traditional physicians in America and around the world.

For long-lasting health, your body must do its own work. HEALTHY HEALING's recommendations help rebalance specific areas of your body so that it can function normally. They work with body functions, not outside them. They are free of harmful side effects that traumatize the body.

About the new look:
There are two columns of categories:
1) DIET AND LIFESTYLE SUPPORT THERAPY (including Bodywork Techniques)

No matter what your health problem is, your diet is your primary "go to" healing tool. The diets I recommend are "real people" diets. People with specific health conditions have used them and have related their experiences to me. Over the years, diseases change - and a person's immune response to them changes. HEALTHY HEALING's diet programs are continually modified to meet new, changing health needs.

2) HERB, SUPERFOOD AND SUPPLEMENT THERAPY

There are many effective recommendations to choose from. You can easily put together the best healing program for yourself. *Choosing one recommendation from each healing target under the interceptive therapy plan, for example, then using your choices together, may be considered a complete healing program.*

All given doses are daily amounts unless otherwise specified. The rule of thumb for natural healing is one month for every year you have had the problem.

Note 1: HEALTHY HEALING 12 states when a recommendation is gender or age-specific.

Note 2: You've told me that the "foot" and "hand" reflexology diagrams in previous editions were just too tiny or too indefinite to be useful. If you like to use reflexology as a healing technique, consult *Reflexology: Health at your Fingertips* by Barbara and Kevin Kunz (includes detailed reflexology charts), or visit http://www.reflexology-research.com/ for detailed reflexology charts you can purchase on line, for more detailed help.

Your Health Care Options Today

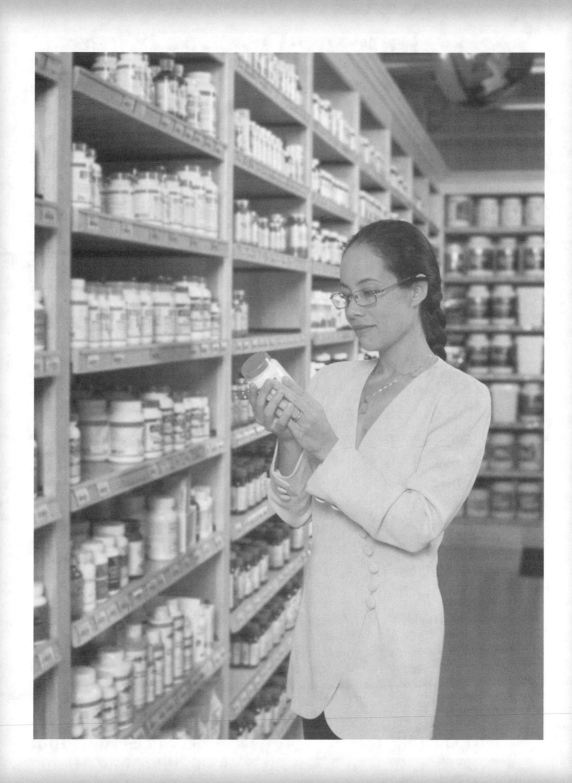

A Clear Look at Your Health Care Options Today

Clearly, Americans want to take more responsibility for their own health care. But what are the real options you have to choose from? How can you judge the pros and cons of conventional and alternative healing systems? Can they work together to complement each other?

What's the difference between drugs and herbal medicines? Can you use them safely together? Can chemical drugs and herbal remedies complement each other? Can you wean yourself off drugs with herbal medicines?

This chapter offers a clear review of the alternative healing systems available today, with a brief analysis of how you can best use each of them.

The important options we'll consider:
- …Naturopathy
- …Homeopathy
- …Chiropractic and Massage Therapy
- …Polarity and Magnet Therapy
- …Hand and Foot Reflexology
- …Acupuncture and Acupressure
- …Biofeedback, Guided Imagery and Hypnotherapy
- …Applied Kinesiology
- …Enzyme Therapy
- …Overheating Therapy
- …Aromatherapy and Flower Essence Therapy
- …Qigong, T'ai Chi Reduce Stress-caused Illness
- …Meditation and Prayer Focus your Healing

We'll also discuss:
- The Pros and Cons of Orthodox and Alternative Medicine
- The Dramatic Rise of Iatrogenic (doctor-caused) Disease
- Fast Healing Techniques after Surgery or Serious Illness
- Drug and Herb Interactions You Should Know About

Your Health Care Options Today

What an explosion of enthusiasm and interest there is in alternative medicine! Sales of herbal products alone have increased by more than 100% since 1994. Researchers estimate that in the next 5 years, up to 96% of all adults in America will be using alternative methods for at least part of their healthcare... even in the medical profession. As orthodox medicine becomes more invasive, and healthcare providers become less in touch with the person who is ill, informed people become more willing to take a measure of responsibility for their own health. The rise of individual, personal health care has begun. But that means lots of answers to thousands of unanswered questions are going to be needed, and America doesn't have a very long history of free and open information about natural healing techniques.

Conventional healthcare today is built upon the pillars of surgery (highly skilled) and drugs (potentially dangerous and open to abuse). Both are literally inaccessible except through a tangled network of third-party red tape, long waits and lots of money. Orthodox medical practice has built a tower of aloofness and indifference that has little to do with intimate care for the individual that must be part of "health care-ing."

Personal health empowerment and traditional healing knowledge in western populations has dropped away as technological advances have become the new health care frontier. Our culture has allowed the entire health care industry to become so powerful and so disproportionately lucrative that it is now in the business of illness rather than health. In one disconcerting example, a cancer physician, returning from an extended vacation, found an empty waiting room. His colleague had been treating his patients nutritionally. The physician wailed, "This is terrible. It took me years to build a long-term, regular patient clientele!"

Thoughtful people everywhere are realizing that much of today's medicine has nothing to do with the quality of our lives.... our doctors receive no reward for maintaining health, only for treating illness. More worrisome still, conventional medicine can only go so far before expense outweighs the value of the treatment. Drug and medical costs, even medical insurance payments, have escalated beyond the reach of most families. After "letting the doctor do it" for decades we are realizing that the doctor can't always do it. A technology based healing system often has to "give up," admitting that there is nothing more that it can do.

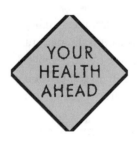

By contrast, alternative natural healing has the goal of giving people a chance to live well.... better than they could without it. It is a philosophy for life. Natural healers never give up. They know you can improve your life no matter what state your health is in. We hear true stories every day of alternative healing methods turning a "death sentence" from modern medicine from days into months and then into years.

Clearly the new twenty-first century finds many people using more natural, less drug-oriented therapies, sometimes as an alternative to conventional medicine, sometimes in a team approach along with it. Health care is personal. To approach it impersonally, through big business and government means that our health is bound to lose.

The problem is that conventional medicine feels that it's losing too. It sees its control of almost a century slipping away, to more personal control (and thus much less revenue). So, it's fighting a rear-guard action. We're bombarded almost daily by self-proclaimed "quackwatchers" dedicated to undermining natural therapies and alternative care practitioners. The media often tells us that there is little scientific evidence to back up the health claims of alternative therapies, particularly herbal remedies. I stand in amazement every time one of these "medical police" comes on CNN and says there's no "hard evidence" that herbs, or other natural remedies, work. They're looking at the picture from the wrong end of the telescope! I'm beginning to wonder if some of these so-called watch dog organizations have had their heads in the sand for the last decade!

In actuality, science is validating herbal medicine by leaps and bounds! People have been demanding more information in spite of government and FDA regulations and bans. And they're getting it! I access a valid study somewhere in the world almost every day from the Internet. The World Health Organization estimates that even today, up to 80% of the world's population still relies on herbal medicine as a primary form of healthcare. Americans shouldn't be the only ones left in the dark.

When you hear that herbal remedies have never been studied or tested, don't believe it. There's an amazing amount of research on every aspect of natural healthcare.... especially herbs. I, myself have participated in some studies with herbal remedies I formulated. The testing was done in a third party lab, funded by the National Institute of Health. Since there aren't enormous monetary rewards to be made from herbal testing results, almost 100% of herbal research is done at universities or third-party labs funded by grants.

But this is not the case for drug tests or studies. They are commissioned and paid for by the drug manufacturing company that stands to benefit from them. This vested interest means that negative information may be rejected, and because the whole process is so horrendously expensive, some aspects of the drug just get overlooked. There's nothing wrong with making money in a business, but after much experience in testing on whole herbs, I believe you can be more confident in testing from the natural healing world. Most companies are small; they don't have big labs. In most instances, they <u>must</u> use third-party, unbiased labs to get their results. In our tests, the results were clear and undeniable... and there was no vested interest bias.

Health is a lifestyle process. It is based in wellness care, not just illness treatment. The best news is that natural remedies work—often far better than prescription drugs for many health conditions.

Orthodox medicine focuses on crisis intervention. Many modern medical techniques were developed during war time, for emergency care, to battle an imminent threat to life. They are at their best in a "heroic mode," bringing up the big guns of surgery and drugs to search out and destroy dangerous organisms. It is the kind of treatment necessary for acute disease, accidents, emergencies and wartime life-saving.

Orthodox medicine is less successful in treating chronic illness. Respected studies show that most illnesses don't just drop out of the sky and hit us over the head. Diseases like arthritis, osteoporosis, high blood pressure, coronary-artery disease, ulcers and hormone imbalances are related to aging and lifestyle. The big guns and emergency measures often don't apply, may be too overwhelming, or even suppress the body's immune response.

Most illness is self-limiting. The human body is a beautifully designed healing system that can meet many of its problems without outside intervention. Even when outside help is needed, healing is enhanced if the patient can be kept free of emotional depression and panic. Emotional trauma impairs immune function by decreasing the body's interleukins, vital immune defense substances. Panic constricts blood vessels, putting an added burden on the heart. Depression intensifies existing diseases, and opens the door to others. There is a direct connection between our mental state and the ability of our immune system to do its job.

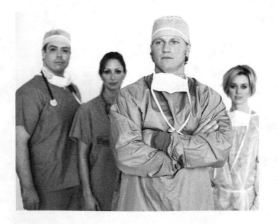

Many U.S. medical schools still don't teach disease prevention, good nutrition or exercise as a part of health. Although alternative techniques are widely accepted in Europe, American physicians downplay the interaction of mind and body, saying that a patient's state of mind does not matter to bacteria or a virus. Objective measures are emphasized—white blood cell counts, blood pressure readings, etc., instead of how the patient feels. For all its brilliant achievements, modern medicine is still pathology oriented. Most doctors see the disease, not the person, and are only trained to use drugs, surgery and laboratory technologies. To paraphrase Abraham Maslow: "If all you're trained to use is a hammer, the whole world looks like a nail."

This approach does not sit well with the informed public today, who want more control over their health problems, and intend to be a part of the decision making process for their health needs.

Conventional medicine teaches that pain means sickness. Pain is treated as a powerful enemy; its symptoms are assaulted with prescription drugs that either mask it or drive it underground — a practice that usually means it will resurface later with increased intensity. We are constantly pressured by the medical community to have exhaustive tests, to be screened for cholesterol, high blood pressure, breast lumps, and cancer cells. If there is acute pain or other symptoms that indicate the need for a doctor, obvious common sense dictates that a doctor should be called, or emergency medical steps taken. But mammography, pap smears, and many other tests are not prevention, simply early detection.

Alternative healers recognize that pain is also the body's way of informing us that we are doing something wrong, not necessarily that something <u>is</u> wrong. Pain can tell us that we are smoking too much, eating too much, or eating the wrong things. It can notify us when there is too much emotional congestion in our lives, or too much daily stress. Pain can be a friend with useful information about our health, so that we can effectively address the cause of a problem.

Many physicians have a financial interest in ordering an array of tests, in performing surgeries, and in prescribing certain medications. Many times, the pressure for testing is driven by these issues rather than for information. The fear of malpractice lawsuits also causes doctors to be overly zealous in ordering tests. Yet medical tests can be hazardous to your health. Faulty diagnoses and inaccurate readings are common in poorly trained, rushed labs. The more tests a person undergoes, the greater the odds of being told, often incorrectly, that something is wrong. Anxiety, even panic, is brought on by needless testing, medication, or treatment, and a brusque or rushed doctor. You can literally worry yourself sick when there is nothing seriously wrong.

Not every problem requires costly, major medical attention. The principles of nature governing health and illness are ageless; they apply equally everywhere at all times. A sensible lifestyle, with healthy food, regular moderate exercise and restful sleep is still the best medicine for many health conditions. Your diet is the most powerful weapon you have for your health. Food nutrients maintain rejuvenative powers, and normalize and rebalance body systems that have gotten out of whack. There is no down time with the laws of nature, and they do not play favorites.

We need to be re-educated about our health—to be less intimidated by doctors and disease. I believe that the greatest ally of alternative medicine will be science itself—not the restricted view of science that assumes its basic concepts are complete, but the open-ended science that sets preconceived notions aside. Today's consumers are not only more aware of alternative health care choices, and more confident in their own healing strength, they also want to do something for themselves to get better. The time has clearly come for a partnership between health care professionals and patients, so that the healing resources from both sides can be optimally employed.

No prescription is more valuable than knowledge. This book is a ready reference for the alternative healthcare choices open to those wishing to take more responsibility for their own well-being. The recommended suggestions are backed up by extensive research into therapies for each ailment, and by contributing healthcare professionals and nutritional consultants from around the country, with many years of eyewitness and hands-on experience in natural healing results.

—I never say throw away your doctor's phone number... We need choices from all kinds of healing. For everyday, non-emergency healing, you may not need to go any further than your own garden or spice rack.

—I do say it's time to return to Mother Nature... I believe that whenever there is a need, Nature provides an answer. Nature's whole, ready-to-use medicines are often the only "prescription" your body needs to get better.

Compare Orthodox and Alternative Medicine

The paradigm shift in medicine at the beginning of this century constituted vast reform for healthcare and medical education. The ability to isolate microbes that cause infectious disease, and to create treatments that would kill those microbes without killing the patient, meant tremendous acceptance for the practice of allopathic medicine, characterizing it as heroic and scientific. But the pendulum swung too far as the sledge hammers of drugs and surgery began to be driven by profit rather than by healing.

Today, there's another paradigm shift in healthcare—one that emphasizes disease prevention instead of disease treatment.

Popular support has changed the way we look at medicine. There is clear evidence that drugs and surgery are often overused, and that human touch is vital to healing. For instance, in the field of mental health, doctors admit that spiritual factors plainly influence disease. An increasing number of MD's now include holistic treatments in their protocols as they see alternative approaches that are more effective, less expensive and safer than drugs.

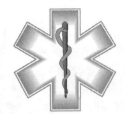 Modern medicine, with drug and laboratory advances as its cornerstones, has had to change its focus because of the enormous rise in chronic diseases. Cancer, diabetes and arthritis (rather than infectious diseases) are the scourge of modern times. Healthcare systems must provide better, safer, less invasive treatments for chronic disorders.

Conventional medicine has so far been devoted to justifying the validity, effectiveness and safety of its science, an emphasis that has resulted in an authoritarian, heavily regulated approach to its action and thinking. Many defend these rigid values and regulations because they have brought about a healthcare system that is arguably the most technologically advanced in the world. Yet, even with the broad medical arsenal available to doctors, they can only cure about one-fourth of the illnesses presented to them.

A report by the U.S. Office of Technology Assessment shows only 10 to 20% of standard medical procedures are effective!

As disease prevention becomes the watchword of wellness, medical strategies need to change. Today's medicine depends on high-tech intervention equipment, surgical procedures, lab tests, a warehouse of antibiotics and powerful biochemicals. Many are hit-or-miss more often than we are willing to admit. They are frequently ineffective, and tend to ignore the person in favor of the illness and its symptoms. Many have serious side effects; some make the patient worse. In spite of a wealth of technology, doctors may have few choices. Drug and surgical treatments can be so dangerous and full of side effects, they are bound to what has been officially approved or authorized. In contrast, alternative medicine methods offer a wide range of choices, often less expensive, and traditionally found effective and much safer.

I feel we need both types of medicine. Clearly, orthodox medicine has saved many lives. Just as clearly, alternative medicine has prevented much illness.

I don't believe there is one "right" path; multi-disciplinary healthcare is a better way. A team approach can take the best tools from each. Most naturopaths believe that building bridges with conventional medicine has tangible benefits. Valuable medical diagnostic tools can monitor a disorder in detail; some drugs can reduce crippling symptoms, often dramatically at first; some new drugs can retard progression of a disease. A study by the New England Journal of Medicine shows American healthcare consumers agree. One in three are using some form of complementary or alternative medicine today.

Alternative medicine is really all about choices, something Americans consider a fundamental right. The realm of alternative medical practice is huge, because there isn't a "one-size-fits-all" for healthcare. Every person is an individual, and different therapies work for different people.

Our bodies are incredibly complicated… our immune systems almost unimaginably complex. Immune response has to rely on thousands of enzymes, delicate fluid balance, interlocking circulatory pathways, as well as our lifestyle, our emotions, and our environment in order to mount an effective defense. Multiply all of this by our personal uniqueness and you can see why we need a wealth of choices for our health.

Core principles distinguish alternative medicine from orthodox medicine.

—Preventive medicine is the best medicine. Alternative healthcare emphasizes prevention over crisis intervention, seeking to improve health rather than simply to extend life by heroic means. Holistic practitioners believe healing originates from the human body, not from medicines or machines, that toxins in the body often cause disease, and that natural remedies which remove toxins help the body regain health.

—The cure and the preventive are often the same. Most alternative healers teach that just as avoiding the causative agents will prevent an illness, removing them will cure the illness. For instance, if obesity is the condition, then the cure, a restricted diet, is the same as the preventive.

—It is important to know the cause of the disease, not just recognize the symptoms. When people seek alternative care, they're asking, "Why do I have this problem? I'm tired of having the doctor just treat the symptoms." Alternative caregivers teach that daily habits create the conditions for health or disease. Alternative practitioners believe that removing disease-causing conditions will prevent disease.

—The person is more important than the disease. Alternative treatments are highly individual. Ten people going to an alternative doctor for a headache may leave with ten different remedies. Medical practitioners often see only the similarities and treat everyone the same.

—The body can heal itself. Alternative medicine practitioners view symptoms such as fever or inflammation, as signs that the body is mounting an immune response to heal itself. Instead of trying to eliminate symptoms, lifestyle therapy treatments work to enhance natural defenses and healing vitality.

—Alternative practitioners are also teachers who can empower you to help yourself. Many adopt the position of coach rather than doctor to give patients the power of their own healing systems.

—Lifestyle is significant to healing. Alternative practitioners look beyond the physical symptoms and take into account that a patient's mental, emotional, even spiritual life as inseparable from physical health. Lifestyle therapy is more subtle than drugs or surgery. You should expect the healing effects of natural medicines to be slower but more permanent — a normal result of your body taking its time to do it right.

The natural healing rule of thumb is one month of healing for every year you've had the problem.

"HEALTHY HEALING," the book you have in your hands, offers you personal empowerment with its wealth of lifestyle choices for health problems…. things you can do for yourself to improve almost every health condition. Even if the condition is serious, even if you are under traditional medical care, there are always significant things you can do to help your body heal. Healing is a physical process *and* an achievement of the spirit. I have seen this to be true in case after case, regardless of the problem or its duration.

"HEALTHY HEALING" details both empirical evidence and clinical studies to offer you choices that are non-invasive, health supporting, body balancing and disease preventing as well as healing. Good information is the key. Most people have plenty of common sense as well as intuitive knowledge about themselves and their health problems. With solid information, people invariably make good choices for their health.

Iatrogenic Disease

The Iatrogenic Disease Review was carefully researched and written by Sarah Abernathy,
the head of our research department

Is "iatrogenic disease" the epidemic of the new millennium? The term "iatrogenic disease" literally means disease caused by doctors, hospitals or drugs. The American media tell us almost daily that it's a skyrocketing problem in today's drug-oriented society. Adverse drug reactions (ADRs) or interactions are now estimated to be between the 4th and 6th leading cause of death in the United States—with a death toll of over 200,000 people each year. The rate at which patients pick up an infection while being treated in a U.S. hospital has also increased …an astounding 36% in the last 20 years! Each year, 90,000 patients die as a result of hospital-acquired infections.

Deepak Chopra, M.D. estimates that "the number of people that die in the U.S. as the result of medical treatment is equivalent to three 747 crashes, with fatalities, every two days." You're actually more likely to be injured or killed by a visit to a physician than by an automobile accident.

Most Americans today either take prescription drugs ourselves or know someone who does. And, the majority of us will spend time in the hospital at some point in our lives. Yet, there is a growing body of evidence which shows that medical prescriptions you trust can be harmful. Further research shows you may leave a hospital sicker than you were when you checked in.

If you have a serious immune disorder like AIDS or cancer, or are undergoing treatments which depress immune response like chemotherapy or radiation, infections that spread through hospitals can spell life or death. Just a few years ago, I lost a friend suffering from leukemia not to his cancer, but instead, to a virulent lung fungus he caught in the hospital while being treated with chemo.

Medical procedures we saw as miracles, like heart bypass surgery, can have serious risks and drawbacks. Nearly 1 in 25 people die during bypass surgery itself. The newest research reveals that many people who do survive the surgery experience a significant decrease in brain function and memory.

Are you filling a prescription for disaster?

Even during these turbulent economic times, the drug industry is the most profitable industry in the U.S. Over 2.5 billion prescriptions are filled each year by people who have little or no idea what the drugs do, the side effects they cause or the consequences of long term use. The elderly are prime targets for drug therapy, often taking two, three, or even more different prescriptions at the same time. Yet, at least 250 available drugs should not be taken by older adults. Parkinson's disease symptoms, memory deterioration, injury accidents, all thought to be a result of aging, are now regularly the result of drug therapy!

Our electronic lifestyle adds to the problem. Today people can easily get their prescriptions over the internet. Just fill out a short on-line questionnaire, and powerful and potentially dangerous drugs arrive in the mail. Literally thousands of web sites advertise the highly controversial drug Viagra, that has now been linked to over 130 deaths. I did some "Viagra Surfing" myself. Many offer Viagra at great discount and without a doctor's prescription.

Americans also spend billions each year on over-the-counter drugs, mostly for heartburn or pain relief. New figures show that Americans take over 85 million aspirin, linked to gastric bleeding, every single day! NSAIDs (non-steroidal anti-inflammatory drugs) like ibuprofen are widely popular for pain relief, but they too are linked to serious gastrointestinal problems and bleeding. The latest statistics show NSAIDs send 76,000 people to the hospital and kill 7,600 people annually in the U.S.!

What's the health result of this massive over-medication in America?

Every year, for thousands of people, adverse drug reactions (ADRs) mean trips to an Emergency Room or even death. For thousands more, drug toxicity is a silent enemy they may never recognize. Drug residues linger in the body for years. You may not even see the consequences of drug overload for a decade! Over time, drugs build up in fatty tissue, the liver or the glands where they are unable to be eliminated through body pathways. As early as our 30s, the liver and kidneys begin to lose their capacity to metabolize and eliminate drugs efficiently. Kidney and liver failure are not uncommon from long-term overuse of over-the-counter pain relievers like acetaminophen and ibuprofen.

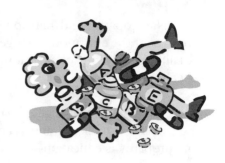

Searching for the Right Blend of Medicine

You may be shocked by this information. Clearly modern medicine isn't all bad. It has saved thousands of lives and made truly wonderful strides. The ability to isolate microbes that cause infectious disease, and to create treatments that would kill those microbes without killing the patient, was a milestone in modern medicine. But even with the vast medical arsenal available to them today, doctors can only cure about one-fourth of the illnesses presented to them.

In response to these limitations, over 50% of Americans now use some form of complementary or alternative medicine. More than half of all medical professionals have tried alternative medicine for their own self-care. An increasing number of MDs are including holistic treatments, adopting some of the practices of natural medicine, in order to offer their patients the best of both worlds.

I believe the best prescription is really a good lifestyle plan: a nutritious diet; regular exercise and mental stimulation; plenty of rest; targeted herbal formulas and supplements for specific imbalances; and a rich spiritual life with loving friends and family. Massage therapy is one of my favorite healing choices. Massage is really therapeutic touch- beneficial for men, women, children, even pets. Not one of the latest "miracle" drugs can replace the basic need to be touched and nurtured.

Today's health care system seems brutal and cold at times. The sick are shuffled around from room to room, waiting… and waiting some more, sometimes just wanting someone who will listen to them. Today's medical tests will never replace the vital communication between doctor and patient. And, a single medical test will never tell the whole picture- the true state of a person's mind, body and spirit.

I feel we need both types of medicine to stay well in today's world. In our fast paced, high stress lifestyle, there may be times when we need to rely on modern medicine for fast symptom relief or to arrest death from a health crisis or injury. Still, modern medicine is no substitute for a sound, nutritious diet regular exercise and the remarkable ability of whole herbs to boost the body's own natural healing response. And, there is no question that health and wellness has a profound spiritual component that is personal for each one of us.

If you've been affected by the shortfalls of modern medicine, natural therapies may be ideally suited to help your body recuperate and regenerate. Although sometimes necessary, drug therapy (particularly long term) and surgical procedures take its toll on even the healthiest of persons. Rebalancing body chemistry, boosting nutrients, restoring foundation strength and immune response should be your focus for a healthy recovery.

Naturopathy

Naturopathy and naturopathic medicine, the fastest growing of all the alternative healing disciplines, represent the enormous change Americans are experiencing in their healthcare. As more people have become disillusioned with conventional health care, naturopathy is seen as a choice gaining respect as a credible healing doctrine.

Today, naturopaths fall into two groups. Traditionally trained naturopaths (N.D.'s) use the naturopathy degree to consult with clients, and as an accreditation to teach, to write and to access research. One of the core beliefs of naturopathy is education—passing on knowledge to empower the client.

A smaller number are trained medically (N.M.D.'s) with an education similar to that of a conventional M.D., with extensive hands-on coursework in anatomy, physiology, biochemistry, pathology, neurosciences, histology, immunology, pharmacology, epidemiology, public health and other conventional disciplines. They add training in therapeutic nutrition training and psychological counseling, subjects that are not required in conventional medical schools. They also learn about herbal therapy, homeopathy, hydrotherapy, massage therapy, chiropractic, and behavioral, as well as Oriental and Ayurvedic medicine systems. All are trained in diet and nutrition as the basic tools of natural therapeutics.

The state laws that govern the practice of naturopathic medicine vary widely. While most states do not yet license naturopathic medicine, as of this writing, licensure is available in eleven states, and many more have begun the legislative debate and process to accredit naturopathic doctors so that they can have standing as valuable contributors in modern healing institutions. Where state laws are liberal, naturopathic medicine covers the full scope of conventional medicine, excluding major surgery and the prescribing of most drugs. Naturopaths in these states can provide diagnostic and therapeutic services including physical exams, lab testing and X-rays. Minor surgery, such as the removal of a mole or wart, is allowed. A few states allow naturopathic medical doctors to deliver babies, specialize in pediatrics, gynecology or geriatrics. They may even work in conventional hospitals. Other states allow naturopathic medicine, but confine it to a more limited scope of practice.

However, many states are clearly becoming aware of the popularity of naturopathic medicine among their citizenry and are considering changes to their current health care regulations. I myself have testified before two state senate committees about the inclusion of more health care disciplines in the medical practice laws they currently have.

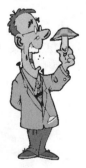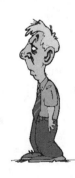

Most states allow traditionally trained naturopaths to consult with clients. Traditional naturopaths specialize in non-invasive, lifestyle consultation, offering an individual approach that educates their clients for long-term health. This approach avoids diagnosing disease and prescribing medication. Rather, because naturopathic principles lead to general improvement in health, it is not unusual for the client to find that long standing health problems have improved or disappeared. In fact, the greatest success of naturopathy is in rebuilding health, in restoring normal body processes. This way, the individual immune system of each person can naturally improve or eliminate chronic and degenerative disease.

Naturopathy is not recommended for severe, acute trauma, like a serious automobile accident, a childbirth emergency, broken bones, or orthopedic problems that need corrective surgery, although it can contribute to faster recovery in these cases.

Because naturopathy sees disease as a manifestation of the natural causes by which your body heals itself, the naturopath seeks to educate his or her clients in how to stimulate the body's own vital healing forces. If the cause of the imbalance is not removed, the disease symptoms will continue either at a lower level of intensity or intermittently, eventually becoming chronic. Fever and inflammation are good examples of the way your body deals with an imbalance that is hindering its normal function.

Although all naturopaths emphasize therapeutic choices based on individual interest and experience, they maintain a consistent philosophy.

Naturopathy is founded on five therapeutic principles.

A typical visit to a Naturopath generally incorporates these beliefs.

1: **Nature is a powerful healing force.**

This is the belief that the body has considerable power to heal itself. The role of the naturopath is to facilitate and enhance this process by educating the client in various approaches to stimulating his or her own internal healing force. Above all, the naturopath must do no harm.

2: **The person is viewed as a whole.**

Understanding the client as an individual is essential. The naturopath must work to understand the patient's complex interaction of physical, mental, emotional, spiritual and social factors.

3: **The goal is to identify and address the cause of the problem.**

Naturopathy does not deal in suppressing symptoms, since symptoms are seen as expressions of the body's attempt to heal itself. Rather it seeks to understand the underlying causes of a disease, which can spring from interacting levels of disharmony in the body, physical, mental, emotional and spiritual.

Some illnesses are the result of spiritual disharmony, experienced as a feeling of deep unease or inadequate strength of will necessary to support the healing process. Naturopaths can play an important role in helping clients to discover the appropriate action for overcoming the disharmony.

Underlying causes, like diet or stress may also play a role in symptoms like ear infections, inflammation or fever. The naturopath can also address the interactive relationships of these conditions and guide the client in finding a natural technique that can alleviate the stress and help to stimulate recovery.

4: **The naturopath is a teacher.**

First and foremost, the naturopath is a teacher, educating, empowering and motivating the client to assume more personal responsibility for his or her own wellness by adopting a healthy attitude, lifestyle and diet. After identifying the conditions that cause the ill health, the naturopath discusses with the client the various methods for creating a return to health.

5: **Prevention is the best approach.**

Prevention is best accomplished by lifestyle habits which support health.

Need to find a good naturopath? Call the California Naturopathic Assn. (530) 676-4842.

Homeopathy

Homeopathy is a kinder, gentler medical philosophy that sees disease as an energy imbalance, a disturbance of the body's "vital force." Its techniques are based on the premise that the body is a self healing entity, and that symptoms are the expression of the body attempting to restore its balance. Homeopathic remedies are formulated to stimulate and increase this curative ability. Each remedy has a number of symptoms that make it unique, just as each person has traits that make him or her unique. Homeopathic physicians are trained to match the patient's symptoms with the precise remedy. Even the highest potencies are non-toxic and do not create the side effects of allopathic drugs. The remedies themselves neither cover up nor destroy disease, but stimulate the body's own healing action to rid itself of the problem.

Homeopathic medicine is based on three prescription principles:

1: **The LAW OF SIMILARS: expressed as "like curing like."** From the tiny amount of the active principle in the remedy, the body learns to recognize the hostile microbe in a process similar to DNA recognition. The LAW OF SIMILARS is the reason that a little is better than a lot, and why such great precision is needed.

2: **The MINIMUM DOSE PRINCIPLE:** means diluting the "like" substance to a correct strength for the individual (strong enough to stimulate the body's vital force without overpowering it). Dilutions are shaken a number of times (3, 6, or 12 times in commercial use) to potentiate therapeutic power through a vibratory effect. Each successive dilution <u>decreases</u> the actual amount of the substance in the remedy. In the strongest dilutions, there is virtually none of the substance remaining, yet potentiation is the highest for healing.

3: **THE SINGLE REMEDY PRINCIPLE:** only one remedy is administered at a time.

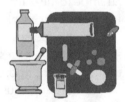

The most effective treatments for the majority of people who use homeopathy to self-treat are combination formulas, which allows for the complexity of different needs. Single remedies work best when administered by a professional homeopath in private practice after an in-depth analysis, where they can be specific to the individual's problem.

About the remedies available in most stores today:

—They work on the antidote principle. More is not better for a homeopathic remedy. Small amounts over a period of time are more effective. Frequency of dosage is determined by individual reaction time, increasing as the first improvements are noted. When substantial improvement is evident, indicating that the body's own healing forces are stimulated and have come into play, the remedy should be discontinued.

—They work on the trigger principle. Start a healing program with a homeopathic medicine. The body's electrical activity, stimulated by the remedy, can mean faster response from other, succeeding therapies.

Homeopathic medicine differs from conventional medicine in two significant ways:

1: Conventional medicines often mask or reduce disease symptoms without addressing the underlying problem. Homeopathic remedies act as catalysts for the immune system to wipe out the root cause.

2: Although both medicinal systems use weak doses of a disease-causing agent to stimulate the body's defenses against that illness (orthodox medicine uses vaccinations; homeopathy uses the antidote principle), homeopathy largely focuses on plants, herbs and earth minerals for this stimulation; conventional medicine uses viruses or chemicals.

Can Homeopathy help AIDS, BioTerrorism and Epidemic Diseases?

The recent worldwide rise in popularity for homeopathy is due to its effectiveness in treating epidemic diseases, such as HIV-positive and other life-threatening viral conditions. Studies show that homeopathy not only treats the acute infective stages, but also reduces the need for antibiotics and other drugs that cause side effects, and further weaken an already low immune response.

In significant Indian tests, the news magazine "Homeopathic Forum," reported 15 of 300 HIV-infected patients who became HIV-<u>negative</u> after homeopathic treatment. Following this and other reports, success with AIDS has been widely experienced by homeopaths in the following areas:

...Prevention - generating resistance to the virus and subsequent infection.
...Support during acute illnesses - reducing the length and severity of the infection.
...Restoration of health - revitalizing the body so that overall health does not deteriorate.

Historically, homeopathy has played an important role in treating epidemic disease. For example, homeopathic remedies were used successfully to treat the flu pandemic of 1918 and scarlet fever outbreaks in the 1800's. Looking at these successes, many experts believe that homeopathic medicine should be considered in the event of a modern biological attack for both prevention and treatment of disease symptoms. Here are a few examples from history of homeopathy's successes in severe epidemics.

Historical Remedies for Epidemic Diseases

—*Belladonna:* Used to treat scarlet fever by homeopathy's founder Samuel Hahnemann.
—*Thuja:* Used to help prevent transmission of smallpox between family members.
—*Baptisia:* Used to prevent Typhus Fever; and used after traditional inoculation in Typhoid carriers.
—*Lathyrus sativa:* Used against polio in Argentina by Francisco Eizayaga.
—*Gelsemium:* Used in the flu pandemic of 1918. Effective for flu when symptoms include: lack of coordination, stupor, and severe weakness. Used in some epidemics of polio.
—*Bryonia and Eupatorium:* Used as a follow-up to Gelsemium in the flu outbreak of 1918.
—*Camphor, Veratrum Album and Cuprum Met:* Used to prevent and cure Asiatic Cholera in 1831.
—*Diptherinum and Diptherotoxinum:* Used successfully as a prophylactic against Diptheria
—*Crotalus Horridus:* Used with good results against Yellow Fever.
—*Variolinum:* A homeopathic nosode used against smallpox. Research by homeopath Dr. Eaton in the early 1900's shows that Variolinum was 97% effective in protecting against smallpox even after disease exposure. (Note: The Homeopathic Pharmacopoeia Convention of the United States (HPUS) has not approved variolinum for modern use because there is no data on which dose or substance was actually proved on these early outbreaks of smallpox.)
—*Tuberculinum bovinum:* A nosode made from tuberculosis bacterium used to confer immunity to children and young adults with inherited tuberculosis.
—*Menningococcinum:* Used in 1974 to help prevent an outbreak of menningitis.

A Modern Homeopathic Approach to BioTerrorism

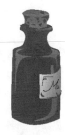

There is no question that we live in troubling times - with threats of biological warfare and terrorist alerts on almost a daily basis. The events of Sept.11, 2001 awakened new fears in many Americans. But, in true American spirit, we have responded with resiliency and determination to fight the new battle and win.

In the fight to protect our health in this new battle, natural therapies should be included as valuable tools. Already one in two Americans use some form of complementary or alternative medicine. Homeopathy has become a favorite for Americans who choose alternative healthcare. The centuries old record of safety for homeopathic medicine cannot be ignored in a world where unknown health threats abound, especially where drug vaccines or antidotes have not been found, or the testing against bioterrorism agents is slight.

As I write this, the large network of natural health care professionals in America are hard at work researching the best adjunctive treatments to bioterrorism threats so we can all be better prepared. In this section, I will be examining a modern homeopathic approach to bioterrorism. Please refer to pg. 474 of this book for my complete lifestyle program with herb, supplement and diet recommendation to help fight supergerms and maintain the strongest immune response.

For your protection:

Biological agents like anthrax and smallpox are very volatile. Seeking medical treatment if you suspect you're infected is critical. Any flu-like symptoms or strange rashes should be checked out by your physician, particularly if there has been any suspicious activity or disease exposure cases in your area. Modern medicine is at its best in life-threatening emergencies, such as arresting death from a bioterrorism infection. Anthrax can often be treated medically with good results.

Homeopathic Remedies for BioTerrorism

Homeopathy uses nosodes (remedies prepared from diseased tissue or products of a disease) to stimulate the body's immune response to the infectious agent. Nosodes work similarly to modern vaccines, but are extremely diluted and far safer. In fact, homeopathic physicians like Samuel Hahnemann were the first physicians ever to develop and use remedies based on the modern vaccine principle. Nosodes can be used to help prevent and treat epidemic disease with some customization for individual symptoms.

Nosodes approved in the Homeopathic Pharmacopoeia Convention of the United States (HPCUS):
Anthracinum, BCG, Candida Albicans, Candida Parapsilosis, Colibacillinum, Hippozaeninum, Influenzinum, Lyssin, Medorrhinum, Morbillinum, Pertussinum, Proteus, Psorinum, Pyrogenium, Sinusitisinum, Staphylococcinum, Streptococcinum, Syphylinum, Tuberculinum, Tuberculinum Bovinum, and Vaccinotoxinum.

Unfortunately, modern science has done little to determine if homeopathic nosodes might be effective against biological agents like anthrax or smallpox. Still, there is no question that homeopathy was used in the 18th and early 19th centuries for epidemic diseases with good results before vaccines or other medicines were readily available. In today's uncertain global climate, it may be wise to consider homeopathic nosodes in case traditional vaccines or prescription drugs are in short supply. A case in point: Testing shows that animals treated with tularemia nosode had 22% greater survival from tularemia infection than animals who weren't treated with the remedy.

To protect against a future biological attack like the anthrax-tainted letters of 2001, many homeopaths developed emergency first aid kits for their personal use. As yet there are no homeopathic remedies approved by the FDA to treat anthrax or smallpox, but here are some examples of remedies a person might consider for an emergency homeopathic first aid kit.

For Skin Anthrax:
Anthracium (anthrax nosode): to help boost immune response to anthrax spores.
Arsenicum album: for skin swelling and burning
Lachesis muta: for inflammation or bleeding
Nitricum acidum: to help eliminate disease toxins
Secale: for pain in the extremities that are worse when sleeping and cold to the touch.

For Inhalation Anthrax:

Anthracium (anthrax nosode): to help boost immune response to anthrax spores. (Some homeopaths only recommend *anthracium* for cutaneous anthrax. Others recommend for both.)

Arsenicum album: for exhaustion, fever and excess heat symptoms.

Bryonia: for chest pain, coughing and inflammation of the mucous membranes; symptoms made worse by moving or talking.

Phosphorous: for coughing, nausea and digestive complaints.

Carbo vegetabilis: for gas, indigestion, and coughing- when symptoms are made worse by heat.

Pyrogenium: for infection, inflammation and fever.

For Stress and Shock:

Aconite: for shock and fright; helpful for fear of flying

Argentum nitricum: helpful for fear of flying accompanied by fear of heights and extreme claustrophobia

Ignatia: for unspoken grief and sadness

Arsenicum: for insecurity about personal safety

Arnica: for bruising, injury, hemorrhaging

Rescue Remedy: A Bach flower essence remedy based on homeopathic principles- effective for any high stress situation, or crisis.

How to take Homeopathic Remedies:

1: For maximum effectiveness, take ½ dropperful under the tongue at a time, and hold for 30 seconds before swallowing; or dissolve the tiny homeopathic lactose tablets under the tongue.

2: Homeopathic remedies are designed to enter the bloodstream directly through the mouth's mucous membranes. Do not eat, drink or smoke for 10 minutes before or after taking. Do not use with chemical medicines, caffeine, cayenne, mint or alcohol; they overpower the remedy's subtle stimulus.

3: Basic dosage: repeat the medicine as needed. You may notice aggravation of symptoms at first as your body restructures and begins to rebuild its defenses, in much the same way as a healing crisis occurs with other natural cleansing therapies. This effect usually passes in a short period of time.

4: Store homeopathic remedies at room temperature out of heat and sunlight, and away from perfumes, camphor, liniments and paints.

Popular Homeopathic Remedies and how to use them:

The right homeopathic remedy can restore health on all levels.
The effects can be quite long lasting.

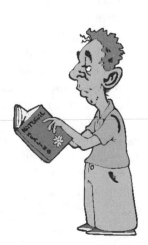

—*ACONITE:* for children's earaches. Helps with trauma of sudden fright or shock.

—*ARSENICUM ALBUM:* for food poisoning accompanied by diarrhea. For allergic symptoms such as a runny nose; for asthma and colds.

—*APIS:* macerated bee tincture. Relieves stinging, burning and rapid swelling after bee sting or insect bites. Good for sunburn and other minor burns, skin irritations, hives, early stage boils, and frostbite. Helps relieve joint pain, eye inflammation and fevers. Apis is effective against pain that is improved by cold and made worse by pressure.

—**ARNICA:** often the first medicine to take after an injury or a fall, to counter bruising and swelling. For pain relief and rapid healing, particular from injuries like sprains, strains, stiffness or bruises. Unlike herbal preparations of Arnica, homeopathic Arnica tablets are safe for internal consumption to relieve contusions, calm someone who has had a great shock, and dispel the distress of accidents and injuries. Use before and after surgery and childbirth to prevent bruising and speed recovery. Apply externally only to unbroken skin.

—**BELLADONNA:** for fast relief of sudden fever, sunstroke or swelling. Used to treat sudden onset conditions characterized by redness, throbbing pain, and heat, including some colds, high fever, earache and sore throat. Recommended for a person who has a flushed face, hot and dry skin, and dilated pupils. A remedy for teething, colds and flu, earache, fever, headache, menstrual problems, sinusitis, and sore throat.

—**BRYONIA:** for flu, fevers, coughs and colds that come on slowly. For some headaches, indigestion, muscle aches and pains. For irritability aggravated by motion. For swelling, inflammation and redness of arthritis when symptoms are worse with movement and better with cold applications.

—**CALENDULA:** promotes healing of minor cuts and scrapes; cools sunburn; relieves skin irritations.

—**CANTHARIS:** treats bladder infections and genito-urinary tract problems, especially where there is burning and urgency to urinate. Good for skin burns, too.

—**CAPSICUM:** a stimulating digestive aid. Apply topically to stop minor bleeding, joint pain and bruises.

—**CHAMOMILLA:** to calm fussy children during teething pain, colic and fever. For childhood cold symptoms of runny nose, tight cough, stringy diarrhea and earache. Treats childhood and adult restlessness, insomnia, toothache and joint pains. Recommended for those who are irascible, stubborn or inconsolable.

—**EUPHRASIA:** an external and internal treatment for eye injuries, especially when there is profuse watering, burning pain and swelling. For abrasions, stuffy headache, and low grade infections that leave constant mucus in the throat.

—**GELSEMIUM:** to energize people with chronic lethargy. To overcome dizziness from colds or flu.

—**HYPERICUM:** used topically and internally to relieve central nervous system pain and and nerve damage trauma. For pain like carpal tunnel syndrome, or an injury that causes shooting pain that goes the length of a nerve, or to an area with many nerve endings, like the fingers and toes. Accelerates healing of jagged cuts and relieves the pain from dental surgery, toothaches, and tailbone injuries. Effective for depression and insomnia. A powerful anti-inflammatory for ulcers, cuts, scrapes, mild burns and sunburn.

—**IGNATIA:** a female remedy to relax emotional tension. Effective during times of great grief or loss.

—**LACHESIS:** for PMS symptoms and menopausal hot flashes, irritability and bloating.

—**LEDUM:** for bruises. Use after Arnica treatment to fade a bruise after it becomes black and blue.

—**LYCOPODIUM:** a mood booster that often increases personal confidence. Favored by estheticians to soothe irritated complexions and as an antiseptic.

—**MAGNESIUM PHOS:** for abdominal cramping, spasmodic back pain and menstrual cramps.

—**NATRUM MURIATICUM:** for water retention and bloating during PMS.

—**NUX VOMICA:** used principally to treat headache, nausea and vomiting due to overeating or drinking. A prime remedy for hangover, recovering alcoholics and drug addiction. Beneficial for gastrointestinal tract problems, like abdominal bloating, peptic ulcer, heartburn, gas, constipation and motion sickness.

—**PASSIFLORA:** a prime remedy for insomnia and nervousness.

—**PODOPHYLLIUM:** helps diarrhea, especially for children.

—**PULSATILLA:** for childhood asthma, allergies and earaches. For runny nose colds, certain eye and ear ailments, skin eruptions, allergies, fainting, and gastric upsets. Effective in homeopathic combination remedies for colds and flu, sinusitis, indigestion and insomnia.

—**RHUS TOX:** a poison ivy derivative, dilutions are taken to alleviate poison ivy and other red, swollen skin rashes, hives, and burns, as well as joint stiffness. A sports medicine for pain and swelling that affects muscles, ligaments, and tendons from sprains and overexertion. A "rusty gate" remedy, for the person who feels stiff and sore at first but better after movement. For stiffness in the joints when the pain is worse with cold, damp weather. Effective in homeopathic combination remedies for back pain, sprains and skin rashes.

—*Sepia:* effective for treating herpes, eczema, hair loss and PMS.

—*Sulphur:* commonly taken for certain chronic (rather than acute) conditions, skin problems, and the early stages of the flu. Treats sore throats, allergies, and earaches.

—*Thuja:* effective for treating warts and moles, and for sinusitis.

—*Valerian:* soothes nerves and eases muscle tension. A good sedative for insomnia.

The Best Combination Remedies I've Used for Self-Treatment:

—**OSCILLOCOCCINUM:** a premiere combination remedy for flu. Symptoms include fever, chills, body aches and pains. Contact Boiron 1-800-264-7661 for information.

—**TRAUMEEL:** for bruises, sports injuries and arthritis. Contact BHI at 800-621-7644 for information.

—**EYE DROPS 1:** for dry, scratchy eyes; sensitivity to light, contact lens irritation and lid infection.

—**EYE DROPS 2:** for allergy-related eye problems like itchiness, burning, watering and redness.

—**EYE DROPS 3:** for computer eye syndrome, eye strain and fatigue, blurry vision and focus, difficulty driving at night, night blindness. Contact Similasan at 800-426-1644 for information on all of these eye drops.

—*Phosphorus 30x:* widely used for animal cataracts, phosphorus also works extremely well for humans in breaking up the film.

—**ENURAID:** a combination designed for incontinence (involuntary urination) and related symptoms. Also good for overactive bladder in women. Contact Hyland's at 800-624-9659 for information.

—**TRACE-LYTE:** a homeopathic electrolyte mineral combination designed to improve the electrical conductivity of the cells and restore body homeostatis. Contact Nature's Path at 800-326-5772 for information. They also make an excellent Trace Lyte product for your pets.

Homeopathic Cell Salts

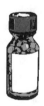

Mineral, or tissue salts in the body can be used as healing agents for specific health problems. Homeopathic doctor, William Schuessler, discovered the twelve cell salts, as well as the Biochemic System of Medicine. He felt that all forms of illness were related to imbalances of one or more of the indispensable mineral salts. His research showed that homeopathically prepared minerals do indeed help maintain mineral balance in our bodies, and in fact, could be used as core nutrients at the cellular level. Cell salts are based on homeopathic remedies and may be used in homeopathic treatment healing programs. As with other homeopathic remedies, mineral salts are used to stimulate corresponding body cell salts toward normal metabolism and health restoration. Essentially, they re-tune the body to return it to its normal healthy balance. Only very small amounts are needed to properly nourish the cells.

The Twelve Cell Salts

Many of today's cell salts are extracted from organic plant sources. These medicines are available both in tinctures and as tiny lactose-based tablets that are easily dissolved under the tongue.

...*Calcarea Fluor:* calcium fluoride - contained in the elastic fibers of the skin, blood vessels, connective tissue, bones and teeth. Used to treat dilated or weakened blood vessels, like those in hemorrhoids, varicose veins, hardened arteries and glands. Helps prevent tooth decay and loose teeth. (The homeopathic preparation, *calcarea fluor* is far safer than the highly toxic calcium fluoride or hydrofluosilicic acid added to toothpastes and city water supplies. See "Water Fluoridation's Tainted History," on pg.119 for more.)

...*CALCAREA PHOS: calcium phosphate* - abundant in all tissues. Strengthens bones, and helps build new blood cells. Deficiency results in anemia, emaciation and weakness, slow growth and poor digestion. Helpful for people who crave lots of fatty, salty foods like ham and bacon.

...*CALCAREA SULPH: calcium sulphate* - found in bile; promotes continual blood cleansing. When deficient, toxic build-up occurs as skin disorders, clogging respiratory mucous, boils and ulcerations, and slow healing. Helps hayfever-prone people.

...*FERRUM PHOS: iron phosphate* - helps form red corpuscles to oxygenate the blood. Treats congestive colds and flu, and skin inflammation. A biochemic remedy for the first stages of inflammation or infections. Great to help reduce children's fevers.

...*KALI MUR: potassium chloride* - deficiency results in coating of the tongue, gland swelling, scaling of the skin, system sluggishness and excess mucous discharge. Used after FERRUM PHOS for inflammatory arthritis and rheumatism.

...*KALI PHOS: potassium phosphate* - found in body fluids and tissues. Deficiency is characterized by intense body odor and tinnitus. Used for mental and nervous system problems like depression, irritability, dizziness, headaches, nervous stomach.

...*KALI SULPH: potassium sulphate* - an oxygen-carrier for the skin. Deficiency causes a deposit on the tongue, and slimy yellow nasal, eye, ear, vaginal and mouth secretions.

...*MAGNESIA PHOS: magnesium phosphate* - an infrastructure constituent. Deficiency impairs muscle and nerve fibers, causing cramps, spasms and neuralgia pain, usually with prostration and profuse sweating. Helpful for sciatica, backaches, colic, spasmodic pain.

...*NATRUM MUR: sodium chloride* - found throughout the body. Regulates moisture within the cells. Deficiency causes fatigue, chills, craving for salt, bloating, profuse secretions from the skin, eyes and mucous membranes, excessive salivation, and watery stools. Useful for dry, cracking skin, cold sores, fever blisters.

...*NATRUM PHOS: sodium phosphate* - regulates the body's acid/alkaline balance. Catalyzes lactic acid and fat emulsion. Imbalance shows a coated tongue, itchy skin, sour stomach, poor appetite, diarrhea and gas. (Symptoms are generally worse after eating fatty foods.)

...*NATRUM SULPH: sodium sulfate* - an imbalance produces edema in the tissues, dry skin with watery eruptions, poor bile and pancreas activity, headaches, and gouty symptoms.

...*SILICEA: silica* - essential to healthy bones, joints, skin and glands. Deficiency produces catarrh in the respiratory system, pus discharges from the skin, slow wound healing and offensive body odor. Successful in the treatment of boils, pimples, for hair and nail health, blood cleansing, constipation, headaches, insomnia and rebuilding after illness or injury.

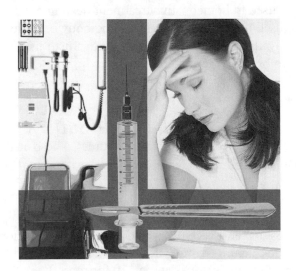

Need to find a good homeopath? Call the National Center for Homeopathy. (703) 548-7790.

Enzyme Therapy

Enzymes are the cornerstones of healing because they are the foundation elements of the immune system. Plant enzymes offer built-in enzyme therapy by providing naturally active antioxidants that fight free-radical destruction.

Enzymes operate on both chemical and biological levels. Chemically, they are the workhorses that drive metabolism to use the nutrients we take in. Biologically, enzymes are our life energy. Your body contains more than 30,000 different kinds of enzymes! Every vitamin, mineral and hormone requires enzyme assistance to perform their functions in the body. Without enzyme energy, we would be a pile of lifeless chemicals.

Each of us is born with a battery charge of enzyme energy at birth. As we age our internal enzyme stores are naturally depleted. A recent study shows that a 60 year old has 50% fewer enzymes than a 30 year old. Enzyme depletion, lack of energy, disease and aging all go hand in hand. Unless we stop the one-way-flow out of the body of enzyme energy, our digestive-eliminative capacities weaken, obesity and chronic illness set in, lifespan shortens. The faster you use up your enzyme supply —the shorter your life.

There are three categories of enzymes:

1: *Metabolic enzymes* like proteases repair cells and stimulate enzyme activity. They help us heal faster by repressing inflammation and breaking up debris in the injury area. They stimulate without repressing immune response (unlike cortisone or hydrocortisone drugs). *Note: If you take enzyme supplements between meals without food, they absorb directly into your body and function as metabolic enzymes in the repair and healing process.*

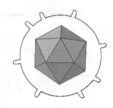

2: *Human digestive enzymes* assimilate our food nutrients. (Digestion actually begins in the mouth when digestive enzymes are secreted in the saliva.) Digestive enzymes are stronger than any other enzymes in human beings and more concentrated than any other enzyme combination in nature. A good thing too, since our processed, over cooked, nutrient-poor diets demand a great deal of enzymatic work!

3: *Fresh plant enzymes* start food digestion, and aid our own digestive enzymes. All foods contain the enzymes required to digest them. Raw foods diets are based on the principle that the more "live" enzyme-rich foods you eat, the better health you will have. The best food sources of plant enzymes for humans are bananas, mangos, sprouts, papayas, avocados and pineapples.

There are three interesting facts about food enzymes:

...All food, whether plant or animal, has its own enzymes that serve it in life. When eaten, these become the property of the eater, are now its food enzymes, and begin immediately to work for the eater's benefit.

...All animals have the proteolytic enzyme, cathepsin, which comes into play after death, and becomes the prime factor for autolysis. In other words, the food helps its own breakdown for the good of the eater.

...Only enzymes from whole foods and whole herbs give the body what it needs to work properly. Our bodies cannot independently absorb food; we must have the help of the food itself.

How does enzyme therapy work to heal? Enzyme therapy uses metabolic enzymes to stimulate immune response. The link between enzymes and immunity comes from lymphocytes, or white blood cells which circulate through the body to attack foreign invader cells. When toxins are detected, white blood cells attack them by secreting enzymes on their surfaces. Diseases like cancer, leukemia, anemia and heart disease can even be diagnosed by measuring the amount and activity of certain enzymes in the blood and body fluids.

Enzyme therapy is regularly recommended for inflammation, pain, blood-thinning and immune support. Olympic athletes from Europe and China are routinely given enzyme preparations to help speed recovery from injuries. Bromelain from pineapples is a good example of a rapid recovery enzyme for sports injuries. Research shows bromelain helps reduce pain and improve function for people with osteoarthritis, too.

Some enzymes clean wounds and control allergic reactions to drugs. Enzyme therapy allows respiratory vessels to unclog, helps degenerative diseases like heart disease, regulates blood sugar, and relieves stomach and colon pain. Pancreatic enzymes (derived from animals) can also be used therapeutically with good results in cystic fibrosis and pancreatic cancer, but are best used under the guidance of a health professional.

The Power of Protease - a remarkable enzyme!

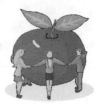

Plant enzyme proteases are a powerful therapeutic agent used in natural medicine. Protease breaks up and assists the body in removing undesirable proteins in the blood- a major cause of chronic illness. Protease, taken on an empty stomach, goes directly to the bloodstream and can reach most body tissues for rapid healing action. Adjunctive therapy with plant protease offers a healing plus for a wide range of conditions.

Here's how protease can help you:

…**Tests show protease promotes healing and recovery from cancer.** Protease can dissolve the fibrin coating on cancer cells, allowing the body's defenses to function better. Proteases also helps shrink tumors by stimulating the removal of dead or abnormal tissue while enhancing healthy tissue growth.

…**Protease boosts immune defenses** fighting viral, bacterial, fungal and parasite infections. Especially helpful for autoimmune disorders like Chronic Fatigue Syndrome, arthritis or fibromyalgia.

…**Protease is a potent antioxidant**. Protease purifies your blood, breaking down protein invaders.

…**Protease accelerates healing from breast and uterine fibroids,** tumors and sebaceous cysts.

…**Protease helps repair scar tissue** in the lungs caused by respiratory disease.

…**Protease reduces food allergies.** Malabsorption of protein is extremely common.

…**Protease reduces swelling and pain of injuries and wounds** and speeds recovery time.

…**Protease helps beautify your skin.** Skin disorders, like acne or rosaceae often greatly improve.

…**Protease reduces risk of kidney stone or gallstone development** in susceptible people.

I've had good results in natural healing programs with PUREZYME, plant protease by Transformation Enzyme, to reduce internal scarring from radiation therapy and to help dissolve sebaceous gland cysts. I have also formulated Crystal Star DR. ENZYME™ with protease and bromelain which is designed to speed healing from infections and take down painful inflammation. It's receiving good reviews from practitioners and consumers alike. *Note: Don't use during pregnancy, if you have a stomach ulcer, before surgery, if using anti-coagulant drugs or with a blood-clotting disorder.*

About Co-enzyme Q-10

Co-enzymes work as catalysts in the body's biochemical reactions. I call CoQ-10 the "holistic enzyme" because it's found in every cell, especially active in body organs — the heart, brain, liver and kidneys. All living foods contain a form of Co-enzyme Q-1 to Q-10. Dark green vegetables, rice bran, wheat germ, beans, nuts, fish and eggs are particularly high in CoQ10. However, the body's ability to synthesize CoQ10 from food begins to decline as early as our twenties. Supplementation is then the best choice for healing results.

CoQ-10 is one of the most powerful antioxidants known. It has a long history of boosting immune response and cardiac strength, increasing energy, reversing high blood pressure, promoting weight loss and healing gum disease (in this regard it has worked when almost nothing else will). CoQ10 is also an anti-aging agent, extending the lifespan of study lab animals an astounding 56%! Like other antioxidant co-enzymes, glutathione peroxidase, and SOD for example, CoQ-10 neutralizes free radicals by turning them into stable oxygen and H_2O_2, then into oxygen and water. CoQ-10 can even prolong the antioxidant activity of vitamin E in the body.

Specific enzyme therapy treatments of CoQ-10 include: congestive heart failure, angina, ischemic heart disease, cardiomyopathy, mitral valve prolapse, infertility caused by low sperm motility, diabetes, tumors, periodontal disease, and candida albicans. Good results have been achieved in specific tests for breast cancer and high blood pressure. In addition, if you're already taking drugs for cancer or high blood pressure, CoQ-10 can alleviate many toxic effects of the drugs.

How much CoQ-10 should you take?

CoQ-10 supplementation only works if there is a clear deficiency. As little as 30mg a day of CoQ-10 is an effective dose for people who are CoQ-10 deficient. Some cancer and heart patients take up to 450mg a day. CoQ-10 is a fat soluble nutrient, so your body assimilates it better if taken along with fatty acids like Omega-3 oils or evening primrose oil. CoQ-10 is only effective as long as it is taken; once discontinued, the illness can return.... especially true in cancer treatment. Take CoQ-10 for up to three months to saturate the tissues.

What reduces healthy CoQ10 levels? An overactive thyroid, aging, some cholesterol lowering drugs, some antidepressants and beta blockers deplete CoQ10.

Do you have enough enzymes?

The first signs of enzyme deficiency are indigestion, gas and bloating after eating meals. Fatigue, premature aging and weight gain are also signs of low enzymes in the body. Most nutrient deficiency problems as we age result not from the lack of the nutrients themselves, but from our lack of enzymes to absorb them.

Nature has designed an interlocking digestive program for us. When our foods don't have enough enzymes for us to digest them, enzymes reserved for metabolic processes get pulled from their normal work to digest food. The pancreas and liver have to use their enzyme stores, too. But even these substitute measures don't make up for the missing food enzymes because we need those enzymes to break down and actually deliver the nutrients.

Low enzymes mean we end up with undigested food in our blood. So, white blood cell immune defenses are pulled from their jobs to take care of the undigested food, and the immune system takes a dive. It's a perfect environment for disease.

Enzyme-rich foods take care of this unhealthy cascade of reactions before it ever starts. Fresh fruits and vegetables (especially bitter greens) have the most plant enzymes. As you increase these foods in your diet, your enzymatic activity also increases. If you don't get enough fresh foods, or you need extra enzyme concentration for healing, plant-based enzyme supplements are the next best choice, especially from herbs and superfoods.

If you can't make them, take them.

Can we maximize daily enzyme benefits?

Enzymes are extremely sensitive to heat. Heat above 120° F. destroys them. Even low degrees of heat can greatly reduce your digestive ability. Enzymes are also affected by excessive sunlight, tobacco, alcohol, caffeine, fluorides, chlorine in drinking water, air pollution, chemical additives and many drugs. Enzyme protection and enzyme therapy are also dramatically reduced by the use of a microwave oven and chronic stress.

High quality enzyme products are available through: Enzymedica, Transformation Enzyme Products, Herbal Products and Development, and Pure Essence Labs as well as Crystal Star® DR. ENZYME™ with protease and bromelain and blended herbs.

For in-depth information on Enzyme Therapy, see The Complete Book of Enzyme Therapy,
by Dr. Anthony J. Cichoke.

Chiropractic

Overwhelming evidence has changed the medical community's attitude toward chiropractic as a method for both healing and normalizing the nervous system. With almost 15 million patients annually, and 35,000 licensed practitioners, chiropractic is now America's second largest health-care system. In fact, the Agency for Health Care Policy and Research now recommends chiropractic therapy as the only safe and effective, drugless form of initial treatment for low back problems in adults.

Meaning "done with the hands," chiropractic therapy uses physical manipulation of the spine to relieve pain and return energy to the body. The central belief of chiropractic is that proper alignment of the spinal column is essential for health, because the spinal column acts as a switchboard for the nervous system. Its practitioners feel that the nervous system holds the key to the body's healing potential because it coordinates and controls the functions of all other body systems.

Today's chiropractors also incorporate physical therapy techniques, nutritional counseling and muscle rehabilitation into their practice. Since nerve obstruction is involved with a wide range of health problems, many also treat fatigue syndromes like CFS, fibromyalgia, lupus, candida albicans yeast, and menstrual difficulties like PMS. Respiratory conditions like asthma, digestive troubles, insomnia and circulatory problems respond well to chiropractic care. It even helps decrease scar tissue formation after injury. Chiropractic adjustment helps prevent wear and tear on joints and ligaments by maintaining their proper positioning. Evidence shows that chiropractic adjustment combined with proper nutrition can relieve joint stiffness, and even reverse arthritis and osteoarthritis in some cases.

Eighty percent of Americans will experience a back problem in their lifetime!

The most common complaint for chiropractic treatment is still lower back pain, mostly from stress-caused constriction which tends to accumulate in the lower back, neck and shoulders. But chiropractors today are no longer just "back crackers." Many use a hand-held activator that delivers a controlled, light, fast thrust to the problem area. The thrust is so quick that it accelerates ahead of the body's tightening-up resistance to the adjustment. A chiropractor locates the fixated area of the spine, makes the adjustment, and corrects the subluxation. Other problems aggravated by the fixation usually begin to heal immediately. The gentleness of this method makes adjustments safer and more comfortable for the patient.

The spinal column and the nervous system work together:

…The spinal column is made up of twenty-four bones called vertebrae that surround and protect the spinal cord. Between each vertebra, pairs of spinal nerves reach to every part of the body, including muscles, bones, organs and glands. Each vertebra also affects and interacts with its neighbor through these nerves.

…The nervous system is comprised of three overlapping systems: the central nervous system, the autonomic nervous system and the peripheral nervous system. Health relies upon the balance and equilibrium of all three interrelated nerve systems, which can be disrupted by misalignment, stress or illness. Almost every nerve in the body runs through the spine, allowing chiropractic adjustments to address many seemingly unrelated dysfunctions, both physical and subconscious.

…Misalignments in the spine, known as subluxations, interrupt the electrical impulse flow from the brain to the nerve structures, resulting in both pain and lower immune response. A subluxation may also have a direct effect on organ function. A chiropractor adjusts spinal joints to remove subluxations in order to restore normal nerve function. Spinal subluxations may not be the sole cause of a given disease, but they are a major predisposing factor to it because they prevent the nervous system from working normally.

Need to find a good chiropractor? Call the American Chiropractic Assn. (800) 986-4636.

Biofeedback

Biofeedback uses high-tech electronic equipment readings to give auditory, verbal, and visual information back to the body about how it is working. Before the advent of the biofeedback machine, conventional medicine held that an individual had no control over heart rate, body temperature, brain activity, or blood pressure. When biofeedback experiments proved, in the 1960's, that people could voluntarily affect these functions, research tests began into how it might be employed for human health.

Here's how biofeedback works: The patient is wired with sensors, and by giving auditory and/or visual signals to his body, learns to control what are usually subconscious responses — like circulation to the hands and feet, tension in the jaw, or heartbeat rate. Biofeedback computers then provide a rapid, detailed analysis of the target activities within the body. Biofeedback practitioners interpret changes in the computer readings which help the patient learn to stabilize erratic and unhealthy biological functions. A normal, healthy reading includes fairly warm skin, low sweat gland activity, and a slow, even heart rate.

Today, biofeedback is used by all kinds of health professionals — physicians, psychologists, social workers and nurses. It is seen as a useful medical tool for controlling health problems like asthma, chronic fatigue, epilepsy, drug addiction and chronic pain. It is a successful specific in the treatment of migraines, cold extremities, and psoriasis, a skin disease that has a psychological foundation.

Biofeedback is used in relaxation therapy to help overcome insomnia and anxiety. Sleep disorders, hyperactivity and other behavior problems in children, dysfunctions stemming from inadequate control over muscles, back pain, temporo-mandibular joint syndrome (TMJ), and even loss of bladder or bowel control due to brain or nerve damage, all show improvement under biofeedback training. Biofeedback often works for bladder incontinence when everything else fails. Studies show it surpasses drug therapy in reducing bladder control problems. National Medicare coverage for biofeedback for incontinence is now <u>mandated</u> by the Health Care Financing Administration (HCFA).

Biofeedback also helps problems like heart malfunction, stress-related disorders like ulcers and irritable bowel syndrome, hiatal hernia, ringing in the ears (Meniere's syndrome), facial tics, and cerebral palsy.

The effects of biofeedback can be measured by:
1: Monitoring skin temperature influenced by blood flow beneath the skin;
2: Monitoring galvanic skin response, the electrical conductivity of the skin;
3: Observing muscle tension with an electro-myogram;
4: Tracking heart rate with an electro-cardiogram;
5: Using an electroencephalogram to monitor brain wave activity.

One of the most common vital signs monitored by biofeedback is *muscle tension*, because this can be used to treat tension headaches, muscle pain, incontinence, even partial paralysis. Another is *skin temperature*, which can be used to treat Reynaud's syndrome, migraines, hypertension and anxiety. Other signs are *perspiration*, which is used to treat anxiety and body odor; *pulse*, which is used to treat hypertension, stress and heart arrhythmia; and *breathing rate*, which is used to treat asthma and anxiety reactions.

Biofeedback is seldom used by itself, but works well with other relaxation techniques and lifestyle changes. Biofeedback's success stories come from people who are willing to make lifestyle improvements.

Visit the Biofeedback Certification Institute of America's website, www.bcia.org, for a biofeedback practitioner

Massage Therapy

A massage can wipe away our blues, reduce our stress, and offer all of us a nurturing human touch. Most of us treasure a self-indulgent massage from our spouse, a friend or a professional massage therapist. But, massage is far more than indulgence and relaxation. Massage therapy has been a recognized healing method for thousands of years. The ancient Romans and Greeks used massage regularly as a healing treatment. In the past decade, overwhelming scientific evidence has shown that massage therapy works. Today massage therapy has joined the alternative medicine techniques of chiropractic and reflexology as a viable health discipline.

…Massage is a godsend for fibromyalgia (yesterday's rheumatism), and major depression. Research shows the anti-depressant effects of a 30 minute massage can last 3 to 36 hours!

…Massage therapy is helpful for pain control, stimulating development of endorphins, the body's natural pain relievers. Special efficacy is reported for back and shoulder pain, and spinal nerve problems. It effectively treats inflammatory conditions by increasing lymphatic circulation, like swelling from injuries.

…Massage therapy is an effective treatment for cardiovascular disorders, actually helping to prevent heart disease. and improving blood circulation throughout the entire circulatory system.

…Massage therapy is often more helpful than drugs for nerve and gynecological problems like PMS.

…Massage therapy helps chronic fatigue syndromes, candida infections and gastrointestinal disorders.

…Massage therapy helps correct poor posture from spinal curvatures and whiplash.

…Massage therapy helps headaches and temporo-mandibular joint syndrome (TMJ).

…Massage therapy helps respiratory disorders like bronchial asthma and emphysema.

…Massage therapy promotes recovery from fatigue, muscle spasms and pain after exercise.

…Massage therapy breaks up scar tissue and adhesions, removing toxins causing eczema or psoriasis.

…Massage therapy is an effective detoxification technique, promoting mucous and fluid drainage from the lungs and increasing peristaltic action in the intestines to promote fecal elimination. Lymphatic massage also fights cellulite by helping to eliminate congested, fatty wastes. I recommend at least one massage treatment during a 3 to 7 day cleanse to stimulate the body's immune response and natural restorative powers.

Two types of massage therapy specifically help the detoxification-body cleansing process:

1: **Deep tissue massage** removes waste in the muscles. Deep tissue therapy uses more direct deep finger pressure across the grain of the muscles to release chronic patterns of tension, and stress accumulation. It also increases circulation to facilitate the movement of waste products out of the muscle tissue. Recent evidence shows that deep tissue massage can break up scar tissue and eliminate it.

2: **Lymphatic drainage** is a highly specialized kneading technique; it's a large surface massage, a unique method that uses precise, complex hand movements to encourage the draining of lymph fluids. In comparison, normal massage techniques are much too forceful to allow drainage in the tissues and may hinder transport.

I call the lymphatic system the body's natural antibiotic. When it is flushed and clean, lymph fluid removes body toxins as part of the auto-immune response to disease. Using slow, gentle strokes with a rhythmic pumping action, the massage technician follows the lymph pathways throughout the body to move the flow of lymph and accelerate detoxification.

Lymphatic massage has four primary effects on your body:
1: It balances the sympathetic and parasympathetic nervous systems.
2: It activates inhibitory reflex cells which decrease or even eliminate pain sensations.
3: It increases lymph flow for a decongestant effect on connective tissue, stimulates blood capillary flow and increases resorptive capacity of the blood capillaries.
4: It boosts immune response by increasing lymph flow and stimulating antibodies.

There are several popular techniques of therapeutic massage today. The choice is limited only by personal preference and desired results. For lasting benefits, use massage therapy as part of a program that includes diet improvement and exercise.

The most popular massage therapy methods:

—Alexander technique - This system strives to improve posture by properly positioning the head and neck. A favorite of actors and singers, the Alexander technique works to expand the chest cavity, improve breathing and body movement. The sessions involve guided body movement as well as table-work massage procedures. To find a practitioner, call (800) 473-0620.

—Feldenkrais - This system believes that to change the way we act, we must change the way we move. Through simple body manipulations and exercises, Feldenkrais practitioners help patients change unbalanced muscle patterns and the thought patterns associated with them. To find a practitioner, call (800) 775-2118.

—Polarity therapy - Besides the muscles, glands and nerves, the human body has a magnetic field that directs these systems and maintains energy balance. A polarity practitioner works to access the magnetic current and its movement patterns to release energy blocks. (See POLARITY THERAPY, page 26.)

—Reflexology - In this system, the feet and hands are seen as end points of energy zones and are associated with organs and glands throughout the body. Specific points are manipulated to open blocked energy pathways. Since the feet serve as reflexes for the entire body, foot reflexology is most often used. Reflexology is best used in conjunction with other massage techniques. (See REFLEXOLOGY, page 35.) For a practitioner, call (727) 343-4811.

—Rolfing - Rolfers attempt to realign the body with gravity by deeply manipulating the connective tissue that contains the muscles and links them to the bones. To find a practitioner, call (303) 449-5903.

—Swedish massage - uses kneading, stroking, friction, tapping and sometimes body shaking to stimulate, cleanse or relax. The techniques help muscles, joints, nerves and the endocrine system. When used before an athletic workout, they can prevent soreness, relieve swelling and tension, and improve muscular performance. By stimulating the body's circulation, a Swedish massage speeds rehabilitation from injury.

Note: As wonderful as massage therapy is, there are some health conditions where massage is not a good idea.
• Don't massage a person with high fever, cancer, tuberculosis or other infections or malignant conditions which might be further spread through the body.
• Don't massage the abdomen of a person with high blood pressure or ulcers.
• Don't massage legs with varicose veins, diabetes, phlebitis or blood vessel problems.
• Massage no closer than six inches near bruises, cysts, skin breaks or broken bones.
• Massage people with swollen limbs gently, only above the swelling, towards the heart.

Massage away the aches and pains of pregnancy....

Massage therapy is especially beneficial during pregnancy. Today more and more women are climbing on the bandwagon and using massage to ease the aches and pains of pregnancy, and facilitate easier childbirth.

Some of massage therapy's benefits during pregnancy....

—Helps release toxins and wastes that overload the circulatory and lymphatic systems, and contribute to fatigue and overall body sluggishness in the mother-to-be.

—Acts as a mood elevator for pregnancy-related depression and anxiety. Stress-reducing activity of massage usually means deeper sleep for moms-to-be and more balanced blood pressure.

—Significantly increases circulation, allowing more oxygen and nutrients to reach the systems of both mother and child for more vibrant health.

—Increases the flexibility of muscles, a definite asset for the birthing experience.

—Stimulates glandular secretions to balance hormone levels.

—Reduces back pain, edema, leg cramps and swollen ankles caused by weight gain and body changes.

—Light lower back massage (near the kidneys) promotes easier bowel movements for pregnant women with constipation. (If you get backaches when you're constipated, your transverse colon is probably blocked up by impacted wastes.)

—May help reduce stretch marks and improve skin elasticity.

Note: There are some pregnant women who should seek advice from a health professional before undergoing massage. Check the following list for risk factors that may apply to you:

• pregnant women at risk for miscarriage
• pregnant women with cancers or tumors
• pregnant women with infectious illness
• pregnant women at risk for early labor
• pregnant women with pre-eclampsia (toxemia)
• pregnant women with gestational diabetes
• pregnant women with placental disorders
• pregnant women with heart disease, high blood pressure or kidney disease

Perineal Massage.... Is it a viable option?

Perineal massage is practiced by midwives and pregnant women all over the country with good results. Some women find they experience less stinging during childbirth after using this technique. Others report that they were able to avoid tears or an episiotomy after perineal masssage treatments.

Perineal massage is normally practiced <u>in the last six weeks of pregnancy</u> to prepare the perineal tissues for the stretching of childbirth. The perineal tissues (between the vaginal opening and the anus) are gently massaged and stretched manually by the midwife, partner or the pregnant women herself. Some studies have disputed the benefits of this technique. One study suggests it is most helpful for women over 30. Ask your midwife, birth attendant or pregnancy massage therapist if perineal massage is right for you and for the best techniques to try.

Three other techniques help prepare the vaginal and perineal tissues for childbirth: 1) Apply hot compresses regularly to help relax vaginal and perineal tissues for easier childbirth; 2) Rub cocoa butter, vitamin E oil or wheat germ oil on the stomach and around vaginal opening and perineum each night to make stretching easier and skin more elastic; 3) Practice Kegel exercises regularly to strengthen pelvic floor muscles.

Polarity Therapy

Polarity therapy is a blend of art and science. Today's technology can show us graphically that the human body consists of electromagnetic patterns, with energy both surrounding the body and coursing through it in a continual flow of positive and negative charges. Expressed in ancient times as an aura, this magnetic field makes up our physical, mental, and emotional characteristics, directs body systems and maintains energy balance.

Healing energies appear to be composed of a combination of subtle electromagnetic fields and quantum fields. Quantum fields propagate without loss of energy. In fact, they have a unique ability to converge their energy, which helps explain how subtle energy devices can focus energy to create healing effects. The combination of the fields seems to boost stress-reducing biochemical mediators. Researchers say healing can never be explained without paying attention to the underlying energy fields that may initiate the healing response.

Randolphe Stone, the founder of polarity therapy, discovered that the human energy field is influenced by many factors—experiences, trauma, relationships, environment, attitudes, nutrition, movement, touch and sound. Today, many respected researchers believe that aberrated electromagnetic fields or wavelengths (such as EMFs) also affect man's energy frequencies. Robert Becker, M.D. author of *The Body Electric* says, "We now live in a sea of electromagnetic radiation that we cannot sense and that never before existed on this earth. New evidence suggests that this massive amount of radiation is producing stress, disease and other harmful effects by interfering with the most basic levels of brain function."

Our society is so dependent on electronics that abolishing electromagnetic radiation is out of the question. But we may be able to protect the body's life force energies with things like Polarity devices which act as "antennas" or "waveguides" to attract and reinforce healthful wave-lengths to the body. Beneficial wave-lengths, first identified by Bell Science Labs have been known since the 1950's.

Is polarity therapy a new technique to reduce stress?

Polarity therapists believe that balancing energy flow in the body is the underlying foundation of health. Popular in holistic spas and detox centers today, a polarity practitioner accesses the magnetic current to release energy blocks. Polarizers reset vortex spins so they are consistent with positive forces. North of the Earth's equator, a toxic vortex spins counter-clockwise; a healthy vortex spins clockwise. South of the equator the reverse is true. Polarizers repolarize or respin the negative vortex action, to either neutralize it or carry it into a beneficial spin. Rooted in Ayurveda tradition, polarity therapy also uses diet and exercise for cleansing tissues, circulation, and preventing illness.

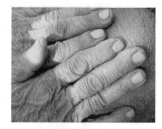

The hands are believed to be viable conductors of energy. Gentle touch induces a relaxed, meditative state to accelerate energy flow through the body. Some polarity therapists just use touch to facilitate energy movement, placing their hands on specific energy pathways on the body. There are three types of touch: rajasic, gentle and stimulating; sattvic, a light, balancing touch; and tamasic touch, which goes deeper into the muscles and tissues. Sessions last anywhere from 60 to 90 minutes, releasing blockages and keeping energy fields open. Frequently, the touch is so light that one doesn't feel anything at all.

There is clinical evidence for the effectiveness of this blend of quantum physics with biology and medicine. When polarity devices are brought in close contact to pain or muscle tension areas, many people report pain relief and a greater sense of well-being. In geriatrics treatment and home health nursing, numerous case studies show that polarizers can make significant health improvement in many patients. Relaxation, reduced fatigue and mental confusion, improved sleep, pain relief, and allergy symptom improvement are just a few of the benefits. Polarity therapy also helps treat migraines, low back pain and other stress disorders.

For polarity devices, SPRINGLIFE POLARIZERS *(888) 633-9233. For polarity practitioners, www.polaritytherapy.org.*

Magnet Therapy

Magnet therapy is an age-old healing technique. The first recorded use of therapeutic magnets dates back to 600 B.C.! Magnet therapy was used in ancient Greece, Persia, Egypt, and in India. There are even reports that Cleopatra slept with a magnet on her forehead to help preserve her beauty. Ancient Chinese physicians used magnetic rock, or lodestone, sometimes even electric eels to treat physical and mental disorders. In the 16th century, the Swiss physician and alchemist Paracelsus advocated magnet use. Magnet therapy was later explored and recommended by the founder of homeopathy, Dr. Samuel Hahnemann.

Modern science has known since the 1950's that a magnetic field is critical to normal body function and coordination. In fact, immune deficiency syndromes like chronic fatigue and fibromyalgia were first identified as magnetic field deficiency syndromes.

Our blood is composed of positively and negatively charged particles. **Magnet therapy balances negative-positive energy.**

A *positive, acid-producing field* may engender health conditions like arthritis, mental confusion, fatigue, pain and insomnia — and encourage fat storage. Refined foods, nicotine, toxic chemicals used in agriculture, auto exhaust, and many prescription drugs are culprits often responsible for this type of field. Emotional stress; hormone fluctuations caused by pregnancy, ovulation, or menopause; nutrient deficiences like iodine; irradiated foods; alcoholism or drug addiction can also cause this type of magnetic imbalance.

A *negative, alkaline-producing field* increases oxygen, encourages deep sleep, reduces swelling and fluid retention, relieves pain, and promotes mental acuity. A negative field acts like an antibiotic, helping destroy bacterial, fungal and viral infections because it lowers body acidity.

Does magnet therapy work? There seems to be no question that magnets can dramatically influence our health. Russians used magnet therapy during World War II to ease pain, specifically from amputation. Today, at least 50 countries including Germany, Japan and Russia have approved therapeutic magnets for healing. Magnet therapy is being enthusiastically rediscovered in the U.S. by health professionals and health conscious consumers looking for non-invasive, non-toxic solutions to chronic pain. Americans spent $500 million on therapeutic magnets in 1997 alone!

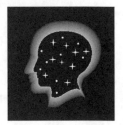

Science is still probing magnet therapy. What we know so far:

1: Magnet therapy increases blood flow, providing more oxygen to body areas that need healing. Magnets also facilitate the body's normal detoxification of the toxic by-products of pain and swelling.

2: Magnet therapy balances pH, restoring an environment unfavorable for disease, favorable for healing.

3: Magnet therapy helps break down scar tissue and release toxins, accelerating recovery from injury.

4: Magnet therapy speeds up the migration of calcium to help heal nerve tissue and bones, and helps eliminate excess calcium in the joints related to arthritis pain.

5: Magnet therapy stimulates enzyme activity, vital to healing.

6: Magnet therapy enlarges blood vessel diameters and reduces inflammation.

7: Magnet therapy helps restore the body's electrical balance, offsetting the effects of free radicals that contribute to degenerative disease .

8: Magnet therapy reduces pain by modulating pain receptors or neuron activity that causes pain. Magnets may stimulate the production of endorphins, our natural pain killers and mood elevators.

9: Magnets can help regulate the pineal gland, and stimulate production of hormones like melatonin.

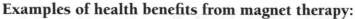

Examples of health benefits from magnet therapy:

—A study in November 1997 Archives of Physical Medicine and Rehabilitation reveals that patients suffering from post-polio pain experienced significant, rapid relief when pressure points were exposed to magnets.

—Studies conducted at John Hopkins, Yale and New York University confirm that magnet therapy reduces pain from tendonitis, arthritis and venous ulcers. Other research finds magnet therapy relieves pain from whiplash, head and knee injuries, and menstrual cramps.

—Magnet therapy is considered a potential treatment for severe depression. An electromagnet is strapped to the left front part of the brain, underactive in depressed people, which induces an electric current in the brain causing brain cells to produce more mood elevating neurotransmitters. The treatment lasts about 5 minutes.

Should you use magnet therapy? Check the following list for people who shouldn't:

…people who have a pacemaker or who have epilepsy
…people who are bleeding externally or internally—magnets promote blood flow
…people who are using an insulin or other drug patch
…pregnant women should not use magnets on the abdomen

Magnetic sleeping pads, cushions, shoe insoles, wraps, adhesives, bracelets and necklaces and massagers are widely available. Use quality magnets with a gauss strength greater than 400 for best results. If you suffer from chronic pain from arthritis, backaches, shoulder and neck pain, repetive strain injuries, migraines or sports injuries, magnet therapy may be a safe, effective alternative to drugs or invasive treatments. In addition, a health practitioner well schooled in magnet therapy can often use magnets supportively to reduce tumors, fibroids and cysts, and to help colitis or chronic constipation.

Consider Encore Technology MAGNELYFE *flexible contour magnets (877-624-6353).*

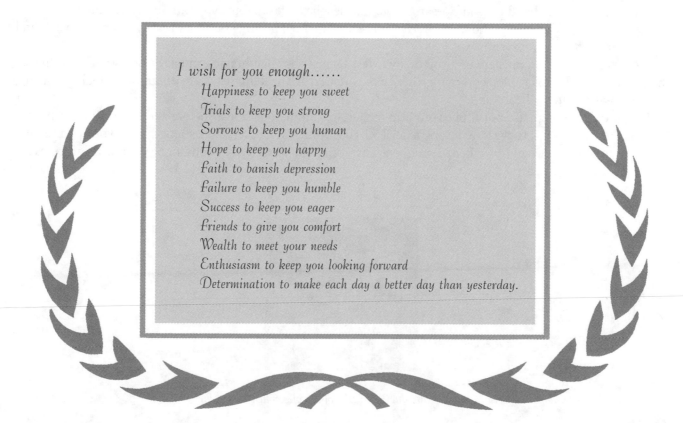

I wish for you enough......
Happiness to keep you sweet
Trials to keep you strong
Sorrows to keep you human
Hope to keep you happy
Faith to banish depression
Failure to keep you humble
Success to keep you eager
Friends to give you comfort
Wealth to meet your needs
Enthusiasm to keep you looking forward
Determination to make each day a better day than yesterday.

Applied Kinesiology
Muscle Testing

Applied kinesiology, or muscle testing is a Traditional Chinese Medicine technique now being enthusiastically rediscovered in America. The word kinesiology means the study of motion, especially the way muscles actually move our bodies. In the natural health field, kinesiology uses principles from Chinese medicine, chiropractic, osteopathy, acupressure and massage to bring the body into balance, and release pain and nerve tension.

Muscle testing is the way most Americans are familiar with applied kinesiology today. Applied kinesiology is based on the premise that muscles, glands, and organs are linked by meridians, or energy pathways throughout the body. Muscle testing is an effective method for detecting and correcting energy movements and imbalances in the body.

Muscle testing detects energy blocks.

Weak muscles indicate an energy flow blockage in one of the body's meridians. Muscle testing reliably identifies weak muscles. A kinesiologist uses stress release techniques to unblock the meridians. The muscles are then retested after visualization, massage techniques and movement exercises; if the muscles have regained strength, the restoration of the energy flow of the meridians is confirmed. Kinesiology does not heal, but rather restores balanced energy flow.

You can use personal muscle testing to determine your own individual response to a food or substance. It's a good technique to use before buying a healing remedy, because it lets you estimate the product's effectiveness for your own body before you buy. You will need a partner for the procedure.

How to use muscle testing:

1: Hold your arm out straight from your side, parallel to the ground. Have a partner place one hand just below your shoulder and one hand on your forearm. Your partner then tries to force your arm down towards your side, while you exert all your strength to hold it level. Unless you are in ill health, you should easily be able to withstand this pressure and keep your arm level.

2: Then, simply hold the item that you desire to test against your diaphragm (under the breastbone) or thyroid (the point where the collarbone comes together below the neck). The item may be in or out of normal packaging, or in its raw state, like a fresh food.

3: Holding the item as above, put your arm out straight from your side as before and have your partner try to press it down again. If the test item is beneficial for you, your arm will retain its strength, and your partner will be unable to force it down. If the item is not beneficial, or could worsen your condition, your arm can be easily pushed down by your partner.

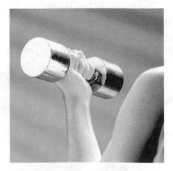

For more information, contact the International College of Applied Kinesiology (913) 384-5336

Hand and Foot Reflexology

Reflexology is an ancient massage therapy that works with the body's energy zones through the feet and hands. It's based on the belief that each part of the body is connected through the nerve system to specific points on the feet and hands. A history of foot massage spans time and place from the Physician's Tomb in Egypt of 2300 B.C. to the Physicians Temple in Nara, Japan of 700 A.D. The ancient Egyptians are believed to have actually developed hand and foot reflexology. Reflexology pictographs have been found in an Egyptian physician's tomb dating back to 2300 B.C.!

The science of reflexology believes that all body parts have energy and share information. Pressure to a particular meridian point brings about better function in all parts of that meridian zone, no matter how remote the point is from the body part in need of healing. Thus, reflexology can also be used for a measure of self-diagnosis and treatment.

Reflexology is often known as zone therapy. Reflexologists look at the feet as a mini-map of the entire body, with the big toes serving as the head, the balls of the feet representing the shoulders, and the narrowing of the foot as the waist area. The hand map is viewed similarly. Ten reflexology zone meridians have been extensively mapped connecting all organs and glands, and culminating in points in the hands and feet. The nervous system is considered an electrical system. Contact can be made through the feet and hands with the electro-mechanical zones in the body to the nerve endings. The nerve endings are called reflex points. The points on the feet are reflexive, like a knee-jerk reaction.... they serve as reflexes for the entire body. Any illness, injury or tension in the body produces tenderness in the corresponding foot (or hand) zone. The points are manipulated to open up blocked energy pathways.

Stress is involved in over 80% of all illness. Reflexology helps the body heal itself by relaxing stress and stimulating the release of pain-relieving endorphins. Its goal is to clear the pathways of energy flow throughout the body, to return body balance, so it's easy to see that reflexology can be helpful for problems like headaches, backaches or stress overload. Reflexology also increases immune response, by stimulating the lymphatic system to eliminate wastes, and the blood to circulate better to poorly functioning areas. Today, reflexology treatments are used for pain relief from injuries and for faster recovery from illness without surgery or heavy medication. In China, over 300 studies show reflexology treatments can improve 95% of 64 different illnesses researched.

Reflexologists rely on an inchworm-like massage motion of the thumb to produce light or deep pressure on each zone, concentrating on the tender spots, which often feel like little grains of salt under the skin.

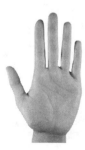

For your own use, picture your hands and feet as your body's control panels. Get a good reflexology chart—available in health food stores. Then use your fingers or a rounded-end tool to locate the reflex points. Some points take practice to pinpoint. The best rule for knowing when you have reached the right spot is that it is usually very tender, denoting crystalline deposits brought about by poor capillary circulation of fluids, or congestion in the corresponding organ. The amount of soreness on the foot point normally indicates the size of the crystalline deposit, and the amount of time it has been accumulating. For most people, the tenderness is usually accompanied by an immediate feeling of relief in the body organ area as the congesting waste deposits break up for removal.

To address specific health problems with reflexology, the following resources offer invaluable help: *Reflexology: Health at your Fingertips* by Barbara and Kevin Kunz, (includes detailed reflexology charts), or visit http://www.reflexology-research.com/ for detailed reflexology charts you can purchase on line.

Both resources show the pressure points for each area, so that you can use reflexology to release energy blocks in your body. Locate the matching point on your own hands and feet and press as directed. In some cases, the points are very tiny, particularly for the glands. They will take practice to pinpoint.

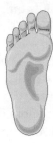

For effective reflexology, press on a reflex point 3 times for 10 seconds each time. Fifteen pounds of applied force on a reflex point is enough to send a surge of energy to remove the obstructive crystals, restore circulation and clear congestion. Use reflexology pressure treatment for twenty to thirty minute sessions at a time, about twice a week. Sessions more often than this will not give nature the chance to use the stimulation or do its necessary repair work. Most people notice frequent and easy bowel movements in the first twenty-four hours after reflexology as the body throws off released wastes.

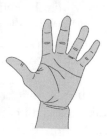

Documented health benefits of reflexology therapy:

...**Reduces PMS.** A study in 1993 in the journal Obstetrics and Gynecology finds women suffering from premenstrual syndrome experience a 40% reduction in symptoms after using reflexology treatments.

...**Improves asthma reactions.** One case study reports a significant improvement in well being and reduction in asthma symptoms after three months of reflexology therapy.

...**Helps balance blood sugar in cases of type 2 diabetes.** Two different studies (one from China; the other from America) reveal reflexology effectively lowers high blood sugar levels in diabetics.

...**Helps restore some movement and sensation for people paralyzed from spinal cord injuries.** Case studies published in the journal Reflexions find some quadriplegic and paraplegic patients respond to reflexology sessions with restored movement. Other effects noted for paralyzed people: some return of bowel and bladder control; induced sweating below the level of the injury; the sensation of bowel rumbling, improved muscle tone; and a decrease in bladder infections.

...**May help remove non-malignant cysts and growths.** Medical doctor Julian Whitaker reports in his book, 199 Health Secrets, that just two weeks of reflexology treatment helped remove a ganglion cyst on his hand.

...**May help dissolve ovarian cysts.** Professional reflexologist Christopher Shirley recounts the story of two women scheduled for surgery to remove ovarian cysts who experienced a mysterious disappearance of the cysts (documented by sonograms) after reflexology treatments.

...**Helps alleviates some symptoms of senility.** Stiffness, restlessness and wandering are reduced in Alzheimer's patients.

...**Reduces pain from labor.** May also help facilitate placental discharge in women who are candidates for surgical delivery.

...**Decreases pain, nausea and anxiety for cancer patients.**

...**Can improve growth rate where degenerative disease has taken a toll.** I have personally seen children with cerebral palsy show marked benefit.

...**Accelerates bowel evacuation in constipation.**

...**Reduces some cardiovascular disease symptoms.** Patients who experienced chest pain, angina and high blood pressure got relief.

...**Lowers stress and anxiety**. Especially for people suffering from nervous exhaustion and menopause associated night panic attacks.

Reflexology can also be part of a good health maintenance program. You don't have to be sick to appreciate the benefits. Many people simply enjoy the tension release a reflexology session gives.

For a reflexologist, call (727) 343-4811 or visit Reflexology Assoc. of America www.reflexology-usa.org

Acupuncture & Acupressure

Acupuncture and acupressure are ancient systems of natural healing from Asia. The central belief of Traditional Chinese Medicine is that the body must be in balance to function at its peak. Both acupuncture and acupressure are considered a means of mobilizing a person's own healing energy and balance, and can positively influence the course of a therapy program.

Traditional Oriental medicine believes that emotional and physical energy, known as qi or chi, flows through the body along specific bio-chemical or energy pathways called meridians. The pathways regulate and coordinate the body's well-being by distributing chi energy through it. Meridian points are connected to specific organs and body functions. When chi energy is flowing smoothly, the body is in perfect balance. When chi energy flow is slowed down or blocked, by factors like injury, poor diet, stress or climate, then physical or emotional illness often results. Chinese medicine sees acupuncture as stimulating the release of blocked energy, which then flows throughout the body allowing it to normalize itself. Because the body meridians are interconnected with the internal organs, Chinese practitioners use acupuncture to treat everything from immune disorders, like chronic fatigue syndrome, to allergies and asthma.

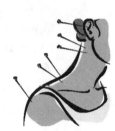

ACUPUNCTURE uses hair thin needles and/or electrodes to direct and channel body energy. Western science believes that acupuncture needling stimulates certain nerve cells to release chemicals in the spine, muscles and brain. These biochemicals allay pain by releasing endorphins, the body's pain-relieving substances. They also stimulate the release of other chemicals and hormones that help normalize body processes. Acupuncture is used in the U.S. mainly for pain relief, but is also valuable in treating environmentally-induced illnesses caused by radiation poisoning or air pollution, is useful in carpal tunnel syndrome, and withdrawal complications from smoking, alcoholism, or drug addiction. Acupuncture is extremely effective in treating rheumatoid arthritis, bringing relief to almost 80% of those who suffer from it.

Surgery and drugs can often be avoided, and there are sometimes spectacular results. The World Health Organization cites 104 different conditions that acupuncture can treat including: migraines, sinusitis, the common cold, tonsillitis, eye inflammation, myopia, duodenal ulcers, neuralgia, Meniere's disease, tennis elbow, paralysis from stroke, speech aphasia and sciatica. The Clinical Journal of Pain shows acupuncture is effective for long term relief of back pain. A new study of 40,000 people shows acupuncture relieves back pain, headaches, and chronic degenerative knee and hip problems for a whopping 90% of people. The state of Maine is funding an acupuncture study to determine its effectiveness in helping drug addicts resist relapse cravings. Acupuncture can also play an important role in reducing post-traumatic stress syndromes, anxiety and panic attacks.

An acupuncture treatment series focuses on individual need and progress, rather than symptoms. They look for lifestyle patterns that affect health and immune response, and place great emphasis on balance and harmony with the patient's environment. Then they try to correct these underlying imbalances to re-establish foundation wellness. Someone suffering acute specific pain may need only a few months of treatments; someone with a chronic disease usually requires a long-term treatment program. Most patients feel relaxed during acupuncture treatment, but response is highly individual, relaxing some, energizing others.

Modern acupuncture uses several adjunct treatments: **moxibustion**, a heat therapy where herbs like Chinese *wormwood* are burned near acupuncture points to radiate through the skin and influence the meridians; **cupping,** a circulation stimulating technique, in which heated glass cups are placed over acupuncture points to draw blood to the area; and **massage therapy** to enhance circulation throughout the body.

Note: Electro-acupuncture should not be used by people with a pacemaker. In addition, if you are hemophiliac or tend towards easy bruising and bleeding, acupuncture may not be the best choice for you.

ACUPRESSURE uses the same principles and meridian points as acupuncture, but works through finger pressure, massage and stroking rather than needles to effect stimulation. Acupressure and massage therapy are frequently combined in a healing stimulation session As with other natural therapies, the aim is to regulate, balance and normalize so the body can function normally. Organ massage, reflexology and deep breathing techniques are frequently used in conjunction with acupressure.

Fourteen primary meridians or channels of energy run through your body. (See diagram.) Each meridian is named for the organ or function connected to its energy flow. Acupressure manually stimulates these points to release blocked energy.

Acupressure is an individualized approach to healing.

A skilled acupressurist works with you as an individual to treat both acute and chronic blockages. Acute blockages are sensitive, usually hot or inflamed. Chronic blockages are cool to the touch, more difficult to find, and the body may have adapted habits (like limping or slouching) to keep from feeling them. A client's trust is integral to the success of a professional acupressure treatment, because the acupressurist must have the body's permission in order to release blocked body meridians and correctly redistribute body chi.

Acupressure can improve cardiovascular disease and reduce depression. It corrects debilitating back pain, organ congestion, and can, in some cases, even reverse serious problems like scoliosis. It is excellent as part of a detoxification program. Acupressure specifically cleanses the lymphatic system of toxins and fluids related to cellulite formation and immune malfunction. (Have at least 3 acupressure treatments before an acupressure lymphatic release to strengthen organs like the liver, kidneys, bladder, lungs and large intestines.)

Use some of the most effective acupressure points yourself:

The primary advantage of acupressure is that it is a self-access therapy. In fact, the Chinese consider acupressure a personal first aid method. Almost every technique can easily be done at home as needed, to relieve pain, and open up body cleansing and healing channels.

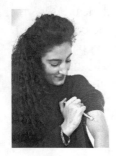

Acupressure is a two-step process.

Step one: find the right pressure point. They are tiny—only about the size of a pin-head—so this may be more difficult than it seems. If you can't find the exact spot on your body at first, poke around a bit—acupressure points are generally more tender than the surrounding area.

Step two: massage the point properly. Use the tip of your index finger, your middle finger, or both fingers side by side. In some spots, it may be easier to use your thumb. Stimulate the point as deeply as can be managed—in a digging kind of massage. A few seconds of pressure, repeated several times, is usually enough. Push until you feel some discomfort.

For optimum benefits, two acupressure points may be simultaneously stimulated at the same time, one with each hand, while the part of the body in between experiences maximum energy flow between the points. Or, you can duplicate the pressure on both sides of the body. Immediately after finding and massaging the point on one side, repeat the technique on the opposite side. In most cases, points only need to be triggered about 15 seconds each to get prompt relief.

Acupressure can be tricky. If you don't experience relief, it may mean one of two things:
1: You did not pinpoint the correct spot. Try another one or try again. Make sure you feel the twinge when you probe and press.
2: You didn't perform the procedure correctly. Remember to use the tip of your thumb or finger, and to apply enough pressure for enough time.

Almost invariably, you'll experience reactions to an acupressure treatment that will let you know you've "hit the spot." Within about 30 seconds of triggering a point, you should feel warmth in that spot and perhaps slight dizziness or a light-headed feeling. Some people report a clammy feeling across the brow or shoulders, breaking out in a sweat, or feeling "electricity" emanating from the acupressure point. These types of reactions are signs that you have found a channel point that needed unblocking; you should feel relief.

Acupressure techniques for common health problems:

…For a sore back, press on the points on either side of the lower spine. (Look for the spot just around the corner from your bottom rib.) Press both sides simultaneously.

…For a backache, apply pressure just below the tailbone.

…For low back pain, apply strong pressure in the middle of the dip on the sides of your buttocks. For the best results, apply pressure to each side simultaneously.

…For a headache, press the point between your eyes.

…For insomnia, press two points, right at the natural hairline on either side of the spine.

…For a sore throat, press the center of your forehead about midway between the eyebrows and the natural hairline. Massage the point until the acupressure reaction occurs.

…For lower abdomen discomfort, such as bowel disorders or indigestion, run your thumb up the inner, rear edge of the shin bone directly in line with your ankle bone toward the knee. At about 3" up, you'll feel the unmistakable tingling that announces the point.

…For weight loss, locate the cleft between the bottom of the nose and top of the upper lip. Pinch it when you're hungry, and within moments your hunger will be gone.

Acupressure as a beauty treatment?

Acupressure can slow down aging and enhance beauty by rebalancing body Qi. Poor Qi drags down circulation, elimination, muscle and nerve tone- all factors that accelerate aging. An acupressure facial works to restore proper Qi flow, stimulating lymph drainage and blood circulation, delivering oxygen to skin cells and reducing muscle tension related to wrinkles. Many people notice improvements in skin tone, fine lines, sagging tissue or dark circles under the eyes after one month of acupressure facial treatments.

An acupressure facial is an effective at-home beauty treatment. A few techniques to try:

…For crows' feet, gently press the points around the orbits of your eyes. Start from the inside orbit point (below the tear duct) and work your way to the outside point (where the upper and lower lid meet).

…To release muscular tension in the jaw, press the point located at the back corner of the jaw. Move finger up and forward. (Most people have tight jaw muscles; this point will likely be tender or sore.)

…For deep creases in the forehead, press on the muscles around the creases; mold the muscles back into the creases. Do light circular massage on the forehead to stimulate lymph flow.

…For laugh lines around the mouth, press the points at the corners of the mouth and the point in the crease between the chin and lower lip.

Acupuncture and acupressure are gaining new respect in the western world as painless, non-toxic therapies for restoring healing energy and for preventing disease. Conventional doctors find that acupuncture and acupressure work well in conjunction with conventional medicine, an unusual benefit for western medicine. Because they are free of toxins and addictive side effects, they have become valuable alternatives for people who used to live on Motrin, Advil and other pain pills that harm the liver.

Animals benefit from acupuncture and acupressure. Both methods are often recommended for hip dysplasia and arthritis in large animals. Acupuncture was successfully used over 3000 years ago in Asia to treat a stomach disorder in an elephant!

Need to find a good acupuncturist? Call (253) 851-6896. To find a veterinary acupuncturist, visit the American Academy of Veterinary Acupuncture on the web - www.aava.org.

Mind-Body Healing
Prayer and Meditation

Meditation practices have been used for thousands of years as a way to bring together mind and body with deep breathing and focused attention. Almost every ancient culture, especially those throughout Asia, the Middle East and the Indian sub-continent included meditation as a part of their religious and spiritual traditions. Meditation is <u>still</u> a regular part of the spiritual life of Chinese Taoists and Zen Buddhists who use it as a way to achieve higher levels of consciousness during ceremonal rites. I myself have been witness to some of these ceremonies. They can be quite intense, with mesmerizing chanting, aromatic burning of incense, and rich harmonics of singing bells. Meditation as a path to greater spirituality has been a part of the life of every monastic and holy order since the beginning of the Roman Catholic church.

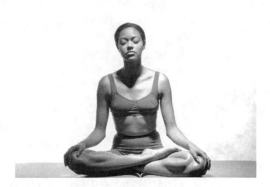

Meditation is the practice of focusing quiet concentration on a religious figure, a positive mantra or affirmation, a chakra center in the body, or the natural rhythm of one's breathing. Most people meditate while sitting, but one can meditate while lying down, standing or even walking slowly. Most people prefer to keep their eyes closed, yet in ancient artwork of Buddha himself in meditation, the eyes are traditionally kept at "half-mast." Meditation can be practiced alone or in groups. For people new to the technique, meditating in groups offers a supportive environment that makes it more effective.

In traditional meditation, the correct posture is just as important as your attention to your mantra and breathing. It can be difficult for new meditators to sit comfortably in the well known Buddha meditation position-- cross-legged with upright posture on a pad or zafu. For people with serious back problems, chairs can make the experience more comfortable, or other sitting positions can be explored. Expert meditators are known to meditate long hours (8 or more hours!) while sitting. Qigong and yoga exercises are regularly recommended to increase strength and flexibility for long meditation sessions.

There are many meditation styles: Zen, mantra meditation, mindfulness, primordial sound and breath awareness. Just sitting quietly in your own home with no distractions can be a form of meditation. More and more people are creating their own home meditation rooms. Adding ritual helpers like aromatherapy, candle burning, soft, relaxing music or chanting personalizes the experience.

I like to think of meditation as a form of mental training that improves concentration and creativity by reducing stress and quieting the mind, important in a world of noise pollution and media overkill. Many healers believe it is one of the best ways to open up communication between the brain and body.

What can meditation do for your health?

Meditation can reduce the stress from today's hectic lifestyles. Modern scientific research reveals meditation boosts the intensity of relaxing, brain alpha waves to levels not seen even during sleep. But, meditation can do much more than calm your nerves. It can be powerful medicine. More than <u>500</u> scientific studies have been done on meditation's health effects.

A few examples of meditation's benefits:

...Saves big money in medical care. The American Journal of Managed Care shows people following a Transcendental Meditation program have 80% fewer hospital admissions and 55% fewer visits to their doctor.

...Slows down aging. Many studies reveal people who meditate live longer, healthier lives.

...Lowers blood pressure. A study in Psychosomatic Medicine in Nov. 1999 shows meditation lowers blood pressure by reducing blood vessel constriction.

...Heals the heart. A 1996 study in the American Journal of Cardiology shows men with coronary artery disease were able to improve their heart rate, blood pressure and work performance by meditating 20 minutes twice daily for six to eight months. Many men were even able to stop their heart medications using <u>only</u> meditation as a lifestyle change. In addition, studies show meditation reduces arterial thickness and plaque linked to heart disease.

...Accelerates recovery from psoriasis. A study published in Psychosomatic Medicine in March 1999 reveals meditation used in conjunction with UV therapy boost healing from psoriasis 4 times faster than UV therapy used alone.

...Improves chronic disorders like PMS, IBS, insomnia, mild depression and tension headaches. There are even reports that meditation speeds recovery from stroke-related paralysis.

Can you pray your way to better health?

Like meditation, prayer is beginning to be seen as a healer today....even in some scientific circles. In studies conducted by the University of Maryland, random groups of people were randomly assigned patients to pray for according to Judeo-Christian principles. Thus, the sources of the prayers were anonymous and the patients receiving the prayers did not know they were being prayed for. A control group of patients did not receive any prayers. In 57% of the studies, prayer had a positive effect on healing. In one study, heart patients were able to breathe better, and reduced their use of diuretics and antibiotics.

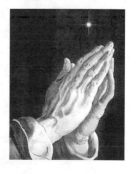

While science will never be able to measure God's response to our prayers, it is clear that faith and spirituality can have a powerful effect on health. Over 200 recent studies show that religious faith speeds recovery from illness and surgery, boosts immune response and extends lifespan. In addition, research reveals amazingly, that prayer can improve the growth rate of cell cultures, seeds, plants, fungi, bacteria, even baby chicks. In one documented case, a prayer circle may have saved the life of a near-death premature infant! Cancer and AIDS have also responded positively to the power of prayer. I recommend including your own blend of spirituality or religious faith into your prescription for better health. Prayer and meditation can be powerful medicine.

Just as your body needs nourishment from healthy foods, your soul needs nourishment from spiritual attention. Never forget... there is always something more.

Qigong and T'ai Chi

Qigong (pronounced Chee gung) was practiced by the Chinese as early as 500 B.C. Ancient drawings of qigong-like exercises are scattered on rock faces throughout China and Tibet. A main pillar of Traditional Chinese Medicine today, qigong is believed to clear the body meridians of obstructions to health, and restore the body's innate healing forces. Taoist and Buddhist philosophies incorporate qigong for mind/body healing.

Qigong provides the structure for all modern martial arts with exercises that can be performed by anyone almost anywhere. In Asia, its slow, shadow boxing movements are practiced by millions every day. Small groups may be seen everywhere in China, morning through evening. Everyone is welcome to join. I have seen, even taken part in, some of these silent, graceful meditative sessions and found them very relaxing. It's no wonder Qigong's popularity is growing in the West for its stress relieving benefits to mind, body and spirit.

Qigong and T'ai Chi are supreme mind-body-spirit healers of Asia

Qi (meaning life energy) and **gong** (meaning practice) is a superior method of balancing the flow of Qi through breathing, gentle movements and thoughtful meditation. With its links to ancient Chinese shamanic beliefs and divine, even magical revelation, the spiritual side of Qigong is mysterious to us in the West. Chinese shamans used qigong exercises and meditations as a way to communicate with the higher powers of Nature and boost their own healing powers. There are documented reports of qigong masters igniting fires by projecting Qi energy!

T'ai Chi (or Taiji) is a popular style of Qigong with slow, dance-like movements that invigorate body and mind. There are over a thousand different exercises, ranging from simple calisthenic movements, meditations and breathing exercises, to more advanced techniques where practitioners affect Qi flow and healing from a distance. Some forms of qigong target specific body systems, health imbalances, stress relief, even health assessment. Enlightened businesses today incorporate qigong exercises as a daily routine to increase productivity and success.

What can Qigong do for you?

Thousands of Asian studies confirm the success of Qigong as a great harmonizer of body and mind with remarkable healing properties. There are reports of people with advanced cancers being cured by qigong, and of lab animals being positively affected by practitioners who project Qi. Amazing!

...**Reduce high blood pressure.** Studies show patients who take blood-pressure lowering drugs and practice qigong have more balanced blood pressure than patients who just take drugs.
...**Accelerate elimination of toxins and wastes** for natural detoxification.
...**Increase circulation**, very helpful for people with angina, migraines and cold hands and feet.
...**Balance brain chemistry and reduce anxiety,** obsessive-compulsive, depression disorders.
...**Improve posture, flexibility, balance and strength.** Prevent or reduce falling injuries in the elderly.
...**Block the damaging effects of free radicals.** Qigong has antioxidant effects, stimulating SOD (Super Oxide Dismutase) production in the body. Qigong also enhances oxygen and nutrient uptake.
...**Fight cancer by boosting immune response.**
...**Relieve chronic pain** from injuries, surgery, arthritis and fibromyalgia.

Work with a skilled Qigong practitioner if you're a beginner. Qigong is not just exercise, it involves lifestyle, diet, emotional wellbeing and spiritual center. Qigong is more than a self-healing therapy, it is a way of life.

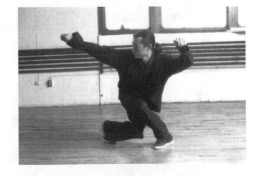

Guided Imagery

Guided imagery uses the mind/body connection to help give people more control over their health. It is a communication technique for accessing the network between mind and body as a source of power for healing. It has its roots in the ancient Greek understanding of how the mind influences the subconscious, and has been employed under many different names throughout the history of medicine, to speed healing by reducing stress and calming the mind.

Imagery is simply a flow of thoughts that you can see, hear, feel, smell, or taste in your imagination. It's the way your nervous system processes information, so it's especially effective for the dialogue between mind and body in the healing process.

Scientifically, imagery works like a computer to program directions into the hypothalamus that a patient wants for his body. This happens almost instantaneously, traveling from the brain through the nervous system, to the endocrine system through the hypothalamus-pituitary adrenal axis, and then through the vagus nerve for both psychological and physical accord.

Everything that is registered in our minds is registered in our bodies. Deepak Chopra M.D., a well-known expert on the mind-body connection, explains that "the mind is in every cell of the body. Every thought we think causes a release of neuropeptides that are transmitted to all the cells in the body."

Messages you send your body through imagery, for example, are immediately translated through the parasympathetic nervous system into neurotransmitters, that direct the immune system to work better against abnormal cells, or the hormone system to rebalance and stop creating abnormal cells.

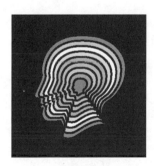

Thoughts of love, for example, cause your body to release interleukin and interferon, body healing elements. On the other hand, anxious thoughts cause your body to release cortisone and adrenaline, immune suppressing elements. Peaceful thoughts release chemicals in your body similar to valium, which help your body relax, adjust and "take a new look" at its health state. The school of imagery believes that the body is in a better position to cope with disease-causing factors if it isn't under stress. When stress levels are high, immune response is reduced, so learning to relax is fundamental to self-healing. Today, guided imagery in one form or another is a part of almost every stress-reduction technique. For many people, imagery is an good way to relax, and its active nature makes it easier to use than other methods.

Guided imagery is a proven method for pain relief, for helping people tolerate medical procedures, for reducing drug side effects, and for stimulating healing response. Guided imagery allows patients to take a much more active role in their own healing process. It's a personal way to help people find meaning in their illness; it offers a way to cope, and accelerates recovery. By helping patients access the images of their unconscious mind, guided imagery may even provide critical information on what is needed for recovery.

Guided imagery helps patients process bottled-up emotional pain, anger, and fear that may be aggravating health problems. Imagery is used to encourage athletes and performers to better performance, minimizing discomfort from all kinds of injuries, including sprains, strains, and broken bones. During healing, it is successful in overcoming chronic pain, addictions, and persistent infections, even in shrinking tumor growths. Even serious, degenerative illness like cancer has responded to guided imagery, with patients showing heightened immune activity as they imagine cancer cells being gobbled up by immune antibodies.

How does guided imagery work for stress and depression?

Stress reduction techniques, like meditation and guided imagery, powerfully affect the progression of disease. It's a proven method for enabling a less painful, faster recuperation. Studies show that both meditation and imagery help people eliminate or reduce the severity and frequency of headaches, dramatically slow the aging process, and can manage the discomfort of lower back pain, heart disease, hypertension, irritable bowel syndrome, even cancer and AIDS.

Experts claim that imagery can help both physical and psychological disorders, from high blood pressure and acne, to diabetes, cancer and addictions.

Stress reactions are an excellent example of an emotional response that manifests itself in the body.... often as illness.

Imagery can help clarify and put in a broader perspective what's really going on in a person's life. If someone under severe stress is able to integrate his or her situation into a broader meaning of life, the feelings of loss, grief or depression will be relatively temporary.

Here's an example: a man might respond to the loss of his wife with a prolonged state of depression. His body, too, will be in a state of depression, making him susceptible to serious health problems. But if he is able to intergrate his loss into his whole life picture, by directly accessing emotions through guided imagery, his loss won't totally overwhelm him, and his grief will lessen over time. Gradually, he can develop a more wholesome view of his life, to again become a participant, rather than a victim of its circumstances.

Two kinds of guided imagery techniques - receptive imagery and active imagery:

—*Receptive imagery* involves entering a relaxed state, then focusing on the area of the body with the ailment. You envision an embodiment of the illness, perhaps a mischievous demon, and ask it why it is causing the trouble. Your unconscious can provide a great deal of information about what your body needs.

—*Active imagery* involves envisioning an illness being cured. This may mean anything from imagining your immune system attacking a tumor, to picturing arm pain as a ball that rolls down your arm and out of your body. I have been part of an active imagery session. It can be dramatic.

How does a guided imagery session work?

Imagery guide therapists use a near-trance condition much like hypnosis, induced through spoken suggestion and soft music to affect healing. Patients are asked to envision themselves in a tranquil place like a quiet woods or a mountain lake, then directed to describe their sensations ....what they see, hear, smell, or feel, in order to reach a deeper state of relaxation. It's a powerful technique (called sensory recruitment) because it summons areas of the brain that control each different sense.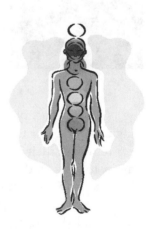

When relaxation has been reached, patients are asked to visualize their immune system as an energy force battling for their health. Their immune responses are analyzed in great detail. They are then asked to join forces with the immune system, by mentally envisioning the illness and then imagining their antibodies and white cells overcoming it. There are 20 different studies showing that people can directly stimulate their immune systems, increasing both natural killer cells and thymus activity using imagery techniques!

Not everyone is capable of working with guided imagery treatment. An active imagination is a must, because the more vivid the image, the more effective the treatment. Successful subjects are those who can understand the value of imagery in helping to solve to their problems, and who do not mentally fight it.

Need to find a good practitioner? Call the Academy for Guided Imagery. (800) 726-2070

Hypnotherapy

The power of suggestion has always played a major role in healing. Today's clinical hypnosis is an artificially induced mental state that heightens receptivity to suggestion. Hypnotherapy uses both suggestion and trance to access the deepest levels of the mind in order to effect positive changes in behavior. It maximizes the mind's contribution to healing by producing a multi-level relaxation state—a state which allows enhanced focus to increase tolerance to adverse stimuli, ease anxiety, or enhance affirmative imagery.

Despite its stage performance history, clinical hypnotherapy does not lead to strange or unethical behavior, nor does hypnosis cause people to divulge deep secrets or do things they wouldn't do normally. The vast majority of people respond to hypnotic suggestions in much the same way they would in their waking lives.

Physiologically, hypnosis stimulates the limbic system, the region of your brain linked to emotion and involuntary responses, like adrenal spurts and blood pressure. Habitual patterns of thought and reaction are temporarily suspended during hypnosis, rendering the brain capable of responding to healthy suggestions.

Research demonstrates that body chemistry does change during a hypnotic trance. The physiological shift can actually be observed, as can greater control of autonomic nervous system functions that are normally beyond one's ability to control. Stress and blood pressure reduction are common occurrences.

In one experiment, a young girl was unable to hold her hand in a bucket of ice water for more than thirty seconds. Her body's blood levels of cortisol were high, indicating she was in severe stress. Under hypnosis, she could keep the same hand in ice water for thirty minutes, with no rise in blood cortisol levels.

Hypnotherapy has healing applications for both psychological and physical disorders.

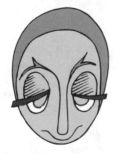

A skilled hypnotherapist can effect profound changes in respiration and relaxation to create enhanced well-being. Hypnotherapy techniques are widely used to help you quit smoking, stop snoring, lose weight, or get a good night's sleep. It helps treat medical conditions like facial neuralgia, sciatica, arthritis, whiplash, menstrual pain and tennis elbow. Migraines, ulcers, asthma, tinnitus, eating disorders, bruxism, nail biting, tension headaches, and even warts respond to hypnotherapy. Professional sports trainers use hypnotherapy to boost athletic performance. Hypnosis helps people tolerate pain during medical procedures, too. It's useful in surgeries where regular anesthesia isn't a good option, in cases like hysterectomies, hernias, breast biopsies, hemorrhoidectomies and Caesarian sections. For minor sugeries, patients who do not tolerate anesthesia well may even undergo surgery without anesthesia using hypnosis. Dentists regularly use hypnosis for root canal patients who can't tolerate anesthesia. A recent study shows that burn victims heal considerably faster with less pain and fewer complications if they are hypnotized shortly after they are injured.

Hypnotherapy dramatically improves symptoms of stubborn Irritable Bowel Syndrome in 80% of people who use it. It's so effective that Adriane Fugh-Berman, MD, of the National Women's Health Network recommends that hypnosis be the treatment of choice for IBS cases that don't respond to conventional therapy.

Scientists are now examining a new aspect of hypnotherapy: its effect on the immune system. Recent research shows that hypnotherapy can be used to train your immune system to fight diseases like cancer.

Hypnotherapy works best as a partnership between doctor and patient. Surprisingly, while most people think they can't be hypnotized, 90% of the population <u>can</u> achieve a trance state, (I have been one of those surprised people myself) and another 30% have a high enough susceptibility to enter a receptive state.

Three conditions are essential for successful hypnotherapy:

…A comfortable environment, free of distraction, so the patient can reach the deepest possible level.

…A trusting rapport between the hypnotist and the patient.

…A willingness and desire by the subject to be hypnotized. People who benefit most from hypnotherapy understand that hypnosis is not a surrender of personal control, but instead, an advanced form of relaxation.

Need to find a good practitioner? Call the American Board of Hypnotherapy. (800) 872-9996

Aromatherapy

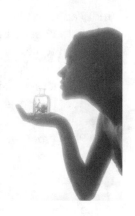

The use of aromatic plant oils has a long legacy in history. The first recorded use of essential oils dates back to ancient Egypt where they were used for embalming the dead. (Jars of plant oils were found in King Tut's tomb.) High born Egyptian women used plant oils in therapeutic baths and aromatic massage. The ancient Greeks and Romans used essential oils for everything from reducing coughs and colds, to stimulating menstruation and fighting off hangovers.

Essential oils were highly valued throughout Bibical times. There are over 188 references to essential oils in the Bible! When the plague hit Europe in the 16th century, people became too afraid to bathe, so aromatic plants were widely used by everybody as natural perfumes to mask body odors. This practice continued up through the middle of the 20th century when modern deodorants came on the scene. By the 18th and 19th centuries, all herbalists, even some traditional doctors used essential plant oils for healing. Modern aromatherapy still stands strong as a powerful therapy—a primary remedy to reduce stress and depression, and is becoming well known for its potential in treating serious problems like Alzhemier's disease.

Volatile oils distilled from plants are the heart of aromatherapy.

The oils are called "essential oils" because they are the regenerating, oxygenating immune defense of the plant, and they act in plants much like hormones do in humans. Seventy-five to 100 times more concentrated than dried herbs and flowers, aromatherapy oils offer high potency for herbal medicines. The molecules of essential aromatherapy oils carry healing nutrients directly to your body's cells.

Essential oils are not oily.

They are non-oily, highly active fluids that evaporate easily and completely. They don't leave marks on your clothing or towels. They may be taken in by inhalation, steams and infusers, or applied topically to the skin. The therapeutic effects of true essential oils are due both to their pharmacological properties and to their small molecule size, which allows easy penetration through the skin, the lymph system, the walls of the blood vessels and body tissues, pathways that impact the body's organ, hormonal, nervous and immune systems.

How does aromatherapy work?

Essential oils affect people first through the sense of smell.

How many times have you smelled something like a perfume or a food and had the taste of it instantly in your mouth? Smell is the most rapid of all your senses because its information is directly relayed to the hypothalamus. Motivation, moods, emotions and creativity all begin in the hypothalamus, so odors affect them immediately. Essential oil molecules work through hormone-like chemicals to produce their sensations. Odors can even influence the glands responsible for hormone levels, metabolism, insulin and stress levels, sex drive, body temperature and appetite.

When inhaled, the odors stimulate a release of neurotransmitters, body chemicals responsible for pleasant feelings and pain reduction. The aromas of apples and cinnamon, for example, have a powerful stabilizing effect on some people, especially those suffering from nervous anxiety. These aromas are even capable of lowering blood pressure, and preventing severe panic attacks.

Scents are also intimately intertwined with thought and memory. Studies on brain-waves show that scents like lavender increase alpha brain waves associated with relaxation; scents like jasmine boost beta waves linked to alertness; other scents enhance your emotional equilibrium merely by inhaling them. Yet, aromatherapy's oils affect different people in different ways, on different levels. Aroma itself is only one of the active healing qualities.

Need to find a good aromatherapist? Call the National Association for Holistic Aromatherapy. (314) 963-2071

Did you know that plants have an electrical frequency?

Essential plant oils carry a bio-electrical frequency expressed as hertz, a term most of us know today from the megahertz rates that drive our electronic equipment. Plants have a frequency from 0 to 15Hz.; dry herbs have a frequency from 15 to 22Hz.; fresh herbs go from 20 to 27Hz.; essential plant oils go from 52Hz to 320Hz. Pure rose oil, extremely rare and expensive, has the highest measured frequency of all plant oils—320 MHz.

Your body has an electrical hertz frequency, too. A healthy body has a frequency between 62 to 78Hz. Disease frequency rates begin at 58Hz. A higher frequency rate destroys an entity of lower frequency. Based on this knowledge, it's easy to see that certain high frequency essential oils can create an environment in which disease, bacteria, viruses and fungus cannot live.

Aromatherapy actually heals through bioelectrical frequency. In fact, a majority of essential oils can affect pathogenic organisms that are resistant to chemical antibiotics. They may turn out to be a good choice for overcoming today's virulent supergerms.

Healing with Essential Oils

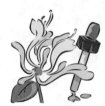

Essential oils have many healing applications. For example, their value for detoxification is quite powerful, clearing certain toxins from the body. When an oil with detoxification properties is applied, toxins like free radicals, heavy metals, fungi, bacteria, viruses and cell wastes actually attach to the essential oil and are then excreted from the body via the skin, kidneys, urine, lungs and bowels.

*An **important word of caution:** Aromatherapy's popularity has spawned many so-called "aromatherapy" products that contain synthetic chemicals which produce the product fragrance- NOT the actual plant essences. These products are not true aromatherapy, and the chemicals in them may actually cause headaches or other reactions. For therapeutic purposes, work with, and buy from, a company that uses only pure, organic essential plant oils. They will cost more. It takes 30 roses to make one drop of essential Otto of Rose; it takes 60,000 roses to make one ounce of real essential Bulgarian rose oil!*

How to use aromatherapy:

1: Most essential oils offer the best results delivered through the skin in a massage or bath oil. In fact, because they're so highly concentrated, I recommend that you ALWAYS dilute them before applying them. Even one drop of pure essential oil applied directly to someone with sensitive skin may cause irritation. Mix about 15 drops of essential oil into 4-oz. of a carrier oil like sweet almond, sunflower, jojoba or a favorite massage oil, then apply to skin or to your bath water.

2: Use a diffuser or a steam inhaler to ease respiratory distress. When inhaled into the lungs, essential oil molecules attach to oxygen molecules, enter the bloodstream and journey through the body with therapeutic action. Inhale essential oils for short periods only; run a diffuser for only 5 to 10 minutes at a time.

3: Uncap oil bottles for a few seconds only or they'll escape. Drop oils into the palm of your hand for blending. Keep bottles tightly capped, away from sunlight and heat when not in use.

4: Use glass containers for all blends of essential oils. Oils can damage plastic containers.

5: Don't shake essential oils. Just gently roll the bottle between your hands.

6: If you experience any irritation, sensitivity, or reaction, discontinue use of the suspect oil.

7: Don't take essential oils internally, except when clearly directed for your needs by a professional.

8: When using essential oils on infants or children, dilute them twice as much as for adults.

9: Follow directions for blending oils carefully; never add more than the recommended number of drops.

A precaution: As always, people with certain medical conditions should be cautious. Some essential oils can trigger asthma attacks or epileptic seizures in susceptible people. Some can elevate or depress blood pressure. Consult a health care professional if you have any of these conditions. Essential oils may also diminish the effectiveness of homeopathic remedies. Check with a homeopathic physician before using essential oils medicinally.

Here's how essential oils assist healing:

…**Essential oils stimulate immune response**, invigorating white blood cell production, and increasing activity of T-cells, NK-cells, alveolar macrophages and serum antibodies. A new study shows all essential oils stimulate phagocytosis, the ability of white blood cells to devour harmful invading microbes. Oils of lemon, peppermint, rosemary and thyme especially enhance immunity.

…**Essential oil's molecules can reach every cell of the body in just 20 minutes.** They cleanse the body by stimulating sluggish circulation to bring oxygen and nutrients to the tissues, and by accelerating disposal of carbon dioxide and other waste products.

…**Essential oil's molecules have an electromagnetic charge** that influences, and balances the charge on our own cell magnetic fields, effective for healing.

…**Essential oils are natural antioxidants which destroy free radicals** and boost the body's resistance to harmful pathogens of all kinds.

…**Essential oils have antibiotic properties**, but each oil is effective against different pathogens. For example, tests show thyme oil, with the component thymol, is a powerful antibiotic agent against micro-organisms in candida and thrush infections. Oregano oil helps guard against seasonal allergies and respiratory infections.

…**Essential oils act as blood purifiers and normalizers**, generally decreasing blood stickiness. For example, rose oil helps counteract the toxic blood effects of alcohol. A rose oil and yarrow combination helps normalize a system invaded by pollen and spore allergens.

…**Essential oils improve lymph system efficiency**, especially the drainage ducts, for better elimination of metabolic residues and toxins. For example, juniper oil enhances the filtration action of the kidneys.

…**Essential oils stimulate the removal of heavy mucous from the lungs and bronchial tubes.** Expectorants herbs like eucalyptus, fennel, frankincense, ginger, peppermint and pine are especially active in a vaporizer.

…**Essential citrus oils help release excess fluid retention.** Oils like lemon, orange or grapefruit, juniper, sandalwood and cypress release fluid and cellulite wastes.

…**Essential oils help normalize body chemistry:** Rose oil and rosemary help normalize particularly against allergens. Thyme oil is an anti-fungal; marjoram promotes blood flow; cedarwood promotes lymph activity. Vetiver and cypress stimulate circulation.

…**Essential oils can pass the blood/brain barrier** - good news for Alzheimer's and Parkinson's disease where so far drugs have not been successful. Frankincense and sandalwood, in particular, boost oxygenation of the limbic system of the brain, increasing the secretion of antibodies, neurotransmitters and endorphins.

…**Essential oils improve skin tone**… try grapefruit, lavender, cypress, basil and juniper.

…**Essential oils can boost energy…** try orange, juniper berry, basil and cinnamon leaf.

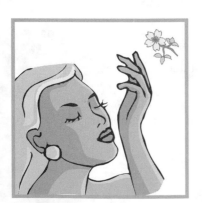

Reducing stress is an aromatherapy specialty

The immediate, profound effect of essential oils on the central nervous system makes aromatherapy a good way to deal with stress. In fact, stress management is aromatherapy's most popular use today, because it promotes mental and physical relaxation while increasing alertness, quality sleep and overall energy. Aromatherapy makes us feel good in part by releasing mood-inducing neurochemicals in our brains. Essential oils like bergamot (geranium oil) also have a normalizing effect on the nervous system, stimulating or sedating according to need. Aromatherapy works well with mega vitamin therapy, to reduce stress in people dependent on powerful tranquilizer drugs.

Relaxing essential oils to reduce stress:

—**Lavender:** induces sleep, exerts a calming and relaxing effect, alleviates stress, reduces depression, tension and hyperactivity. Can also be used to calm animals. Balances nerves and emotions. Pain relief for headaches. Calms the heart and lowers high blood pressure. Rub on stomach for painful menstrual periods.

—**Marjoram:** calms anxiety and reduces grief. A warming analgesic for pain, stiff joints, colds, asthma, painful periods. A tonic for the heart, lowers high blood pressure. Promotes blood flow in skin. Note: Take a break after one month of usage.

—**Chamomile:** a mild sedative for anxiety and chronic stress. Good for dry, sensitive skin. Helpful for asthmatics whose symptoms worsen with stress.

—**Sandalwood:** good for relaxing before meditation and sleep. Stimulates immune response. Heals cracked, dry skin; relieves itching and inflammation. Massage over kidney area for cystitis and kidney problems. Many call sandalwood an aphrodisiac.

—**Clary sage:** calms edgy nerves, brings feelings of well-being, lifts the mind and reduces stress. A hormone balancer, sage is helpful for PMS cramps and muscle spasms. Reduces hyperactivity in kids. Useful for all types of skin inflammations, and for aging skin and wrinkles. Helps rebalance liver activity.

Stress reduction and relaxation blends:

—**Soothing Massage Oil:** to 2 ounces sweet almond oil, add 4 drops bergamot oil, 4 drops chamomile oil, 4 drops lavender oil, 4 drops sandalwood oil, 2 drops coriander oil and 2 drops frankincense oil.

—**Anti-Stress Diffuser Oil:** combine 15 drops lavender oil, 10 drops sage oil, 10 drops elemi oil, 10 drops geranium oil, 8 drops bergamot oil, 8 drops orange oil, 8 drops jasmine oil, 6 drops ylang ylang oil and 5 drops coriander oil. Add a few drops to your diffuser or lamp bowl.

Essential oils for depression:

—**Bergamot:** an uplifting anti-depressant; relaxes nervous system; good for anxiety. Eases digestion. Helps with eczema, psoriasis and acne. An antiseptic for wounds and urinary tract infections. Precautions: May cause photosensitivity. Avoid hot sun right after use on skin.

—**Geranium:** both a stimulant and calmer, depending on the body's need. Acts as an antidepressant and tonic to the nervous system to reduce stress. Helpful in overcoming addictions and anorexia. Helps the pituitary gland to regulate endocrine and hormone balance. Helps menopause, PMS and through its astringent action, stems heavy periods. Enhances circulation to the skin. Helpful for eczema, burns and shingles. Precautions: Avoid during pregnancy. It's a good skin cleanser, but test first for skin sensitivity.

—**Lemon:** uplifting to the psyche. Also cleanses the skin and balances overactive sebaceous skin glands related to acne and dandruff.

—**Neroli:** relieves stress, depression, anxiety, nervous tension and insomnia. Helps headaches. A heart tonic to improve circulation and help nerve pain. Useful for dry, sensitive skin.

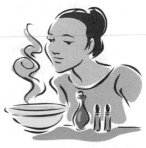

—**Rose (Damask):** influences hormonal activity and glandular function; stabilizes mood swing and reduces postpartum depression. Aphrodisiac qualities make rose useful in impotence and frigidity treatment. Especially good for skin dryness and wrinkling.

—**Jasmine**: uplifting, soothing, very good for depression; a hormone balancer, known for erogenous qualities. Helpful for menstrual pain and uterine disorders. Helpful for respiratory difficulties, bronchial spasms, catarrh, cough and hoarseness. Especially good for dry, sensitive skin.

—**Ylang Ylang**: uplifts the mood, eases anxiety, diminishes depression, eases feelings of anger, shock, panic and fear. Balances women's hormones. Helps high blood pressure and insomnia. Balances sebum flow to stimulate the scalp for hair growth.

—**Frankincense**: a rejuvenating oil to reduce tension and anxiety. I myself have used this oil with good results for SAD (seasonal affective disorder) and reduced immune response.

Essential oils for energizing and motivating:

— **Lavender**: can either stimulate or sedate, according to one's physiological needs. (See previous page).

—**Cypress**: calms irritability, and stress reactions like sweating. Balances body fluids, and helps release cellulite. Helps nose bleeds, heavy periods and incontinence. Soothes sore throats. An astringent for oily skin, hemorrhoids and varicose veins. Precautions: Avoid in pregnancy.

—**Ginger**: sharpens senses and aids memory. Helps settle indigestion. Aids colds and flu, and reduces fever. Helps motion sickness, nausea and gas pain. Add to massage rubs for rheumatic pain and bone injuries, sores and bruises. Precaution: May irritate skin. **Ginger and fennel** stimulate circulation from your heart to your fingertips.

—**Rosemary**: encourages intuition, enlivens the brain, clears the head and enhances memory. Reduces exhaustion, weakness and lethargy. A sinus decongestant. Pain relieving properties for arthritis or gout. A heart tonic, normalizes low blood pressure. Avoid during pregnancy, with high blood pressure or epilepsy.

—**Lemon**: cools the body and awakens the mind. Add a few drops of lemon oil to your after shower moisturizer to increase your energy during the day.

—**Peppermint**: relieves depression and gives the brain a noticeable lift; eases headache pain and improves memory, too. In one case, the aroma of peppermint oil was used successfully to help awaken a 17-year old boy in a coma for three months. Like lemon, peppermint balances oily skin problems such as acne and fights bacterial infections. A few drops are excellent used in a water-based face and body spritz for hot flashes.

Energy stimulation blends:

•**Revitalizing Oil**: mix, then massage into skin in the morning, 2 oz. sweet almond oil, 6 drops lavender, 4 drops rosemary, 3 drops geranium, 3 drops orange, 2 drops coriander, and 2 drops patchouli oils.

•**Invigorating Inhalant Oil**: in a small glass bottle, combine 8 drops rosemary oil, 6 drops cinnamon oil, 4 drops peppermint oil, 3 drops basil oil, 1 drop ginger oil. Inhale directly from the bottle.

•**Fatigue-Busting Diffuser Oil**: in a glass bottle, combine 15 drops rosemary oil, 12 drops cedar oil, 10 drops <u>each</u> lavender and lemon oil, 2 drops peppermint oil. Add a few drops to your diffuser.

•**Rejuvenating Bath**: to your bath add 4 drops rosemary oil, 2 drops each orange and thyme oil.

Essential oils and blends are available from your health food store or
from Wyndmere Naturals (800) 207-8538 or Aromaland (800) 933-5267

Color Therapy and Essential Oils

Only recently has the color of essential oils received mainstream attention. Essential oils have vibrant colors which are degraded by UV light. This is the traditional reason why aromatherapy preparations come in brown glass bottles. But, the color of an essential oil is actually a good indicator of its quality. In addition, in energetic medicine, the colors of essential oils can be used to determine how oils may affect the seven chakras or energy pathways in the body.

Some interesting examples: the reddish color of rose, sage and jasmine oils connect to the red base chakra (linked to home and family) that is believed to help energize, warm and stimulate. The orangy color of ginger, patchouli and sandalwood connect to the orange sacral chakra (linked to sexuality and community) thought to help boost lymphatic flow and enhance creativity. The blueish color of chamomile and tea tree connect to the blue third eye chakra (linked to intuition and motivation) that may help improve clarity, focus and ambition. One company, NHR Organic Oils, manufactures their essential oils in clear glass bottles (protected by a metal container) so you can see their vibrant healing colors. (866) 562-0890.

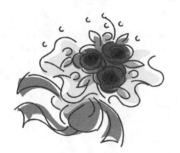

Flower Essence Therapy

Flower essences are part of an emerging field of life-enhancing therapies that work to address emotional health and mind-body well-being through human energy fields. Although new to America's complementary medicine repertoire, the art of flower essence healing strikes a responsive chord in almost every healing discipline—medical and naturopathic health practice, homeopathy, massage therapy, chiropractic, psychotherapy through guided imagery, even dentistry and veterinary work.

Like homeopathy and acupuncture, flower essences stand apart from standard western type science. Like homeopathic remedies, flower essences are highly diluted. Yet also like homeopathy, they are powerful healers, potentiated vibrational tinctures from the patterns of biomagnetic energies discharged by flowers. Flowers are the highest concentration of a plant's life force, the crowning act of its growth, its energy and its allure. Flower essences are captured at the highest moment of the plant unfolding into blossom. The essence is generally prepared from a sun infusion of blossoms in a bowl of water, which is potentiated, then preserved with brandy.

The application of flower essences for specific emotions and attitudes was developed by Dr. Edward Bach, an English physician and homeopath in practice in the 1930's. Bach's research showed that flowers discharge specific patterns of biomagnetic energies that can be harnessed for healing power through emotional balance. Bach's work on the relationship of stress to disease showed that the link between the mind and body is most evident during stress. He also showed the significance of destructive emotions like depression, hate and fear.

Bach was one of the first modern healers to realize that true healing means the manifestation of one's higher spiritual force. He saw that emotional balance strengthened the body's ability to resist disease and he used flower essences as a healing tool to assist in that balance. In the last decade, modern medicine is also beginning to see the connection between negative emotions and lower disease resistance. "What Bach was doing with his vibrational essences was working to increase his patients' resistance by creating internal harmony and amplifying the higher energetic systems that connect human beings to their higher selves." Richard Gerber, M.D. Vibrational Medicine.

Bach documented scientifically the clinical criteria used today in flower essence research. His compound, **Rescue Remedy**, is still the most widely used of all flower essences, a gentle, effective remedy which restores emotional balance during stress or anxiety for people and pets. It can also be used in emergency situations or at any time of upset, illness, shock or trauma, like impending events which produce anxiety. RESCUE REMEDY contains essence of cherry plum for fear of losing control, clematis for resignation and fatalism, impatiens for anxiousness, rock rose for panic, and star of Bethlehem for fright. It is also available in a skin creams to help soothe stress reactions that show up on the skin.

For more, contact Nelson Bach, Wilmington Technology Park, 100 Research Drive, Wilmington MA 01887-4406, (800) 319-9151

Can you use aromatherapy to ignite your sex life?

Aromatherapy is one of the best ways to stimulate a loving mood. Essential oils have been used for thousands of years to enhance the sexual experience and also to lure lovers. Aromatherapy oils have deep subconscious effects on our feelings, triggering memory, lifting emotions and altering attitudes. Aromatherapy experts believe essential oils act like hormones in plants, and have hormone balancing action in people when used therapeutically.

Men and women have different preferences when it comes to just about everything- including their choice of aromatherapy oils. Sexuality-enhancing aromatherapy oils men prefer include cinnamon, sandalwood, lavender, patchouli, coriander, jasmine and cardamom. Oils especially nice for women are ylang ylang, rose, clary sage, neroli and rosewood. I like to use an old fashioned aromatherapy burner, but a few drops of your favorite oil sprinkled on a pillowcase will do just fine to enhance sexual feelings and enjoyment.

Good news:

Essential plant oils can be used to help treat specific sexual problems in men and women. Just a few drops of rose oil in vitamin E oil or aloe vera gel is an effective topical treatment for vaginal dryness. One drop of ylang ylang oil taken in a honey/royal jelly blend can be helpful for low libido in women and impotence in men.

Aromatherapy can help treat underlying problems that lead to low libido. Tea tree or lavender oil can be used topically (diluted) to treat men who have scrotal eczema problems. A drop of lavender oil applied to the temples can relax men and women who can't "get in the mood" due to stress or irritability. For adrenal exhaustion (a big cause of low libido in women), inhaling the aroma of clary sage is a good choice (helps hot flashes, too).

Aromatherapy massages or baths are a good choice to enhance sexuality. The combination of ylang ylang and sandalwood is wonderful in an aromatherapy massage, inhaler or bath. Neroli and jasmine oil have mild aphrodisiac qualities and can be used in baths, inhalers or massage oils. Use the oils according to your preference.

While aromatherapy normally serves to enhance the sexual experience, sometimes it can evoke more powerful sexual feelings. In Robert Tisserand's book, Aromatherapy To Heal and Tend the Body, he tells the story of an aromatherapist treating a man who had been impotent for some years. After following her recommendations, the man began making sexual advances on her! Perhaps, ditching the Viagra for a sensual sandalwood massage is worth a try after all.

Aromatherapy makes sense in a natural sexuality program. Unlike powerful prescription drugs like Viagra (linked to over 130 deaths), aromatherapy is gentle, non-invasive and acts as a natural stimulant to the senses.

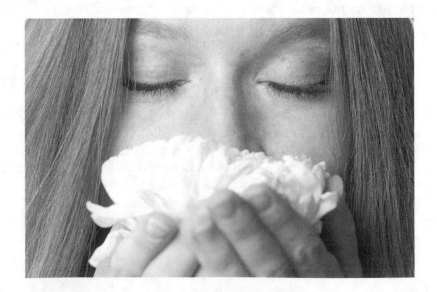

Holistic Recovery From Surgery

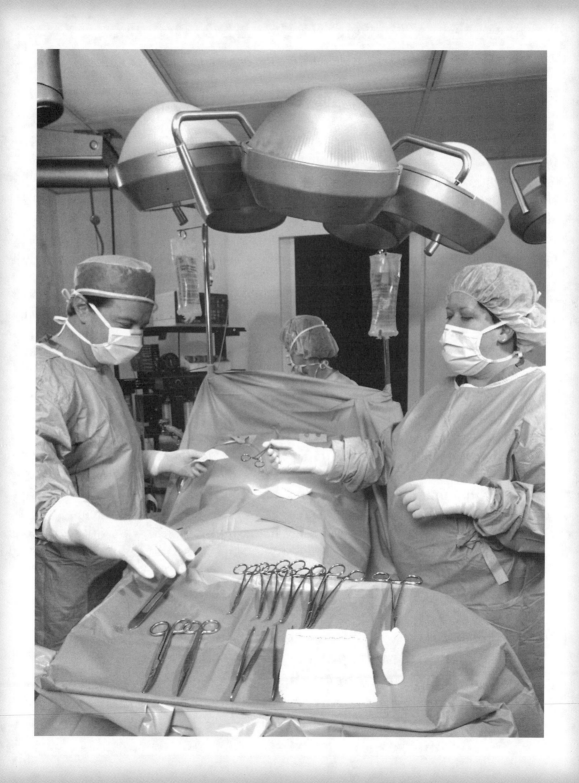

Holistic Recovery From Surgery

Target your Diet and Supplements
to Heal Better and Faster

Already the 21st century offers a wealth of new surgical advances. New health plans provide coverage for more surgical techniques. As many as 40 million Americans every year have in-patient surgery procedures. Yet, surgery is always traumatic on the body, and as more and more Americans go under the knife, I see a disconcerting trend. Patients are rushed in and out of operating rooms, and then rushed out of the hospital with no tools on how to recover. Most doctors provide little or no information on how diet choices and supportive therapies can jumpstart healing from surgery and get you on the fast track back to health.

Regardless of the advances, surgery is still invasive, still highly stressful. The body's healing response is still painful as it is in any injury. Even new state-of-the-art anesthesia drugs used in surgery today can severely tax an exhausted liver as it works to detoxify from the drugs. Both research and common sense tell us to eat the best diet possible before a known surgery date. Adding supplements like zinc, vitamin K and vitamin C, is another smart step, because they're known to speed wound healing and recovery.

What about herbs? Are they safe to take before surgery?

The beneficial effects of whole herbs and whole herb formulas on recovery and tissue healing are undeniable, often dramatic. Reports of interactions of <u>whole</u> herbs with drugs, especially blood thinning or anesthetic drugs, reported in an extremely small number of cases, don't always show clear evidence that the whole herb was the problem.

Many nutritional supplements, foods and herbs (which in their whole form *are* foods), make great sense as a way to fortify your body for the stress and trauma of surgery and healing. Consult your doctor, anesthesiologist or surgeon if you feel doubts or uncertainty.

Important information in this chapter about better healing:

...**Recovering from surgery or serious illness**
...**Normalizing after chemotherapy and radiation**
...**Best results with minimal scarring after cosmetic surgery**
...**Herb interactions with surgery procedures and drugs used during surgery**

Healing Naturally After Surgery

When your body is in crisis, orthodox medicine is at its best. It plays a heroic role with emergency intervention technology that can stabilize a crisis condition, or arrest a life-threatening disease long enough to give your body an opportunity to fight, a chance to heal itself. But whether your visit to an operating room is elective or unplanned, surgery and major medical treatments are always traumatic on body systems..... and the recovery period is often the most difficult part.

I've seen it happen over and over again.... preparing your body well before surgery, and following up with a good post-op program makes an enormous difference in accelerating your recovery. Your body has the power to heal itself, but its vital recuperative forces need extra nutritive help after surgery to do it; a speedy recovery calls for more concentrated nutrients than a normal diet provides. Take healing steps *before and after* your surgery to strengthen your system, alleviate body stress, and increase your chances of rapid recovery and healing.

Note: Advise your doctor of any supplements or herbs you're taking well before your scheduled surgery. While whole herb combinations are generally safe and have few known interactions, <u>standardized</u> herbs may cause reactions to prescription drugs, anesthesia, even surgery itself. Please refer to my list of suspect herbs on pg. 69.

Pre-op techniques to build up your body's defenses before surgery

Start 2 to 3 weeks before your scheduled surgery, include daily:
—Extra vegetable protein. You must have protein to heal. Eat brown rice, other whole grains, sea greens.
—Vitamin C 3000mg with bioflavonoids and rutin for tissue integrity.
—B Complex 100mg with pantothenic acid 500mg for adrenal strength.
—A multivitamin/mineral with antioxidants, beta-carotene, zinc, calcium, magnesium for tissue repair.
—Take a full spectrum, pre-digested amino acid compound drink, about 1000mg daily.
—OPC's, pycnogenol or grape seed, 50mg 2x daily, as powerful antioxidants.
—Garlic capsules, 4-6 daily until 3 days before surgery, a natural antibiotic that enhances immunity.

Strengthen your ability to heal. Include daily:
—Bromelain 750mg twice daily (with Quercetin 250mg to curb inflammation).
—CoQ-10, 120mg daily and/or germanium 150mg capsules daily - as free radical destroyers.
—CHLORELLA 15 tablets, 1 packet powder, or Crystal Star ENERGY GREEN RENEWAL™ drink.
—*Centella asiatica* (gotu kola) capsules, 2 caps 2x daily for nerve tissue repair and collagen development.
—Crystal Star FEEL GREAT NOW!™ with ginseng caps, 2 daily for recuperation strength.
—Vitamin K for blood clotting. Food sources: leafy greens, blackstrap molasses, alfalfa sprouts. *Note: The best source of vitamin K is made by your own "friendly" intestinal bacteria. Supplementing with a good probiotic (like Crystal Star DR. PROBIOTICS™ with FOS) is one of the best ways to synthesize vitamin K in your body.*
—Take a potassium juice (page 291), a potassium supplement liquid, or a protein-mineral drink daily.

Note 1: The medical community uses information and testing results from synthetic, rather than naturally-occurring vitamin E sources, like wheat germ and soy. Thus, many doctors insist that no vitamin E be taken four weeks prior to surgery in an effort to curb post-operative bleeding. I have not found this to be a problem with natural vitamin E, but suggest that you consult your physician if you are in doubt.

Note 2: Immediately prior to surgery, take a pinch of ginger powder (or 8 - 10 drops ginger extract) in water to relieve nausea after surgery. Don't take garlic 2 to 3 days before surgery (it's a slight blood thinner.)

Post-Op techniques to help you recover faster when you come home.

Eat a very nutritious diet. Include frequently:
—AloeLife ALOE GOLD drink, one 8-oz. glass daily.
—A potassium broth (page 291), or a mixed vegetable drink.
—A protein drink, like Nature's Life SUPERGREEN PRO 96, or Nutri-Tech ALL ONE multi drink.
—Plenty of fresh fruits and vegetables. Have a green salad every day.
—Daily sushi (at least 6 pieces), or daily sea veggies for vitamin B_{12} and new cell growth.
—Brown rice and other whole grains with tofu for protein complementarity and more B vitamins.
—Yogurt and other cultured foods re-establish normal, friendly intestinal flora.
—Bromelain 1500 with quercetin 500mg daily (or Crystal Star® DR. ENZYME™ with protease and bromelain) to reduce bruising, swelling, pain and tenderness.
—*Evening Primrose oil* caps 3000mg daily for EFA's that rebuild and nourish delicate post-op skin.
—*Gotu kola*, fast acting to repair nerve damage, reduce numbness and promote collagen synthesis.

Accelerate Healing After Surgery

Herbal combinations can contribute much to the success of surgery—nurturing, normalizing and supporting healing.

Specific systems that herbs can help in healing:
•**Cardiovascular System and Blood Vessels** - *hawthorn, garlic and ginkgo (best used after surgery)*
•**Respiratory System** - *mullein and coltsfoot*
•**Digestive System** - *chamomile and lemon balm*
•**Glandular System** - *panax ginseng*
•**Bowel/Urinary System** - *corn silk for the bladder; yellow dock for the bowel*
•**Reproductive System** - *women: black cohosh, false unicorn root. men: saw palmetto and damiana*
•**Nervous System** - *oats, gotu kola and St. John's wort*
•**Musculo-Skeletal System** - *aloe vera, oatstraw, sarsaparilla*
•**Skin** - *sea vegetables, nettles, red clover, and calendula, St. John's wort oil or cream for scarring*
•**Immune System** - *nettles, cleavers, red clover*
•**Drug and Liver detoxification** - *milk thistle seed*

Note: Dairy foods and iron supplements interfere with some antibiotics. Acid fruits (oranges, pineapples, grapefruit) may inhibit penicillin and aspirin action. Avocados, bananas, cheese, chocolate, colas and fermented foods interfere with monoamine oxidase (mao), an anti-depressant drug. Avoid fatty foods; they slow nutrient assimilation.

Clean the body and vital organs, to counteract infection. Include daily for one month:
—High potency, multi-culture like UAS DDS-Plus with meals.
—Crystal Star LIVER RENEW™ capsules, or LIVER CLEANSE FLUSHING™ tea.
—REISHI MUSHROOM extract helps clear toxicity and provides deep body tone.
—Fight infection with Lane Labs BENEFIN cartilage caps 6 daily for 1 to 2 weeks.
—Enzyme therapy like Crystal Star DR. ENZYME™ with protease and bromelain, or Prevail VITASE.
—Fresh carrot juice, or one can of BE WELL juice daily.

Build up the body tissues. Include daily for one month:
—Crystal Star RESTORE YOUR STRENGTH™ drink, with ADRENAL ENERGY BOOST™ caps.
—Vitamin C with bioflavonoids and rutin 500mg only, with pantothenic acid 1000mg.
—Carnitine 250mg with CoQ-10, 60mg 3x daily, or Siberian Eleuthero, 2000mg daily, as antioxidants.

—Zinc 30-50mg, Futurebiotics VITAL K potassium, or Flora VEGE-SIL to help rebuild tissue.
—Regrow hair and nails with sea veggies and Co-enzymate B complex sublingual, 3x daily.
—AloeLife ALOE SKIN GEL or Crystal Star SCAR REDUCER™ gel to heal skin and scars.

Important recovery and recuperation tips:
—If you are taking antibiotics, take them with bromelain 750mg for better effectiveness,
     and supplement with B Complex, Vitamin C, Vitamin K and calcium.
—If you are taking diuretics, add Vitamin C, potassium and B complex, to strengthen kidneys.
—If you are taking aspirin, take with vitamin C for best results.
—If you are taking antacids, supplement with Vitamin B_1 and/or calcium.
—If your surgery involved bone and cartilage, take Crystal Star OCEAN MINERALS™ caps 4 daily.
—If you smoke, add Vitamin C 500mg, E 400IU, beta-carotene 50,000IU and niacin 100mg.
—***Considering chelation therapy?*** It works in your body like a magnet collecting heavy metals and triglycerides. It is <u>not</u> recommended if you have weak kidneys; too many toxins are dumped into the elimination system too fast, stressing a healing body. Try CARDIO-CHELATE by Metabolic Response Modifiers.

Normalize after Chemotherapy and Radiation

Chemotherapy and radiation treatments are widely used by conventional medicine for several types, stages and degrees of cancerous growth. While some partial successes have been proven, the effects of both chemotherapy and radiation can be worse than the disease itself in terms of healthy cell damage, body imbalance, and reduced immunity. Cancer experts at Duke University estimate that 40% of cancer patients actually die from malnutrition, largely as a result of the severe nausea, vomiting, lack of appetite and poor nutrient uptake that follows chemotherapy treatment. Amazingly, analysis of more than <u>100</u> clinical studies published in *Surgical Forum* showed no benefits, but did show significant damage when chemotherapy 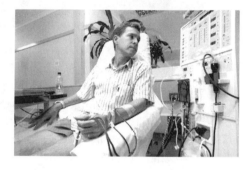 was the sole treatment for breast cancer patients! Radiation treatment, given to about 60% of cancer patients, has debilitating side effects, too. Painful swallowing, unusual fatigue and skin reactions are acute side effects. Long-lasting ulcers, painful sores, reproductive malfunction and chronic diarrhea are frequently reported. Many patients actually develop *other* cancers because the risk for leukemia is so much higher. Doctors and therapists do recognize the drawbacks to chemotherapy and radiation, but under current government and insurance restrictions, neither they nor their patients have insurer-approved alternatives.

Bewilderingly, even with all of the new information on alternative methods and new, less invasive procedures, surgery, chemotherapy, radiation and a few extremely strong drugs are still the only protocols approved by the FDA in the United States for malignant disease. The cost for these treatments is beyond the financial range of most people, who, along with physicians and hospitals must rely on health insurance to pay the expense. Medical insurance will not reimburse doctors or hospitals if they use other healing methods. Thus, exorbitant medical costs and special interest regulations have bound medical professionals, hospitals, and insurance companies in a vicious circle where no alternative or new measures may be used to control cancer. Everyone is caught in a political web where it comes down to money instead of health. This is doubly unfortunate, since there is advanced research being done and new choices available in Europe and other countries to which Americans are denied access. (Unfortunately, recent 2002 legislation passed in Europe denies Europeans access, too, banning over-the-counter ability to purchase many supplements, forcing EU citizens to get remedies like high potency vitamins and herbal supplements only through their doctors.)

Scientists admit that current treatments have been pushed to their limits. But new testing and research are extremely expensive. Even today, the vast majority of funds provided by the National Cancer Act supports research to improve the effectiveness of existing therapies—radiation, surgery and chemotherapy. This practice is easier and cheaper, but it leaves patients with the same three therapies, just more precise use of them. Even when a new treatment is substantiated, there is no reasonable investment certainty that government (and therefore health insurance) approval can be obtained through the maze of red tape and politics.

Some of this is changing as cancer patients refuse to become victims of their medical system as well as the disease. The American people are demanding access, funding and insurance approval for alternative health techniques and medicines. Slowly, state by state, especially in the western states, legislators and regulators are listening, health care parameters are expanding, and insurance limitations are becoming more inclusive.

Conventional medicine rarely treats cancer as a systemic illness, defining it instead only by location and symptomatology. It's the way lab science and our left brains work, breaking things down into one-for-one causes and effects, assaying, isolating, identifying… in consequence, hardly ever looking at the whole person or the whole picture.

By contrast, alternative healers regard cancer as a reflection of the whole body state rather than a localized disease in one part. Naturopaths believe that a healthy body with strong immune response can prevent, even destroy abnormal cells. Alternative therapists seek to strengthen the immune system of the cancer patient, generally avoiding highly toxic modalities like radiation and chemotherapy, rather using a multifaceted, non-toxic treatments which rely on bio-chemistry, metabolic, nutrition and herbal therapies.

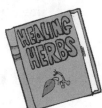

You can help your body clean out drug residues, minimize damage to healthy cells, rebuild strength after chemotherapy and radiation, and get over the side effects.

For three months after chemotherapy or radiation, take the following daily:
—Take *Turkey Tail* mushroom daily to rebuild immune defenses against tumor growth.
—Crystal Star RESTORE YOUR STRENGTH™ broth — 1 heaping tsp. in 8-oz. hot water.
—CoQ$_{10}$ capsules, 60mg 3x daily, and/or germanium 150mg daily.
—Vitamin C crystals with bioflavonoids, ¼ tsp. in liquid every hour, about 5 to 10,000 mg daily.
—800mcg folic acid to normalize DNA synthesis, especially if methotrexate was used in your treatment.
—Floradix HERBAL IRON, 1 tsp. 3x daily, or Crystal Star ENERGY GREEN RENEWAL™ drink to
    counteract the anemia that causes such extreme fatigue after chemo treatments.
—An herbal anti-inflammatory to reduce swelling: *turmeric* (curcumin) or Crystal Star ANTI-FLAM™ caps.
—HAWTHORN or GINKGO BILOBA extract, 30 drops daily under the tongue as a circulatory tonic.
—Aloe vera concentrate, like AloeLife ALOE GOLD for detoxification and to ease nausea.
—A liver support capsule or tea, like Crystal Star LIVER RENEW™ capsules.
—Sea veggies 2 tbsp. dry snipped daily, or Co-enzymate B complex sublingual 3x daily for hair regrowth.

And consider:
—Medicinal mushrooms rebuild immunity, and may help prevent cancer reoccurrence-
    Maitake D-Fraction, *Agaricus, Reishi, Cordyceps* and *Turkey Tail*, available from Maitake Products.
—For chemo-induced stomatitis, consider BHI's TRAUMEEL (Found effective by injection in recent studies.
    Injectable TRAUMEEL is available by prescription).
—*Ashwagandha* (extract) 30 drops daily to rebuild immune white blood cells.
—*Chamomile* tea or Lane Labs NATURE'S LINING™ for inflammation of mucous membranes.
—For chronic dry mouth, add *flax seed* oil to your diet; try Crystal Star WOMAN'S DRYNESS™ extract.
—Keep your diet about 60% fresh foods for the first month after chemotherapy.
—Exercise with a morning sun walk and some stretches on rising and retiring.

Facial Surgery Healing Program

We all want to look great at every age. The plastic surgery industry is booming! As cosmetic surgery technology has raced ahead, Americans are racing to reclaim their youth under the knife. An amazing 6.6 million cosmetic surgery procedures were performed in 2002 and the figure is growing. In 2002, over 100,000 face lifts were performed—up from 36,981 procedures in 1990!

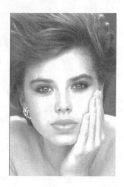

I've worked closely with Dr. Harry Mittelman of Menlo Park, CA. to develop a comprehensive program to boost healing from facial surgery. My own mother-in-law used the program from start to finish and became one of the oldest women at age 87 to undergo a full face lift. The results were amazing. The doctors said her skin actually healed faster than most young people! If you choose to have cosmetic surgery, consider this Healthy Healing Facial Surgery Healing Program to boost the benefits.

PRE-OP: daily - 2 to 3 weeks before surgery:
—Bromelain 1500mg to reduce inflammation.
—*Evening Primrose oil* caps 1000mg for skin healing essential fatty acids.
—Royal Jelly/Siberian ginseng tea drink or Prince of Peace ROYAL JELLY-GINSENG vials.
—Ester C - 5000mg with bioflavonoids 500mg to increase collagen production.
—Vitamin K, sea greens and-or plenty of alfalfa sprouts for capillary integrity.
—Crystal Star ZINC SOURCE THROAT RESCUE™ drops, IODINE-POTASSIUM-SILICA drops or OCEAN MINERALS™ caps.
—Brown rice and a green salad every day.
No aspirin or alcohol 1 week before to 2 weeks after surgery; they increase bleeding tendency and reduce healing ability.

POST-OP: pre-suture removal, daily for 1 week: (*Apply ice packs hourly for 3 days to reduce swelling*)
—Crystal Star ANTI-FLAM™ capsules 4 at a time as needed, for pain relief or swelling
—Bromelain 1500mg with quercetin, or Crystal Star DR. ENZYME™ with protease to reduce bruising.
—Co-Q10, 150mg daily, for enzyme therapy tissue repair.
—*Gotu kola*, for nerve damage repair and reducing numbness.
—Ester C - 5000mg w. bioflavonoids for new collagen production, tissue tightening, capillary healing.
—*Evening Primrose oil* caps 1000mg daily, for essential fatty acids.
—ROYAL JELLY + GINSENG VIALS by Prince of Peace.
—Vitamin K, sea veggies, 2 tbsp. daily, or plenty of alfalfa sprouts, (for bruising and bleeding).
—Brown rice and a green salad every day, for B vitamins (skin) and chlorophyll healing (blood).

POST-OP: post-suture removal, daily for 3 weeks:
—Bromelain 1500mg with Ester C - 5000mg with bioflavonoids - reduce inflammation, boost collagen.
—Evening Primrose oil caps 2000mg with a Royal Jelly-Siberian ginseng tea combination.
—Apply Crystal Star BEAUTIFUL SKIN™ gel and/or AloeLife SKIN GEL, for scar and scab healing.
—Yoanna OXYGEN FIRMING C COMPLEX with DMAE and ALOE PEARL cream for skin renewal.
—Co-Q10, 150mg daily and *Centella Asiatica* (gotu kola), capsules by Solaray for nerve restoration.
—Brown rice and a green salad every day. Add sea vegetables for skin tone and texture.

2 Months later:
—Try TOKI, Lane Labs collagen drink for 6 months for beautiful skin tone and texture.
—Seaweed-aloe mask if you've had a face lift: mix 1 tsp. kelp granules, 1 tsp. aloe vera gel, drops jojoba oil.
—Continue with Ester C and royal jelly to rebuild and nourish delicate post-op skin on the face.

Herbs, Drugs and Surgery

Do herbs and the drugs used in surgery procedures interact? If they do, are you risking your health during or after surgery?

These are legitimate questions today, and you should be informed about the answers because the medical world is changing at light speed. Drugs, especially pain-killing and tissue rejection drugs used in surgery, are far more sophisticated than they were even a decade ago. Surgical techniques have made huge advances, transplanting, even replacing whole body parts successfully. Herbs have changed too, with the widespread introduction of standardized herbal products (see page 66), the laboratory concentration and potentizing of certain compounds from herbs in an attempt to provide a more natural alternative to drugs.

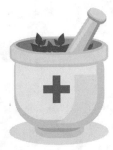 ***So what's the story on herbs?*** Should you feel safe taking herbs before and after surgery to help you heal and recover faster? We are frequently warned by the American medical world that herbs may have dangerous interactions with drugs. Clearly, herbs are both foods and medicines; many have strong therapeutic propeties on their own. Much of Europe and most of Asia commonly prescribe herbs to help recovery.... even for advanced surgical procedures. Milk thistle seed extract, for example, is especially helpful to reduce drug toxicity to the liver caused by anesthetics and other prescription drugs.

After talking with many surgery patients, and my own experience, here's my opinion: clearly, people who took specific supplements and herbs before and after their surgeries tolerated the surgery better and recovered faster with less scarring. (See preceding pages.) There was a difference in the risk of interaction when using a whole herb formula and a standardized herb, or an herbal formula where the natural balance of the plants had been changed. Whole herbs are generally much gentler (not weaker), because they have protective benefits built into the make-up of the plant.

Which herbs and supplements are most controversial in the surgery?

•**Ginkgo Biloba** may increase the risk of bleeding: Ginkgo's blood-thinning ability has raised concerns about abnormal bleeding during surgery, especially if a patient is also taking *warfarin,* a drug blood thinner. I agree that care should be used before taking ginkgo if you are taking *warfarin.* However, ginkgo is a powerful antioxidant that neutralizes free radicals (generated in large amounts by surgery trauma) that can be helpful after your procedure. As a circulation enhancer, it helps accelerate healing and convalescence.

•**Garlic** may increase the risk of bleeding: A mild blood thinner, patients are now commonly warned not to take garlic just prior to surgery to avoid the risk of excess bleeding, especially if already taking blood thinners like *warfarin, heparin* or aspirin. Clearly, care should be taken if you are taking blood thinning drugs. However, garlic is a very mild blood thinner, and as a powerful antioxidant and anti-infective, it can help prevent free radical cascades and infections after surgery. It's a good liver detoxifier that helps eliminate drugs from your system after surgery. Garlic contains germanium, a known wound healer; and increases glutathione levels for better immune response.

•**Kava** may increase anesthesia's effects: Kava's muscle-relaxing, pain killing qualities seem to over-potentiate the effects of some tranquilizers used in surgery procedures, as well as cause interactions with certain long term antidepressants and anti-convulsants. Avoid this possibility by avoiding kava 2 to 3 days before your surgery. After your surgery, kava's pain killing qualities are beneficial against body stress, and may reduce your need for toxic drug analgesics.

•**Vitamin E** (synthetic): may increase the risk of bleeding: doctors warn against this blood thinning vitamin for up to a week before surgery, especially if the patient is taking *warfarin, pentoxifylline, heparin* or aspirin. Study cases showing increased hemorrhagic stroke caused by bleeding, used synthetic vitamin E instead of natural vitamin E from soy or wheat germ oil; even in these studies, however, the risk of more common types of stroke was reduced. (There was a definite cumulative effect in the vitamin E- aspirin cases). In my experience, especially when vitamin E is part of a natural multi-vitamin or other multi-supplement formula, or as natural vitamin E from soy or wheat germ, there has not been appreciable extra bleeding. Post-operatively, vitamin E can be protective against the side effects of some drugs and for faster skin healing.

•**St. John's Wort** may decrease the effectiveness of anesthesia and other drugs: I agree with the medical community that St. John's Wort, especially the standardized products and in concentrated formulas, has numerous unhealthy interactions with a fairly wide spectrum of current drugs. It should be avoided for 1 to 2 weeks before surgery; and the anesthesiologist should know that you are taking it.

•**Ephedra** can cause irregular heartbeat and spikes in blood pressure: I agree that you should avoid high dose ephedra formulas before surgery.

•**Feverfew** may inhibit blood coagulation: Anesthesiologists warn that feverfew interferes with blood coagulation ability, especially when used with blood thinning drugs like *warfarin, heparin* and aspirin. People who use the herb post-operatively for drug-induced headaches report no adverse effects.

•**Panax Ginseng (American and Asian)** may elevate blood pressure and heart rate in some people: One of the best herbs for enhancing recovery energy and stamina, ginseng has gotten a bad rap based on one report of interference with the anticoagulant *warfarin.* Another unconfirmed report, 24 years ago, in JAMA stating that ginseng at high doses raises blood pressure and increases heart rate, nervousness, sleeplessness and diarrhea, has been thoroughly discredited, yet is still widely believed in many quarters.

•**Ginger** in high doses may increase the risk of bleeding: Recommended by European physicians for decades to curtail nausea after surgery, drug reports show that ginger, like feverfew may increase the risk of abnormal bleeding, especially if taken along with some of the blood thinning drugs like *warfarin, heparin* or aspirin. So far, the effects seem to be based on theory or don't seem to be significant, especially in the cases of ginger-containing foods like ginger ale, or cookies like ginger snaps.

•**Gotu Kola** may increase the effects of anesthesia: Some reports show that gotu kola has an additive effect for some anesthetics. If you decide to stop taking it because of this before your surgery; consider taking it after surgery for its noticeable, sometimes dramatic ability to accelerate nerve and tissue repair.

•**Nightshade plants (potatoes, tomatoes, eggplant, peppers and tobacco):** Compounds in nightshade plants inhibit two enzymes that help break down anesthetic drugs, interfering with the body's ability to clear anesthetics from the bloodstream. Patients who eat, or smoke, nightshade plants within 24 hours of surgery have up to 80% of the compounds in their blood at surgery time and have a more difficult time waking up and moving after surgery. Keep this in mind for at least two days before your surgery.

•**Valerian** may increase the effects of anesthesia: but helps after surgery to ease and relax stress.

•**Echinacea** may increase allergies in some people; may increase risk of poor wound healing: It helps mightily after surgery in accelerating nerve and tissue repair and decreases infection.

Note: For more information on how to use your diet to help heal and recover faster, see Section 4.

Herbal Medicine Today

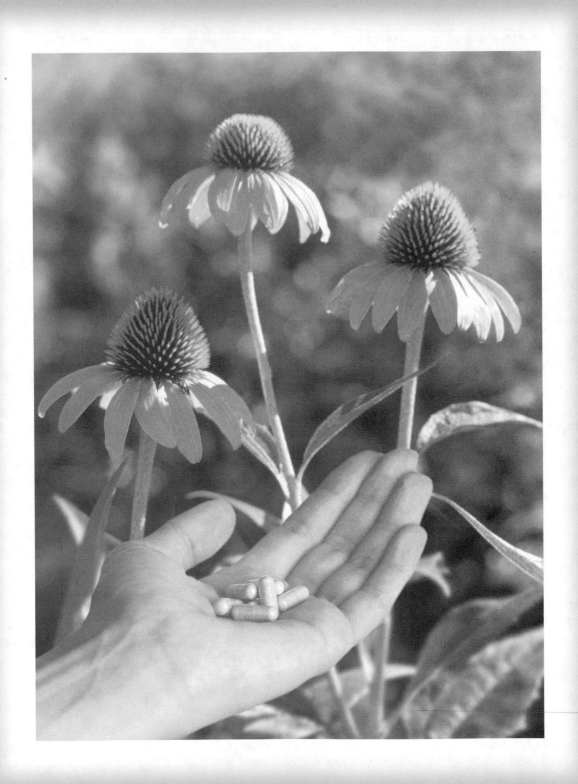

Herbal Medicine Today
*Herbs have a Unique
Healing Spirit*

Americans are rediscovering herbal healing with enthusiasm. Using herbs for healing brings us back to one of the basics of human life. Herbs give you respect for the wonders of our planet. They are highly complex, intelligent plants....living medicines....one of the powers of the universe.

Herbal healing exemplifies universal truth at its highest level. It is both a science and an art, with qualities we would all like to represent, and the ones we value most in ourselves. In a very grasping world, herbs are always giving. They show us how health care ought to be... conscious of the whole person, easy to use, gentle, safe, inexpensive, always available, and able to handle any problem.

Herbs work better together than they do by themselves, and they bring people together because they help us care for each other with Mother Earth.

Herbal medicines are products for problems. They can be used in the first line of defense against disease, and at every stage of healing. I believe that except for emergency or life-threatening situations, herbs deserve a place in your primary health care.

Herbs work integrally with each person's body. Each of us can draw from an herb's wonderful complexity the elements we need in order to heal.

Although herbs respond to scientific methods, they are much more than a scientific, or even a natural healing system. Their healing work goes on automatically, whether it is analyzed or not. Our bodies know how to use the body balancing nutrients of herbs without our brains having to know why.

Like all great realities of nature, there is so much more than we shall ever know.

Important considerations:

...Herbal medicine choices today
...The controversy over standardizing herbal elements
...Using herbs safely - herb-nutrient-drug interactions
...plus a little about my philosophy of herbal healing

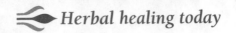

Your Herbal Medicine Choices Today

Medical science is changing fast. In many ways in America, indeed around the world, we are in a time of paradigm shift.... especially in the global approach to healing. Americans are enthusiastically increasing their use of herbs as natural complements to drugs and drugstore medicines. Researchers estimate that in the next five years, up to 96% of all adults in America will be using herbal remedies for at least part of their healthcare..... even in the medical profession — an astounding number when you consider the media, and government regulatory agency campaigns waged against them!

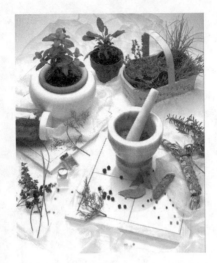

How does the tradition of herbal healing fit into modern medicine?
As our world grows undeniably smaller, people interact more, changing long-held beliefs. Many enlightened medical physicians say the threat they once saw as "alternative" health care is now viewed as an additional choice for them, as well as their patients. Herbs are becoming part of an "integrated medicine" that encompasses all types of healing methods. The slow but steady acceptance of herbs as ideal self care for preventing illness, and home care for addressing daily, non-emergency or moderate health problems is underway within health care regulatory agencies, insurance companies, hospitals, even drug companies.

Immune strength is where natural, complementary medicines, like herbs and homeopathic compounds are important. Each of us is individual; our healing supports need to be able to work with us in a personal way for permanent health. Natural remedies involve the cooperation of our own bodies in the healing that takes place. Herbs let your body do its own work better.

If we think about it for a minute, we realize that medicinal foods like herbs aren't the alternative healing system, drugs are the alternative system. Even the latest chemical drugs aren't the answer. In fact, it seems that new drugs are becoming *less* instead of more effective, against a number of powerful viruses. Recent research shows that even the latest, most robust antibiotics hardly survive a year before the microbe they were designed to arrest, develops, mutates and grows stronger against them...... a good example of a non-living agent like a drug trying to control a living thing.

While we must be respectful of all ways of healing, we haven't fully realized that we have a choice. All the advances made by modern medicine still don't address chronic illness, or disease prevention very well.

Today's allopathic medicine is "heroic medicine," developed originally in wartime for wartime emergencies. But this type of medicine often hits our bodies with a heavy hammer, preventing us from being able to rebuild against slow-growing, degenerative diseases. Many doctors admit that drugs are really a patching up system of medicine. There is no such thing as an essential drug, so drugs can't combine with your body to restore and revitalize; drugs can't help stimulate immune response either. In fact, most drugs and all surgeries, create body trauma, along with their corrective benefits, that requires additional rounds of healing.

Further, many people today see our Earth as a being of great, essential intelligence, evolving and growing, even as as mankind evolves and grows. The microcosmic world of pathogenic organisms that cause disease is changing, too—often replicating at enormous rates. Both organisms and diseases are becoming more virulent, environmental pollutants are becoming more widespread and our immune defenses are becoming weaker.

Herbs can point out a path that shows us how we might best succeed on our planet. We know we can count on the safety and effectiveness of herbs. Drug can't achieve that confidence. We know that herbs reach out to us with their marvelous abilities to help us address the health problems of today, just as they addressed ancient ones. Herbs may be our best hope to bring the balance back between the healing forces and diseases.

I have long believed that herbs are a path to the wider universe — an eye of the needle through which we can glimpse the wonders of creation and what it's really all about. God shows us his face in herbs, because they seem almost miraculous in their benefits to mankind. So, I see herbal medicines as part of a larger wellness picture..... they are worldwide, alive, big enough and intelligent enough to grow along with us.

Herbs are without a doubt... UNIVERSAL. They do not discriminate, but embrace humans of all sorts and animals of all kinds, with their benefits. While it seems, on a day-to-day basis that we are hopelessly divided — in the end we are all one. Our hopes and dreams are the same.

Herbs help us care for each other. Worldwide herbal healing knowledge is a force to bring humans together for the good of us all. Herbal medicines of old traditions like the Ayurvedic philosophy, Native American and rainforest medicines, long thought to work only for the people of their own cultures, are now available to grateful people everywhere. Old tribal traditions, once so entirely separate, are sharing their knowledge and their herbs.

Western herbal formulas now include herbs from every corner and every herbal culture in the world. Native American cleansing herbs and techniques like herbal smudging and therapeutic sweating are now used to relieve modern pollution problems. We use Chinese and Rainforest herbs successfully for Western diseases, even though the healing tradition that originated them had a different cultural viewpoint. Western herbalists are learning how to use time-honored Ayurvedic herbs in combination with our own herbs, for western health problems.

On a recent trip to Asia, I could see that herbal knowledge is going both ways, as Western herbs flow east to Asian healers. (Still, I was also surprised to see that even today, many Chinese pharmacies carry no drugs. According to workers in the pharmacies, their customers don't believe in drugs—only herbs and fortifying animal extracts.)

If man, an intelligent being, is changing, might not herbs, intelligent plants, be changing, too? Herbs are intricate plants, filled with long memory. They have intelligently adapted to the Earth's changes as we have, and they have always interacted with humans. Perhaps they are moving along the universal continuum with us - always available for us, with a highly complex structure able to match our own complexity of need.

Where is herbal healing going from here?

The winds of change are blowing once more as we begin a new millennium. There is clearly an enormous rebirth of interest in the ways of Nature and holistic healing. I believe modern medical technology and the holistic approach can come together for the good of mankind. The holistic approach is the prevalent one in most societies. Western herbal thought has taken a detour through technology. Yet, useful knowledge has surfaced that otherwise might not have been found. If we can put aside the greed and politics that have surrounded our healthcare, the best of both worlds may surface... a time when holistic medicine can be supported by scientific studies, and scientific analysis can be validated by its relevance to human lifestyles.

Notable healer Albert Schweitzer said "the doctor of the future will be oneself."
If we are to become the doctor, where is our medicine?
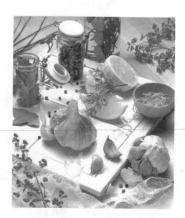
Our medicine is all around us.
Our food is our pharmacy.
Herbs are our medicine.
The oceans are our healers.
Our very breathing can bring us real health.

These things are truly healthy healing... balancing the body from the inside out, naturally and safely. They don't need pages of warnings and lists of dangers. Everyone can use them.

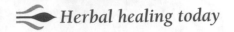

Using Herbs Safely: A Practical Guide

If you read nothing else in this book about herbs, read this. It's the foundation for getting the most out of herbal healing...

People have been using herbal medicines for thousands of years to meet their health needs. Self treatment is still the primary use of herbs today, even though enlightened clinics and practitioners are beginning to incorporate herbal remedies as complementary medicines.

We're often taught to think of herbs as natural drugs. While we must recognize and respect the power of herbal medicines, they are really foods with medicinal qualities. They combine with our bodies as foods do, so they are able to address both the symptoms and causes of a problem.

As nourishment, herbs offer the body nutrients it may not always receive, either because of poor diet, or environmental deficiencies in the soil and air. As medicine, herbs are essentially body balancers that work with the body functions, so that it can heal and regulate itself.

Herbs work like precision instruments in the body, not like sledge hammers.
Herbal medicines can focus on a special problem or be broad-based for overall support.

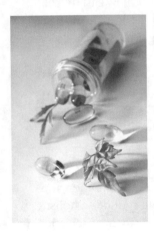

Most herbs, as edible plants, are as safe to take as foods. Herbs offer a rich variety of healing elements with almost no side effects. Occasionally, a mild allergy-type reaction may occur as it might occur to a food, a personal response to a certain plant. This could happen because an herb has been adulterated with chemicals in the growing or storing process, or in rare cases, because incompatible herbs were used together. The key to avoiding an adverse reaction is moderation. Anything taken to excess can cause side effects. Use common sense, care, and intelligence when using herbs for either food or medicine.

Drugs on the other hand, are not nourishing. They work exactly the opposite from foods. Drugs run powerful interference against a harmful process that's happening in your body in order to stabilize it. They disrupt a cascade of harmful events in order to arrest a serious conclusion.

But make no mistake, drugs can't normalize or nourish you. Only your own immune powers, herbs or food can do that, through your body's enzyme activity. Drugs keep the interference process going. Sometimes that's what's needed to help you arrest disease, but over the long term, they tend to work against your body, hitting its delicate balance with a disruptive hammer. (That's one of the reasons you might have gotten good results from a drug at first, and poorer results as time went on.)

Your body, especially your immune system, always tries to normalize itself. But as the disruption process over time takes your body further from normal, your immune system finally doesn't know what normal is - and ends up attacking the wrong elements, or everything, in confusion.

That's where immune-compromised illness comes in. America is at a crisis point with immune-imperiled diseases like candida, chronic fatigue syndrome, Hashimoto's, fibromyalgia and lupus. They affect a woman's delicate body balance most. They are way under-diagnosed by our health care system, and they're reaching epidemic proportions.

It's a big reason we're having so much trouble with our health care system today.
Are we looking at medicine from the wrong end of the telescope? Modern medicine is only concerned with sickness. All drugs are formulated for, and marketed to, someone who is sick. All lab testing is done on infected cells. We never see how a drug might affect healing cells or healthy cells, or someone who is not sick.

Two-thirds of the drugs on the American market today are based on medicinal plants.

...But modern herb-based drugs are not herbs; they are chemicals. Even when a drug is derived from an herb, it is so refined, isolated and purified that only a chemical formula remains. Chemicals work in our bodies far differently than herbs. Chemical drugs cause many effects—only some of which are positive. Eli Lilly, a pharmaceutical manufacturer, once said "a drug isn't a drug unless it has side effects."

...Herbs in their whole form are not drugs. Do not expect the activity or response of a drug, which normally treats only the symptoms of a problem. In general, you have to take more and more of a drug to get continuing therapeutic effect.

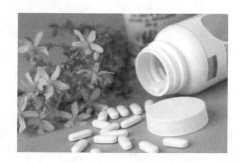

...Herbal medicines work differently in the body. Herbs are foundation nutrients. They nourish the body's deepest elements, like the brain, glands and hormones. Herbs work to normalize and support at the cause of a problem, for a more permanent effect. Results seem to take much longer. Even so, some improvement from herbal treatment can usually be felt in three to six days. Chronic or long standing problems take longer, but herbal remedies tend to work more quickly with each new infection, and new cases of infections grow fewer and farther between. *Rule of thumb: expect one month of healing for every year you have had the problem.*

Balance is the key to using herbs for healing.

Herbal combinations are not addictive, but they are powerful foods that you should use with care. It takes a little more attention and personal responsibility than mindlessly taking a prescription drug, but the extra care is worth far more in the results you can achieve for your well-being.

As with other natural therapies, there is sometimes a "healing crisis" during an herbal healing program. This is known as the "Law of Cure," and simply means that you may seem to get worse before you get better. The body generally eliminates toxic wastes heavily during the first stages of a cleansing therapy. This is especially true in the traditional three to four day cleansing fast that many people use to begin a serious healing program. Temporary exacerbation of symptoms can range from mild to fairly severe, but usually precedes good results.

Herbal therapy without a fast works more slowly and gently. Still, some weakness may be felt as disease poisons are released into the bloodstream to be flushed away. Strength shortly returns when this process is over. Watching this phenomenon allows you to observe your body at work healing itself... an interesting experience indeed.

Herbs work better when taken along with a natural foods diet.

Everyone can benefit from an herbal formula, but results increase dramatically when fresh foods and whole grains form the basis of your diet. Subtle healing activity is more effective when it doesn't have to labor through excess waste material, mucous, or junk food accumulation. (Some congested people carry around over 10 pounds of excess density.)

Interestingly, herbs themselves can help counter the problems of "chemicalized foods." They are rich in minerals, the basic elements missing or diminished in today's quick-grow, over-sprayed, over-fertilized farming. Minerals and trace minerals are a basic element in food assimilation, providing not only the healing essences to support your body in overcoming disease, but also the foundation minerals that allow it to take them in!

Your body has its own unique, wonderful mechanism. It has the ability to bring itself to its own balanced and healthy state. Herbs simply pave the way for the body to do its own work, by breaking up toxins, cleansing, lubricating, toning and nourishing. **Herbs promote elimination of waste matter and toxins from the system by simple natural means. They support nature in its fight against disease.**

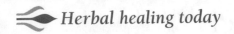

Herbs work better in combination than they do singly.
Like the notes of a symphony, herbs work better in harmony than standing alone.

A good herbal formula gives your body a wealth of subtle healing essences from which to choose. Herbs work synergistically together… one and one can make three. As I formulate an herbal combination, I work from the point of view of the illness or health condition, and I work with the way herbs combine together to get the desired effect, not just the properties of each herb.

Why herbs work better in combination:

1: Herbs work synergistically and more efficiently in a combination. The value is in the formula, not simply one or two chemicals within it, no matter how potent they are. Synergy plays an important role in safety, too. (Look at what happens when we refine wheat, extract sugar cane, distill alcohol, isolate ephedrine from ephedra or cocaine from coca leaves - incredible health problems for both the user and society.)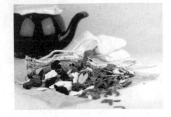

2: A good combination contains two to five primary herbs for specific healing purposes. Since all body parts, and most disease symptoms, are interrelated, it is wise to have herbs which can affect each part of the problem. For example, in a prostate healing formula, there would be herbs to dissolve sediment, anti-inflammatory herbs, tissue-toning and strengthening herbs, and herbs with antibiotic properties.

3: Herbs are foods, full of nutrients… and nutrients always work best as a team. Thus a combination of herbal nutrients gently stimulates the body as a whole, encouraging body balance rather than a large supply of one or two focused properties.

4: A good combination includes herbs that can work at different stages of need. A good example of this is an athlete's formula, which includes herbs for short term energy, long range endurance, muscle tone, glycogen and glucose use, and reduction of lactic acid build-up.

5: A combination of several herbs with similar properties increases the latitude of effectiveness, not only through a wider range of activity, but also by reinforcing herbs that were picked too late or too early, or grew in adverse weather conditions. No two people, or their bodies, are alike. Good response is augmented by a combination of herbs.

6: Finally, certain herbs, like *capsicum, lobelia, sassafras, mandrake, tansy, Canada snake root, wormwood, woodruff, poke root, and rue* are beneficial in small amounts and as catalysts, but should not be used alone.

How should you take herbs for the most benefit?

—Herbs are not like vitamins. I see herbs as healers and vitamins as insurance policies.
The value of herbs is in their wholeness and complexity, not their concentration.

—Herbs should not be taken like vitamins.
Vitamins work best when taken with food. Herbs <u>are</u> foods… so it's not necessary to take herbal formulas with food. Herbs combine and work with the body's enzyme activity as foods do. Herbs have their own plant enzymes that work with yours. Except for some food-grown vitamins, vitamins are partitioned substances. Vitamins work well to shore up nutrient deficiencies, but they do not combine with the body in the same way as foods or herbs do; excesses are normally flushed from the system.

Unlike vitamins, herbs provide their own digestive enzymes for the body to take them in. In some cases, as in a formula for mental acuity, the herbs are more effective if taken when body pathways are clear, instead of concerned with food digestion.

Taking herbs all the time is like eating large quantities of a certain food all the time. Your body may receive imbalanced nourishment from nutrients that are not in that food. This is also true of multiple vitamins. They work best when strengthening a deficient or weak system, not as a substitute for a good diet. However, superfood plants like green grasses, sea plants, aloe, and green algae, and adaptogen tonics like ginsengs and bee products can be taken for longer periods of body balancing. **Therapeutic herbs work best when used as needed. Dosage should be reduced and discontinued as the problem improves.**

Herbal effects are often specific; take the best formula for your particular goal at the right time—rather than all the time—for optimum results. Rotating and alternating herbal combinations according to your changing health needs allows your body to remain responsive to their effects. Reduce dosage as the problem improves. Allow your body to pick up its own work and bring its own vital forces into action. If you are taking an herbal remedy for more than a month, discontinue for one or two weeks between months to let your body adjust and maintain your personal balance.

Achieve best results by taking herbal capsule combinations in descending strength: 6 the first day, 5 the second day, 4 the third, 3 the fourth, 2 the fifth, and 2 the sixth for the first week. Rest on the 7th day. When a healing base is built in the body, decrease to the regular dose recommended for the formula. Most combinations should be taken no more than 6 days in a row without a break.

Take only one or two herbal combinations at the same time. Address your worst problem first. Take the herbal remedy for that problem—reducing dosage and alternating on and off weeks as necessary to allow the body to thoroughly use the herbal properties. One of the bonuses of a natural healing program is the frequent discovery that other conditions were really complications of the first problem, and often take care of themselves as the body comes into balance.

Herbs are amazingly effective in strengthening your body's immune response. But the immune system is a fragile entity. It can be overwhelmed instead of stimulated. Even when a good healing program is working, and obvious improvement is being made, adding more of the medicinal agents in an effort to speed healing can aggravate symptoms. Even for serious health conditions, moderate amounts are the way to go, mega-doses are not. Much better results can be obtained by giving yourself more time and gentler treatment. It takes time to rebuild health.

Herb effectiveness usually goes by body weight, especially for children. Child dosage is as follows:

> *½ dose for children 10-14 years*   *¼ dose for children 2-6 years*
> *⅓ dose for children 6-10 years*   *⅛ dose for infants and babies*

Herbs can be ideal for self treatment in maintaining health. They are potent medicines, yet clearly have few, if any, side effects, and are almost always safe when used in their whole (food) form. They often work well in a complementary role with more conventional medicines, especially after an emergency problem is arrested and stabilized. But be smart. Learn about the herbs you are taking. You'll be able to use them more effectively. *See the following section for specifics on standardized herbs and drug interactions.*

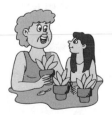

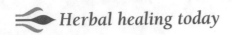
Today's Herbal Medicine Choices

Whole-Herb Healing or Standardized Plant Constituents?

Clearly, American health care consumers are increasing their use of herbs as natural alternatives to drugs. Standardizing separate herbal constituents for potency is popular today as herbal manufacturers enter drug-oriented health care markets. But, when we standardize herbs or use isolated plant constituents, aren't we making medicinal herbs (which are really healing foods), into drugs? This has become the center of the debate between the drug world and natural whole herb healing.

What do we sacrifice when herbal constituents are "standardized"?

Americans need safe, effective, alternative medicines. In order to meet this demand, government regulators and orthodox medicine try make herbal remedies fit into a laboratory drug mold in order to have a reliable measurement of effectiveness. But setting arbitrary benchmark requirements for herbal potency, as well as their ability to perform, is a slippery slope, far more difficult than it appears.

Here's why: when we say that certain standardized elements are all there is to herbal healing, we lose. Herbs are incredibly intricate, living medicines… medicines whose value lies in their complexity, and their ability to

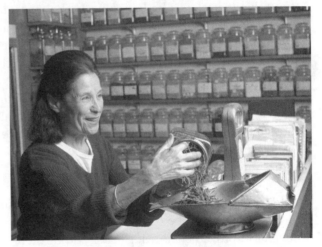

combine with our bodies—not in the concentration or potency of any one element. Standardizing an herb for only one or two isolated "active ingredients" attempts to use limited laboratory procedures to convince the AMA, the FDA and medical scientists of the value of herbal therapy. Some companies see standardizing as a way for herb products to challenge negative media campaigns, by measuring some "active constituents" of a plant. It's also considered a way to deal with FDA regulations that require drug measurability, and demand that active ingredients be stated on product labels. We must not fall into the same wrong-headed, self-defeating pit of fifty years ago, when the regulations for standardizing drugs nearly killed all herbal medicine.

As a traditional naturopath and herbalist, I believe that standardization short-changes the full spectrum of whole-herb healing.

Throughout the 6,000 year tradition of herbal healing, in every culture, herbalists have effectively used whole herbs for healing. There is tremendous value in the knowledge gained through empirical observation and interpretive understanding of real people with real problems and natural solutions.

The immense success of herbal healing rivals modern day allopathic medicine. Yet in today's health care world, laboratory yardsticks are the only measurements science understands or governments approve. Herbal healing fell out of favor not because it was ineffective, or even because something better was discovered, but because science and technology had little understanding of Nature. Medical market economics had no incentive to investigate herbs, because no one could "patent a plant."

Quality and consistency are legitimate concerns for effectiveness. Herbal product suppliers must integrate herbal traditions, ethical commitments, FDA regulations and consumer concerns. A way must be found to work with regulations that were never intended to deal with the complex effects of herbal healing.

Herbs have rejuvenative, tonic qualities entirely missed by standardization.

Herbal healing is due not just to herbal bio-chemical properties, but also to their unique, holistic effects, and significantly, to their interaction with the human body.

…Recent tests are beginning to prove it. For example, substantial new research has been done with the "active constituents" isolated from the lapacho tree (pau d'arco herb). Time after time, the therapeutic actions of the isolated elements proved inferior to the whole plant. Further refinement and purification only resulted in declining activity of the isolated constituent's activity.

The reason for this is that whole herbs work best as body balancers and transformers, especially facilitating the immune system, providing the groundwork for the body to begin healing itself. The results of whole herb healing may take much longer than drugs, but the effects are usually long lasting.

A drug-like approach neglects one of the main benefits of herbs.

Herbs have the unique healing ability to address multiple problems simultaneously. It's almost impossible to chase the intricate principles that really make herbs heal. In most cases, the full medicinal value of herbs is in their internal complexity. Each herb has dozens of biochemical constituents working synergistically. There are many complementary elements in each herb… some similar to the "main" one, some catalyzing, and so on. Even further, many of the constituents within a whole herb are unknown; and internal chemical reactions within a combination of herbs are even less understood.

Research often shows that the chosen "active ingredient" to be standardized may have been the wrong one, or not the best choice, or the even most powerful. Using a standardized herb is like using a "natural drug," with one property for one problem. The resulting product often misses the full range of benefits offered by the whole herb. Potentiating a single property only gives you part of the picture, and can lead to problems.

Today, scientists determine almost arbitrarily how much of an active ingredient being studied is needed, and then measure it as they would a drug. When a lab test or drug company with a marketing agenda is allowed to decide which herbal element is worthwhile, which one will be marketed to the public, hundreds of others may never be brought to light—with the certain consequence that valuable healing knowledge will be lost by default. We can see this in examples like St. John's wort and Lily of the Valley.

Many herbal constituents actually serve to boost the solubility and the activity of each other—*sometimes up to a dramatic 500 times increase of bioavailability and activity*—for longer, stronger effectiveness. Factoring in even just the complementary and booster elements (and we know there are a wide range of *other* catalyzers), and we can see that a whole herb can actually be *stronger* than a standardized herb… a proven instance where the whole is more than the sum of its parts.

In fact, many botanical agents work ONLY in their whole form. Thus, important vitamins, minerals, enzymes and amino acids available that have a function in whole herbs are lost through the standardizing process.

We also see many of the same unwanted side effects, adverse reactions, drug interactions, even addictions that are the downside of drugs. One more plus, because of the whole herb potency phenomenon, smaller doses can be used to get the same effect with less chance of safety issues.

Some popular herbs that have suffered standardization drawbacks...

Ginseng: a popular body balancer and energizer ingredient in many herbal products. One highly publicized lab test identified two of its 22 known ginsenosides (Rb1 and Rb2), in an attempt to isolate ginseng's ability to lower cholesterol. Yet hundreds of world-wide studies, with well-documented evidence (but without the publicity budget), show that ginseng has dozens of *other* actions that control disease and promote wellness, functions entirely missed by this test. Should we deny people the ultimate value of ginseng's activity simply because a laboratory hasn't tested, or understood, even a fraction of its broad activity range yet?

As a formulator of whole herb compounds, I've experienced the best results with a combination of ginsengs—like American, Chinese, Ashwagandha, and *Siberian Eleuthero* ginseng types which work to tonify and strengthen the body against stress reactions and some degenerative disease. In another standardized ginseng drawback, many people I talk to are uncomfortably stimulated by high potency, standardized ginseng products.

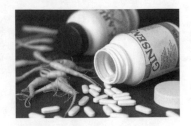

St. John's wort: a popular herb, taken today for depression. Most manufacturers standardize only for the *hypericin* content of St. John's wort, yet even modest scientific testing shows that depression responds to more than just this one St. John's wort constituent. For example, a recent German study finds *hyperforin* in St. John's wort modulates serotonin, a brain chemical linked to mood disorders, which acts as a mild anti-depressant. There is more than one "magic bullet" constituent that helps reduce mild to moderate depression in St. Johns' wort. Whole St. John's wort also has a long tradition of safe, effective use as an herbal anti-viral, a capability becoming more valuable as modern supergerms become more virulent.

However, *standardized* St. John's wort has noticeable side effects and it interacts with a long list of prescription drugs. (For the latest list of known interactions and side effects, see pg. 69.) I find a whole herb combination that includes St. John's wort in combination with other whole herbs works better, addressing more symptoms and body imbalances related to the primary problem, with far less potential for interactions and side effects.

Licorice: a popular herb for sore throat. Licorice is a delicately balanced plant where I believe standardization does the public health injustice. Licorice is standardized for glycyrrhizin (also known as glycyrrhizic acid or glycyrrhizinic acid) which helps protect the liver and stimulates aldosterone, a key adrenal hormone. However, too much of this one constituent can disrupt the body's sodium and water balance, leading to serious disruptions in body chemistry and dangerously elevated blood pressure. Whole licorice root offers inherent protection against this type of reaction. An Italian study with lab animals reveals using whole licorice root extract results in far less incidence of side effects and is far safer than using just glycyrrhizin alone.

In addition, whole licorice root contains over <u>400</u> phytochemicals, many of which have healing and immune boosting activity. Whole licorice extract soothes irritated mucous membranes and is especially beneficial for sore throat, hoarseness or bronchitis. Further, isoflavonoids in licorice work with its glycyrrhizin to balance estrogen levels in women. When we standardize licorice, we lose this natural balance and many healing actions of the plant.

Ephedra: an herbal bronchodilator (also called ma huang). Ephedra is another herb that has fallen prey to the drawbacks of herbal standardization. When used properly according to herbal tradition, ephedra can be a godsend for asthma, and as a thermogenesis stimulant, a natural aid for weight loss. But when an ephedra consituent, ephedrine, is misused or standardized, it can be a recipe for disaster. Concentrated, standardized extracts of ephedrine have a much more powerful effect than the whole herb in combination formulas. (See pg. 70 for a list of known risks, contraindications and interactions with standadrized ephedrine products.) A few rules of thumb to aid in your ephedra purchases: Responsible ephedra products should contain a very minimal amount of ephedrine (from .1 to 2 mg.). 25mg ephedrine or <u>much more</u> is used in some preparations, and can be dangerous. Use whole herb ephedra products only as directed and avoid them altogether if you have any of the contraidications.

Kava Kava: a relaxing, stress relieving herb. Kava kava is on the media "radar screen" today, for its interaction with alcohol, and for its potential liver toxicity. Has kava been unfairly accused? Is this a case where standardization leaves us with an overly refined product that resembles a drug more than a plant? The jury is still out on kava. We have much more to learn about what type of kava preparations or dosages may cause problems like skin rashes and scaling. New research centers on how high doses of kava may interact with other drugs or alcohol that affect the liver. For more information on kava interactions, see pg. 70.

Facts You Need to Know
Herb-Nutrient-Drug Interactions
This Review was carefully researched and written by Sarah Abernathy, the head of our research department

Do you worry that the herbal remedies, high potency vitamins, and supplements you're taking could interact with prescription drugs? You're not alone. Nearly every day, someone contacts my research department to ask whether they can use herbal therapies with prescription drug treatments.

As the lines blur between supplements, natural remedies and drugs, the answers aren't simple. Opinions on the topic vary widely in both the natural healing and medical worlds. Some practitioners advise against using herbs and supplements altogether while on drug therapy; others routinely recommend them, especially if a drug is leaching nutrients from the body or causing side effects. Adding to the confusion, almost every day brings a new media report, oftentimes biased or incomplete, on the hazards of combining herbs with drugs.

Confused about a safe choice? Here's the scoop on drug-herb-nutrient interactions....

Investigating how herbs and nutrients interact with drugs is a new research area with few qualified experts. Knowledge comes slowly and laboriously. Drug and herbal companies move in different worlds, so information is hard to gather and analyze. The learning curve on the safety of each herb-nutrient-drug combination is complex. Much of the information we have on herb-nutrient-drug interactions comes from anecdotal reports or small tests. It's a detailed, complex subject that will eventually need millions of university grant dollars to determine which herbs and nutrients interact with which drugs. **One major obstacle?** Neither orthodox medicine nor the natural healing world has a vested interest in funding such research.

More confusing, much of the information is based on theory about <u>potential</u> interactions, but with no reports actually <u>confirming</u> the interaction. Since drugs as chemicals work outside the system, and herbs as foods are processed through our enzyme system, a theorized interaction often never occurs or is neutralized.

It's important to remember that whole herbs are really foods (albeit powerful foods). We don't normally expect an herb to interact with a drug anymore than we expect a food to interact with a drug. Think about it for moment, would you stop eating mushrooms or spinach just because you're taking antibiotics?

In many cases, herbs and supplements can be used supportively, to maintain health while a person is on drug therapy. For instance, *ginkgo biloba* may be taken to help counteract the sexual side effects of anti-depressant drugs. B-complex vitamins are widely known to reduce drug-induced nutrient depletion from medications like oral contraceptives, estrogen replacement drugs, and methotrexate.

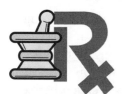

Herb-Nutrient-Drug Interactions to be aware of....

Herb, nutrient, drug interactions are rare but can happen. The following list is a good sampling of the known negative interactions between the herbs, nutrients, and prescription medications you may be taking.

St. John's Wort: St. John's wort has become an herbal boon for depression in the modern world. Some research shows this herb's anti-depressant effect rivals conventional anti-depressant drugs for mild to moderate depression! This is certainly good news for people who want a natural alternative to drugs like Prozac which can cause side effects like low libido, agitation or fatigue.

However, <u>standardized</u> St. John's wort can interfere with many prescription medications. New research reveals St. John's wort can decrease effectiveness of HIV drugs, drugs for organ transplants and cancer, digoxin, statin drugs, warfarin, chemotherapy drugs, tricyclic antidepressants, asthma medicines, even oral contraceptives. Some doctors advise against using the herb before surgery because it reduces effectiveness of the new anesthetics.

Don't use St. John's wort if you're taking antidepressant drugs. The combination of St. John's wort and SSRI antidepressants may lead to "serotonin syndrome," a condition marked by confusion and cardiovascular irregularities. Several documents report this interaction. St. John's wort is also contraindicated for people taking anti-depressant MAO inhibitors (monoamine oxidase inhibitors) because it is believed the herb may interact with them, too. New research from Ireland concludes these interactions are rare, and that St. John's wort actually has fewer side effects and health risks compared to conventional antidepresssant drugs (McIntyre 2000).

Standardized St. John's wort products can cause side effects. Photosensitivity is a big problem; fatigue and gastrointestinal upset occur in some people. Avoid standardized St. John's wort if you use tanning beds or take drugs that cause photosensitivity. (You might get burned!) Preliminary research suggests high doses of St. John's wort may also increase the risk of sun-induced cataracts. (Wear sunglasses when using it!) **I find St. John's Wort works best** *in whole herb combinations* **which are less likely to cause side effects or have interactions.**

Kava Kava: Kava Kava helps calm the mind and relax the muscles without causing side effects like over-sedation or addiction. However, kava is not safe for everyone. ***If you're drinking alcohol, don't take kava.*** Kava can intensify the effects of alcohol. In addition, kava may interact with anti-anxiety medications like buspirone (Buspar), benzodiazepines and anesthetics. Kava should also be avoided by people taking anti-psychotic drugs and Levodopa for Parkinson's disease.

Recent media reports say kava causes liver damage. However, the reported liver problems in these cases may have been due to alcohol abuse or the simultaneous use of medications that damage the liver. (In the South Pacific where kava is used regularly in high doses, there are few reports of liver toxicity.) A 2003 study shows pipermethystine, found primarily in kava's stem peelings has hepatotoxic effects in vitro. While traditional healers use only the root in preparations, widespread production of the herb means that some manufacturers use stem peelings and leaves in products due to cheaper costs. Experts speculate this has led to current toxicity problems. Still, until we know more, avoid kava when you drink alcohol, or if you have liver problems, or if you take drugs that affect the liver. Note: Discontinue kava use if you experience warning signs of jaundice like yellowing of the eyes.

Ephedra: Bad press has now stopped the sale of ephedra (ma huang) in the U.S.. I believe the ephedra controversy is a case of a plant being judged for one of its constituents instead of as a whole. Most of the health problems associated with ephedra are actually due to one of its constituents—ephedrine. When used properly, ephedra is the best herbal bronchodilator for respiratory problems like asthma, and a natural thermogenic aid for weight loss.

Some companies used concentrated, standardized extracts of ephedrine, which have a stronger effect on the body than the whole herb. Others used synthetic ephedrine, a drug derived from the plant, and combined it with caffeine or other stimulating drugs in "herbal ecstasy" compounds. This type of preparation caused dangerous spikes in blood pressure and heart rate, especially in combination with illicit drugs!

Even with whole herb ephedra products, use precautions. Don't use ephedra if you have heart problems or high blood pressure. Don't use ephedra continuously because of potential long-term strain on the adrenal glands. Don't use if you're pregnant or nursing; taking a MAO inhibitor, stimulant drugs or decongestants; or if you have heart or thyroid disease, prostate enlargement, or diabetes. If these contraindications don't apply to you, I recommend using ephedra only as a whole herb, in combination with other herbs in expert herbal formulations, or as a weak tea for a limited span of time.

Ginkgo biloba: Widely used to help reduce age-related problems like poor circulation, heart disease, tinnitus and impotence, ginkgo is best known as a memory aid. While generally very safe, ginkgo's blood-thinning effects can interact with some anticoagulants like Warfarin, and over-the-counter drugs like aspirin or ibuprofen. Don't take ginkgo before surgery without medical supervision.

Note: Many herbs and supplements have mild blood thinning effects and should be used with caution if you're taking blood thinning drugs or preparing for surgery. High doses of vitamin E, garlic, ginger, bromelain, protease and feverfew may affect bleeding, and should be used with caution. CoQ10 may reduce the effectiveness of blood thinning drugs like Warfarin. Consult with your doctor on the remedies you're taking.

Licorice: Licorice has a long tradition of safe use as a natural antibiotic and antiviral in both Western and Chinese herbal medicine. It's an American favorite for female hormone balance and adrenal exhaustion. Most people can take licorice without problems, but avoid it if you have high blood pressure. In very high doses, the licorice constituent, *glycyrrhizin*, can cause potassium loss, fluid retention and elevated blood pressure. Licorice is not advised for people with a history of renal failure or who take heart medication or steroid drugs.

Feverfew: Traditional herbalists turn to feverfew for migraine relief. Five different studies reveal feverfew is more effective than a placebo at relieving migraine pain, even reducing migraine-related symptoms like nausea, vomiting and sensitivity to light. Some theorize that a combination of NSAIDs (non-steroidal anti-inflammatory drugs) and feverfew may increase the risk of stomach irritation because both substances affect prostaglandins that protect the stomach lining. (NSAIDs by themselves are a clear risk factor for stomach ulcers.) Feverfew can also affect blood clotting. Use with caution if you take like Warfarin or Heparin.

Vitamin A: Supplemental vitamin A is used to counteract night blindness, as an antioxidant in natural cancer treatment, and in creams to prevent wrinkles. But high doses of vitamin A can be toxic and should definitely be avoided during pregnancy. Don't take vitamin A if you take the prescription drug Accutane for acne. Accutane is structurally similar to vitamin A and has similar toxicities. Avoid vitamin A if you're under treatment for thyroid cancer. Beta carotene, which is converted to vitamin A in the liver as needed, is a much safer choice for people concerned with vitamin A toxicity.

Grapefruit juice: **Grapefruit juice is one of the few foods that interacts with prescription drugs.** Grapefruit juice causes some drugs to be absorbed too quickly - a dangerous effect for people taking drugs with high potential for toxicity or serious side effects. Don't drink grapefruit juice if you take calcium channel blockers for high blood pressure. The combination can be fatal! Grapefruit juice can also have dangerous interactions with drugs for allergies like Claritin and Allegra, and antihistamines like Benadryl. Grapefruit juice may interact with organ transplant drugs, estrogens and oral contraceptives, anti-anxiety medications, Methadone, Viagra, HIV drugs, seizure drugs and statin drugs for high cholesterol. Note: While grapefruit juice has the reputation for interactions, the fruit may have the same effect if consumed in large amounts.

_____*A note on antidepressant MAO drugs (mono amine oxidase inhibitors): MAO's are a rare class of drugs known to have interactions with foods. People taking MAO inhibitors for depression should avoid foods high in tyramine like cheese, sausage, alcohol, legumes, fish, sauerkraut, soups, and yeast extracts, and the herbs ginseng and scotch broom.*

My final word on interactions between drugs, herbs and nutrients?

We have much to learn about how herbs and nutrients interact with powerful prescription drugs. Still, I believe most negative interactions occur when people use highly potent standardized herbs, take extremely large doses of herbs or nutrients, or combine herbs and nutrients with drugs that have innate toxic properties and serious side effects.

There's no such thing as an essential drug. Drugs don't play a normal role in human biology. Health problems are not caused by drug deficiencies. Drug side effects occur for this very reason.... because they aren't part of the normal workings of the body.

Supplements and whole herbs will always be gentler and easier to take than drugs. Sometimes short-term drug therapy may be necessary to stabilize a serious health problem so that immune response can take over for long term health. If you're on drug therapy or preparing for a medical procedure, talk to your doctor about the natural remedies you're using and ask about possible interactions. Working with a knowledgeable health professional trained in both natural and conventional approaches is by far the best choice. Finding the right blend of medicine for you is worth this extra effort.

More information: •Lininger, Schuyler, D.C., Alan Gaby, M.D., Steve Austin, N.D., Forrest Batz PharmD, Eric Yarnell, N.D., Donald Brown, N.D., George Constantine Rph, Ph.D. *A-Z Guide To Drug-Herb-Vitamin Interactions.* Healthnotes, Inc. 1999. •Harkness, Richard, Pharm.,FASCP & Stephen Bratman, M.D. *Drug-Herb-Vitamin Interactions Bible.* Prima Health, 2000.

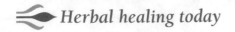

Herbal Preparation & Delivery Methods

Today, herbs are available at all quality levels. Worldwide communications and improved storage allow us to simultaneously obtain and use herbs from different countries and different harvests, an advantage ages past did not enjoy. However, because of the natural variety of soils, seeds, and weather, every crop of botanicals is unique. Every batch of a truly natural herbal formula is slightly different, and offers its own unique benefits and experience.

There must be a firm commitment to excellence from growers and suppliers, because herbal combinations are products for problems. For therapeutic success, herbs must be BIO-ACTIVE and BIO-AVAILABLE.

If you decide to make your own herbal preparations, buy the finest quality herbs you can find. There is a world of disparity between fairly good herbs and the best. Superior stock must go into a medicinal formula so that the herbal product can do its job correctly. Superior plants cost far more than standard stock, but their worth in healing activity is a true value for the health care customer.

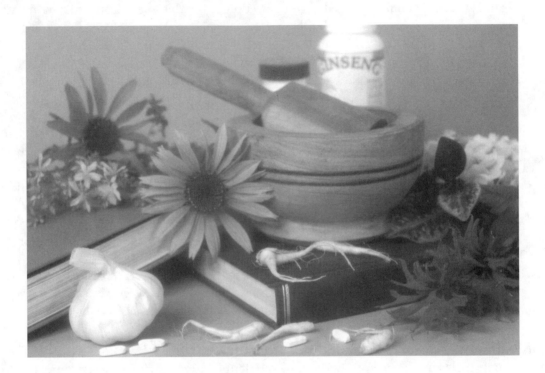

Which preparation form should you choose?

Whichever herbal preparation form you choose, it is generally better to take greater amounts at the beginning of your program, to build a good internal healing base, and to stimulate your body's vital balancing force more quickly. As the therapeutic agents establish and build, and you begin to notice good response, reduce your dose gradually, finally reducing to long range preventive amounts.

"Parts" are a good way to set a common denominator for building an herbal compound. For personal use, one tablespoon is adequate as one part when using powdered herbs for filling capsules; one handful is common as one part for cut herbs in a tea or bath blend. (See HOW TO MAKE AN HERBAL EXTRACT for quantity information for an extract or tincture.)

Herbs can be applied to almost any necessity of life. It's simply a matter of knowing their properties, how they work together and how to use them correctly. Herbs are foods, and your body knows how to use them. Give them time. Give yourself a good diet, some rest and relaxation for the best results.

...**Herbal teas** are the most basic of all healing mediums — easily absorbed by the body as hot liquid. They are the least concentrated of all herbal forms, but many herbs are optimally effective when steeped in hot water. The hot brewing water releases herbal potency and provides a flushing action that is ideal for removing toxic, loosened wastes. Although teas have milder, more subtle effects than capsules or extracts, they are sometimes the only way for a weakened system to accept therapeutic support, and often work synergistically with stronger medicinal forms to boost their value.

NOTE 1: Volatile essential oils are lost during cutting of herbs for tea bags. For best results, buy cut herbs or crumble leaves and flowers, and break roots and barks into pieces before steeping for best results.

NOTE 2: Medicinal teas may have bitter tasting properties. Where taste is unpleasant, I add mint, lemon peel, spices, or stevia (sweet herb) to improve taste without harming therapeutic qualities.

Tips on taking herbal teas:

1: Use 1 packed small teaball to 3 cups of water for medicinal-strength tea. Use distilled water or pure spring water for increased herbal strength and effectiveness.

2: Bring water to a boil, remove from heat, add herbs and steep covered off heat; 10 to 15 minutes for a leaf-flower tea; 15 to 25 minutes for a root-bark tea. Keep lid down during steeping so volatile oils don't escape.

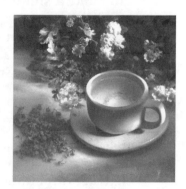

3: Use a teapot of glass, ceramic or earthenware, not aluminum. Aluminum can negate the effect of the herbs as the metal dissolves into the hot liquid and gets into the body.

4: Drink medicinal teas in small sips throughout the day rather than all at once. One-half to 1 cup, taken 3 or 4 times over a day allows absorption of the tea, without passing before it has a chance to work.

...**An infusion** is a tea made from fresh, dried or powdered herbs. Use directions above, or pour 1 cup of boiling water over 1 tablespoon of fresh herb, 1 teaspoon of dried herb, or 4 opened capsules of powdered herbs. Cover and let steep 10 to 15 minutes. Never boil. A cold infusion can be made by simply allowing the herbs, especially powders, to stand in cool water for an hour or more.

...**A decoction** is a tea made from roots and barks. Use directions above, or put 2 tablespoons of cut herb pieces into 1 cup cold water. Bring to a light boil, cover, and simmer gently for 20 to 30 minutes. Strain. For best results, repeat the same process with the same herbs. Strain again and mix both batches.

...**Sun tea** is a cold infusion where herbs are put in a covered jar and allowed to stand in the sun.

...**Herbal broth**, rich in minerals and enzymes, are made by grinding dry ingredients in a blender. Simply mix 2 tbsp. of dry mix to 2 cups hot water. Let flavors bloom for 5 minutes. Add 1 tsp. BRAGG'S LIQUID AMINOS to each broth for a flavor-nutrient boost if desired. Sip over a half-hour period for best assimilation.

...**Herbal capsules** are generally four times stronger than teas, more concentrated, yet bypass any herbal bitterness and are convenient to take. Capsules make both oil and water soluble herbs available through stomach acid and enzyme alteration. Freeze-dried powdered herbs, with all the moisture removed, are also available in capsules, and are four times more concentrated than regular ground herbs. As noted with herbal teas above, grinding herbs into powders creates facets on the whole herb structure causing potential loss of volatile oils. Effective potency for powdered herbs is six months to a year. (See page 65 for more information on how to take herbal capsules.)

...**Herbal extracts** are 4 to 8 times stronger than capsules. They are effective used as a spray where all the mouth receptors can be brought into play, or as drops held under the tongue, bypassing the digestive system's acid-alkaline breakdown. Their strength and ready availability make extracts reliable emergency measures. Small doses may be used repeatedly over a period of time to help build a strong base for restoring body balance.

For treatment during the first week of an acute condition, hold an extract dose in the mouth for 30 seconds, 3 or 4 times daily. After the first week, the vital force of your body will often be sufficiently stimulated in its own healing ability, and the dose may be reduced so your system can take its own route to balance. As with other herbal preparations, take extracts 6 days in a row with a rest on the seventh day before resuming. As the body increases its ability to right itself, the amount, frequency and strength of the dosage should be decreased.

Herbal tinctures are also extractions, are made using a 25% alcohol and water mixture as the solvent. Tinctures are generally extracted from individual herbs rather than compounds. When a commercial compound is made, each separately prepared tincture is added rather than made from the beginning as a compounded extract. Commercial tinctures use ethyl alcohol, but diluted spirits are suitable for home use; vodka is ideal.

Extracts are more concentrated than tinctures, because they distill or filter off some of the alcohol. A tincture is typically a 1:10 or 1:5 concentration (10 or 5 units of extract come from 1 unit of herbs), while a fluid extract is usually 1:1. Even stronger, a solid or powdered extract has the solvent completely removed. Powdered extracts are at least 4 times as potent as an equal amount of fluid extract, and 40 times as potent as a tincture. One gram of a 4:1 solid extract is equivalent to ⅐ of an ounce of a fluid extract, and 1½ ounces of a tincture. *Note: Homeopathic liquid formulas are not the same as herbal tinctures or extracts, and their use is different.*

To make a simple herbal extraction:

Alcohol, wine, apple cider vinegar, and vegetable glycerine are common mediums for extracting herbal properties. Alcohol releases the widest variety of essential herbal elements in unchanged form, and allows the fastest sublingual absorption. Alcohol and water mixtures can resolve almost every relevant ingredient of any herb, and also act as a natural preserver for the compound. Eighty to one hundred proof (40-50%) vodka, is an excellent solvent for most plant constituents. It has long term preservative activity and is easily obtainable for 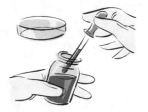 personal use. The actual amount of alcohol in a daily dose is about ⅓₀ oz., but if alcohol is not desired, extract drops may be placed in a little warm water for 5 minutes to allow the alcohol to evaporate before drinking. Most extracts are formulated with 1 gram of herb for each 5ml of alcohol.

Extract directions:

1: Put 4-oz. dried chopped or ground herb, or 8-oz. of fresh herb, into a quart canning jar.

2: Pour about one pint of 80 to 100 proof vodka over the herbs and close jar tightly.

3: Keep the jar in a warm place for two to three weeks, and shake well twice a day.

4: Decant liquid into a bowl; then pour slurry residue through several layers of muslin or cheesecloth into the bowl. Strain liquid through the layers once again to insure a clearer extract.

5: Squeeze out all liquid from cloth. (Sprinkle solid residue around your houseplants as herb food. I have done this for years, and they love it.)

6: Pour the extract into a dark glass bottle. Stopper, seal tightly, and store away from light. An extract made in this way will keep its potency for several years.

Herbal wine infusions are a pleasant, effective method of taking herbs, especially as digestive aids with meals. Take as warming circulatory tonics by-the-spoonful in winter. The alcohol acts as a transport medium and stimulant to the bloodstream.

To make a simple wine infusion, use fresh or dried herbs:

…*Method 1:* For a warming winter circulation and energy tonic, pour off ¼ cup of a fortified wine, such as madeira, cognac or brandy. Place chosen herbs and spices in the wine and recork the bottle. Place in a dark cool place for a week or two. Strain off the solids, and combine the medicinal wine with a fresh bottle. Mix well, and take a small amount as needed for energy against fatigue.

…*Method 2:* For a nerve and brain tonic, steep fresh or dried herbs in a bottle of either white or red wine for about a week. Strain off herbs, and drink a small amount as needed.

Herbal syrups are well accepted by children, and can greatly improve the taste of bitter herbal compounds. They are also excellent treatment forms for throat coats and gargles, or bronchial, chest-lung infections. Syrups are simple and quick to make.

Two simple ways to make an herbal syrup:

…*Method 1:* Boil ¾ lb. raw or brown sugar in 2 cups of herb tea until it reaches syrup consistency.

...*Method 2:* Make a simple syrup with ¾ lb. raw sugar in 2 cups of water, boiling until it reaches syrup consistency. Remove from heat, and while the syrup is cooling, add an herbal extract or tincture—one part extract to three parts of syrup.

Herbal pastes and electuaries (mediums that mask the bitter taste of medicinal herbs) are made by grinding or blending herbs in the blender with a little water into a paste. The paste is then mixed with twice the amount of honey, syrup, butter, or cream cheese for taste. Other good electuaries include fresh bread rolled around a little of the paste, or peanut butter.

Herbal lozenges are an ideal way to relieve mouth, throat, and upper respiratory conditions. Make them by combining powdered herbs with sugar and a mucilage herb, such as marshmallow or slippery elm, or a gum, such as tragacanth or acacia. Both powdered herbs and essential herbal oils may be used. Proper mucilage preparation is the key to successful lozenges.

To make an herbal lozenge:

1: Soak 1-oz. powdered mucilage herb (listed above) in water; cover for 24 hours; stir occasionally.
2: Bring 2 cups of water to a boil and add the mucilage herb.
3: Beat to obtain a uniform consistency and force through cheesecloth to strain.
4: Mix with enough powdered herb to form a paste and add sugar to taste. Or, mix 12 drops essential peppermint oil (or other essential oil) with 2-oz. of sugar and enough mucilage to make a paste.
5: Roll on a board covered with arrowroot or sugar to prevent sticking. Cut into shapes and leave exposed to air to dry. Store in an airtight container.

External use preparations:

The skin is the body's largest organ of ingestion. Use topical herbal preparations as needed.

Herbal baths provide a soothing gentle way to absorb herbal therapy through the skin. In essence, you soak in a diluted medicinal tea, allowing your skin to take in the healing properties instead of your mouth and digestive system. The procedure for taking an infusion bath is almost as important as the herbs themselves.

Two good therapeutic bath techniques:

...*Method 1:* Draw very hot bath water. Put bath herbs in an extra large tea ball or small muslin bath bag (sold in natural food stores). Steep in the bath until the water cools slightly and is aromatic, about 10 to 15 minutes.

...*Method 2:* Make a strong tea infusion on the stove as usual with a full pot of water. Strain and add directly to the bath. Soak for at least 30 to 45 minutes to give your body time to absorb the herbal properties. Rub all over your body with the solids in the muslin bag while soaking for best herb absorbency.

Herbal douches are an effective method of treating simple vaginal infections. Simply steep the herbs as for a strong tea, strain, and pour the liquid into a douche bag. Sit on the toilet, insert the applicator, and rinse the vagina with the douche. Use one full douche bag for each application. Most vaginal conditions need douching three times daily for 3 to 7 days. If the infection does not respond in this time, see a qualified health professional.

Herbal suppositories and boluses are an effective way to treat rectal and vaginal problems, acting as carriers for the herbal medicine. Herbal suppositories generally serve one of three purposes: to soothe inflamed mucous membranes and aid the healing process; to help reduce swollen membranes and overcome pus-filled discharge; and to work as a laxative, stimulating normal peristalsis to overcome chronic constipation.

To prepare a simple suppository:

Mix about a tablespoon of finely powdered herbs with enough cocoa butter to make a firm consistency. Roll into torpedo shaped tubes about an inch long. Place on wax paper, and put in the freezer to firm. Remove one at a time for use and allow to come to room temperature before using. Insert at night.

Herbal ointments and salves are semi-solid preparations, that allow absorption of herbal benefits through the skin. They may be made with vaseline, UN-Petroleum Jelly or cocoa butter for a simple compound; or in a more complex technique with herbal tea, oils and hardening agents like beeswax, lanolin or lard.

To prepare a simple ointment or salve:

...*Method 1:* Warm 6-oz. of vaseline, petroleum jelly or lanolin in a small pan with 2 tbsp. cut herbs; or stir in enough powdered herbs to bring the mixture to a dark color. Simmer gently 10 minutes, stirring. Then filter through cheesecloth, pressing out all liquid. Pour into small wide-mouth container when cool but still pliable.

...*Method 2:* Best used as a carrier base for volatile herbal oils in chest rubs or anti-congestive balms (the base itself is not absorbed by the skin). Steep herbs in water to make a strong tea. Strain off the liquid into a pan. Add about 6-oz. total of your choice of almond, sesame, wheat germ or olive oils, or cocoa butter to the strained tea. Simmer until water evaporates, and the herbal extract is incorporated into the oils. Add enough beeswax to bring mixture to desired consistency; use about 2-oz. beeswax to 5-oz. of herbal oil. Let melt and stir until blended. Add 1 drop tincture of benzoin, available at a pharmacy, for each ounce ointment to preserve mixture against mold.

Herbal compresses and fomentations draw out waste residue like cysts or abscesses, via the skin, or release them into your body's elimination channels. Make a compress by soaking a washcloth in a strong herb tea, then applying it as hot as possible to the affected area. The heat boosts the activity of the herbs and opens the skin pores for fast assimilation. Use alternating hot and cold compresses to stimulate nerves and circulation. Apply the herbs to the hot compress — leave the cold compress plain. *Cayenne, ginger* and *lobelia* work well for the hot compress.

To make an effective compress:

...Add 1 tsp. powdered herbs to a bowl of very hot water. Soak a washcloth and apply until the cloth cools. Then apply a cloth dipped in ice water until it reaches body temperature. Repeat several times daily.

...Green clay compresses, for growths, may be applied to gauze, placed on the area, and left for all day. Simply change as you would any dressing when you bathe.

Herbal poultices and plasters are made from either fresh herbs (crushed and blender blended with a little olive or wheat germ oil), or dried herbs (mixed with water, cider vinegar or wheat germ oil into a paste). Either blend may be spread on a clean cloth or gauze, and bound directly on the affected area. Cover the whole application with plastic wrap to keep from soiling clothes or sheets, and leave on for 24 hours. There is usually throbbing pain while the poultice is drawing out the infection and neutralizing the toxic poisons. This stops when the harmful agents are drawn out, and signals the removal of the poultice. A fresh poultice should be applied every 24 hours.

To make a plaster:

Spread a thin coat of honey on a clean cloth, and sprinkle it with an herbal mixture such as cayenne, ginger, and prickly ash, or hot mustard or horseradish. The cloth is then taped directly over the affected area, usually the chest, to relieve lung and mucous congestion.

Herbal liniments are used as warming massage mediums to stimulate and relieve sore muscles and ligaments. They are for external use only. Choose heat-inducing herbs and spices like *cayenne*, *ginger, cloves* and *myrrh*, and drops of heating oils like *eucalyptus, wintergreen* and *cajeput*. Steep in rubbing alcohol for two to three weeks. Strain and decant into corked bottles for storage.

Herbal oils are used externally for massage, skin treatments, healing ointments, dressings for wounds and burns, and occasionally for enemas and douches. Simply infuse the herb in oil instead of water. Olive, safflower or almond oil are good bases for an herbal oil.

To make an herbal oil for home use:

...*Method 1:* Cut fresh herbs into a glass container and cover with oil. Place in the sun and leave in a warm place for three to four weeks, shaking daily to mix. Filter into a dark glass container to store.

...*Method 2:* Steep powdered herbs directly into the oil. Let stand for one or two days. Strain and bottle.

Foods For Your Healing Diet

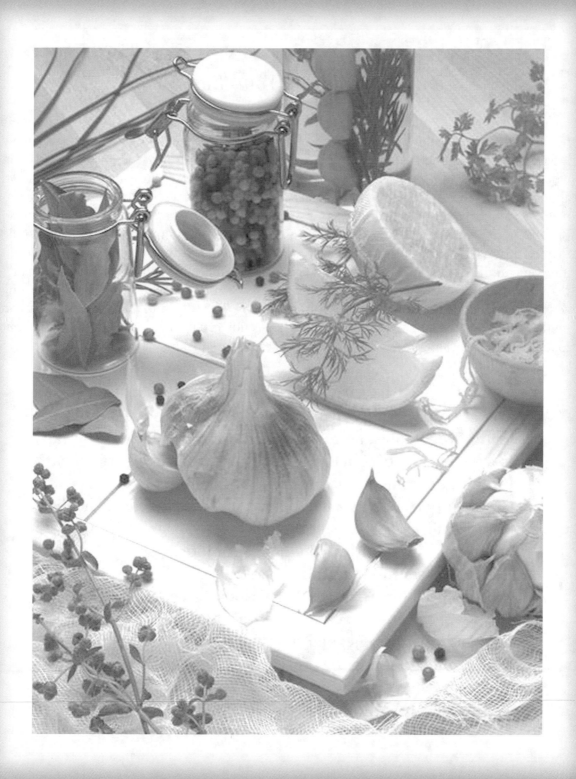

Food and Diet Choices for Healing
Your Diet may be Your Best Healer

Your food may be your best medicine, but, following the standard USDA food pyramid is not enough to stay healthy in today's world. Now antiquated, the food pyramid we use today leaves out important details, like the <u>right</u> fats to include in your diet, the difference between whole grains and refined grains, and which foods offer the most antioxidant protection. An abundance of new research on nutraceuticals and the phytonutrients in our foods shows dramatic evidence that our diets can heal as well as nourish us.

Diet improvement is a major weapon against disease, from common colds to cancer. Whole food nutrition allows the body to use its built-in restore and repair abilities. A healthy diet can intervene in the disease process at many stages, from its inception to its growth and spread.

However, foods aren't equal in their healing abilities. Some foods don't contribute to healing activity at all, others actually deter or arrest the healing process… and there are a lot of urban myths about food that add to the confusion. This section can help you sort out the facts about foods, especially healing foods and food categories that are making news today.

Important diet options that affect healing:

…The case for eating organic foods. Are GE foods really so bad?

…Fruits, vegetables, and chlorophyll for plant enzyme therapy

…Is a vegetarian diet better? What's the truth about red meat?

…Protein: how much do you need for healing?

…Green superfoods and healing mushrooms for faster healing

…Macrobiotics for serious healing: balancing your body chemistry

…Soy foods and cultured foods for probiotics

…Water is essential for healing

…Caffeine in a healing diet? What about green and black teas?

…Does wine fit into a healing program?

…Fats and oils: there's good news and bad news

…Dairy foods in a healing diet? Are butter and eggs okay?

…Sugar and sweeteners: are they all bad? Low salt or no salt?

…Sea greens and iodine therapy

…Powerhouses of the desert: bee nutrients, jojoba, aloe vera

The Case for Eating Organically Grown Foods

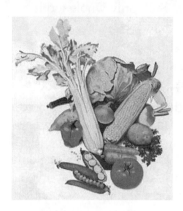

America's agriculture is the best and biggest on earth. Our grocery stores and food markets offer the most beautiful, delectable food in the world. But there's a catch. Almost 80% of the 4.5 billion pounds of pesticides we dump yearly in the U.S. are used in agriculture to produce our food! Pesticide by-products are even used in our water! (See page 116.) In 1997 alone, pesticide costs totalled over 12 billion dollars. Although our government has recently taken steps to reduce pesticide use by "phase out" programs, it may be too little, too late, because so many of these chemicals have already contaminated our food and water supply. Pesticides can remain in the food chain for decades. DDT, chlordane and heptachlor are found in soils more than 20 years after their use was discontinued. Even worse, the pesticides used today are 10 to 100 times more potent than the chemicals used just 25 years ago.

More than 2 *million* synthetic substances are known, 25,000 are added each year—over 30,000 are produced on a commercial scale, some so widespread we are unaware of them. A recent report from the Pesticide Action Network of North America reveals that Americans are exposed to toxic pesticides from foods up to 70 times a day! They work their way into our bodies faster than they can be eliminated, and they're causing allergies and addictions in record numbers. Only a tiny fraction are ever tested for toxicity, and those that come to us from developing countries have few safeguards in place. A recent report from the Pesticide Action Network of North America reveals that Americans are exposed to toxic pollutants from foods up to 70 times a day!

Recent World Health Organization studies show that chemical and environmental factors are responsible for 80 to 90% of all cancers. Canadian research shows that pesticide sprays encourage life-threatening bacteria to grow on food crops, posing a real threat for people who eat fresh commerical produce- especially strawberries, raspberries and lettuce. New studies also link pesticides and pollutants to hormone dysfunctions, psychological disorders and birth defects. The molecular structure of many chemical carcinogens interacts with human DNA, so long term exposure can result in metabolic and genetic alteration that affects immune response.

The chemical industry points out that DDT and some other harmful pollutants containing environmental hormones are illegal in America. Yet, the U.S. is still the largest seller of DDT to the rest of the world. Many food-producing countries that supply America do not have pesticide bans, so imported foods from them still carry a toxic threat to us. Even if we ban the sprayed foods at our ports, the Earth's winds circle the globe and all the Earth's waterways are connected, so pesticides with environmental hormones reach the entire world's food supply.

The newest statistics come from breast cancer research. The dramatic rise in breast cancer in the last decade is consistent with the increased accumulation of organo-chlorine (PCB) residues. In Long Island, for instance, women living in areas previously sprayed with DDT have one of the highest breast cancer rates in the U.S.

Israel's pesticide experience offers even more dramatic evidence of the pesticide-breast cancer connection. Until twenty years ago, breast cancer rates and contamination levels of organo-chlorine pesticides in Israel were among the highest in the world. An aggressive phase-out of these pesticides has led to a sharp reduction in contamination levels… and to breast cancer death rates.

Here's how the link between pesticides and breast cancer seems to work.
Pesticides, like other pollutants, are stored in fatty tissue areas like breast tissue. Some pesticides (including PCB's and DDT) compromise immune function, overwork the liver and disrupt the glands the way too much estrogen does. A recent study showed up to 60% more *dichloro-diphenyl-ethylene* (DDE), DDT, and *polychlorinated bi-phenols* (PCB's) in the bodies of women who have breast cancer than in those who don't. Some researchers suggest that the reason today's older women have a higher than normal rate of breast cancer may be that these women had greater exposure to DDT before it was banned.

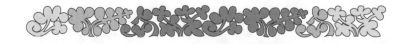

What can we do to overcome these environmental health threats? It's a quandary. The healthy fruits and vegetables we're all encouraged to eat are likely to contain unhealthy pesticides. Should you stop eating fresh produce? Of course not; fruits and vegetables clearly protect against cancer and heart disease. Still, only whole foods are wholesome. A healthy detox twice a year is a good way to rid yourself of dangerous chemicals.

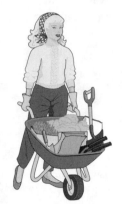

Start with the foods you eat.

Take steps to protect yourself from chemical residues in your food.

1: Almost 50% of U.S. consumers now use organic foods when they have a choice! They're a first line of protection for you and your family against chemical overload. Organic food standards require that no food labeled organic can be treated with chemical pesticides, radiation, genetic engineering, or have any contact with sewage sludge. In a recent study of 96 school children, the only child who had *no measurable pesticides* in his urine lived in a home where the family ate organic food exclusively. Fix organic food yourself for the best results if you're on a healing diet. A rapidly growing group of Americans are seeking out farmer's markets and produce stands.... even growing some of their own foods. Grocery stores and markets now offer affordable organic products to meet the growing consumer demand.

2: Buy seasonal, local produce whenever you can. Avoid imported foods as much as possible. Foreign countries have different regulations for pesticide use, so produce from other countries typically contains higher levels of pesticides than U.S. grown. Developing countries have few regulations. Mexico, for instance, has only recently begun phasing out DDT and chlordane which have been banned in the U.S. for decades. Imported produce also carries the threat of dangerous microbes, like those found in Guatemalan and Mexican strawberries in 1997.

3: Eat fruits and vegetables that have low PCB residues - like avocados, onions, broccoli, bananas, cauliflower, sweet potatoes, corn, watermelon. Eat a wide variety of foods to keep your exposure to any one pesticide low. Always wash foods with high residues: strawberries, cherries, spinach, bell peppers, cucumbers and grapes.

4: What about sea foods? America's coasts are in crisis. The ecosystem of our planet has been drastically upset by overfishing and by incredible amounts of waste dumped into our waters. Over one-third of U.S. shellfish beds are closed due to contamination from chemicals like PCB's and methyl mercury. Should you stop eating seafood? Of course not. Fish, seafoods and sea greens are some of the healthiest foods our planet offers. Fish like salmon and tuna are loaded with Omega-3 fatty acids that clearly decrease risk of heart disease and cancer. Sea greens like nori, wakame and dulse are some of the few non-animal sources of B-12, needed for cell and nerve development. They are rich in natural iodine to strengthen poor thyroid function, at the root of many energy and weight problems. Just 2 daily tablespoons of dried sea greens in rice, soups and salads boost metabolism and energy.

Some seafoods are not safe to eat today. Striped bass, rock cod, ocean perch, catfish, walleye, shark, caviar and lake trout, langoustinos and Maine lobster may have high residues of DDT, chlordane, dioxin and PCB's. Tuna, shark and swordfish from Connecticut aren't safe for pregnant women or children because of high mercury levels. At this printing, the safest seafoods to include in your diet are farmed abalone, Dungeness crab, halibut, Pacific wild salmon and shrimp. Wild abalone and swordfish are both so scarce they are on the endangered species list.

6: Be extra careful of your water supply. There's reason for concern. More than 100 million people in the U.S. get their drinking water from groundwater, but only half of that water is disinfected before it reaches their homes. In addition, experts estimate that 50% of the U.S. water supply is contaminated with giardia, which unlike bacteria, is not killed by chlorination. Giardia waterborne bacteria sickened 300,000 people and killed more than 100 in Milwaukee in 1993. Twenty-two American cities in 1996 were served by public water systems that violated minimum safety levels for contaminants.

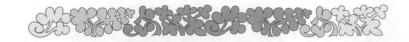

There are new concerns about pharmaceutical drugs in water supply. Here's the problem: Drugs pass though the body via normal urination. Water treatment plants inevitably receive some of these wastes, but they are not equipped to remove them. Hormones, caffeine, antidepressants and painkillers have all been found in rivers that receive water from treatment plants. Science is still determining how drug pollutants may affect human health. Preliminary results indicate both animals and humans living near drug contaminated water show hormone disruption!

Should you stop drinking water? Of course not. Water is critical to your very existence. But you can be sure your water is as clean as possible. —Drink quality water. Buy bottled water, distilled water or invest in a purification system. Reverse osmosis systems are expensive (about $1,000), but they are the best at eliminating impurities. Carafes and pitchers are much cheaper (about $25). They remove some organic pollutants and lead. —Investigate your drinking water quality. Read the review on water safety on page 116. Ask your water utility for its latest contamination review. *Call the Safe Water Hotline at 800-426-4791 for information about water safety.*

7: Avoid environmental hormones coming in from pesticide-laden foods and polluted water. Only in the last five years has anyone realized how common environmental estrogens are in our world. How do environmental hormones affect you? Exogenous (outside the body) estrogens and androgens affect your vital endocrine systems. Nearly 40% of pesticides used in commercial agriculture are suspected endocrine disrupters. They contain hormone-like substances, especially estrogens and androgens (major male and female hormones), that spell disaster for our health. People who live in high pesticide agricultural areas, who eat a high fat diet or hormone-injected meats, or who use placenta-containing hair care products are most at risk.

Science is just beginning to accept, even though naturopaths have known for some time, that man-made estrogens can stack the deck against women by raising their estrogen levels hundreds of times over normal. Some experts still believe that there is no significant difference between man-made and natural hormones, but it seems apparent from the evidence of thousands of women that even if a lab test can't tell the difference their bodies can.

Women's diseases linked to long exposure to synthetic estrogens: • breast and reproductive organ cancer; • breast and uterine fibroids, ovarian cysts; • endometriosis, pelvic inflammatory disease (PID).

More evidence of abnormally high estrogenic activity? American girls are reaching puberty at earlier and earlier ages. Nearly half of African American girls and fifteen percent of white girls start to develop sexually by age *eight*. A 2000 study links breast development in female babies 6 to 24 months old to a high number of hormone-disupting phthalates (in plastics, personal care products and lubricants) circulating in the blood!

Women aren't the only ones endangered by the estrogen-imitating effects of these substances. Alarming statistics relating to sperm count and hormone-driven cancers show substantial evidence that man-made estrogens threaten male health with reproductive disorders, too.

Environmental androgens (substances that mimic male sex hormones) in chemicals are even more widespread and may reveal even more frightening results. Research on synthetic androgens is too new to know all the hormonal implications, but early indications show widespread involvement in some cancers. One in vitro study found that out of ten pollutants, five bound to human androgen receptors while only two bound to estrogen receptors.

Men's health problems linked exposure to environmental hormones: • a 50% average decrease in male sperm counts over the past 50 years; • a 32% rise in undescended testes, small penis size and male fertility problems; • a dramatic rise in prostate disease, testicular cancer and male cancer deaths.

More bad news: For the first time in history, large numbers of people worldwide are having trouble conceiving children. In America today, one in six married couples of child-bearing age has trouble conceiving and completing a successful pregnancy. Chemical pollutants seem to be a factor in the birth rise of female and intersex babies where males would normally be born. Both humans and animals are now being born with both male and female genitalia, a frightening sign that our hormonal health, and that of future generations, is in jeopardy. Other effects include birth defects, impaired immunity, diabetes, and liver damage.

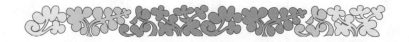

About Genetically-Engineered Foods
Are they "superfoods" or a disaster in the making?

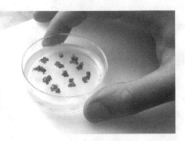

Food technology is expanding almost at the rate of the "big bang"! GE foods are everywhere. Today, up to 70 percent of the foods on American grocery shelves are genetically engineered (a number expected to grow to 90% by 2012). Most of the soy, corn, potatoes, tomatoes, dairy foods and yellow squash at your market is genetically engineered.Over one-third of U.S. farmland is planted with genetically-engineered seeds. *All* food is expected to be genetically engineered in the next ten years. At the end of the twentieth century, there were enough GE crops to cover Great Britain, Taiwan and New York's Central Park!

You may be shocked but should you be worried? Genetically engineered foods may contain DNA from widely different species. Plant, animal, insect, even bacterial or viral DNA make up new "improved" foods.

Pros and Cons of the New Millennium Food Supply
Are GE foods really "Franken-foods?"

There are benefits from genetic engineering:
• Proponents of GE foods insist that genetic engineering can boost resistance to pests, decreasing the need for harsh pesticide sprays and incidence of plant disease.
• Genetic engineering improves shelf life by altering genes which lead to spoilage.
• GE companies hope to create "super crops" that will feed the Earth's exponentially growing population for generations to come. However, a new United Nations Food and Agriculture Organization report reveals industrialized countries will be able to produce enough food to feed the entire world by the year 2030 <u>without</u> the use of genetically modified organisms. Still, genetic engineering is already here for some animal foods. "Super salmon" now grow to 10 lbs. in only 14 months.
• GE foods offer an easy delivery route for drugs and vaccinations. Genetically modified chickens now lay drug-enriched eggs to fight certain diseases. (***Warning: For people who rely on natural therapies, drug delivery through foods is not desirable because it leads to nutrient imbalances.***)

There's also a downside risk to GE foods... a price to pay:
• Allergens are transferred at the molecular level. As we add genes into foods from substances that aren't normally in our food chain, new allergies could (indeed already have) run rampant. We simply won't know which GE foods will cause reactions until it's too late. New reports show that soy allergies have gone up 50% since genetically engineered soy came into the food supply in 1997.
• Using genes in GE foods from already known allergens (like peanuts) can trigger severe reactions in allergic people. Eating a GE food that contains an allergen could mean life or death for an allergic person! A 1996 study in the New England Journal of Medicine revealed that splicing soybean genes with Brazil nut genes causes the same allergy reaction as eating the Brazil nut itself.
• Cross-pollination means pollen from GE crops will likely transfer into organic crops located nearby, so even organic foods may be exposed to genetically altered organisms. In Canada, two organic farmers recently filed class action lawsuits against GE giants, Monsanto and Aventis, claiming that their GE canola has spread so rapidly across Canadian prairies that organic farmers there can no longer even try to grow organic canola.
• Crops that are genetically engineered to build resistance to pesticides may transfer into neighboring weeds creating "superweeds" which can't be killed by herbicides. Further, biotech's ability to increase a crop's resistance to pesticides means commercial farmers will use <u>ever more toxic pesiticides and herbicides</u> which ultimately increase the pollution of our environment and food.

• Research shows bioengineering may destroy healing properties and reduce nutrient content of foods! A 1999 study in the Journal of Medicinal Food shows that cancer-fighting phytoestrogens in genetically engineered soybeans are 14% *lower* than in natural soybeans.

• Genetic engineering means animal by-products make their way into vegetarian foods. Fish genes (which improve shelf life) are routinely added to GE tomatoes, outraging vegetarians who assumed that at least their fruits and vegetables were free of animal products.

• GE foods developed to create their own insecticides or herbicides are especially precarious. A GE food that can kill another living organism could be dangerous for consumption by both animals and people. Even the ability to kill a so-called harmful plant or insect is risky. Mother Nature has many pathways to the health and survival of the Earth's species; we know only a tiny portion of how nature really works. As our own Native Americans have long known.... we are all one.... unnaturally changing ANY species has far-reaching consequences for others.

• Genetic engineering may prompt the development of "super" insects, that can resist normal methods of eradication and disturb the ecosystem. We already see disruptions in insect populations from GE technology. A European study shows ladybugs who eat aphids that dine on genetically engineered, insect-resistant potatoes live far shorter lives and produce one-third fewer eggs. California studies report monarch butterflies dying from eating GE corn pollen!

Should we slow down technology until we get a better handle on the health implications?

We might like to put the breaks on but studies are showing it may be too late. We know some critical GE dangers already. For example, once you alter plant DNA you run the risk of risk of causing mutations that lead to cancer. Yet only 1% of the USDA's molecular biology budget is spent on exploring the risks of genetic engineering on our foods!

Case in point: the "Flavr Savr" tomato, introduced in 1994 has become an example of a GE food failure. The "Flavr Savr" produced fewer yields, and the tomatoes themselves were too soft, and bruised too easily. Moreover, genes in the tomatoes conferred resistance to the antibiotics *kanamycin* and *neomycin* in the people who ate them. Antibiotic marker genes are used throughout the genetic engineering process today. Yet, over 150 genetically engineered foods were approved for sale in the year 2000, virtually none of them tested for this type of risk. If we continue to rely on these techniques, genetic engineering may cause the rates of antibiotic-resistant bacteria coming from foods to skyrocket, making people even more susceptible to supergerms than they are now!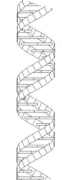

The massive genetic pollution of our population may be the ultimate price we pay for disrupting the natural balance within plant and animal species through genetic engineering. Once a living organism is genetically modified, it can reproduce, mutate and migrate at will and is almost impossible to control. Even innocent mistakes could have disastrous consequences, let alone attacks on our foods devised by terrorists.

Darwin may have been right after all. Natural selection may be the ultimate key. Nature never does anything without good reason. Plants and animals change naturally with time to adapt to a changing environment. For instance, we know many plant species have lengthened their growing season to better use the effects of global warming. Over time, we know plants may become more resistant to certain diseases or the effects of pollution. Documented studies show some tomatoes growing in polluted areas actually become stronger, boosting their antioxidant nutrients to protect themselves from harsh conditions.... in the process, becoming a more powerful medicinal food..... without genetic engineering!

Nature is the world's premier biochemist, making biological adjustments that keep humans and plants protected from changing conditions and diseases strains.

Today we are breaking Nature's laws almost without thought to the consequences.... simply because we can do it, or because, to our limited way of thinking, we think we can improve on nature.

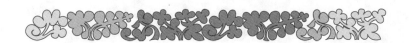

Never before have we so upset the boundaries set by Nature between species as we have with genetic engineering. Europe and Japan have already rejected "franken-foods." Other foreign markets threaten to stop buying U.S. foods until they are free of GMO's (genetically modified organisms). Americans are slowly waking up to the dangers of genetic engineering. Gerber baby foods has announced they will be "GE-free."

For industry giant Monsanto, genetic engineering means new GE species will be patented for enormous profit. According to its own Director of Corporate Communications, Monsanto believes it is the FDA's responsibility to assure the safety of the foods they sell.

At this writing (2003), the FDA does not require labels on GE foods, feeling that labels will frighten consumers. So, there's no way to be sure whether the foods you buy are genetically altered. The FDA says GE foods don't need labelling because they are no different than hybrids created by cross breeding. Yet hybrids are vastly different from GE foods. Hybrids result from cross breeding two or more varieties of the same species. Genetically engineered foods have no species boundaries. Genes from entirely different species can be used. Animal, viral and bacterial genes can all be inserted in a GE plant or animal. In reality, the FDA has no policy on how GE foods should be regulated because they are clearly not natural foods!

Surveys show that over 80% of Americans want GE foods to be labeled. Congress introduced a bill in December 1999 that may eventually force manufacturers to label GE foods to allow consumers a choice. U.S. agricultural groups now warn member farmers about the consequences of genetic engineering in terms of consumer dissatisfaction and "massive lawsuit liability."

What can we do to protect ourselves? If you want GE foods to be labeled as I do, write to Jane Henney M.D., FDA Commissioner, at 5600 Fishers Lane, Rockville, MD 20857.

Protective measures you can take to avoid GE foods:

1: Stick with certified organic foods which are less likely to be affected by genetic tampering. The Organic Standards Board does allow processed organic food to contain 5% non-organic ingredients which could theoretically be genetically engineered although the vast majority of the industry opposes the practice.

2: Buy seasonal fruits and vegetables from organic local farmers when possible. Buying with the seasons in your community helps strengthen small organic farmers. Always ask if genetically engineered seeds are used.

3: Especially avoid non-organic foods routinely genetically engineered - soy, canola oil and corn foods. Non-organic rice, beans, tomatoes, potatoes and papayas are also regularly genetically engineered.

4: Consider organic dairy. Most commercial dairy is injected with rBGH, a GE hormone. Research in a 1995 Cancer Letter shows cows treated with GE hormones have higher levels of insulin growth factor, a risk factor for breast and prostate cancer and child leukemia.

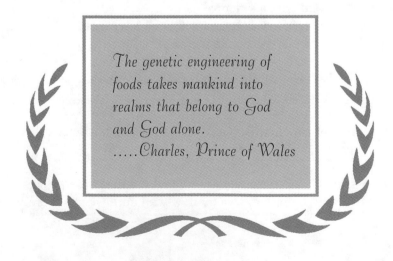

The genetic engineering of foods takes mankind into realms that belong to God and God alone.
.....Charles, Prince of Wales

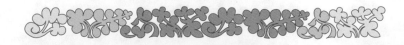

Fresh Fruits and Vegetables

Plant Chlorophyll provides critical Enzyme Therapy

Fruits and vegetables top the list of healing foods!

Massive research is validating what natural healers have known for decades. The more fruits and vegetables you eat, the more nutrition you get... and the less your risk of disease becomes. Sadly, less than 25% of Americans get the recommended daily 5 servings of fruits and vegetables that protect against disease. The news is even worse for our kids, who have largely stopped eating fruits and vegetables altogether — a major factor in the rise and prevalence of childhood allergies and asthma today!

Fresh fruits and vegetables are treasure chests of miracles for your healing diet.

Fruits and vegetables do what natural healers do best..... work with your body so it can use its built-in restorative powers. Even if your genetics and lifestyle are against you, your diet still makes a tremendous difference in your health and healing odds. Fresh fruits and vegetables accelerate body cleansing, and help normalize body chemistry. I emphasize a detoxifying fresh vegetable juice diet as part of almost every healing program that I develop.

Fruits and vegetables are full of nutraceuticals, the natural chemicals in plants with pharmacologic action. Scientists are enthusiastically embracing the healing possibilities of plant nutrients in fresh foods. Green leafy vegetables, for example, have almost *20 times more* essential nutrients, ounce for ounce <u>than any other food</u>! What's more, the nutrients in greens make the nutrients in other foods work better for healing.

The preventive medicine possibilities are astounding, too. Studies show that people who eat plenty of vegetables have less than half the cancer risk of people who eat few vegetables. Even moderate amounts of vegetables make a big difference. For instance, eating fresh vegetables twice a day, instead of twice a week, cuts the risk of lung cancer by 75%, even for smokers. One National Cancer Institute spokesman said it is almost most mind-boggling that common foods can be so effective against a potent carcinogen like tobacco!

There's more. Certain body chemicals must be "activated" before they can initiate cancer cell growth. Fresh foods can block the activation process, because food chemicals in cells can determine whether a cancer-causing virus, or a cancer promoter like excess estrogen, will turn tissue cancerous.

Fruits and vegetables may intervene even if you already have cancer. When cells mass into tumors, food compounds in cruciferous vegetables can restrain further growth by flushing certain carcinogens from the body, or shrinking patches of precancerous cells. Antioxidant foods can snuff out carcinogens, nip free radical cascades in the bud, even repair some cellular damage.

Although less powerful at later stages, a good diet can help prolong your life even after cancer takes hold. Fresh foods foster a healthy environment that deters wandering cancer cells from attaching to unhealthy tissues. The evidence is so overwhelming that researchers are starting to view fruits and vegetables as powerful preventatives that might wipe out cancer — an about-face for cancer study!

Fresh fruits and vegetables are far more than powerful cancer protectors. They are medicine for most, if not all, human ailments. You can always use your food as medicine for your health problems.

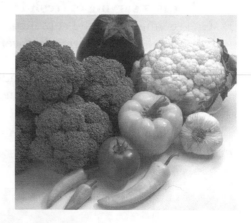

Three examples: 1) Research shows cherries can reduce pain and inflammation even better than aspirin. 2) Many women know that cranberry juice helps control bladder infections. The cranberry phytochemical, D-mannose, helps flush the infecting *E.coli* bacteria from the urinary tract. 3) Green leafy vegetables act as sweepers and scourers for the intestinal tract, keeping it free from toxins that could otherwise cause disease.

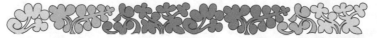

Fresh fruits are Nature's smiles.

Fruits are wonderful for a quick system wash and cleanse. A short fresh fruit cleansing diet is especially beneficial for heavy meat eaters whose systems may be clogged with fermented wastes. It is also an excellent way to purify the body in the spring because it slightly thins the blood after a long winter of eating rich, dense foods. Fresh fruit's natural water and sugar content speeds up metabolism to release wastes rapidly. Fresh fruit has an alkalizing effect in the body- beneficial for acid-related conditions like arthritis. Its easily convertible natural sugars transform to give us quick energy and speed up the calorie burning process.

But these advantages are only true of fresh fruits. The way that you eat fruit is as important as what fruit you eat. Fruits have their best healing and nutrition effects when eaten alone or with other fruits, as in a fruit salad, separately from grains and vegetables. With a few exceptions, both fruits and fruit juices should be taken before noon for best energy conversion and cleansing benefits.

Cooking fruits changes their properties from alkalizing to acid-forming in the body. This is also true of sulphured, dried fruit, and of combining fruits with vegetables or grains. When you eat fruit in any of these ways in excess, digestion slows down because the fruits stay too long in the stomach; gas forms, because the fruit sugars become concentrated, resulting in fermentation instead of assimilation. (Note: dried fruits, in moderation, can be a great source of fiber... especially for older people whose digestions can't take a lot of fresh fruits.)

New studies on fruits show more amazing benefits. Citrus fruits possess fifty-eight known anti-cancer compounds, more than any other food! Some researchers call citrus fruits a total anti-cancer package because they contain every class of nutrient — carotenoids, flavonoids, terpenes, limonoids, coumarins, and many more known to neutralize chemical carcinogens. Yet, citrus fruits act more powerfully <u>as a whole</u> than any of the separate anti-cancer compounds they contain. One phytochemical, for example, in oranges, is the potent antioxidant glutathione, a confirmed disease combatant. Commercially processed orange juice, unlike whole oranges, loses its glutathione concentration. Oranges are also rich in beta-carotene and vitamin C, and they're the highest food in glucarate, a powerful cancer-inhibitor. *TIP: Eat organically grown fruits whenever possible. The pesticides from sprayed fruits can enter your body very rapidly because of quick fruit sugar metabolism.*

Fresh vegetables are Nature's superfoods.

The healing power of vegetables works both raw and lightly cooked. It's not always true that raw vegetables are better. Some fragile anti-cancer agents, like indoles and vitamin C, are destroyed by heat, but a little heat makes beta-carotene, for example, more easily absorbed. Lightly cooked vegetables are gentler, especially if your digestion is impaired. If you have trouble digesting fresh fruits and vegetables, taking a high quality digestive enzyme or Hcl supplement helps minimize discomfort and maximizes nutrient assimilation.

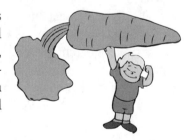

What is a serving of fresh fruits or vegetables?
One serving is about ½ cup of cooked, chopped veggies; 1 cup of raw leafy vegetables; 1 medium piece of fruit, or 6-oz. of fruit or vegetable juice. Only 10 percent of Americans eat that much every day.

The following pages detail astounding new studies which show that the same phytochemicals that protect plants from pests and disease also protect our bodies from cancers and heart disease.

See my new cookbook, DIETS FOR HEALTHY HEALING, for all the details on using food as your best medicine.

 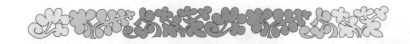

1: Organic sulphur compounds, like the allylic sulfides in garlic and onions, contain more than 30 different anti-carcinogens. Quercetin and ajoene can block the most feared cancer-causing agents like nitrosamines and aflatoxin, linked specifically to stomach, lung and liver cancer. Ajoene in garlic is three times as toxic to malignant cells as to normal cells. Interleukin in garlic boosts macrophages and T-lymphocytes, your body's own immune agents responsible for destroying tumor cells.

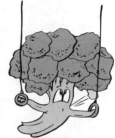

—*Allylic sulfides* in garlic also provide cardiovascular protection by suppressing cholesterol synthesis in the liver, by reducing LDL cholesterol, while keeping good high density lipoproteins at normal levels. Garlic may even reverse arterial blockages of atherosclerosis, and is a valuable weapon against tuberculosis, HIV, sickle cell anemia and ulcers.

—*Sulforaphane,* a compound in cruciferous vegetables, mustard and horseradish, induces protective phase II enzymes, which detoxifiy carcinogens. Sulforaphane delays onset of cancer, and inhibits both size and number of tumors. Tests show sulfarophane also fights *H. pylori* bacteria linked to stomach ulcers and some stomach cancers.

2: Antioxidants in foods like wheat germ, soy, yellow or green vegetables, green tea, citrus and olive oil help normalize pre-cancerous cells by snuffing out carcinogens and nipping free radical cascades in the bud.

—*Allylic sulfides* (see above) are also powerful antioxidants, defending cells against damage by oxidizing toxins. Allylic sulfides in garlic and onions inhibit the growth of a wide spectrum of bacteria and viruses, including *staphyloccus, streptoccocus* and *salmonella.* Garlic particularly fights funguses and parasites, making it a specific for candida albicans yeast overgrowth and HIV related conditions.

—*Green leafy vegetables* exhibit extraordinarily broad cancer protective powers, largely because they are so rich in antioxidants. Alpha, beta and other carotenes, folic acid and zeaxanthin in greens offer potent cancer protection. (Lutein, a little known antioxidant, is more potent than beta-carotene against cancer.) The darker the green color a vegetable has, the more cancer-inhibiting carotenoids it has. Dark greens like spinach, collard greens and kale are also well known today for their role in preventing age-related macular degeneration. Eat a green salad every day!

3: Organic acids: metabolic compounds with significant antioxidants and far reaching anti-cancer effects.

—*Phytic acid,* an antioxidant compound from rye, wheat, rice, lima beans, sesame seeds, peanuts and soybeans, appears to prevent colon cancer and enhances immune killer cell activity. It may be a better antioxidant than vitamin C, because it also naturally chelates both iron and zinc to help prevent heart disease.

—*Folic acid,* a B vitamin in wheat, wheat germ, leafy vegetables, beets, asparagus, fish, sunflower seeds, and citrus fruits is critical to normal DNA synthesis — so healthy cells stay healthy. Folic acid reduces the risk of birth defects like spina bifida, lowers the risk of atherosclerosis and, potentially, cancer. Today folic acid is counted as an important weapon against heart disease because it reduces homocysteine levels.

Note: While folic acid is seen as a cancer protector after menopause, excess folate can be tumor promoting. The key is getting plenty of folic acid from your food instead of just taking supplements. For example, people who eat lots of leafy greens have a low incidence of lung cancer. People who merely take folic acid supplements but do not eat leafy greens still lack protective folic acid in their lungs.

—*Vitamin C,* an antioxidant in citrus fruits, cherries, tomatoes, green peppers, strawberries, leafy greens, hot red peppers and broccoli, reduces both LDL cholesterol and triglyceride levels. Vitamin C's antioxidants also promote wound healing and boost interferon immune response and T-cell production. A vitamin C body flush (see page 193) is one of my favorite healing tools against allergies, colds and flu. Research shows that taking vitamin C supplements helps reduce both duration and severity of colds, and may also prevent secondary bacterial and viral complications. Antioxidants in C, E and carotenoids lower the common cataract risk of oxidative stressors like ultraviolet light. Vitamin C also improves blood sugar levels in non-insulin dependent diabetics. Some scientists believe that America's high rates of asthma are a result of a marked decrease in vitamin C antioxidants. Unlike other mammals, humans can't manufacture vitamin C on their own; we must obtain it from eating vitamin C rich foods or taking vitamin C supplements.

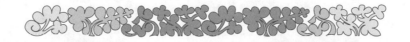

4: Bioflavonoids, initially called vitamin P (for their rapid permeability), are a significant part of the vitamin C complex for healing. Biolfavs help vitamin C keep your collagen, your body's intercellular cement, healthy. Bioflavonoids strengthen capillaries, connective tissue and blood vessel walls to reduce hemorrhages and ruptures which lead to spider and varicose veins, and bruises. (The first signs of deficiency in vitamin C and bioflavonoids are a tendency to bruise easily, varicose veins, or noticeable purplish skin spots.) Find bioflavs in the skins and pulp of citrus fruits, grapes, cherries and berries. Good herb sources: buckwheat greens, peppers, yellow dock, elder, hawthorn, horsetail, rosehips, shepherd's purse, sea plants and nettles.

Some of the benefits bioflavonoids have for you:

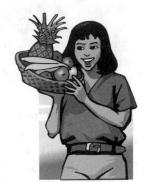

•bioflavs build an antibiotic-antiviral barrier against infections and boost immunity
•bioflavs have potent anti-inflammatory action without the side effects of aspirin
•bioflavs help prevent allergies and asthma
•bioflavs reduce excessive internal bleeding, promote healing of cuts and bruises
•bioflavs help detoxify carcinogenic chemicals, radiation and heavy metals
•bioflavs assist in preventing cardiovascular disease
•bioflavs act much like estrogens to curtail menopausal symptoms
•bioflavs help prevent cataracts and macular degeneration
•bioflavs help prevent easy bruising, especially in the elderly.

5: Genistein, a flavonoid in soy and cruciferous vegetables like broccoli, impedes angiogenesis (the growth of blood vessels that feed tumors), and deters cancer cell development by inhibiting enzymes that promote tumor formation. New tests on soy genistein show that it promotes the positive effects of estrogen while preventing many of estrogen's bad effects, especially hormone-driven cancers like breast and ovarian cancers. Other research suggests very large doses of soy isoflavones may aggravate breast cancer. Until we know, I believe moderation (2-3 servings a week of fermented soy foods) is the way to go with soy. *Note:* New research suggests large doses of genistein may block the anti-cancer activity of the estrogen-blocking drug, Tamoxifen. Ask your physician if you're unsure.

6: Quercetin, a flavonoid in garlic, cherries, dark berries and superfoods like chlorella, is one of the strongest anti-cancer food agents known. Quercetin blocks cell changes that initiate cancer, and stops malignant cells from clumping together to become tumors. An antioxidant, quercetin inhibits free radicals to prevent them from oxidizing LDL cholesterol. Quercetin also controls sticky blood, a risk factor for arteriosclerosis and coronary artery disease, by preventing platelet build-up and removing excess iron in the blood. Quercetin is one of Nature's most powerful protectors against allergy attacks. It is a powerful natural antihistamine and anti-inflammatory. Quercetin works best when a healing base is allowed to build up in the body.

7: Carotenoids, found mainly in fruits, vegetables and sea plants, are critical to your successful healing program. Carotenoids are present in virtually every cell of the human body. We're familiar with beta-carotene, but there are over 600 other carotenoids, some even more important in decreasing degenerative disease and boosting immune response. New studies on carotenes like alpha-carotene, lycopene, lutein, zeaxanthin, and beta-cryptozanthin show a 3 to 1 reduction in strokes and other heart risks when they're added to your diet.

Some of the newest healing benefits attributed to carotenes:

•**Cataracts** — eating less than 3 servings of carotene-rich foods increases risk of cataracts.
•**Immune system** — carotenes enhance both infection-fighting functions and immunity against tumors.
•**Heart disease** — drops almost 50% in men who take beta-carotene every other day for five years.
Note: Carotenes are most effective when working together as they do in nature. Different body organs selectively store different carotenoids depending on need. There is mounting evidence that high doses of one carotenoid can result in depressed levels of other carotenoids. Too much supplementation of any one carotene may reduce the protective level of other carotenes.

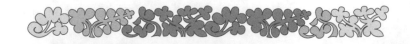

—Lycopene, a carotene found in tomatoes, red grapefruit, apricots and watermelon protects plants from the harmful effects of UV rays. It protects the human body in the same way. Lycopene is the body's most common carotene; it's concentrated in the prostate gland and is commonly used successfully as a natural preventative for prostate cancer. Lycopene also protects against mouth, lung, stomach, pancreas, bladder, colon and rectum cancers. Lycopene is 56% more powerful than beta-carotene and 100 times more efficient than vitamin E as a free radical scavenger. A high lycopene diet may cut heart attack risk in half! Lycopene is fat-soluble, so when lycopene-rich tomatoes are cooked with oil, as in spaghetti sauce, their bio-availability improves. Watermelon actually has 60% more lycopene than raw tomatoes. For best results, eat (or drink) lycopene-rich watermelon before a meal that includes some fat. (Watermelon is also rich in the amino acid, *citrulline,* for natural diuretic action for water retention.)

—Lutein is the most abundant carotenoid in fruits and vegetables, especially dark leafy greens like spinach, kale and broccoli, and in egg whites. Lutein and zeaxanthin are potent antioxidants, especially concentrated in the macula of the eye, responsible for detailed vision. The macula is covered by a layer of lutein and zeaxanthin, natural sunscreens which selectively filter out visible blue light. If blue light is allowed to reach the retina, it can cause photodamage that contributes, over time, to degeneration of the macula. Lutein and zeaxanthin help protect against retinal damage and strengthen blood vessels that supply the macular region. A new study shows high lutein diets are protective against colon cancer, too.

—Beta carotene, in red, yellow and dark green vegetables and fruits, and sea plants, protects against cancer, heart disease, cataracts, low immune response and high cholesterol. Beta carotene reduces tumor cell proliferation and free radical activity in the tumor. Even after they form, studies show tumors exposed to beta carotene are substantially smaller than tumors not exposed. Harvard studies say that beta carotene acts like a chemotherapy agent on squamous carcinoma tumor cells. Tufts University studies show that beta carotene changes into a substance called retinoic acid which can treat bladder cancer with considerable success.

—Alpha carotene, found in apricots, carrots, peaches and sweet potatoes, is 30% more powerful than beta carotene in preventing cancer. Alpha carotene animal studies show it especially inhibits cancers of the skin, liver and lungs.

—Canthaxanthin, a carotene in mushrooms can decrease skin cancer risk and boost immunity.

8: Plant polyphenols: are a form of bioflavonoids. Active polyphenols appear in grapes, pomegranates, raspberries, huckleberries, strawberries and green tea. Some experts believe that polyphenols in the famous early 1900's "Grape Cure" for cancer were key factors in its success. Polyphenols inhibit the growth of cancer tumors, and lower the risk of heart attack by decreasing the likelihood of blood clots and cholesterol plaques.

—Catechin, the most abundant plant polyphenol breaks up free radical cell chains of fats, prevents DNA damage, helps block carcinogens, protects against digestive and respiratory infections.

—Green tea catechins show excellent antioxidant effects on fatty foods. Antioxidant properties of green tea catechins are 30 times more powerful than vitamin E and 50 times more potent than vitamin C. Green tea catechins have been used with good results for viral hepatitis, and may help prevent stomach cancer. Note: Don't miss these benefits from Green Tea, page 154.

9: Ellagic acid: a phenol in walnuts, berries (esp. raspberries), grapes, apples, tea and pomegranates is an antimutagen against nicotine-induced lung tumors, an anticarcinogen for skin tumors and for chemically-induced cancers. Research finds that ellagic acid from raspberries arrests cancer cell division and induces cancer cell death (apoptosis) within 72 hours for breast, pancreas, esophageal, skin, colon and prostate cancer cells.

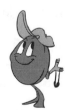

10: Saponins: abundant steroids in plants like beans, spinach, tomatoes, potatoes, oats, alfalfa and sea foods. They are significant in many herbs, like ginsengs and licorice root. Ginseng saponins lower cholesterol by binding to cholesterol in the gastrointestinal tract. Saponins fight infections by forming disease-specific antibodies. They effectively ward off microbial and fungal infections, even viruses and cancerous growths.

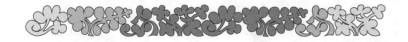

11: Glycyrrhizin: a hormone-like saponin in licorice root, is effective for normalizing menopausal hormone levels. It appears to deter hormone-driven tumors (like those of breast cancer) by acting as a natural estrogen blocker. Glycyrrhizin has anti-viral properties — for example, it is able to slow progression of the HIV virus by inhibiting cell infection and inducing interferon activity for immune response. Glycyrrhizin encourages production of hydrocortisone for anti-inflammatory activity. Like cortisone, but without the side effects, it relieves arthritic and allergy symptoms,and those that accompany *candida albicans* yeast infections.

12: Indoles: like indole-3 carbinole from broccoli, cabbage, radishes, turnip or mustard greens are natural antioxidants with tumor preventing activity. Indoles also alleviate some symptoms of fibromyalgia and related chronic fatigue syndrome.

—*Indole-3-carbinole* also prevents cancer in two other amazing ways: 1) Indoles improve the enzyme pathways through which our bodies get rid of cancer-causing agents. Indole-3-carbinole changes the metabolism of carcinogenic toxins by producing phase 1 and phase 2 detoxification enzymes. The enzymes make toxins water soluble.... your body can easily rid itself of water soluble substances, thus reducing the risk of cancer. 2) These same detox enzymes also inhibit certain carcinogenic materials from binding with DNA. When the materials cannot attach to DNA, cancer can't get started. In one of Nature's miracle pathways, the by-products formed when indole-3-carbinole reacts with stomach acids are more bioactive than indole-3-carbinole itself. The by-products even help clear the body of bad cholesterol.

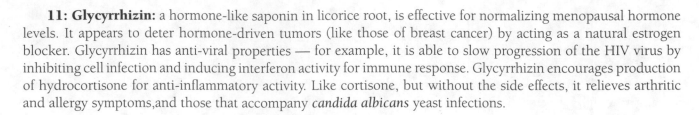

—*DIM (di-indolylmethane),* the most biologically active cruciferous indole known, improves estrogen metabolism and our ability to eliminate excess estrogens, especially from sources like pesticides and synthetic hormones. Structurally similar to estrogen, DIM increases estrogen conversion into "good" estrogen metabolites-2-hydroxy estrogens with antioxidant properties that protect the brain and heart. Women who eat plenty of vegetables containing DIM, lower their risk of breast and uterine cancers, and cervical dysplasia. Early reports find DIM reduces PMS symptoms like breast pain and moodiness, and may improve endometriosis. Proper estrogen metabolism also means the burning of more stored fat for menopausal women. Men who eat plenty of vegetables containing DIM enhance the activity of testosterone and muscle growth, and have a substantially lower risk of colon cancer. DIM even improves the safety of superhormones like DHEA and HRT drugs by metabolizing excess estrogen that may result from supplementation.

13: Isoprenoids: fat soluble antioxidants that neutralize free radicals by anchoring themselves to fatty membranes, then grabbing free radicals that attach to the membranes and pass them to other antioxidants.

—*Vitamin E,* from almonds, wheat germ, wheat germ oil, leafy veggies, salmon, soy foods, and organ meats, is an antioxidant isoprenoid. There's a clear correlation between vitamin E, a lower risk of heart disease and Alzheimer's, and better body balance for women during menopause or menstrual difficulties. I believe the best vitamin E comes from dietary sources—foods and herbs. Many doctors say synthetic vitamin E may increase hemorrhaging during surgery; they don't recommend it for a pre-op or post-op nutritional program. I have found this not to be a problem for dietary vitamin E, which is safe before and after surgery.

—*CoQ-10,* an isoprenoid also known as ubiquinione or uniquinol, is available mainly through protein sources like fish, meats, sea vegetables and some of the green superfoods. CoQ-10, an extremely important anti-oxidant enzyme, does a lot more than just protect us from free radical damage. It actually targets particular diseases with its powerful enzyme therapy. Highly successful against gum disease, ulcers, even some AIDS related diseases, CoQ-10 strengthens your cardiovascular system against coronary artery disease, especially if you've had a previous heart attack. It helps lower high cholesterol and high blood pressure. It helps overcome fatigue. It reduces the risk of breast and prostate cancers; I have seen myself that it can even reduce the rate of tumor growth once the cancer has begun.

Note: for more about CoQ-10, see **Enzymes & Enzyme Therapy**, page 92.

Chlorophyll
A Key to Healing from Green Vegetables

Green foods are power plants for humans. Our body chemistry comes from plant nutrients because plant chlorophyll (one of the most powerful nutrients on Earth) transmits the energies of the sun and the soil to our bodies. The sun is the energy source of the Earth—plants constitute the most direct method of conserving the energy we receive from the sun. Fruits, vegetables, grains and grasses reach out to us on branches and stems, making themselves beautiful and nourishing to attract us. Plants have no fear of being eaten as animals do. The life energy of plants simply transmutes into higher life form of mankind.

Chlorophyll offers amazing healing benefits for humans. The most therapeutic ingredient in green foods is chlorophyll, the basic component of the "blood" of plants. Chlorophyll is the pigment that plants use to carry out photosynthesis - absorbing the light energy from the sun, and converting it into plant energy. This energy is transferred into our cells and blood when we consume fresh greens. Chlorophyll is in all green plants, but is particularly rich in green and blue-green algae, wheat grass, parsley, and alfalfa.

Our blood has a unique affinity to chlorophyll. The chlorophyll molecule is remarkably similar to human hemoglobin in composition, except that it carries magnesium in its center instead of iron. Eating chlorophyll-rich foods helps our bodies build oxygen-carrying red blood cells. In my opinion, eating green foods is almost like giving yourself a little transfusion to help treat illness and enhance immunity.

Chlorophyll is a better tonic than Geritol for tired blood. It calms the nerves, so it's helpful for insomnia, exhaustion and nervous irritability. It's beneficial for skin disorders used topically and internally, helps you cope with deep infections, and dental problems like pyorrhea. Its anti-bacterial qualities are a proven remedy for colds, ear infections and chest inflammation.

Chlorophyll detoxifies your liver and is a potent antioxidant. It helps neutralize and remove drug deposits, and purifies the blood. Even the medical community sees chlorophyll as a means of removing heavy metal buildup, because it can bind with heavy metals to help remove them. A new U.S. Army study reveals that a chlorophyll-rich diet doubles the lifespan of animals exposed to radiation. Since the days of Agent Orange and Gulf War Syndrome, chlorophyll is being considered as protection against some chemical warfare weapons.

Chlorophyll is rich in vitamin K, necessary for blood clotting. Naturopathic physicians use chlorophyll for women with heavy menstrual bleeding and anemia. Vitamin K helps form a compound in urine that inhibits growth of calcium oxalate crystals, so chlorophyll helps with kidney stones. Vitamin K also enhances adrenal activity, so chlorophyll-rich foods help maintain steroid balance for a more youthful body.

Chlorophyll improves body detoxification and digestion. It helps reduce chronic bad breath and body odor.... even in pets! Add it to your detox juices during a cleanse to help keep blood sugar levels stabile.

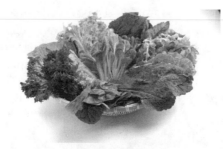

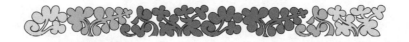

Boost Your Enzymes for Better Healing Results

Enzymes are the catalysts for every body process. None of your vitamins, minerals or hormones can work without the right enzymes. Each of us is born with a battery charge of enzymes at birth, but as we age our internal enzyme stores are naturally depleted. In fact, a 60-year-old has 50% fewer enzymes than a 30-year-old. This is why eating enzyme-rich foods is so critical as we age.

Where have all the enzymes gone?

Most of us are enzyme deficient today. Our processed food diet means we're getting few enzymes from foods. Enzymes are highly sensitive to heat, too. Heat above 120 F. destroys them- a reason why microwaving food can have disastrous effects on your health. Chemical additives, tobacco smoke, chlorine in drinking water, fluorides and air pollution also sap body enzymes. Many prescription drugs, caffeine and alcohol deplete enzymes. The result: An inadequate enzyme supply that burdens both digestion and metabolism, and may even lead to fatigue, weight gain, skin disorders, degenerative disease and <u>accelerated aging</u>.

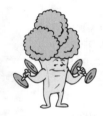

Add more enzymes to your diet.

Fresh foods contain the highest amount of enzymes to work with yours. Some enzyme enthusiasts say a raw foods diet is the only way to reap the benefits of enzyme therapy. I find lightly *cooked* foods along *with* enzyme booster foods works better for most people....especially for people with serious diseases like cancer or AIDS whose digestive systems may not be able to tolerate a completely raw foods diet. Some nutrients like lycopene (a carotenoid in tomatoes) are actually better used by the body when they're slightly cooked.

What can enzyme therapy do for you?

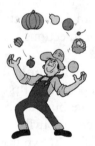

1) **Improve problems** like heartburn, indigestion, lactose intolerance and gas.
2) **Speed healing from wounds, surgery, or injuries.** Studies show enzyme therapy promotes recovery from ankle joint distortion, the most common sports' injury.
3) **Reduce pain and inflammation in arthritis and ulcerative colitis.** Some patients are even able to completely avoid surgery for colitis by using supplemental enzymes.
4) **Relieve sinusitis.** In one study, the enzyme bromelain from pineapple resolved sinus infection in 85% of patients after 9 days of treatment.
5) **Heal shingles.** Research reveals enzymes greatly reduce neuralgia reoccurrence in shingles patients.
6) **Boost weight loss.** Research shows animals fed raw potatoes (high in enzymes) lose significantly more weight than those fed cooked potatoes.
7) **May enhance sexuality.** Enzymes are high in pheromones linked to sexual attraction. A male sperm enzyme is responsible for dissolving a spot on the female egg so sperm can successfully fertilize it.
8) **The enzyme protease is amazing.** Protease boosts immune response, fights infection, reduces scar ring, unclogs arteries, even shrinks tumors. Try Crystal Star® DR. ENZYME™ with protease and brome lain or Transformation PUREZYME protease.

High enzyme foods to include in your healing diet: fresh fruit and vegetable juices; fermented foods like miso, yogurt, kefir and raw cultured vegetables; sprouted seeds; cruciferous vegetables like broccoli, cabbage, and cauliflower (boosts production of phase two enzymes which remove carcinogens from cells); pineapple, papaya, bananas and mangos; superfoods like barley grass, alfalfa and chlorella. Some experts say green barley extract contains all the enzymes necessary for life... even contains the enzyme superoxide dismutase, which prevents free radical damage. *To learn more about the healing power of enzymes, consult The Complete Book of Enzyme Therapy, written by my esteemed colleague, Anthony J. Cichoke M.A., D.C., D.A.C.B.N.*

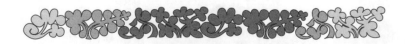

Is a Vegetarian Diet Better?

Vegetarian eating is seen today as a practice of enlightenment, of increased understanding of responsibility for mankind's place on the Earth, perhaps even of higher consciousness. Decades of study clearly demonstrate that a balanced vegetarian diet may be one of the healthiest diets we can follow. I believe moving towards a plant-based diet may be one of the best ways to save our personal and global environments.

We see the horrors on our daily news, and start to shrink from every kind of violence. Some people say that killing of any kind is wrong. Others say killing is reserved for our "enemies." But who, as our world grows smaller, and we see that people everywhere are just like us, is our enemy? Certainly not the Earth's animals. Our views of our ancient ancestors are changing as our view of ourselves changes. The stereotype of early humans as "Man the hunter" is today more often seen as "Man the gatherer."

Today's vegetarian culture is not the first. It was widely practiced by the ancient Greeks and Romans. But the fall of Rome led to "dark ages" in vegetarian thought much as it did in the arts. Scientific rationale dominated western ideas..... reasoning that animals were placed on earth for the convenience and use of humans and could be killed, eaten, and exploited as necessary. Vegetarianism was not practiced by the general populace for over 1500 years. Only the Christian abbeys kept vegetarian principles alive.

Darwin's theory of evolution challenged the scientific justification for eating animals. Darwin believed that both humans and animals were part of a continuum of life, separated only in degree, not in kind. His work began the vegetarian "renaissance" of the late 18th and 19th centuries.

Many people today become vegetarians for similar environmental and spiritual reasons. Even people who enjoy eating meat are going "veg," in response to the severe animal cruelty and horrific sanitation problems of today's factory farms. More than compassion for animals, the growing problem of antibiotic and hormone-loading on food animals, and the spread of Mad Cow disease in humans from contaminated beef has inspired health conscious people to switch to a plant-based diet.

What is a vegetarian? Good question.

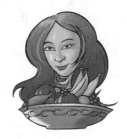

When we try to apply the different social foundations and ideas from around the world to vegetarianism, an accepted definition becomes confusing if not impossible. Food and diet are inextricably intertwined in both the religion and culture to which they belong. Different kinds of foods are seen differently by different peoples.

Ways vegetarians are classified today.
—Semi vegetarian: eats poultry, fish, eggs and dairy foods, but not red meats or pork
—Pesco vegetarian: eats fish, eggs and dairy foods, but not poultry, red meats or pork
—Lacto ovo vegetarian: eats eggs and dairy foods, but no animal food that "has eyes"
—Ovo vegetarian: eats eggs, but no other animal food product
—Vegan: excludes all animal derived foods (some eat bee products)

Becoming a vegetarian affects both body and mind.... indeed the very core of our being. When they change their diet, people find their point of view about life changes, too. Nutrition awareness and knowledge increases. Most vegetarians support a "green" lifestyle—consciously trying to preserve instead of thoughtlessly wasting the Earth's bounty—as their consciousness of the planet heightens.

The benefits of a vegetarian diet?
...Vegetarians live longer... an average of 6 to 10 years longer than the rest of the population.
...Vegetarians are better hydrated from the high water content of fresh foods.

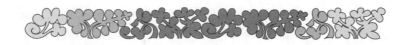

...A vegetarian diet is low in fat, so it's heart smart. Vegetarians have a well documented history of lower risk for high blood pressure, heart attacks, coronary artery disease, heartburn, obesity, gallstones, kidney disease, diabetes, osteoporosis, colon disease, and several types of cancer.

...Vegetarians are energetic. Energy comes from carbohydrates and healthy fats from grains, legumes, fruits and vegetables. Energy also comes from vitamins, minerals and amino acids, plentiful in plant foods.

...Vegetarians report better body balance, especially protein balance. Vegetable protein abounds in grains, legumes like beans and lentils, soy foods, potatoes, green vegetables, nuts and seeds, pasta and corn. Animal proteins are known to raise cholesterol, while protein from soy has been found to lower cholesterol. One of the big problems with today's high meat "Zone" weight loss diets is that they rely largely on caloric restriction for weight loss, and ignore the cardiovascular implications of a high meat diet.

...Vegetarians regularly have lower concentrations of pesticide residues in their bodies. Red meat is one of the highest food sources of pesticides. Our meat animals don't eat organically grown foods!

...Being a vegetarian is easier on your pocket book than a meat-based diet. A vegetarian diet also takes the least toll on our environment and conserves natural resources.

How long does it take to become a vegetarian if you've been a lifelong meat-eater? Transition time varies widely. Only 30% of newly converted vegetarians stop eating meat immediately; 70% eliminate meat from their diets over months, even years. Make the transition a new adventure in eating. Vegetarian cuisine is incredibly diverse and interesting. Get a new cookbook or two and tantalize your taste buds!

What's the truth about red meat?

I believe eating red meats puts us a step away from environmental harmony. The human digestive system is not easily carnivorous. Our bodies have to struggle to use red meat energy. Eating red meat is a lot like extracting oil out of the ground. It can cost more to get the oil out than it's worth on the market. Meat protein, which the body can use, is often cancelled out by lengthy digestion time and after-dinner lethargy.... a disproportionate amount of energy goes to the task of assimilation. Too much of the highly concentrated protein in red meat can create toxicity from unused nitrogens—hard for your kidneys to cope with. Kidney and gallstones are far more frequent in heavy red meat eaters.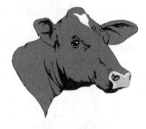

Animals are closer to us on the bio-scale of life. They experience fear when killed. They don't want to be eaten. On the other hand, when we eat plants, there is an uplifting transmutation of energy. Red meats make our bodies become denser, with more internal fermentation and body odor. Commercial red meats today are shot through with hormones and slow-release antibiotics (stock yard animals are often sick and over-medicated), and preserved with nitrates or nitrites. These substances are passed into us at the dinner table.

Red meat is our biggest diet contributor of excess protein and saturated fat levels. No one argues that less fat in the diet is healthier, or that saturated fats are the most harmful. Knowing this, livestock growers and butchers have made some changes. Beef now has 27%, and pork 43% less trimmable fat than cuts sold in the supermarket in the 1970s and 1980s. (There's still a lot of saturated fat in the meat marbling, however.) Cooked red meats are acid-forming in the body; when red meat is cooked to well-done, chemical compounds are created that are capable of causing many diseases.

Finally, meat eating promotes more aggressive, arrogant behavior—a lack of gentleness in personality. From a spiritual point of view, red meat eating encourages ties to life's material things, expansion of territory, and the self-righteous intolerance that makes adversaries.

Most of us eat more meat than we need. A 100 gram serving of meat is the size of a deck of cards, smaller than your computer mouse. A small can of salmon or tuna is two servings. Half a chicken breast, or a small hamburger patty is one serving. A small boneless roast weighing just over 2 pounds provides 10 servings.

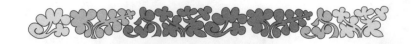

About Red Meat and a Healing Diet

Many recent scientific studies find that eating red meat increases the risk of degenerative diseases like heart disease, stroke and cancer. The American Heart Association, American Cancer Society, National Academy of Sciences, and American Academy of Pediatrics are just a few of the scientific organizations recommending less consumption of red meat and other animal foods, and a shift to a more vegetarian diet.

I don't believe red meat should be part of a healing diet. Here's why:

Health implications begin immediately after slaughter as meat starts to decompose. Salt preservation and re-frigeration retard spoilage, but even slight putrefaction produces toxins and amines that accumulate in your liver, kidneys and intestines. These destroy friendly bacteria cultures (especially those that synthesize B vitamins), and degrade small intestine villi where food is absorbed into the blood. Saturated animal fats gather around organs and blood vessels, leading to cysts, tumors, cholesterol build-up and clogged arteries. Experts say that excess absorption of meat proteins may overstimulate immune response, resulting in immune tolerance.

Meat is significantly harder to digest than plant foods, taking 4 to 4½ hours to be absorbed in the intestines versus 2 to 2½ hours for grains and vegetables. Meat requires more oxygen in the bloodstream for digestion than plant digestion.

There's even more recent bad news about red meat.

—**Pesticides:** Beef contains the highest concentration of herbicides of any food in America. Eighty percent of all herbicides used in the U.S. are sprayed on corn and soy beans, which are used primarily as feed for cattle. The National Research Council (NRC) of the National Academy of Sciences cites pesticide-tainted beef as nearly 11 percent of the total cancer risk from pesticides to consumers. The chemicals accumulate in the cattle and are passed onto consumers in finished cuts of beef.

—**Irradiation:** There are still no long term studies to prove that food irradiation is safe, but tainted meats are now so wide-spread in America, the FDA has approved irradiation of red meat to destroy deadly bacteria like *E. coli*. For pennies a pound, hamburger or sausage can be zapped with radiation (the equivalent of 10 to 70 million chest X-rays) to kill pathogens by altering the genetic make up of the harmful bacteria. Benzene, a potent carcinogen, is created when red meat is exposed to irradiation. Just one molecule of benzene absorbed into the body is enough to cause cancer. Some experts believe that food irradiation may also lead to fetal malformations, kidney problems and cardiac disease. Numerous studies show irradiation causes bleeding in the heart! Nor does it seem that food irradiation actually solves the underlying problem: unsanitary slaughterhouse and factory farm conditions, which give birth to the food borne illnesses that irradiation "treats."

—**Hormones:** More than 95 percent of all feedlot-raised cattle in the U. S. receive growth hormones, antibiotics or other drugs. (Europe rejects our hormone-injected beef, and has, in fact, banned the practice since 1995.) In order to speed weight gain and time-to-market, hormone levels are increased two to five times through anabolic steroids. Time-release synthetic estradiol, testosterone and progesterone slowly seep into the animal's blood. These hormones then become part of the hormone assault on people now implicated in increased cancer risk and other hormone-driven diseases.

—**Antibiotics:** In 1990, more than 15 million pounds of antibiotics were given to U.S. livestock to fight diseases which were running rampant in cramped feedlots and contaminated pens. The beef industry says it has discontinued automatic use of antibiotics in beef cattle, but antibiotics are still given to dairy cows, which account for 15% of the beef eaten in the America. Veal calves become so sick in their tiny pens that antibiotics are routinely used to keep them alive until slaughter. Contrary to veal industry claims, no drugs have been approved by the U.S. FDA for formula-fed veal calves. Some of the drugs used routinely, like sulfamethazine, are carcinogenic and residues may be present in consumer veal.

An amazing fact: In 2001, the Union of Concerned Scientists reported that the antibiotics used in factory farms account for <u>over 50%</u> of all antibiotic use in the U.S. Further, according to the Institute of Medicine, the overuse of antibiotics in factory farms is <u>responsible</u> for the huge increase in antibiotic-resistant, food borne illness. The problem is so out of control that in 1997, the World Health Organization called for a ban on the routine feeding of antibiotics to livestock. Unfortunately, as of this writing, the animal agriculture industry continues to load up food animals with heavy doses of antibiotic meds.

—**Inadequate inspections:** Since 1985, the National Academy of Sciences has reported that federal meat inspections were inadequate to protect the public from meat-related diseases. However, recommended corrective steps were never adopted. Instead, an experimental inspection system, virtually eliminating the federal meat inspector, and increasing online meat production by up to 40 percent was developed. It placed responsibility for carcass inspection on packing house employees. Thousands of carcasses pass through this inspection system with pneumonia, measles, peritonitis, abscesses, cancer, tumors, fecal or insect adulteration, and contaminated heads (called "puke heads"), on their way to American dinner tables. The amount of meat that is recalled because of contamination has skyrocketed in the last decade. Single recalls regularly include more than 10 million pounds of contaminated meat! Even more frightening, current USDA records indicate that much of the meat that is recalled is never actually taken out of the U.S. marketplace!

—**Disease:** There appears to be a new link between cattle diseases and disease in humans. Bovine leukemia virus (BLV), an insect-borne retrovirus that causes malignancy in cattle, is found in 20% of cattle and 60% of U.S. herds. It may cause some forms of human leukemia, since BLV antibodies have been found in leukemia patients. Bovine immunodeficiency virus (BIV), widespread in American herds since the 1980's, genetically resembles human HIV virus, and like HIV in humans, appears to suppress the immune system in cattle. One study suggests that BIV "plays a role in either malignant or slow viruses in humans." Scientists now overwhelmingly accept that Mad Cow Disease in cattle is able to cross the species barrier with humans when diseased beef is eaten. At least 143 people in Britain have already died from Mad Cow Disease. In a disturbing turn of events, mad cow disease has also recently been detected in U.S. cattle herds.

Are there enough benefits from red meat to add it back to your diet <u>after</u> healing?

In order to build human protein, we need 22 amino acids. Clearly, red meat has complete protein and all the amino acids. Our bodies make amino acids, except for the eight essential amino acids that must be obtained from our foods. Plant proteins have more amino acids, but no plant on its own has enough of the essential amino acids.

Can vegetarians get enough amino acids for protein building?

Plant protein combinations are good choices—like beans with rice or corn, tofu with whole grains, and legumes like peanuts and beans with whole wheat or corn. Bee pollen and sea plants contain all the essential amino acids and are considered complete foods by many vegetarians.

Can vegetarians get enough absorbable iron?

Red meat has long been considered the best source of food iron. Hemoglobin, the plasma of red blood formation, is part of red meat tissue, and delivers from 2 to 10 times more iron than any other source. Yet, new research shows us that body absorption of red meat iron may not be very efficient, because <u>vegetarians</u> have almost the same levels of iron in their blood as people who eat one or more servings of meat daily.

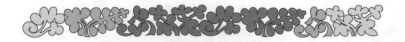

Legumes, whole grains, nuts, spinach, clams, asparagus, poultry, prunes, raisins, pumpkin seeds, beets and soy foods all provide easy-to-use iron. Note, too that most iron supplements are not as well absorbed as food iron and are constipating, especially for children and pregnant women. I recommend herbal iron in combinations that include yellow dock root, dandelion, alfalfa, sea greens like spirulina and nettles.

Can vegetarians get enough zinc for proper growth?

Red meat is a good source of zinc, needed for growth and immunity. Other good food sources include: chicken, seafood, spirulina, whole wheat and wheat germ, lima beans, legumes, soy foods, nuts and eggs.

Can vegetarians get enough B vitamins, especially B-12, essential for new red blood cells?

Red meat is a good source of B-complex vitamins like riboflavin, thiamine and niacin. B vitamins help muscle tissue use food energy, so it's not surprising that animal muscle is a good source. Red meat is a good source of B-12, responsible for cellular growth and repair. A B-12 deficiency takes a long time to notice and can cause serious health problems. For B vitamins, whole grains, like brown rice, and sea greens are primary sources. For critical Vitamin B-12, consider sea greens, soy foods, eggs, brewer's yeast, cereals and supergreens like chlorella, spirulina and especially barley grass. If you eat few of these foods, take a vitamin B-12 supplement.

Can vegetarians get enough calcium for strong bones?

Clearly, calcium is gaining in importance for the aging baby boomer population, especially for osteoporosis prevention, stress reduction and weight loss. Red meat and dairy foods are a good source of calcium for strong teeth and bones. But, are they really the best sources of calcium? High protein from meat consumption is known to leach calcium from the body. An estimated 28 mg of calcium is lost for every hamburger that a woman eats. In addition, new research reveals that diets high in animal protein may lead to increased bone loss and risk of osteoporosis.

Calcium from herbs and vegetables (especially leafy greens) are superior in my mind. They come with the proper balance of magnesium, and without the concentrated animal protein that offsets mineral absorption. Calcium is plentiful in root vegetables, broccoli, nuts and seeds, dark leafy greens, brussels sprouts, legumes like peas and beans, soy foods, whole grains, and supergreens like chlorella and spirulina. Some herbs are actually quite high in calcium, too. Lambs quarters contains a whopping 1500mg per oz.! Carrot juice is another excellent source of calcium. Organic is best for high calcium content. One 8-oz glass of fresh, organic carrot juice has 300-400mg of bioavailable calcium. 1 8-oz. glass of fortified milk only has about 250mg- with LOW ASSIMILATION.

Note: If you decide to include red meat in your diet, consider ostrich meat as a healthier red meat in America. Ostrich meat tastes, looks and feels like beef. It is comparable to beef in iron and protein content. But ostrich meat has less than half the fat of chicken, and two-thirds less fat and calories than beef and pork.

I believe vegetarians play a key, active role in conserving precious water, topsoil, and our Earth's resources that are wasted by an animal-based diet. Avoiding red meats may become one of most important things you can do for your own health and that of the planet.

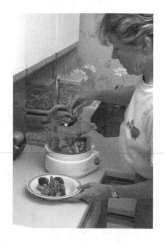

Albert Einstein, whom we know as a great mathematician, was also a passionate vegetarian. He once said of his commitment, "Nothing will benefit human health and increase the chances for survival of life on Earth as much as the evolution to a vegetarian diet."

Note: An outstanding resource on the benefits of a vegetarian diet that I referred to often in the writing of this book: *The Food Revolution: How Your Diet Can Help Save Your Life and the World*, by longtime vegetarian and environmentalist, John Robbins.

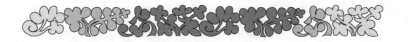

Protein: *How Much Do You Need?*

You must have protein to heal. Next to water, protein is your body's most plentiful substance, its primary source of building material for muscles, blood, skin, hair, nails, and organs like the heart and brain. All body tissues depend on protein. Blood can't clot without protein. Protein and its precursors, amino acids, work at hormonal levels to control basic functions like growth, sexual development and metabolism. The enzymes for immune and antibody response are formed from protein, too.

The human body doesn't make protein, it must be obtained through diet. But since protein is available from a wide range of sources, usually only people with severe malnutrition are protein deficient. Even people in less industrialized countries, get plenty of protein from foods like lentils, tofu, nuts, peas, seeds and grains. Protein deficiency usually means low stamina, mental depression, low immune resistance and slow wound healing. Surgery, wounds, or prolonged illness are stresses that use up protein fast. At times of high stress, you'll want to take in extra protein to rebuild worn-out tissues.

Protein is at the heart of the debate between a vegetarian diet and a meat-based diet. There's no agreement among experts about how much protein is best. Protein requirements differ according to your health, body size and activity level. The American Journal of Clinical Nutrition says adults need 2.5% of their calorie intake in protein. World Health sets adult protein needs at 4.5% of calorie intake. The National Academy of Sciences recommends 6%. The National Research Council recommends 8%. The FDA says protein should make up 10% of your total daily calories. A 2,000-calorie diet allows for 50 grams of protein. The official RDA for adult men and women is 0.8g for each kg of body weight per day (about 55 grams of protein for 150 pound person). American's average consumption of protein is about 90 grams daily.

How much protein do you really need? The rule of thumb is to simply divide your body weight by 2; the result is the approximate number of grams of protein you need each day. An easy way to translate protein grams into your diet is to eat an amount of protein food that covers the palm of your hand at each meal; vegetarians double the amount to two palmfuls.

The problem with too much protein.

Experts say that Americans eat too much protein for good health. Unlike carnivorous animals, whose digestive and metabolic systems are adapted to a meat-based diet, humans who consume more than half their calories as meat protein are at risk for protein poisoning (a serious watch word for dieters on the new extra high-protein "zone" diets). The National Academy of Sciences now recommends that Americans reduce their protein intake by 12 to 15 percent and switch from animal to plant protein sources.

Protein is the least efficient of the body's cellular engines—fats, carbohydrates and protein. To burn protein the body must boost its metabolic rate by 10%, straining the liver's ability to absorb oxygen. Protein does not burn cleanly, leaving behind nitrogen waste that your body must eliminate, a taxing process on your kidneys. It's why excessive protein consumption is linked to urinary tract infections. For diabetics, the extra workload increases the risk of serious kidney disease. John's Hopkins Hospital now treats and cures severe kidney disease with a very low protein diet and amino acid supplements.

—**Too much protein is linked to high cholesterol.** Protein that is not used for building tissue or energy may be converted by the liver and stored as fat.

—**Too much protein irritates the immune system**, keeping it in a state of overactivity.

—**Too much protein can cause fluid imbalance**; calcium and other minerals are lost through the urine.

—**Too much animal protein actually contributes to osteoporosis**, heart disease and cancers like renal cancer and lympho-sarcoma through loss of critical minerals.

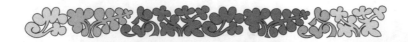

Scientific opinion about protein is changing. 1) In the past, animal source proteins were considered superior because they were the highest in protein. Today many experts believe they actually have too much protein for good health, because it's stored in the body as toxins or fat. 2) Animal source protein was thought to be complete protein, supplying necessary amino acids. Now we know it also includes unhealthy inorganic acids. 3) Animal protein was seen to supply more iron and zinc, but is now seen as also supplying cholesterol, fat and calories. An important study by Baylor College of Medicine in Houston showed men on diets high in <u>soy</u> protein experienced a drop in cholesterol, compared to men on diets high in animal protein. The study concluded that men should replace up to 50% of meat protein with vegetable protein.

Does your body know the difference between animal and vegetable protein? *Does your body work differently depending on the type of protein you eat? Amazingly, it appears that it does.*

Research shows that eating lots of high protein animal foods may cause your body to extract calcium from your blood and excrete it, a cause of osteoporosis. Research from China shows that osteoporosis is rare in Chinese people with a plant-based protein diet, only appearing in Chinese cities where people live more western lifestyles. The same tests show that when animal protein in the diet increases, so does the risk of coronary heart disease, arteriosclerosis, kidney stones, arthritis, cataracts, and cancer. In contrast, Eskimos, with a meat-based diet, *and twice the RDA of calcium*, have the highest rate of osteoporosis in the world.

Women need more protein per pound of body weight than men to attain the same health level. A woman's body works best with lean protein like seafood, whole grains, and legumes rather than higher fat meat protein. Depression, PMS, menopause symptoms and chronic fatigue can disappear when lean protein is increased.

Can vegetable protein satisfy your body's needs? Protein is formed from combinations of the 22 amino acids, drawn from an amino acid pool in our blood. Early nutritional opinion held that vegetable proteins had to be carefully combined so that all essential amino acids and proteins were available at each meal to create complete protein, and maximum utilization of amino acids. Today's research shows that our bodies break down proteins into amino acids and redistribute them, so even meals with incomplete protein have the same effect as a complete protein.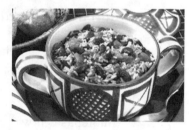

Plant foods team up to make complete protein - a process called protein complementarity. Beans and rice are an example of good protein balance - the incomplete, low lysine protein of rice is balanced by the higher lysine protein of beans. Beans like soy and black beans contain equal or *greater* protein than beef. Eating a wide variety of plant protein foods is the secret. Vegetarians typically eat less protein than meat eaters, but their diets still meet or exceed the protein RDA.

Consider these good vegetable protein sources for your healing diet:

—Whole grains, nuts, seeds, legumes, and soy foods are good sources of protein and essential fatty acids. The ancient grain quinoa is a rich source of lysine and an especially good source of protein because its amino acid profile closely resembles the pattern usable by the body.

—Green, leafy vegetables like kale and chard, and cruciferous vegetables, like broccoli, cabbage and cauliflower, have easily absorbed protein (about 8%) plus EFA's.

—Superfood plant protein sources include the blue-green algae, sea greens, spirulina and chlorella.

—Nutritional yeast, a key immune-enhancing food, is an excellent source of protein, B vitamins, amino acids and minerals. Chromium-rich, nutritional yeast improves blood sugar metabolism, substantially reduces cholesterol and speeds wound healing by boosting collagen production.

—Sprouts are a natural source of protein and almost every other nutrient - vitamins, enzymes, essential fatty acids, antioxidants and minerals that strengthen immune response and protect from toxic buildup.

—Flax, sesame, sunflower, pumpkin (for zinc and EFA's), almonds, and chia are my favorite nuts and seeds for protein. Roasting or heating deactivates enzyme inhibitors that reduce digestability.

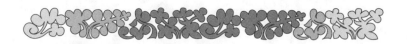

Nature's Superfoods Help You Heal Faster

Green "superfoods" are superior sources of essential nutrients—nutrients we need but can't make ourselves. We may all be adding more salads and vegetables to our diets, but concern for the quality of foods grown on mineral-depleted soils makes green superfoods like chlorella, spirulina, barley and wheat grass popular. They are nutritionally more potent than regular foods, and are exceptional food antioxidants for healthy healing.

Green and blue-green algae (phyto-plankton) are almost perfect superfoods.

They have rich high quality protein, fiber, chlorophyll, vitamins, minerals and enzymes. Use them therapeutically to stimulate immune response, accelerate healing and tissue repair, help prevent degenerative disease and promote longer life.

Take a look at their dramatic statistics:
- **They are the most potent source of beta carotene available in the world today.**
- **They are the richest plant sources of vitamin B-12.**
- **Their amino acids are virtually identical to those needed by the human body.**
- **Their protein yield is greater than soy beans, corn or beef.**
- **They are the only food source, other than mother's milk, of GLA, an essential fatty acid.**
- **They are natural detoxifiers to protect against chemical pollutants and radiation.**

Chlorella alone has a higher concentration of chlorophyll than any known plant.

It is a complete protein food, with all the B vitamins, vitamin C and E, lipoic acid and many minerals high enough to be considered supplemental amounts. The list of chlorella benefits is long and almost miraculous, from detoxification to energy enhancement, to immune system restoration.

…Chlorella's cell wall material is especially beneficial for intestinal and bowel health, detoxifying the colon, stimulating peristaltic activity, and promoting friendly bacteria.

…Chlorella eliminates heavy metals, like lead, mercury, copper and cadmium. Other studies show that chlorella binds to harmful pesticides and insecticides like PCBs and DDT, involved in breast cancer, and carries them out of the body.

…Chlorella is an important source of carotenes in healing tumors.

…Chlorella strengthens the liver, your body's major detoxifying organ, to rid you of infective agents.

…Chlorella reduces arthritis stiffness.

…Chlorella helps reduce fatigue from viral infections like Epstein-Barr and Herpes.

…Chlorella normalizes blood pressure.

…Chlorella relieves indigestion, hiatal hernia, gastritis and ulcers.

…Chlorella decreases menopausal complaints by assisting with estrogen production in the body.

…Chlorella is effective in weight loss programs. It has cleansing ability, rich nutrition that keeps energy up during dieting, and maintains muscle during lower food intake.

…Chlorella's most important benefits come from a unique biochemical combination of molecules called the Controlled Growth Factor, a composition that provides noticeable increase in immune health.

…Chlorella is a key addition to your anti-cancer arsenal. Tests published in the journal Ethnopharmacology show chlorella prevents cancer in 80% of lab animals. In another test at the Medical College of Virginia, chlorella was given to twenty human patients with an advanced form of conventionally incurable brain cancer. Two years after the treatment, seven of the patients were still alive with no traces of cancer in their bodies!

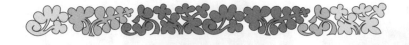

Spirulina is the original green superfood.

Microscopic algae like spirulina were the first organisms to use photosynthesis to make their own food. The ancient Aztecs, Mayans and Toltecs all harvested lake spreads of spirulina as a high nutrient food source. Spirulina is an ecological wonder because it grows in both ocean and lake waters and can be cultivated in extreme environments useless for conventional agriculture. Big business isn't necessary for spirulina. Small scale community farms are spirulina's biggest producers. It grows in such a variety of climates and conditions that some consider it the nutrition answer for whole populations on the brink of starvation. Amazingly prolific, spirulina doubles its bio-mass every two to five days, and doesn't deplete any topsoil—a true miracle food for our modern era! Researchers say that spirulina alone could double the protein available to people on a fraction of the world's land, while helping restore the environmental balance of the planet.

Acre for acre, spirulina yields 20 times more protein than soybeans, 40 times more protein than corn, and 400 times more protein than beef. And it's a complete protein, with all 22 amino acids, the entire vitamin B-complex, including B-12 (with more than liver), carotenes, naturally chelated minerals, and essential fatty acids like gamma linolenic acid (GLA). Digestibility is high, for both rapid and long range energy.

Recent discoveries show spirulina reduces your risk of cancer, especially mouth cancers. Spirulina can also be used as a rich source of nutrients to help the body heal and overcome the damaging effects of chemotherapy. It is an especially rich source of iron (28 times higher than beef liver) to help rebuild red blood cells, and high quality protein to accelerate healing. Spirulina boosts production of infection-fighting cytokines for enhanced immune protection. Spirulina demonstrates amazing activity against AIDS, preventing viral replication early tests. Spirulina is also good choice for weight loss, for stamina strength, and to lower cholesterol.

Green grasses are some of the lowest-calorie, most nutrient-rich foods on the planet.

Green grasses are the only plants on earth that can give sole nutritional support to an animal throughout life. Yet they are some of the most underused. Grasses have the extraordinary ability to transform inanimate elements from soil, water and sunlight into living cells. Grasses contain all the known minerals and trace minerals, balanced vitamins and hundreds of enzymes. The small molecular proteins and chlorophyllins in grasses are absorbed directly through our cell membranes.

Their rich chlorophyll helps humans, as it does plants, to resist the destructive effects of air pollution, carbon monoxide, X-rays and radiation. Studies on barley, wheatgrass and alfalfa show they have the capacity to aid a wide range of health problems: high blood pressure, diabetes, gastritis, ulcers, liver disease, asthma, eczema, hemorrhoids, skin infections, anemia, constipation, body odor, bleeding gums, burns, even cancer. Good sources of vitamin K for blood clotting, green grasses are effective for bone strength and varicose veins, too.

Barley grass has highly concentrated nutrients.

It has ten times more calcium than cow's milk, five times more iron than spinach, and seven times more vitamin C and bioflavonoids than orange juice. Its significant contribution to a vegetarian diet is 80mcg of vitamin B-12 per 100grams of powdered juice.

First used by Roman gladiators for stamina, modern barley grass research shows results for DNA damage repair and delaying aging. It's is the richest food source of the antioxidant isoflavone, *2-0-GIV*, which experts think accounts for its DNA repair success. Barley juice also has anti-viral activity and neutralizes heavy metals like mercury. University of California, Davis tests show an enzyme-rich barley extract can even neutralize the toxicity of several pesticides. Barley is an ideal anti-inflammatory for healing gastrointestinal ulcers, hemorrhoids and pancreatic infections. Dr. Kubota of Tokyo Pharmacy Science says, "barley grass has effects measurably stronger than either steroid or non-steroid drugs, and few if any side effects."

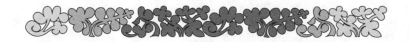

Alfalfa is one of the world's richest mineral-sources

Its long roots pull up earth minerals from depths as great as 130 feet! Alfalfa's high chlorophyll content and rich plant fiber make it a good spring tonic, infection fighter and natural body deodorizer. It is a restorative in treating cases of narcotic and alcohol addiction. It is a specific therapy for arthritis, skin disorders and liver problems. Because of its high vitamin K content, alfalfa encourages blood-clotting. It is also used to treat bladder infections, colon disorders, anemia, hemorrhaging and diabetes. Alfalfa's recognized phytohormones are effective in normalizing estrogen production. It is also a good food source of CoQ10.

Wheat grass liquid has clear curative powers for cancerous growths

Made famous in the clinics of health pioneer Anne Wigmore, wheat grass rectal implants have particular success in colon cancer cases. Like all green grasses, wheat grass provides protection from carcinogens through its chlorophyll capacity to strengthen cells, detoxify the liver and blood, and biochemically neutralize pollutants. Wheat grass also normalizes the thyroid gland to stimulate metabolism which is helpful in correcting obesity problems. Wheat grass ointment is used for disorders like skin ulcers, impetigo and itching. Fifteen pounds of fresh wheat grass has the nutritional value of 350 pounds of vegetables with all their enzyme activity.

Green Kamut is an excellent new choice for green superfood lovers.

The young tender leaves of the grass Kamut, an ancient wheat plant from Egypt's nile region, are higher in B vitamins, vitamin E, magnesium, zinc, amino acids, and chlorophyll than today's wheat. Kamut is also richer in protein, beta carotene, potassium, calcium, iron and antioxidants than wheatgrass powder. Kamut works best when grown together with alfalfa. Alfalfa increases nitrogen in the soil which, in turn, boosts the chlorophyll content of kamut. Green Kamut powders are sweet tasting, and easily added to juices.

Medicinal mushrooms are powerful immune protectors.

Mushrooms are the great recyclers of nature, thriving off decaying matter on forest floors, and enriching the soil to feed other plants. They play much the same role in your health. They are a powerful healing food. Natural healers now use mushrooms to help prevent and treat cancers, even to help the sickest cancer patients in easing the dying process and, some believe, their transformation to the spirit world.

Mushrooms have long held a sacred place in Chinese medicine. Ancient Taoists used mushrooms as a food to promote spiritual enlightenment. The medicinal mushroom, reishi, was believed by many ancient Chinese to confer long life, even immortality. Many of today's Chinese "superior" drugs—those that increase resistance to disease agents - are derived from mushrooms. An amazing American mushroom fact: In 1928, a mushroom mold was used to create penicillin and, later, an entire class of lifesaving antibiotic drugs.

Mushrooms have a clear place in natural medicine today. They are used to combat everything from heart disease and cancer, to Syndrome X and AIDS. You can add them to your diet as well as take them supplementally. Medicinal mushrooms like shiitake and maitake are delicious immune tonics, boosting your resistance to toxic chemicals, bacteria and viruses while you enjoy their meaty taste.

Maitake are the strongest tumor growth inhibitors of all mushrooms.

They are also highly effective against hormone driven cancers like breast, prostate and endometrial cancer, and even high mortality cancers like lung, liver, pancreas and brain cancer. Maitake (*Grifola Frondosa*) has a most unusual synergistic effect with chemotherapy. Most natural therapies do not co-exist well with either chemotherapy or radiation, but patients taking maitake along with chemotherapy report a lessening of side effects such as loss of appetite and nausea. Maitake also appears to protect healthy cells from becoming cancerous, and prevent the spread of cancer once it has taken hold.

Maitake's chemical structure stands apart from other mushrooms. Known as D-fraction, researchers say it's Nature's most effective agent for targeting foreign substances and stimulating immune response. D-fraction has powerful anti-tumor activity, deterring the formation of new tumors, arresting tumor spread. Research on prostate cancer by New York Medical College shows D-fraction induces apoptosis (cell death) of cancer cells. D-fraction is now FDA approved for phase 2 clinical trials against advanced breast and prostate cancer. Researchers document anti-hypertension, anti-obesity and anti-hepatitis activity, as well as success against Chronic Fatigue Syndrome for maitake.

Maitake can help fight AIDS. Almost 40% of AIDS patients develop Kaposi's Sarcoma, a malignant skin cancer. Conventional medicine has not developed an effective treatment. Studies by Japan's National Institute for Health and the U.S. National Cancer Institute show that maitake works rapidly to prevent destruction of T-cells by HIV. Naturopaths report improvement in just a few days when maitake extract is <u>applied</u> to KS lesions.

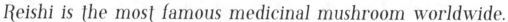

A new extract from maitake, SX Fraction is currently in use for its role in normalizing sugar imbalances. Preliminary reports show SX-fraction enhances insulin sensitivity and improves insulin/glucose metabolism- good news for people with diabetes or Syndrome X.

Maitake is effective taken orally, an advantage over other mushrooms where extracts often need to be injected, or where the therapeutic benefit is lost when taken orally.

Reishi is the most famous medicinal mushroom worldwide.

Used in China for over 5000 years, reishi was regularly collected as a tonic for the Chinese royal family. Its Chinese name, *Ling Zhi* translates into "spirit," a clear tribute for their high opinion of this healing mushroom. Reishi mushrooms (*ganoderma*) are in the highest class of adaptogen tonics for promoting longevity. They have strong antioxidant protection and free radical scavenging activity for deep immune support. They are especially effective for recovery from serious illness. Reishi is an excellent cardiotonic, even significantly lowering blood pressure in those individuals with hypertension who were unresponsive to ACE inhibitors.

Reishi is used therapeutically against fatigue, to relieve allergy symptoms, liver toxicity (especially hepatitis), bronchitis and carcinoma. New research shows success against chronic fatigue syndrome. Reishi may be used daily to lower cholesterol and triglycerides, induce sound sleep and increase resistance to infections. Reishi is also a superior nervous system tonic for people affected by chronic stress, and is believed to "calm the mind" in Chinese medicine. Note: Reishi works best in extracts or powdered forms.

Shiitake are a culinary treat and a therapeutic wonder.

Shiitake mushroom extracts can protect the body from cancer risk, even help shrink existing tumors. Research showing strong anti-tumor power has been done on two components of shiitake, *lentinan* and *lentinula edodes* mycelium (LEM). These constituents enhance the body's natural ability to eliminate a tumor rather than by possessing direct anti-tumor activity. Japanese research reveals chemotherapy patients who received lentinan injections twice a week had longer survival times with less tumor growth, than patients who just received chemotherapy.

Shiitakes (*Lentinus edodes*) are especially effective in treating systemic conditions related to early aging and sexual dysfunction. Shiitakes help lower cholesterol levels, reduce blood pressure and fight viruses and bacteria by producing a virus that stimulates immune interferon. They help reduce environmental allergies and candida yeast overgrowth, soothe bronchial inflammation, and regulate bladder incontinence.

Studies with HIV patients show that LEM may be more effective at preventing the spread of the HIV virus in the body than AZT, the most commonly prescribed AIDS treatment drug — possibly because LEM works by blocking the initial stages of HIV infection, while AZT merely slows replication of the virus, and generally becomes less effective over time. LEM also shows results for hepatitis and chronic fatigue syndrome.

Add shiitakes frequently to your diet... a little goes a long way.

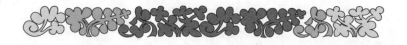

Royal Agaricus is the richest source of Beta Glucan.

Royal agaricus is called the "mushroom of God" in its native Brazil. Like the modern re-discovery of many ancient healing secrets, rainforest researchers in Brazil saw that native people who lived where *Agaricus* grew were much healthier than the rest of the population, and had especially low cases of cancer. Subsequent tests attributed this to the high content of Agaricus' immune boosting polysaccharide, beta glucan. Like other mushrooms, it also helps regulate blood sugar, and lower blood pressure and cholesterol levels. Research shows promise in natural cancer treatment, viral diseases, and as a bactericide against *salmonella*.

Lion's Mane may help inhibit Alzheimer's disease.

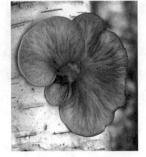

Named for its white cascading tendrils, lion's mane is new to western markets. Studies reveal lion's mane stimulates the growth of neurons, and may play a role in inhibiting brain dysfunction caused by Alzheimer's disease, senility, or traumatic injury. In TCM, it's used as a body strengthener for the five organs to promote general vigor, and as a specific for constipation, indigestion, high blood pressure, and the nervous system.

Tremella is a specific for bone health.

Tremella enhances calcium absorption and provides bone-protective vitamin D. It's popular in Chinese cuisine and regularly used in TCM in herbal cough syrups for asthma and coughs. Tremella is valued for its ability to strengthen chi and reduce fevers. It can help lower cholesterol, balance blood sugar, protect against radiation poisoning, and has anti-tumor activity. One added benefit… tremella offers real benefit for smooth healthy skin.

Turkey Tail can boost recovery from chemotherapy and radiation.

Widely used in Japan for immune boosting activity, turkey tail improves T-cell balance and may inhibit HIV infection and hepatitis. Like other medicinal mushrooms, turkey tail has anti-cancer activity, can boost recovery from chemo and radiation therapies, and has mild antibiotic action. Turkey tail isn't recommended for cooking. Simmer the mushroom, and take as a healing broth; or use turkey tail capsules.

Poria Cocos is a unique body chemistry balancer.

Unlike the other medicinal mushrooms, poria cocos has a tonic rather than an immune enhancing effect — it has a unique ability to balance body chemistry, especially mineral balances. Poria is a mushroom amphoteric (with both alkaline and acidic properties). A Traditional Chinese Medicine herb, poria cocos works on the heart, spleen, and kidney meridians, indicated by poor appetite, diarrhea and lethargy. TCM specialists believe that poria replenishes the spleen, thus strengthening the body against dizziness, and balancing body fluids. American naturopaths also use poria to prevent excess water retention and toxic build-up. Poria cocos is used in herbal remedies for sleep disorders, liver tone, restlessness, fatigue, tension and nervousness.

Cordyceps is a dramatic oxygenator and energizer.

First brought into the modern spotlight by Chinese runners who broke nine world records in 1993, Cordyceps sinensis (caterpillar mushroom) is used in Traditional Chinese Medicine as a tonic and energizer that supports the kidneys and lungs. For athletes, these effects can mean increased lung capacity and stamina, and shorter recovery times. Research shows that cordyceps also enhances immunity by increasing activity of helper T-cells and natural killer cells, accelerates spleen regeneration, increases SOD (superoxide dismutase) activity, enhances oxygen uptake to the heart and brain, possesses testosterone-like effects, improves libido and sperm count, and is effective in reducing uterine fibroids. Cordyceps is recommended for better energy levels in health problems like CFS and fibromyalgia. It is a proven choice for people who feel too tired to exercise. Trials with people are limited, but cordyceps has been widely tested on animals with good results.

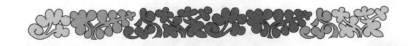

Macrobiotics: A Choice for Serious Healing

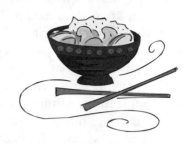

Macrobiotics is a 4000 year old diet and lifestyle philosophy based on the ancient principles of traditional oriental medicine The term "macrobiotics" was coined by Hippocrates in Greek times - "macro" meaning "long" and "bios" meaning "life." In America, macrobiotics has become a popular, purifying diet approach for serious, degenerative illness like cancer, diabetes and heart disease. Most notably, macrobiotics is seen as an effective method of improving body chemistry against cancer and has for most of this century, been part of the natural healing tradition for cancer. It is an effective technique because it works to normalize body chemistry, not only to remove toxins, but also to rebuild healthy blood and cells.

It teaches that our health is continually influenced by our environment, including our climate, geography, social ties and the foods we eat. A macrobiotic way of life focuses on the understanding that we create our health through our lifestyle choices. Macrobiotics views illness as the body's natural attempt to regain internal balance as well as harmony with the external world. People who have given up on drugs and even natural alternatives often end up finding healing success in the macrobiotic way of life.

There is no single macrobiotic diet… rather macrobiotics is a way of eating, low in fat, non-mucous-forming, rich in plant protein and fiber. It stimulates the heart and circulation through Asian foods like miso, green tea and shiitake mushrooms. It is alkalizing with umeboshi plums, sea greens and soy foods. It is nutrient rich—especially high in potassium, natural iodine, magnesium, calcium, and B-complex vitamins. The majority of the foods are from the center of the food spectrum—vegetables and whole grains—with a minimum of foods from the extremes; fruits and sugars are more cooling, meat and dairy foods are more stimulating as are some aromatic spices, like garlic, cayenne and mint teas.

Even in its strict form, a macrobiotic diet is nutritionally balanced with adequate protein and low fat. Harvard's School of Public Health analyzed the standard recommendations of a macrobiotic diet. The results showed that the diet exceeded the recommended daily nutrient allowances of both the FDA and the World Health Organization, without having to take extra protein, vitamins or minerals. From a macrobiotic perspective, supplements other than whole herbs are thought to interfere with the nutrients in the whole foods themselves.

For most Americans, becoming macrobiotic requires a major shift in the way we look at life; indeed, it is usually a complete lifestyle change. A strict macrobiotic diet is usually too rigid to fit in with the demands of today's lifestyles, but macrobiotic principles can be tailored to meet your individual needs.

1: The first diet change is to eat organic whole foods whenever possible. This is often a greater change than it might seem, because it means seeking these foods out, changing shopping habits and-or grocery stores to find your sources. One of the cornerstones of macrobiotic body balancing is eating with the seasons. Yet, America's worldwide, market driven culture stands at the opposite end of this principle. We import our foods any time of the year without regard to our own seasons. Buying organically grown seasonal produce is a good way to ensure this fundamental element of macrobiotics.

2: The second change is to gradually eliminate foods not at ease in a macrobiotic diet. This means a lot of label reading to identify highly processed, chemicalized foods, frozen, irradiated and canned foods, and foods with colorants and preservers. Avoid animal protein and fat, including dairy products (except fertile eggs). Eliminate fried foods and high sugar foods, hot spices and strong alcoholic beverages. Use sweeteners like rice syrup and barley malt in small amounts instead. Limit sweet, tropical fruits, fruit juices, carbonated sodas and caffeine. Buy fresh and packaged food from your health food store to avoid genetically modified foods.

3: The third change is learning to prepare foods in their whole form. It's a big change for people who are used to pre-prepared foods. It means buying fresh foods, and preparing them simply in order to keep the greatest value of the nutrients.

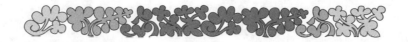

4: The fourth change is to include foods in harmony with macrobiotic principles. The most apparent difference between macrobiotics and other diet approaches is its reliance on whole grains. At least half of the daily food intake is whole grains—brown rice, whole wheat, oats, barley, millet, buckwheat, rye, amaranth, kamut and corn. In modern modified macrobiotic diets, small amounts of pasta, non-yeasted breads and partially processed whole cereal grains are allowed. Cook grains with a little sea salt or season with sea veggie granules.

Locally-grown, organic vegetables, both raw and cooked, are the second most important foods for macrobiotics, comprising about 30% of the diet. Steam, sauté in olive or sesame oil, parboil or bake them. Good vegetables for healing include: green cabbage, bok choy, dark leafy greens, broccoli, cauliflower, parsley, watercress, burdock root, carrots, turnips, pumpkin, winter squash, onions and scallions. Cucumbers, celery, lettuce and herbs like chives and dill are recommended seasonally, 2 to 3 times a week. Vegetables like potatoes, tomatoes, eggplant, peppers, spinach, beets and zucchini are not recommended for the regular diet because they are thought to aggravate body acidity.

Beans and sea greens, comprising about 5-15 percent of a macrobiotic diet, are considered supplementary, rather than daily foods. For Americans used to more protein in their diet, I find that eating beans like black beans, chickpeas, soy and lentils makes changing to macrobiotics easier. Sea greens like kombu, dulse, kelp, sea palm, wakame, hijiki, arame, mekabu and nori can be used with any grains, beans, and vegetables, especially in soups. Soups may make up 10 to 15% of an initial macrobiotic diet. A daily bowl of miso soup starts the alkalizing, immune-boosting process right away.

Other foods in order of their importance in a macrobiotic diet are vegetable oils, nuts, fruits, fish and occasional fertile eggs. Although many macrobiotic followers prefer to avoid all animal foods, macrobiotics is not a vegetarian system. White meat fish, like flounder, cod, sole, trout and halibut are recommended 2 to 3 times a week. Fruits are eaten only occasionally as desserts or snacks 2 to 3 times a week. Nuts and seeds, like pumpkin, sesame and sunflower seeds are occasional snacks. Therapeutic foods, like white tea, green tea, shiitake, maitake and reishi mushrooms, raw sauerkraut, and umeboshi plums should be included regularly.

5: The fifth change is to eat only when hungry and to learn to chew your food well - about 50 times per bite for the best nutrient absorption. Chewing is the cornerstone of a grain-based macrobiotic diet because grains are by nature acidic; saliva which is alkaline, counteracts the acid. The acid-alkaline balance of your blood is crucial to your body's healing ability as well as to mood and emotion. Americans, who generally lead fast-paced, high stress lives, sometimes find this change the hardest to make.

Can you tell if macrobiotic changes are helping your healing program? Here is the usual sequence for normalizing body chemistry: It takes ten days for plasma to recycle, so improvements become noticeable after ten days. It takes 30 days for white blood cells to renew, so immune function begins to improve after a month. It takes 120 days for red blood cells to renew, so true healing begins in 4 months. Most people notice healthier emotional and mental patterns around this time as well.

Is macrobiotics for you?

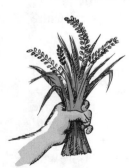

A macrobiotic diet's greatest benefit is that it is cleansing and strengthening at the same time. I view macrobiotics a little differently than the traditional Asian model. I see macrobiotics not as a "no deviation" regimen, but as a way of life based on a whole foods diet and an active lifestyle in harmony with nature.

After an initial macrobiotic detox diet, I believe in a light, modified macrobiotic diet, one that emphasizes the principles of macrobiotics for longer term health, with more individual flexibility rather than a set pattern. For most people, this means a diet high in vegetable fiber and protein, low in saturated fats and trans fats that can alter body chemistry and enhance cancer potential.

Macrobiotic counseling sessions can help you structure a macrobiotic diet and lifestyle geared to your needs. *For more information, contact the Kushi Institute at 1-800-975-8744 or visit www.kushiinstitute.org.*

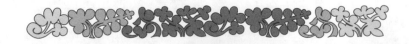

Cultured Foods Offer Healing Probiotics

What are probiotics? Why are they so important for your healing diet? Probiotics are beneficial micro-organisms like *Lactobacillus, Bifidobacteria*, and *Streptococcus* residing in your intestinal tract. They manufacture vitamins, especially B vitamins like biotin, niacin, folic acid and B-6, that detoxify chemicals and metabolize hormones. They empower enzymes that maximize food assimilation and digestion.

<u>Probiotics</u> (as opposed to <u>antibiotics</u>), are an amazing fighting force. These disease fighters compete at a basic level with harmful microorganisms in your body.

—First, probiotics deprive undesirable bacteria of nourishment thus preventing their growth.

—Second, probiotics attack specific pathogens by changing your body's acid/alkaline balance to an *anti-biotic* environment. (Probiotic activity against vaginal yeast infections is a good example of this.) If you are taking long courses of drug antibiotics, remember that they kill *all* bacteria, both bad and good. *All* intestinal flora are severely diminished. For most people, poor digestion, diarrhea or constipation, flatulence, bad breath, bloating, tiredness, migraines, even acne are a result of long antibiotic treatment.

Probiotic organisms prevent disease, even treat infections by restoring micro-organism balance in your intestinal tract. It doesn't matter how good your diet is if your body can't use it. There are up to 4 lbs of bacteria in the human intestinal tract. Your body must maintain an ecological balance of these bacteria to protect your health. Our modern lifestyle destroys normal body balance. Health experts say most people have around 15% "good" bacteria and 85% "bad" bacteria... an environment ideal for disease development. Stress, alcohol, chemicalized foods, environmental pollutants, antibiotic and steroid drugs all hamper our ability to use nourishment. When unfriendly bacteria get the upper hand in the balance, the door opens to infections.

The best way to get probiotics in your diet? Add them through foods like yogurt, kefir or raw sauerkraut.

Think of probiotic supplements as an insurance policy for your health. Most supplements have *lactobacillus acidophilus* (which attaches in the small intestine), *bifidobacterium* (which attaches in the large intestine), and *lactobacillus bulgaricus* (three protective strains of flora). Together they produce hydrogen peroxide, a byproduct that helps maintain protective microbial balance and protects against pathogens.

What probiotics can do for you:

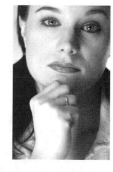

—Probiotics boost immune response, inhibiting growth of pathogenic organisms

—Probiotics detoxify the intestinal tract by protecting intestinal mucosa levels

—Probiotics develop a barrier to food-borne allergies

—Probiotics neutralize antibiotic-resistant strains of bacteria

—Probiotics reduce cancer risk

—Probiotics reduce risk of inflammatory bowel disease, IBS and diverticulosis

—Probiotic synthesize needed vitamins (like vitamin K) for healing

—Probiotics prevent diarrhea by improving digestion of proteins and fats

Important new discoveries about probiotics:

Probiotics from foods and supplements are a viable way to improve your health. Probiotics play a key role in preventing osteoporosis. Bone loss is one unfortunate result of a lack of friendly microorganisms in the gastrointestinal tract. Vitamin K, a vital building block of healthy bones, is a byproduct of lactobacilli.

New research shows new benefits for acidophilus. Lactobacilli acidophilus, part of the normal flora in your urinary tract and vaginal tissue, helps you digest dairy foods, prevents most yeast infections and restores intestinal

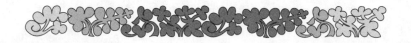

balance especially for traveler's and antibiotic-induced diarrhea. Acidophilus is highly successful for children's diseases. Children have naturally strong immune systems and may only need the gentle body balancing of friendly flora instead of a harsh drug or chemical antibiotic.

Important note: Experience with many people has shown me that acidophilus is very effective as a healing medicine when it is sprinkled directly on food ..... particularly for low immune response conditions, like candida albicans, eating disorders and HIV infection where nutrient assimilation is seriously compromised. Pets with digestive problems or system weakness also benefit from the addition of acidophilus on food. *Note: Don't cook with acidophilus. It negates its healing properties.*

Acidophilus benefits:
—helps synthesize B vitamins and produces essential enzyme stores
—helps overcome lactose intolerance by digesting milk sugars
—reduces blood fat and cholesterol levels
—improves elimination — contributing to sweet breath and normal body odor
—kills pathogens that contribute to cancer; helps block tumor development. A 1997 study showed the growth of breast cancer cells slowed by up to 85% after exposure to *Acidophilus.*
—found to be as effective as the drug Neomycin Sulfate against *E. Coli.*
—especially beneficial for people with antibiotic-induced diarrhea
—inactivates some harmful viruses
—helps detoxify the gastrointestinal tract and improves G.I. health
—prevents yeast infections
—prevents urinary tract infections

As beneficial as they are, not everyone can use probiotics. Each person's digestive system is highly individual, like the immune system to which it is a gateway. Many experts question whether single strain probiotic supplements survive the digestion process which can't always differentiate between good and bad bacteria.

...Test your probiotic products: Add 3 to 4 capsules of a probiotic product to 6-oz. of milk. If the product is active, the milk will ferment into a yogurt-like substance in 24-48 hours.

Pre-biotics **like FOS may be a more practical approach.** Pre-biotics feed the beneficial bacteria you already have in your gastrointestinal tract. Fructo-oligo-saccharides (FOS) are naturally-occurring carbohydrates in vegetables like artichokes, bananas, onions, garlic, barley and tomatoes. The FOS saccharides can't be digested by humans, but are easily used by our intestinal flora. Competition for food and attachment sites in our intestines is fierce between hundreds of microorganisms, both good and bad. FOS supplements give your friendly bacteria a competitive edge and actually increase your body's population of beneficial bacteria.

HSO's (homeostatic soil organisms) are the latest probiotic craze. HSO's may be more effective than traditional probiotics because they can withstand heat, cold, chlorine, fluorene, ascorbic acid, stomach acids, even pH changes. HSO's are probiotics that supercharge immune defenses. Naturally present in the Earth's soil, HSO's are friendly bacteria which protect plants from disease and help them digest nutrients. Some experts believe they are a key to human immunity and proper digestion, too. Our heavy pesticide use means our soil, and therefore our food is largely devoid of HSO's. Supplemental HSO's are now available to help solve this problem.

Here's how HSO's help: 1) They flush waste matter lodged in the intestines. 2) They improve nutrient absorption by breaking down hydrocarbons (hydrocarbons split food into basic elements). 3) They produce lactoferrin- a potent natural immune stimulant. 4) They inhibit pathogens (viruses, fungi, bacteria, parasites). 5) They increase immune response by raising B-cells and antibodies.

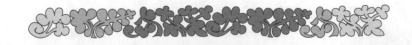

Cultured Soy Foods in Your Healing Diet
How to get the benefits of soy while avoiding the pitfalls...

Soyfoods are nutritional powerhouses. Even if soy isn't a magic bullet for preventing heart disease or curing cancer, it still has amazing health benefits. Soy protein compares in quality to animal protein — it's a good alternative to meat or dairy foods. Soy foods offer complete protein, with all nine essential amino acids necessary for protein synthesis in the body. Further, soy protein is much easier for the kidneys to process than meat protein. Just one cup of cooked soybeans (edamame) contains about 20g protein. A pound of tofu contains about 30g. Soy foods are rich in other essential nutrients, too, like calcium, iron, zinc and B vitamins.

What can cultured soy foods do for you?

1: **Soy protein helps lower cholesterol.** Numerous studies show that when animal protein is replaced by soy protein, there is a significant reduction in both total blood cholesterol and LDL (bad) cholesterol. Adding as little as 25 to 50 grams of soy protein daily to your diet for one month can result in a cholesterol drop.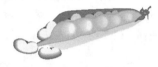

2: **Soy amino acids can lower high insulin levels.** In fact, the latest research shows soy can control diabetes in women as well as some drugs. Having low insulin levels also means your liver makes less cholesterol.

3: **Soy foods help maintain normal vascular function.** Studies find soy isoflavones can reduce arterial plaque. Soy antioxidants help stop atherosclerosis by preventing oxidation to LDL cholesterol.

4: **Soy contains rich diet sources of five known anticancer agents:**
   a. protease inhibitors that arrest development of colon, lung, liver, pancreas and esophagus cancers.
   b. compounds that block formation of nitrosamines leading to liver cancer.
   c. phytosterols that inhibit cell division and proliferation in colon cancer.
   d. saponins that slow the growth of cancerous skin cells.
   e. isoflavones that slow osteoporosis and lower risk of hormone-related cancers, like breast and prostate cancer. (One study finds that pre-menopausal females who rarely eat soy foods have twice the risk of breast cancer as those who frequently eat soy foods. The test showed that just one serving a day of soy protein led to significant lengthening of the menstrual cycle, suppressing the midcycle surge of gonadotrophins and luteinizing hormones —effects that decrease the risk of breast cancer.) A recent study in the March 2000 issue of Cancer Research reveals that isoflavones help prevent the growth of breast cancer cells. Phase 1 testing is going on right now with soy isoflavones for breast and prostate cancer prevention by the National Cancer Institute. The Japanese, with low rates of hormone-driven cancers, eat five times more soy products than Americans. The typical U.S. diet yields 80 milligrams of phytosterols a day, the Japanese eat 400 milligrams a day. Western vegetarians eat about 345 milligrams a day.

Soy contains genistein. How can genistein help your health?

—Genistein is an abundant soy isoflavone that works much like human estrogen. Genistein helps balance your body's estrogen supply, acting both as an estrogen and as an estrogen blocker, depending on your need. Like many phytohormone herbs, it promotes the positive actions of estrogen, and prevents many of its bad effects by competing for both estrogen and progesterone receptors to prevent their availability for tumor growth.

—Genistein has benefits for men's health. Research on 8,000 Hawaiian men found that the men who ate the most tofu had the lowest rates of prostate cancer, kidney disease and diabetes complications.

—Genistein also inhibits angiogenesis, the formation of new blood vessels that nourish tumors.

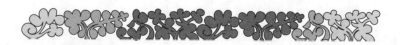

New research reveals concerns about eating too much soy…

In spite of all its benefits, new evidence shows that eating too much soy can have some drawbacks. Most of the problems occur for vegetarians who rely too heavily on soy for their protein, eating large servings of soy foods (especially *non-cultured* soy foods) many times a day.

Potential problems with soy you'll want to avoid:

—Soy foods are hard to digest for a lot of people. The tummy upsetting culprits? Heavy processing, and enzyme (trypsin) inhibitors, that are present in all beans. I always prefer *cultured soy foods* like tempeh, miso, tofu, soy milk and soy sauce in a healing diet because their healthy bacteria improves their digestibility.

—Phytates in soybeans can bind to minerals like zinc, calcium and iron in the digestive tract and prevent their absorption. Note: Fermented soy foods contain the least phytates. Soaking soy beans for 12-24 hours before cooking also reduces levels of phytates.

—Soy foods are routinely genetically engineered, posing a problem for many people ethically and health wise. People with food sensitivities are especially affected.

—A recent Hawaiian study suggests that eating a lot of tofu may speed up the aging process, even affect your brain. Researchers speculate that soy's plant hormones act as an anti-estrogen in the brain, but more research needs to be done to determine if this is true. (*Note:* Factors like the normal aging process itself, a history of stroke, and a good education play a much more significant role in the risk for mental decline than soy intake.)

—One study shows that genistein may actually increase the growth of estrogen-dependent breast cancer cells in vitro. Other studies dispute these findings, but it may be possible that very high doses of soy isoflavones can aggravate certain types of breast cancer.

—Eating a lot of soy can disrupt thyroid activity, leading to symptoms like weight gain, bloat, and fatigue that menopausal women dread! Some research shows that 40mg of soy isoflavones a day can slow down the production of thyroid hormone. (One should note that isoflavone supplements usually contain 40mg. A tablespoon of soy powder contains about 25mg. of isoflavones.) A Japanese study reveals that eating soy may even trigger hypothyroidism and goiter. Cooking your soy food helps deactivate these properties.

—Animal studies suggest that a soy-based diet may lead to infertility problems. However soy's long history of moderate consumption in the Japanese and American cultures does not confirm this risk.

—Soy may not be the best choice for infant formulas. According to the Maryland Nutritionists Association, babies on soy-based formulas receive the equivalent of 5-6 birth control pills every day from soy's plant estrogens! Because of the potential impact on hormonal health, researchers and experts are now advising caution when considering soy based infant formulas—unless there is a clear allergy to cow's milk.

My final word on soy?

   Eat soy in moderation. Soy foods (especially *cultured* soy foods) have confirmed benefits for our health. Enjoy soy foods in a balanced diet rich in fruits, vegetables, legumes, whole grains, sea foods and sea greens. Soy overload (4-5 servings a day) and high doses of isolated soy isoflavones may potentially lead to problems for some people. Whenever possible, choose organic fermented soy products that are less affected by genetic engineering.

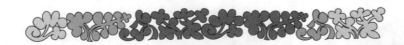

Soy foods that benefit a healing diet:

Tofu: a nutritionally balanced food made from cooked, curdled soybean milk, water and nigari, a mineral-rich seawater precipitate. It is the soy food highest in both total isoflavones and genistein. Combined with whole grains, tofu yields a complete protein, providing dairy richness without the fat or cholesterol, yet with all the calcium and iron. Cooked, tofu is easy to digest, full of fiber, and a non-mucous-forming way to add a rich creamy texture to recipes. Ironically, nearly all the soybeans raised in the U.S. are earmarked for animal feed. Most of the rest is shipped to Japan.

Popular in America, fresh tofu has a light, delicate character that can take on any flavor, from savory to sweet. It comes firm-pressed, in soft cubes, or with a custard-like texture. It is smoked or pre-cooked in seasonings or deep-fried in pouches called age (pronounced "ah-gay") for stuffing. It is both aseptically packaged and freeze-dried to keep at room temperature and reconstitute for later use, camping and travel.

Tofu by the numbers:

…Tofu is low in calories. Eight ounces has only 164 calories.

…Tofu provides highly absorbable organic calcium. Eight ounces supplies the same amount of calcium as 8-oz. of milk, about 12% of the adult calcium RDA.

…Tofu is high in iron. Eight ounces supplies the same amount of iron as 2-oz. of beef liver or 4 eggs.

…Tofu contains all 8 essential amino acids and has almost 8% quality protein. Eight ounces supplies the same amount of protein as 3¼ oz. of beef, 5½ oz. of hamburger, 1⅔ cups of milk, 2-oz. of cheese, or 2 eggs. It is lower in fat than all of these. Unlike most animal protein, cooked tofu has a digestion rate of 95%.

…As little as 4-oz. of tofu a month offers women breast cancer prevention benefits.

…Tofu may help fight prostate cancer. A study of 8,000 Hawaiian men shows men who eat the most tofu have the lowest rates of prostate cancer.

Miso: a tasty food made from fermented soybean paste. It's body alkalizing, lowers cholesterol, represses carcinogens, helps neutralize allergens and pollutants, lessens the effects of smoking, and provides an immune-enhancing environment, even to the point of rejuvenating damaged cells. Miso also attracts and absorbs environmental toxins like radioactive elements in the body and helps to eliminate them.

Take a look at miso's benefits:

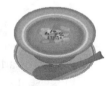

…Miso has even stronger antioxidant effects than soy itself. As miso ages, its color turns deep brown from melanoidine. Melanoidine suppresses the production of fat peroxide in the body. Fat peroxides (oxidized fats) become free radicals, which destroy normal cell functions and are a cause of aging.

…Miso's essential fatty acid, linoleic acid, stimulates sebaceous glands for baby soft skin texture. LA also significantly inhibits the production of melanin, the pigment that causes dark spots on the skin, by repressing synthesis of the enzyme tyrosinase that synthesizes melanin.

…Miso's fatty acid, ethyl linoleate, has an anti-mutagenic effect against carcinogens found in scorched foods like charcoal barbecued meats and French roasted coffee.

…Miso's linoleic acid, plant sterols and vitamin E work synergistically to suppress cholesterol, inhibiting cholesterol absorption in the small intestine and promoting excretion of serum cholesterol. Vitamin E, a component of HDL (good cholesterol), helps transport harmful cholesterol and increase HDL levels.

…Miso is a healthy substitute for salt or soy sauce. There are many kinds, strengths and flavors of miso, from chickpea (light and mild) to hatcho (dark and strong). Delicious natto miso is a sweet mix of soybeans, barley and barley malt, kombu, ginger and sea salt.

…Miso is naturally fermented for your healing diet. Miso is still a living food, with its active enzymes and beneficial microorganisms intact to aid digestion.

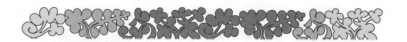

Miso is highly concentrated; use ½ to 1 tsp. of dark miso, or 1 to 2 tsp. of light miso per person. Dissolve in a small amount of water to activate the beneficial enzymes before adding to a recipe. Omit salt from the recipe if you are using miso. Unpasteurized miso found in the refrigerated section is the best choice. (Pasteurization kills its active cultures.) I especially like miso in tonic broths with vegetables and immune boosting herbs, and in dipping sauces for seafood.

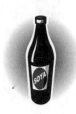

Soy Sauce: is a fermented blend of soy wheat, water and salt. Universally loved for almost every type of cuisine, its mild flavor works better in recipes than Tamari (see below). In America, the low sodium version is preferred.

Tamari: is a wheat-free soy sauce, lower in sodium and richer in flavor than regular soy sauce. (Dilute to use in recipes.) Bragg's LIQUID AMINOS, an energizing protein broth sold in health food stores, is of the tamari family, but unfermented, even lower in sodium, with all 8 essential amino acids.

Soy milk: nutritious, smooth, delicious, and versatile, is simply made by pressing ground, cooked soybeans. It's lactose and cholesterol free, with less calcium and calories than cow's milk, but more protein and iron. Use it cup for cup like milk in cooking. It adds a slight rise to baked goods. It's often used in treatment diets for diabetes, anemia and heart diseases. Soy milk formulas have long been used for infants allergic to cow's milk. Experts are now concerned large amounts of phytoestrogens from soy formulas may cause disruptions in future hormonal health. There are no studies which confirm this theory. But, experts currently advise non-GMO soy-based formulas to be used only if there is a clear allergy to dairy formulas.

Tempeh: is a meaty, high texture Indonesian soy food, with complete protein and all essential amino acids. Tempeh differs from tofu—it has a denser firmer composition, a mushroom-like aroma and is higher in fiber. Tempeh is enzyme-active, predigested and cultured, making it highly absorbable. It's rich in B vitamins (especially B-12), low in calories and fat, and cholesterol free. Tempeh has the highest quality protein of any soyfood, with over 19% protein (about as much as beef and chicken), and *50% more* protein than ground beef. It's a great choice for meat eaters trying to go vegetarian because it's so hearty and filling. I especially like tempeh squares premarinated in teriyaki or spicy Szechwan sauce.

Soy foods to include in small amounts....
...**Soy cheese:** made from soy milk, is lactose and cholesterol free. (A small amount of calcium caseinate, milk protein, is added to allow soy cheese to melt.) Mozzarella, cheddar, jack and cream cheese types are widely available. Use it cup for cup in place of any low-fat or regular cheese.
...**Soy ice cream, pudding, frozen desserts and yogurt:** widely available for dessert enthusiasts.
...**Soy mayonnaise:** the taste, consistency and fat content of regular mayonnaise.
...**Soy nut butter:** a fast, easy way to get complete plant protein before workouts or when on the run. Spread on whole grain crackers or breads.

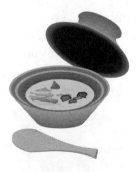

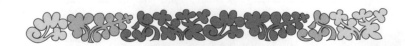

More Cultured Foods to add to your healing diet....

Soy foods are not the only cultured foods to choose from. All cultured foods help promote acid/alkaline balance (important for disease prevention), strengthen the digestive system and build immune response. They are a specific for Candida albicans, lactose intolerance and all malabsorption problems. Here are a few more of my favorite cultured foods for healing.

Kombucha: although known as a "mushroom," kombucha is not a mushroom at all, but a symbiotic culture of yeast and microorganisms. It is a popular natural tonic of Russian origin, for lowering blood pressure, raising immune T-cell counts and increasing vitality. It is noted for its dramatic antibiotic and detoxifying activity.

—To make kombucha tonic, place a small amount of kombucha culture into sweetened black or green tea. The culture feeds on the sugar and like a tiny biochemical factory, produces glucuronic acid, glucon acid, lactic acid, vitamins, amino acids, antibiotic substances, and more to make it a healthful cultured drink.

However, I recommend buying Kombucha tea from the refrigerated section of your health food store. I have personally known several cases where making kombucha culture at home was unsuccessful, and became contaminated with unsafe organisms.

The benefits of kombucha culture tonic:

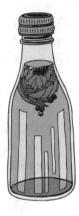

—helps the liver bind up toxic substances so they can be eliminated from the body
—cleanses the colon; relieves constipation and colitis; arrests simple diarrhea
—relieves arthritis pain and carpal tunnel syndrome
—helps return gray hair to its natural color; thickens hair and strengthens nails
—relieves bronchitis and asthma
—helps overcome candida albicans yeast infections
—reduces menopausal hot flashes, headaches and migraines
—reduces cravings for fatty foods
—improves eyesight, cataracts and floaters
—relieves acne, eczema and psoriasis
—acts as a mild diurectic for edema and PMS bloat
—vitalizes flagging libido and sexual energy

Note: A small number of people experience cleansing reactions like headaches, rashes, intestinal gas or insomnia when they first start drinking kombucha. Increasing water intake can help eliminate or minimize the symptoms.

Vinegar: a known elixir for health since the Stone Age, Greek and Roman soldiers and Japanese Samurai warriors used vinegar as a source of strength and power. Vinegar is an excellent, cultured food, full of beneficial organisms that help digest heavy foods and high protein meals. Brown rice, balsamic, apple cider, herbal, raspberry, ume plum and aged wine vinegars have been used for 5000 years as health enhancers. The most nutritious vinegars are not overly filtered (they look slightly cloudy) and still contain the "mother" mix of bacteria and enzymes in the bottle.

Vinegar has an array of health benefits:

— loaded with gallbladder enhancing enzymes and essential acids that aid digestion
—assists in killing infections, both bacterial and fungal
—a powerful remedy for resolving liver stagnation and indigestion
—a vinegar hair rinse treats dandruff and seborrhea
—successfully used in vaginal douches for feminine problems for years. Just add 2 tsp. of vinegar (apple cider is best) to one cup of warm water for the best results.

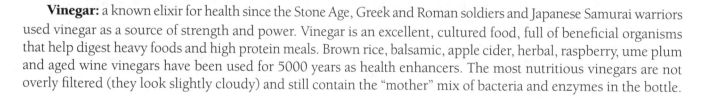

—remarkable effects in the treatment of arthritis, osteoporosis and memory loss
—high potassium helps balance body sodium, encourages bowel regularity and sustains nerve health
—large amounts of pectin and potassium help a healthy, relaxed heartbeat and blood pressure
—a vinegar footbath softens hard callouses, and a footbath is an effective treatment for athlete's foot
—diluted vinegar eardrops can ward off and gently relieve children's ear infections

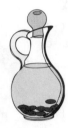

Apple Cider Vinegar: a well known health tonic containing over 30 important nutrients, apple cider vinegar enhances memory, fights arthritis and promotes weight loss. It contains natural antibiotics and antifungals that can fight ear infections, dandruff and athlete's foot when used externally. It helps soothes sore throats used in a gargle. A warm apple cider vinegar drink has remarkable detoxifying effects. Mix 1 tsp. apple cider vinegar, 1 tsp. maple syrup, and warm water. Drinking this blend a half hour before each meal helps ease heartburn and chronic indigestion, soothes throat irritation, halts hiccups, and boosts mental clarity.

Yogurt: an intestinal cleanser that helps balance and replace friendly flora in the G.I. tract. Yogurt is nutrient-dense, providing a wealth of proteins, vitamins, and minerals (more protein and calcium than milk). The culturing process makes yogurt a living food. Most yogurt contains the beneficial bacteria lactobacillus bulgaricus and streptococcus thermophilus; some have extra lactobacillus acidophilus. Yogurt is dairy in origin, but is far better tolerated than regular dairy foods, because yogurt itself stimulates lactase activity. Bacterial fermentation elements in yogurt actually substitute for the missing enzyme lactase. *Note: If you have frequent bladder infections or dairy intolerance, avoid full-fat yogurt products. Non-fat yogurt is better tolerated.*

Yogurt has wide-ranging health benefits:
—a good source of absorbable calcium, yogurt strengthens against osteoporosis
—yogurt's lactic acid bacteria lower the enzymes responsible for developing colon cancer
—studies show people who eat yogurt with active cultures produce four times more gamma interferon, a natural immune booster with anti-viral action.
—eating just one cup of yogurt daily reduces Candida albicans yeast living in the
    vagina by 30%. (Can also be applied to a tampon and inserted to stop itching.)
—helps lower bad cholesterol and raise protective lipoprotein levels (HDL's)
—yogurt culture enzymes help lessen intolerance for lactase-deficient people
—fights diarrhea caused by antibiotic overload, especially in children
—spoonable yogurt with fruit (or even veggies) is well adapted for older infants (after three months)
    through toddlers. Introduce it gradually into the diet when the child begins to eat solid foods, usually
    between four and six months.

Yogurt cheese: is delicious, creamy, meltable, widely available in health food and gourmet stores. It's easy to make from regular plain yogurt, is much lighter in fat and calories than sour cream or cream cheese, but has the same richness and consistency.
    …*To make yogurt cheese:* Spoon about 16-oz of plain yogurt onto a piece of cheesecloth or into a sieve-like plastic funnel (available from kitchen catalogs or hardware stores). Hang the cheesecloth over a kitchen sink faucet, or put the funnel over a large glass. It takes 14 to 16 hours for yogurt whey to drain out. Store in a covered container in the refrigerator; it keeps well for 2 to 3 weeks.

Low-fat cottage cheese: a cultured dairy product, but usually still okay for those with a slight lactose intolerance. It is a good substitute for ricotta, cream cheese, and chemical-filled cottage cheese foods. Mix with non-fat or low-fat plain yogurt to add the richness of cream or sour cream to recipes without the fat.

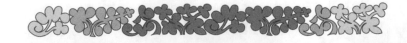

Kefir: a traditional Bedouin drink originally made with camel's milk, is today made from kefir grains or mother cultures prepared from grains. Kefir is a complete protein. It's full of biotin, B vitamins, especially B-12, calcium, magnesium and the amino acid tryptophan, for natural calm. Russian healers use kefir medicinally to treat metabolic and gastric disorders, tuberculosis, atherosclerosis, allergies, even cancer.

Kefir replenishes beneficial intestinal bacteria, producing lactic acid which balances stomach pH. Kefir is acidic when made, but becomes alkaline once ingested. Kefir's friendly bacteria contain partially digested proteins along with the minerals which contribute to the assimilation of proteins essential to healing.

Kefir may actually be a better cultured dairy choice than yogurt because it contains twice its "friendly bacteria" and has more nutrients. Kefir's curd size is small, making it easy to digest for babies, invalids and the elderly. Kefir, like yogurt, boosts immunity, and is used with success to help AIDS, herpes, cancer, candida and chronic fatigue syndrome. A natural tranquilizer, kefir is a good food choice for children with ADD, too.

…Kefir cheese: a delicious cultured food, low in fat and calories, similar to sour cream. Kefir cheese has a slighty tangy rich flavor that really enhances snack foods and raw vegetables like celery, cauliflower and carrots. Use it cup for cup in place of sour cream, cottage cheese, cream cheese or ricotta.

Cultured vegetables: commonly called sauerkraut, from the Austrian words sauer (sour) and kraut (greens), are fresh veggies changed by fermentation into one of the richest cultured foods for healing. They're loaded with vitamin C and minerals. Because they're pre-digested, raw cultured vegetables improve digestion (especially of animal proteins and grains), and re-establish your inner ecosystem. The enzymes in cultured vegetables boost your own enzymes, particularly those essential to cell rejuvenation, toxin elimination and immune response. They are alkaline-forming for better body balance.

Raw sauerkraut is one of the richest sources of enzymes and lactobacillus available. The *lactobacilli* in cultured veggies are star players in beating Candida albicans yeast overgrowth and controlling the cravings for sugary foods that are so common in candidiasis. Raw sauerkraut is also effective in treating peptic ulcers, ulcerative colitis, colic, various food allergies, cystitis, vaginal infections, constipation and digestive disorders. Further, it regenerates the blood, improves digestion and boosts metabolism for ongoing health.

However, the healing power of sauerkraut's probiotics and enzymes is only in *unpasteurized* sauerkraut. The sauerkraut that most Americans find on supermarket shelves is highly salted and pasteurized, with its *lactobacilli* and enzymes destroyed. Find effective cultured veggies instead at your health food store (in the refrigerated section) from *Rejuvenative Foods, P.O. Box 8464, Santa Cruz, CA 95061, 800-805-7957.*

If you can't find cultured veggies, here's how to make your own:

Cabbage is the main element of unheated, fresh sauerkraut. You can use green cabbage alone, or make a half-and-half blend of green and red.

For mixed cultured vegetables: chop or shred a small head of green cabbage and set aside. Use a food processor or blender for finer consistency. Chop a blend of other vegetables—like 1 beet, 2 carrots and 1 green bell pepper. Or make a Kim Chee blend of carrots, onions, red or yellow bell pepper, some fresh grated ginger and a little chili pepper. Place the veggies in a sanitary glass or stainless steel pot (never use plastic) and let sit for about 7 days at a moderate room temperature (59° to 71°). The naturally present enzymes, lactobacillus acidophilus, lactobacillus plantarum, and lactobacillus brevi in the vegetables proliferate, transforming the sugars and starches in the vegetables into lactic and acetic acids.

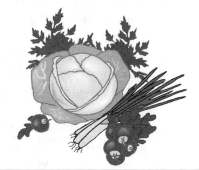

Refrigerate your cultured vegetables and eat them within six months. They'll hold their flavor, enzymes and lactobacillus cultures. Raw sauerkraut works well in salads, on sandwiches (a natural Reuben), rice cakes and pizzas, and in omelette dishes.

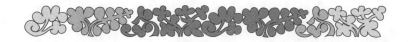

Water is Essential for Healing

Your body goes down fast without water. Second only to oxygen in importance for your health, just a few short days without water can be fatal! Water is almost 75% of the body....every cell is regulated, monitored and dependent on an efficient flow of water. Your body's "navigable waterways" are the pathway for every nutrient..... minerals, vitamins, proteins, salts and sugars to get to where it needs to go for your health. Even messages from your brain cells are transported on waterways to your nerve endings.

When your body gets enough water, it works at its peak. Water maintains your body's equilibrium and temperature, lubricates tissues, flushes wastes and toxins, moisturizes your skin, and acts as a shock absorber for joints, bones and muscles. When you get enough water, fluid retention *decreases*, gland and hormone functions improve, the liver breaks down and releases more fat, hunger is curtailed.

Should you drink more water?

A new nationwide survey say yes. Dehydration is a cause of ailments like chronic constipation and urinary tract infections, problems like hemorrhoids and varicose veins, kidney stones, even diseases like arthritis. New evidence shows that dehydration plays a role in some cancers, too. Water may be especially protective against cancers of the urinary tract, colon and breast, flushing out carcinogens before they make you sick.

Experts tell us that thirst is an evolutionary development designed by Nature to indicate severe dehydration. But drinking liquids only if you're thirsty isn't enough to keep your skin moist and supple, your brain sharp or elimination systems regular. Your body water can even keep you beautiful. Many Americans have reduced their intake of fats (including good Omega-3 fats and other essential fatty acids) to the point that their bodies aren't able to hold or use the water they take in. Try adding sea veggies to your diet for moister skin, shining eyes and lustrous hair.... known benefits of sea plants since ancient Greek times.

Current estimates conclude that more than 1 billion people worldwide do not have access to safe water! Water-borne illness accounts for a staggering 80% of diseases in the world. Even in the U.S., 7 million Americans become sick (some die!) from contaminated drinking water. **Fluoridated water is especially dangerous,** increasing absorption of aluminum from deodorants, pots and pans, etc. by 600%, a possible concern for Alzheimer's dementia. Chemicals used by industry and agriculture find their way into our ground water, adding more pollutants. Most U.S. tap water is chlorinated, fluoridated, and treated to the point where it is an irritating, disagreeable fluid instead of a healthy drink. City tap water may contain as many as 500 *different* disease-causing bacteria, and parasites. Some tap water is so bad, that without the enormous effort our bodies exert to dispose of these chemicals, we would ingest enough of them to turn us to stone by the time we turn thirty! Bottled water has become a major industry, but even some bottled water may be contaminated. A Natural Resources Defense Council study reveals that up to 25% of bottled water samples violate state limits for arsenic or carcinogenic compounds! *(For a full report report, check out the web, www.nrdc.org/water/drinking/default.asp)* Purifiers or a purifier hooked to your fridge will make your tap water more drinkable.

Most Americans suffer from some degree of dehydration! Our bodies use a lot of water every day. Our kidneys receive and filter our entire blood supply 15 times each hour! If we get overheated, our 2 million sweat glands perspire to cool our skin and our internal organs, using 99% water. We use a small amount of water during breathing and our tear ducts lubricate our upper eyelids 25 times per minute. Crying and laughing release water from our eyes and nose. Just normal activity requires 3 quarts of replacement water each day. Strenuous activity, a hot climate or a high salt diet increases this requirement.

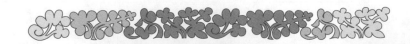

What happens when you don't get enough water? A chain reaction begins.

1: a water shortage message is sent from your brain;
2: your kidneys conserve water by urinating less (constipation and bloating occur);
3: at 4 percent water depletion, muscle endurance diminishes—you start to get dizzy;
4: at 5 percent water loss, headaches from mild to quite severe begin—you get drowsy, lose the ability to concentrate and get unreasonably impatient;
5: at 6 percent water loss, body temperature is impaired—your heart begins to race;
6: at 7 percent body water depletion, there is a good possibility of collapse.

Check your urine to tell if you're drinking enough water. The color should be a pale straw and you should urinate every few hours. If your urine color is dark yellow, start drinking more water!

Other common signs that you might be dehydrated:

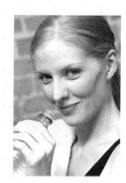

—unexplained headaches (mild to severe), usually with some dizziness and fatigue
—unexplained irritability, impatience, restlessness and difficulty sleeping
—unusually dry skin and loss of appetite along with constipation
—dull back pain that is not relieved by rest
—unexplained weight gain and swollen hands and-or feet (from water retention)
—mitral valve prolapse (MVP) may be linked to dehydration.
   Sufferers report reduced symptoms when they increase their water intake.
   allergy and asthma reactions can be minimized by boosting water intake.

Loss of body water accelerates aging. Water hydration at all levels, from body cleansing to skin beauty is a protection against accelerated aging. It is a major complication when you're sick. Dehydration is now one of the top 10 causes of hospital stays among the elderly, costing Medicare up to $450 million annually! Sadly, half of all dehydrated seniors who are admitted to the hospital die within one year. Studies show many elderly people fear urinary incontinence so they drink less liquid. Other research shows the sense of thirst is so impaired in some seniors that they do not even seek water when they need it.

Water is critical for any successful detoxification program because it dilutes and eliminates toxin accumulations in the bloodstream, and cleanses the kidneys. Add half a squeezed lemon to each glass of water for the best cleansing effects. The best time to detoxify is at night, while you sleep.

Water is your most important catalyst in losing weight and keeping it off. In fact, we often mistake thirst for hunger because our thirst mechanism is so poor. Before you give into temptation and dig into the snack foods, have a glass of water. Water naturally suppresses appetite, helps you feel full, and helps your body metabolize stored fat. Low water intake causes fat deposits to increase—more water intake actually reduces fat deposits. If you are overweight, the more body fat you have, the less system water you have. Larger people have larger metabolic loads—they need more water.

Thirst is not a reliable signal that your body needs water.

By the time you feel thirsty, you're probably already suffering from some degree of dehydration. Thirst is an evolutionary development, controlled by a part of the forebrain called the hypothalamus, (which also controls sleep, appetite, satiety, and sexual response) designed to alert us to <u>severe</u> dehydration. So you can easily lose a quart of water during activity before thirst is even recognized.

Can we solve the dehydration problem? Human bodies have some strange anomalies. From early adulthood our thirst sensation begins to fail, putting us inexplicably at risk for dehydration. So we have to plan for our water supply. Stranger still, our thirst signal shuts off before we have had enough for well-being.

Where does your body get its daily replacement water? Plain cool water is the best way to replace body fluids but other healthy liquids besides water also count as replenishment. Unsweetened fruit juices diluted with water or seltzer, and vegetable juices should be considered. Foods provide up to 1½ quarts. Fruits and vegetables are more than 90% water. Even dry foods like bread are about 35% water. Digestive processes yield as much as a pint a day for metabolism.

Drinks that don't count as good water replenishment
—Alcohol and caffeine drinks are counter-productive for water replacement because they are diuretic.
—Drinks loaded with dissolved sugars or milk increase water needs instead of satisfying them.
—Commercial sodas leach several important minerals from your body.

Even though most of us don't get enough water, drinking *too much* water can have some adverse health effects. It can severely depress electrolytes, imperative to vibrant energy, pH balance and mineral uptake. Purified water, such as distilled or reverse osmosis techniques compound this problem.

What's enough? It sounds like a lot, but eight to ten 8-ounce glasses of water daily is a sufficient amount. If you are physically active or working under hot weather conditions, you'll need more. Replace lost electrolytes with electrolyte drinks like Alacer EMERGEN-C or ELECTRO-MIX, or Nature's Path TRACE-LYTE.

Are you worried about retaining too much water, or getting water logged? Believe it or not, drinking more water is the best treatment *against* retaining fluid! Here's why: When you don't get the water you need, your body holds onto the water it has. Diuretics are only a temporary solution because you'll end up ravenously thirsty as your body tries to replace the water that the diuretics flush out. (See "What happens when you don't get enough water," previous page.) Diuretics also have a compromising effect on important nutrients like potassium. Solve a water retention problem by giving your body what it needs—plenty of water. When your body has the right amount, it will naturally release the excess.

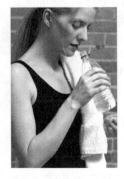

Hydrate before, during and after exercise- even if you're not sweating or thrsty. You may not be pushing yourself to the brink of collapse, but even 30 minutes of exercise can put you at risk for dehydration. Humans sweat more than any other mammal; normal exercise causes a loss of one to two quarts of fluid every hour of a workout. Sweat acts as your body's air conditioner, keeping muscles (which generate 8 to 10 times more heat during exercise), cooled. Take in water, juice or an electrolyte drink during your workout to maintain fluid needs.

If you're exercising in hot weather, drink about 20-ounces of fluid two hours before your workout, even if you aren't thirsty. This gives your body time to absorb what it needs. Drink another 8-oz. about 15 minutes before you exercise. During exercise, drink 8-oz. of water or an electrolyte drink every 20 minutes. Don't wait until you feel thirsty. You may already be low. When your workout is over, weigh yourself. The scale may show some weight loss, but it's not fat loss — it's water. Conditioned athletes drink a pint of water for every pound lost during a workout.

For a healing program, several types of water are worth consideration.

—**Mineral water** comes from natural springs with varying mineral content and widely varying taste. The natural minerals are beneficial to digestion and regularity. In Europe, bottled mineral water has become a fine art, but in the U.S., it isn't tested for purity except in California and Florida.

—**Distilled water** can be from a spring or tap source; it is de-mineralized so only oxygen and hydrogen remain. Distilling is accomplished by reverse osmosis, filtering or boiling, then converting to steam and recondensing. It is the purest water, so naturopaths use it in detox programs and in herbal formulas.

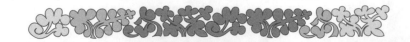

—**Sparkling water** comes from natural carbonation in underground springs. Most bottles are also artificially infused with CO_2 to maintain a standard fizz. This water aids digestion, and is excellent in cooking to tenderize and give lightness to a recipe.

—**Artesian well water** is the Cadillac of natural waters. It always comes from a deep uncontaminated source, has a slight fizz from bubbling up under rock pressure, and is tapped by a drilled well.

—**Micro-clustered bottled water** is the latest technology for rehydrating fast. Regular water molecules enter cell membranes slowly through small aquaporin water channels. Micro-clustered water passes through these channels quickly, greatly accelerating hydration rates. Research shows athletes who used Penta micro-clustered bottled water for three days significantly increased their performance. Microclustered water also enhances absorption of herbs, supplements and food nutrients. Penta costs more than other brands, but may be worth it, especially for athletes, the elderly and others at high risk for dehydration.... It's guaranteed chlorine free, arsenic free, fluoride free, chromium free and MTBE free. *Visit www.pentawater.com for more.*

Water fluoridation's tainted history

Water fluoridation is historically mandated by governments but rejected by citizens. The controversy has raged since fluoride was introduced in 1945. Most developed countries have banned fluorides in their water. Japan has rejected fluoridation. Europe is 98% fluoridation-free and is actively opposed in Britain, Australia and New Zealand. Yet, our federal government continues to push for mass fluoridation of America's water supply.

Even many government officials don't think it's a good idea. In July 1997, after an 11 year review of evidence showed that fluoride was linked to cancer, nerve impairment, bone pathology and low IQ scores in kids, the union representing all toxicologists, chemists, biologists and other professionals at the Environmental Protection Agency in Washington, D.C., went on record against adding fluoride to public drinking water. It said "As the professionals who are charged with assessing the safety of drinking water, we conclude that the health and welfare of the public is not served by the addition of fluoride to the public water supply."

The fluoridated water controversy affects every city and county in America. The evidence has stacked up for decades. Water fluoridation causes adverse environmental and health effects.

Finding out the truth about our public water supply can be a shock. Extensive research into the history of fluoride use over the last two decades, and conversations with scientists and knowledgeable dentists, convince me that fluoride added to food or water poses a major health risk for Americans. Even fluoride proponents, like Dr. Harvey Limeback, are changing their minds about fluoride's safety. According to Limeback, "Children under three should never use fluoridated toothpaste. Or drink fluoridated water. And baby formula must never be made up using Toronto tap water (which is fluoridated). Never."

In the first decade of the millennium, our country's water supply is in a grave situation. Fluoride is in almost all commercial toothpastes and regularly added to 75% of public drinking water. Could massive fluoridation cause massive fluoride poisoning in the U.S. population? I equate it to something like the widespread lead poisoning that decimated the health of Romans, especially the children, 2000 years ago.

We need to dispel the myths about fluoride. It could mean your health....
Fiction: **Fluoride is safe for humans.**

Fact 1: Fluoride is more toxic than lead, and even in minute doses, is damaging to brain/mind development of children. In areas where fluorosis (fluoride poisoning) is prevalent, a higher concentration of fluoride is found in fetal brain tissue of unborn children.

Fact 2: Some studies show that fluoride is linked to Alzheimer's and senile dementia, perhaps through a fluoride-aluminum combination in the brain. A new study shows fluoride increases the body's absorption of aluminum from deodorants, or pots and pans by over 600%! The aluminum concentration in the brains of Alzheimer's patients is 15 times higher than in healthy individuals.

Fact 3: Hip fracture rates are much higher in people living in fluoridated communities. The U.S. Dept. of Health and Human Services said in its Toxicological Profile (1993) that "postmenopausal women and elderly men in fluoridated communities may be at increased risk for bone fractures." Fluoride's cumulative effect on bone density is devastating.

Fact 4: Menopausal women, people over 50, and people with cardiovascular (particularly high cholesterol), thyroid and kidney problems are especially affected by fluoride exposure. Fluoride reduces thyroid and metabolism activity, so some experts lay America's unusually high blood cholesterol levels, and our current epidemic of obesity, at least partially at fluoride's door. Research shows that after World War II when widespread fluoride exposure began, widespread hypothyroidism also began. More work is being done on the question, but already reports say that thyroid problems lessen when fluoride exposure is removed.

Fact 5: New concerns have risen over how fluoride affects the pineal gland. 11 cadavers analyzed in the U.K. were found to have extremely high levels of fluoride in the calcium crystals produced by the pineal gland. The levels averaged from 9000 ppm to 21,000 ppm—levels as high or higher than those found in bones of people with skeletal fluorosis. Experts theorize that high levels of fluoride in the pineal gland may cause a drop in melatonin production, signalling early onset of puberty, a growing problem today. Fluoride's role in early puberty is currently under investigation. There is already historical evidence that shows girls living in fluoridated communities begin menstruating earlier than girls in non-fluoridated communities.

Fiction: <u>Calcium fluoride found naturally in water is safe</u>.
Fact 1: All forms of fluoride are poisonous. The most toxic forms are those with a higher solubility of free fluoride ions such as in hydrofluosilicic acid, a hazardous by-product of the phosphate fertilizer industry which is the substance routinely added to fluoridate water.

Fiction: <u>Water fluoridation helps provide dental care to poor children</u>.
Fact 1: National survey data by the National Institute of Dental Research shows that children living in fluoridated areas have tooth decay rates almost identical to those living in non-fluoridated areas. Even large-scale studies show no difference in decay rates of permanent teeth in fluoridated and non-fluoridated areas. In fact, a recent study by the New York Department of Health showed that children who drink fluoridated water have more cavities and tooth discoloration than children who drink non-fluoridated water. 2000 studies in the Journal Caries Research show that the rates of cavities actually declined when cities in Europe stopped fluoridating their water. Moreover, the latest research from the pharmaceutical company Sepracor, reveals the levels of fluoride found in fluoridated toothpaste may actually cause and exacerbate gingivitis, and other gum diseases.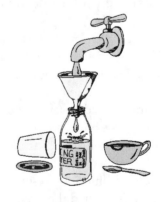

Fact 2: The U.S. National Research Council admits that dental fluorosis (fluoride poisoning causing teeth to become brittle and chip easily) affects from 8% to 51% of children drinking fluoridated water. Dental fluorosis has steadily increased since the introduction of fluoride to drinking water in 1945.

Fact 3: Poor children, more likely to be malnourished than other kids, are most vulnerable to fluoride's toxicity. Fluoride toxicity strikes the malnourished harder than other populations. Further, the primary cause of tooth decay in poor communities is baby bottle tooth decay (BBTD), caused by babies sucking on bottles of fruit juice, sugar water or milk for extended periods of time. <u>Even fluoride proponents admit that fluoride does not solve BBTD.</u>

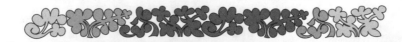

Fiction: <u>Mandatory water fluoridation is safe for the American population</u>.

Fact 1: Evidence from animal and human epidemiology studies links fluoride exposure to cancer, genetic damage, nervous system dysfunction and bone diseases. Fluoride exposure is also linked to low IQ in children. A University of Arizona study finds that the more fluoride a child drinks, the more cavities appear.

Fact 2: The poison control center receives over 11,000 calls a year for poisoning from ingesting fluoride toothpaste. In 1997, the FDA even mandated a poison warning label on fluoride toothpaste! Small children, who tend to swallow toothpaste are most at risk. Signs of fluoride poisoning include vomiting and muscle cramps. Look for non-fluoridated toothpastes like Nature's Gate SPEARMINT or CINNAMON TOOTHPASTE at your health food store. Try Ayurvedic herb peelu (literally "tree for tooth care"). Peelu is a natural antibacterial that removes tartar and has natural chlorine to help whiten teeth. Xylitol gum (made from birchwood chips or plum) helps reduce cavities by neutralizing mouth acids, and enhances tooth remineralization. Xlear Xleardent is a good choice.

Can you do anything to protect yourself from fluoride's risks?

Mandatory water fluoridation throughout the U.S. is either about to begin or has already been instituted. Americans need to work hard to stop mandatory water fluoridation before it's too late. It isn't just the water we drink, it's the food we eat, too. Crops watered with fluoridated water mean fluoride is leeched into our fruits and vegetables. Not even organic produce is safe from fluoride in the water supply.

After forced fluoridation by its public health service, Natick, Mass mailed its water bills with a warning that pregnant women, parents of children under 3 years, and anyone with fluoride sensitivity should consult their physicians before drinking city water. Santa Cruz, California became the first city in California (following the state fluoridation mandate of Oct. 1995) to pass an ordinance to prevent its water fluoridation. Other California cities feel they've been hoodwinked by the massive public health telemarketing campaigns on fluoride's supposed "health benefits." Some are already embroiled in lawsuits to stop the fluoridation process; others like Wastonville and Redding California are jumping on the "no fluoridation" bandwagon as their citizens become aware and alarmed about water safety.

If you want to help stop mandatory water fluoridation, contact David C. Kennedy, D.D.S. @ Citizens for Safe Drinking Water 2425 3rd Ave, San Diego, CA 92101, 800-728-3833.

For more information about fluoride, check the internet: *www.keepersofthewell.org*; *www.sonic.net/~kryptox/fluoride.htm*; *www.nofluoride.com*; or *www.fluoridation.com*.

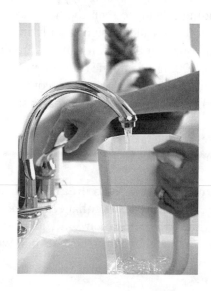

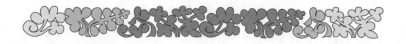

Foods for your healing diet

Caffeine in a Healing Diet?

What's the real scoop on caffeine? Like most of mankind's other pleasures, there is good news and bad news about caffeine. Caffeine is America's favorite stimulant. A broad spectrum of our society say they can't function without their morning fix. Coffee and caffeine containing foods are widely heralded for the strong antioxidant phenols they contain.

In fact, moderate use of caffeine has been hailed for centuries for its therapeutic benefits. Every major culture uses some food form of caffeine to overcome fatigue, handle pain (especially migraine headaches), open breathing passages for asthmatics, control weight and jump-start sluggish circulation after rich food or drink. Caffeine is a plant-derived nutraceutical—it's a food with medicinal attributes. Coffee, black tea, colas, sodas, chocolate and cocoa, analgesics like Excedrin, and over-the-counter stimulants like Vivarin, all have caffeine. Taking regular aspirin or an herbal pain reliever with a caffeine drink increases the pain relieving effects.

Caffeine absorbs rapidly into the bloodstream. In just a few minutes, it enters all organs and tissues. Within an hour after ingestion, it is distributed in body tissues in proportion to their water content. Caffeine stays in the body for about three hours, then is excreted in the urine; it does not accumulate in body tissue.

Caffeine is an effective short-term energy booster. It mobilizes fatty acids into the circulatory system, allowing greater energy production, endurance and work output. It has a direct potentiating effect on muscle contraction for both long and short-term sports and workout activity.

Caffeine shows solid evidence for clearer mental performance and shortened reaction times. Caffeine stimulates serotonin, a brain neurotransmitter produced by tryptophan, that increases the capacity for intellectual tasks and alertness by releasing adrenaline into the bloodstream. The net effect also decreases drowsiness and improves mood. There is new evidence that caffeine may protect against Parkinson's disease. (Researchers speculate that caffeine reduces the release of transmitters like glutamate that can kill brain neurons.) Other studies suggests that caffeine can reduce colon cancer risk through its laxative action. Further, the latest report in the Journal of the American Medical Association reveals that drinking 2-3 cups of caffeinated coffee a day may reduce gallstone risk by up to 40%!

Caffeine's benefits for weight loss have long been known. Caffeine promotes weight control because it enhances thermogenesis, converting stored body fat to energy. For dieters who don't burn enough calories to produce normal heat during dieting, adding caffeine to their diet produces greater thermogenesis response. Even relatively small, commonly consumed doses of caffeine significantly influence calorie burning, actually raising metabolic rate... the rise lasts for several hours, far beyond its direct stimulation.

One study shows that a single dose of 100mg. of caffeine (the amount in one cup of coffee) increases metabolic rate 4% for up to three hours! If the same amount of caffeine was consumed at two-hour intervals for 12 hours, metabolic rate increased between 8 to 11%. These metabolic increases seem small, but over several months there is steady, substantial weight loss.

The same study shows that low doses of caffeine help weight control after initial weight loss because caffeine blocks appetite while keeping calorie-burning efficient.

Caffeine stimulates the nervous system and heart action, relaxes smooth muscles in the digestive tract and blood vessels, increases urine flow, enhances stomach acid secretion and boosts muscle strength. Research in India reports that caffeine, taken with antioxidant supplements, offers powerful protection against free radical DNA damage by altering the behavior of a gene-damaging chemical.

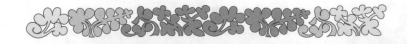

The DNA-protective effect was stronger with the combined coffee-antioxidant regimen than with either coffee or antioxidants alone.

Interesting note: Olfactory hallucinations are an unexpected effect of new caffeine research. When given caffeine intravenously, sleeping volunteers awoke recalling smells of wet hay, dirty socks and ammonia from their childhood.

Caffeine's health problems are also well known. In excessive amounts, caffeine has drug-like activity, causing jumpiness, nerves and heart palpitations. Excessive amounts of caffeine actually reduce mental performance by elevating cortisol levels, taxing the hippocampus involved in memory and learning. In excessive amounts, caffeine produces oxalic acid in the system, causing health problems waiting to become diseases. It can restrict liver function, and constrict arterial blood flow. It leaches B vitamins from the body, particularly thiamine, which is needed for stress control. It depletes essential minerals, including calcium and potassium.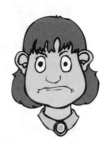

As an addictive substance, caffeine is difficult to overcome, but if you have caffeine-related health problems it's worth going through the temporary withdrawal symptoms. Improvement in the health condition is often noticed right away.

Decide for yourself. Here are the caffeine links to specific health concerns:

…Caffeine and Bone Health: excessive caffeine causes calcium depletion increasing risk of osteoporosis. Women with osteoporosis should limit caffeine for optimum mineral assimilation. (Moderate amounts do not cause calcium depletion or contribute to bone loss.)

…Caffeine and Fertility: caffeine seems to affect women's health more than men's. Some experts say the more coffee a woman drinks the less likely she is to conceive, but new studies show there is no relationship between a morning cup of coffee and infertility.

…Caffeine and Pregnancy: avoid caffeine during pregnancy and nursing. Like alcohol, it can cross the placenta and affect the fetus' brain, central nervous system and circulation. HIGH DOSES (more than 300mg per day) are linked to spontaneous abortion and low birth weight.

…Caffeine and PMS: reduce, rather than avoid caffeine during menses. Caffeine causes congestion through cellular overproduction of fibrous tissue and cyst fluids. Yet low-dose caffeine intake improves memory and alertness during menses.

…Caffeine and Breast Disease: the link between caffeine and breast fibroids isn't official, but there is almost immediate improvement when caffeine is decreased or avoided. Today, even many medical professionals advise their patients to cut down on coffee to help shrink breast and uterine fibroids.

…Caffeine and Menopause: caffeine is a trigger for hot flashes in menopausal women, and can provoke night time panic attacks in some women.

…Caffeine and Sleep: caffeine consumed late in the day or at night disrupts brain wave patterns. You'll take longer to get to sleep. A 1998 Australian study shows regular caffeine users sleep longer and more soundly when caffeine is cut from their diets.

…Caffeine and Severe Blood Sugar Swings: caffeine causes the liver to release glycogen which triggers insulin release, and a sharp blood sugar drop within 1 to 2 hours.

…Caffeine and Exhausted Adrenal Glands: excessive caffeine exhausts the adrenals by releasing too much adrenaline, so you have less resistance to stress and are more vulnerable to hormone imbalances that affect health in both men and women.

…Caffeine and Cancer: studies on caffeine and cancer, particularly bladder and organ cancers, show a link but no definite causal relationship. **Further, the carcinogenic effects blamed on caffeine are now thought to be caused by the hydrocarbon roasting process used in making coffee, since decaffeinated coffee is also implicated in some organ cancers.** I believe the acidic body state promoted by coffee is not beneficial to the healing process as the body works to normalize its chemistry during healing.

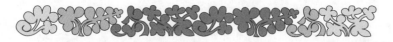

...Caffeine and Heart Disease: heavy coffee drinking (more than 4 cups a day), has been directly implicated in heart disease. New research shows caffeine may increase homocysteine, an amino acid whose high levels contribute to heart disease. In addition, research shows brewed coffee contains cholesterol-raising oils. Moderate caffeine does not appear to increase heart disease risk.

...Caffeine and High Blood Pressure: excessive caffeine can elevate blood pressure significantly and produce nervous anxiety. Watch out when caffeine is combined with phenyl-propanolamine, the appetite suppressant in most commercial diet pills.

...Caffeine and Ulcers: caffeine is not linked to gastric or duodenal ulcers, but it stimulates gastric secretions, sometimes leading to a nervous stomach or heartburn. On the good side, caffeine is a "bitter" food, stimulating bile secretion for good digestion.

...Caffeine and Headaches: caffeine causes headaches in some people — and withdrawal headaches when eliminated after regular use. Strangely enough, coffee is a niacin-rich healing remedy for temporary relief of migraine headaches (the niacin content of coffee increases when the beans are roasted).

...Caffeine and Asthma: caffeine reduces asthma symptoms by dilating lung and nasal passages. Regular caffeine consumption reduces wheezing considerably. Some researchers believe this is why asthma symptoms decrease when children become adults.

Caffeine in common foods: (a pharmacologically active dose of caffeine is about 200 mg)

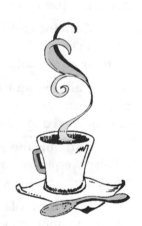

Coffee — 5-oz. cup Decaf	4mg
Coffee — 5-oz. cup Instant	65mg
Coffee — 5-oz. cup Percolated	110mg
Coffee — 5-oz. cup Drip	135mg
Tea — 5-oz. cup Bag, brewed 3 minutes	45mg
Tea — 5-oz. cup Loose, black, brewed 3 minutes	55mg
Tea — 5-oz. cup Loose, green, brewed 3 minutes	35mg
Tea — 5-oz. cup Iced	30mg
Cola — 12-oz. glass	45mg
Chocolate/Cocoa — 5-oz. cup	10mg
Milk chocolate — 1-oz	10mg
Bittersweet Chocolate — 1-oz	30mg

You can break the caffeine habit with herb teas, caffeine-free coffee substitutes like roasted chicory, barley or dandelion root, and energy supportive herbal pick-me-ups with no harmful stimulants of any kind. I recommend green tea, maté tea and kola nut as bio-active forms of caffeine for weight loss and mental clarity. They don't have the heated hydrocarbons of coffee.

If you just can't give up your morning cup of joe, consider organic, shade-grown coffee as a healthier alternative to commercial coffee blends. Commercial coffee is loaded with pesticides and herbicides linked to cancer and other numerous health problems. Organic, shade-grown coffee is a much healthier choice for your body and for the environment. Over 150 species of migratory birds are found in shaded coffee farms, compared to just 5 to 20 species in unshaded coffee farms. To find out how to order shade-grown coffee, contact *Thanksgiving Coffee Co. at 800-648-6491*.

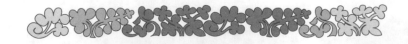

Tea and Your Healing Diet

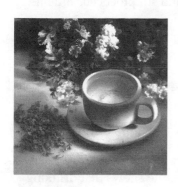

All black, white, green and Oolong teas come from one plant, *camellia sinensis*, an incredibly productive shrub that ranges from the Mediterranean to the tropics. Tea leaves can be harvested every 6 to 14 days for 25 to 50 years! Tea is defined by the way its leaves are processed. For green tea, the first tender leaves of spring are picked, rolled, steamed, crushed and dried with hot air. Green tea leaves are not fermented. Oolong tea leaves are semi-fermented for one hour. Black tea is fermented for 3 hours, then dried and scented with spices to strengthen aroma and reduce bitterness. White teas are the newest tea rage in the West. White tea leaves are picked from only the youngest leaves, which are still covered with short white hairs. They are quickly steamed and dried with minimal processing. White teas offer a very delicate, sweet flavor highly prized by serious tea connoisseurs, preferred for purifying and detoxification.

How does tea fit into a healing diet? White tea, green tea and black tea have enzymes that promote digestion and help our bodies resist harmful bacteria, like *Staphylococcus aureus*. High flavonoids in all three teas reduce harmful blood clotting linked to heart attacks. They contain polyphenols (not tannins as commonly believed) that act as antioxidants, yet do not interfere with iron or protein absorption. (Whole leaf teas may be healthier than bag-cut teas because they contain more antioxidants.)

Green tea has been the most widely studied tea for health benefits. It contains larger amounts of healing nutrients, including twice as much vitamin C, more than twice the amount of bioflavonoid activity (two cups a day of green tea can meet your body's daily needs for bioflavonoids), and six times the free radical fighting antioxidants of black tea. Green tea is highly enzyme-active to help you burn calories for weight loss. It is a good fasting tea, providing energy support and clearer thinking during cleansing. Green tea is a vasodilator and smooth muscle relaxer with theophylline for bronchial dilation against asthma.

Should you be drinking a daily cup of green tea for better health? Science validates green tea's health benefits. Most studies center around the over 200 different catechin polyphenol compounds that comprise up to 35% of green tea. The polyphenols reduce cholesterol to lower the risk of heart attack, and protect against cancer by thwarting nitrosamines that produce cancer-causing substances. Research at the American Health Foundation in N.Y. shows that green tea's anticarcinogens are anti-mutants "preventing activation of carcinogens so that free radicals never even form."

One green tea compound, EECG (epigallocatechin-3 gallate), has formidably high levels of free-radical-scavenging activity. Green tea's EECG is 30 times more powerful than vitamin E against DNA-destroying attacks. Black tea loses its EECG and other beneficial polyphenols entirely during fermentation.
Scientists also believe EECG is the substance that inhibits the enzyme urokinase, crucial for cancer growth and metastasis. EECG attaches to urokinase and prevents it from invading cells to form tumors. Some cancer tests show that EECG may even engender a process called apoptosis, in which cancer cells shrivel and die.

Both black and green teas have caffeine. Is the caffeine in tea different from that in coffee or chocolate? The natural, bioactive caffeine contained in black tea (50 to 80mg per cup), white tea (about 15 to 25 mg. per cup) and green tea (about 30 to 35mg per cup) helps combat mental fatigue. The latest research from Israel shows drinking tea (green or black) may significantly extend lifespan for people with heart disease. Compare this to one cup of regular coffee at 110 to 135mg per cup.

More amazing, research shows that green tea's caffeine may be the synergistic delivery system for therapeutic catechins like EECG. A cup of green tea contains 100-200mg of EGCG. Scientists believe two to four cups per day could provide cancer protection.

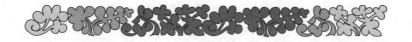

Green tea has an astounding catalog of curative applications.

…Green tea is antibacterial, a quality known for 5,000 years ago by the Chinese, who used it to purify water. Green tea polyphenols have wide-ranging antimicrobial action against food poisoning, and streptococcus mutans, a mouth bacterium that causes tooth decay and may cause serious illness if it establishes in the heart valve. Tea polyphenols bind to mouth bacteria as a shield to strengthen tooth enamel against plaque. Note: Don't add milk to green tea. Milk inhibits absorption of the protective polyphenols.

…Green tea also provides a protective effect against both esophageal and oral cancers, according to the American National Cancer Institute. Note: To fully benefit from green tea's anti-cancer properties, pour hot, not boiling water over the tea leaves. In addition, consider blending green tea with turmeric. New research reveals they work synergistically for oral cancer prevention.

…A dual study by the Shanghai Cancer Institute and the U.S. National Cancer Institute shows that drinking green tea once a week for six months means less risk for colorectal and pancreatic cancers, with benefits stronger for women. (The same study showed that green tea increased female fertility through its body-balancing effects.)

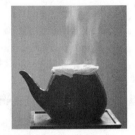

…Green tea may reduce the risk of several forms of environmentally-induced cancers. Research in Japan on stomach, skin and lung cancers (where people drink large amounts of strong green tea) show a low incidence of these cancers. A recent large Japanese study recorded that drinking several cups of green tea on a daily basis was effective in reducing lung cancer death rates even in men who smoked two packs of cigarettes a day. Smoking is far more prevalent in Japan than in the U.S., but the instance of lung cancer is much lower, indicating to researchers that green tea protects against lung cancer.

…Green tea may protect our skin against radiation damage. As the ozone layer thins and UV radiation increases, skin cancers have risen throughout the world. In a Rutgers University study, green tea showed good results against skin cancer when it was taken before and during exposure to UV rays.

…Green tea is an antimicrobial skin refresher. Acne, cuts, sunburn and athlete's foot all benefit from a cool green tea foot bath.

…Green tea is a significant heart health protector. Its catechins are potent inhibitors of blood clumping which leads to atherosclerosis. The catechins also suppress the formation of the angiotensin I conversion enzyme which contributes to high blood pressure.

…Green tea stabilizes and increases elimination of harmful blood lipids to prevent oxidation of LDL cholesterol. University of Kansas research shows that green tea is over 100 times more effective than vitamin C at protecting cells from damage from heart disease, and is 25 times more effective than vitamin E as a heart protecting antioxidant. The Japanese, who favor green tea, clearly have lower blood fat levels and reduced heart disease risk.

…Green tea helps dieters because it promotes fat burning, regulates blood sugar and insulin, and has a satiating and tension calming effect during dieting. A 2000 study published in the Journal of Obesity shows green tea increases thermogenesis by whopping 28 to 77% in lab animals!

White tea may be the most potent tea for cancer protection....

The newest reports reveal white tea has a higher polyphenol content than both green or black teas; just one cup of white tea has the antioxidant capacity of 12 glasses of orange juice! Like green tea, white tea is a very rich source of EGCG (epigallocatechin-3 gallate), known for its antioxidant, anti-cancer effects. A 2000 study from

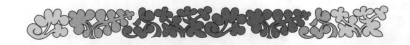

Oregon State University shows white tea is 3 <u>times</u> more protective against DNA mutations linked to cancer than green tea. Because it can only be picked a few days during springtime, white tea is very rare, and very expensive. Republic of Tea carries Silver Rain White Tea. Crystal Star uses a blend of high quality green and white teas in DR. VITALITY™ caps and tea. Many fine white teas are also available on *www.specialteas.com*

I regard white tea as an outstanding choice for detoxification programs of all kinds. People report to me that white tea shows an especially noticeable difference in a skin detox, offering a lovely clear texture to the skin. I include white tea for just this effect in Crystal Star BEAUTIFUL SKIN™ caps and tea.

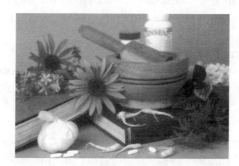

Tea nomenclature can be confusing. Names like oolong, black or jasmine tea refer to how the tea leaf is processed. Names like Assam, Darjeeling or Ceylon, etc., refer to country or region where the tea is grown. Names like pekoe, orange pekoe, etc., refer to leaf size.

- Green tea (bancha) - tender spring leaves of the Japanese tea plant. (See above.)
- Green tea (kukicha) - made from roasted twigs rather than the leaves of the tea plant. Kukicha is a favorite in macrobiotic diets for its blood cleansing qualities, high available calcium and mellow, smooth flavor.
- Silver Needle- a rare, delicate tea made from white tea leaves. The large size of the leaves means they cannot be measured by tsp.
- White Peony - a rare tea made from white tea leaves, darker than the Silver Needle, with the same sweetness. Cannot be measured by tsp.
- Darjeeling - the finest, most delicately flavored of the black Indian teas.
- Earl Grey - a popular, hearty, aromatic black tea scented with bergamot oil.
- English Breakfast - a connoisseur's rich, mellow, fragrant black tea.
- Ceylon - a tea grown in Sri Lanka with an intense, flowery aroma and flavor.
- Irish Breakfast - a combination of Assam and Ceylon flowery orange pekoes.
- Jasmine - a black tea scented with white jasmine flowers during firing.
- Lapsang Souchong - a fine black tea with a strong, smoky flavor.
- Oolong - a complex, delicate tea, semi-fermented, steam-fired in baskets over hot coals.

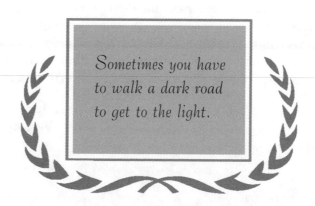

Sometimes you have to walk a dark road to get to the light.

Does Wine Fit into a Healing Diet?

Naturally fermented wine is still a living food. It is a complex biological fluid possessing definite physiological values. Records dating back 4,000 years refer to wine as a food, a medicine, a part of religious ceremonies and a pleasing element in social life. Wine is much more than an alcoholic beverage—vastly more complex than beer or spirits; it is never boiled, so its biologically active compounds are not destroyed or altered by heat. Many small, family owned wineries make chemical-free, additive-free wines that retain their nutrients, including B vitamins, and minerals like potassium, magnesium, calcium, organic sodium, iron and phosphorus.

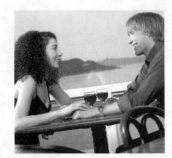

Wine has significant health benefits. In moderation, it is a mild tranquilizer for the heart and blood pressure. Further, wine boosts levels of "good" HDL cholesterol and helps prevent "bad" LDL cholesterol from damaging arteries. U.C. Davis research on wine tannins shows that a glass or two of wine a day may cut coronary heart disease risk by 50%, by subtly decreasing blood clot formation, and considerably reducing stress. Danish research reveals that drinking wine reduces stroke risk, too. A study released in the journal Epidemiology reveals that drinking 2-3 glasses of wine a day reduces death rates from <u>all causes</u> 30%.

…As a cultured food like yogurt and other fermented foods, wine helps digestion. (For more, see my chapter on "Cultured Foods" pg. 107) Wine boosts circulation, relieves pain and reduces excess body acid production. It is superior to tranquilizers or drugs for nervous tension. It is important in a weight loss program, because a glass of wine relaxes. When you are relaxed, you tend to eat less.

…Wine is full of antioxidants. Studies at U.C. Berkeley show that red wine is rich in polyphenols, powerful antioxidants that help neutralize free radicals which damage DNA and alter body chemistry. Wine antioxidants, along with its carotenes like lutein and zeaxanthin, are significant protectors for the eyes. A new study reveals that just drinking 2 to 4 glasses of wine a month can cut the risk of macular degeneration (the leading cause of blindness in people over 60) by over 20 percent. A study of wine antioxidants by the journal Epidemiology shows that its polyphenols even help prevent hepatitis A virus replication.

…Wine is a more powerful anti-microbial against common bacteria than some drugs. It can, for example, reduce the growth of some harmful stomach bacteria colonies within 20 minutes. Bismuth salicylate, a pharmaceutical remedy for traveller's diarrhea, takes two hours to do the same job. The latest research shows wine can successfully address the food and water-borne micro-organisms that cause digestive havoc and upset tummies referred to as "Delhi belly" and "Montezuma's revenge."

There's much more…
—*Quercetin*, an antioxidant flavonoid in red wine may be one of the most powerful anticancer agents ever discovered. Early results show that quercetin reverses tumor development by blocking the conversion of normal body cells to cancer cells. Quercetin activity is boosted by the wine fermentation process and by friendly flora in our intestinal tracts. Quercetin also normalizes insulin release levels, so it prevents some complications of diabetes like cataracts, diabetic retinopathy (blindness), neuropathy (nerve damage) and nephropathy (kidney damage). Doctors use quercetin in wine as a potent free radical scavenger against HIV infection, because wine also relieves AIDS pain and stress.

—*Resveratrol*, a compound in red grape skins, is a key to wine drinkers' healthy cholesterol levels. Resveratrol also seems to prevent blood platelet aggregation, keep blood vessels open and flexible, and reduce blood clotting

 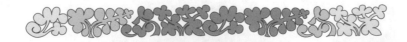

in arteries narrowed by years of heavy fat consumption. In nature, resveratrol fights off fungal disease for the grape plants. In animal tests, resveratrol stops production of abnormal cells, like cancer cells at three separate stages of development—inhibiting the enzyme cyclo-oxygenase that stimulates tumor growth.

Note: Resveratrol has mild estrogenic effects and may aggravate hormone dependent tumors, or add to high estrogen stores in women already using HRT drugs. Preliminary results find resveratrol offers protection against liver and oral cancers.

Are sulfites in wine really a health hazard? Sulfur dioxide (SO_2) is a naturally occurring sulfite that protects the wine's character by inhibiting the growth of molds and bacteria. Wine yeasts naturally produce up to 20 parts per million of SO_2 during fermentation. (Human bodies produce about 1,000mg of sulfites a day in our normal biochemical processes.) Top European winemakers have counted on sulfur dioxide to prevent wine spoilage for centuries. In a method used since Roman, even Egyptian times, today's winemakers use mined SO_2 heated into a liquid, to protect wine from oxidizing.

What is organic wine? Sadly, the grapes which produce our wines are one of the most heavily sprayed fruits in America. Grape skins also have a notable affinity for fluoride, a highly toxic substance used in pesticides and regularly added to the water supply. (For more, see my chapter on "WATER," pg.116)

Wines made from organically grown grapes are increasingly popular in both Europe and California. Organic wine means wine made from organically-grown grapes, without using sulfites, yeast, bentonite, egg whites, gasses like N_2 or CO_2 in the process. Added sulfites, rather than naturally-occurring sulfites, have been known to cause allergic reactions like congestion and stuffy nose for many people.

In 1988, following a food-borne sulfites scare, the U.S. ATF required alcoholic beverages of all kinds, both imported and domestic, to carry a "CONTAINS SULFITES" label if there were more than 10 parts per million sulfites in the beverage, regardless of whether sulfites had actually been added. This hasty ruling became, and still is, a major problem for winemakers, especially when wine has naturally-occurring sulfites at this level.

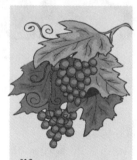

Wine was created from the beginning to make men joyful, not to make men drunk.

Wine enjoyed in moderation is a pleasure of the soul and the heart.

Are both red and white wines healthy? Research shows that phenol compounds in both red and white wine reduce LDL oxidation, platelet formation and fat buildup in your arteries. However, the benefits of wine consumption are especially notable among red wine drinkers. The reason for this seems to be the resveratrol contained in the skin of the grape. As a potent antioxidant and source of mild plant estrogen, resveratrol may afford extra protection for women against menopausal heart disease.

Still, as with most of mankind's pleasures, a little is good, a lot is not. Drinking more than two glasses of wine (or any alcoholic beverage) a day increases the risk of heart disease and adds to hypertension. And as many menopausal women will tell you, your capacity for alcohol changes markedly as your hormones change. Certain cancers, like mouth, esophageal, stomach, breast and colon cancer, increase markedly if you regularly have more than one or two alcoholic drinks a day, including wine. If you're at high risk, switch to purple grapes and grape juice instead. In addition, eating foods high in folate like dark greens, asparagus, and beans helps reduce breast cancer risk for women who drink wine regularly.

Note: I don't recommend liquor other than wine, even in cooking, during a healing program. Although most people can stand a little hard liquor without undue effect, and alcohol burns off in cooking, concentrated sugar residues won't help your recovering body.

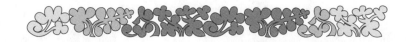

Fats and Oils in a Healing Diet

The great fat debate has filled the American media for more than a decade, but much of the information is contradictory and inaccurate. Most people today know that there is a direct relationship between the quantity of fat we consume and the quality of health we can expect. Yet, in the last 50 years, Americans have increased their intake of fat calories (especially Omega-6 fats) by over 33%.

The link between high salt and fat intake on health has also become clear. Too much salt inhibits the body's capacity to clear fat from the blood. Yet, in the last thirty years, Americans have consumed more salt than ever before, largely because we eat 50% more restaurant and pre-prepared foods than our parents did. Much of this food is fried and salty, or salt-preserved (animal foods), and full of spicy or salty condiments.

Are the new fat replacements like Olestra a good choice for health?
The latest research on olestra has some medical doctors seriously concerned.

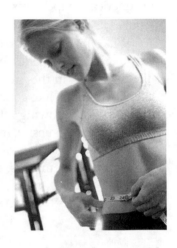

As they try to cut back on fat intake, more Americans are turning to fat replacements like Olestra snack foods. Olestra is a non-calorie fat replacement synthesized from sugar and fatty acids. It's special function for weight loss is that is not digested or absorbed in the body, passing through rather than being stored. Painful diarrhea and loss of bowel control (anal leakage throughout the day) are documented side effects of Olestra consumption! Further, Olestra inhibits the absorption of fat soluble vitamins and other nutrients. Fake fat manufacturers know this and have temporarily curbed this outflow by boosting Olestra products with vitamins A, D, E and K. But, olestra robs the body of key cancer fighting carotenoids too, and those are <u>not</u> added to Olestra products. Walter Willett, M.D., Department of Nutrition Harvard School of Public Health, and Meir Stampfer, M.D., Professor Nutrition and Epidemiology, reveal three startling estimates on the potential health impact of reduced carotenoid levels from olestra consumption.

1) A 15% reduction in blood lycopene (a carotenoid) levels from light olestra snacking. Just 3 snack bags a week could potentially cause 15,900 additional cases of prostate cancer each year.
2) A 10 to 15% reduction in the levels of blood carotenoids lutein and zeaxanthin from light olestra snacking could cause up to 600 cases of blindness from Age Related Macular Degeneration (AMD) each year.
3) A 15% decrease in total carotenoid levels from light olestra snacking could cause up to 50,000 additional deaths each year from coronary heart disease!

As a result of their findings, Dr.'s Willett and Stampfer urged the FDA not to subject the American public, including children and pregnant women, to the potential health hazards of olestra in the food supply calling it a "massive uncontrolled experiment, with potentially disastrous consequences." Sadly, their advice was not heeded. Olestra, FDA approved in 1995 for limited use in snack foods, is now widely available in the U.S.

Are fat-free foods any better?

Fat-free foods aren't much better. They may be fat-free, but these foods are commonly loaded with sugar. Sugar, corn syrup and fructose are usually three of the first five ingredients on any box label of fat free sweet snacks. It's well known that too much sugar can wreak havoc on blood sugar levels, especially for diabetics or hypoglycemics, an ever-growing segment of Americans. Over-consumption of sugary treats also triggers the production of insulin- your body's signal to make fat! Fat-free but loaded with sugar, is a poor choice for a dieter and for

general health! Many fat-free snacks are also loaded with salt as Americans try to make up for the taste loss in fat free foods. Highly salted foods contribute to blood pressure disturbances and water retention. There's more bad news: fat-free snacks are often laced with fillers, preservatives, artificial flavors and colors - many with known toxicity.

As debatable as they are, Americans still clamor for fat-free foods - eating them occasionally is unlikely to cause any ill effects. Just remember that many of these foods are highly refined, chemicalized "non food foods." The unnatural nature of many of these foods makes them an unhealthy choice for everyday eating.

*The Truth about Fat...*We clear up the confusion so you can make the best choice for a healing diet.

Not all fats are alike. Regardless of its "bad press," our bodies need fat to keep warm, protect our tissues and organs, and supply us with energy. Fat is the most concentrated source of energy in our diets, providing nine calories per gram of energy compared to four calories per gram from carbohydrates or protein. Fat even helps us use carbohydrates and proteins more efficiently by slowing down digestive processes. I never recommend a "no fat" diet to anyone.

Like protein supplies essential amino acids, fat supplies essential fatty acids, (see page 133) We need some fat for healthy skin and hair, to metabolize cholesterol, for brain health and emotional wellness, and for prostaglandin balance. Fat releases a hormone in the stomach called cholecystokinin that sends the brain a "full" message when we have satisfied hunger so we don't overeat. We need fat in order to absorb critical fat-soluble vitamins A, D, E and K. Fats elevate calcium levels and transport calcium for strong bones and elastic muscles. Adding a little fat to high carbohydrate meals helps prevent rises in blood sugar and insulin levels. Some fats actually help you lose fat by increasing metabolic rate and activating caloric burning.

What's the difference between saturated, polyunsaturated and monounsaturated fats?

The difference is in molecular structure. All fat molecules are composed of carbon and hydrogen atoms. A saturated fatty acid has the maximum possible number of hydrogen atoms attached to every carbon atom—hence the term "saturated." An unsaturated fatty acid is missing one pair of hydrogen atoms in the middle of the molecule—a gap called an "unsaturation." A fatty acid with one gap is said to be "monounsaturated." Fatty acids missing more than one pair of hydrogen atoms are called "polyunsaturated."

Animal foods have more saturated fat, and except for palm and coconut oil, plant foods have more unsaturated fats. Saturated fats, like butter, meat and dairy fats, shortening and lard, are solid at room temperature. They are the culprits that clog the arteries, and lead to heart disease. Saturated fats tend to thicken the blood, causing blood pressure to rise, increasing the work load on your heart. They also promote blood stickiness, exaggerate plaque build up on the arteries and reduce oxygen availability to your heart muscle.

Not all saturated fat is created equal. The saturated fats in coconut and palm oil contain medium chain triglycerides which do NOT clog the arteries like the long chain triglycerides in animal fats. For more information on coconut and palm oils, see pg. 137.

Unsaturated fats, both mono and polyunsaturated, like seafood, plant or nut oils, are liquid at room temperature. While tests show unsaturated fats help reduce cholesterol, just switching to unsaturated fats without increasing dietary fiber will not bring about better health. For the best benefits, eat moderate amounts of unsaturated fats, if desired, small amounts of medium chain saturated fats along with a high fiber, balanced whole foods diet.

Is there a health difference between polyunsaturated and monounsaturated fats?

—Monounsaturated fats, as in seafoods, avocados, nuts, olive oil, canola and peanut oil, are considered the healthiest fats. Monounsaturated oils are rich in fatty acids and important for normalizing prostaglandin levels. Tests show that moderate amounts of unrefined, mono-unsaturated oils considerably lower allergy reactions.

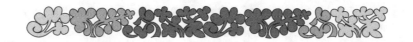

—**Polyunsaturated fats,** like those in walnuts, vegetable oils and seafood, are healthier than saturated fats, but not as healthy as monounsaturated fats. Polyunsaturated vegetable oils are good sources of essential fatty acids (linoleic, linolenic, arachidonic) necessary for cell membrane function, balanced prostaglandin production and metabolic processes. Good polyunsaturates include: sunflower, safflower, sesame and flax oils. Note: Balance is the key for polyunsaturated fats. Too many polyunsaturated fats without enough monounstaurated fats may contribute to asthma and other health problems.

Are all plant oils unsaturated fats?

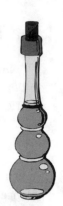

All plant oils are cholesterol-free, but commercial oils are highly processed to prevent rancidity.

—*Refined oils* are degummed, de-pigmented through charcoal or clay, deodorized under high heat, and chemically preserved. Unfortunately, processing also destroys healthy antioxidants and forms hazardous free radicals. Refined oils are clear, odorless..... and almost totally devoid of nutrients.

—*Unrefined vegetable oils* are the least processed and most natural. They are mechanically pressed and filtered (cold pressing applies only to olive oil). They have small amounts of sediment, and taste and smell like the nut, seed or fruit they came from.

—*Solvent-extracted oil* is a second pressing from the first pressing residue. The petroleum chemical hexane is generally used to get the most efficient extraction; it is still considered an unrefined oil.

Note 1: Vegetable oils are traditionally seen as top dietary sources of essential fatty acids. New research shows this to be true only of cold pressed oils. Commercial oils contain such a large number of contaminants and are so heavily processed that they can no longer be regarded as good sources of EFAs.

Note 2: Heat and air exposure easily cause unrefined oils to spoil, so store them in an air-tight container in a cool dark cupboard (65°F) or the fridge. Purchase small bottles if you don't use much oil in your cooking.

What are hydrogenated fats?

All fats, especially unsaturated fats, tend to break down when exposed to air. Largely to prevent rancidity and extend shelf life, manufacturers use chemical processes to change the biochemical composition of fats. They hydrogenate, partially hydrogenate and poly-unsaturate, so that the processed fats are not water-soluble when bound to protein. Hydrogenation bubbles hydrogen molecules through a poly-unsaturated oil to reconstruct its chemical bonds for more stability. For example, hydrogenation converts liquid corn oil to a semi-solid form—margarine. Some tests show that these altered fats are comparable to animal fats in terms of saturation and effects in the body.

What are trans fats? *Why are they such a problem for our health?*

Trans fatty acids are byproducts of hydrogenation. When hydrogen molecules are added back to a polyunsaturated fatty acid, some of the hydrogenated fatty acids take on a "straight" structure, and become trans fatty acids. While originally only used for foods like shortening and margarine, today trans fats are part of most snack foods, pastries and desserts. Some researchers think they may be real villains in health problems.

Here's why:

Trans fatty acids have proven to raise blood cholesterol almost as much as saturated fat. Some trans-fat actions in the body may even be worse. Where saturated fats increase both LDL and HDL cholesterol levels, trans fats increase LDL cholesterol (bad), and *decrease* HDL cholesterol, the good cholesterol which actually helps clear arteries. Trans fats have been linked to increased cancer risk, premature skin aging and lowered immune response from impaired prostaglandin and cell functions. Most significant, they interfere with the metabolism of natural fats and with your body's ability to use critical essential fatty acids.

The American Journal of Public Health says that trans fats may be responsible for up to 30,000 heart disease deaths each year in the U.S.! European studies find that women with breast cancer have higher levels of trans fatty acids in their bodies than women who do not. High levels of trans fats raise breast cancer risk an astounding 40%! Trans fats interference at the metabolic level may affect the nervous system, brain health, even your skin texture.

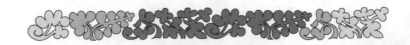

How do you know if trans fats are part of the foods you buy?

You don't. Trans fats are neither saturated, monounsaturated, or polyunsaturated, so food labels don't have to disclose how much a food contains. Foods with "partially hydrogenated oil" in their ingredient lists do contain trans fats, but some foods have only slightly hydrogenated oils with tiny amounts of trans fats. Other foods contain heavily hydrogenated oils. The FDA limits the saturated fat in foods labeled "no-cholesterol" or "low-cholesterol." And, a trans fat content line on product labels will be *mandatory* by January 2006.

Hydrogenated and trans fats are difficult for your body to process. They end up blocking circulation, inhibiting cell renewal, impeding the free flow of blood and lymph fluids. The whole body shows a losss of electrical energy that is replenished only when active lipids, like omega oils are added to the diet. It may take *a year or two* before trans fats are released from your body fat. Start today to reduce trans fats in your diet!

Here are some pointers:

**REDUCE intake of fast foods and deep fried foods- they are loaded with trans fats.

**AVOID buying foods that contain vegetable shortening or partially hydrogenated oils. There are plenty of healthy and delicious snack foods that don't contain these health offenders at natural foods store.

**COOK WITH natural unrefined oils like olive oil, flaxseed oil (great in salad dressings) or canola oil instead of margarine or shortening. Butter, in small amounts, is okay, too. No scientific studies have ever clearly linked butter consumption with heart disease. It should be used sparingly, however, especially for people watching their weight or who have high cholesterol. Coconut butter (made from coconut oil) is another good choice. To find out more about coconut oil, see pg 137.

**STORE oils in a dark cupboard or in the refrigerator. Natural unrefined oils are fragile and can become rancid quickly. Purchase small bottles if you don't use much oil in your cooking. Omega Nutrition, Health from the Sun and Spectrum Essentials all manufacture quality, organic, unrefined natural oils that I like.

What about margarine? We used to think it was healthier than butter. Is it?

Margarine products today are lower in calories, total fat, saturated fat and trans fats than ever before. Many are made from soy oil, so they are cholesterol-free and contain vitamin E. Most are sold in a squeeze tube, soft and liquid, meaning they have low amounts of trans fatty acids. Yet margarine manufacturers are currently allowed to omit trans fats from their labels (presumably because the amounts are small). Hopefully, this consumer information problem will soon be solved with new trans fat label requirements in Jan. 2006.

Note: Looking for a low saturated fat alternative to margarine or shortening? Blend equal amounts of warm butter and vegetable oil. Good for all types of cooking. Nut oils, perilla oil and grape seed oil... all work well.

Essential fatty acids.... we know they're the good fats and they're important. What are they?

1: Essential fatty acids (EFA's), are the healthy fats that protect our bodies from degenerative disease and boost our brain power. EFA's help us maintain energy, insulate our body, and protect our tissues and organs.

2: Essential fatty acids and the essential amino acids from which protein is made, form lipoproteins, the organic compounds that make up our bodies. They are indispensable to each other and work synergistically.

3: Essential fatty acids like other essential nutrients, are nutrients your body needs but cannot make for itself. Fatty acids include AA-arachidonic acid, ALA-omega 3, LA-omega 6, DHA-docosahexaenoic acid, EPA-eicosapentaenoic acid and GLA-gamma linolenic acid. A healthy body can make GLA from linoleic acid (LA), the most common fatty acid in foods, but that ability is impaired if your body is deficient in zinc, magnesium and vitamins A, B_6, B_3 and C. A diet high in saturated fats or hydrogenated oils also block this conversion.

4: Essential fatty acids are significant components of nerve cells in the "hormone-prostaglandin cascade" which converts cells into hormone-like messengers known as prostaglandins—instrumental in energy production, essential to circulatory health, integral to good metabolism. Low EFA's disconnect the cascade.

5: Essential fatty acids are major components of hemoglobin production and cell membranes; without them, the membranes would become stiff and lose their ability to function.

6: Essential fatty acids play an important role in regulating blood triglyceride levels.

7: Essential fatty acids impact our growth, vitality, and mental state, by connecting oxygen, electron transport, and energy in the body's vital oxidation processes.

An amazing amount of scientific research has been done on the effects of essential fatty acids for specific ailments. Here are some of the positive results:

…EFA's are a big part of your brain. 60% of your brain is made up of fatty material! If you aren't getting enough of these good fats in your diet, your brain suffers first, in terms of learning impairment and recall capacity. Recent studies find high EFA's in breast milk even increases IQ in children. Conversely, a lack of essential fatty acids appears to be a regular problem of children with attention deficit hyperactive disorder.

…EFA's inhibit harmful blood clots in the arteries, and help prevent cardiovascular damage through significant antioxidant and anti-bacterial activity.

…EFA's reduce the risk of breast and colon cancer and inhibit tumor growth.

…EFA's show remarkable results in reducing the inflammation of rheumatoid arthritis and osteoarthritis as well as that found in Parkinson's and M.S.

…EFA's are significant for healthy skin and hair. In fact, EFA deficiency is involved in most serious skin diseases like eczema, dermatitis, psoriasis, acne and hair loss. Borage oil, rich in GLA, shows especially good results for relieving chronic skin disorders.

…EFA's reduce irritability and depression associated with PMS and menopause through their involvement in the hormone-prostaglandin cascade process.

EFA treatment research shows promise for many health problems:
- Autoimmune disorders—chronic fatigue syndrome, Lupus (SLE) and fibromyalgia
- Childhood infections, especially recurrent respiratory problems like asthma
- Neurologic conditions like M.S. or Guillain Barre syndrome
- Raynaud's disease (unexplained colds hands and feet)
- Hypertension and high blood pressure
- Some cases of schizophrenia and autism
- Adult onset diabetes
- Scleroderma
- Less incidence of anaphylactic shock and allergic reactions
- Colon and bowel inflammatory conditions like Crohn's disease and I.B.S.
- Chronic headaches especially from drug, caffeine or alcohol withdrawal symptoms
- Slows or reverses progression of Huntington's disease, an untreatable, inherited brain disorder.

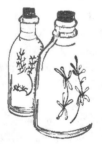

Do you have enough essential fatty acids?

The first signs of deficiency are usually in the form of red, dry, scaly skin that appears first on the face, clustered in the folds of the nose, lips, forehead, eyes and cheeks. Dry, rough areas may also appear on the forearms, thighs and buttocks. If you experience reduced vision and unexplained mood swings, you may be suffering from an EFA deficiency. A diet rich in plant foods results in low levels of saturated fat and higher levels of essential fatty acids. *Warning: If you're on a serious weight loss diet, a very low-fat diet may cause a deficiency in EFAs.*

We hear a lot about Omega-3, Omega 9 and Omega-6 health oils today. *What are they?*

Omega oils contain a family of fatty acids—EPA (eicosapentaenoic acid), DHA (docosahexaenoic acid), CLA (conjugated linoleic acid), LNA (alpha linolenic acid) and GLA (gamma linolenic acid). Omega-3 and Omega-6 fatty acids differ in bio-chemical structure, but both are important in proper body fat balance. They are equally

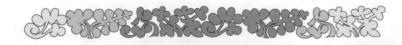

important in the development of prostaglandins, the essential hormone-like substances that control reproduction, inflammation reactions, immunity and cell communications. Find Omega oils in walnut, perilla, canola and wheat germ oil, dark greens like spinach, and herbs like evening primrose oil, ginger and flax, but the richest Omega oils come from the sea. Omega oils are synthesized by plankton at the base of the ocean food chain. They are in the tissues of all sea life, both plant and animal.

Clinical results show a long list of benefits for Omega oils:

—Omega oils mean smoother skin, smoother muscle action and better digestion. Their PGE 3 prostaglandins enhance lymph function for immune response, and protect against cancer growth by suppressing malignant cell division. Health problems like PMS and rheumatoid arthritis improve with omega fatty acids.

—Omega oils are an effective diet remedy for the 30% of America's population who need to lower their cholesterol levels. Omega-3 oils are precursors for series 3 prostaglandins (PGE 3), which help balance cholesterol by raising HDLs and decreasing triglycerides. In fact, recent research shows that they reduce excess blood fats of all kinds, slowing down the rate at which the liver produces harmful triglycerides.

—Omega oils help prevent artery blood clots, inhibiting excess production of thromboxane which promotes clotting. They arrest platelet aggregation to fight atherosclerosis, improve circulation by letting more blood reach the muscles, and increase oxygen supply. Enhanced blood flow is important in lowering high blood pressure, may even repair some damage caused by clogged arteries, and relieve chest pain of coronary heart disease.

Omega-6 fatty acids are found in black currant seed, borage, flaxseed, walnut, chestnut, soy, hemp and primrose oil. Omega-6 oils are precursors for series 1 prostaglandins (PGE1) needed for T-lymphocyte immune function, kidney health, tumor protection, low cholesterol and inhibiting blood platelet stickiness.

Omega-3 oils are abundant in cold water fish and sea greens, flaxseed oil, perilla oil arugula, spinach and purslane (the number one dark green vegetable containing omega 3's). Omega-3 oils are precursors for series 3 prostaglandins (PGE 3), which help balance cholesterol by raising HDLs (high density lipoproteins, the "good" cholesterol) and decreasing triglycerides (body fats). PGE 3 prostaglandins also enhance lymph function for immune response, inhibit platelet aggregation to fight atherosclerosis and protect against cancer growth by suppressing malignant cell division. Omega 3's 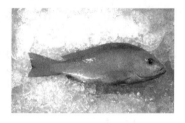 are critical to proper retinal function and vision. Australian research links low omega 3 fatty acids body levels to severe depression. A new study published in Archives of General Psychiatry finds omega 3 fatty acids in fish oil can even stabilize mood for people with manic depression. You can even fight fat with omega 3's. Omega 3 fatty acids actually increase metabolic rate, rid the body of excess fluid and heighten energy levels.

Omega 9 fatty acids are found in olive oil, and like Omega 3 fatty acids, are credited for reducing inflammation and vasoconstriction. Omega 9's are not essential for health, but they support proper Omega 3 and Omega 6 fatty acid activity in the body.

A closer look at some of the beneficial fatty acids in omega oils.

The Omega-3 fatty acids, DHA and EPA are naturally found in fish, sea vegetables, marine algae and eggs; they are synthesized from LNA in the body. Experts have known for years that fish eaters suffer less heart disease and have lower cholesterol and triglyceride levels than those who don't eat fish. A primary study of 80,000 nurses shows stroke risk due to blood clotting could be reduced by 50% just by eating omega 3 rich fish 3 times a week!

Both DHA and EPA support coronary health. However, EPA from salmon and herring, has major medical backing for heart protection, improving cholesterol levels, and thinning the blood to prevent re-clogging of arteries after balloon angioplasty. EPA treatment is most promising for the elderly who regularly experience re-clogging within 6 months of an angioplasty.

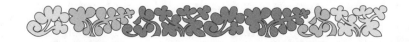

DHA is the most predominant EFA in brain tissue. DHA is a large part of the retina of the eye and is critical for good eye function. DHA is the most abundant fatty acid in breast milk (see page 215). It's a big reason mother's milk is best for a newborn's health, supplying the full range of EFA's needed for proper development of a child's central nervous system, brain and retina. Breast feeding your baby may make your baby smarter. A new 18 year

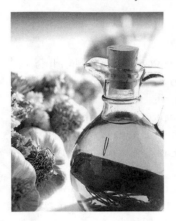

study finds that breast-fed infants have an academic advantage! The determining factor seems to be the high content of DHA (*docosahexaenoic acid*) in breast milk. Sadly, American women have the lowest levels of DHA in the world and pregnancy depletes stores even further.

America's "diabetes epidemic" has focused attention and controversy on treating non-insulin dependent diabetes with fish oil EPA. Studies are conflicting. EPA seems like a good choice for diabetics who suffer from high blood fat levels and are at high risk of heart disease, but early 90's studies showed that fish oil might raise blood sugar levels, (a health risk for type II diabetes), and that large doses of fish oil supplements might lead to insulin resistance. New data in the American Journal of Clinical Nutrition reports that fish oil supplements are NOT linked to higher blood sugar or insulin. *If you have blood sugar imbalances, use EPA supplements under professional supervision.*

More EPA-DHA news:

Both EFA's help overcome food allergies and rheumatoid arthritis. Both help clear inflamed skin diseases like eczema and psoriasis. Both have significant normalizing effects on high cholesterol and triglyceride levels. Low levels of both are linked to mental problems like depression, memory loss, attention deficit/hyperactivity disorders, hostility, and senility. Studies show that both DHA and EPA help protect against Alzheimer's and promote clearer thinking; they may also help cardiac arrhythmias. Research on EPA and DHA shows they may eliminate binging and help burn fats during dieting. Our body's ability to make both EPA and DHA decreases as we age.

Do you know about CLA? It's an important new discovery getting a lot of attention.

CLA (conjugated linoleic acid) occurs naturally in dairy products like cheese, lamb, sunflower oil and beef. (Its discovery during scientific studies on cancer-causing substances in beef showed actually inhibited cancer growth.) It plays a role in muscle growth and nutrient-energy conversion. CLA converts the most energy from the least amount of food, making it popular among athletes for increasing muscle mass and burning fat. Like all fatty acids CLA contains powerful antioxidants for immune health and shows remarkable results for lowering cholesterol.

CLA studies were the first to show that fats can help you lose fat. CLA especially inhibits the body's mechanism for storing saturated fat by boosting its ability to use fat reserves for energy. The more saturated fat you eat, the more CLA you need. Since Americans are eating more vegetable oils, chicken and fish, and reducing their dairy and meat intake, our CLA intake has dropped over the last 20 years. Some researchers say that the marked increase in body fat in the American population may be due to CLA decrease.

Is GLA the most bioactive fatty acid? *My healing observations indicate that it is.*

GLA (Gamma Linolenic Acid - an omega-6 fatty acid) is made in the body from LA (linoleic acid). LA itself is an omega-6 fatty acid found abundantly in most vegetable oils. GLA can also be obtained from evening primrose oil (perhaps the most bio-active), black currant and borage seed oil.

GLA is a source of cellular energy and helps the body burn fat instead of storing it. It's part of the team of structural fats that form the brain, bone marrow, cell membranes and muscles. It acts as electrical insulation for nerve fibers, is regarded as an anti-coagulant and has anti-inflammatory qualities. GLA is a significant precursor of prostaglandins which regulate hormone and metabolic functions.

GLA is therapy for breast tenderness during PMS, for vaginal dryness during menopause, for better nerve transmission in M.S. cases, for weight loss, for pain and morning stiffness of arthritis, chronic fatigue syndrome, heart health, diabetes, eczema, hyperactivity in children, schizophrenia and skin or hair dryness. A powerful anti-

inflammatory, GLA can work wonders to relieve cramping, sunburns and headache pain. A Canadian study in the Journal of Human Hypertension finds that students who take a GLA borage oil supplement have reduced stress levels, so GLA may be a wonderful tool for resisting "stressed out" reactions.

What about hemp seed oil? *Experts say it has the most remarkable fatty acid profile of all.*

It has GLA, absent from the fats we normally eat. Hemp contains a perfect balance of omega and gamma fatty acids — a ratio of 3:1. Hemp has been used for thousands of years as a valuable resource of edible seeds and oil, as a medicine and as fiber for clothes and rope. It's popularity is rising again as people learn about its rich nutritional properties. Hemp seeds contain 25% high quality protein and 40% fat with high amounts of EFA's — Omega-6, (Linoleic Acid- 58%), Omega-3, (Alpha-Linolenic Acid-20%), Omega-9, (Oleic Acid-11%), saturated Fatty Acids-9% and GLA, (Gamma Linolenic Acid- 2%).

Research shows that hemp oil has anti-inflammatory properties, so it's great first aid for wounds and burns. It stimulates the growth and health of the skin, hair and nails. Today's cosmetic manufacturers use hemp's rich EFA's as a primary ingredient in skin products. Try Hemphoria's FOOT FRENZY and HELPING HANDS CREAMS.

Hemp is not good for cooking because it shouldn't be heated above 120°F/49°C. But it has a distinct, nutty flavor, good in salad dressings, spreads, dips and baked potato mixed with fresh herbs. Keep hemp oil refrigerated. Buy unrefined, unfumigated, residue-free oil like Omega Nutrition VIRGIN HEMP SEED OIL.

Does hemp seed oil alter your consciousness? *No, you can't get high by eating foods containing hemp.*

Hemp contains <u>trace</u> only amounts of THC, the psychoactive compound in marijuana. Hemp seed oil is perfectly legal and not psychoactive. Canada passed an Industrial Hemp Act in 1998 so that this remarkable plant could be used for its nutritional benefits. Hemp is still illegal to grow in the U.S. Legal battles over the inclusion of hemp as a food rather than a controlled substance (like heroin or cocaine) are ongoing.

What about coconut oil, palm oil and other tropical oils?

Coconut oil, a much maligned tropical oil, long under attack by the American Soybean Association, is making a comeback for its taste and therapeutic value. The soy sponsored studies were used to promote polyunsaturated oils and replace use of tropical oils. Coconut oil was falsely accused. Scientists now know that the studies were flawed and the stud's conclusions were incorrect. The true villains were actually hydrogenated oil products along with a lack of healthy EFA's in the diet. For over forty years, however, the negative publicity caused a coconut oil scare and set fire to the foundation of its popularity.

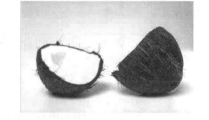

You may have heard that coconut oil is over 90% saturated fatty acids (SFA), and believe that it is unhealthy. The truth is there are two kinds of saturated fats — long chain and medium chain. Long chain saturated fats (LCT's) are associated with "bad" cholesterol; Medium chain saturates or triglycerides (MCT's) like those found in coconut oil, provide energy, are easily digested and do not clog arteries like the long chain group.

MCT's help your body metabolize fat efficiently, so that the fats provide energy instead of being stored. MCT's are easily digested, so coconut oil is useful for people who have trouble digesting fat. Natural practitioners use a formula with coconut oil MCT's for patients with malabsorption problems, like those with eating disorders. Infant formula with coconut MCT's can be a lifesaver for premature babies. The healthy fats in coconut and other tropical fruits deserve at least partial credit for the glowing, wrinkle-free skin of native Hawaiians.

Common misconceptions of coconut oil are that it raises cholesterol, causes heart disease and obesity. Yet, coconut oil does not cause heart disease. Polynesian islanders, who have gotten most of their fat calories from coconut oil for centuries have an exceedingly low rate of heart disease. It does not raise blood cholesterol. Studies show coconut oil has a neutral effect on blood cholesterol. Coconut oil is actually a good choice if you are a dieter or body builder concerned about body fat. It's less likely than other oils to cause obesity, because the body easily converts its calories into energy rather than fat. I recommend Health Support COCONUT OIL capsules.

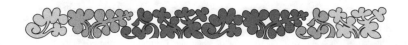

Coconut oil is one of the few plant sources of lauric acid (almost 50% of its fatty acid content), a rare disease fighting fatty acid. It is naturally found in mother's milk and protects an infant from viral and bacteria infection. For example, natives who live in the tropics, an ideal environment for parasites, are protected from infections through their traditional diet. Lauric acid has proven effective for immune-compromised conditions like HIV, fibromyalgia and lupus, respiratory infections like chronic bronchitis, pneumonia or severe flu, and as an immune booster.

Coconut oil is a good cooking oil with a sweet, tropical flavor. Compared to flax oil, which has alpha-linolenic acid easily oxidized by heating, the SFA's of coconut oil are 300 times more resistant to oxidation. It is a healthy alternative to refined oils and hydrogenated vegetable oils, like margarine. It may be used in place of butter - use three-quarters the amount of coconut butter to obtain the same baking results. Try Omega Nutrition COCONUT BUTTER—100% organic, unrefined coconut oil.

Coconut oil is still one of the best kept nutritional secrets. Forty years of false dietary information have taken their toll. But the general public is catching on to the truth. More balanced information will help this healthy oil to rise out of the ashes of unfair publicity and take its place in our healing pantheon.

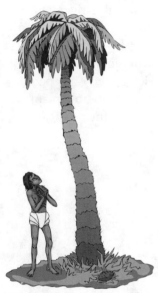

Is palm oil okay? It's another tropical oil that's received a great deal of negative publicity, falsely accused under the same series of polyunsaturated oil tests. Once again, all the evidence wasn't taken into account. Like coconut oil, palm oil is high in saturated fats, but no discernment was made between the *two kinds* of saturated fats — long chain and medium chain. (See previous page.) Palm oil, too, was accused of hiking blood cholesterol levels and clogging arteries. (Several new studies show that even a diet high in palm oil doesn't boost cholesterol in people with normal levels.)

In fact, of all the commonly used vegetable oils, palm oil is the most versatile. Even after refining, palm oil doesn't need hydrogenation — the big health culprit, for its use. Palm oil is a rich source of alpha and beta carotene and vitamin E tocotrienols. A National Cancer Institute study reveals that alpha carotene in palm oil is 10 times more powerful at cancer inhibition than beta carotene alone! Still, palm oil is usually heavily refined (coconut oil is not) which depletes its nutrient value and makes it harder for the body to digest. For this reason, I recommend avoiding commercial palm oil in a healing diet. Use high quality palm oil supplements instead. They're a good choice for people who want palm oil's benefits without the refinement of commercial products.

I have worked with and recommend Lane Labs PALM VITEE, a palm oil byproduct especially rich in tocotrienols. **Tocotrienols** help lower high cholesterol, thin sticky blood, and reduce risk of atherosclerosis. Tocotrienols combined with CoQ10 help treat congestive heart failure, the type women commonly experience after menopause. They are potent antioxidants, too. Palm Vitee's tocotrienols neutralize free radicals 40 to 60 times more effectively than vitamin E.

Further, products like Palm Vitee should be included as part of any natural program to help prevent stroke. In one clinical trial, 28% of patients who had suffered one previous stroke showed significant improvement after taking Palm Vitee for 12 months. Their arteries actually became less blocked. (The other 64% remained stabile; just 8% had progression of their disease taking Palm Vitee. In the control group, 0% improved, 60% remained unchanged and 40% actually worsened.) See Product Resources Directory for information on how to order Lane Labs PALM VITEE GEL CAPS.

The best news about these good fats? They actually fight the bad fats!

Essential fatty acids, especially linoleic acid, CLA (conjugated linoleic acid) and LNA, fight harmful fat deposits in your body fat. They protect against damage from hard fats, because they repel their stickiness and disperse them in the body. Forget about losing weight. Good fats are truly vital for us to even survive! The more saturated fats you eat, the more EFA's you need.

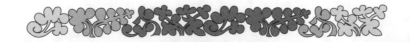

Active fats play a critical role in the functioning of the entire body. They are vital for cell renewal, brain and nerve activity, and the body's adjustment to temperature change. Active lipid metabolism is critical to our energy resources. Our cells need live electron-rich, true polyunsaturated lipids to absorb proteins and oxygen, and pump them through our systems. Lipids are only water soluble and system active when they are bound to protein where they are protected and available on demand when the body needs energy.

So eat more essential fatty acids like Omega 3s (cold water fish and flax).... they encourage more anti-inflammatory prostaglandins.

How do you maintain the right balance of fats in your diet?

As we fight the battle of the bulge in America, we have seriously disrupted our fat balance. We've cut back on saturated fat from meats and dairy foods, and increased our intake of omega-6's from corn and soybean oils. In the U.S., we eat the highest amount of omega-6 fatty acids of any population on Earth! And, the animals we eat are fed a diet high in Omega-6 oils, so we get even more omega 6's when we eat them.

A good ratio of Omega-6 to Omega-3 fatty acids may be about 1:1, (the ratio our primitive forebears lived on), but diet amounts for modern man are 10 to 20 parts Omega-6 oils to 1 part Omega-3's, a highly imbalanced ratio. Americans are eating 10:1 to even 40:1! The result for health? Experts believe that an overload of Omega-6 fatty acids leads to body chemistry changes that increase our risk for heart disease. Further, an overload of Omega 6's causes the body to overproduce prostaglandins that have pro-inflammatory and pro-clotting effects!

Take a look at your diet. If you eat a lot of vegetable oils and animal foods, you may be getting too many Omega 6's. Reduce your ratio of these foods for better fat balance.

It's easy. Simply increase your intake of omega-3 fatty acid foods like fish, flaxseed and green vegetables. They help your body compete with the production of Omega-6 prostaglandins and reduce their adverse effects. If you need more Omega-3 fatty acids, try this healthy treat: SPINACH SALAD, with flaxseed oil/lemon dressing and a little smoked salmon to top. The flaxseed oil dressing (I only use about 1 tbsp.), spinach and salmon all contain high omega 3 fatty acids. Top with a few walnuts if desired. Walnuts are a balanced source of omega 3 and 6 fatty acids.

I highly recommend my "Intense Fat and Sugar Cleanse" once or twice a year to help rid your body of unhealthy fats and sugar that can contribute to weight gain, poor energy and reduced immune response. It's a great way to get your fats back in balance! See pg.179 for more information.

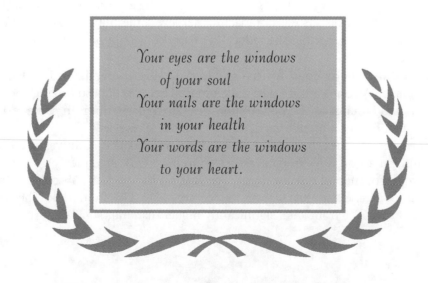

*Your eyes are the windows
of your soul
Your nails are the windows
in your health
Your words are the windows
to your heart.*

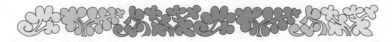

Dairy Foods in a Healing Diet

I believe you should avoid dairy foods during a cleansing diet, especially a mucous cleansing diet. Dairy products interfere with the cleansing-healing process because their density and high saturated fats challenge both digestion and metabolism. Dairy foods are tremendous mucous producers that burden the respiratory, digestive and immune systems. Cow's milk in particular has clogging properties for many people. Pasteurized milk is a relatively dead food as far as nutrition is concerned. Even raw milk can be difficult to assimilate for someone with respiratory problems.

Over one-quarter of Americans are intolerant to dairy foods.

They experience allergic reactions, poor digestion and mucous build-up. In addition to a lactose sensitivity, many people process some proteins like casein in cow's milk poorly, throwing off excess from cheeses, cream, ice cream and milk. Milk-digesting lactase levels are at their highest immediately after birth, decreasing after weaning. Dairy foods become harder to digest as we age, causing strain and accumulating mucous clogs on eliminative organs. Even people without great sensitivity to dairy foods report an energy rise when they reduce their dairy intake.

Children are especially susceptible to dairy reactions.

An Italian study reveals that two-thirds of children with chronic constipation experience relief just by switching to soy milk (for some children, rice milk is even better). Besides constipation and early allergy reactions, cow's milk can cause a loss of iron and hemoglobin in infants by triggering loss of blood from the intestinal tract. Small children who drink a lot of cow's milk may fall prey to vitamin D toxicity. Some research shows that iron absorption is blocked by as much as 60% after a meal that includes dairy foods. Recent studies in the New England Journal of Medicine show that children who are not given cow's milk products during infancy have a dramatically lower risk of diabetes later in life. The culprit appears to be a cow's milk protein, bovine serum albumin, which differs just enough from human proteins to cause an anti-body reaction. The antibodies attack and destroy insulin producing beta cells in the pancreas, increasing the likelihood of childhood or Type II diabetes.

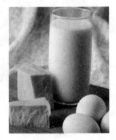

When dairy foods are removed from the diet of mucous clogged children, enlarged tonsils and adenoids shrink, a clear sign of immune system relief. Doctors who put children on dairy-free diets often report a marked reduction in colds, flu, sinus and ear infections.

Women do not handle dense, building foods like dairy products, as well as men. Their systems back up more easily, so less dairy (especially cheese) usually means easier bowel movements for women. Female problems, like fibroids, fatty cysts, bladder and kidney ailments can be improved by avoiding dairy. A sugar in dairy products, galactose, may even be fatal to a woman's eggs, impacting her level of fertility. When a women is having trouble getting pregnant, I usually recommend that she reduce her dairy consumption first.

Isn't calcium from dairy foods good for us?
Contrary to advertising, dairy products are not a very good source of calcium for people. We don't absorb dairy calcium well because of pasteurizing and homogenizing, high protein and fat content, and an unbalanced ratio of phosphorus to magnesium. In cattle tests, calves given their own mother's milk that had first been pasteurized, didn't even live six weeks!

Bovine growth hormone residues, pesticides, herbicides, fertilizers and additives used in cattle-raising also inhibit calcium and mineral absorption. In contrast, calcium from dark green leafy greens is easily absorbable. One study compares the absorption of calcium from vegetable sources with the absorption from cow's milk. The absorption of calcium from brussels sprouts was 63.8%, compared to 32% from milk. The absorption of calcium from broccoli was 52.6% and 50% from kale, significantly higher than milk's 32%.

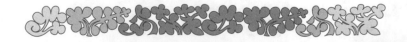

Besides leafy greens, other vegetables, nuts, seeds, fish and soy foods have measurable amounts of absorbable calcium, along with minerals like magnesium, potassium and zinc that are easy for us to assimilate. Herbs, like sea plants, lamb's quarters (a delicious watercress-like green), borage seed, pau d' arco, valerian, wild lettuce, nettles, burdock and yellow dock offer healing concentrations of calcium.

Dairy foods aren't a very usable source of protein for humans, either. Cow's milk contains proteins that are harmful to our immune systems, (see previous page). Repeated exposure to these proteins disrupts normal immune response. Fish and poultry proteins are much less damaging; plant proteins pose the least hazard.

The truth about milk for strong bones? Most of us are told from childhood to drink milk for strong bones. The dairy industry floods us with advertisements featuring sports stars and celebrities touting milk's bone building benefits. However, new research reveals dairy consumption is not a bone protector after all. Homogenized milk has very low magnesium and is a poor source of absorbable calcium. Milk protein can actually CAUSE calcium loss via the urine. A twelve year study of 78,000 women (Harvard Nurses' Health Study) finds that high intake of milk and other dairy foods does NOT reduce bone breaks or osteoporosis. The study found instead that hip fracture risk was 1.45 times *higher* in women who drank 2 or more glasses of milk a day compared to women who drank one glass or less per week. The Journal of Epidemiology shows elderly people with high dairy intake have double the risk of hip fractures than those with the lowest intake!

How specific dairy foods can affect your healing diet:

What about butter? Surprise! Butter is okay in moderation. Although a saturated fat, butter is relatively stable, and like raw cream, it is a whole, balanced food, used by the body better than its separate components. When butter is needed, use raw, unsalted butter, not margarine or shortening. Don't let it get hot enough to smoke. If you want less saturated fat, use the new butter-yogurt blends or ghee (clarified butter), a body balancing food recommended in Ayurveda. Simply melt the butter and skim off the top foam. Let it rest a few minutes and spoon off the clear butter for use. Discard whey solids that settle to the bottom, and the foam. Soy margarine is a vegan alternative for baking.

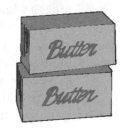

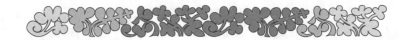

There's good news about eggs, too! "Eggsperts" are finally realizing what many of us in the whole foods world have long known. Although high in cholesterol, eggs are also high in balancing lecithins and phosphatides, so they don't add to the risk of atherosclerosis. In fact, phosphatidylcholine in eggs can actually help prevent cholesterol from entering your bloodstream. Nutrition-rich fertile eggs from free-run chickens are a perfect food. The difference in fertile eggs and eggs from commercial egg factories is remarkable; the yolk color is brighter, the flavor fresher, the workability in recipes better. The distinction is most noticeable in poached and baked eggs, where the yolks firm up and rise higher. Cook eggs lightly for the best nutrition - poached, soft-boiled, hard boiled or baked, never fried. Eggs are concentrated protein; use them with discretion.

Is cheese OK? Americans eat over 28 pounds of cheese per person each year! Saturated fats in cheese make it hard for a healing diet to succeed. Commercial cheese, like milk, is poorly digested by many Americans. Commercial cheeses, even when labeled "natural" contain bleaches, coagulants, emulsifiers, moisture absorbants, mold inhibitors and rind dyes that visibly leak into the cheese itself. Many restaurant and pizza cheeses add synthetic flavors, colors and preservatives. Processed cheese foods (like Velveeta) get their texture from hydrogenated fats rather than natural fermentation. Even if you're not on a healing diet, limit your cheese consumption to small amounts of low-fat or raw cheeses that provide usable proteins with good mineral ratios. Low sodium, low fat cheeses are easy to find, and are a better choice for healing. Raw cheeses are superior in taste and health value to pasteurized cheeses, which have higher salts and additives.

Options to make your cheese choice healthier:

...**Rennet-free cheeses** use a bacterial culture, instead of calves' enzymes to separate curds and whey. Rennet, the dried extract of the enzyme rennin, is derived from the stomach of a suckling calf or a lamb. It speeds up the separation process of cheese making.

...**Real mozzarella cheese** is from buffalo or sheep's milk - low fat, and delicious!

...**Raw cream cheese** is light years ahead of commercial cheese that have gums, fillers and thickeners.

...**Goat cheese (chevre) and sheep's milk cheese (feta)** are both lower in fat than cow's milk cheeses, higher in nutrients like calcium, potassium and magnesium, and more easily digested. There is a world of difference in taste.

...**Rice cheese**, made from cultured rice milk is the newest entry into the healthy cheese market. It's meltable and delicious.

...**Lowfat cottage cheese**, is a good substitute for ricotta, cream cheese and processed cottage cheese foods that are full of chemicals. Usually okay for those with a slight lactose intolerance, cottage cheese mixes with non-fat or low-fat plain yogurt to add the richness of cream or sour cream to recipes without the fat.

...**Yogurt cheese** is easy to make, lighter in fat and calories but with all the richness of sour cream or cream cheese. See page 114 for how to make fresh yogurt cheese. It's also widely available in gourmet stores.

...**Kefir cheese** is an excellent replacement for dairy foods in dips and other recipes. (I like it better.) Available in health food stores, kefir cheese is low in fat and calories and has a slightly tangy, rich flavor that really enhances snack foods. Use it cup for cup in place of sour cream, cottage cheese, cream cheese or ricotta.

...**Tofu** is a white digestible cheesy curd made from fermented soybeans. Tofu is a good replacement for cheese, in texture, taste and nutritional content. It is high in protein, low in fat, extremely versatile, and may be used in place of sour cream, cheese, milk and cottage cheese in cooking. Tofu can even be used in place of eggs in quick breads, cakes, custard-based dishes, quiches and frittatas.

...**Soy cheese**, made from soy milk, is a non-dairy cheese free of lactose and cholesterol. A minute amount of calcium caseinate (milk protein) is added for melting. Mozzarella, cheddar, jack and cream cheese are available. Use it cup for cup in place of cheese.

Apart from the way dairy foods affect your healing ability, there are controversial issues surrounding the manufacture of dairy foods that influence your health.

There is a whirlwind of controversy about rBST (*recombinant bovine somatotrophin*) and rBGH (*recombinant bovine growth hormone*), genetically engineered hormones which increase milk production (some call the tecnique the first use of cloning). However, since America always has a surplus milk supply and long-standing dairy subsidies, it's hard to see why an American dairy farmer would use a potentially harmful hormone in order to produce even more surplus milk. We know little about the long-term effects of these hormones. We do know they increase mastitis infections (inflammation, infection or even cancer) in treated cows, leading to increased use of antibiotics to treat the mastitis. This leads to higher levels of antibiotics and toxins in the milk, widely questioned by scientists and concerned consumers alike. A 1997 study in the International Journal of Health Services, suggests that genetically engineered rBGH may promote breast and colon cancer, acromegaly, hypertension, diabetes and breast growth in men. Even the milk itself from hormone-treated cows is not very wholesome. It has less protein and higher levels of saturated fat. Further, lab animals fed BGH develop thyroid cysts and prostate problems, clear signs of hormone disruption. Research published in The Cancer Letter in 1995 shows that cows who've been treated with hormones have higher levels of insulin growth factor, a known risk factor for breast and prostate cancer, and childhood leukemia. It is an issue that has the whole world divided. Already Europe and Canada have banned the use of growth hormone in dairy cows.

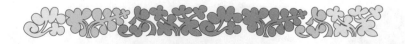

The European Commission has suspended all imports of beef and bovine liver from the U.S. until they become satisfied these imports are produced without the use of hormones. Although our U.S. FDA maintains hormone-injected foods are safe for consumption, I advise caution.

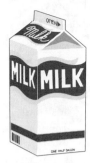

What about antibiotic loading in factory farms? Modern medicine is clearly losing the battle against the onslaught of new drug-resistant pathogens. The Union of Concerned Scientists estimates that an astounding <u>24.6</u> million pounds of antibiotics are fed to animals every year to help fight illness that breaks out in overcrowded, unsanitary feed lots. Antibiotic loading in factory farms means we get low dose antibiotics when we consume commercial dairy products. Today there is a growing body of evidence showing that antibiotic overuse in factory farms is a major contributor to the growing problem of antibiotic-resistance supergerms (particularly antibiotic-resistant foodborne illnesses) in humans.

More worrisome news:

...Pesticides seem to concentrate in the milk of both farm animals and humans. A study by the Environmental Defense Fund found widespread pesticide contamination of human breast milk among 1,400 women in forty-six states (1997). The levels of contamination were twice as high among meat-and-dairy-eating women as among vegetarians.

...Ovarian cancer rates parallel dairy-consumption patterns around the world. The culprit is galactose, a milk sugar from lactose. Women with ovarian cancer often have trouble breaking down galactose. In tests, animals fed galactose develop ovarian cancer. Unlike lactose intolerance, there are no clear signs of digestive upset, but a new series of enzyme tests can tell you whether you lack the proper enzymes.

...Cow's milk is associated with insulin-dependent diabetes. The milk protein bovine serum albumin (BSA) somehow leads to an autoimmune reaction in the pancreas impairing its ability to produce insulin. Exposure to large amounts of cow's milk in the diet may lead to juvenile diabetes.

...Dairy proteins may play a major role in the development of non-Hodgkin's lymphoma, a cancer of the immune system. A 1989 study and a growing consensus among scientists shows that high levels of the cow's milk protein beta-lactoglobulin are found in the blood of lung cancer patients as well.

...Bovine leukemia virus is found in 3 out of 5 dairy cows in the U. S.! In about 80% of U.S. dairy herds, a large percentage are contaminated when the milk is pooled for distribution. Pasteurization, if done correctly, kills the virus, but the issue continues to haunt, because the percentage of cattle with the virus is so large.

Are there good dairy alternatives?

Today there are. I use rice or soy milk and cheese, tofu and nut milks in place of dairy foods. At the least, consider organic, low-fat or non-fat dairy foods, and goat's milk, and raw cheeses instead of pasteurized dairy. (Farmer's markets have raw dairy foods in many states; Georgia and California are the only states who sell raw milk in stores.) Kefir and yogurt, although made from milk, don't have the absorption problems of dairy foods. Unless lactose intolerance is severe, these cultured foods don't cause a lactose reaction, and their friendly flora cultures help you heal without the downside of dairy.

For a long term diet, consider most dairy products as good for taste, but questionable for nutrition. A little is fine.... a lot is not. Small changes in your cooking habits and point of view are all it takes - mostly a matter of not having dairy foods around the house, and substituting dairy-free alternatives in your recipes. (See FOOD EXCHANGES section pg. 259.) Reducing your dairy intake usually means some weight loss, too, with lower blood pressure and cholesterol levels. Soon, you won't feel deprived at all, just delighted.

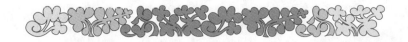

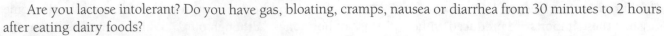
Are you lactose intolerant? Do you have gas, bloating, cramps, nausea or diarrhea from 30 minutes to 2 hours after eating dairy foods?

Some good dairy substitutes.

…**Kefir** is a cultured food made by adding kefir grains (natural milk proteins available at health food stores), to milk and letting the mixture incubate overnight at room temperature to milkshake consistency. Kefir has 350mg of calcium per cup. Use the plain flavor, cup for cup, as a replacement for whole milk; buttermilk for half and half; and use fruit flavors in sweet baked dishes.

…**Soy milk** is nutritious, versatile, smooth and delicious. It is lactose and cholesterol free, (substituting soy milk for dairy milk in your diet can help reduce serum cholesterol). Soy milk contains less calcium and calories than milk, but more protein and iron. It adds a slight rise to baked goods. Use it cup for cup as a milk replacement in cooking; plain flavor for savory dishes; vanilla for sweet dishes or on cereal.

…**Almond milk** is a rich, non-dairy liquid. Use it 1 for 1 in place of milk in baking, sauces, gravies, cream soups and protein drinks. For 1 cup almond milk: place 1 cup blanched almonds in a blender; add 2 to 4 cups water, depending on consistency desired. Add 1 tsp. honey; whirl until smooth. Other nut milks are okay; I like almond the best.

…**Sesame tahini** is rich, creamy, ground sesame seed butter. Use tahini as a dairy replacement in soups, dressings or sauces without the cholesterol yet with all the protein. Mix tahini with water to milk consistency as a milk substitute in baking. Use it in healthy candies and cookies, and on toast in place of peanut butter. Mix tahini with oil and seasonings for an excellent salad topping to greens and salad ingredients.

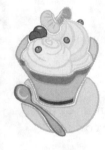

…**Yogurt** helps balance and replace friendly flora in the G.I. tract. Yogurt's culturing process makes it a living food. Yogurt contains more bioavailable protein and easily absorbed calcium than milk, a good thing for people at risk for osteoporosis. Even if you have a lactase enzyme deficiency, bacterial fermentation elements in yogurt actually substitute for the missing enzyme to help you digest lactose. Yogurt also kills the bacteria which causes most ulcers and gastritis. Yogurt boosts blood levels of gamma interferon, a component of the immune system that rallies killer cells to fight infections. The lactic acid bacteria in yogurt lowers levels of enzymes responsible for the development of colon cancer.

Yogurt is a remarkably good food treatment for children with diarrhea, especially if the child's diarrhea is aggravated by antibiotics. Many parents introduce spoonable yogurt to their children early - after about four and six months of age - as soon as the child begins to eat solid food.

What's really low-fat? Here's the strange low-down on low-fat milk.
—Two percent (reduced fat) milk is actually 35% fat.
—One percent (low-fat) milk is actually 25% fat by calories.
—Skim milk is called "fat free" or "non-fat."

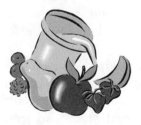

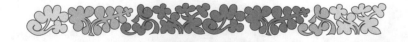

Sugar and Sweeteners: Are They All Bad?

Is the bad health rap on sugar too extreme?

Sugar in America is synonymous with fun, good times and snacking. Our culture instills the powerful urge for sweetness from an early age. Americans eat sugar to "cope" in times of stress and tension.

For the average American, almost 20% of daily calories come from refined white sugar. That works out to about 150 pounds of sugar per year — a substantial amount when you realize that sugar often replaces more nutritious foods in our diets. The news is even worse for our kids who are regularly overdosed on sugar. Today's kids eat enough sugar to count for half of their daily calories! The problem is so out of control that over 46 health advocacy groups signed a letter to the U.S. government in 1998, urging it to commission more funds for studies on sugar before the problem gets worse.

Sugar has so infiltrated our food supply that most of us hardly notice it's there. In fact, in August of 1999, the Center For Science in the Public Interest filed a petition to our FDA to require more explicit labeling of added sugar in foods. Almost all snack foods and pre-prepared foods have added sugar in their ingredients.

Today, sugar qualifies as America's favorite but most poorly understood drug. It's easily the most addictive because it affects so many body systems and is so highly concentrated. (It takes 16 feet of 1-inch diameter sugar cane to produce just 1 teaspoon of refined sugar) Refined sugar only entered into our food supply at the turn of the 18th century.

There's some good news about sugar. It offers quick energy and helps metabolism. In small amounts, sugar offers a brain boost for kids and older adults. It also "closes" our digestive processes. A little sugar actually suppresses appetite, reducing the likelihood of overeating. It's the reason we traditionally eat sweet things at the end of a meal. Sugar can also improve the taste of complex carbohydrate foods, better for us than fatty foods. Actually, some of the warnings about sugar have been overstated. For instance, the sugar in most snacks and desserts is a less-fattening culprit than fat. Fat not only contributes more calories, but the calories are metabolized differently in the body, causing more weight gain than sugar.

Still you should know the problems sugar can cause to your health.

Refined sugar is sucrose, the ultimate naked carbohydrate - stripped of all nutritional benefits. Refined sugars include: white, raw, brown and turbinado, yellow D and sucanat. All sugars can be addictive. Like a drug or alcohol, sugar affects your brain first, with a false energy lift that eventually lets you down lower than when you started. Most sugars add nothing but calories to your body.

A high sugar diet is linked to kidney stones and chronic dental problems. Studies show that sugar accelerates aging by altering cellular proteins and nucleic acids. Too many sugary foods raise insulin production resulting in problems like diabetes and hypoglycemia, high triglycerides and high blood pressure.

Raised insulin is also the body's signal to store fat. Sugar needs insulin for metabolism. Eating a lot of sugar means some of those calories become fat instead of energy. Excess metabolized sugar is transformed into fat globules, and distributed over body storage areas like the stomach, hips and chin.

Too much sugar upsets mineral balances, like magnesium and zinc, too. Sugar especially drains calcium, which advances aging and overloads your body with acid-ash residues responsible for much of arthritic stiffening.

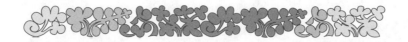

Arthritis and fibromyalgia pain are regularly worsened by a diet high in refined sugar. In addition, a recent animal study shows a diet high in sugar causes osteoporosis, even when calcium intake is adequate. Sugar ties up and dissolves B vitamins, producing over-acid conditions that become gout, nerve, gum and digestive problems. Sugar also robs the body of the trace mineral, chromium. Taking chromium supplements can help reduce sugar cravings and balance blood sugar levels. Hyperactivity and Attention Deficit Disorder (ADD), affecting up to 10% of children today, are clearly aggravated by a high sugar diet.

A high sugar diet raises your risk for infection because it provides a breeding ground for staph and yeast infections. Bacteria, candida, cancer, fungi and parasites thrive on sugary foods. Excess sugar depresses immune response to fight these problems, too. Sugar destroys the ability of white blood cells to kill germs for up to 5 hours after consumption!

Refined sugar is linked to high cholesterol, heart disease and coronary thrombosis. New data implicates sugar in nearsightedness and skin problems like eczema, psoriasis and dermatitis. A study at the University of Alabama shows that people suffering from depression have less symptoms when sugar is removed from their diets. Other research shows that when women switch from a diet high in sugar to a sugar-free, high nutrient diet, their food addictive behavior stops.

Unfortunately, it doesn't stop there.

Personality-changing, mental and emotional signs of too much sugar:
— irritability, irrational mood swings
— chronic or frequent bouts of anxiety and panic attacks
— unexplained depression with manic-depressive tendencies
— poor concentration, hyperactivity, forgetfulness or absentmindedness
— loss of enthusiasm and motivation
— uncharacteristic undependability, inconsistent thoughts and actions
— moody personality changes with emotional outbursts

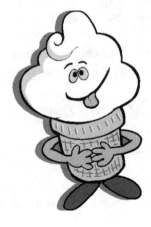

Physical effects of eating too much sugar:
— anxiety episodes and panic attacks
— bulimia eating disorder
— candidiasis and chronic fatigue syndrome
— diabetes and-or hypoglycemia
— food addiction with loss of B-vitamins and minerals
— menopausal mood swings and unusual low energy periods
— obesity (sugar raises insulin, your body's signal to make fat)
— shakiness; excessive, unexplained sweating
— high cholesterol and triglycerides leading to risk of atherosclerosis
— excessive emotional swings and food cravings, especially before menstruation
— tooth decay and gum disease

Sugar does interfere in a healing program. Foods that affect your sugar balance have a major impact. Glucose is the main sugar in the blood and brain. Under ideal conditions, glucose is released into the bloodstream slowly to maintain balanced blood sugar levels. (Eating small amounts of sugary foods after a meal or in combination with foods high in protein and essential fatty acids slows their absorption.)

Small blood sugar fluctuations disturb one's feeling of well being. Large blood sugar fluctuations cause feelings of depression, anxiety, mood swings, fatigue, even aggressive behavior. Today, millions of Americans can't use glucose correctly. Over 60% of the population suffers from some degree of the "blood sugar blues." At least twenty million of us suffer from diabetes (high blood sugar) or hypoglycemia (low blood sugar).

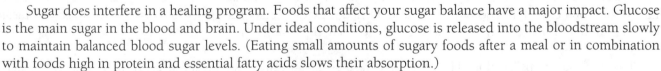

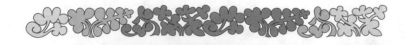

Hypoglycemia, often called a "sugar epidemic" in America is widespread in every industrialized country today. It's a direct effect of too much sugar and refined carbohydrates, coupled with low fiber foods. The pancreas reacts to too much sugar by producing too much insulin. The excess insulin lowers blood sugar too much as the body strives to achieve normal glucose-insulin balance. Hypoglycemia results.

Hypoglycemia is marked by dozens of unpleasant symptoms, especially in the way the brain functions. The brain requires glucose as an energy source to think clearly, and is the most sensitive organ to blood sugar levels. Worst case scenario reactions of hypoglycemia can even range to unconsciousness or death.

Diabetes, another "sugar epidemic" rising by leaps and bounds, also results from too much sugar, refined carbohydrates and caffeine. The number of 30 year olds diagnosed with diabetes has increased 70 percent, in just the last ten years! Chronic hypoglycemia often precedes diabetes. When your body doesn't use carbohydrates correctly, it may produce too little insulin, so blood sugar levels stay too high. The pancreas can't work properly; and glucose can't enter the cells to provide energy. Instead, it accumulates in the blood, resulting in serious symptoms from mental confusion to uncontrollable obesity, blindness, even coma.

While seeming to be opposite problems, diabetes and hypoglycemia really stem from the same cause — an imbalance between glucose and oxygen in the body. Poor nutrition, the common cause of both disorders, can be improved with a high mineral, high fiber diet, adequate protein, small frequent meals, and regular mild exercise. If you have either condition, there must be diet and lifestyle change for there to be a real or permanent cure. Alcohol, caffeine, refined sugars and tobacco must be avoided.

Note: Even though poor sugar metabolism is the cause of both diabetes and hypoglycemia, the different effects of each problem call for specific modifications. Get better body response by addressing low blood sugar and high blood sugar separately. See Diabetes and Hypoglycemia Diets, pages 396 and 463 in this book.

There are good, healthy alternatives to refined sugar.

Just because you follow a sugar-free diet doesn't mean you have to give up good taste or sweet comforts. In moderation, your body easily metabolizes whole food sweeteners like honey, molasses, maple syrup, fruit juice or barley malt which can satisfy your sweet tooth. Clinical tests on crystalline fructose, and the herbs stevia and gymnema sylvestre, are good news for sugar disorders. These natural sweeteners are heros in the effort to control sugar balance and sugar cravings. But they do not eliminate hypoglycemia or diabetes. Only a better diet and regular exercise can make a permanent difference.

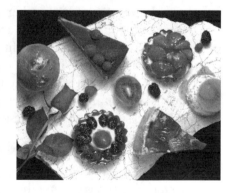

Note: Always look for the least processed sweetener. Most commercial sweeteners bear no resemblance to their natural counterpart. For example, before cane sugar (the worst culprit), is refined and bleached, it is rich in vitamins and minerals.

Sweet choices to consider for your healing diet:

Fructose is a commercial sugar with the same molecular structure as that in fruit. It is called fruit sugar, but it's usually made from corn starch. It has a low glycemic index, releasing its glucose into the bloodstream slowly. Fructose produces liver glycogen rapidly making it a more efficient energy supply than other sweeteners. It is almost twice as sweet as sugar, so less is needed for the same sweetening power.

Fructose may be the sweetener of choice in a weight loss diet. In clinical tests, people who drank liquids sweetened with fructose before meals ate 20 to 40% fewer calories than normal, more than compensating for the 200 calories in the fructose. Those who drank liquids sweetened with table sugar ate 10 to 15% fewer calories; those who drank liquids sweetened with NutraSweet, Equal or aspartame (chemical sweeteners widely used in drinks and snack foods), ate the same calories as normal. Fructose also helps people pick foods with less fats. Dental health studies report less plaque and tarter with fructose than with sugar.

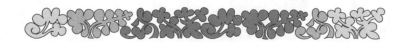

Fructose is so easy to use and so efficient in its sweetening power that it is as common in commercially prepared foods today as sucrose. Does it have the same drawbacks? Fructose chemical stucture has highly reactive molecules which bind to protein molecules, sometimes altering the structure of critical enzymes and their proteins. This protein-fructose interaction may cause major organ damage if you have diabetes. Fructose labeling can be a problem as well. Fructose products can be pure fructose, or 90% fructose, or high fructose corn syrup (55% fructose that has a high percentage of glucose requiring insulin for metabolism). Fructose also inhibits copper absorption, essential to the production of hemoglobin which is linked to coronary problems. Studies in Israel reveal that rats fed a high fructose diet age faster and show deteriorating collagen changes that relate to premature skin wrinkling and sagging. Fructose may also stimulate high cholesterol levels.

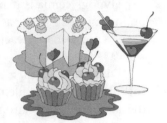

Bottom line? There are some advantages to fructose used in moderation, but if you are hypoglycemic or diabetic, fructose is still sugar and should be avoided.

Stevia rebaudiana (sweet herb), has been used as a natural sweetener in South America for over 1500 years. It is non-caloric, and about 25 times sweeter than sugar when made as an infusion with 1 tsp. leaves to 1 cup of water. Two drops of the infusion equal 1 tsp. of sugar in sweetness. In baking, 1 tsp. finely ground stevia powder equals 1 cup of sugar. If you decide to use stevia (I recommend it), experiment with it. Adding too much stevia to meals can produce a licorice-like after taste; adding too little won't sweeten adequately.

Tests show stevia helps regulate blood sugar. In South America, stevia is sold as a health aid to people with diabetes and hypoglycemia, because it helps lower high blood pressure but does not affect normal blood pressure. Many stevia users say it inhibits tooth decay, aids mental alertness, counteracts fatigue and improves digestion. Most stevia users say they have less desire for tobacco and alcohol.

Experts say that stevia may soon be regarded as one of the Earth's good-for-you sweeteners. Clinical studies show it safe even in cases of severe sugar imbalance. In the 1970's, the Japanese refined the glycosides from stevia to make a product called Stevioside, 300 times sweeter than sugar. Stevioside is widely used as a non-calorie sweetener in South America and Asia where it enjoys a 42% share of the food sweetener market. Still, while Stevioside does not affect blood glucose levels and is a good sweetener for both diabetics and hypoglycemics, it does not retain the extraordinary healing benefits of whole stevia leaves and extract.

Stevia is effective for weight control because it contains no calories, yet significantly increases glucose tolerance. Research shows that stevia may block fat absorption, too. People whose weight loss problems stem from sugar cravings benefit most from stevia. They experience reduced desire for sugary foods.

Today, stevia is sold on the market as a dietary supplement after a decade-long FDA ban, heavily influenced by Nutrasweet politics.

Luohan fruit: Found in the mountainous region of southern China, luohan is a low glycemic, non-caloric sweetener 20 times sweeter than sugar. Luohan has been used for centuries in Traditional Chinese Medicine (TCM) to help treat coughs, colds, bronchitis, constipation, even diabetes. According to TCM, luohan promotes the proper flow of energy (Qi), and has a harmonizing, balancing effect on the spleen and stomach. It is rich in minerals (esp. zinc and selenium), essential fatty acids and amino acids. In addition, luohan promotes fat burning, does not affect blood sugar adversely, and is safe for diabetics and hypoglycemics. Preliminary tests indicate luohan fruit can inhibit tooth decay and pathogenic bacteria that lead to stomach problems. About ¼ of the whole fruit can be used to sweeten 8-oz. of water. Luohan concentrates are also available, and are convenient and easy to use. I've tried, and like Herbasway HerbaSwee luohan liquid.

Date sugar is ground, dried dates. It is the least refined, most natural sweetener. It has the same nutrient values as dried dates—about half as sweet as sugar. Use like brown sugar. In baking, mix with water before adding to the recipe to prevent burning, or add as a sweet topping after removing your dish from the oven.

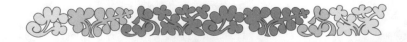

Gymnema sylvestre is an herb that curbs cravings for sweet foods and reduces blood sugar levels after sugar consumption. Gymnema's molecular structure, similar to that of sugar, can block absorption of up to 50% of sugar calories. Both sugar and gymnema are digested in the small intestine, but the larger molecule of gymnema cannot be fully absorbed. So, taken before sugar, the gymnema molecule blocks the passages through which sugar is normally absorbed.... far fewer sugar calories get assimilated. If you eat a 400 calorie, sugary dessert, only 200 of the sugar calories are absorbed. The remaining sugar is eliminated as waste.

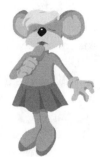

Take the gymnema taste test. Taste something sweet, then swish a sip of gymnema sylvestre tea in your mouth. Now taste something sweet again. You will not be able to taste the sugar, because gymnemic acid prevents the taste buds in your mouth from being activated by sugar molecules in the food. Gymnema blocks the taste of the sugar in your mouth in the same way it blocks sugar in digestion.

Gymnema has obvious uses for diabetes. It helps lower glucose significantly for diabetics, and may help lower their cholesterol and triglycerides. Gymnema can actually enhance insulin production in both Type I and Type II diabetics to regenerate pancreatic cells. Gymnema is regularly recommended to help control diabetes in India. Take with GTF Chromium for best results.

FOS (Fructo-oligo-saccharides) are compounds found naturally in foods like bananas, onions, garlic, artichokes, barley, tomatoes, rye, honey, and asparagus. They're only half as sweet as sugar. FOS are not digested in the stomach, they pass untouched into the large intestine where friendly intestinal flora consume them as nourishment. More significant, the by-products of FOS consumption are healthy EFA's, which are absorbed by the walls of the large intestine and used for energy. Studies show no harmful links for FOS. They do not affect DNA nor promote cancer. Try Crystal Star DR. PROBIOTICS™ with FOS.

The advantages of FOS:
...FOS feeds beneficial bacteria, while starving harmful bacteria
...FOS relieves constipation
...FOS stops antibiotic-induced yeast
...FOS lowers cholesterol and triglyceride levels
...FOS inhibits formation of cavities
...FOS lowers blood sugar levels in diabetics

Note: Use FOS as a partial replacement for sugar in recipes. Too much (more than 40 grams) can cause loose stools, since FOS are not digested. Use FOS as a nutritional enhancement rather than a replacement.

Blackstrap molasses is the liquid sludge after sucrose is extracted from the cane sugar refining process. Rich in minerals and vitamins, molasses has more calcium, ounce for ounce, than milk, more iron than eggs, and more potassium than any other food. The amounts of B vitamins, pantothenic acid, iron, inositol and vitamin E make it an effective treatment for restoring thin and fading hair.

Sorghum molasses is concentrated sorghum juice, a grain related to millet. It is similar to molasses but with lighter, milder flavor. Sorghum is made by crushing the plant stalks then boiling the juice into a syrup.

Corn syrup is commercial glucose made from chemically purified cornstarch with everything removed except the starch. Most corn syrup has sugar syrup added to it because glucose is only half as sweet as white sugar. It is highly refined and absorbed into the bloodstream very quickly.

Fruit juice concentrate is a highly processed product with about 68% soluble sugar. It contains measurable vitamins and minerals, and promotes slower digestion. Refined sugars raise serotonin levels in the brain, which can make you feel drowsy. Unrefined fruit sweeteners have less impact on brain chemistry because natural fruit sugars do not affect serotonin levels.

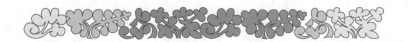

Barley malt and brown rice syrups are mild, natural sweeteners made from barley sprouts, or cultured rice and water cooked to a syrup. Only 40% as sweet as sugar, barley malt's blood sugar activity is a slow, complex carbohydrate release that does not upset insulin levels. **Amazake** is a pudding-like sweetener made from organic brown rice. The rice is cooked, then injected with koji, the *Aspergillus* enzyme culture used in miso and shoyu. Amazake is 21% sugar, mainly glucose and maltose, and is high in B complex and iron.

Turbinado sugar is raw sugar refined by washing in a centrifuge so that surface molasses is removed. It goes through the same refining process as white sugar, just short of the final extraction of molasses, and is essentially the same as white sugar.

Honey is a mixture of sugars formed from nectar in the bodies of bees. A natural sweetener with bioactive, antibiotic and antiseptic properties, honey contains all the vitamins, minerals and enzymes necessary for proper metabolism and digestion of glucose and other sugars. Still, honey is almost twice as sweet as sugar. Avoid it if you have candidiasis or diabetes; use it with great care if you are hypoglycemic.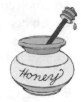

Maple syrup is made from sugar maple tree sap. It takes 30 to 40 gallons of sap to make one gallon of syrup. Unless labeled pure maple syrup, it may be mixed with corn syrup or other additives to cut its cost. **Maple sugar** is crystallized maple syrup.

Sucanat, (an acronym from <u>su</u>gar <u>ca</u>ne <u>nat</u>ural) is the trade name for a sweetener made from dried granulated cane juice, available in health food stores. Its average sugar content is 85%, with complex sugars, vitamins, minerals, amino acids and molasses retained. Use 1 to 1 in place of sugar. It is still a concentrated sweetener; use carefully if you have sugar balance problems.

Xylitol, a sweetener derived from plums, birchwood chips, strawberries, and corn which is safe for diabetics and hypoglycemics. Just as sweet as table sugar but with ⅓ fewer calories, xylitol works well to sweeten cereals and hot drinks, but doesn't work well for baking. Apart from its sweetening ability, xylitol is becoming well known today for its role in fighting infections, tooth decay, and sinusitis (esp. in a nasal spray). It can cause diarrhea in susceptible people; Use xylitol sparingly until you become used to it.

The following chart helps you convert your favorite recipes from sugar to natural sweeteners. If you have serious blood sugar problems, like diabetes or hypoglycemia, consult the appropriate diet pages in this book or your healing professional, about the kind and amount of sweets your body can handle.

Sweetener substitution amounts are for each cup of sugar:

Substitute Sweetener	Amount	Reduce Liquid in the Recipe
•Fructose	⅓ to ⅔ cup	....
•Maple Syrup	⅓ to ⅔ cup	¼ cup
•Honey	½ cup	¼ cup
•Molasses	½ cup	¼ cup
•Barley or Rice Syrup	1 to 1¼ cups	¼ cup
•Date Sugar	1 cup	....
•Sucanat	1 cup	....
•Apple/Pear Juice	1 cup	¼ cup
•Xylitol	1 cup	....

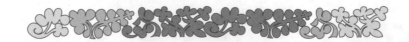

What about aspartame, and its brand names, Nutrasweet and Equal?

The FDA has received more complaints about adverse reactions to aspartame than any other food ingredient in the agency's history! In fact, 75% of the complaints reported to the FDA's Adverse Reaction Monitoring System are for aspartame-related symptoms. Yet, we get an incredible amount of these chemical sweeteners in our food. At least 30% of the U.S. population is sensitive to even moderate doses of aspartame and may suffer several symptoms.

Health problems related to synthetic sweeteners are not new. They've been a market-submerged health risk for decades. Saccharin has been used for 100 years, even though its involvement in bladder cancer from the 50's to the 70's was undeniable. NutraSweet and Equal have taken the place of saccharin in pre-prepared foods and drinks. Americans are consuming more of these sweeteners than ever.

Aspartame, 200 times sweeter than sugar, is a combination of two amino acids with neurotransmitter effects — phenylalanine and aspartic acid. PKU seizures (phenylketonuria) result when the body can't effectively metabolize phenylalanine. High levels of the amino acid phenylalanine in body fluids can cause brain damage in anyone. All aspartame products include a warning that the sweetener contains phenylalanine.

Aspartame is clearly linked to blood sugar use problems — high blood pressure, insomnia, hypoglycemia, diabetes, ovarian cancer and brain tumors. One study shows that the more NutraSweet consumed, the more likely tumors are to develop. Aspartame is also associated with brain damage in fetuses.

There are immediate, serious reactions to aspartame..... severe headaches, extreme dizziness, attention difficulties, memory loss, slurred speech, throat swelling, allergic effects, and retina deterioration (generally attributed to methyl-alcohol, a substance released when aspartame breaks down.) Dangerous side effects are worse when NutraSweet is used hot or cooked, as it is in pre-prepared foods. Adverse effects are reversible when NutraSweet consumption is stopped.

Over time, methanol toxicity from aspartame can mimic the symptoms of multiple sclerosis and lupus, both diseases common for diet soda drinkers. In fact, many cases of M.S. and lupus are actually misdiagnosed. Sometimes just eliminating aspartame can cause a complete remission of symptoms.

More recent worrisome news:

1: Aspartame may be a cause of Gulf War Syndrome! Diet soda sweetened with aspartame was left sitting in the blistering desert heat for weeks at a time for our troops in Desert Storm. By the time our soldiers drank them, aspartame's chemical structure was so altered by the heat it made people sick right away.

2: Grand mal seizures are another side effect of aspartame, especially serious for pilots or people flying. Aspartame contains 10% methanol which can cause oxygen deprivation. At high altitudes, this effect is magnified, sometimes causing sudden memory loss, visual problems and epileptic seizures. Reports in the magazines Flying Safety and Navy Physiology recounted several instances where pilots who had Equal in their coffee went into epileptic convulsions!

3: Although marketed as a weight control aid, aspartame can actually <u>increase</u> appetite, and cravings for sweets, especially for people with blood sugar disorders. Especially avoid aspartame sweeteners if you have sugar sensitivities, genetic PKU, advanced liver disease, are allergy-prone or pregnant.

Despite a huge health outcry, the synthetic sweetener problem isn't going away. It's just changing. Here's how the next generation of sweeteners can affect you:

—**Acesulfame K, acesulfame potassium**, an organic salt, entered the U.S. market in 1988, under the brand names Sunette, Sweet One and Swiss Sweet table sweeteners. It is 200 times sweeter than sugar and boosts the sweetening effect of other sweeteners. It passes through the human digestive system unchanged, and therefore is non-caloric. Ninety studies on its safety were submitted to the FDA.

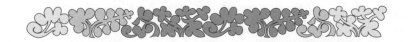

Some of this research indicates that acesulfame potassium may not be so safe after all. Animal tests show it aggravates reactive hypoglycemia, produces lung tumors, breast tumors, thymus tumors, some forms of leukemia, and respiratory disease even when less-than-maximum doses were given. In fact, the Center for Science in the Public Interest petitioned the FDA in l988 for a stay of approval because of "significant doubt" about acesulfame potassium's safety.

—**Sucralose, chlorinated sucrose (Splenda)**, 400 to 800 times sweeter than sugar, has recently been approved in the U.S.and is heavily advertised. Sucralose is seen as a chemical by your body, not as a carbohydrate, so it has no effect on insulin secretion or carbohydrate metabolism. However, recent evidence suggests sucralose may disrupt glucose levels for diabetes. While the manufacturer states the absorption of sucralose is very limited, research from the Japanese Food Sanitation Council reveals that up to 40% of this sweetening chemical is absorbed, and may concentrate in the liver, kidneys and gastrointestinal tract. It could be unsafe to try and convert this concentrated sweetener to sugar amounts in baking.

Original FDA studies concluded sucralose was not carcinogenic and did not cause significant genetic change, birth defects, brain or nerve damage. Forty studies determined it was biodegradable, safe for plant and aquatic life. However, some experts feel the original data was flawed, and that sucralose may pose hazards to human health and to the environment. In animal tests, sucralose is linked to a 40% shrinkage of the thymus gland; atrophy of the lymph follicles in the spleen and thymus; enlarged liver and kidneys; decreased red blood cell count; aborted pregnancy; and diarrhea.

—**Alitame, brand name ACLAME**, is formed from the amino acids l-aspartic acid and L-alanine, chemically similar to aspartame. It is 2,000 times sweeter than sucrose. Alitame is hydrolyzed to release aspartic acid, metabolized normally in the body, then excreted in urine and feces. Fifteen studies indicate that alitame is safe at a dose of 100 mg/kg per day. However, the FDA, bowing to the negative publicity from aspartame (alitame is even more concentrated), is delaying approval in the U.S. pending further tests. Alitame is already being used in foods and beverages in Australia, New Zealand, Mexico and China.

Beware of these chemical sweeteners on food labels if you have sugar-related problems:

• **Dextrose**, a plant monosaccharide, synthetically derived from cornstarch.
• **Lactose, milk sugar**, a di-saccharide sweetener mainly in infant foods and baked goods. May cause gastrointestinal disturbances in lactose intolerant people.
• **Maltose, malt sugar**, a disaccharide often synthetically derived from corn syrup. It does not normally stimulate insulin production.

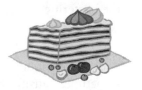

• **Sorbitol,** derived from corn, is absorbed slowly. It is used in diabetic foods because it needs little insulin and does not promote tooth decay. Can cause diarrhea.
• **Raw sugar**, a granulated, evaporated sugar cane juice product. It is 98% sucrose.
• **Saccharin,** made of petroleum and toluene, a solvent used to stop knocks in gasoline engines, is 300 times sweeter than sugar and calorie free, but is linked to bladder cancer. The FDA tried to ban saccharin in 1977, but relented under industry pressure. It is now sold with a warning label, but has largely been replaced by Nutrasweet and Equal. It does not metabolize, is excreted quickly and does not build up in the body.
• **Agave Nectar** is a new, high fructose sweetener. It's 90% solids, a percentage much greater than traditional high fructose corn syrup. (This amount of fructose may aggravate a copper deficiency linked to coronary problems.) Agave tastes like honey, but has a lower glycemic index. More testing is being done, but agave nectar is a new generation sweetener to look for soon.

Is there a healthy diet that won't stimulate over-production of insulin but will allow normal blood sugar activity? Can we control hunger all day, and manage our weight without starving?

A ***low glycemic diet*** is a good answer, both to regulate blood sugar and to control a sugar craver's weight. What is a low glycemic diet? It's a diet that keeps insulin levels low meaning fewer calories are turned into fat and more are burned for energy, resulting in weight loss. A low-glycemic diet is low in fats and total calories, largely vegetarian, with most proteins from vegetable sources. It includes mono-unsaturated oils like olive or canola oil.

Whole foods, especially whole grains and fresh vegetables, have a low-glycemic index. They don't elevate blood sugar after a meal like sugary, high-glycemic index foods which put blood sugar on a roller coaster and elevate it too rapidly. Insulin responds immediately to stimulate fat production. Too much insulin also causes too much sugar storage, which then results in low blood sugar. Low blood sugar causes stress-hormone release, fatigue and ultimately ravenous hunger. The process begins all over again.

Plant fiber from whole foods also regulates digestion for more balanced blood sugar levels. Plant fiber binds with most fats to prevent their absorption. In addition, plant fiber foods speed up bowel transit time to take stress off your liver so it can metabolize fats efficiently. Eat whole grains, legumes, fresh fruits and vegetables, seafood, sea greens, soy foods and brown rice frequently. They are high fiber foods that will help stabilize blood sugar swings and lessen cravings for sugar. Seafood, soy foods and legumes offer high quality protein which is essential to sugar balance. Some spices like cinnamon, clove and bay leaf also help control both blood sugar levels and sugar cravings.

By combining low glycemic foods, like high fiber foods, along with exercise and certain nutritional supplements that help balance your blood sugar, you can optimize brain biochemistry. You'll feel more comfortable while dieting, and can diet without binging.

Nutrients that help reduce sugar cravings and withdrawal are B vitamins, vitamin C, zinc, trace minerals, the amino acid L-glutamine and chromium. Chromium helps insulin work more efficiently at removing sugar from the blood. Glutamine is used directly by the brain and is helpful in reducing sugar craving.

For longer life and better health, use sugar sparingly, on special occasions.

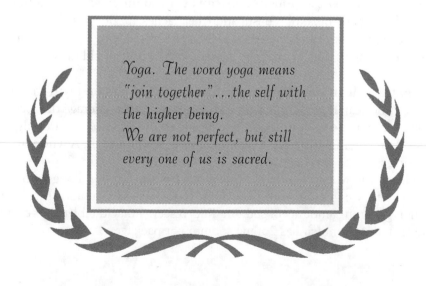

Yoga. The word yoga means "join together"...the self with the higher being.
We are not perfect, but still every one of us is sacred.

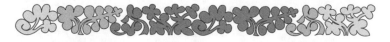

A Low Salt Diet for Healing

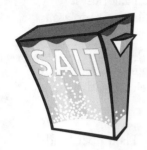

In the past generation, Americans have consumed more NaCl than ever before—too much restaurant food, too many refined foods and too many animal foods. Heart disease, hypertension and high blood pressure have increased correspondingly, so most people are aware that excessive salt is a diet problem. Too much salt constricts circulation, and causes kidneys to retain fluid and migraines to occur frequently. Like too much sugar, salt is a cause of hyperactivity and aggressive behavior. The average American adult consumes between 8,000 and 10,000mg of sodium a day.

Nutrition and medical studies are replete with the negative effects of salt. Yet, sodium is a necessary nutrient for good health and essential to human existence. In ancient times, salt was so valuable that men traded it for its weight in gold. Today's media medicine teaches us that salt is dangerous and that the public should avoid it. But, while certain individuals who are salt-sensitive must curb their intake, most Americans do not suffer ill effects when they use salt sensibly in their diets.

Naturally occurring sodium, accompanied by its partner mineral, potassium, regulates blood pressure, transmits nerve impulses and maintains muscle activity. Together, sodium and potassium pump nutrients into the cells to nourish them, and drain waste products out of them to clean. The sodium-potassium relationship also helps maintain fluid balance, so you don't retain excess fluid or get dehydrated.

We need salinity for good body tone because sodium is necessary for muscles to contract. It is needed for strong blood.... without sodium, the body cannot use calcium. Sodium helps keep body pH balanced. It transports nutrients and nerve impulses. It keeps glands and organs healthy, and produces hydrochloric acid so we can digest our food. Too little sodium leads to low vitality, stagnate blood and loss of clear thinking, because the brain depends on good fluid circulation.

Sodium is critical to blood pressure balance. Table salt is 40% sodium and 60% chloride; it's the sodium that affects blood pressure. A sodium-restricted diet for hypertension ranges from 1,000 to 3,000mg a day. Our bodies need about 500 milligrams (¼ teaspoon) of sodium to help regulate the distribution of body fluids. Sodium restriction has no effect on the blood pressure of people who have normal blood pressure.

Do you have too little salt? Signs of sodium deficiency include <u>low</u> blood pressure, weakness, flatulence, diarrhea, and unexplained nausea. Tissue dehydration causes wrinkles and sunken eyes. Poor fluid circulation in the brain causes confusion, irritability and heightened allergies. Diuretics, excessive sweating, fever, diarrhea, heat, even exercise can cause severe sodium imbalance, and make your body lose too much salt.

The overwhelming evidence shows most Americans eat too much salt..... up to 6,000mg a day! PMS symptoms like breast tenderness and bloating, constipation, headaches, dizziness, asthma, fatigue, increased urinary excretion of calcium (increased risk of kidney stones and osteoporosis), ringing in the ears and body weakness. Beyond extra salty food, cortisone drugs or anabolic steroids causes us to build up salt.

Where does the extra salt in our diets come from? It is a common myth that table salt is the major source of sodium in the American diet. Ten percent of the sodium in the average diet occurs naturally in food, 15 percent comes from salt you add to your food, (one teaspoon of salt = about 2,000mg of sodium). But most salt is added during food processing - up to 4,000 milligrams of sodium a day. A whopping 75 percent is added to food during processing.

Junk and fast foods are the worst offenders. A steady diet of these foods along with high blood pressure is an explosive health situation. We get salt from medicines, too. Over-the-counter drugs like antacids, laxatives, and sleeping aids contain generous amounts of sodium. Effervescent antacid tablets, for example, contain 276mg sodium per tablet and Instant Metamucil has 250mg sodium per package.

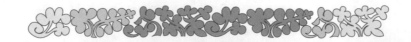

Sodium-containing ingredients that you may not recognize on a label include: sodium caseinate, monosodium glutamate, trisodium phosphate, sodium bicarbonate and sodium sterol lactate.

The Average American consumes 8000 - 10,000mg of salt a day.
1: Ten hard, salted pretzel twists 2400mg
2: 1 large dill pickle 1700mg
3: Macaroni and cheese (1 cup)...1343mg
4: 1 cup Campbell's Tomato-Rice soup 1480mg
5: 1 tablespoon tamari soy sauce 960mg
6: Stouffer's Chicken Stir-Fry with Veggies 630mg
7: 1 cup canned French cut green beans 780mg
8: Cottage cheese (¼ cup) 457mg
9: One shake of the salt shaker...250mg
10: 6 large black olives..230mg
11: Light tuna (½ can) 287mg

Fat-free foods usually have even more salt to compensate for the lack of flavor from fat. Fat-free mayonnaise, margarine and cream cheese, for example, can have double the sodium content of their fattier counterparts.

There are many good ways to get the good salts that your body needs:
1: Sea greens' salty taste is really a balanced mineral chelate.
2: Herb salts and seasonings provide plant enzymes to make salts absorbable.
3: Sea salt contains traces of magnesium, iron, potassium and many minerals besides sodium.
4: Tamari is a wheat-free soy sauce, lower in sodium and richer in flavor than soy sauce.
5: Umeboshi plums are highly alkalizing, excellent for a macrobiotic diet.
6: Naturally fermented foods like pickles, relishes and olives are also healthy cultured foods.
7: Bragg's LIQUID AMINOS is an energizing protein broth, with valuable amino acids.
8: Miso is a salty-tasting soy paste made from cooked, aged soybeans.
9: Gomashio blends sesame seeds and sea salt, a delicious staple in oriental cooking.
10. Sea salt is higher in trace minerals, tastes good and is a good substitute in moderation for regular table salt. Sea salt contains little iodine, so add sea greens and sea foods, rich in iodine, for your ongoing diet.

A salt-free diet may be desirable for someone who eats too much salt. However, once the body's salinity normalizes, some salt should be brought back into the diet quickly.

LOW SALT, NOT NO SALT, is best for a permanent way of eating.
Don't worry about sodium deficiency; even a low sodium diet has 2,400mg.

Sea Greens....Therapy from the Ocean

In the West, we eat land vegetables for our main source of greens, but vegetables from the sea are nutritious foods and powerful healers. Sea greens are some of the oldest living species on Earth. Biologists say that marine algae are the ancestors of literally <u>every</u> land vegetable we know today! We have remnants of Stone Age sea greens meals from Australia. We have medicinal records using sea greens from 3000 B.C. in China. The Greeks did, and still do use sea greens as dietary healers. When we eat sea greens, we are tapping into the ancestral and restorative source of all life- the ocean.

Sea greens are really large, multicelled algae with superior nutritional content. They transmit the energies of the sea to your body as a rich source of nutrients. Ounce for ounce, along with herbs, they are higher in vitamins and minerals than any other food. Sea greens are one of nature's richest sources of vegetable protein, and they provide full-spectrum concentrations of beta carotene, chlorophyll, enzymes, amino acids, fiber, and octacosonal for tissue oxygenation. The distinctive salty taste is not just "salt," but a balanced, chelated combination of sodium, potassium, calcium, magnesium, phosphorus, iron and trace minerals.

Sea greens help re-mineralize us. They convert inorganic ocean minerals into organic mineral salts that combine with amino acids. Our bodies use this combination as an ideal way to get usable nutrients for structural building blocks. In fact, sea greens contain all the necessary trace elements for life, many of which are depleted in the Earth's soil.

The same 56 elements that circulate in sea water course through our veins. Sea plant chemical composition is so close to human plasma that perhaps the greatest benefit from sea greens is promoting our internal rebalance. Sea greens act as the ocean's purifiers, and they perform many of the same functions for our bodies. Their rich antioxidant qualities are effective toxin scavengers for detoxification. Sea greens help normalize our bodies from the effects of a modern diet. They strengthen us against disease, and reduce excess stores of fluid and fat.

Sea greens are powerful healers. They have anti-inflammatory, antiviral, antimicrobial, antifungal, and anticancer activity. Sea greens algin is the element largely responsible for sea plant's success in treating obesity, asthma and arteriosclerosis. Algin absorbs toxins from our digestive tracts in much the same way that a water softener removes the hardness from tap water. Less toxins enter our bloodstream because of algin's activity.

Sea greens are the most nutritionally dense plants on the planet.
They access all the nutrients in the ocean, acquiring nourishment across its entire surface through wave action and underwater currents. Sea greens are rich in fiber and packed with vitamins, with measureable amounts of vitamins K, A, D, B, E and C, and a broad range of carotenes. Sea greens are almost the only non-animal source of vitamin B-12 for our cell development and nerve function. They are full of amino acids, up to 20% protein, active enzymes and essential fatty acids to rejuvenate us. They contain 10 to 20 times the minerals of land plants. Beyond their mineral quantities, their mineral balance is a natural stabilizer for sound nerve structure and good metabolism. Sea plant iodine, for example, helps control and prevent gland disorders like breast and uterine fibroids, prostate inflammation and adrenal exhaustion.

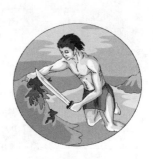

Some of the things sea greens can do for you:

1: **Sea greens and our destructive environment:** Sea greens cleanse and purify all the world's oceans- they can do the same for your body. Sea plants can protect us from a wide range of toxic elements in the environment, including heavy metals (most dental fillings still contain them) and radiation by-products, converting them into harmless salts that our bodies can eliminate. The natural iodine in sea greens can reduce by almost 80% the radioactive iodine-131 absorbed by the thyroid. Sea greens are so effective that the U.S. Atomic Energy Commission recommends that people consume two to three ounces of sea greens a week (or 2 tbsp. of algin supplements a day) for maximum protection against radiation poisoning. Still, although seaweeds contain the compounds that directly counteract carcinogens, most researchers believe that they have even more value in boosting the body's immune system so it can combat the carcinogens itself. Japanese studies reveal that seaweed extracts boost immune response by stimulating white blood cells found in the lymph nodes, spleen, thymus and tonsils.

2: **Sea greens and cancer:** Sea greens carry powerful antioxidant and anti-cancer activity, to arrest the proliferation of cancer cells. Some experts consider them more potent than the drugs used to treat breast and prostate cancer, especially as interceptive measures. Over 47 different varieties of sea greens are known to possess anti-cancer activity. Japanese studies show that a diet with as little as 5% sea greens inhibits cancer growth, even causing remission of some active tumors. Green laver, a sea lettuce, in particular, contains oligosaccharides which may prevent cancer cell replication.

Increased breast cancer risk is clearly linked to iodine deficiency and hypothyroidism. Japanese women have less than one-sixth the breast cancer rate of American women of similar age. Japanese women who live in rural areas have a much lower breast cancer rate than Japanese women in urban areas. The determining factor seems to be diet. The rural Japanese women routinely eat sea plants.... a food uncommon in the diets of American and urban Japanese women who eat many processed foods. In animal studies, rats exposed to chemicals known to cause breast cancer were fed sea greens and were protected against getting cancer. One in vitro study shows L-tryptophan from kelp, not normally associated with cancer protection, inhibits breast cancer.

Women with low iodine levels often have cervical hyperplasia and breast fibroids, too. In clinical trials, hyperplasia lesions have been corrected by sea plants. My own experience with sea plant iodine shows that it reduces both breast and uterine fibroids, with significant anti-inflammatory and anti-scarring effects.

3: **Sea greens and bone health:** Sea greens are loaded with body building minerals like calcium, iron, iodine and potassium. Just one-half cup of cooked hijiki contains more iron than two eggs and the same amount of calcium as a half-cup of milk! Magnesium, essential for the absorption of calcium, is rich in sea greens. Magnesium stimulates production of calcitonin, the hormone which increases calcium in the bones. Sea greens are a good source of natural vitamin D, also essential for calcium absorption, bone health and muscle function. Many people don't store vitamin D very well; our indoor lives don't let us get out in the sun as much as in times past. Forty percent of Americans (especially women) are deficient in vitamin D. Even many who take vitamin D supplements show a deficiency.

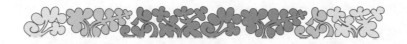

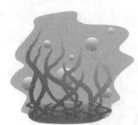

4: **Sea greens and your thyroid:** In our era of processed foods and iodine-poor soils, sea greens and sea foods stand alone as potent sources of natural, balanced iodine. Iodine is essential to life; the thyroid gland cannot make thyrozin, the enzyme that regulates metabolism, without it. Iodine is an important element of alertness and rapid brain activity, and a prime deterrent to arterial plaque.

Thyroid hormones are made from iodine and the amino acid tyrosine. Thyroglobulin, the mixture of tyrosine and iodine stored in the thyroid gland, is transformed into hormones that regulate our metabolism, protein, carbohydrate and carotene use, and cholesterol (sea greens help lower cholesterol). The amount of thyroid hormone released into the bloodstream determines the body's base energy level and along with the adrenal glands, the rate that sex hormones are made. Sea plants nourish an underactive thyroid and normalize adrenal functions to trigger increased libido.

Preventive measures may be taken against iodine deficiency problems or disease risk by adding just 2 tablespoons of chopped, dried sea greens to your daily diet.

Goiter, a thyroid disorder, develops when the pituitary gland stimulates the thyroid to make more hormones but the thyroid can't do it because of an iodine deficiency. It enlarges in the attempt and goiter develops. The rate of goiter in the U.S. is relatively high — 6% of the population in some areas. It's a strange situation, since few people in the U. S. are iodine deficient (the average American intake of iodine is estimated at over 600 micrograms daily from iodized salt). Since the recommended adult allowance for iodine is quite small, 150 micrograms, experts believe that at least some of the high rates of goiter are really connected to too much sugar, alcohol, fats and caffeine, or to eating a lot of goitrogen foods, which block iodine absorption.

Goitrogen foods are cruciferous vegetables like broccoli, cauliflower or cabbage, legumes like beans, peas and peanuts, beets, and nuts like almonds, which may cause a mild hypothyroid state when eaten raw. Cooking neutralizes the thyroid-blocking components. If you have a tendency to goiter or hypothyroidism, cook these healthy foods lightly.

5: **Sea greens and pregnancy:** Iodine deficiency has a profound effect on the health of the fetus early in conception. I recommend that a woman who wants to become pregnant consider adding sea greens to her diet while she is trying to conceive, rather than waiting until she realizes that she is pregnant. Most American women get enough iodine from fish and seafood, but in developing, landlocked countries, where iodine is not plentiful in food, infants are often born with cretinism which results in stunted growth, mental deficiency, puffy facial features and lack of muscle coordination, all signs of low iodine.

Sea greens in a pregnant woman's diet help the health of the mother, too.
—Hemoglobin counts rise from 65% to 83%
—Colds decrease in number and severity; arthritic conditions improve
—Hair color and quality improve; fingernails grow stronger
—Skin texture improves; capillary strength increases, so there is less bruising
—Eye conditions improve, especially if there is eye redness or inflammation
—Constipation lessens and a sense of well-being increases
—Stretch marks are less during pregnancy and skin heals better afterwards. Many estheticians
   recommend topical use of a sea greens and aloe vera gel to prevent stretch marks during pregnancy.

6: **Sea greens are a valuable treatment for candida albicans.** Their high mineral content, especially selenium, builds up immunity against candida. Enzymes use the rich iodine in seaweeds to produce iodine-charged free radicals, which deactivate yeasts. Other immune-compromised diseases like chronic fatigue, HIV infection, arthritis and allergies respond to sea plant treatment, too.

7: **Sea greens and vaginal infections:** Iodine-rich sea plants are effective against a wide range of harmful organisms like trichomonas, candida and chlamydia. A douche solution with 1 tablespoon dried sea vegetables to 1 quart of water, used twice daily for 7 to 14 days, is effective against most of these pathogens.

8: **Sea plants effectively lower blood pressure and cholesterol:** Nutrition studies show that they help deter arteriosclerosis and reduce toxins in the liver and kidneys.

9: **Sea greens and herpes:** Studies from the 1970's and 80's reveal that certain forms of red marine algae exhibit powerful anti-viral activity against herpes 1 & 2. The red marine algaes Dumontiaceae, Gigartina, Dillwyn and Nothogenia offer the most protection. *Vibrant Health and Pure Planet offer high quality anti-viral red marine algae products for your anti-herpes arsenal. See the Product Resources pg. 624 for contact information.*

10: **Sea greens and menopause:** Sea greens are a rich source of fat-soluble vitamins D and K that assist with production of steroid hormones like estrogen and DHEA in the adrenal glands. This is especially important during menopause because the adrenals glands play a key role in shoring up hormone production when estrogen production slows down. Vitamin K in sea greens, in particular, boosts adrenal activity, meaning that eating them can help maintain female hormone balance for a more youthful body for years to come.

11. **Sea greens boost weight loss and deter cellulite build-up.** Virtually fat-free (mostly healthy EFA's) and with low calories, sea plants help your thyroid normalize metabolism, especially as you age. Sea plant fiber and algin lower bowel transit time to aid weight loss. Sea plant antioxidants increase your body's fat-burning ability. Sea greens organic iodine boosts thyroid activity, so food fuels are used before they turn into fatty deposits.
Both eating sea greens and bathing in them help reduce cellulite. The detoxifying qualities of sea plant algin stimulate lymphatic drainage, and help your skin and fat cells absorb minerals to discourage cellulite. Sea minerals act like electrolytes to break the chemical bond that seals fat cells. The fat cells open temporarily to allow trapped wastes to escape into the lymph system and be eliminated by the kidneys and bladder. The best spas apply a sea plant solution as part of a body wrap, or bath, to do this very thing. It's called thalassotherapy, and it's been used for centuries to speed up metabolism and increase circulation to cellulitic areas.

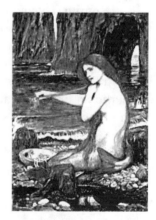

12: **Sea greens are a beauty treatment:** Seaweeds add amazing luster to the skin. Ancient sea-loving Greeks said that Aphrodite, the goddess of love who rose out of the foaming sea, owed her supple skin, shiny hair, and sparkling eyes to the plants of the sea. A seaweed face mask increases circulation, stimulates lymphatic drainage and dilates capillaries to tone your skin. Applying seaweed can speed recovery from minor burns, clear acne and heal scars. Seaweed returns mineral salts to your skin that stress and pollution deplete. Skin cells hold moisture better when they absorb the mineral salts, making the skin more supple and elastic. By retaining moisture, the skin plumps, removing the look of lines and wrinkles. Many women report smoother skin and better skin texture after a seaweed treatment. Amino acid, mineral and vitamin content help nourish the skin, too. Some seaweeds possess molecules similar to collagen.

A seaweed bath is a great way to get the benefits of sea plants.
Seaweed baths are Nature's perfect body-psyche balancer. Remember how good you feel after a walk in the ocean? Seaweeds purify and balance the ocean; they can do the same for your body. Noticeable rejuvenating effects occur when toxins are released from your tissues. A seaweed soak is like a wet-steam sauna, only better, because sea greens balance body chemistry instead of dehydrating it. The electrolytic magnetic action of the sea plants releases excess body fluids from congested cells and dissolves fatty wastes through the skin, replacing them with key minerals. Vitamin K, a fat-soluble vitamin in seaweeds, aids adrenal activity, so a seaweed soak also helps maintain hormone balance for a more youthful body.

If an ocean near you has unpolluted waters, you can collect your own sea greens. Gather them from the water, (not the shoreline), in buckets or clean trash cans, and carry them home to your tub. If you don't live near the ocean, dried sea greens sold in health food stores work, too.

Whichever type of seaweed you choose, run very hot water over the seaweed in a tub, filling it to the point that you will be covered when you recline. The water will turn rich brown as the plants release their minerals. As you soak, the gel from the seaweed transfers onto your skin. This coating increases perspiration to release toxins from your system, and replaces them by osmosis with minerals. Rub your skin, especially cellulitic areas with the sea leaves during the bath to stimulate circulation, smooth and tone the body, and to remove wastes coming out on the skin surface. When the sea greens have done their work, the gel coating dissolves and floats off the skin, and the leaves shrivel - a sign that the bath is over.

Each bath varies with the individual, the seaweeds used, and water temperature, but the gel coating release is a natural timekeeper for the bath's benefits. Forty-five minutes is usually about right to balance the acid-alkaline system, encourage liver activity, cellulite release and fat metabolism. Skin tone, color, and better circulation are almost immediately noticeable. To get the most from a seaweed treatment, dry brush cellulitic skin before your seaweed bath to exfoliate dead skin, and open up pores for waste elimination and blood flow to the affected area.

Note: A seaweed soak is one of the most effective treatments in natural healing, but use it with care. If you are under a doctor's care for heart disease or high blood pressure, check with your physician to see if a seaweed bath is okay for you.

Sea plants come in green, brown, red and blue-green algae. A quick profile:

...**Kelp** (*Laminaria*), a brown sea plant, containing vitamins A, B, E, D and K, is a good source of vitamin C, and is rich in minerals. Kelp proteins are comparable in quality to animal proteins. Kelp's sodium alginate (algin), helps remove radioactive particles and heavy metals from the body. Algin, carrageenan and ager are kelp gels that rejuvenate gastrointestinal health. Kelp works as a blood purifier, relieves arthritis stiffness, and promotes adrenal, pituitary and thyroid health. Kelp's iodine can normalize thyroid-related disorders like obesity and lymph system congestion. It is a demulcent that helps eliminate herpes outbreaks. Kelp is rich—a little goes a long way.

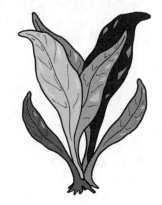

...**Kombu** (*Laminaria digitata, setchelli, horsetail kelp*), has a long tradition as a Japanese delicacy with great nutritional healing value. It is a decongestant for excess mucous, and helps lower blood pressure. Kombu has abundant iodine, carotenes, B, C, D and E vitamins, minerals like calcium, magnesium, potassium, silica, iron and zinc, and the powerful skin healing nutrient germanium. Kombu is a meaty, high-protein seaweed, higher in natural mineral salts than most other seaweeds. Add a strip of kombu to your bean pot to reduce gas.

...**Hijiki** (*Hizikia fusiforme*) is a mineral-rich, high-fiber seaweed, with 20% protein, vitamin A, carotenes and calcium. Hijiki has the most calcium of any sea green, 1400mg per 100gr. of dry weight. Japanese studies reveal hijiki boosts natural killer T-cells for more disease protection.

...**Nori** (*Porphyra, Laver*) is a red sea plant with a sweet, meaty taste when dried. It contains nearly 50% balanced protein, higher than any other sea plant. Tests find that protein and carbohydrates from Japanese nori are 70% assimilable- very high for a vegetable. Nori's fiber makes it a perfect sushi wrapper. Nori is rich in all the carotenes, calcium, iodine, iron, and phosphorus.

...**Arame** (*Eisenia bycyclis*), is one of the ocean's richest sources of iodine. Herbalists use arame to help reduce breast and uterine fibroids, and, through its fat soluble vitamins and phytohormones, to normalize menopausal symptoms. Arame promotes soft, wrinkle-free skin, enhances hair's glossiness and prevents hair loss.

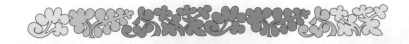

...**Sea Palm** (*Postelsia palmaeformis*), American arame, grows only on the Pacific Coast of North America. One of my favorites, it has a sweet, salty taste that goes especially well as a vegetable, rice or salad topping.

...**Bladderwrack** (*Fucus vesiculosus*) is packed with vitamin K .... an excellent adrenal stimulant. It is still used today by native Americans in steam baths for arthritis, gout and illness recovery.

...**Wakame** (*Alaria, Undaria*) is a high-protein, high calcium seaweed, with carotenes, iron and vitamin C. Widely used in the Orient for hair growth and luster, and for skin tone.

...**Dulse** (*Palmaria palmata*), a red sea plant, is rich in iron, protein, and vitamin A. It is a supremely balanced nutrient, with 300 times more iodine and 50 times more iron than wheat. Tests on dulse show activity against the herpes virus. It has purifying and tonic effects on the body, yet its natural, balanced salts nourish as a mineral, without inducing thirst.

...**Irish moss** (*Chondrus crispus, Carrageen*) is full of electrolyte minerals: calcium, magnesium, sodium and potassium. Its mucilaginous compounds help you detoxify, boost metabolism and strengthen hair, skin and nails. It is traditionally used for a low sex drive.

Sea greens are tasty and widely available today.

Crush, chop, snip or crumble any mix of dry sea greens, just as they are, into soups, sauces, casseroles, rice or noodles, rice and let them blend into your recipe. Roast them into pizzas, nachos or focaccias. Pan toast them with Chinese noodles and ginger... yum. If you like them in salads, remember that a vinegar dressing tenderizes sea greens as well as cooking them does. If you add sea veggies, no other salt is needed, an advantage for a low salt diet. Sundried, they are convenient to buy, store, and use as needed. Store them in a moisture proof container and they keep indefinitely.

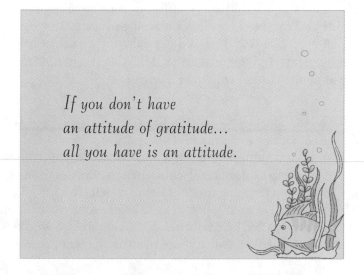

*If you don't have
an attitude of gratitude...
all you have is an attitude.*

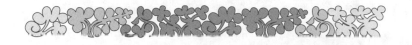

Healing Powerhouses of the Desert

Aloe vera, the lily of the desert, is a unique, potent healing superfood. Today it's the subject of a wealth of new research. Over seventy-five healing compounds have been identified in aloe, including steroids, antibiotic and anti-carcinogenic agents, amino acids, minerals and enzymes (one enzyme has been isolated to treat burns). It has excellent transdermal properties, allowing it to penetrate deep skin levels.

...Aloe gel has been used since ancient Egyptian times as a skin lubricant and healer for cuts, bruises, insect bites, sores, acne, eczema and burns. Research shows healing results for skin cancers, hemorrhoids and varicose veins. Surgeries use aloe gel for post-op healing, because it's a natural antiseptic, astringent and lymphatic stimulant that boosts antibody formation against infections. Aloe is an amazing wound healer, fighting infection, increasing collagen production, and dramatically reducing scar tissue. An 18-month study reveals applying aloe vera gel results in 100% resolution of wounds and diabetic ulcers (stages 1-4).

...Aloe juice, a traditional herbal bitter, is widely popular today because it boosts the body's self-cleansing action — balancing rather than causing harsh irritant effects. Aloe juice has anti-inflammatory EFA's that help the stomach and colon. Aloe juice alkalizes digestive processes to prevent overacidity, a common cause of indigestion, acid reflux, digestive tract irritations like IBS, colitis, Crohn's disease and ulcers. Ulcer patients taking aloe juice show up to 80% reduction in the number of ulcers being formed. Even if ulcers have already formed, healing is three times faster.

Aloe is a core healer in the alternative arsenal with unique nutritional and body balancing properties. It helps normalize fat metabolism to reduce cholesterol and triglycerides. New research shows it's effective for immune disorders like candida, parasite invasions, fatigue syndromes like fibromyalgia, allergies, arthritis, eczema and psoriasis.

I call aloe vera an intelligent plant, because it can differentiate between normal cells, mutated cells (cancer) or diseased cells (HIV). It stimulates normal cell growth, while inhibiting cancer cell division (even lymphocytic leukemia) and virus spread. Aged aloe vera juice is widely used in AIDS treatment to block the HIV virus movement from cell to cell. Acemannan, an aloe derivative with powerful anti-viral effects, shows promise against herpes viruses.

Aloe vera is loaded with mucopolysaccharides, phytochemicals with profound healing qualities. Mucopolysaccharides are credited with aloe's immune enhancement qualities, antiviral and antibacterial activity, and its ability to eliminate toxic wastes. Rich in organic silicon, MPS's are a vital component of cell and artery walls, mucous membranes, and the connective tissues of bones, teeth and cartilage. They link with collagen and elastin to maintain tissues and organs, alleviate joint problems and rebuild degenerating cartilage. Essentially mucopolysaccharides and collagen hold our tissues together. MPS's also reduce inflammation and blood clotting time, lessening the risk for cardiovascular disease.

Nature's most energizing superfoods come from high desert beehives.

Royal jelly is a powerhouse containing every nutrient necessary to support life. No other food source compares nutritionally to royal jelly, and it can't be duplicated in a lab. The exclusive food of the queen bee, royal jelly transforms a "cinderella" worker bee into a queen bee. Her life expectancy rises to an astounding 6 years, compared to a worker bee's 6 week life span — an amazing result of her royal jelly diet!

Royal jelly's rejuvenative powers have been seen for centuries as a fountain of youth for us, too. Herbalists say royal jelly is a fabulous nutrient for skin and hair, nourishing the skin to ease wrinkles, dryness, even adult acne. It is effective for gland and hormone imbalances that mean menstrual, menopause and prostate problems.

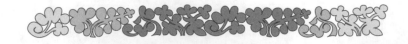

Chinese herbalists advocate royal jelly as a natural antibiotic, for liver disease, arthritis and anemia. Royal jelly has extraordinary powers to strengthen the human immune system. It is a rich source of B vitamins (especially B-5, pantothenic acid), minerals, sex hormones, enzyme precursors... and *all eight* essential amino acids. Success stories show royal jelly is effective against fatigue, stress, insomnia and depression. Royal jelly may even offer a super boost to fertility. A study from Cornell University reveals chickens fed royal jelly lay twice as many eggs as other chickens. Even older hens started laying eggs again on a royal jelly diet!

Royal Jelly is quite difficult to harvest and commands high prices because of its scarcity and consumer demand. Highest quality royal jelly products are preserved in their whole, raw, "alive" state for the best absorption. As little as one drop of pure, extracted fresh royal jelly delivers a daily supply.

I find that **PANAX GINSENG - ROYAL JELLY VIALS** are one of the best ways to take these two dynamos for a healing diet. The attributes of ginseng and royal jelly have synergistic activity in combination.

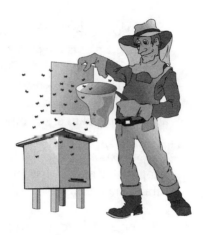

Propolis is one of the most powerful antibiotics in nature. Bee hives have been called "the most antiseptic places in nature," because propolis neutralizes harmful organisms that enter the hive. Bees are prone to bacterial and viral infections; propolis protects the bees from these infections. The powerful antibiotic properties of propolis can also protect humans — specifically against *staphylococcus aureus*, a bacteria that causes serious infections, blood poisoning and a type of pneumonia. (Interestingly, *staph. a.* has become resistant to all but <u>one</u> pharmaceutical antibiotic.) But, studies show that propolis <u>inhibits</u> the streptococcal bacteria that causes strep throat and dental cavities. Propolis even works well with two anti-staph drugs, streptomycin and cloxacillin. Performing much like a prescription antibiotic, propolis prevents bacteria cell division and break down of bacteria cell structure. However, unlike conventional antibiotics, propolis also works against viruses, has anti-inflammatory effects, and may even prevent blood clots.

Bees collect the base for propolis from the leaf buds on the bark of trees, then convert it with their enzymes to a sticky material of 50-55% resin and balsam, 30% wax and 10% pollen. Rich in immune defense vitamins, minerals and amino-acids (all 22 of them), bees paste a propolis shield on the inner hive walls to guard against harmful microorganisms as well as to patch holes or cracks in the hive. Nature is incredibly efficient.

Propolis creates a natural antibiotic shield for humans, too. Research shows that taking propolis during high risk cold and flu seasons reduces colds, coughing, and inflammation of mouth, tonsils and throat membranes. Look for a supplement that contains propolis, vitamin C and zinc for the best results. Further, propolis is rich in flavonoids and B-vitamins that work both internally and externally to heal scars, bruises and blemishes.

Bee pollen is called Nature's perfect survival food because it's nutritionally complete. It has all 22 amino acids, 27 minerals, the full span of vitamins, complex carbohydrates, essential fatty acids, enzymes and co-enzymes. Bee pollen has 5 to 7 times more protein than beef! Bee pollen is so nutrient rich, it's been used worldwide for centuries to rejuvenate and rebuild the body after illness. I've experienced this healing ability myself.

The West discovered pollen's long life benefits by accident during a 1950's investigation of native Russian bee keepers who regularly lived past 100 years of age, and who ate raw honey, rich in bee pollen, every day.

Pollen is a valuable aid to weight control. It's ability to normalize body metabolism and stoke metabolic fires helps keep calories burning and weight stable. Bee pollen also acts as a natural appetite suppressant through its amino acid phenylalanine (for people who need to gain weight, phenylalanine produces the opposite effect).

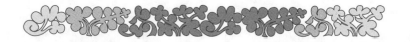

There's more. Bee pollen also:

…increases energy levels and strength for athletes
…helps the body normalize from diarrhea and constipation
…tranquilizes without side effects
…increases blood hemoglobin
…rids the body of toxins from drugs, alcohol, smoking, and chemicalized food
…chelates and flushes out artery-clogging biochemical deposits
…reduces the negative effects associated with radiation
…protects against skin dehydration and stimulates growth of new skin tissue
…helps reduce upper respiratory infections

Note: Bee pollen has shown great effectiveness for the relief of allergy symptoms. However, a small percentage of the population may be allergic to bee products.

Jojoba benefits are attracting more and more Americans.

Desert plants are always full of long-lasting moisturizers. For us, this means they are wonderful cosmetics as well as soothing healers. The jojoba plant is no exception. Jojoba nut oil has been used by Native Americans for hundreds of years—treating sores, cuts, bruises, and burns. As a diet supplement and appetite suppressant, they roasted the nuts to make a coffee-like beverage when food was scarce. As a skin conditioner, it was used to soothe and heal the skin after sun or wind burn. As a hair restorative oil, it is an effective scalp treatment.

Jojoba oil is actually like a liquid wax with rich antioxidant properties to keep it from turning rancid. For people, this means that jojoba oil is a natural mimic of sebum oil secreted by the human skin. So it is an effective lubricant and protector in protecting human skin from aging and wrinkling.

Fortunately for the world's sperm whale population, jojoba oil is virtually identical to sperm whale oil, with a melting temperature close to that of the human body. It is an ideal natural base for the cosmetics in which whale oil was used until the mid 1950's.

Jojoba oil is rapid, penetrating, hypo-allergenic skin therapy. Besides moisturizing and soothing skin, jojoba gives your skin a healthy glow because it restores natural pH balance. Studies show that just one hour after application, jojoba oil increases skin softness by as much as 37 percent, reducing superficial lines and wrinkles, especially around the eyes, by as much as 25 percent! Because of its purity and antioxidant freshness, herbal healers use jojoba to treat skin problems like adult acne, psoriasis, and neurodermatitis that are not responsive to chemical medicines.

Jojoba oil is the most effective natural scalp cleansing substance discovered so far. As in Native American medicine, jojoba helps restore non-hereditary hair loss that is linked to dandruff or clogged scalp follicles. Each hair is lubricated by sebum, manufactured by sebaceous glands that lie next to the hair follicles. Healthy hair grows about one half inch per month for 2 - 4 years unless there is sebum balance interference, because of a nutrient deficiency, illness or excessive stress. When too much sebum collects, hair follicles clog, resulting in poor hair texture and growth, and shortened hair life. Jojoba dissolves excess sebum deposits, opens up hair follicles and encourages healthy hair growth.

Jojoba, like other cactus type plants, has notable appetite suppressing activity from its constituent called *simmondsia*. Taken as a weight control liquid by native peoples, jojoba is made today into many weight control aids from a tasty candy bar to a chocolate-y beverage.

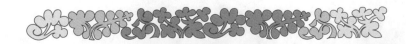

A Special Guide to Detoxification

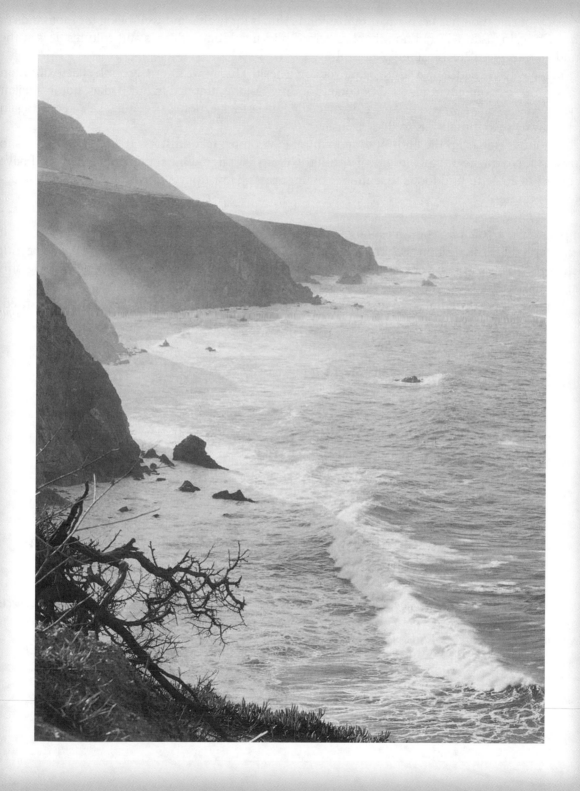

A Special Guide to Detoxification

Body purification has been a part of mankind's rituals for health and well-being for thousands of years. Cleansing is a rich tradition that has helped humans through all ages and cultures. It is at the foundation of every great healing philosophy.

You may have tried a juice fast to better your own health. Today, we normally think of detoxification as a way to clean out environmental pollutants or drug residues trapped in our bodies, but in ancient times, it was used as a way to reconnect with the divine. Detoxification is becoming valued once again as a pathway to spirituality as well as cleansing.

No one is free from the enormous amount of environmental and stress toxins assaulting us in our world. No one is immune to every unhealthy lifestyle option. One report I read said we'd have to return to 1904 to find foods that are free of impurities. How do we remain healthy in a destructive environment?

This chapter answers your questions about body cleansing. It discusses detoxification in detail. It defines a good detoxification program, how it works in the body, and the benefits you can expect. It includes visible signs that your body might need a good cleansing, and the types of detox programs you can use to best suit your needs.

Step by step instructions are included for the initial diets, supplements, and herbs you'll need, along with tips that can give you the best results.

Detoxification programs included:

...**Colon and bowel cleansing**

...**Bladder and kidney cleansing**

...**Lung and chest congestion cleansing**

...**Liver and organ cleansing**

...**Lymphatic cleansing**

...**Skin cleansing**

...**Blood cleansing: for heavy metal toxicity, alcohol, drug addictions**

...**Detox from Fats and Sugars**

For more information, see my book, DETOXIFICATION ©1999-2004, a comprehensive book on all aspects of cleansing for a safe, effective personal detox program. Over 250 pages, it includes delicious green cuisine cleansing recipes, detox plans for specific health problems, and easy-to-use detox charts.

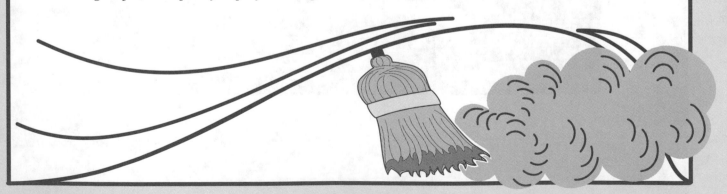

Understanding Detoxification

What is detoxification? Our bodies do it naturally every day..... It's one of our most basic automatic functions. Detoxification is the normal body process of eliminating or neutralizing toxins through the colon, liver, kidneys, lungs, lymph and skin. Just as our hearts beat nonstop and our lungs breathe continuously, so our metabolic processes continuously dispose of accumulated toxic matter. But today, our bodies are fighting a losing battle.... systems and organs that were once capable of cleaning out toxic material are now completely overloaded; much of it stays in our tissues. Our bodies try to protect us from dangerous material by setting it aside, surrounding it with mucous or fat so it won't cause imbalance or trigger an immune reaction. (Our bodies store foreign substances in fatty deposits — a significant reason to keep your body fat low. Some people carry around up to 15 extra pounds of mucous that harbors this waste!)

We mourn yesterday's pollution-free environment, whole foods and pure water. But, since humans are born with a "self-cleaning system," this ideal probably never existed. Today, we control our environment even less. The best thing is to minimize pollution and to periodically get rid of toxins through detoxification.

Detoxifying with special cleansing diets may be a missing link to disease prevention, especially for immune-compromised diseases like cancer, arthritis, diabetes and candida albicans. Our chemicalized-food diet, with too much animal protein, too much fat, too much caffeine and alcohol radically alters our internal ecosystems. Even if your diet is good, a body cleanse can restore vitality against environmental toxins that pave the way for disease-bearing organisms and parasites.

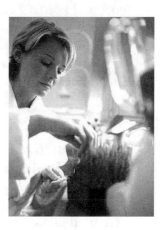

A detox program aims to remove the cause of disease before it makes us ill. It's a time-honored way to keep immune response high, elimination regular, circulation sound and stress under control, so your body can handle toxins it encounters. In the past, detoxification was used clinically for recovering alcoholics and drug addicts, or as a personal "spring cleaning" for general health. Today, a regular detox program twice a year still makes a big difference for health, and for the quality of our lives.

Should you detoxify?

Western societies are exposed to chemicals on an unprecedented scale. Industrial chemicals pollute our water through run-offs; pesticides and additives are in our foods; heavy metals, anesthetics, residues from drugs, and environmental hormones are trapped within our bodies today in greater concentrations than at any other point in history. Every body system is affected, from tissue damage to sensory deterioration.

Many chemicals are so widespread that we are unaware of them. But they have worked their way into our systems faster than they can be eliminated, and are causing allergies and addictions in record numbers. More than 2 million synthetic substances are known, 25,000 are added each year, and over 30,000 are produced on a commercial scale. Only a tiny fraction are ever tested for toxicity. A lot of them come to us from developing countries that have few safeguards in place. This doesn't even count the second-hand smoke, caffeine and alcohol overload, or daily stress that is an increasing part of our lives.

The molecular structure of some chemical carcinogens interacts with human DNA, so long term exposure may result in metabolic and genetic alteration that affects cell growth and behavior. World Health Organization research implicates environmental chemicals in 60 to 80% of all cancers today. Hormone-disrupting pesticides and pollutants are linked to hormone problems, psychological disorders, birth defects, still births and most recently breast cancer.

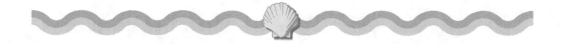

When toxic matter saturates our tissues, antioxidants and minerals in vital body fluids are reduced, immune defenses are thrown out of balance. Circumstances like this are the prime factor in today's immune compromised diseases like candidiasis, lupus, fibromyalgia, and chronic fatigue syndrome (CFIDS).

Chemical oxidation is the other process that allows disease. The oxygen that "rusts" and ages us also triggers free radical activity, a destructive cascade of incomplete molecules that damages DNA and other cell components. And if you didn't have a reason to reduce your animal fat intake before, here is a critical one: *oxygen combines with animal fat in body storage cells and speeds up the free radical process.*

Almost everyone can benefit from a cleanse. It's one of the best ways to remain healthy in dangerous surroundings. Not one of us is immune to environmental toxins, and most of us can't escape to a remote, unpolluted habitat. In the last few decades, technology has become seriously able to harm the health of our entire planet, even to the point of making it perilous for life. We must develop our culture further. Mankind and the Earth must work together, take larger steps of cooperation in order to save it all for us all.

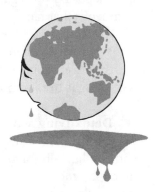

It has to start with us. We can keep our own body systems in good working order so that toxins are eliminated quickly. We can also take a closer look at our air, water and food, and keep a watchful eye on the politics that control our environment. Legislation on health and the environment follows two pathways in America.... the influence of business and profits, and the demands of the people for a healthy habitat and responsible stewardship of the Earth. (*See "Fluoridation — An unnecessary poison in our drinking water," page 119*).

Does detoxification play a role in mind-body health?
From the beginning of healing on Earth it seems the answer has been a resounding yes!

In ancient Native American cultures, detoxification was regarded as a religious practice. Cleansing methods were used as a way to purify the body as a living temple to God. Purification rituals were used to clear out both bad influences and spirits as well as body toxins. In sweat lodges, first famous as places for purification prior to religious rituals like the vision quest (and still widely used today), both spiritual cleansing and body cleansing are felt to take place. I myself have participated in a traditional sweat lodge on a recent herbal tour to the Southwest. I was amazed that even as an uninitiated person I could so quickly feel the power of this cleansing ritual.

In Ayurvedic healing, toxins (called *ama*) are deemed one of the main causes of disease, creating imbalances that must be resolved to restore health. Ayurvedic practitioners believe *ama* results from poor digestion and elimination. Ama is also felt to be created through negative emotions (anger, fear, greed, resentment), unwholesome forms of entertainment (like violent movies), chronic stress, and being around negative people. Ayurvedic cleansing techniques like *panchakarma* (involving the use of laxatives, sweat treatments, and therapeutic enemas) are recommended seasonally by healers to remove these mental and physical impurities. Music therapy, massage and meditation are regularly used as ways to rebalance the mind, body and spirit.

On a recent herbal tour to Hawaii, I saw that cleansing rituals are deeply rooted in Polynesian traditions, too. Ancient Hawaiians used sweat lodges for mind, body, and spirit purification. Still today, Hawaiians believe a sweat lodge raises consciousness, increases mind-body awareness and boosts capacity for healing.

The evidence is undeniable.... a cleanse is a great way to strengthen mind-body connections. Cleaning out mental and physical impurities allows the body to better hear those "cell phone calls" from the spirit that mean it's time for a change in lifestyle, relationships or career. Some people find their entire lives improve after a cleanse, because a cleanse opens the door to new ways of thinking and experiencing the world.

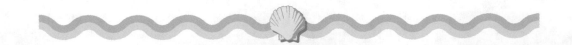

Is your body becoming toxic? **Body signs can tell you that you need to detoxify.**

Each of us has different "toxic tolerance" levels. Listen to your body when it starts giving you those "cellular phone calls." If you can keep the amount of toxins in your system below your toxic level, your body can usually adapt and rid itself of them.

Signs you might have reached your toxic tolerance level:

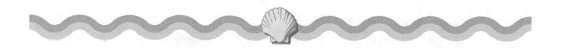

—Frequent, unexplained headaches, back or joint pain, or arthritis?
—Chronic respiratory problems, sinus problems or asthma?
—Abnormal body odor, bad breath or coated tongue?
—Chronic stress from an unhealthy work environment or home life?
—Environmental sensitivities, especially to odors?
—Food allergies, poor digestion or constipation with intestinal bloating or gas?
—Unusually poor memory, chronic insomnia, depression, irritability, chronic fatigue?
—Brittle nails and hair, psoriasis, adult acne, unexplained weight gain over 10 pounds?

Lab tests like stool, urine, blood or liver tests, and hair analysis can also shed light on the need for a detox.

What benefits can you expect from a good detox?

A detox cleans out waste deposits, so you aren't running with a dirty engine or driving with the brakes on. After a cleanse, the body starts rebalancing, energy levels rise physically, psychologically and sexually, and creativity begins to expand. You start feeling like a different person — because you are. Your outlook and attitude change, because cleansing and diet improvement have changed your actual cell make up.

1) You'll clean your digestive tract of accumulated waste and fermenting bacteria.
2) You'll clear excess mucous and congestion from the body.
3) You'll purify the liver, kidney and blood, impossible under ordinary eating patterns.
4) You'll enhance mental clarity, impossible under chemical overload.
5) You'll be less dependent on sugar, caffeine, nicotine, alcohol or drugs.
6) You'll turn around bad eating habits; your stomach will have a chance to reduce to normal size.
7) You'll release hormone secretions that coupled with essential fatty acids from plant sources can strengthen your immune system.

You've decided your body needs a cleanse. Next decide on the time factor for your detox. It's important. How long can you give out of your busy lifestyle to focus on a cleansing program so that all the processes can be completed? 24 hours, 2 or 3 days, or up to ten days? It's important to allocate your time ahead of time, to prepare both your mind and your body for the experience ahead.

A good detox program is in 3 steps: cleansing, rebuilding, maintaining.

Years of experience with detoxification convince me that if you have a serious health problem, a brief 3 to 7 day juice cleanse is a good way to release toxins from the system. Shorter cleanses don't get to the root of a chronic problem. Longer cleanses upset body equilibrium more than most people are ready to deal with outside a clinical environment. A 3 to 7 day cleanse can clean your pipes of systemic sludge - excess mucous, old fecal matter, trapped cellular and non-food wastes, or inorganic mineral deposits that are part of arthritis.

A few days without solid food can be an enlightening experience about your lifestyle, too. It's not absolutely necessary to take in only liquids, but a juice diet increases awareness and energy availability for elimination. Fresh juices literally pick up dead matter from the body and carry it away. Your body becomes easier to "hear," telling you via cravings what foods and diet it needs — for example, a desire for protein foods, or B vitamin foods like rices, or minerals from greens. This is natural biofeedback.

A detox works by self-digestion. During a cleanse, the body decomposes and burns only the substances and tissues that are damaged, diseased or unneeded, like abscesses, tumors, excess fat deposits, and congestive wastes. Even a relatively short fast accelerates elimination, often causing dramatic changes as masses of accumulated waste are expelled.

You will know your body is detoxing if you experience the short period of headaches, fatigue, body odor, bad breath, diarrhea or mouth sores that commonly accompany accelerated elimination. However, digestion usually improves right away as do many gland and nerve functions. Cleansing also helps release hormone secretions that stimulate immune response and encourages a disease-preventing environment.

What about a water fast? I don't recommend it. Here's why:

Water fasting was used by ancient Greek and Roman healers, by medieval monks, and up through the early 20th century by healers of all kinds. Juice cleansing is a far better evolution in detoxification methods. Detoxification experts agree that fresh vegetable and fruit juice cleansing is superior to water fasting. Fresh juices, broths and herb teas help deeply cleanse the body, rejuvenate the tissues and guide you to a faster recovery from health problems than water fasting.

You may have heard that a traditional water fast is the "purest" way to detoxify, but a water fast was harsh and demanding on the body, even before our diets and environment changed. Today, it can even be dangerous. Today, people in western societies eat huge amounts of food and environmental toxins are part of the picture. Pollutants and chemicals deeply buried in our tissues release into elimination channels too rapidly during a water fast. Your body is essentially "re-poisoned" as the chemicals move through the bloodstream all at once. Sometimes, the physical and emotional stress of a water fast even overrides the healing benefits.

On the other hand, vegetable and fruit juices are alkalizing, so they neutralize uric acid and other inorganic acids better than water, increasing healing effects. Juices support better metabolic activity, too. Metabolic activity slows down during a water fast as the body attempts to conserve dwindling energy resources. Juices are easy on digestion — easily assimilated into the bloodstream. They don't disturb the detoxification process.

Step one: elimination. You'll clean out mucous and toxins from the intestinal tract and major organs. Everything functions more effectively when toxins, obstructions and wastes are removed.

Step two: rebuilding healthy tissue and restoring energy. With obstacles removed, your body's regulating powers are activated to rebuild at optimum levels. Eat only fresh and simply prepared, vegetarian foods during the rebuilding step. Include supplements and herbal aids for your specific needs.

Step three: keeping your body clean and toxin-free. Modifying lifestyle habits is the key to a strong resistant body. Rely on fresh fruits and vegetables for fiber, cooked vegetables, grains and seeds for strength and alkalinity, lightly cooked sea foods, soy foods, eggs and low fat cheeses as sources of protein, and a little dinner wine for circulatory health. Include supplements, herbs, exercise and relaxation techniques.

What type of cleanse do you need?

Cleanses come in all shapes and sizes. You can easily tailor a cleanse to your individual needs. Unless you require a specific detox for a serious illness, or recovery from a long course of drugs or chemical therapy, I recommend a short cleanse twice a year, especially in the spring, summer or early autumn when sunshine and natural vitamin D can help the process along.

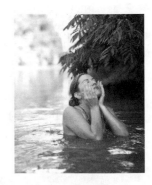

Check out the types of cleanses on the following pages to see which is right for your needs.

Try a Spring Cleanse

A "Spring Cleanse" is a breath of fresh air for your body after a long winter.

A mild spring cleanse is an important, vitality technique no matter how healthy you are. Even though you may exercise during the winter to keep trim, most people still feel at an energy low during the cold, dark months. Our bodies still reflect the ancient seasonal need to harbor more fat for warmth and survival. In a time when people were closer to Nature than we are today, the great majority farmed the land from spring to fall, and lived lives of demanding physical labor. Winter was a time of inactivity, with a natural tendency towards rest. Harvest foods stored in the autumn lost much of their nutrition value through the winter, so people had to eat denser foods, and more of them, to receive the same nutrition. Even in modern times, many days without sunshine and vitamin D mean that our bodies are less able to use nutrients efficiently.

Cold weather prompts people to eat heavier, fattier, comfort foods, too. Old winter "hibernation" patterns also mean that metabolism slows, sometimes by as much as 10%. So, much to the dismay of many of us, fall and winter are the most difficult times of the year to control body weight.

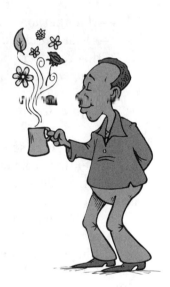

Nature has designed the perfect time for a spring cleanse. Winter weather illnesses like colds, bronchitis and flu leave our bodies with accumulated toxins. Heavy winter clothing, especially thick waterproof coats, hinders normal breathing and perspiration of our skin. When spring finally arrives, new green leafy vegetables liven up our metabolism. Cleansing, antioxidant-rich herbs promote a feeling of new life and restoration of well-being. Nature starts chuckling in the spring. (Laughter is a good cleanser for people, too. It boosts our beta endorphins for a sense of euphoria.) Warmer weather lowers our appetite needs (we tend to shed pounds along with congestion), prompts more activity and movement, and stimulates cleansing.

A "spring cleanse" is actually a very light diet. It focuses on digestion, elimination of accumulated wastes, and improving body functions. Try a spring or summer cleanse for a long weekend. That's enough time to fit comfortably into most people's lives, and it doesn't become too stressful on the body. The best way is to start on Friday night with a pre-cleansing salad, then follow with a cleansing diet like the one in this book, and end with a light Monday morning fruit bowl. Amplify the purifying effect with a stimulating, circulation bath or sauna.

Is your body showing signs that you need a Spring Cleanse?
—Do you feel bloated, constipated and congested? (a sign that your diet is heavier and richer than usual)
—Have you gained weight even though you aren't eating more food? (a sign of winter fat storage)
—Do you feel slow and low energy most of the time? (a sign of cold weather body slowdown)
—Has your digestion worsened? (a sign your body isn't using its nutrients well)
—Do your lungs feel clogged and swollen? (a sign of shallower breathing, perhaps a low-grade infection)

Benefits you can expect from a Spring Cleanse
—Your digestive tract gets a "wash and brush" of accumulated waste.
—Your liver, kidney and blood are purified, impossible under ordinary eating patterns.
—Your mental clarity receives a boost, impossible under an overload of food chemicals.
—You'll relieve dependency on habit-forming sugars, caffeine, nicotine, alcohol or drugs.
—Bad eating habits get a break..... with a new chance to improve your diet patterns.
—Your stomach has a chance to reduce its size for weight loss and better weight control.

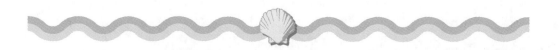

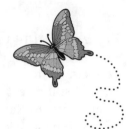

Spring Cleanse Detox Plan

Start with the 3-day nutrition plan below:
The focus is on fresh plant foods: 1) high chlorophyll plants for enzymes; 2) fruits and vegetables for fiber; 3) cultured foods for probiotics; 4) eight glasses of water a day.

The evening before your spring cleanse.....
—Have a light salad with plenty of greens. Take your choice of gentle herbal laxatives.

The next 3 days....
—*On rising:* take a cleansing flushing tea like Crystal Star DR. VITALITY™, or 1 heaping tsp. fiber mix in juice. Add 3000mg vitamin C with bioflavs daily to raise glutathione levels, an important detox nutrient.
—*Breakfast:* take your choice of fruit juices.
—*Mid-morning:* take a small glass of potassium broth (pg. 290), or 2 tbsp. aloe juice concentrate in juice or water, or a superfood green drink (see suggestions below); or a cup of green tea or Crystal Star DR. VITALITY™.
—*Lunch:* fresh carrot juice; or raw sauerkraut or a seaweed salad (in natural or Asian food stores)
—*Mid-afternoon:* take a glass of fresh apple juice; or an herbal cleansing tea.
—*About 5 o' clock:* take another small potassium broth, a fresh carrot or vegetable juice like Knudsen's VERY VEGGIE, or a superfood green drink (suggestions below).
—*Supper:* take miso soup with 2 tbsp. dried sea vegetables (dulse, nori, etc.) snipped over the top. (Note: Finish your cleanse with a small green salad with fresh sprouts on the last night.)
—*Before Bed:* repeat the herbal cleansers that you took on rising, and take a cup of mint tea.

Spring cleanse supplement suggestions: Choose 2 or 3 cleansing boosters.
...**Gentle herbal laxatives:** Crystal Star LAXA-TEA™, Zand CLEANSING LAXATIVE tabs, Yogi GET REGU-LAR TEA, or AloeLife ALOE GOLD. After your initial juice detox, Zand HERBALS QUICK CLEANSE Kit for the intestinal tract and liver.
...**Cleansing boosters:** Crystal Star DETOX BLOOD PURIFIER™ with goldenseal, Transformation PUREZYME clears accumulations of an inactive winter, or Planetary RED CLOVER CLEANSER.
...**Flushing boosters:** Nature's Secret SUPERCLEANSE, Planetary TRIPHALA, Crystal Star DR. VITALITY™.
...**Chlorophyll-rich plants — spring's great gift to us:** Pure Planet CHLORELLA, Futurebiotics COLON GREEN caps, Crystal Star ENERGY GREEN RENEWAL™, Green Foods GREEN MAGMA, Wakunaga HARVEST BLEND; NutriCology PRO-GREENS WITH EFA's or Nature's Secret ULTIMATE GREEN.
...**Enzyme support:** Transformation Enz. RELEASEZYME; Herbal Products POWER-PLUS ENZYMES, Crystal Star DR. ENZYME™ with Protease and Bromelain.
...**Electrolytes help detoxify cells:** Nature's Path TRACE-LYTE MINERALS; Arise & Shine ALKALIZER.
...**Probiotics replenish healthy bacteria:** UAS DDS-PLUS WITH FOS, Nutricology SYMBIOTICS powder, Wakunaga KYO-DOPHILUS or Crystal Star DR. PROBIOTICS™ WITH FOS.
...**Antioxidants defeat pollutants:** Biotec Foods CELL GUARD; NutriCology ANTIOX FORMULA II; Rainbow Light MULTI CAROTENE COMPLEX; Solgar OCEANIC BETA CAROTENE.
...**Fiber:** Crystal Star BIOFLAV, FIBER & C™ drink, Jarrow GENTLE FIBERS drink; AloeLife FIBERMATE.

Spring cleanse bodywork suggestions: Techniques to accelerate and round out a cleanse.
Irrigate: Take an enema the first, second and the last day of your spring cleansing program.
Exercise: Take a walk for ten minutes the first day of your cleanse. Each day increase by five minutes.
Sauna: Take a hot sauna or a long warm bath with a rubdown, to stimulate circulation. Dry brush your body before your sauna to help release toxins coming out through the skin.
Massage therapy: Get one good lower back and pelvis massage during your cleanse.

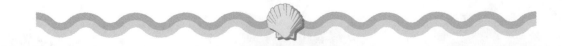

Aromatherapy supports detoxification: Try stress-reducing flower remedies: Natural Labs STRESS/TENSION or CLEANSING REMEDY, or Nelson Bach RESCUE REMEDY. Aromatherapy bath: add 8 to 10 drops of essential oil to a bath. Stir water briskly to disperse. Lavender and chamomile are good choices.

Deep Breathing helps your cleanse: Remove stress, increase energy, compose your mind, improve your mood: Take a deep breath. Exhale slowly.... slowly. Take another deep breath. Release slowly. And again. Maintain a quiet rhythm, exhaling more slowly than you inhale. Close your eyes. As you exhale, visualize toxins dislodging and leaving your body. As you inhale, visualize nutrients rebuilding your vibrancy.

24-Hour Cleanse

A "24-Hour Cleanse" is an invaluable healing tool.

Put this cleanse into action as soon as you realize you aren't feeling well. Pull this jewel out of your pocket at the first signs of unexplained low energy, poor skin or congestion. It's a great way to recover quickly from a cold or flu. It's also an easy first step before making a significant diet improvement or change.

A 24-hour detox is a juice and herbal tea cleanse that lets you go on with your normal activities, and "jump start" a healing program. Even though it's quick, without the depth of vegetable juices needed for a major or chronic problem, it's often enough, it's definitely better than no cleanse at all, and can make a difference in the speed of healing. Even if your program is only going to consist of lifestyle changes aimed at better health, a 24 hour cleanse can point you in the right direction.

Is your body showing signs that it needs a twenty four hour cleanse?

—Do you feel "toxic"? Are you tired a lot for no reason?

—Do you feel congested? Do you have the first signs of a cold or flu? (Go right into this cleanse.)

—Is your skin dry or flaky? Is your skin tone sallow? Is your hair dull, dry and brittle?

—Are the soles of your feet or your palms often peeling?

—Do you frequently get mouth herpes? yeast infections? urinary tract infections? unusual allergies?

24-Hour Detox Plan

The evening before you begin... have a green leafy salad to give your bowels a good sweep. Dry brush your skin before you go to bed to open pores for the night's cleansing eliminations. Take an herbal laxative.

The next day, over the next 24 hours take fresh juices, herbal drinks, water, and a long walk.

—**On rising:** take 2 tbsp. fresh lemon or lime juice, 1 tbsp. maple syrup and 1 pinch cayenne in water.

—**Breakfast:** fresh juice: 1 pear, 2 apples, 4 oranges, 1 grapefruit; or cranberry juice from concentrate.

—**Mid-morning:** have a Zippy Tonic: 1 handful dandelion greens, 3 fresh pineapple rings and 3 radishes; or a cleansing, energizing tea with antioxidants like Crystal Star GREEN TEA CLEANSER™.

—**Lunch:** juice 4 parsley sprigs, or a handful of dandelion greens, 3 tomatoes, ½ green bell pepper, ½ cucumber, 1 scallion, 1 lemon wedge; or a glass of apple juice with 1 packet chlorella granules dissolved.

—**Mid-afternoon:** a cup of Crystal Star CLEANSING & PURIFYING TEA™ or Flora PURIFICATION tea

—**Dinner:** take a glass of papaya-pineapple juice for enzymes; or try a HIGH MINERAL BROTH: 7 carrots, 7 celery stalks, beet tops from 1 bunch, 2 potatoes, 1 onion, 4 garlic cloves, 3 zucchini, 1 handful of parsley. Place in a large soup pot, cover with water, bring to a boil, simmer 30 minutes. Remove and discard veggies.

—**Before Bed:** have a cup of mint tea, or I tsp. Red Star NUTRITIONAL YEAST BROTH or miso soup.

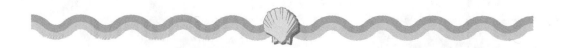

24-Hour cleanse supplement suggestions:
…**Cleansing boosters:** Crystal Star CLEANSING & PURIFYING TEA™; Crystal Star LIVER RENEW™ caps or Planetary BUPLEURUM LIVER CLEANSE.
…**Electrolyte boosters for removal of toxic body acids:** Nature's Path TRACE-LYTE Liquid Minerals.
…**Probiotics:** Wakunaga KYO-DOPHILUS; New Chapter ALL FLORA.
…**Vitamin C:** Take 1,000mg of vitamin C 3x per day with bioflavonoids.

Pointers for best results from your Twenty-four Hour Cleanse:
…Drink 8 to 10 glasses of water a day to hydrate, and flush wastes and toxins from all cells.
…Focus on chlorophyll-rich foods (leafy greens, sea greens) and juices (super green foods like chlorella, barley grass or spirulina). Chlorophyll is the most powerful cleansing agent in nature.

Stress Cleanse Detox Plan

Start with a 3 day juice-liquid diet and follow with 1 to 4 days of a diet with plenty of fresh vegetables and fruits. Add high fiber foods like whole grains and beans. Especially avoid unhealthy fats, like trans fats. But make a point to get plenty of essential fatty acids from sea veggies, and herbs like ginger, ginseng or evening primrose oil. Drink plenty of water.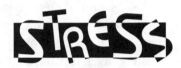

—*On rising:* take a glass of 2 fresh squeezed lemons, 1 tbsp. maple syrup and 8-oz. of pure water.
—*Breakfast:* nutrient-dense Kick-Off Cleansing Cocktail: juice 1 handful fresh wheat grass or parsley, extremely rich in chlorophyll and antioxidants, 4 carrots, 1 apple, 2 celery stalks w. leaves, ½ beet with top.
—*Mid-morning:* a glass of fresh carrot juice or fresh apple juice. Add 1 tbsp. of a green superfood like Crystal Star ENERGY GREEN RENEWAL™ drink; Green Kamut GREEN KAMUT; Vibrant Health GREEN VIBRANCE.
—*Lunch:* have a liquid salad: juice 4 parsley sprigs, 3 large quartered tomatoes, ½ green or red bell pepper, ½ cucumber, 1 scallion, 1 lemon wedge.
—*Mid-afternoon:* a cup of Crystal Star CLEANSING & PURIFYING TEA™, green or white tea, or mint tea.
—*Dinner:* have a warm Potassium Essence Broth (page 291), for mineral electrolytes. Or try Super Soup, with antioxidants, antibiotic properties and immune boosters: 1 cup broccoli florets, 1 leek (white parts, a little green), 2 cups fresh peas, ½ cup sliced scallions, 4 cups chard or bok choy leaves, ½ cup diced fennel bulb, ½ cup fresh parsley, 6 garlic minced cloves, 2 tsp. astragalus extract (or ¼ cup broken pieces astragalus bark), 6 cups vegetable stock, a pinch of cayenne, 1 cup diced green cabbage, ¼ cup snipped sea vegetables. Bring all ingredients to a boil, then simmer for 10 min. Let sit for 20 minutes. Strain and use broth only.

Stress cleanse supplement suggestions: Choose 2 or 3 cleansing boosters.
…**Cleansing boosters:** Crystal Star DETOX BLOOD PURIFIER™ caps with goldenseal stimulates the body to eliminate wastes rapidly, or Planetary RED CLOVER CLEANSE.
…**Cleansing support:** New Chapter LIFE SHIELD; Futurebiotics OXY-SHIELD protects the body against oxidative damage. When solid food is again introduced, use Nature's Secret ULTIMATE CLEANSE.
…**Enzyme support:** Transformation EXCELLZYME; Crystal Star DR. ENZYME™ w. Protease.
…**Antioxidants help remove toxins:** Biotec Foods CELL GUARD; Source Naturals ASTAXANTHIN.
…**Probiotics:** UAS DDS-PLUS + FOS; Jarrow JARROW-DOPHILUS; Pure Essence FLORALIVE.
…**Electrolytes dramatically boost energy:** Alacer EMERGEN-C; Nature's Path Trace-Lyte LIQUID MINS.
…**Green superfoods:** Crystal Star ENERGY GREEN RENEWAL™; Vibrant Health GREEN VIBRANCE.
…**Detoxing flower remedies:** Natural Labs STRESS & TENSION; Nelson Bach RESCUE REMEDY.

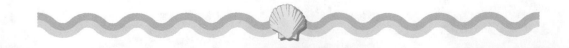

Stress cleanse bodywork suggestions: Techniques to accelerate and round out a cleanse.

...**Enema:** Enemas can be a best friend to your cleansing program. Flushing your colon on the first, the second and the last day of your stress detox gives your body a giant step forward in releasing toxins.

...**Especially helpful:** Guided imagery, biofeedback and aromatherapy techniques.

...**Exercise:** Repeat this body stretch at least 5 times each morning and each evening before bed during your cleanse. Stand tall—raise your hands above your head. Reach your arms and fingers for the sky—move your hands and fingers as if you are trying to climb up into the sky. As you reach, inhale deeply through your nostrils while rising on your toes. Exhale slowly; gradually letting your arms hanging loosely at your sides. Follow your stretch with a brisk walk.

...**Deep Breathing:** Deep, relaxed breathing removes stress, induces relaxation, composes the mind, improves mood and increases energy. 1. Take a deep, full breath. Exhale, slowly. Slowly. 2. Take another deep, full breath. Release slowly. 3. And again. 4. Maintain a quiet rhythm, exhaling more slowly than you inhale.

...**Massage:** Have a massage therapy treatment to further remove toxins and stimulate circulation.

Lung and Chest Congestion Cleanse

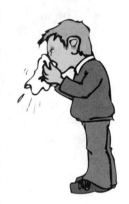

Mucous is unhealthy when it congests us and obstructs our breathing during a sinus infection, asthma or a cold. But that same mucous is also a body lubricant and an important body safeguard. Human beings take about 22,000 breaths a day, and along with the oxygen, we take in dirt, pollen, disease-causing germs, smoke and other pollutants. Mucous gathers up these irritants as they enter the nose and throat to protect the mucous membranes that line the upper respiratory system. So mucous build-up may be a sign that your body is trying to bring itself to health. The problems start when your body holds on to too much. Some of us carry around up to 10 to 15 pounds of excess mucous!

Body systems work together, of course. Extra pressure of disease or heavy elimination on one body part puts extra stress on another. Supporting your kidneys, for example, takes part of the waste elimination load off your lungs so they can recover faster. Similarly, promoting respiratory health also helps digestive and skin cleansing problems. The lungs, though, are on the front line of toxic intake from viruses, allergies, pollutants, and mucous-forming congestives.

A program to overcome any chronic respiratory problem is usually more successful when begun with a short mucous elimination diet. This allows the body to rid itself first of toxins and accumulations that cause congestion before an attempt is made to change eating habits. Foods that putrefy quickly inside your body are the same foods that spoil easily in the air — like meat, fish, eggs and dairy products. These same foods are the ones most likely to produce excess mucous, too, which in turn slows down transit time through your gastrointestinal tract and colon. so you end up feeling logy and congested.

Is your body showing signs that you need a congestion cleanse?

Respiratory system congestion, a cold or flu is a sure sign of excess mucous in the body, especially in the colon and intestinal tract. A mucous cleanse helps release excess mucous in the respiratory system and colon.

Pointers for best results from your lung and chest congestion cleanse:

...Herbal supplements are a good choice for a mucous congestion cleanse. They can break up mucous and act as premier broncho-dilators and anti-spasmodics to open congested airspaces. They soothe bronchial inflammation and coughs. They are expectorants to remove mucous from the lungs and throat.

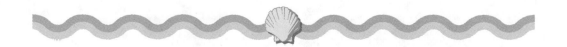

...Drink 8 to 10 glasses of water daily to thin mucous and aid elimination.

...Take 10,000mg ascorbate vitamin C crystals with bioflavonoids daily the first three days —just dissolve ¼ tsp. in water or juice throughout the day, until the stool turns soupy, and tissues are flushed. Take 5000mg daily for the next four days.

...Take a brisk, daily walk. Breathe deeply to help lungs eliminate mucous.

...Take an enema the first and last day of your detox diet to clean out excess mucous.

...Apply wet ginger-cayenne compresses to the chest to boost circulation and loosen mucous.

...Take a hot sauna or a long warm bath with a rubdown to stimulate circulation.

Benefits to notice as your body responds to a mucous congestion cleanse.
—Congestion clear up as the mucous cleansing diet and supportive supplements go to work.
—If there is bronchial inflammation and/or cough it will give way to relief as the cleanse progresses.
—Mucous from the lungs and throat will break up and be eliminated from the body.
—Mucous from the colon may also be expelled from the body.
—Discomfort from colds or flu, allergies or asthma will clear faster as the cleanse speeds up recovery.

Lung and Chest Congestion Cleanse Detox Plan

The night before your mucous cleanse...
—Mash 4 garlic cloves and a large slice of onion in a bowl. Stir in 3 tbsp. honey. Cover, let macerate for 24 hours; remove garlic and onion and take only the honey-syrup infusion — 1 tsp. 3x daily.

The next 3 days....
—*On rising:* take 2 squeezed lemons in water with 1 tbsp. maple syrup.
—*Breakfast:* have a water-diluted grapefruit juice or pineapple juice as natural expectorants with 1 tbsp. green superfood, such as Crystal Star RESTORE YOUR STRENGTH™; Barleans GREENS or Nature's Secret ULTIMATE GREEN; take 2 or 3 garlic capsules and ¼ tsp. ascorbate vitamin C or Ester C powder in water.
—*Mid-morning:* have a glass of fresh carrot juice; or a cup of congestion clearing tea, like Crystal Star D-CONGEST™ extract, to aid mucous release, or Yogi BREATHE DEEP tea, an aid in oxygen uptake.
—*Lunch:* have a vegetable juice like V-8, or a potassium broth (page 291); or make this Mucous Cleansing Tonic by juicing: 4 carrots, 2 celery stalks, 2-3 sprigs parsley, 1 radish and 1 garlic clove.
—*Mid-afternoon:* have a mixed veggie drink, or a packet of Pure Planet CHLORELLA granules in water; or a greens and sea vegetable drink like Crystal Star ENERGY GREEN RENEWAL™ drink.
—*Dinner:* apple or papaya/pineapple juice.
—*Before Bed:* take a hot vegetable broth, add 1 tbsp. nutritional yeast. Have a small fresh salad on the last night of the cleanse.
—*The next day...* begin with small simple meals. Have toasted muesli or whole grain granola for your first morning of solid food, with a little yogurt or apple juice; a small fresh salad for lunch with lemon/oil dressing; a fresh fruit smoothie during the day; a baked potato with butter and a light soup or salad for dinner.

Mucous cleanse supplement suggestions: Choose 2 or 3 cleansing boosters.
...**Deep body cleanser for intestinal tract and lungs:** Use Nature's Way 5 SYSTEM CLEANSE caps after juice cleansing to help pull intestinal mucous and clear mucous congestion from the respiratory system. Nature's Secret ULTIMATE RESPIRATORY CLEANSE for longstanding respiratory-mucous congestion problems.
...**Mucous cleansers:** Use Crystal Star D-CONGEST™ spray to aid mucous release; Herbs Etc. LUNG TONIC to loosen and remove mucous; Baywood Dr. Harris' ORIGINAL ALLERGY FORMULA, herbal antihistamines and enzymes which digest excess mucous secretions, allowing the body to safely eliminate them.

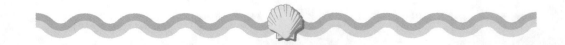

...**Herbs relieve mucous:** mullein loosens / expels mucous; slippery elm removes excess mucous, soothes mucous membranes; sage helps mucous discharge; white pine, an antioxidant expectorant, reduces mucous.

...**Oxygen uptake:** Crystal Star DR. VITALITY™, Yogi BREATHE DEEP, NutriCology Germanium.

...**Enzyme support:** Herbal Products and Development POWER-PLUS ENZYMES; Transformation Enzyme GASTROZYME relieves bouts of mucous congestion.

...**Electrolyte boosters** help digestive efficiency up to 80%: Nature's Path TRACE-LYTE liquid minerals.

...**Probiotics** maintain proper mucous levels: UAS DDS-Plus + FOS; Ethical Nutrients INTESTINAL CARE.

Mucous cleanse bodywork suggestions: Techniques to accelerate, round out your cleanse.

Enema: Take an enema the first, second and last day of your juice fasting to help thoroughly clean out excess mucous. Or, irrigate: have a colonic for a more thorough colon cleanse.

Exercise: Take a brisk walk each day of your cleanse. Breathe deep to help lungs eliminate mucous.

Massage therapy with percussion: a rubdown loosens mucous. Most people have several congestion-releasing bowel movements and expectoration incidences within 24 hours after massage treatment.

Compress: Apply wet *ginger-cayenne* chest compresses to increase circulation and loosen mucous.

Essential oils: Eucalyptus (inhale) — antiviral action loosens mucous. Tea tree oil (inhale) — antiviral, antibacterial decongestant. Oregano oil (inhale) — antiviral, antibacterial helps eradicate infection.

Deep Breathing Exercise: Do this deep breathing exercise often during your cleanse to remove stress, compose your mind, improve your mood and increase your energy: Take a deep, full breath - engage the diaphragm so that the lungs are filled to capacity. Exhale it slowly.... slowly. Take another deep, full breath. Release slowly. And again. Maintain a quiet rhythm, exhaling more slowly than you inhale.

Bathe and Sauna: long warm baths and saunas help loosen mucous congestion. Add to your bath 5 drops of eucalyptus, tea tree oil or oregano oil.

Brown Rice Cleanse

A brown rice diet is a good cleanse for weight loss.

A brown rice cleanse is especially useful for dropping a few quick pounds, and it's a great way to transition from an unhealthy diet into a better diet. A brown rice cleanse is based on macrobiotic principles for body balance. It's cleansing, yet filling. You don't feel like you're on a cleanse at all, yet it does the trick. It's a diet that uses rice as a nutrient building food, and vegetables and vegetable juices as concentrated cleansing supplements. A brown rice cleanse is high in potassium, natural iodine, and other minerals, so most people notice improvement in their hair, skin texture and nail growth.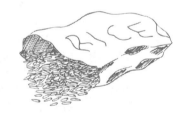

A brown rice diet is the best cleansing diet for colder times of the year. Brown rice adds a building, warming factor to a cleanse, making your meals more satisfying, ensuring that you get plenty of fiber and minerals. It's an effective option to a juice cleanse and much easier to fit into your lifestyle.

Almost everybody loses some weight during this cleanse. Many people experience a 2 to 5 pound weight drop. Most people notice an improvement in vitality and energy levels right away, too. People with heart problems regularly notice a more stable heartbeat and better circulation. A fiber-rich cleansing diet with sea veggies, that eliminates meat and dairy protein, almost invariably lowers the risk of cardiovascular problems.

Is your body showing signs that a brown rice cleanse would help you?

—Is your immune response low?

—Do you feel like you need to clear cobwebs from your brain? Are you feeling logy and out-of-sorts?

—Do you need to lose about 10 pounds?

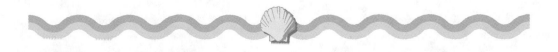

7-Day Brown Rice Detox Plan

The night before your brown rice cleanse....
A green leafy salad for dinner sweeps your bowels. Take an herbal enema the night before your cleanse.

The next day....
—*On rising:* take a glass of 2 fresh squeezed lemons, 1 tbsp. maple syrup and 8-oz. of pure water.
—*Breakfast:* have an energy green drink: 6 carrots, 1 beet, 8 spinach leaves and ¼ cup fresh parsley.
—*Mid-morning:* take a cup of Crystal Star CLEANSING & PURIFYING TEA™ or Yogi PEACH DETOX Tea.
—*Lunch:* have a veggie juice like Super V-7: 2 carrots, 2 tomatoes, a handful of spinach leaves and parsley, 2 celery ribs, ½ cucumber, ½ green bell pepper. Add 1 tbsp. green superfood, like Wakunaga HARVEST BLEND, Body Ecology VITALITY SUPERGREEN, or Nutricology PRO-GREENS.
—*Mid-afternoon:* have a glass of carrot juice.
—*Dinner:* have steamed brown rice and mixed steamed vegetables. Sprinkle with sea veggies like dulse or kelp, easily purchased in flakes or granules. Use 1 tbsp. flax or olive oil, and 1 tbsp. Bragg's LIQUID AMINOS.
—*Before Bed:* have a cup of herbal tea such as peppermint, spearmint or chamomile.
—*The next 6 days:* have 2 to 3 glasses of mixed vegetable juices throughout the day. Don't eat any solid food during the day. Have steamed brown rice and mixed vegetables for an early dinner each evening.

7-day brown rice cleanse supplement suggestions: Choose 2 or 3 cleansing boosters.
...**Cleansing boosters:** Crystal Star FIBER & HERBS COLON CLEANSE CLEANSE™ caps stimulate rapid waste elimination; Nature's Secret ULTIMATE CLEANSE helps detoxify all five channels of elimination.
...**Cleansing teas:** Yogi PEACH DETOX Tea; DAILY DETOX by M.D. gentle enough to take on a daily basis.
...**Enzymes**, a dieter's best friend: Crystal Star DR. ENZYME 2 FAT & STARCH BUSTER™.

7-Day Chemical Pollutant Cleanse

Chemical pollutants and toxic by-products affect every facet of our lives.....our water and food supply, the workplace, our homes. Heavy metal poisoning and pollutant toxicity are major health problems of the American culture. We have moved from fetid air to undrinkable water to severe allergy reactions and serious diseases caused by pollution. There seems to be no way to avoid toxic exposure. The main influence of an unhealthy environment is the damaging effect on immune response, especially the impact on filtering organs, like liver and kidneys. Periodic detoxification can help our bodies defend us.... against yet more pollutants. (An astounding twenty-five thousand NEW chemicals enter our society every year.) A hair analysis can help determine nutrient deficiencies related to chemical overload, and which heavy metals are lodged in your body.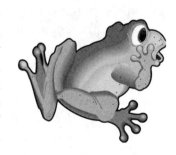

Is your body showing signs that it needs a pollution/heavy metal cleanse?
—Are you far more sensitive to odors like perfumes and strong cleansers than most people?
—Do you have an unusually small tolerance for alcohol?
—Are there medications you can't take, or some vitamins or other supplements that make you feel worse?
—Do you have small black spots along your gum line? Unusually bad breath or body odor?
—Is your reaction time when driving noticeably poorer in city traffic?
—Do you have unexplained seizures, memory failure or psychotic behavior?
—Have you become infertile or impotent?

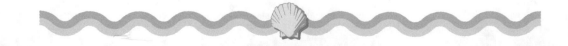

7-Day Chemical Pollution Detox Plan

Note: A heavy metal, pollutant detox is one of the most likely cleanses for a "healing crisis" to occur. You may feel head-achy, with a slight upset stomach as toxins release. Drink more water to help reduce symptoms. The feelings should pass quickly, usually within 24 hours. I don't recommend an all-liquid diet if you're trying to release heavy metals or chemicals. They may enter the bloodstream too fast and heavily for your body to handle safely. Eat solid cleansing foods instead to release the toxins more slowly and safely.

—*On rising:* 2 tbsp. cranberry concentrate in water with ½ tsp. vitamin C crystals or 1 tsp. liquid MSM; or Crystal Star GREEN TEA CLEANSER™; or blend 2 tsp. lemon, 1 tsp. honey, 1 cup water and 1 tsp. acidophilus in 8-oz. aloe vera juice.

—*Breakfast:* have a glass of fresh carrot juice with 1 tsp. green superfood like Barleans GREENS or Pines MIGHTY GREENS, and whole grain muffins or rice cakes with kefir cheese; or a cup of soy milk or plain yogurt blended with a cup of fresh fruit, walnuts, and ½ tsp. acidophilus) in 8-oz. aloe vera juice.

—*Mid-morning:* take a cup of green tea, with ½ tsp. ascorbate vitamin C crystals; or a fresh vegetable juice with 1 tbsp. green superfood such as Nutricology PRO-GREENS or Wakunaga KYO-GREEN.

—*Lunch:* have a leafy salad with lemon-flax oil dressing; or a cup of miso soup with brown rice; or steamed veggies with brown rice; and green tea with ½ tsp. vitamin C and ½ tsp. acidophilus powder.

—*Mid-afternoon:* have a carrot juice with 1 tsp. spirulina or a packet of chlorella.

—*Dinner:* have a baked potato with Bragg's Liquid Aminos and a fresh salad with lemon-flax dressing; or a black bean or lentil soup; or a Chinese steam/stir fry with vegetables, shiitake mushrooms and brown rice.

—*Before Bed:* an 8-oz. glass of aloe vera juice with ½ tsp. vitamin C and another carrot juice.

7-day chemical-pollutant cleanse supplement suggestions:

…**Pollutant/Heavy Metal cleansers:** Crystal Star TOXIN DETOX™ caps, or sea greens 2 tbsp. daily; Bernard Jensen LIQUI-DULS; New Chapter CHLORELLA REGULARIS; N-Acetyl-Cysteine 600mg. daily.

…**Enzyme support:** Protease binds to heavy metals, sparing metabolic enzyme destruction. Transformation Enzyme PUREZYME (high doses effective in lowering blood mercury toxins).

…**Liver enhancers:** Planetary BUPLEURUM LIVER CLEANSE; *Milk Thistle Seed* extract or *dandelion* extract.

…**Antioxidants defeat pollutants:** Alpha Lipoic Acid is one of the most powerful liver detoxifiers ever discovered. Jarrow Formulas ALPHA LIPOIC or ALPHA-LIPOIC by MRI; NutriCology ANTIOX FORMULA II.

…**Oral chelation rids heavy metals:** Metabolic Response Modifiers CARDIO CHELATE; Golden Pride FORMULA ONE w/ EDTA. PSP Marketing DESTROXIN (Zeolite) detoxifies heavy metals and petrochemicals (highly recommended by holistic health practitioner, Howard Peiper, N.D.)

Fat and Sugar Cleanse

Is your body showing signs that it needs a fat and sugar cleanse?

—Is cellulite, a mixture of fat, water and wastes, collecting on your hips, thighs or tummy?

—Are your upper arms slightly flabby, your waistline, wrists and ankles noticeably thicker?

—Does your face look jowl-y or puffy?

Try my light fat and sugar detox. It makes you feel terrific and it's so easy. Sugary foods, fried foods and fast foods are so devoid of digestive enzymes that they collect as excess fat. Your body also dumps its congestive metabolic wastes to get them out of the way — one of the places that receives metabolic wastes is fat. Start the night before with a green leafy salad to sweep your intestines. Dry brush your skin all over for five minutes before you go to bed to open your pores for the night's cleansing eliminations.

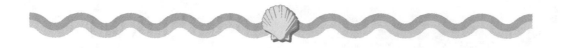

1 to 3 Day Intense Fat and Sugar Cleanse

—*Upon rising:* have a cup of green tea to cut through and eliminate fatty wastes. For maximum results, add drops of ginseng extract to control sugar cravings, or licorice extract for maximum sugar stabilizing.

—*Breakfast:* have a Fat Melt Down Juice: juice 2 apples, 2 pears, 1 slice of fresh ginger to help reduce fat from places where it is stored in cellulite. The ginger stimulates better blood circulation.

—*Mid-morning:* have a daily superfood drink. Green superfoods help cleanse the body of fatty build-up.

—*Lunch:* enjoy a mixed vegetable juice, like Knudsen's VERY VEGGIE. Even regular V-8 juice works fine.

—*Mid-afternoon:* Enzymes are a dieter's best friend! Take a glass of papaya-pineapple juice, or green tea.

—*Dinner:* Have some miso soup with snipped sea greens. Seaweeds add minerals and improve sluggish metabolism. Add spices like cinnamon, cayenne, mustard and ginger to speed up the fat burning process.

—*Before bed:* have apple juice, or licorice or peppermint tea to rebalance and restore normal body pH.

Watchwords:

•Add more fiber from whole grains and vegetables to get rid of excess sugar. High fiber foods improve glucose metabolism, promote weight loss and reduce sugar cravings.

•A 15 minute dry sauna 3x a week really helps balance sugar levels. When I worked at a European spa, we used this technique for weight loss and blood sugar problems with great results!

•Expert dieters drink 8 glasses of water a day. Water naturally suppresses appetite and helps a high metabolic rate. Water is the most important catalyst for increased fat burning. It enhances the liver's ability to detox and metabolize so it can process more fats. Don't worry about fluid retention; high water intake <u>decreases</u> bloating, because it flushes out sodium and toxins.

1-3 Day Intense Fat and Sugar Cleanse supplement suggestions:

…**Essential fatty acids**: Without essential fatty acids (EFA's), poor fat metabolism is certain. Control excess fluid retention with EFA's. Flax Oil -1 or 2 tbsp. over a salad; Crystal Star *Evening Primrose Oil*, 2000mg daily; CLA, an Omega-6 fatty acid with fat-burning properties, 1800mg daily.

…**Appetite suppressants:** Crystal Star DETOX-FAT & SUGAR RELEASE™ formula especially helps prevent overeating fatty and sugary foods while your body releases the excess it has; Gaia Herbs DIET SLIM; Source Naturals DIET-PHEN.

…**Special tips:** Source Naturals GLUCO SCIENCE, 3x daily. Acupressure for sugar willpower: pinch the little bud of cartilage above your ear canal for 1 minute to short-circuit nerve impulses that cause cravings.

Intense Fat and Sugar cleanse bodywork suggestions:

<u>Enema</u>: Take an enema the first day of your excess fat cleanse to help release toxins out of the body.

<u>Exercise</u>: Exercise promotes an "afterburn" effect, raising metabolic rates for up to 24 hours. Exercise before a meal raises blood sugar levels and decreases appetite for several hours. Exercise for women with the little tummy bulge that appears at menopause? 100 hard tummy sucks each morning. It works!

<u>Dry brushing</u>: Fatty wastes get trapped beneath the skin's surface easily (especially in women) when the liver or lymphatic systems are sluggish. Use a natural bristle brush - brush vigorously 5 to 10 minutes in a rotary motion and massage in this order: feet and legs, hands and arms, back and abdomen, chest and neck.

<u>Massage</u>: Have a massage therapy treatment at the end of your cleanse to move excess fluid wastes and unattached fats into elimination systems, and to stimulate skin circulation.

<u>Bathe away excess fats</u>: Crystal Star HOT SEAWEED BATH™; or a sea salt bath: add 1 cup Dead Sea salts, 1 cup Epsom salts, ½ cup regular sea salt and ¼ baking soda to a tub; swish in 3 drops lavender oil, 2 geranium drops oil, 2 drops sandalwood oil and 1 drop neroli oil.

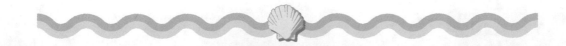

About detoxification juices....

Detoxification drinks have a powerful effect on your body's recuperative powers because of their rich, easily absorbed nutrients. Fresh juices contain proteins, carbohydrates, chlorophyll, mineral electrolytes and healing aromatic oils. But most importantly, fresh juice therapy makes available to every cell large amounts of plant enzymes, an integral part of the healing and restoration process.

Nothing gets done in our bodies without enzymes. Digestion, assimilation and elimination are all instigated or assisted by enzymes. Enzymes play a vital part in breaking down foreign matter like toxins, as well as food. Enzymes and mineral electrolytes (which restore bowel peristaltic activity) are major contributors to moving toxins out of the body instead of building up and poisoning us. When your diet is full of cooked foods without enzymes, or low residue, processed foods (which tend to putrefy), internal decay develops far more rapidly.

Our bodies are designed to be self-healing organisms. Healing is allowed to occur through cleansing. Cleansing foods and juices can optimize your detox program. In fact, they are crucial to its success in three ways:

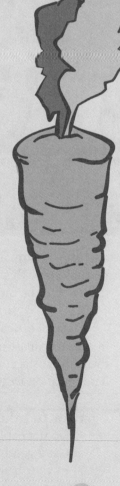

1) They keep your body chemistry balanced and body processes stable while you detox, so you don't become uncomfortable. Remember... Mother Nature is cleaning house during a detox. You may eliminate accumulated poisons and wastes quite rapidly, causing headaches, slight nausea and weakness as your body purges. (These reactions are usually only temporary and disappear along with the waste and toxins.)

2) They regulate the speed of your detox so your body doesn't cleanse too fast or dump too many toxins into your bloodstream all at once that your body can't handle.

3) They support your nutrition and energy levels while you detox, so you don't become too hungry or too tired. New healthy tissue starts building right away when you take in detoxification juices. Gland secretions stimulate the immune system during a cleanse to set up a disease defense environment.

Should you get a juicer?
Juicers are expensive, but they really boost the nutrient power of your cleansing drinks. A good juicer essentially predigests fresh fruits and vegetables for fast assimilation by your body. A juicer can juice all of a fruit or vegetable (rinds, stems, peels, seeds) to give you up to 95% of the plant's nutritive value.
Champion, JuiceMan and Acme are all good juicers for a detox program.

Need good recipes for detox drinks, juices and foods?
Check out my new COOKING for HEALTHY HEALING COOKBOOKS and my DETOXIFICATION BOOK for loads of Green Cuisine recipes to make your detox a success!

Bodywork Techniques for Detoxification

Detoxing is lifestyle therapy. Bodywork is a big part of body cleansing. This chapter has step-by-step instructions for bodywork techniques you can do to acclerate and enhance your detox program.

Overheating therapy can realize enormous health benefits

Overheating therapy has been known throughout history. It's really <u>hyper</u>thermia used as a healing technique. Ancient healers knew that a slight fever was a powerful healing tool against disease. Greek physicians raised body temperature in healing centers as an immune defense against infection. I've visited such an ancient center near Pergamum in modern Turkey, that still exists. It was amazingly modern to my eyes. The Romans had elaborate bath complexes for cleansing and healing. The Scandinavians use healing steam baths today. Native Americans and Hawaiians still use sweat lodges for spiritual and cleansing rituals. On a recent herbal tour I led to the Southwest, I participated in a sweat lodge ceremony. Even that short experience showed me how powerful overheating therapy can be.

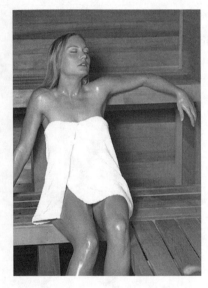

High heat procedures, like overheating baths, saunas and steam rooms are reemerging therapeutically today as health care professionals find that a non-life-threatening fever can have exceptional healing activity. Slightly raising body temperature creates a natural defense and healing force by the immune system to rid the body of harmful pathogens... to literally burn out invading organisms. Ancient herbalists used heat-producing herbs as protective healing measures against colds and simple infections, even against serious degenerative diseases like skin tumors. Today, alternative healing clinics use artificially induced fevers to treat infections like acute bronchitis, pneumonia, arthritic conditions like fibromyalgia and lupus, even cancers like leukemia.

Despite skepticism by conventional medicine, for supergerms like the HIV virus with no effective drug therapies, other methods must be tried. AIDS syndromes like cytomegalovirus respond to blood heating. CNN Health News reported on a blood heating procedure for AIDS in treating Kaposi's sarcoma, a cancer that produces severe skin lesions in HIV-infected patients. The sores vanished in about four months after the therapy, along with other symptoms. Since 1997 many AIDS sufferers with sarcoma have undergone hyperthermia with success. In some cases, the blood has even tested negative for the HIV virus! (Researchers warn that even if the blood tests HIV free the virus may still be in the bone and re-surface.)

How overheating therapy works as a detoxification mechanism: When exposed to heat, blood vessels in the skin dilate to allow more blood to flow to the surface, activating sweat glands which then pour water onto the skin's surface. As the water evaporates, it draws both heat and toxins out through the skin becoming a natural detoxification treatment as well as a cooling system and immune response stimulant.

How to take a simple overheating therapy bath in your home:
1: Do not eat for two hours before treatment. Empty your bladder and colon if possible.
2: Get a good thermometer so that your water temperature can be correctly monitered.
3: In your bathtub, plug the emergency outlet to raise the water to the top of the tub. You must be totally immersed for therapeutic results — with only nose, eyes and mouth left uncovered. Start slowly running water at skin temperature. After 15 minutes raise temperature to 100°F, then in 15 minutes to 103°F. Even though the water temperature is not high, heat cannot escape from your body when you are totally covered, so body temperature will rise to match that of the water, creating a slight healing fever.

Can't find a recommended product? Call the 800 number in Product Resources for the store nearest you.

4: A therapy bath should be about 45 minutes. If you have any discomfort, sit up in the tub for 5 minutes.

5: Gentle massaging with a skin brush during the bath stimulates circulation, brings cleansing blood to the surface of the skin and relieves the heart from undue pressure.

A sauna is another way to use overheating therapy principles.

Today, alternative physicians and clinics use saunas as an easy way to help people release toxins like pollutants and heavy metals. A 30 minute sauna raises body temperature enough to induce a mild, cleansing fever, and a therapeutic sweat. A good sweat allows your skin to eliminate body wastes through perspiration. It dramatically increases the detoxification capacity of your skin and optimizes the skin's ability to normalize its protective mantle and pH. Finish each sauna with a cool shower and a brisk rubdown to remove released toxins on the skin. Note: Dry sauna heat can aggravate rosacea, but benefits most other skin disorders.

To use a sauna as a healing technique, and to enhance immune response, especially during high risk seasons, take a sauna once or twice a week. Like an overheating therapy bath, a sauna also inhibits the advance of infective organisms that cause diseases like flu and bronchitis. A sauna reaches deeper into body processes, boosting organ and gland activity. I personally have seen people with blood sugar disorders like hypoglycemia benefit dramatically from a bi-weekly sauna.

Cleansing benefits of a dry sauna:
—creates a fever that inhibits the replication of pathogenic bacteria and viruses
—increases the number of leukocytes in the blood to strengthen the immune system
—provides a prolonged, therapeutic sweat that flushes out toxins and heavy metals
—stimulates vasodilation of peripheral blood vessels to relieve pain and speed healing
—accelerates cardiovascular activity, reduces high blood pressure, promotes relaxation and well-being

Steam baths go back to the prehistoric hot springs of early man.

Our first ancestors, like primates today in both Japan and Russia, used hot springs to clean and warm himself, and to remove parasites. As with dry heat saunas, ancient Greeks and Romans used them to sweat for health. But the benefits of a steam bath are different than those of a sauna. Hot steam particularly helps respiratory diseases and rheumatic pain. The humid heat of a steam bath is ideal for skin tone and texture.

A steam bath works quicker than a sauna, too, cleansing the body in about 15 minutes compared to 30 to 40 minutes in a sauna. The powerful detoxification process of hyperthermia does not take place until the body reaches a temperature of 101-103° F. In a dry heat sauna, your body's cooling mechanism retards hyperthermia by natural evaporation. In a steam bath, evaporation is not possible so there is no loss of body heat. In fact, steam condensation actually becomes the heat transfer mechanism on the body.

Note: Overheating is one of the most effective treatments in natural healing. Inducing a "fever" is a natural, constructive means the body also uses to heal itself. Heat methods are powerful and should be used with care. If you are under medical supervision for heart disease or high blood pressure, a heart vitality check-up is advisable. If you are, or have been recently ill, supervision is needed during an overheating bath, and reactions must be monitored closely. The pulse should not go over 130 or 140. Some people who are seriously ill lose the ability to perspire; this should be known before using overheating therapy. Check with your physician to determine if overheating therapy from a sauna or a seaweed bath is all right for you.

Can't find a recommended product? Call the 800 number in Product Resources for the store nearest you.

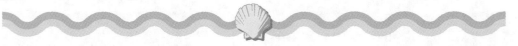

Water therapy helps your cleanse in many ways

1: A detox bath is pleasant, easy and stress free.

Healing clinics and spas are famous all over the world for their therapy baths. They use mineral clays, aromatherapy oils, seaweeds and enzyme herbs to draw toxins out of the body through the skin, and to put restorative nutrients into the body through the skin. During a detox program, take a daily therapy bath to remove toxins coming out on the skin. The procedure for an effective healing bath is important, because you're soaking in an herbal tea, letting your skin take in the healing nutrients instead of the digestive system.

There are two good ways to take a therapeutic bath:

1: Draw very hot bath water. Put the herbs and seaweeds into a large teaball or muslin bath bag. Add mineral salts directly to the water. Steep until water is aromatic. Rub your body with the solids in the muslin bag during the bath.

OR

2: Make a strong tea infusion in a large teapot, strain and add to hot bath water. Soak as long as possible to give the body time to absorb the healing properties.

Note: Before your bath, dry brush your body all over for 5 minutes with a natural bristle, dry skin brush to remove toxins from the skin and open pores for nutrients. After your bath, use a mineral salt rub, such as Trillium BODY POLISH, a spa "finishing" technique to make your skin feel healthy for hours.

2: Thalassotherapy uses the sea for cleansing and health.

Thalassotherapy is an ageless, cleansing, health-restorative technique. Thalassa is the ancient Greek word for sea. The Greeks indeed used the sea for their health care and well-being. I myself have seen 2500 year-old healing sites on the Greek islands of Rhodes and Corfu, and the ancient Greek healing center at Pergamum in what is now Turkey. Even judging by the therapeutic centers still known to us, much of the population of the ancient world soaked in sea water tubs and hot seaweed baths, drank and inhaled sea water for health, got sea water massages, had seaweed facials and and used sea water pools for hydrotherapy and detoxification. Today, we are learning once again, about the ability of the sea to reduce tension and de-stress us, detoxify our bodies, improve circulation, relieve allergies and congestion, and ease arthritis symptoms.

Seaweed baths are Nature's perfect body/psyche balancer.

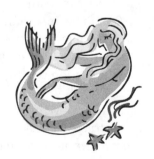

Remember how good you feel after an ocean walk? Seaweeds purify and balance the ocean — they can do the same for your body. A hot seaweed bath is like a wet-steam sauna, only better, because the sea greens balance body chemistry instead of dehydrating. Electro-magnetic action of the seaweed releases excess fluids from congested cells, and dissolves fatty wastes through the skin, replacing them with minerals, especially potassium and iodine. Iodine boosts thyroid activity, so food is used before it turns into fatty deposits. A seaweed bath once a week stimulates lymph drainage and fat burning so you can keep off excess weight and reduce trapped cellulite waste. Vitamin K in seaweed boosts adrenal activity to maintain hormone balance for a younger body.

How to take a seaweed soak:

If you live near the ocean, gather seaweeds from the water, (not the shoreline) in buckets or trash cans; carry them home to your tub. Or buy dried seaweeds from your health food store. Crystal Star packages dried seaweeds, gathered from pristine waters around Maine, in a made-to-order HOT SEAWEED BATH™.

Can't find a recommended product? Call the 800 number in Product Resources for the store nearest you.

Place the seaweeds in a tub and run very hot water over them, filling the tub to the point that you will be covered when you recline. The water turns rich brown as the plants release their minerals. Add an aromatherapy oil if desired, to help hold the heat in and boost your detox program. Let the bath cool enough to get in. As you soak, the gel from the seaweed transfers onto and coats your skin. Your skin perspires under the coating to release system toxins, which are replaced with sea minerals by osmosis. Enhance this process by rubbing your skin with the seaweed during the bath to stimulate circulation and remove wastes coming out on the skin surface. When the sea greens have done their work, the gel coating dissolves and floats off the skin, and the seaweeds shrivel - a sign that the bath is over.

Note: The release of the gel coating is a natural timekeeper for the bath. Forty-five minutes is long enough to balance body pH, encourage liver action and fat metabolism. You'll see better skin texture and color almost immediately. After the bath, take a cayenne - ginger capsule to assimilate the seaweed minerals.

No time for a soak? Seaweed facials are great tonics for your skin.

The ancient Greeks said that Aphrodite, goddess of love, rising out of the foamy sea, owed her supple skin, shiny hair and sparkling eyes to the ocean's plants. Human body makeup is a lot like that of the ocean, so taking in things from the sea helps replace nutrients we may have lost. Sea plants especially contain minerals that stress and pollution deplete from the skin. Sea plant cell structure allows your skin to easily absorb the minerals. A seaweed facial stimulates lymphatic drainage and dilates capillaries for better tone. Sea plant mineral salts help your skin hold moisture and plump up, smoothing out fine lines and wrinkles. Sea plants contain elements similar to collagen that make the skin more supple and elastic, and add amazing luster.

Thalassotherapy seaweed wraps are premier restorative body conditioners.

Top spas use thalassotherapy seaweed wraps to rapidly cleanse the body of toxins, and to elasticize and tone the skin. The sea plant mineral solution easily enters skin pores to break down unwanted fatty cells and cellulite deposits stored in fluids between cells. Wraps are most successful when used along with a short detox program that includes 8 glasses of water a day to flush out loosened fats and wastes.

I have seen astounding benefits from thalassotherapy wraps during my work with sea herbs in European spas. The results were so amazing I formulated two gel wraps you can use at home.

__Here's how:__ Mix 10 drops of _each_ herbal extract for each wrap in aloe vera gel; slather on your torso, upper arms and thighs to the knee. Have a partner wind plastic wrap several times around your thighs, upper arms and torso to just _under_ the breasts. Lie down on towels, cover yourself with towels or a cotton blanket, turn on soft music and relax for an hour.

1) Tightening and toning wrap to improve muscle, vein and skin tone:
   Extracts of *Kelp, Cranesbill, White Oak, Marshmallow, Angelica, Rosemary, Lemon Balm, Hawthorn.*
2) Thermogenesis wrap to enhance metabolism, boost circulation and reduce puffiness:
   Extracts of *Bladderwrack or Kelp, Alfalfa, Ginger Root, Dandelion, Spearmint, Capsicum, Cinnamon.*

3: Hot and cold hydrotherapy stimulates vital healing energy.

Alternating hot and cold showers increase lymph drainage, discharge toxins, improve blood flow, stimulate metabolic activity, relieve cramps, tone muscles, relax bowel and bladder tightness, and boost energy.

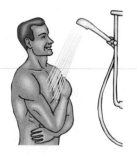

—Home hydrotherapy is easy. Begin with a hot shower for three minutes. Follow with a sudden change to cold water for 2 minutes. Repeat this cycle three times, ending with cold. Brush with a natural bristle brush or loofa your skin during the cold cycle. Follow your shower with a full or partial massage, or a brisk towel rub, and then finish with some mild stretching exercises.

Can't find a recommended product? Call the 800 number in Product Resources for the store nearest you.

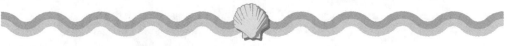

4: What are ozone pools? How do they help your body purify?

Ozone, or "activated oxygen" (O₃) is the fresh, clean scent you smell in the air after a thunderstorm. Ozone is the most powerful natural oxygenator available and one of the fastest, safest and most thorough methods of purification known. Professional spas use ozone pools in their detox treatments today to destroy water and airborne viruses, cysts, bacteria and fungi on contact. Ozone pool baths are actually the next generation of oxygen baths that you can use in your own home detox plan. They noticeably increase energy and tissue oxygen uptake.

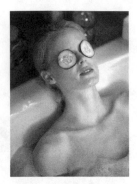

Take an oxygen bath once a day each day of your cleanse.

Start with a food grade 35% hydrogen peroxide. Pour in 1 cup per bath. (Alternate bath: add ½ cup food grade H_2O_2, ½ cup sea salt, and ½ cup baking soda to bath.) Soak for about 30 minutes. Oxygen baths are stimulating rather than relaxing. Most people notice a significant energy increase within 3 days. Other benefits include body balance and detoxification, reduction of skin cancers and tumors, relief of asthma and lung congestion, as well as arthritis and rheumatism.

Use herbs that supply oxygen through the skin. *Rosemary, peppermint* and *mullein* are very effective. Pack a small muslin bath or tea bag with the herb, drop it in the tub or spa, and soak for 20 minutes. Use the bag as a skin scrub during the bath to tone and smooth skin.

Home use protocol for food grade hydrogen peroxide:

For external use, purchase 35% food grade H_2O_2, or magnesium peroxide from your local health food store. Do not use household, beauty supply or any other form of peroxide for internal use - many of these products have added chemicals to stabilize the H_2O_2. You will also need an eye dropper.

Watchwords for using H_2O_2: Don't take with carrot juice, carbonated drinks or alcohol. Take on an empty stomach 1 hr. before or 3 hours after meals. If you get the 35% H_2O_2 on your skin, rinse it under running water a few minutes. Do not ever take 35% H_2O_2 internally without diluting. Buy 3% H_2O_2 from the health food store instead. If your stomach is upset at any level from 3% H_2O_2, go back one level for a day or two. Then proceed again.

As your body releases dead bacteria or various forms of poisons from your tissues, you may experience cleansing effects as they are eliminated through the skin, lungs, kidneys and bowels. Some reactions to the cleansing effect could include skin eruptions, slight nausea, headaches, sleepiness, unusual fatigue, diarrhea, head or chest congestion, ear infections, boils or other ways the body uses to loosen toxins. This is natural cleansing of the body and should be of short duration.

For infections or funguses, I find it more beneficial to use H_2O_2 in an alternating series - usually 10 days of use, and then 10 days of rest, or 3 weeks of use, and 3 weeks of rest, in more serious cases.

An easy chart to determine number of days, drops and times per day to take H_2O_2:

Count Day	Number of drops	Times per day
1	3	3
2	4	3
3	5	3
4	6	3
5	7	3
6	8	3
7	9	3
8	10	3
9	11	3
10	12	3

Can't find a recommended product? Call the 800 number in Product Resources for the store nearest you.

...**Douche:** mix 6 tbsp. of 3% solution to a quart of warm distilled water. Do not exceed this amount.

...**Colonic enema:** add 1 cup 3% solution to 5 gallons warm water. Do not exceed this amount.

...**Regular enema:** add 1 tablespoon of 3% solution to a quart of warm distilled water.

...**Detox bath:** add about 2 quarts 3% H_2O_2 to a tub of warm water.

...**Foot soak:** add 3% H_2O_2 to a gallon of warm water as needed.

...**For animals:** 1-oz. of 3% H_2O_2 can be added to 1 qt. of your pets drinking water if they are ill.

...**Humidifiers and steamers:** mix 1 pint 3% solution to 1 gallon of water.

...**Vegetable soak:** add ¼ cup 3% H_2O_2 to a sink of cold water. Soak light skinned vegetables (like lettuce) 20 minutes, thicker skinned (like cucumbers) for 30 minutes. Drain, dry and chill to prolong freshness. If time is a problem, spray produce with a solution of 3%. Let stand for a few minutes, rinse and dry.

...**To freshen kitchen:** use a spray bottle of 3% to wipe off counter tops and appliances. It will disinfect and give the kitchen a fresh smell. Works great to clean a musty refrigerator and kids' school lunch boxes.

...**House and garden plants:** put 1-oz. of 3% in 1 quart water. Mist plants with this solution to deter pests.

For topical therapeutic use: at a 3% solution, H_2O_2 can effectively be used externally. Make a 3% solution by mixing 1 part 35% H_2O_2 with 11 parts of water. Place in a spray bottle or dip a cotton ball in the solution and use as a facial freshener after bathing, being careful to avoid the eyes, eyebrows and hair.

Earth's Bounty O_2 gel, mixed with aloe vera juice, vegetable glycerine and red seaweed extract, is useful as a topical antiseptic and antifungal. Apply to affected areas, or massage into the soles of the feet.

5: A baking soda alkalizing bath balances an over-acid system.

It is a simple but remarkable therapeutic treatment for detoxification. It is especially helpful if you suffer from too little sleep, high stress, too much alcohol, caffeine or nicotine, chronic colds or flu, or over-medication. Baking soda balances an over-acid system leaving you refreshed and invigorated, with extra soft skin.

How to take a baking soda bath:

Fill the bath with pleasantly hot water to cover you when you recline. Add 8-oz. baking soda and swirl to dissolve. Soak for 30 minutes. When you emerge, wrap up in a big thick towel and lie down for 15 minutes to dispel any weakness or dizziness that might occur from the heat and rapid toxin release. Use this rest time for a face mask — the hot water will have opened up the pores for maximum benefits.

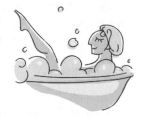

6: An arthritis sweat bath releases a surprising amount of toxic material.

Inorganic sediment residues can aggravate your joints. Epsom salts or Dead Sea salts, and herbs with a diaphoretic action, can play a big part in the success of the bath.

How to take the arthritis bath: Improvement after an arthritic sweat bath experience is notable.

For best results, take this bath at night before retiring. *Note: Protect your mattress with a sheet of plastic.* Make a tea of *elder flowers, peppermint* and *yarrow*. Drink it hot before the bath. Pour 3 pounds Epsom Salts or enough Dead Sea salts for 1 bath into very hot bath water. In the bath, rub arthritic joints with a stiff brush for 5 to 10 minutes — stay in the bath for 20 to 25 minutes. On emerging, do not dry yourself. Wrap up immediately in a clean sheet and go straight to bed, covering yourself with several blankets. The osmotic pressure of the Epsom salt solution absorbed by the sheet will draw off heavy perspiration. The next morning the sheet will be stained with wastes excreted through your skin — sometimes the color of egg yolk. *Note: This is a strong detox procedure and it happens relatively quickly. Take extra care if you have a weak heart or high blood pressure.* Repeat the bath once every two weeks until sheet is no longer stained, a sign that the body is cleansed. Drink pure water throughout the procedure to prevent dehydration and loss of body salts.

Can't find a recommended product? Call the 800 number in Product Resources for the store nearest you.

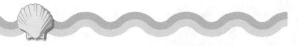

7: A sitz bath puts herbal help where you need it most.

A sitz bath is a healing technique for increasing circulation in the pelvic and urethral area. It's a good way to relieve anal and vaginal irritations, and improve the pelvic muscle tone if you suffer from incontinence (a fast growing group of people in America). The best sitz baths combine herbs with astringent, antiseptic, emollient, and hemostatic properties that assist the natural healing process. Sitz baths help women recover from hemorrhoids and vaginal infections. They help men strengthen the prostate, urinary and anal area.

How to take a sitz bath:
—*For a cold sitz bath*, use cool water at a temperature anywhere from 40° to 85°F. Make a strong, strained tea with your choice of herbs. A good combination includes herbs like *goldenseal root, marshmallow root, plantain, juniper berry, saw palmetto berry, slippery elm* and *witch hazel leaf*. Add the tea to 3" of water in a tub. Soak in the bath for 5 minutes with enough water to reach your navel, once a day for 5 minutes until healed. Use the strained herbs as a compress on the affected area after the bath.

OR

—*For a hot sitz bath*, start with water about 100°F and increase the heat by letting hot water drip continuously into the tub until the temperature reaches about 112°F. The water should cover your hips when seated. Add Epsom salts, Breh or Batherapy bath salts, *ginger powder, comfrey* or *chamomile* to the bath water. Place your feet at the faucet end of the tub so that they are soaking in slightly hotter water as the water drips in. Cover your upper body with a towel, and your forehead with a cool, wet washcloth. After 25 minutes, take a cool shower rinse before drying off to stimulate circulation.

Enemas use water flushing to cleanse your insides

Enemas are an important part of a congestion cleansing detox. They release old, encrusted colon waste, discharge parasites, freshen the G.I. tract and make the cleansing process easier and more thorough. Enemas accelerate any cleanse for better results. They are especially helpful during a healing crisis, after a serious illness to speed healing, or to remove drug residues. Migraines and skin problems like psoriasis are relieved with enemas. Adding herbs to the enema water serves to immediately alkalize the bowel area, control irritation and inflammation, and provide healing action to ulcerated or distended tissue.

Herbs for specific enemas. *Use 2 cups strong brewed tea to 1-qt. water per enema.*
—**Garlic** helps kill parasites, harmful bacteria, and cleanses mucous congestion. Blend 6 garlic cloves in 2 cups water and strain. For small children, use 1 clove garlic to 1 pint water.
—**Catnip** is effective for stomach and digestive conditions, and for childhood diseases.
—**Pau d'arco** normalizes body pH against immune deficient diseases like yeast and fungal infections.
—**Spirulina** helps detoxify both blood and bowels. Use 2 tbsp. powder to 1-qt. water.
—**Wheat grass** boosts immune response; helps eliminate blood toxins; stimulates the liver and colon.
—**Lobelia** neutralizes food poisoning especially if vomiting prevents antidote herbs being taken by mouth.
—**Aloe vera juice enemas** heal tissues in cases of hemorrhoids, irritable bowel and diverticulitis.
—**Lemon juice enemas** rapidly neutralize an acid system, cleanse the colon and bowel.
—**Acidophilus enemas** relieve gas, yeast infections and candidiasis. Mix 4-oz. powder in 1-qt. water.
—**Coffee enemas** detoxify the liver, stimulating both liver and gallbladder to remove toxins, open bile ducts, increase peristaltic action, and produce enzyme activity for healthy red blood cell formation and oxygen uptake. Use 1 cup of regular strong brewed coffee to 1-qt. water. Also often effective for migraine headaches.

Can't find a recommended product? Call the 800 number in Product Resources for the store nearest you.

How to take an effective detox enema:

Place warm enema solution in an enema bag. Hang the bag about 18 inches higher than the body. Attach the colon tube, and lubricate its attachment with vaseline or vitamin E oil. Expel a little water to let out air bubbles. Lying on your left side, slowly insert the attachment about 3 inches into the rectum. Never use force. Rotate attachment gently to ease insertion. Remove kinks in the tubing so liquid will flow freely. Massage abdomen, or flex and contract stomach muscles to relieve any cramping. When all solution has entered the colon, slowly remove the tube and remain on the left side for 5 minutes. Then move to a knee-chest position with your body weight on your knees and one hand. Use the other hand to massage the lower left side of the abdomen for several minutes.

Massage loosens old fecal matter. Roll onto your back for 5 minutes, massaging up the descending colon, over the transverse colon to the right side and down the ascending colon. Then move onto your right side for 5 minutes, in order to reach each part of the colon. Get up and quickly expel into the toilet. Sticky grey-brown mucous, small dark crusty chunks or tough ribbony pieces are usually loosened and expelled during an enema. These poisonous looking things are obstacles and toxins interfering with normal body functions. An enema removes them from you. You may have to take several enemas until there is no more evidence of these substances.

Fresh wheatgrass juice enemas stimulate the liver to cleanse. Wheatgrass enema nutrients are absorbed by the hemorrhoidal vein, just inside the anal sphincter, then circulate to the liver where they increase peristaltic action of the colon, and attract waste and old fecal matter like a magnet to be eliminated from the body. Wheatgrass juice tones the colon and is absorbed into the blood, adding oxygen and energy to the body.

—Use pure water for an initial enema rinse of the colon.
—Then use about a cup of water to 4 ounces of fresh wheatgrass juice.
—Hold the juice for ten minutes while massaging colon area. Then, expel.

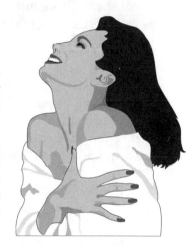

Herbal implants are concentrated enema solutions for more serious health problems, like colitis, arthritis or prostate inflammation. For best results, prepare for an implant by taking a small enema to clear out the lower bowel. You'll be able to hold the implant longer.

Implant procedure: Mix 2 tbsp. herbal powder like spirulina, or wheat grass in $\frac{1}{2}$ cup water and add to a syringe. Lubricate the tip of the syringe with vaseline or vitamin E oil, get down on your hands and knees and insert the nozzle slowly and gently into the rectum. Squeeze the bulb to insert the mixture into the rectum, *but do not release pressure on the bulb before withdrawing*, so the mixture stays in the lower bowel. Hold 15 minutes before expelling.

A colonic irrigation is a "super enema."

Both colonics and enemas are effective in detox programs. Benefits are a matter of degree, but they're dramatically different in terms of waste removed and body improvement. Your colon is over five feet long. If you want to cleanse all of it, you need a colonic irrigation.

A colonic irrigation, administered by a practitioner, uses special equipment and gravity (or oxygen for more control) to give your colon an internal bath.

To take a colonic, lie on a special colema-board placed about three feet below a temperature-controlled water flow. A speculum is gently inserted in your rectum; the practitioner releases a gentle flow of water from a small water tube. There is no discomfort, no internal pressure, just a steady gentle water flow in and out of the colon through the evacuation tube, carrying with it impacted feces and mucous. Unlike an enema, a colonic irrigation does not involve the retention of water. As the water flows out of the bowel, the practitioner gently massages the abdomen to help the colon release its contents, recover its natural shape, and normalize peristaltic wave action. A view tube lets you see the colonic material being released — an edifying experience. You do nothing but lie back and relax while the entire colon is cleansed.

Can't find a recommended product? Call the 800 number in Product Resources for the store nearest you.

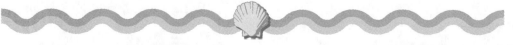

Special guide to detoxification

A colonic irrigation uses about 40 gallons of water and takes about forty-five minutes. The colonic procedure is not offensive or painful. The first things most people feel after a colonic irrigation is a sense of lightness, energy and an improved sense of well-being. Skin condition, digestion and immune response improve, usually within days. Body odor and bad breath essentially disappear, as does belly distension. Colonics are best done in the evening so that you can relax and retire for healing rest. For a better result, take an herbal green drink before and after the colonic.

Bentonite Clay Colonic:

Bentonite clay is a mineral substance with powerful absorption qualities to pull out suspended impurities from body tissues. It helps prevent proliferation of pathogenic organisms and parasites, and sets up an environment for rebuilding healthy tissue. It is effective for lymph congestion, cellulitic fatty tissue, blood cleansing and reducing toxicity from environmental pollutants. It may be used orally, anally, or vaginally. It works like an internal poultice, drawing out toxic materials, then draining and eliminating them through evacuation. Note: Bentonite clay is a powerful cleanser and should be only used short-term as directed. Bentonite clay packs are also effective applied topically to varicose veins and arthritic areas.

To take bentonite as an enema:

1: Mix ½ cup clay to an enema bag of water. Use 5 to 6 bags for each enema set to replace a colonic. Follow normal enema procedure, or the directions with your enema apparatus.

2: Massage across the abdomen while expelling toxic waste into the toilet.

Exercise has significant influence on detoxification.

—Exercise speeds up removal of toxins through perspiration. Sweating helps expel toxins through the skin. Exercising to the point of perspiration offers overheating therapy benefits, too. In sweat tests on athletes, potential cancer causing elements, like heavy metals and pesticide PCBs were excreted from their bodies through perspiration.

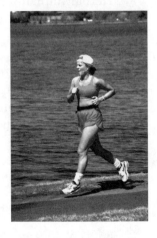

—Exercise stimulates removal of toxins through deep breathing. Low impact aerobics help build a stronger diaphragm and elasticize your lungs.

—Exercise stimulates metabolism, especially before you eat, to aid weight loss. Exercise uses up stored body fat. Calories are burned at a greater pace for several hours after you exercise.

—Exercise stimulates circulation, lowering blood pressure and preventing heart disease by increasing blood flow. Heart endurance tests show exercise strengthens your circulatory system right down to your capillaries.... even forming new ones!

—Exercise stimulates your lymphatic system. Blood is pumped through your body by your heart, but lymphatic fluid depends solely on exercise for circulation. Good lymph function is critical to your body's ability to cleanse itself.

—Exercise reduces stress improves your mood by increasing oxygen levels. It. Vigorous exercise releases endorphins, our "feel good" hormones into the brain, explaining the "high" people experience after exercise.

—Disease often results from an underactive body. Exercise transports oxygen and nutrients to your cells while it carries away toxins and wastes to elimination organs.

Can't find a recommended product? Call the 800 number in Product Resources for the store nearest you.

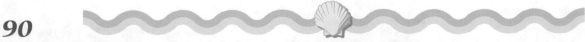

Exercise recommendations for your cleanse:

1: During initial, heavy cleansing — simple, body-balancing, stretching exercises.

2: During the rest of your cleanse — low-impact, aerobic exercise, like a walk or an easy swim.

3: For your maintenance program, strengthening exercise, like daily walking for better circulation and lymph activity. An exercise program that raises your heart rate for 20 to 30 minutes offers the most benefits.

Yoga accelerates detox results.

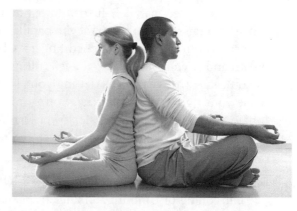

In the 80's, everyone was signing up for aerobics classes. In the 21st century yoga is the fitness byword, attracting baby boomers and Gen X'ers alike. Today, more than 12 million Americans practice yoga. Physicians are even recommending yoga to their patients. But yoga is not new at all. It's a 5,000 year-old Eastern practice, involving special postures called "asanas" which experts believe allow energy to flow unimpeded through the body.

Yoga literally means "union," and it's considered one of the best bodywork techniques to harmonize, and unite mind, body and spirit. Physically, yoga can range from a gentle to rigorous workout. It works all the major muscle groups- including the hips, thighs, abdominals, arms and back. It strengthens, tones the body, and increases flexibility. On a mental level, yoga sharpens focus and concentration, and helps remove fear-based blocks to learning. Spiritually, practicers often notice a change in their outlook as yoga opens the door to new ways of thinking and experiencing the world.

Yoga is powerful medicine for healing, too. Research published in the Journal of the American Medical Association reveals yoga reduces carpal tunnel syndrome more than wearing wrist splints alone. Studies show good results for arthritis and fibromyalgia pain reduction. A 1990 study by Dr. Dean Ornish finds yoga in combination with regular aerobic exercise, stress reduction therapies, and a low fat vegetarian diet stabilizes and, in some cases, reverses arterial blockages.

Amazingly, the newest research shows yoga is as effective as drug therapy in lowering blood pressure. Digestive problems can clear up with yoga practice because yoga increases blood flow to the intestines and stimulates peristalsis (intestinal contractions). It also helps cut stress reactions that are a big part of digestive problems. People who have been in serious accidents, have been diagnosed with cancer, hypothyroidsim and Crohn's disease have all attested to yoga's healing powers.

By boosting circulation and metabolism through deep breathing and "asanas" (yoga postures), yoga accelerates the results of your detox program. Further, yoga helps re-establish body balance after toxins and negative emotions are released. Bikram yoga classes are especially recommended for detoxification; Bikram intsructors turn up the heat to 85 degrees or higher in their classrooms to induce a cleansing sweat.

Try these yoga postures at home: *Posture instructions reprinted with permission by www.yogasite.com.*

<u>The Cobra</u> (stretches the spine, strengthens the back and arms, opens the chest and heart): Lie down on your stomach. Keep your legs together, arms at your side, close to your body, with your hands by your chest. Step One: Inhaling, slowly raise your head and chest as high as it will go. Keep your buttocks muscles tight to protect your lower back. Keep your head up and chest and heart out. Breathe several times and then come down. Repeat as necessary. Step Two: Follow the steps above. When you've gone as high as you can, gently raise yourself on your arms, stretching the spine even more. Only go as far as you are comfortable. Your pelvis should always remain on the floor. Breathe several times and come down.

Can't find a recommended product? Call the 800 number in Product Resources for the store nearest you.

__Dog and Cat__ (increases the flexibility of the spine): This is really two poses, one flowing into the other. Begin on your hands and knees, with your hands just in front of your shoulders, your legs about hip width apart. Inhale, tilting the tailbone and pelvis up, letting the spine curve downward, dropping the stomach low, lift your head up. Stretch gently. Exhale, moving into cat by reversing the spinal bend, tilting the pelvis down, drawing the spine up and pulling chest and stomach in. Repeat several times, flowing smoothly from dog into cat, and cat back into dog.

__The Triangle__ (stretches the spine, opens the torso, improves balance and concentration): Start with your spread 3-4 feet apart, feet parallel. Turn your left foot 90 degrees to the left and your right foot about 45 degrees inward. Inhale and raise both arms so they're parallel with the floor. Exhale, turn your head to the left and look down your left arm toward your outstretched fingers. Check that your left knee is aligned with your left ankle. Take a deep breath and stretch outward to the left, tilting the left hip down and the right hip up. When you've stretched as far as you can, pivot your arms, letting your left hand reach down and come to rest against the inside of your calf, while your right arm points straight up. Turn and look up at your right hand. Breathe deeply for several breaths. Inhale and straighten up. Exhale, lower your arms. Put your hands on your hips and pivot on your heels, bringing your feet to face front. Repeat the posture on the other side.

Ear Coning for Ear Cleansing

Ear coning or candling, an ancient healing process used by almost every healing tradition, is a comfortable way to clean out excess wax and other accumulations. Chinese Traditional Medicine, Native American and Mayan societies, even the ancient Egyptians all used ear candling to gently remove ear wax, fungus, and yeast from ear canals. Ear coning was even considered a spiritual practice to clear the mind and senses.

Ear candles are strips of muslin dipped into a mixture of wax and herbs that have natural antibiotic and decongestant activity like sage, cedar, spearmint, echinacea, goldenseal and rosemary. The muslin is formed into a tapered cone, and the narrow end of the candle is gently placed at the ear canal, while the opposite end is lit. The spiral design of the cone creates a vacuum which draws the soothing smoke into the ear canal. The smoke goes through the eustachian tube into the lymphatic system, then by osmosis, draws accumulations out into the cone. The process is soothing, and takes about 45 minutes.

The benefits of ear coning:
—stimulates and detoxifies the lymph system.
—helps remove excessive wax and allows better hearing, usually immediately.
—clears "swimmers ear," where ear wax stops water clearing from the ear, allowing bacteria to fester.
—relieves pain and pressure from mucous blown into the ear from the Eustachian tube.
—helps clear itching mold caused by candida yeast allergy.
—helps remove parasites growing in the ear.

Your skin is a key organ for detoxification.

I frequently use herbal compresses to draw out waste and waste residues, like cysts or abscesses, through the skin and release them into the body's elimination channels. Many of the itchy skin rashes and break-outs such as adult acne and histamine reactions on the rise in so many people today are linked to the body's attempt to detoxify from drug overload, high sugar diets, high stress lifestyles (confirmed in studies) and liver exhaustion. The body's normal cleansing mechanisms are thrown way out of whack and the skin is a fairly easy exit organ.

Alternating hot and cold compresses produce the best results. Apply the herbs to the hot compress, and leave the ice or cold compress plain. I regularly use *cayenne*, *ginger* and *lobelia* effectively for the hot compresses.

Can't find a recommended product? Call the 800 number in Product Resources for the store nearest you.

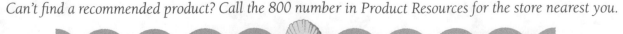

Effective herbal compresses I use:
1: Add 1 tsp. powdered herbs to a bowl of very hot water. Soak a washcloth and apply until the cloth cools. Then apply a cloth dipped in ice water until it reaches body temperature. Repeat several times daily.

2: Green clay compresses are effective toxin-drawing agents for growths. Apply to gauze, place on the area, cover and leave all day. Change as you would any dressing when you bathe.

Dry skin brushing helps remove toxins during a detox and opens pores for better assimilation of nutrients. Dry skin brushing removes the top layer of old skin, helping to eliminate uric acid crystals and mucous residues. Dry skin brushing stimulates circulation, cleanses the lymph system and increases cell renewal. Dry brushing your skin every 24 hours rejuvenates your skin during detoxification. After your detox, dry brushing before your shower once a week will keep your skin beautiful and keep cellulite build-up down.

Good technique for skin brushing can make all the difference to its success:
—Use a natural bristle brush, not synthetic — it scratches skin surface.
—Do not wet your skin. It stretches the skin and will not have the same effect.
—Especially brush the bottoms of your feet, nerve endings here affect the whole body.
—Do circular, counter-clockwise strokes on the abdomen; lighter strokes over and around the breasts.
—Dry brush before you bathe in the mornings (before bed, it can cause too much stimulation).
—Brush the whole body, for best results. Wash your brush every few weeks in water and let it dry.

Give your body a detoxifying ascorbic acid flush.
Vitamin C (ascorbic acid) accelerates detoxification, changing body chemistry to neutralize allergens, fight infections, promote rapid healing and protect against illness.

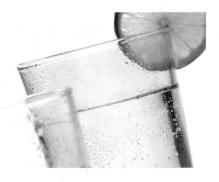

Here's how:
1. Use non-acidic vitamin C or Ester C powder with bioflavonoids.
2: Take ½ tsp. every 20 minutes until a soupy stool results. (Use ¼ tsp. every hour for a very young child; ½ tsp. every hour for a child six to ten years old.)
3: Then, slightly reduce amount taken so that the bowel produces a mealy, loose stool, but not diarrhea. The body will still continue to cleanse. You will be taking about 8-10,000mg of vitamin C daily depending on body weight and make-up. Continue for one to two days for a thorough flush.

An herbal "vag pac" can detox the vaginal area.
A cleansing herbal combination may be used as a vaginal pack by placing it against the cervix, or as a bolus inserted in the vagina. The pack acts as an internal poultice to draw out toxic wastes from the vagina, rectum or urethral areas. A "vag pac" is effective for cysts, benign tumors, polyps and uterine growths, and cervical dysplasia. It takes 6 weeks to 6 months for complete healing to take place, depending on the problem such as the shrinking of a tumor. I myself have seen success with tumors with this method.

How to make a pack:
—Formula #1: Mix 1 part of each herb with cocoa butter to form a finger-sized suppository: *squaw vine, marshmallow root, slippery elm, goldenseal root, pau d'arco, comfrey root, mullein, yellow dock root, chickweed, acidophilus* powder.

Can't find a recommended product? Call the 800 number in Product Resources for the store nearest you.

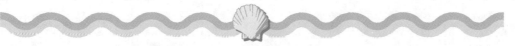

—Formula #2: Mix 1 part each with cocoa butter to form a finger-sized suppository: *cranesbill powder, gold-enseal root, red raspberry leaf, white oak bark, echinacea root, myrrh gum* powder.

Place suppositories on waxed paper in the fridge to chill and harden slightly. Smear a suppository on cotton tampon and insert, or insert as is, and use a sanitary napkin to catch drainage. Use suppositories at night; rinse out in the morning with white oak bark tea, or yellow dock root tea to rebalance vaginal pH. Repeat for 6 days. Rest for one week. Resume and repeat if necessary.

Chelation therapy cleans out your arteries.

Chelation therapy was developed in Germany in the early 1930's and introduced into the United States in 1948 as a method of preventing or reversing heart and artery pathology (hardening of the arteries) from diminished blood circulation. Today chelation is used by medical authorities around the world as a cleansing treatment for heavy metal and radiation toxicity, digitalis intoxication, lead and snake venom poisoning and heart arrhythmias. A chelating, synthetic amino acid, protein called EDTA, (ethylene-diamine-tetracetic acid) has the unique property of binding with divalent metals that are clogging arteries. When EDTA is injected, it flushes the cells of ionic minerals, especially calcium, and travels with them out of the body through the kidneys.

Oral chelation refers to specific foods and nutritional supplements that help cleanse the blood vessels of accumulated detritus (waste) and improve blood flow. While experience among chelating physicians indicates that oral chelates take about eight times longer to show health benefits than IV chelates, oral chelation is successful in improving circulation, reversing heart disease, stroke and sexual impotency due to poor circulation. I use oral chelation as a preventive against atherosclerosis and many degenerative diseases. Metabolic Response Modifiers CARDIO-CHELATE is a premier oral chelation product with EDTA that I've used with good results.

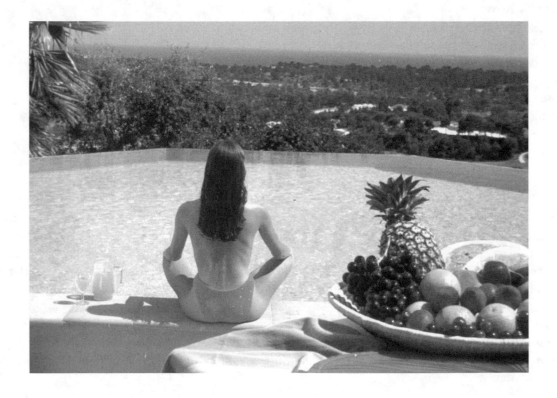

Can't find a recommended product? Call the 800 number in Product Resources for the store nearest you.

Which Body System Cleanse do You Need?

You can target your detox to focus on a specific body system. Each body system has tell-tale signs when it becomes overloaded with pollutants or congestion. Directing your detox to the body system that needs it goes to the heart of a problem right away, and frequently clears up other related conditions as well. This chapter details the seven body systems that make a noticeable difference in your health after a cleanse.

Do you need a colon cleanse?

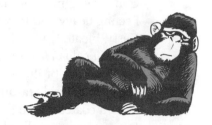

A colon elimination cleanse is a cleanse most of us need. The latest estimates show that over 90% of disease in America is directly or indirectly attributable to an unhealthy colon. As the solid waste management organ for the entire body, your colon is also the easiest breeding ground for putrefactive bacteria, viruses and parasites. (A nationwide survey reveals that one in every six people have parasites living somewhere in the body.)

Hardly any healing program will work without a colon cleanse as part of it. Problems like headaches, skin blemishes, bad breath, fatigue, arthritis and heart disease are linked to a congested colon. Colon and bowel malfunctions are one of the biggest factors in accelerated aging, too. Cleansing your colon lightens the toxic load on every other part of your body.... even your mind (mental dullness is a sign of colon congestion). When colon health is compromised, waste backs up, becomes toxic, and releases the toxins into the bloodstream. Real healing takes place at the deepest cellular levels. Your cells are fed by your blood. The nutrients that reach your blood get there by the way of the colon. So a clogged, dirty colon means toxins in your blood.

Is your colon toxic? **Ask yourself these questions:**

...Is your elimination time slow? Bowel transit time should be approximately twelve hours. Slow bowel transit time allows wastes to become rancid. Blood capillaries lining the colon absorb these poisons into the bloodstream, exposing the rest of your body to the toxins.

...Do you eat too much fast food? highly processed, chemical laced food? synthetic foods? A clean, strong system can metabolize or eliminate many pollutants that come into your body, but if you are constipated, they are stored in your system. As more and different chemicals enter your body they tend to inter-react with those that are already there, forming second generation chemicals more harmful than the originals. Colon cancer, now the second leading cancer in the United States (slightly behind lung cancer in men and breast cancer in women), is a direct result of accumulated toxic waste. Colitis, irritable bowel syndrome, diverticulosis, ileitis and Crohn's disease, are all signs of waste congestion. They're on the rise, too. Over 100,000 Americans have a colostomy every year! An incredible fact.

...Is your digestion poor? The most common sign of toxic bowel overload is poor digestion. If you're eating a lot of rich, red meats and cheeses, white bread, sugary, salty foods or fried foods, they're robbing your body of critical electrolytes and they have almost no fiber for digestion. A high fiber diet is both cure and prevention for waste elimination problems. Eating high fiber means you're moving food through your digestive system quickly and easily. A low residue diet causes a gluey state — your intestinal contractions can't work efficiently. You can picture this if you remember the hard paste formed by white flour and water when you were a kid. A lot of the food we eat today is simply crammed into the colon, never fully excreted.

Media attention has been focused for decades on high fiber foods. Everybody in America must have changed their diet to a more colon-healthy pattern....right?. This is simply not the case. Americans target their diets to reduce fat at all costs, often at the expense of a fiber-rich diet. A gentle, gradual change from low fiber, low residue foods helps almost immediately. In fact, a gradual change is better than a sudden, drastic change, especially when the colon is inflamed.

Can't find a recommended product? Call the 800 number in Product Resources for the store nearest you.

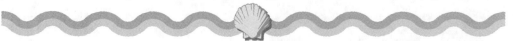

Check your fiber. The protective level of fiber in your diet is easily measured:
—The stool should be light enough to float.
—Bowel movements should be regular, daily and effortless.
—The stool should be almost odorless, signalling less bowel transit time.
—There should be no gas or flatulence.

Could your body use a colon cleanse?
—Constipated most of the time? (*a colon cleanse softens, removes colon congestion*)
—Feeling heavy and logy? (*a colon cleanse helps you lose colon congestive weight*)
—Gassy, bloated, audible bowel rumbling and discomfort after you eat?
    (*a colon cleanse removes gluey materials impairing digestion*)
—Catch a cold, or flu every few weeks? (*a colon cleanse releases excess mucous that harbors viruses*)
—Tired for no real reason? (*a colon cleanse boosts immune and liver response for more energy*)
—Have a coated tongue, bad breath, body odor? (*a colon cleanse clears rancidity that causes smells*)
—Do you feel mentally slow and tired? (*a colon cleanse lets more blood circulation get to your brain*)
—Skin unusually sallow and dull? (*a colon cleanse removes toxin that come out through your skin*)
—Have a degenerative disease like cancer, arthritis or lupus? (*a colon cleanse removes toxic elements*)
—Cholesterol numbers too high? (*a colon cleanse increases absorption of cholesterol-lowering foods*)

Colon Elimination Detox Plan
Start with this 3 to 5 -day nutrition plan: The 4 keys: 1) high chlorophyll plants for enzymes; 2) fruits and vegetables for fiber; 3) cultured foods for probiotics; 4) eight glasses of water a day.

The night before your colon cleanse...
—Take your choice of gentle herbal laxatives.
—Soak dried figs, prunes and raisins in water; add 1 tbsp. molasses, cover, leave over night.

The next 2-4 days...
—*On rising:* take a cleansing booster product, or 1 heaping teaspoon of a fiber drink in juice or water.
    Take 1000mg vitamin C with bioflavonoids to raise body glutathione levels.
—*Breakfast:* discard dried fruits from soaking water and take a small glass of the liquid.
—*Mid-morning:* take 2 tbsp. aloe juice concentrate in a glass of juice or water and 1000mg vitamin C.
—*Lunch:* take a small glass of potassium broth (page 291); or a glass of fresh carrot juice.
—*Mid-afternoon:* take a large glass of fresh apple juice; or an herbal colon cleansing tea.
—*About 5 o' clock:* a small glass of potassium broth, or fresh carrot juice, or a mixed vegetable drink.
—*Supper:* take a glass of apple or papaya juice and 1000mg vitamin C.
    (Note: Finish your cleanse with a small raw foods salad on the last night.)
—*Before Bed:* repeat the herbal cleansers that you took on rising, and take a cup of mint tea.

Colon cleanse supplement suggestions: Choose 2 or 3 cleansing boosters.
...**Gentle herbal laxatives:** Zand CLEANSING LAXATIVE tabs. Note: If you have a sensitive colon or irritable bowel disease (IBS), heal your colon before you cleanse. Avoid products with senna or cascara sagrada. Use a gentle herbal cleansing formula, with peppermint oil, like Crystal Star BWL-TONE I.B.S.™, to lessen inflammation and irritation of bowel mucosa which make the bowel more permeable to toxins.

...**Cleansing boosters:** Planetary TRIPHALA; Nature's Secret SUPERCLEANSE; Crystal Star FIBER & HERBS COLON CLEANSE™; *una de gato* extract drops in water.

Can't find a recommended product? Call the 800 number in Product Resources for the store nearest you.

...**Chlorophyll sources:** Crystal Star ENERGY GREEN RENEWAL™ drink; Pure Planet CHLORELLA; Future-biotics COLON GREEN; Wakunaga KYOGREEN™ drink; Green Foods GREEN MAGMA if you have IBS.

...**Enzymes:** Transformation Enzyme DIGEST-ZYME with meals; Use PUREZYME or Crystal Star DR. ENZYME™ with Protease and Bromelain between meals if you have food allergies, too.

...**Electrolyte speed up a cleanse:** Nature's Path TRACE-LYTE Liquid Minerals; Arise & Shine ALKALIZER.

...**Probiotics replenish healthy bacteria:** Jarrow JARRO-DOPHILUS.

...**Antioxidants defeat pollutants:** Country Life SUPER 10 ANTIOXIDANT; NutriCology ANTIOX.

...**Fiber support:** Planetary TRI-CLEANSE; AloeLife FIBERMATE.

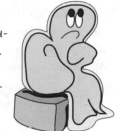

Note 1: Drugstore laxatives aren't really cleansers. They offer only temporary relief, are usually habit-forming, destructive to intestinal membranes, and don't get to the cause of the problem. The laxative so irritates the colon that the bowels expel whatever loose material is around.

Note 2: Bowel elimination problems are often chronic and may need several rounds of cleansing. If doing more than 1 colon cleanse, alternate with periods of eating a healthy diet

Colon cleanse bodywork suggestions: Techniques to enhance your cleanse.

Irrigate: a colonic irrigation is a good way to start a colon/bowel cleanse. (See how to take a colonic, page 189) Grapefruit seed extract (15 to 20 drops in a gallon of water) is effective, especially if there is colon toxicity along with constipation. Or, take a catnip or diluted liquid chlorophyll enema every other night during the cleanse. Note: Enemas may be given to children. Use smaller amounts according to size and age. Allow water to enter very slowly; let them expel when they wish.

Exercise: take a brisk walk for an hour every day to help keep your elimination channels moving.

Bathe: take several long warm baths during your cleanse. A lower back and pelvis massage and dry skin brushing will help release toxins coming out through your skin. Lemon Detox Bath: add into warm bath — 5 drops lemon and 2 drops geranium essential oil.

Massage therapy: get one good lower back and pelvis massage during your cleanse.

Visualize your detox: Close your eyes; inhale and exhale long and slowly. As you exhale, visualize toxins dislodging and leaving your colon. As you inhale, visualize nourishing nutrients rebuilding vibrancy.

Do you need a bladder-kidney cleanse?

Kidney function is vital to health. The kidneys are largely responsible for the elimination of waste products from protein breakdown (such as urea and ammonia). If the movement of salts, proteins or other bio-chemicals goes awry, a whole range of health problems arises, from mild water retention, to major kidney failure, and mineral loss. Concentrated protein wastes can cause chronic inflammation of the kidney filtering tissues (nephritis), and can overload the bloodstream with toxins, causing uremia.

But your bladder and kidneys do more than just remove water wastes. Channeling pollutants and chemicals out of our systems before they build up in the tissues and contaminate our cells is obviously crucial to the body's internal hygiene. The bladder and kidneys are primary removal sites for toxic and potentially toxic chemicals in the bloodstream.

The urinary system is also part of a complex process that maintains your body's fluid stability. Urinary controls are involved with the brain, hormones, and receptors all over the body. They are smart controls that register what your body needs for fluids. Sometimes, they remove very little salt or water; at other times, they remove a lot. By the way.... dehydration is the most common stress on the kidneys. Natural medicine emphasizes the importance of ample, high-quality water for kidney health.

Can't find a recommended product? Call the 800 number in Product Resources for the store nearest you.

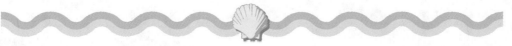

Could your body benefit from a bladder-kidney cleanse?

Do you have chronic lower back pain, irritated urination, frequent unexplained chills, fever, or nausea or unusual fluid retention? A gentle, natural, three to five day cleansing course might be just the thing to keep you from getting a full-blown, painful bladder infection.

Bladder-Kidney Detox Plan

Start with this 3-day nutrition plan: Water is the key. Drink 8 to 10 glasses of water each day. Bladder and kidneys operate efficiently only if there is sufficient water volume flowing through them to carry away wastes. Avoid dietary irritants on the kidneys, such as coffee, alcohol, and excessive protein.

Note: Avoid commercial antacids during healing. Some NSAIDS drugs are implicated in kidney failure cases.

The night before your bladder cleanse....

—One cup of bladder cleansing herb tea, like Crystal Star BLADDER-KIDNEY COMFORT™ tea; Herbal Magic URINARY TEA or *uva ursi* tea. Add ¼ tsp. non-acidic C crystals.

The next 3 days....

—*On rising:* take 1 lemon squeezed in a glass of water, with 1 tsp. acidophilus liquid; or 3 tsp. cranberry concentrate in a small glass of water, add ¼ tsp. non-acidic vit. C crystals. (Cranberry juice reduces ionized calcium in the urine by over 50% to create an unfavorable environment for urinary tract infections.)

—*Breakfast:* have a glass of watermelon juice or cranberry juice, or Crystal Star BLADDER-KIDNEY COMFORT™ tea, with ¼ tsp. non-acidic vitamin C crystals or a glass of organic apple juice with ¼ tsp. acidophilus powder.

—*Mid-morning:* take 1 cup watermelon seed tea (grind seeds, steep in hot water 30 minutes, add honey); or a potassium broth (page 291) with 2 tsp. Bragg's LIQUID AMINOS; or an herbal bladder cleansing tea.

—*Lunch:* have a carrot-beet-cucumber juice, or a chlorophyll-rich drink, or a glass of carrot juice.

—*Mid-afternoon:* a cup of bladder herb tea, (*parsley/oatstraw, plantain, watermelon seed* tea or *cornsilk*).

—*Dinner:* have a carrot juice, add 1 tsp. spirulina powder; or another cranberry juice, add ¼ tsp. ascorbate vitamin C crystals.

—*Before Bed:* take a glass of papaya or apple juice with ¼ tsp. acidophilus powder.

Bladder-Kidney cleanse supplement suggestions:

Liquid supplements are best with this cleanse. Herbal remedies provide excellent support for a kidney cleanse. Take them as liquids (drinks or teas) for best results.

...**Superfoods:** Take a liquid green superfood each day of your cleanse: Crystal Star ENERGY GREEN RENEWAL™ drink; Sun Wellness CHLORELLA; Wakunaga KYOGREEN; *spirulina* powder in juice.

...**Bladder/kidney cleansers:** Crystal Star BLADDER-KIDNEY COMFORT™ tea; Planetary CRANBERRY BLADDER DEFENSE tabs; *cornsilk* tea; Natural Balance CRAN-MAX caps.

...**Antibiotic-anti-infective-anti-inflammatory:** Crystal Star ANTI-BIO™; Gaia ECHINACEA-GOLDENSEAL phyto-caps; *marshmallow* tea; vitamin C-1,000mg 3x a day; Nature's Plus AQUAACTIN.

...**Enzyme support:** Transformation PUREZYME (a protease supplement that breaks apart protein-based viscid matter that cements salts into stones). Use with Transformation KIDNEY DRAINAGE drops (assists protease in eliminating excessive wastes from the kdneys).

...**Bladder/kidney healing tonics:** Herbs Etc. KIDNEY TONIC; Gaia Herbs PLANTAIN/BUCHU SUPREME; Nature's Apothecary KIDNEY SUPPORT; Crystal Star GREEN TEA CLEANSER™; *dandelion* tea; *parsley* tea.

...**Electrolyte mineral support:** Nature's Path TRACE-LYTE Liquid Minerals; Arise & Shine ALKALIZER.

...**Probiotic support:** UAS DDS-PLUS, Jarrow's JARRO-DOPHILUS EPS.

...**Fiber supplements reduce risk of stones:** All One FIBER COMPLEX; Nature's Secret ULTIMATE FIBER.

Can't find a recommended product? Call the 800 number in Product Resources for the store nearest you.

Bladder cleanse bodywork suggestions: Techniques to accelerate, round out your cleanse.

Exercise: Take a daily brisk walk to keep kidney function flowing.

Enemas: Take a spirulina or catnip enema at least one day of your kidney cleanse to help release toxins. See enema instructions (page 180) in this book.

Heat therapy: Hot saunas release toxins and excess fluids, and flush acids out through the skin.

Compresses: Apply wet and hot to lower back to speed cleansing. Combine your choice — *ginger* and *oatstraw*, or *cayenne* and *ginger*, or *mullein* and *lobelia.* Or, take alternating hot and cold sitz baths.

Massage therapy: Have at least one massage during your cleanse to stimulate circulation.

Bladder-Kidney Baths: Add 8-10 drops of essential oils to your bath — a combination of two or three oils, like juniper, cedarwood, sandalwood, lemon, chamomile, eucalyptus or geranium. Stir the water to disperse. (Or use about 15 drops essential oil in 4-oz of jojoba oil and rub on kidney area).

Note: After your cleanse, add sea foods and sea vegetables, whole grains and vegetable proteins. Continue with a morning green drink or Crystal Star GREEN TEA CLEANSER™. Kidney healing foods include garlic and onions, papayas, bananas, watermelon, sprouts, leafy greens and cucumbers. Take these frequently for the rest of the month. Avoid heavy starches, red or prepared meats, dairy foods (except yogurt or kefir), and salty, fatty and fast foods. They all inhibit kidney filtering.

Improvement signs that your body is responding to the cleanse:
• The flow of urine is increased.
• Bladder infections and-or irritated urination abate.
• You'll feel lighter and cleaner as your kidneys detoxifies free of congestion.

Need a liver cleanse? **The liver is your most important organ of detoxification.**

Your life depends on your liver. To a large extent, the health of your liver determines the health of your entire body. The liver is really a wonderful chemical plant that converts everything we eat, breathe and absorb through the skin into life-sustaining substances. The liver is a major blood reservoir, forming and storing red blood cells, and filtering toxins at a rate of a quart of blood per minute. It manufactures natural antihistamines to keep immune response high.

More than any other organ, the liver enables us to benefit from the food we eat. Without the liver, digestion would be impossible and the conversion of food into living energy nonexistent. It is the primary metabolic organ for proteins, fats and carbohydrates. It synthesizes and secretes bile, a substance that not only insures good food assimilation but also is critical to the excretion of toxic material from the gastrointestinal tract. Blood flows directly from the gastrointestinal tract to the liver, where it deals with toxic substances from our food before they are distributed through our blood. Blood also keeps returning to the liver, processing toxins again and again through the lymph system until they are excreted by the bile or kidneys.

Liver congestion and exhaustion interfere with these vital functions. Unfortunately, since the common American diet is high in calories, fats, sugars and alcohol, with unknown amounts of toxins from preservatives, pesticides and nitrates, almost everybody has liver malfunction to some extent. Health problems occur after many years of abuse, when the liver is so exhausted it loses the ability to detoxify itself. Still, your liver also has amazing rejuvenative powers, continuing to function when as many as 80% of its cells are damaged. More remarkable, the liver can regenerate its own damaged tissue, so that even in life-threatening situations, such as cirrhosis, hepatitis, acute gallstone attacks, mononucleosis or pernicious anemia, the liver can be rejuvenated, and major surgery or even death averted. You can help your liver take a "deep cleansing breath"... something I've found you can almost feel as its miraculous powers of recovery begin to flow.

Can't find a recommended product? Call the 800 number in Product Resources for the store nearest you.

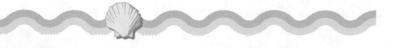

A liver detox is often the first vital step for the body to begin to heal itself. Gland function and digestion often improve right away. You will notice this in terms of fewer instances of swollen glands during cold and flu season, and less lower back fatigue (adrenal swelling). Weight and cellulite control difficulties may be solved, especially if you notice unusual stomach distension, a clear sign of a swollen liver. Both gallstone and kidney stone accretions lessen. Drug and alcohol cravings reduce. Most women notice that PMS and other menstrual difficulties like endometriosis are far less severe. Seemingly unrelated problems like breast and uterine fibroids or infertility, even osteoporosis may be corrected. Male impotence is normally improved. Inflammatory conditions like shingles flare-ups, neuritis pain, and herpes outbreaks are helped. Brown skin spots and spots before the eyes (signs that the liver is congested and eliminating poisons by other body avenues) begin to fade.

Would your body benefit from a liver cleanse?
—Unexplained fatigue, listlessness, depression or lethargy, lack of energy; numerous allergy reactions?
—Unexplained weight gain and the appearance of cellulite even if you are thin?
—A distended stomach even if the rest of your body is thin?
—Mental confusion, spaciness?
—Sluggish elimination, general constipation alternating to diarrhea?
—Food and chemical sensitivities, accompanied by poor digestion, sometimes unexplained nausea?
—PMS, headaches and other menstrual difficulties; bags under the eyes?
—Yellowish tint and/or liver spots on the skin; poor hair texture, slow hair growth; skin itching?
—Anemia and large bruise patches indicate severe liver exhaustion?

Liver Detox Plan
Your liver is probably the most stressed in the spring and early summer (one of the reasons that people with skin problems get more flare-ups in the spring). As upward energy movement in the spring is mirrored in the human body, outgoing energy more readily rids us of wastes we collected during the fall and winter. I recommend a short liver detox twice a year — spring and fall, using the extra vitamin D from the sun to help.

Start with this 3-day plan: Drink 8 glasses of water each day. Add ¼ tsp. vitamin C crystals to each drink you take. It's a natural heavy metal toxin chelator. Have a dark green leafy vegetable salad every day.

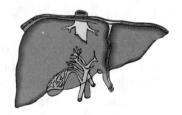

The Liver

The night before your liver cleanse...
—One cup of miso soup with sea greens snipped on top.
—Make up a liver tonic: 4-oz *hawthorn berries,* 2-oz. *red sage (salvia),* 1-oz. *cardamom seeds.* Steep 24 hours in 2 qts. water. Add honey. Take 2 cups daily.

The next 3 days....
—*On rising:* take 1 lemon squeezed in a glass of water; or 2 tbsp. cider vinegar in water with 1 tsp. honey.
—*Breakfast:* take a potassium broth, (page 291) or carrot-beet-cucumber juice; or Crystal Star RESTORE YOUR STRENGTH™ drink. Add 1 tsp. *spirulina* to any drink.
—*Mid-morning:* take a green veggie drink; or a green superfood powder in water or vegetable juice like Crystal Star ENERGY GREEN RENEWAL™ drink mix, *spirulina* or *chlorella* in water or vegetable juice.
—*Lunch:* have a glass of fresh carrot juice, or organic apple juice, or a cup of liver tonic tea (above).
—*Mid-afternoon: mint* or green tea, Crystal Star LIVER CLEANSE FLUSHING™ tea or Flora's BILIV tea.
—*Dinner:* have another carrot juice or a mixed vegetable juice; or have a hot vegetable broth.
—*Before Bed:* a pineapple/papaya juice with 1 tsp. royal jelly.

Can't find a recommended product? Call the 800 number in Product Resources for the store nearest you.

 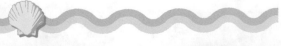

Note: Keeping fat intake low is crucial to liver regeneration and vitality. Beets, artichokes, radishes and dandelions are good liver foods because they promote the flow of bile, <u>the major pathway for chemical release from the liver</u>. A permanent diet for liver health should be lacto-vegetarian, low in fats, rich in vegetable proteins, with plenty of vitamin C foods for good iron absorption. A complete liver renewal program can take from 3 to 6 months..... it's worth it.

Liver cleanse supplement suggestions: Choose 2 or 3 cleansing boosters.
...**Bitters herbs stimulate liver and bile flow:** Crystal Star BITTERS & LEMON™ extract; Floradix GAL-LEXIER; Gaia SWEETISH BITTERS; Solaray turmeric caps; *dandelion* tea.

...**Cleansers:** Crystal Star LIVER RENEW™, Planetary BUPLEURUM LIVER CLEANSE.

...**Liver tonics and vitality support:** *Milk thistle seed* extract (accelerates liver regeneration by a factor of four); Zand MILK THISTLE FORMULA; Herbs Etc. LIVER TONIC.

...**Enzyme support:** Transformation Enzyme LYPOZYME contains the highest amount of lipase (digests fats) found in any product. It also aids in the breakdown of gallstones.

...**Lipotropics prevent fatty accumulation:** Phosphatidyl Choline or choline 600mg, or Solaray LIPOTROPIC PLUS; sea greens (any kind) every day; *dandelion* tea; *gotu kola* or *fennel seed* tea.

...**Liver antioxidants:** ALPHA-LIPOIC ACID by MRI. (Lipoic acid is one of the most powerful liver detoxifiers ever discovered); CoQ_{10} 60mg 3x daily; Solaray ALFA-JUICE caps; Transformation Enzyme EXCELLZYME.

Liver cleanse bodywork suggestions: Techniques to accelerate and round out your cleanse.
Adequate rest: the liver does some of its most important work while you sleep!

Enema: take a coffee enema (1 cup coffee to 1 qt. water) the first and last day of your liver cleanse.

Massage therapy: Have a massage to stimulate circulation.

Improvement signs that your body is responding to the cleanse: Many skin conditions trace back to liver problems, so skin conditions show signs of clearing and skin becomes more radiant. Stiff, aching muscles experience relief. Warmth may return to cold hands and feet. Recurring headaches or migraines may disappear.

Do you need a lung-respiratory cleanse?

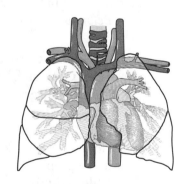

Lung and respiratory diseases of all kinds have increased dramatically in just the last decade. Air, water and environmental pollutants may have finally reached an overload point on the general population where congestion is more common than breathing free. During high risk seasons, almost a third of Americans have a congestive cold every two or three weeks. Cold symptoms are frequently your body's attempt to cleanse itself of wastes and toxins that have built up to the point where natural immunity cannot handle them. Your glands are always affected. Since the endocrine system works on a 6 day cycle, a cold usually runs for about a week as the body works through all its detoxification processes.

Your lungs are on the front line of toxic intake from viruses, allergies, pollutants, and mucous-forming congestants. An occasional lung cleanse supports your respiratory system in releasing pollutant-caused infections. But your body works together. Extra pressure of disease or heavy elimination on one part of the body puts extra stress on another. Cleansing your kidneys, for example, takes part of the waste elimination load off your lungs so they can recover faster. Similarly, promoting respiratory health through a lung cleanse also helps digestive and skin problems.

Any program to overcome chronic respiratory problems is more successful when begun with a short mucous elimination plan like a lung cleansing diet. This allows the body to first rid itself of toxic accumulations that cause congestion before an attempt is made to change eating habits.

Can't find a recommended product? Call the 800 number in Product Resources for the store nearest you.

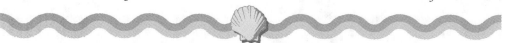

Could your body benefit from a lung and respiratory cleanse?
—Do you have a chronic phlegmy cough? Do you wheeze with asthma?
—Do you have a runny nose in any weather? Are you a cigarette smoker?
—Is your head stuffy with congestive allergies?
—Do you have bronchitis or severe sinusitis?
—Are you highly sensitive to chemicals and pollutants?

Lung and Respiratory Detox Plan

Alkalize your body during a lung cleanse. Acid-forming foods aggravate or prolong colds and other respiratory problems. During a lung detox, use alkalizing foods like fresh fruits, high chlorophyll greens and sea greens, and non-gluten grains like brown rice or millet in a ratio of about 4:1 over acid-forming foods. Begin with a 3 day juice diet and follow with 1 to 4 days of a diet of 100% fresh foods. Drink plenty of non-dairy fluids, like water, juices, herb teas or broth to hydrate and flush. Milk congests and constipates.

The night before your lung cleanse....
—Take your choice of gentle herbal laxatives.

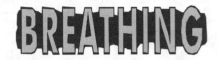

The next 3 days....
—*On rising:* take 2 squeezed lemons in water with 1 tbsp. maple syrup or a cup of green tea.
—*Breakfast:* take diluted grapefruit or pineapple juice natural as expectorants with 1 tbsp. green superfood, like Crystal Star ENERGY GREEN RENEWAL™, or Barleans GREENS .
—*Mid-morning:* take a carrot juice or mixed fresh vegetable juice like Knudsen VERY VEGGIE juice.
—*Lunch:* have a Potassium Juice (page 291) or another cup of green tea.
—*Mid-afternoon:* have a cup of mucous cleansing tea, or a few sprays of Crystal Star D-CONGEST™ extract with *mullein, marshmallow, pleurisy root, wild cherry, osha, ginger, horehound and peppermint.*
—*Dinner:* have a warm Potassium Essence broth (page 291); or try this broth, rich in zinc, vitamin A, C, potassium and magnesium electrolytes: In 2½ cups water, cook 1½ cups fresh mixed vegetables with 1 tbsp. miso. Strain and take broth. Blender blend veggies, broth and 4 tbsp. sunflower seeds for a hearty version.
—*Before Bed:* have cranberry or celery juice or a cup of miso soup.

Lung cleanse supplement suggestions: Choose 2 or 3 cleansing boosters.
...**Deep Cleansing:** Zand CLEANSING LAXATIVE tabs; Planetary TRI-CLEANSE drink mix.
...**Lung cleansers clear congestion:** Yogi BREATHE DEEP tea; Zand DECONGEST caps.
...**Anti-infectives for lungs:** Nutricology PROLIVE with antioxidants (olive leaf extract). Oregano oil, with antiviral and antibacterial properties that help eradicate lung infection while thinning excessive mucous secretion, helps conditions like asthma, colds, flu, bronchitis and pneumonia. Tea Tree has decongestant, antiviral and antibacterial properties.Crystal Star D-CONGEST™ spray, an expectorant aids mucous release.
...**Chlorophyll-rich superfoods:** like *chlorella, spirulina* and *barley grass* speed up lung cleansing.
...**Herbal lung support:** Herbs Etc. LUNG TONIC caps maximize lung capacity and oxygen absorption.
...**Immune support herbs:** *panax ginseng, echinacea, ashwagandha, astragalus, Siberian ginseng, goldenseal, licorice, suma, pau d' arco, red clover.* Immune-enhancing mushrooms, like *reishi, maitake, shiitake.*
...**Enzymes:** Transitions GASTROZYME (clears mucous congestion), PUREZYME (strengthens immunity).
...**Electrolyte increase oxygen uptake:** Trace Minerals' TRACE-LYTE Liquid Minerals.
...**Probiotics inhibit pathogens:** Jarrow Formulas JARRO-DOPHILUS.
...**Antioxidants and lung function:** Vit. C 1000mg 3x day raises body glutathione levels to protect lungs; Beta Carotene 150,000IU with extra lycopene 5-10mg; Source Naturals PROANTHODYN.

Can't find a recommended product? Call the 800 number in Product Resources for the store nearest you.

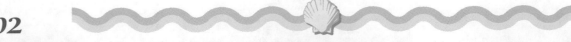

Lung cleanse bodywork suggestions: Techniques to accelerate and round out your cleanse.

Deep Breathing Exercise: Do this exercise often during your cleanse to reduce stress, increase energy, compose your mind, improve your mood: Take a deep, full breath. Exhale slowly... slowly. Take another deep, full breath. Release slowly. And again. Maintain a quiet rhythm, exhaling more slowly than you inhale.

Exercise: If you are cleansing your lungs and not ill with a cold, flu, or other respiratory infection, take a brisk, daily walk on each day of your cleanse. Breathe deep to help the lungs eliminate mucous.

Compress: Apply wet ginger/cayenne compresses to chest to increase circulation, loosen mucous.

Essential oil support: To assist your lung cleanse, use oregano, tea tree, and eucalyptus oils (singly or in combination). Put a total of 15 drops essential oils in 1-oz of a carrier oil (such as jojoba) and rub on the chest. As an inhalant: add 6 drops of the essential oils to one quart hot water—inhale the steam. Eucalyptus especially has antiviral action to loosen mucous, and treat asthma, bronchitis and sinusitis.

Bath or Sauna: Take a hot 20 minute bath or sauna at the onset of a cold, flu or beginning of a respiratory cleanse to stimulate your body's defenses and increase toxin elimination.

Note: Steer clear of environmental and heavy metal pollutants like chlorofluorocarbons and tobacco smoke (even secondary smoke). They contribute greatly to respiratory problems and can undo all your hard cleansing work.

Do you need a blood purifying cleanse?

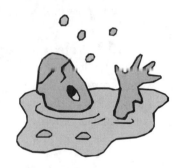

Your blood is your river of life. Healthy blood is critical. The blood must supply oxygen to your body's sixty trillion cells, transport nutrients, hormones and wastes, warm and cool the body, ward off invading organisms, seal off wounds and much more. It is your body's chief neutralizing agent for bacteria and toxic wastes. Toxins ingested in sublethal amounts can eventually add up to disease-causing amounts. For example, slow viruses like those that lead to MS, a nerve disease, can enter the cells and remain dormant for years, feeding on toxic wastes, then reappearing in a dangerous form. While the body has a self-purifying complex for maintaining healthy blood, the best way to protect yourself from disease is to keep those cleansing systems in good working order. Follow a modified blood purifying diet for 1 to 2 months, or longer if your body is still actively cleansing, or needs further balancing. You can return to a blood cleansing regimen as needed.

Cautionary note for people who suffer from severe blood toxicity: Most immune deficient diseases are the result of blood toxins. You'll benefit from a blood purifying diet to boost immunity. However, where there are large amounts of toxins and pollutants in the blood (in serious conditions like AIDS, lupus, or fibromyalgia for example), an all-liquid fast is not recommended. It may be too harsh for an already weak system, and may dump more toxins out into the bloodstream than your body can handle. In these severe cases, keep your initial diet as pure as possible in order to be as cleansing as possible..... vegetarian, free of all meats, dairy foods, fried, preserved and fried or fatty foods.

Would your system benefit from a blood cleanse?

—a simple blood-color test monitors blood improvement. Make a small, quick, sterilized razor cut on your finger. If the blood is a dark, bluish-purplish color, it is not healthy. Healthy blood is a bright red color.

    —a deep, choking, chronic cough

    —depression, memory loss or unusual insomnia, schizophrenic behavior, seizures, periodic black-outs

    —sexual impotence or dysfunction

    —black spots on the gums, bad breath or body odor, unusual, severe reactions to foods and odors

    —loss of hand/eye coordination, especially when driving

Can't find a recommended product? Call the 800 number in Product Resources for the store nearest you.

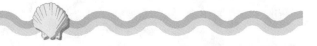

Blood Cleansing Detox Plan

Begin with a 3 day juice-liquid diet; follow with 1 to 4 days of 100% fresh solid and liquid foods.

The night before your blood cleanse.....
—Take your choice of gentle herbal laxatives, like Yogi GET REGULAR tea.

The next 3 days....
—*On rising:* Take 2 to 3 tbsp. cranberry concentrate in 8-oz. water with ½ tsp. ascorbate vitamin C crystals, or use a green tea formula like Crystal Star GREEN TEA CLEANSER™; or cut up a half lemon with skin and blend with 1 tsp. honey, and 1 cup water; or ½ tsp. Natren TRINITY in 8-oz. aloe vera juice.
—*Breakfast:* a glass of fresh carrot juice; or an 8-oz. aloe vera juice with ½ tsp. acidophilus powder.
—*Mid-morning:* take a potassium broth (page 291), add ½ tsp. ascorbate vitamin C crystals; and another fresh carrot juice, or *pau d'arco* tea.
—*Lunch:* have a glass of Knudsen's VERY VEGGIE juice, or a carrot or apple juice. Mix in 1 tbsp. green superfood such as Crystal Star RESTORE YOUR STRENGTH™ drink mix or Barleans GREENS.
—*Mid-afternoon:* Vegetable juice: handful spinach, 4 romaine leaves, 4 sprigs parsley, 6 carrots, ¼ turnip.
—*Dinner:* a cup of miso soup with 2 tbsp. dried sea greens (any kind) snipped over the top.
—*Before Bed:* a glass of aloe vera juice with ½ tsp. ascorbate vitamin C, and ½ tsp. Natren TRINITY.

Blood cleanse supplement suggestions: Choose 2 or 3 cleansing boosters.
Note 1: Vegetable and fruit juices stimulate rapid, heavy waste elimination, a process that can generate mild symptoms of a "healing crisis." Slight headache, nausea, bad breath, body odor and dark urine occur as the body accelerates release of accumulated toxins. If you are detoxifying from alcohol or drug overload, 5,000 to 10,000mg. of ascorbate vitamin C is recommended daily, to help alkalize and encourage oxygen uptake. In addition, sprinkle ½ tsp. lactobacillus powder over any food for body chemistry improvement.

Note 2: One of the most potent blood cleansing formulas available is Crystal Star DETOX BLOOD PURIFIER™ blend. This formula has been used successfully for over two decades to rebalance blood and body chemistry. It is strong and fast-acting. Should you decide to use it, take it alone.... not with other herbal formulas, or even vitamins other than vitamin C.

...**Herbal blood cleansers:** Crystal Star GREEN TEA CLEANSER™ and LIVER RENEW™ capsules; Planetary RED CLOVER CLEANSER capsules; M.D. Labs DAILY DETOX II tea; Herbal Magic COL-LIV HERBAL BASE; Nature's Way DANDELION with Goldenseal.
...**Blood purifiers with immune boosters:** Nature's Answer BLOOD SUPPORT; Herbal Magic PURIFY HERBAL.
...**Enzyme support:** Transformation PUREZYME, breaks down protein invaders in the blood supply leaving them open to destruction by the immune system; Use with Transformation HEMO DRAINAGE drops (assists protease in improving blood flow, thus ridding the body of excessive proteins in the blood).
...**Electrolytes establish healthy blood and strengthen immunity:** Arise & Shine ALKALIZER; Nature's Path TRACE-LYTE Liquid Minerals.
...**Probiotics provide nutrients for building blood:** Crystal Star DR. PROBIOTICS™ with FOS, UAS Labs DDS-PLUS; Source Naturals LIFE FLORA; or Nutricology SYMBIOTICS.
...**Chlorophyll enhances blood cleansing:** CHLORELLA by Sun Wellness; Pure Planet CHLORELLA.
...**Antioxidants strengthen white blood and T cells:** MICROHYDRIN 1000mg daily; Solgar Advanced ANTIOXIDANT FORMULA; Jarrow Coenzyme Q_{10}; Enzymatic Therapy GRAPE SEED Phytosome 100.
...**Antioxidant blood cleansers:** germanium 150mg; Vitamin E 1000IU with selenium 200mcg; CoQ_{10} 200mg daily; Vit. C-3000mg w. bioflavs. daily; Quercetin and bromelain 1500mg daily, for auto-immune reaction; Lane Labs BENEFIN shark cartilage 1200mg to stimulate interferon, interleukin and lymphocytes.

Can't find a recommended product? Call the 800 number in Product Resources for the store nearest you.

Blood cleanse body suggestions: Techniques to accelerate and round out your cleanse.

Enema: Take an enema (page 180) the first, second and last day of your blood cleansing program.

Irrigate: Take a colonic or Nature's Secret SUPERCLEANSE once a week to remove infected feces.

Exercise: Exercise daily in the morning, if possible.

Massage therapy: Have a massage to stimulate blood circulation.

Bathe or sauna: Take several saunas or long hot baths during a blood cleanse for better detoxification. Stir in 15 drops of rosemary, cypress and vetiver essential oils to your bath to assist your blood cleanse.

Do you need a lymph cleanse?

The lymphatic system includes lymph vessels and nodes, thymus gland, tonsils and spleen. It's really a network of tubing that drains waste products from tissues, produces disease-fighting white blood cells (lymphocytes) and antibodies, and carries the bulk of the body's waste from the cells to the elimination organs. Experts call the lymphatic system a secondary circulatory system, because it assists the bloodstream throughout the body to collect tissue fluid not needed by the capillaries or skin and return it to the heart for recirculation. Your lymph system is also a key to your immune defenses, because special filtering lymph nodes along the lymph ducts remove infective organisms.

Liver health is a key to lymphatic health. The liver produces the majority of body lymph. Lymph is a major route for nutrients from the liver and intestines, so it's rich in fat-soluble nutrients, especially protein. Lymph system integrity depends on special immune cells that filter out harmful bacteria and yeasts. The spleen is the largest mass of lymphatic tissue. It destroys worn-out red blood cells, and serves as a healthy blood reservoir for new red blood. During times of demand, such as a hemorrhage, the spleen can release its stored blood and prevent shock from occurring.

An amazing fact: Physical exercise and deep breathing are critical to healthy lymph and immune response. The valves of the lymph system transport waste-filled fluids to be flushed and filtered. But since there is no pump, as there is with the heart, lymph circulation depends solely upon breathing and muscle movement.

Would your body benefit from a lymph cleanse?

—you're under chronic stress; constantly tired (indicating liver exhaustion)

—your skin is very pale; you are extremely thin; your memory is noticeably failing

—you have low immune response with frequent colds

—your body looks uncharacteristically soft and pudgy or has newly noticeable cellulite (indicating too many saturated fats and sugary foods), you probably need a lymph-draining cleanse.

Lymph Cleansing Detox Plan

Poor nutrition is the most frequent cause of sluggish lymph. Immune-boosting vegetables are cabbage, kale, carrots, bell pepper, collards, garlic. Lymph-enhancing fruits are apple, pineapple, blueberry and grape. Start your lymph cleanse: with a 4 to 7 day cleanse; follow with 1 to 4 days of a diet of 100% fresh foods.

—**On rising:** take a glass of lemon juice and water regularly in the morning for lymph revitalization.

—**Breakfast:** have a fresh mixed vegetable lymph juice builder: handful parsley, 1 garlic clove, 5 carrots, 3 celery stalks. Add 2 tbsp. green superfood like Crystal Star ENERGY GREEN RENEWAL™, or Green Kamut.

—**Mid-morning:** have 2 cups Crystal Star LIVER RENEW™ tea for liver and lymph flushing; or a lymph tea blend of *white sage, astragalus, echinacea root, Oregon grape root and dandelion root*.

Can't find a recommended product? Call the 800 number in Product Resources for the store nearest you.

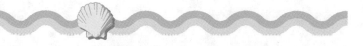

—*Lunch:* A vitamin A/carotene/C drink: 3 broccoli flowerets, 5 carrots, 1 garlic clove, 2 celery stalks and ½ bell pepper. Add 2 tbsp. green superfood: Vibrant Health GREEN VIBRANCE or Green Foods VEGGIE MAGMA.

—*Mid-afternoon:* a glass of apple or grape juice.

—*Dinner:* have a Potassium Essence Broth (page 291), for mineral electrolytes. Or, a broth rich in zinc, vitamin A and C, potassium and magnesium electrolytes: In 2½ cups water, cook 1½ cups mixed carrots, broccoli, dark leafy greens, celery and parsley and 1 tsp. miso. Strain, use broth. Hearty version: blend warm broth and vegetables. Add 4 tbsp. sunflower seeds.

—*Before Bed:* have a glass of papaya juice.

Dietary pointers for best results from your lymph cleanse:

—Drink 8-10 glasses of bottled water each day of your cleanse.

—Include potassium-rich foods regularly — sea vegetables, broccoli, bananas and seafood.

—Avoid caffeine, sugar, dairy foods and alcohol during your cleanse. They add to lymphatic stagnation.

—Spicy foods like natural salsas, cayenne pepper, horseradish and ginger stimulate sluggish lymph.

Lymph cleanse supplement suggestions: Choose 2 or 3 cleansing boosters.

…**Lymphatic cleansers:** An *echinacea-goldenseal-myrrh* combination like Crystal Star ANTI-BIO™ caps for white blood cell formation; Herbs Etc. LYMPHATONIC - with echinacea to reduce lymphatic congestion; red root, a powerful lymphatic cleanser, synergistic with echinacea and ocotillo to flush lymph congestion; Nature's Apothecary LYMPH CLEANSE; Gaia Herbs ECHINACEA-RED ROOT Supreme a lymphatic and liver cleanser. Note: Echinacea extract and astragalus extract are highly successful deep lymph cleansing single herbs.

…Herbal lymph immune support: Maitake Products REISHI capsules.

…Immune support: Silica decisively increases immune phagocytes: Eidon SILICA; Flora VEGE-SIL.

…Supporting lymph nutrients: Vitamins A, C, E, B-complex, carotenes, iron, zinc and selenium.

…Enzyme support: Protease is a powerful lymph booster. Transformation Enzyme PUREZYME, used with LYMPHATIC DRAINAGE (assists protease in removing lymphatic wastes); shark cartilage, such as Lane Labs BENEFIN for leucocyte production.

…Electrolyte boosters: Mineral electrolytes play a major role in detoxifying the lymph glands, helping to remove acid crystals. Nature's Path TRACE-LYTE Liquid Minerals.

…To overcome lymph deficiencies: Protein and vitamin B-12.

Lymph cleanse bodywork suggestions: Techniques to accelerate, round out your cleanse.

Irrigate: take a colonic irrigation or a Sonné BENTONITE CLAY CLEANSE once a week to remove lymph congestion and infected feces from the intestinal tract.

Exercise: it's critical to lymphatic flow. Activate muscles with regular exercise and stretching. Start each exercise period with deep breathing. Mini-trampoline exercise clears clogged lymph nodes.

Massage therapy: elevate feet and legs for 5 minutes every day, massaging lymph node areas.

Essential oil support: use geranium, juniper and black pepper. Use one or a combination of all three oils. Put a total of 15 drops essential oil in 1-oz. of a carrier oil (such as jojoba) and rub on the skin.

Boost lymph circulation: with an alternating hot and cold shower at the end of your daily shower.

Bathe: a lymph-cleansing mineral bath — add 1 cup Dead Sea salts, 1 cup Epsom salts, ½ cup regular sea salt and ¼ baking soda to a tub; swish in 3 drops lavender oil, 2 drops *chamomile* oil, 2 drops *marjoram* oil and 1 drop *ylang ylang* oil. Or, try a Crystal Star HOT SEAWEED BATH™ (great for cellulite, too).

Eliminate aluminum: cookware, food additives, alum-containing foods like relishes and commercial condiments, and deodorants.

Can't find a recommended product? Call the 800 number in Product Resources for the store nearest you.

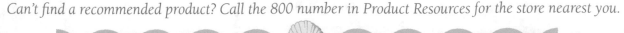

Improvement signs show that your body is responding to the lymph cleanse:
—Most people notice an increase in their daily energy.
—You'll no longer catch every cold that comes your way; illnesses you do get won't last as long.
—Most people notice far fewer stress reactions as body chemistry normalizes.
—Better weight control, if you were overweight; with less cellulite formation as congestion lessens.

Do you need a skin cleanse?

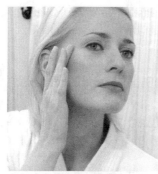

Your skin is the surest mirror of your lifestyle. Almost everything that's going on inside you shows on your skin. Your skin is your body's largest organ of elimination and detoxification, and it acts as a backup for every other elimination organ. When your colon becomes overloaded with toxins, or your liver cannot efficiently filter impurities coming from the digestive tract, your skin tries to compensate by releasing the toxins from your body. It sweats them out, or throws them off through rashes or boils. Your skin is the essence of renewable nature.... it sloughs off old, dying cells every day, and gives your body a clean, new start.

Your skin is also your body's largest organ of absorption and ingestion—both for nutrients and toxins. Good dietary care and habits show quickly. By the same token, chemicalized food toxins and nutritional deficiencies from a poor diet show up first on your skin. For example, toxins eliminated through the oil glands in the skin, show up as acne. The skin mirrors our emotional state and our hormone balance, too. So, stress reactions and hormone disruption show up as poor skin texture, or spots and blemishes.

Would your body benefit from a skin cleanse?

—Do you have sallow skin? Poor skin coloring may indicate build-up from liver wastes or drug residues.
—Do you have age spots? Brown mottled spots on the hands or face may reflect liver waste accumulation.
—Do you have adult acne, or uneven skin texture? Waste build-up from environmental pollutants, poor diet, liver exhaustion and stress allow increased free radical formation which attack skin cell membranes.
—Do you have wrinkles, or sagging skin contours? Free radical activity also affects skin collagen and elastin proteins, resulting in wrinkling and dry skin. Poor skin tone is a sign of antioxidant deficiency.
—Do you have puffy or swollen eyes, dark circles under eyes, or crusty, mucous formations in your eyes?
—Is your breath bad? Does your mouth feel coated instead of clean and fresh? Do you have body odor? These are pretty solid signs your body is overloaded with wastes.
—Do you have a skin disorder? Psoriasis, dermatitis and seborrhea all indicate its time for a skin cleanse.
—Do you have skin sores or rashes that aren't healing? or hard skin bumps? Your body may be overloaded with wastes you're not eliminating.
—Do you have unusually oily skin? or scaly, itchy skin? or chronically chapped and red skin?
—Is your circulation poor with chronically cold hands and feet? Are your ankles noticeably swollen? Your body lacks tissue oxygen uptake.

Benefits you may notice as your body responds to skin cleansing:
…Most people experience noticeable appearance improvement in about 3 weeks.
…Your face will look rested, rejuvenated and revitalized.
…Your skin's natural glow will return as capillary circulation and lymphatic drainage improve.
…Skin blemishes, blotches and spots diminish or disappear.
…The whites of your eyes will become whiter; dark circles will disappear.
…Your skin texture will appear smoother and softer; fine lines will appear less noticeable.

Can't find a recommended product? Call the 800 number in Product Resources for the store nearest you.

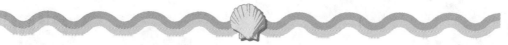

Skin Cleansing Detox Plan

1: Your diet is the fastest way to change your looks. Soft smooth skin depends on fresh fruits and vegetables. Skin tissues need a rich, oxygen blood supply and plenty of mineral building blocks. Silica, sulphur, calcium and magnesium are specific minerals for your skin. Plants are the best way for your body to get them.

2: Beautiful skin tone needs vitamin A, vitamin C, minerals and vegetable protein foods for collagen and interstitial tissue health. Eliminate or limit sugary foods, fried foods and trans-fats, like those in milk and dairy foods, margarine, shortening and hydrogenated oils. Avoid red meats and refined foods of all kinds.

3: Drink at least 8 glasses of bottled water each day of your cleanse—herbal "skin" teas are fine, too. Water keeps your body flushed so wastes and toxins won't be dumped out through the skin as blemishes or rashes. Fluoridated water may leach vitamin E out of your body.

My gentle skin cleanse offers skin cleansing diet recommendations, and targeted herbs and supplements to help treat specific problems or deficiencies.

Keys to the plan's success:

1. High in vitamin C foods to stimulate collagen production.
2. High in minerals. Mineral-rich foods are superior skin tonics, rapidly improving skin texture and tone in cases of deficiency.
3. High in essential fatty acids (EFA's) for soft supple skin with less wrinkling.
4. Includes gentle cleansers like green tea, ginger and chlorophyll to help clear toxins from the bloodstream before they can damage the skin.
5. Highly alkalizing and hydrating. An overacid, dehydrated body sets the stage for skin disorders and premature skin aging.

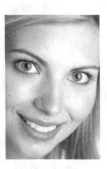

Begin your skin cleanse with this 3-day liquid diet and follow with 4 days of a diet of fresh foods.

—*On rising:* take a glass of lemon juice and water; add New Chapter GINGER WONDER syrup if desired.

—*Breakfast:* make a Complexion Booster: juice 2 slices of pineapple and 2 apples. add 1 tsp. nutritional yeast and 1 tsp. wheat germ oil. Or try 1 tbsp. Crystal Star BEAUTIFUL SKIN™ tea or caps.

—*Mid-morning:* have watermelon juice when available (rich in natural silica), or a skin tonic drink: juice 1 cucumber, 1 handful fresh parsley, 1 4-oz. tub fresh sprouts and sprigs of fresh mint. Or, have a superfood green drink, like Crystal Star ENERGY GREEN RENEWAL™, or Barleans GREENS drink mix.

—*Lunch:* have a fresh carrot juice; or a skin drink: juice 5 carrots, 2 apples, add 15 drops Ginger Extract.

—*Mid-afternoon:* have a carrot/beet/cucumber juice once a week for the next month for a clean liver.

—*Dinner:* have a warm Potassium Essence Broth (page 291) for mineral electrolytes. Or, make a high luster skin broth: In 2½ cups water, cook 2 cups chopped fresh mixed vegetables, add 1 tsp. miso and 2 tbsp. chopped dried sea vegetables. Vegetable protein aids faster healing for damaged skin.

—*Before Bed:* have Crystal Star BEAUTIFUL SKIN™ tea, or white tea or green tea for skin texture improvement; or a pineapple-papaya, papaya or apple juice; or VEGEX yeast broth for high B-complex vitamins.

Skin cleanse supplement suggestions: Choose 2 or 3 cleansing boosters.

...**Deep skin-blood cleansing:** Planetary YELLOW DOCK SKIN CLEANSE, Crystal Star RED SKIN RELIEF™ caps; sage or *burdock root* tea. White tea daily. *Note: I regard white tea as an outstanding choice for detoxification programs of all kinds. It shows an especially noticeable difference in a skin detox, offering a lovely clear texture to the skin. I use white tea for just this effect in Crystal Star BEAUTIFUL SKIN™ caps and tea.* Include a green superfood daily during your skin cleanse.

...**Smoothing/hydrating herbs for skin:** Crystal Star BEAUTIFUL SKIN™ caps and tea for blemishes and skin maintenance; Immudyne REJUVENATING SERUM with beta glucan; Source Naturals SKIN ETERNAL caps and serum; Nature's Apothecary SKIN SUPPORT - blood purifiers and mineralizers; Herbs Etc. DERMATONIC -

Can't find a recommended product? Call the 800 number in Product Resources for the store nearest you.

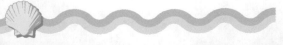

stimulates waste elimination; *burdock root* normalizes the skin's beneficial oils; *chamomile* tea or CAMOCARE Facial Therapy; Yoanna Oxygen Firming C Complex or *lavender* aromatherapy oil to reduce puffiness, MyChelle PERFECT C SERUM provides skin-absorbable vitamin C to enhance collagen production.

...**Skin nutrients:** New Chapter MULTIMINERAL caps; Maine Coast Organic Sea Vegetables; Diamond HERPANACINE for superior skin support; Futurebiotics HAIR, SKIN & NAILS - results in just 2 weeks.

...**Antioxidants essential for skin health:** Beta carotene protects against sun's free radicals; vitamin E protects against lipid peroxidation caused by UV rays; Bioflavonoids improve vascularization of the skin.

...**Essential fatty acids reduce skin dehydration and wrinkling:** Spectrum Organic ESSENTIAL MAX EFA OIL or EVENING PRIMROSE OIL 3000mg caps daily.

...**Enzymes:** Protease heals skin disorders; Transformation PUREZYME, Crystal Star DR. ENZYME.

...**Silica:** a mineral for collagen support, reduces dry, wrinkled skin. Eidon SILICA Mineral Supplement; Flora VEGESIL; Crystal Star IODINE, POTASSIUM, SILICA drops; Body Essentials SILICA GEL

...**MSM** (*Methyl Sulfonyl Methante*): enhances tissue pliability and helps repair damaged, scarred skin: Nature's Path MSM-LYTE.

Skin cleanse bodywork suggestions: Techniques to accelerate and round out your cleanse.

The healthiest skin needs some sunlight every day. Early morning sunlight on the body for natural vitamin D is a key. Exercise to get skin circulation flowing is another key.

Dry brushing: Use a natural bristle brush. Start with the soles of your feet - brush vigorously making rotary motions and massage every part of your body — work up to the neck.

Facial massage: Skin circulation for better tone.

Sauna: one of the best ways know to purify your skin quickly. Twenty minutes in a sauna 3 times a week during your skin cleanse can do wonders!

Healing skin application treatment: Add 1 tsp. of kelp granules to 1 tbsp. high quality aloe vera gel. Apply on face and neck. Leave on 10 minutes before rinsing. A natural mini face lift!

Skin Beauty Face tea: steep chamomile, calendula, rosehips, juice of 1 lemon and 2 tsp. rose water. Strain; apply with cotton balls to the face. Nature's Path SKIN-LYTE a liquid electrolyte spray.

Aloe vera: Herbal Answers HERBAL ALOE FORCE Gel boosts circulation and new cell growth.

Fruit acid treatment: Rub face with the insides of papaya or cucumber skins (natural AHA's) to neutralize wastes that come out on the skin.

Essential oil support: Lavender, geranium, sandalwood and neroli. Use one or a combination of all three oils. Put a total of 15 drops essential oil in 2-oz of a carrier oil (such as jojoba) and rub on the skin.

Skin mineral bath: Add 1 cup Dead Sea salts, 1 cup Epsom salts, ½ cup regular sea salt and 4 tbsp. baking soda to a tub; swish in 3 drops lavender, 2 drops geranium, 2 drops sandalwood and 1 drop neroli oil. Or, try a high iodine-potassium Crystal Star HOT SEAWEED BATH for soft, silky, glowing skin all over.

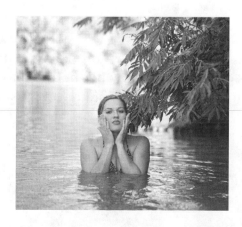

Can't find a recommended product? Call the 800 number in Product Resources for the store nearest you.

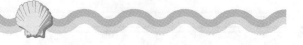

Lifestyle Healing Programs
for
People with Special Needs

Do you have special lifestyle therapy requirements?

—If you are pregnant, your diet needs are different, your nutritional supplement and herbal choices may have to be modified, your exercise regimen will have to change at least temporarily, and you'll have special health problems to address.

—If you are a kid, children's health requirements are different than an adult's. Childhood diseases are often unique to children; your immune system will probably need much less stimulation. Certain natural remedies seem to just work better for small people in their childhood years.

—If you are in your golden years, your diet and exercise needs change as your metabolism and glandular functions change. Herb and nutritional supplement choices need a different focus to fight the symptoms of aging, and immune response enhancement becomes far more important.

—If you are an athlete, active sports enthusiast or body builder, you are using up nutrients at a far greater rate than most people. More than likely you'll need far more herbal or nutritional supplementation. Normal dosage is usually not enough, either, for an athlete's higher metabolic needs.

Finally...
—If you are a family pet, you probably know how wonderful Mother Nature's remedies can be for your health problems. But you may not have access to the remedies or your mom may not be around to help. The special natural therapies for animals in this section may be just the ticket for you.

Having a Healthy Baby

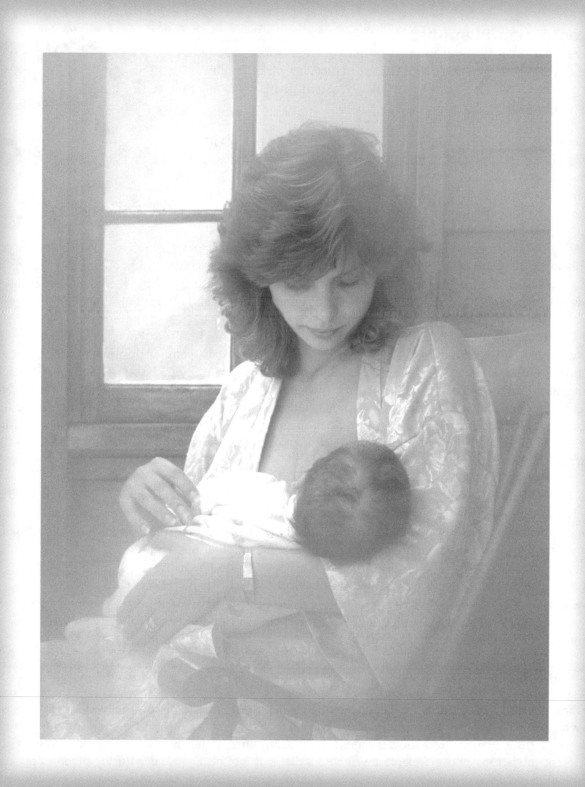

Having A Healthy Baby
Optimal Pregnancy Choices

Pre-conception Planning:

In America today, 20% of married couples of child-bearing age have trouble conceiving and completing a successful pregnancy. The fertility industry grosses $2 <u>billion</u> a year! Unfortunately, current fertility treatments have serious drawbacks.

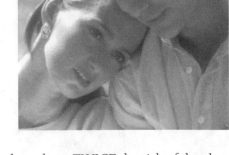

—Research shows Intracytoplasmic Sperm Injection (ICSI), introduced in 1993 to boost sperm count in infertile men, may cause abnormalities in embryos and even slow development in children.

—In vitro fertilization regularly results in multiple pregnancies and tough decisions for expectant parents. A new technique called "blastocyte transfer" is in the works to reduce risk of multiple births.

—A 1999 study in the journal Lancet shows women treated with fertility drugs have TWICE the risk of developing breast cancer - and over 5 TIMES the risk for uterine cancer as other women! Another study reports women who have not been pregnant before increase their risk for ovarian cancer <u>27 times</u> when they use fertility drugs. Moreover, women regularly report drug side effects like mood swings and chronic bloating.

Up to 40% of the time, the man is the infertile one in conception problems. For men, conception is affected by a zinc deficiency, a fast food diet, long term exposure to solvents like paint or printing presses, chronic infections and too much alcohol. For women, conception inhibitors are great emotional stress, being underweight, and severe anemia. Further, hormone imbalance problems like endometriosis, polycystic ovary syndrome, and fibroids routinely lead to infertility in women. Non-steroidal anti-inflammatory drugs (NSAIDS) like ibuprofen, and milk consumption (rBGH milk shows clear signs of hormone disruption) have also been linked to women's infertility. New research implicates hormone mimics from pollutants, estrogen exposure in the womb, chemical residues in food, water and plastics to infertility in both sexes.

Note: If you're worried by the studies linking herbs like St. John's wort, ginkgo biloba and echinacea to infertility, know that the herbs were only tested in a test tube on hamster eggs. It is highly improbable that the same herbs used in a living animal or human would have the same effect. Herbs, as gentle healing foods, are processed by our enzymatic systems.... neutralizing, in the majority of cases, potential for toxicity.

Diet is a critical key to successful conception... for both partners:

I've seen over and over again that a good diet and lifestyle is critical for at least six months before trying to conceive for both partners. Nature tries in every way possible to insure the survival of a new life....but the poor nutrition and stress of today's culture seems to be at the base of most fertility problems.

—A **"virility nutrition"** program for a man includes a short cleansing diet, then zinc-rich foods, healthy omega-3 fats, protein rich foods, minimal sweets and dairy foods, and plenty of whole grains. **Organic foods are important. A study reported in Lancet shows men who eat organic foods produce 43% more sperm than those who don't!** Take natural vitamin E, 400IU daily. New studies show vitamin E significantly improves sperm motility and fertility in men. Tests show the amino acid L-carnitine, 500mg daily, boosts sperm quality in subfertile men. Unless you're grossly overweight, a weight loss diet may <u>not</u> be a good idea during preconception. Severe food limitation has a direct impact on the testicles. A man's fertility rise may take place in as little as 2 months after his diet improvements. For a complete, step-by-step fertility enhancing diet for men, please consult my book, *Do You Want To Have A Baby? Natural Fertility Solutions & Pregnancy Care,* co-authored with Sarah Abernathy.

Can't find a recommended product? Call the 800 number in Product Resources for the store nearest you.

—A **"fertility nutrition"** program for a woman includes plenty of salads and greens, very low sugars, and a smaller volume of whole grains and nuts. Her diet should be low in saturated fats, but rich in essential fatty acids from sea greens and Omega-3 oils. I recommend fish and wild seafoods (from uncontaminated waters) during pre-conception, rather than meat, (unless certified organic, because much of America's meat and poultry is antibiotic and hormone laced). Limit dairy foods. Eating too much dairy clogs the female system. Drink a cup of green tea every morning. A new study shows that women who drink a cup of green tea daily get pregnant faster! Important: A woman's fertility rise may take 6 to 18 months after her diet change. Normalize your body weight before conception! Being overweight magnifies pregnancy problems like back and knee pain. Overweight women also increase their risk of developing toxemia or high blood pressure during pregnancy. Severely underweight women may risk premature births or low birth weight babies. For a complete, step-by-step fertility enhancing diet for women, please consult my book, *Do You Want To Have A Baby? Natural Fertility Solutions & Pregnancy Care, co-authored with Sarah Abernathy*.

Both men and women should limit their saturated fat intake to about 10% of the diet. Especially reduce sugary foods (artificial sweeteners like aspartame are particularly hazardous for your unborn child) and meats that are regularly laced with nitrates and-or hormones, like red meats, and smoked, cured and processed meats.

Lifestyle habits are important for fertility.

Avoid or reduce consumption of tobacco, caffeine, and alcohol. (Moderate wine is ok until conception.) Get light exercise, and morning sunshine every day possible. Take alternating hot and cold showers or apply alternating hot and cold compresses to the abdomen or scrotum to increase circulation to the reproductive areas. Massage therapy sessions, and deep breathing exercises, especially during long walks together, are very beneficial. Acupuncture and deep tissue massage has also been very successful in overcoming fertility problems for women and men.

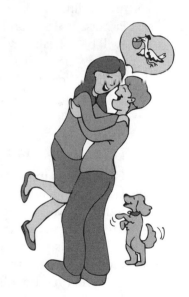

Herbs are a good choices for infertility problems because they address a multitude of infertility causes: hormone imbalance; body toxicity; stress; female obstructions and scarring. Crystal Star CONCEPTIONS Tea is a broad spectrum formula that helps maximize conception potential without the side effects or risk of fertility drugs. (See stress, ovarian cysts, fibroids and endometriois pages in this book for information on how to overcome these problems.)

Vitamins, minerals and herbs can help, too. There is a link between infertility and lack of vitamin C in both sexes. Today's new home tests can help you determine your most fertile periods, too, so you'll have a better chance of becoming pregnant. OVU-TEC fertility detector (saliva method) is a good choice. Call 800-528-0559 to learn more.

When is it time to consider an infertility workup?

Infertility is defined as the inability to conceive for 12 consequent months of trying. So, if you are at this point, you may want to consider a workup. An infertility workup to help understand the cause of infertility may be useful. It can allow you to target the problem and address it quicker. A workup normally includes a complete physical, sexual history, semen analysis for the man, a blood hormone evaluation for the woman, and a test showing compatibility of the man's sperm and the woman's vaginal secretions. Please note that formerly "infertile" couples have been able to conceive after following natural therapies.

Note: Over use of NSAIDs (Non-steroidal anti-inflammatory drugs) like ibuprofen can induce "luteinized unruptured follicle syndrome," a syndrome in which eggs are never released for conception. In fact, some "infertile" women have been able to complete successful pregnancies after stopping NSAID use!

Can't find a recommended product? Call the 800 number in Product Resources for the store nearest you.

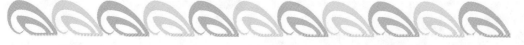

Optimal Eating for Two During Pregnancy

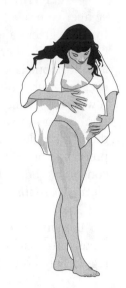

A woman's body changes so dramatically during pregnancy and childbearing that her normal daily needs change. The body takes care of some of these requirements through cravings. During this one time of life, the body is so sensitive to its needs, that the cravings you get are usually good for you. We know that every single thing the mother does or takes in affects the child. Good nutrition for a child begins before it is born, actually even before it is conceived. New research shows that when a child reaches adulthood, his or her risk for heart disease, cancer, and diabetes can be traced to poor eating habits of the parents as well as genetic factors. The nutritious diet suggestions in this section will help build a healthy baby, minimize the mother's discomfort, lessen birth complications and reduce excess fatty weight gain that can't be lost after birth.

A good diet also minimizes pregnancy risk and discomforts.... preventing miscarriage and high blood pressure, supporting your body against toxemia, fluid retention, constipation, hemorrhoids and varicose veins, gas and heartburn, morning sickness, anemia, even hormone adjustment. After pregnancy, a good diet is important for sufficient breast milk, reducing post-partum swelling, and healing stretched tissue.

Promise yourself and your baby that at least during the months of pregnancy and nursing, your diet and life-style will be as healthy as you can make it. A largely vegetarian diet of whole foods along with seafood and organic poultry provide a nutritional powerhouse. Base your pregnancy diet on whole grains, leafy greens and fresh fish. Avoid shark, mackerel and swordfish, notorious for high mercury levels dangerous to a developing fetus; (eat canned fish only in moderation). Turkey, eggs, legumes, nuts, seeds, vegetables, nutritional yeast (food-source B-vitamins), bananas and citrus fruits assure the best possible nutrition for your baby.

Diet Keys: **Eat small frequent meals instead of large meals.**

1: **Protein is important.** Experts recommend 60 to 80 grams of protein daily during pregnancy, with a 10 gram increase each trimester. Focus on vegetable protein — whole grains, beans, peas, lentils, seeds, sprouts, with fish, seafood or hormone-free turkey 3 times a week. Take a high quality protein drink 3 times a week for optimal growth and energy. It's the quality, not the quantity of protein that prevents and cures toxemia.

Try this proven protein drink: Mix ½ cup vanilla rice milk, ½ cup yogurt, ½ cup orange juice, 2 tbsp. nutritional yeast, 2 tbsp. toasted wheat germ, 2 tsp. molasses, 1 tsp. vanilla, one pinch cinnamon.

2: **Have a fresh fruit or green salad every day.** Eat plenty of fiber foods, like apples, pears and prunes for regularity. Have whole grain cereals and vegetables like broccoli and brown rice for strength.

3: **Drink plenty of healthy fluids:** pure water, mineral water, and juices throughout the day to keep your system free and flowing. Carrot juice at least twice a week is ideal. Include pineapple and apple juice.

4: **Eat folate rich foods:** like fresh spinach, other leafy greens, sea greens, and asparagus for cell growth.

5: **Boost your essential fatty acids (EFA's):** from fish, spinach and arugula, flax seed, and especially from sea greens (2 tbsp. per day of snipped dry sea greens do the trick) for your baby's healthy brain and skin.

6: **Eat carotene-rich foods:** like carrots, squashes, tomatoes, yams, and broccoli for disease resistance.

7: **Eat vitamin C foods:** like broccoli, bell peppers and fruits for connective tissue.

8: **Eat bioflavonoid-rich foods:** like citrus fruits and berries for capillary integrity.

9: **Eat alkalizing foods:** like miso soup and brown rice to combat and neutralize toxemia.

10: **Eat mineral-rich foods,** like sea veggies, leafy greens, and whole grains for baby building blocks. Include silica-rich foods for bone, cartilage, connective tissue. For zinc, consider foods like pumpkin and sesame seeds. For collagen and elastin formation - try brown rice, oats, green grasses and green drinks. Calcium is especially important. If calcium is in short supply, it will be leached from the mother's teeth and bones to help support the fetus. Eat calcium-rich green vegetables, cooked kale, carrot juice, and yogurt *often*. Highly bioavailable calcium from herbs is a good choice, too, like Crystal Star CALCIUM-MAGNESIUM SOURCE™ and Floradix CALCIUM liquid.

Can't find a recommended product? Call the 800 number in Product Resources for the store nearest you.

Important diet watchwords you should know during pregnancy and nursing.
See my book Do You Want To Have A Baby? for a complete, detailed pregnancy diet.
—Don't drastically restrict your diet to lose weight. Low calories may mean low birth weight for the baby.
—Eat a wide range of healthy foods to assure the baby access to all nutrients. Avoid cabbages, onions, and garlic. They can upset body balance during pregnancy. Broccoli, cauliflower, cabbage, onion, milk and chocolate (the worst!) have all been found to aggravate colic in nursing babies. Avoid red meats.
—Don't fast - even for short periods where fasting might be helpful, like constipation, or to overcome a cold. Food energy and nutrient content may be diminished.
—Avoid chemicalized, smoked, preserved, and artificially colored foods.
—Avoid alcohol, caffeine (5 or more cups of coffee daily is linked to spontaneous abortion) and tobacco.
—Avoid chemical solvents, and CFCs such as hair sprays, and cat litter. Your system may be able to handle these things without undue damage; the baby's can't. Even during nursing, toxic amounts occur easily.
—Avoid smoking and secondary smoke. Your baby, like you, metabolizes the harmful cancer-causing residues of tobacco. The chance of low birth weight, SIDS and miscarriage is much more likely if you smoke. Smoker's infants have a mortality rate 30% higher than non-smoker's. Nursing babies take in small amounts of nicotine with breast milk, and become prone to chronic respiratory infections.
—Exposure to alcohol is the most common cause of mental retardation in the U.S. Avoid alcohol to reduce risk of Fetal Alcohol Syndrome, mental retardation and motor-skill problems.

More diet watchwords:
•During labor: Refrain from solid food. Drink fresh water, or carrot juice; or suck on ice chips.
•During lactation: Add almond milk, nutritional yeast, green drinks and green foods, avocados, carrot juice, goat's milk, soy milk and soy foods, and unsulphured molasses, to promote milk quality and richness. Fennel seed tea promotes breast milk in lactating women and reduces colic in nursing infants. Earth Mama Angel Baby MILKMAID tea with fenugreek helps increase breast milk quickly (good results with our tester). *Vitex* extract also improves poor milk quality. Wayne State University studies show that exposure to pollutant PCBs from breast milk can lower a child's IQ score by as much as 6 points. Your focus on organic foods can minimize exposure.
•During weaning: Drink papaya juice to slow down milk flow.

About Breast Feeding

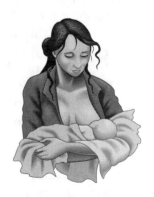

Mother's milk is best. The baby who is not breast fed loses Nature's "jump start" on immune response and may face health disadvantages that last a lifetime. Unless there are unusual circumstances, your breast milk should be your baby's only food during the first six months of life. Despite all the claims made for fortified formulas, nothing can take the place of breast milk. Today's pediatricians recommend breast feeding your baby for up to a year. The first thick, waxy colostrum is extremely high in protein, essential fatty acids needed for brain and nervous system development, and protective antibodies. A child's immune system is not fully established at birth, and the antibodies in breast milk are critical. They fight early infections and create solid immune defenses that prevent the development of allergies.

Breast-fed babies have lower risk of SIDs (Sudden Infant Death Syndrome), Crohn's disease, lymphoma, and respiratory infections. Breast-fed babies also have less colic. Breast milk is loaded with bifidobacteria, the beneficial micro-organisms that make up 99% of a healthy baby's intestinal flora — extremely important for protection against salmonella poisoning and other intestinal pathogens.

Mother's milk is best for boosting and balancing your baby's fats. It contains the full range of EFA's needed for proper development of a child's central nervous system, brain and eyes. The Journal of Pediatrics says that breast-feeding your baby may even make him or her smarter, giving your child an academic advantage!

Can't find a recommended product? Call the 800 number in Product Resources for the store nearest you.

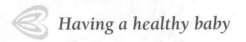

The determining factor seems to be the high content of DHA (docosahexaenoic acid) in breast milk, an essential fatty acid which comprises over 50% of the brain. DHA, vital in infant development, increases 3 to 5 times in the last trimester of pregnancy and triples <u>again</u> in the first 12 weeks of life. Note: If you work out.. research shows that immune antibodies passed through breast milk drop 50% after intense workouts. Wait an hour to breast feed after workouts to ensure that your baby gets the maximum nutrients.

Note: If you are unable to breastfeed long term, try to breastfeed for at least the first month to ensure that your child benefits from colostrum and critical nutrients that establish strong immune defenses.

Supplements help nutritional deficiencies during pregnancy

During pregnancy, illness, body imbalance, even regular supplements need to be handled differently, even if your healing method is holistically oriented. A mother's body is very delicately tuned and sensitive at this time; imbalances occur easily. Mega-doses of anything are not good for the baby's system. Doses of all medication or supplements should almost universally be about half of normal, to allow for the infant's tiny system capacity. Ideal supplements are food-source complexes for best absorbability.

Avoid all drugs during pregnancy and nursing — including alcohol, aspartame (Nutrasweet), tobacco, caffeine, MSG, saccharin, X-rays, aspirin, Valium, Librium, Tetracycline and harsh diuretics. Even the amino acid L-Phenylalanine can adversely affect the nervous system of the unborn child. Especially stay away from recreational drugs—cocaine, PCP, marijuana, meth-amphetamines, Quaaludes, heroin, LSD.

Supplements that can help you during pregnancy:

…**A superfood green drink.** A green drink is a good nutrition "delivery system" during pregnancy because it is so quickly absorbed with so little work by the body. Crystal Star's ENERGY GREEN RENEWAL™ drink mix or capsules contains land and sea greens, grasses and herbs full of absorbable, potent chlorophyllins, complex carbohydrates, minerals, proteins, and amino acids. Other good ones: Body Ecology VITALITY SUPER GREEN, Green Foods VEGGIE MAGMA.

…**A good prenatal multi-vitamin supplement**, starting six to eight weeks before the expected birth. Clinical tests show that mothers who take nutritional supplements during pregnancy are far less likely to have babies with neural tube and other defects. Be sure your prenatal formula contains 350 to 500mg of magnesium. Body demands for magnesium increase during pregnancy. Pre-eclampsia, marked by elevated blood pressure, fluid retention and protein loss through urine, premature labor and poor fetal growth are all tied to magnesium deficiency during pregnancy. Try Pure Essence MOTHER TO BE Formula (highly effective) New Chapter PERFECT PRENATAL.

…**An absorbable, food source multi-mineral supplement** (not just calcium or iron). Nature's Path TRACE-MIN-LYTE or Crystal Star OCEAN MINERALS™ caps offer good body building blocks. Beta-carotene 10,000mg, with vitamin C 500mg, niacin 50mg, and available plant iron are better for skeletal, cellular and connecting tissue development than calcium supplements alone.

…**Extra folic acid, 800mcg daily to prevent neural tube defects**. Timing is essential. Supplementing folic acid *after* the first three months of fetal development *cannot* correct spinal cord damage.

…**Vitamin B$_6$ 50mg for bloating, leg cramps and nerve strength**; also prevent proneness to glucose intolerance and seizures in the baby.

…**Bioflavonoids daily.** Over 50% of women who habitually miscarry have low vitamin C and bioflavonoid levels. Bioflavonoids enhance vein and capillary strength, and help control bruising and internal bleeding from hemorrhoids and varicose veins. Bioflavonoids are a "deep tissue tonic" that support and maintain tissue integrity, tighten and tone skin elasticity. They minimize skin aging and wrinkling due to pregnancy stretching. Bioflavs are fiber-rich for regularity — a definite pregnancy advantage! Take citrus bioflavonoids 600mg with vitamin C daily, or bioflavs from herbs and gentle foods, like apricots, berries, cantaloupes, cherries, grapefruits, grapes, oranges and lemons.

Can't find a recommended product? Call the 800 number in Product Resources for the store nearest you.

Bioflavonoids help control excess fatty deposits, too. Herbs and citrus fruits are some of the best bioflav sources. BILBERRY EXTRACT is one of the single richest yet gentlest sources of herbal flavonoids in the botanical world, especially helpful for pregnant women suffering from distended veins, hemorrhoids, weak uterine walls and toxemia.

...DHA, an Omega 3 fatty acid found in seafood and sea greens. Pregnant women pass large amounts of DHA in utero to their babies to ensure proper brain and nervous system development. As a result, many new moms are deficient, leading to problems with forgetfulness and even postpartum depression. I recommend New Chapter Supercritical DHA100 to help meet high DHA demand during pregnancy. It works!

...Kelp tablets, 6 daily, or Crystal Star OCEAN MINERALS™ capsules, for natural potassium and iodine. A lack of these minerals means mental retardation and poor physical development. Kelp is widely used in agriculture (animal feed) to help with fertility, healthy births and lactation, and it can help people, too!

...Natural vitamin E, 200-400IU, or wheat germ oil, to help prevent miscarriage and reduce the baby's oxygen requirement, lessening the chances of asphyxiation during labor. Discontinue 1-2 weeks before delivery date.

...EFAs, (omega-3 rich flax oil, borage seed, evening primrose oils), for baby's brain development. Udo's PER-FECTED OIL BLEND is a good choice.

...Calcium lactate with calcium ascorbate vitamin C for collagen development.

...Zinc, 10-15mg daily. Zinc deficiency results in poor brain formation, learning problems, low immunity.

Important supplement watchwords:

<u>During the last trimester</u>: Rub vitamin E or wheat germ oil on your stomach and around vaginal opening to make stretching easier and skin more elastic. Earth Mama Angel Baby STRETCH OIL and Magia Bella ULTRA-IN-TENSIVE ANTI-STRETCH MARK CONCENTRATE (belly only) are recommended. Begin to take extra minerals as labor approaches.

<u>During labor</u>: Take calcium-magnesium to relieve pain and aid dilation.

<u>During nursing</u>: Nutritional supplements like iron, calcium, B vitamins or a prenatal multiple, should be continued during nursing. Increase dose slightly to recover normal strength. Breast milk is a filtered food supply that prevents baby from overdosing on higher potencies. Apply vitamin E oil to ease breast crusting. Apply a *marshmallow* fomentation to relieve pressure in engorged breasts.

Herbs for a healthy pregnancy **Good and easy for you; gentle for the baby.**

Herbs have been used during pregnancy for centuries to ease the hormone imbalances and discomforts of stretching, bloating, nausea and pain without impairing the health of the baby. They still do today. A study in Obstetrics and Gynecology 2001 reports that 91% of the women surveyed were using herbal remedies during pregnancy. Herbs are mineral-rich foods, perfect for the extra growth requirements of pregnancy and childbirth. They are easily-absorbed and non-constipating. Ideal supplements affecting a developing child's body should be from food source complexes. Herbs are identified and accepted by the body's enzyme activity as whole food nutrients, lessening the risk of toxemia or overdose, yet providing gentle nutrition for both mother and baby.

Important: Early pregnancy and later pregnancy must be considered separately with herbal medicinals. If there is any question, always use the gentlest herbs and consult your health care professional.

HERBS YOU CAN TAKE DURING PREGNANCY:

• Many women prefer body balancing teas during pregnancy. They are the gentlest way to overcome morning sickness and hormone adjustment. Take two daily cups of red raspberry tea, high in iron, calcium and other minerals; or Earth Mama Angel Baby MORNING WELLNESS tea (for nausea), or Earth Mama Angel Baby THIRD TRIMESTER tea (<u>only for third trimester</u>) strengthen the uterus and birth canal, guard against birth defects, long labor and afterbirth pain, and tone the uterus for a quicker return to normal.

Can't find a recommended product? Call the 800 number in Product Resources for the store nearest you.

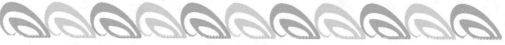

• Iodine-rich foods are a primary deterrent to spinal birth defects, and also help protect against mental retardation risk. Take kelp tablets, a sea greens sprinkle on your daily salad or rice, Crystal Star OCEAN MINERALS caps™, or New Chapter OCEAN HERBS.

• Many pregnant women need extra calcium and iron, minerals that are easily depleted during pregnancy. Herbal sources of absorbable calcium and iron are one of the best ways to get these minerals because they absorb through the body's own enzyme system. Herbal minerals provide the best bonding agent between your body and the nutrients it is taking in. They are also rich in other nutrients that encourage the best uptake by the body. Take Crystal Star CALCIUM MAGNESIUM SOURCE™, a calcium-rich compound of herbs with magnesium for optimum uptake, and naturally-occurring silica from gentle herbs like oatstraw, nettles and dark greens help form healthy tissue and bone — a prime factor in collagen formation for connective and interstitial tissue. Crystal Star IRON SOURCE BLOOD BUILDER™ extract drops in warm water, or Floradix IRON PLUS HERBS are absorbable, non-constipating herbal iron sources with measurable amounts of calcium and magnesium, along with naturally-occurring vitamins C and E for optimum iron uptake.

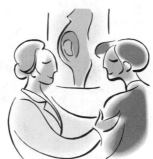

• Consider a mineral-rich pre-natal herbal compound during the 1st and 2nd trimester, for absorbable minerals and toners to elasticize tissue and ease delivery. A good formula might include herbs like *red raspberry, nettles, oatstraw, alfalfa, chamomile, peppermint, yellow dock root* and dairy free acidophilus (Try UAS DDS plus or Jarrow JARRO-DOPHI-LUS with FOS.) During the last trimester, I recommend a broad activity herbal mineral compound, like Crystal Star OCEAN MINERALS™ caps, or CALCIUM-MAGNESIUM™ caps, loaded with highly absorbable plant minerals, or Floradix CALCIUM-MAGNESIUM liquid with vitamin D, zinc and herbs.

• Five weeks before the expected birth date, an herbal formula to help your body prepare for parturition, aid in hemorrhage control and uterine muscle strength for correct presentation of the fetus might contain herbs like *red raspberry, false unicorn, cramp bark, squaw vine* and *bilberry*.

HERBS YOU CAN TAKE DURING LABOR:
—Earth Mama Angel Baby LABOR EASE tea, Red Earth Herbal Drops LABOR-EASE drops (use with midwife guidance) Crystal Star PMS RELIEF™ drops for fast acting relief of contraction pain. Put 15 to 20 drops in water and take small sips as needed during labor. Try Crystal Star STRESS OUT MUSCLE RELAXER™ drops in warm water for afterbirth pain (excellent results), an analgesic formula that helps the lower back and spinal block area, often within 20 minutes.

—For false labor, magnesium therapy helps. If there is bleeding, go to a hospital and call your midwife. 2 capsules, cayenne, can be helpful to curtail flow.

HERBS YOU CAN TAKE DURING NURSING:
—Add 2 tbsp. nutritional yeast to your diet, along with *red raspberry, marshmallow root*, or *fenugreek* tea to promote and enrich milk after the child is born.
—Take VITEX extract, Motherlove MORE MILK or Earth Mama Angel Baby MILKMAID tea to promote an abundant supply of mother's milk.
—*Fennel seed, alfalfa, red raspberry, cumin, fenugreek* teas help keep baby colic free.
—For infant jaundice, Hyland's NATRUM SULPHURICUM.

HERBS YOU CAN TAKE FOR WEANING:
—*Parsley-sage* tea to help dry up milk.
—Amazake rice drink can help wean from breast milk.

Can't find a recommended product? Call the 800 number in Product Resources for the store nearest you.

Safe herbs you can use during pregnancy:
Take herbs in the mildest way, as relaxing teas, during pregnancy.

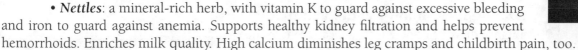

• **Red Raspberry**: the quintessential herb for pregnancy - an all around uterine tonic. It is anti-abortive to prevent miscarriage, antiseptic for protection against infection, astringent to tighten tissue, rich in calcium, magnesium and iron to help prevent cramps and anemia. It facilitates birth by improving natural contractions, and is hemostatic to reduce risk of hemorrhaging. Assists with plentiful milk production, too.

• **Nettles**: a mineral-rich herb, with vitamin K to guard against excessive bleeding and iron to guard against anemia. Supports healthy kidney filtration and helps prevent hemorrhoids. Enriches milk quality. High calcium diminishes leg cramps and childbirth pain, too.

• **Peppermint**: use after the first trimester to help digestion, soothe the stomach and overcome nausea. Contains highly absorbable amounts of vitamin A, C, silica, potassium and iron.

• **Ginger root**: excellent for morning sickness; has lots of needed minerals.

• **Bilberry**: strong, gentle astringent, rich in bioflavonoids to fortify veins and capillaries. A hematonic for kidney function and a mild diuretic for bloating.

• **Burdock**: mineral-rich, hormone balancer, liver booster. Prevents water retention and baby jaundice.

• **Yellow dock root**: improves iron assimilation; helps prevent infant jaundice (small amounts only).

• **Dong quai root**: a blood nourisher, rather than a hormone stimulant. Use in moderation.

• **Echinacea**: an immune system stimulant to help prevent colds, flu and infections.

• **Chamomile**: relaxes for quality sleep, lifts the spirit, and helps digestive and bowel problems.

• **Vitex**: normalizes hormone balance for fertility. Discontinue when pregnancy is realized.

• **False unicorn**, black and blue cohosh: for final weeks of pregnancy only, to assist child labor and delivery. To avoid risks, use with midwife guidance only.

• **Wild yam**: for general pregnancy pain, nausea or cramping; lessens chance of miscarriage.

• **Alfalfa**: highly nutritive, rich in enzymes, full of vitamin K to reduce postpartum hemorrhage.

• **Dandelion greens and root**: a gentle diuretic that reduces pregnancy-related water retention; reduces fatigue and system sluggishness.

• **Sea greens**: exceptional source of vitamins and minerals to prevent birth defects; balances thyroid.

• Aromatherapy essential oils of **lavender and chamomile** alleviate nausea.

• Aromatherapy essential oils of **fennel seed and anise** reduce heartburn.

HERBS TO AVOID DURING PREGNANCY: Medicinal herbs should always be used with common sense and care, especially during pregnancy. Some herbs are not appropriate.

Contra-indicated, cautionary herbs:

–**Aloe vera**: can be too strong as a laxative. Dilute aloe vera juice with 4 parts water if you decide to use it, or use an aloin-free brand like Herbal Answers HERBAL ALOE FORCE juice.

–**Angelica and rue**: stimulate oxytocin that causes uterine contractions.

–**Barberry, buckthorn, rhubarb root**, *mandrake, senna and cascara sagrada*: too strong as laxatives.

–**Black cohosh**: can stimulate uterine contractions. Blue cohosh also affects uterine sloughing. (Some health professionals use it to induce labor.)

–**Buchu, uva ursi and juniper**: too strong diuretics.

–**Licorice rt.**: can exacerbate water retention and high blood pressure in susceptible persons. In large amounts, licorice may lead to preterm deliveries.

–**Coffee**: too strong a caffeine and heated hydrocarbon source - a uterine irritant. In extremely sensitive individuals who take in excessive amounts, may cause miscarriage or premature birth.

–**Comfrey**: pyrrolizides (carcinogenic) cannot be commercially controlled for an absolutely safe source.

–**Ephedra, Ma Huang**: contains ephedrine alkaloids that can overstimulate the heart.

–**Horseradish**: too strong for a baby.

–**Male fern**: too strong a vermifuge.

Can't find a recommended product? Call the 800 number in Product Resources for the store nearest you.

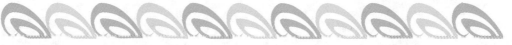

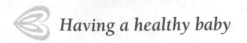

–*Goldenseal, lovage, mugwort, southernwood, wormwood*: emmenagogues that cause uterine contractions. *Mistletoe, thuja, tansy and wild ginger* also act to cause uterine contractions.

–*Hyssop*: its volatile oil is too strong for a developing fetus;

–*Pennyroyal*: stimulates oxytocin that can cause abortion.

–*Yarrow and shepherd's purse*: strong astringents and mild abortifacients.

Preventing SIDS: Sudden Infant Death Syndrome

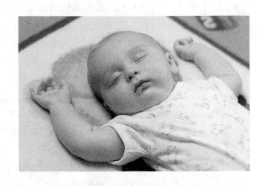

Every year, 3,000 infants die of Sudden Infant Death Syndrome (SIDS) in the U.S. If your baby has a weak system, or poor lung tissue development (signs that he or she is a candidate for SIDS) a weak ascorbate vitamin C, or Ester C with bioflavs solution is an option that you may want to explore with your pediatrician. (The US RDA for vitamin C for infants is 35 mg.). Routinely feeding babies iron-fortified weaning foods to prevent anemia may <u>increase</u> the risk of SIDS, according to the British Medical Journal. Evidence indicates that infant pillows filled with foam polystyrene beads cause babies to inhale toxic gases and suffocate. Just putting your child to sleep on his back cuts SIDS risk in half because it helps prevent accidental suffocation! In fact, modern doctors now recommend <u>parents only place infants on their backs to sleep</u>.

New research done by Barry Richardson suggests that toxic gases emerge from the interaction between household fungi and baby mattress chemicals or flame retardants. Using a chemical-free mattress cover like DR. D'S CRIB LIFE MATTRESS COVER may help reduce your child's SIDS risk. (Call 800-528-0559.) Avoid loose blankets, too. Wearable blankets are a safer choice.

Exposure to second-hand smoke greatly increases the risk of SIDS because it reduces an infant's ability to withstand low oxygen levels if his/her face and head get covered. Even when a baby is merely in rooms where smoking occurs, its risk of dying from SIDS can increase 800%! A newly identified SIDS risk is a heart abnormality called a prolonged QT interval which can be detected by an EKG and treated with up to 90% success rate. Some new research shows that taking low doses of carnitine (less than 100mg) during the last trimester can help protect the baby from SIDS. Evidence from seven different studies suggests that babies who use pacifiers have lower risk for SIDS. Further, the same *H. pylori* bacteria linked to ulcers may be linked to SIDS. Scientists recommend avoiding transmitting adult saliva to very tiny babies to prevent *H. pylori* transmission.

If you feel your child is at risk, a high tech T shirt to monitor heartbeat and breathing is now available.

Bodywork for Two

1: Get some mild daily exercise, such as a brisk walk for fresh air, more tissue oxygen and circulation. Take an early morning, or half hour sun bath when possible for vitamin D, calcium absorption and bone growth.

2: Consciously set aside one stress-free time for relaxation every day. Yoga stretches and pregnancy massage are especially helpful. The baby will know, thrive, and be more relaxed itself.

3: If you practice reflexology, do not press the acupressure point just above the ankle on the inside of the leg. It can start contractions.

4: Rub cocoa butter, vitamin E oil or wheat germ oil on the stomach and around the vaginal opening every night to make stretching easier and the skin more elastic during delivery. Many women swear that it makes an enormous difference. Gently stretch perineal tissues with your fingers to prepare for the birthing experience.

5: Get adequate sleep. Body energy turns inward during sleep fo repair, restoration and fetal growth.

Can't find a recommended product? Call the 800 number in Product Resources for the store nearest you.

Special Problems during Pregnancy

Reduce standard dosage of any medication, orthodox or natural, to allow for the infant's tiny system. To learn more about natural therapies for special problems during pregnancy, please consult my book, *Do You Want To Have A Baby? Natural Fertility Solutions & Pregnancy Care,* co-authored with Sarah Abernathy.

AFTERBIRTH PAIN: take STRESS OUT MUSCLE RELAXER™ extract, especially after a long labor, to tone and elasticize uterus; Earth Mama Angel Baby POSTPARTUM RECOVERY tea to restore vitality, tone the uterus and reduce tension; *una da gato* tea for quicker return to normal. For post-partum tears and to heal sore perineal muscles, use a sitz bath: *1 part uva ursi, 1 part yerba mansa rt., and 1 part each comfrey leaf and root.* Simmer 15 minutes, strain, add 1 tsp. salt, pour into a large shallow container; cool slightly. Or use Mother Love's SITZ BATH or Earth Mama Angel Baby POSTPARTUM BATH HERBS. Sit in the bath for 15 to 20 minutes twice daily. Use Earth Mama Angel Baby NEW MAMA BOTTOM SPRAY to aid healing from episiotomies.

ANEMIA: take a non-constipating herbal iron, such as Pure Planet CHLORELLA, *yellow dock* tea, Crystal Star IRON SOURCE BLOOD BUILDER™ caps, or Floradix IRON plus herbs. Have a green drink often, such as apple-alfalfa sprout cucumber juice, Green Foods CARROT ESSENCE. Add vitamin C and E to your diet, eat plenty of dark leafy greens.

BREASTS:
  -**for infected breasts:** 500mg vitamin C every 3 hours, 400IU vitamin E, and beta-carotene 10,000IU daily; chlorophyll from green salads, green drinks, or green supplements — Crystal Star ENERGY GREEN RENEWAL™ or Green Foods GREEN MAGMA. For mastitis - redness, fever, flu-like symptoms, consult a health care professional.
  -**for caked or crusted breasts:** simmer *elder flowers* in oil and rub on breasts. Wheat germ oil, almond oil and cocoa butter are also effective, or use Earth Mama Angel Baby NATURAL NIPPLE butter.
  -**for engorged breasts during nursing:** lie on your back to drain excess flow. Allow baby to nurse until breasts soften (if possible), and pump breasts if you miss a feeding. Apply ice bags to the breasts to relieve pain; or use a *marshmallow root* fomentation with ½ cup powder to 1 qt. water. Simmer 10 minutes. Soak a cloth in mix and apply to breast. Try Motherlove BREAST COMPRESS or Earth Mama Angel Baby BOOBY TUBES.
  -**for sagging breasts <u>after</u> weaning:** MagiaBella BUST SUPPORT or Baywood BREAST MAXIMIZING LOTION.

CONSTIPATION: Increase fluid intake. Add fiber fruits, like prunes and apples, and 1 tbsp ground flax seeds to the daily diet. *Red clover* infusion is a specific. Kelp tabs lubricate and move the bowels without risks.

FALSE LABOR: catnip tea or red raspberry tea will help. See also MISCARRIAGE pg. 498 in this book.

GAS and HEARTBURN: Take papaya or bromelain chewables or papaya juice with a pinch of *ginger*. After meals, a weak tea with *fennel, spearmint, peppermint* or *chamomile*, or Earth Mama Angel Baby HEARTBURN TEA.

HEMORRHOIDS: apply: Crystal Star HEMR-EZE™ gel, or Mother Love's RHOID BALM, or Earth Mama Angel Baby BOTTOM BALM (all highly recommended). Keep topical treatments in the refrigerator for the best results.

INSOMNIA: Crystal Star CALCIUM MAGNESIUM SOURCE™ or Flora CALCIUM MAGNESIUM. Nervine herbs like *scullcap,* and *passion flower* or *chamomile* tea help. A pregnancy body pillow can work wonders for support.

LABOR: for nausea during labor, take *ginger* tea or miso broth, or Alacer EMERGEN-C with a little salt added to prevent dehydration. For labor pain, take *crampbark extract, or lobelia, scullcap or St. John's wort extract* in water. For nerve pain, apply St. John's wort oil to temples and wrists; or use *rosemary/ginger* compresses. Acupressure treatments during labor reduce stress and increase dilation. Changing positions helps; take short walks or stand on hands and knees. Hypnosis helps stop the flow of catecholamines, stress hormones that hinder the birthing process. *For more information on HypBirth, check out hypbirth.com or call 818-248-0888.* For post-partum bleeding: *shepherd's purse* or *nettles* tea. For sleep during long labor: use *scullcap* tincture. (*Scullcap* may be used throughout labor for relaxation.) Hydrate with cool drinks even if you feel nauseated. Take bromelain to relieve pain and swelling after episiotomy.

Can't find a recommended product? Call the 800 number in Product Resources for the store nearest you.

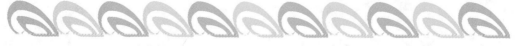

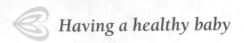

MORNING SICKNESS: *Ginger* works in clinical trials: 1 gram daily. Use homeopathic IPECAC and NAT. MUR, add vitamin B-6, 50mg 2x daily; sip mint tea when queasy. See MORNING SICKNESS page 506 in this book.

MISCARRIAGE: for prevention and hemorrhage control, drink *raspberry* tea every hour with ¼ tsp. ascorbate vit. C powder added, and take drops of *hawthorn* extract every hour. Avoid physical strain at the time of conception to aid successful implantation of the fertilized egg. See MISCARRIAGE program, page 498 for complete information. According to John Lee M.D., transdermal progesterone 40mg. per day can help prevent miscarriage caused by luteal phase failure. Ask your healthcare professional.

POST-PARTUM SWELLING and DEPRESSION: use homeopathic ARNICA. Make a post-partum cordial with 4 slices of *dong quai rt.*, ½ oz. *false unicorn rt.*, 1 handful *nettles*, ½ oz. *St. John's wort* extract, 1 handful *motherwort herb*, ½ oz. *hawthorn berries*, and 2 inch-long slices of fresh *ginger*. Steep herbs in 1 pint of brandy for 2 weeks, shaking daily. Strain an add a little honey if desired. Take 1 tsp. daily as a tonic dose. Good results.

Depression is helped by B vitamins - Nature's Secret ULTIMATE B. Progesterone deficiency may be indicated. Consider progesterone balancing herbs like *sarsaparilla rt.* and *wild yam*, or an herbal formula like Crystal Star PRO-EST™ BALANCE roll on. Recent research from the National Institutes of Health reveals that women with low DHA levels are more likely to suffer from postpartum depression. Consider New Chapter Supercritical DHA100, 1 daily. Aromatherapy eases "baby blues"- Earth Mama Angel Baby HAPPY MAMA Spray.

STRETCH MARKS: apply wheat germ, avocado, sesame oil, vitamin E, or A, D & E oil. A *comfrey-calendula* beeswax salve also works well. Take vitamin C 500mg 3 to 4 times daily for collagen development. Earth Mama Angel Baby STRETCH OIL. Use on bellies, bottoms and breasts. See STRETCH MARKS program pg. 543 in this book.

SWOLLEN ANKLES: use Nature's Apothecary BILBERRY extract in water.

TOXEMIA, Eclampsia: toxemia is caused by liver malfunction and disease. The liver cannot handle the increasing load of the progressing pregnancy. There is a marked reduction in blood flow to the placenta, kidneys and other organs. Severe cases result in liver and brain hemorrhage, convulsions and coma. Toxemia is indicated by extreme swelling, accompanied by high blood pressure, headaches, nausea and vomiting.

Vegan women have reduced risk. Avoid red meat and excess salt, especially. Green drinks, like apple-alfalfa sprout-cucumber or Green Foods GREEN MAGMA offer a "chlorophyll cleanout." Include dandelion greens as a mild diuretic to the diet 3-4 times weekly. Add vitamin C 500mg every 3 to 4 hours, 10,000IU beta-carotene, BILBERRY extract in water, and B Complex 50mg daily. Iodine therapy via daily *kelp* tablets produces good results.

UTERINE HEMORRHAGING: take *bayberry/cayenne* capsules, and get professional help immediately. Take *bilberry* extract daily with strengthening herbal flavonoids for tissue integrity. Use *dong quai* tea to help normalize uterine contractions or *shepherd's purse* extract for heavy bleeding. Use under the care of a clinical herbalist.

VARICOSE VEINS: take vitamin C 500mg with bioflavonoids, 3 daily; or *bilberry* extract 2x daily in water; or *butcher's broom* tea daily (also helpful for leg cramps during pregnancy). Natural Balance GREAT LEGS reduces leg heaviness and varicose veins (ask your health care provider first). Take Crystal Star VARI-VEIN™ caps for relief of spider veins after you give birth. For very dark spider veins postpartum, sclerotherapy (saline injections) can be useful.

Note: Baby diapers have been a huge cause for concern for mothers and families who are ecologically minded. Most diapers are still non-biodegradable, and most are impregnated with chemical polymer salts to absorb moisture. Use a diaper service, or your own washing machine, or use all-cotton Rmed TUSHIES if you're concerned.

NOTE: For more detailed fertility and pregnancy-related information along with natural baby care tips, please consult my book, *Do You Want To Have A Baby? Natural Fertility Solutions & Pregnancy Care,* co-authored with Sarah Abernathy.

Can't find a recommended product? Call the 800 number in Product Resources for the store nearest you.

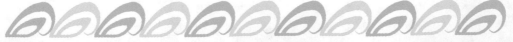

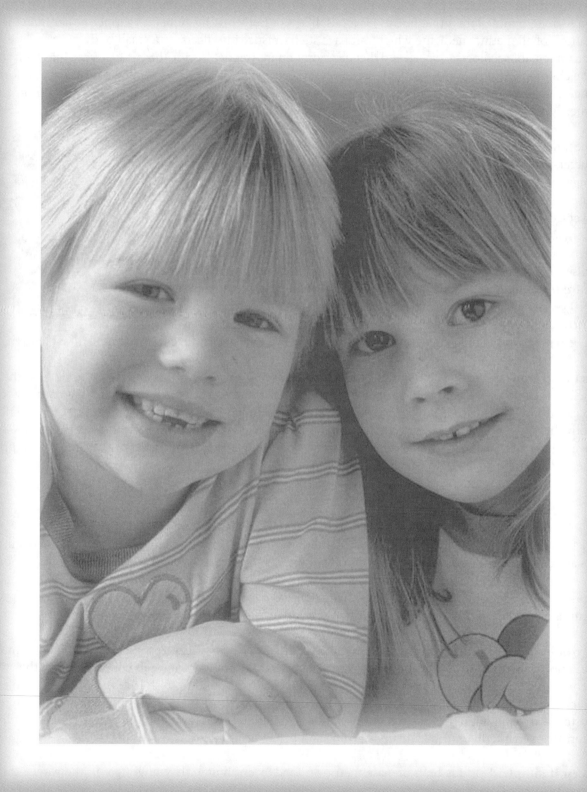

Alternative Healing Options For Children

Healthy children develop powerful immune systems in infancy. Unless unusually ill, a child often needs only the body-strengthening forces that nutritious foods, herbs or homeopathic remedies supply, rather than the strong medications of allopathic medicine which can have such drastic side effects on a small body.

The undeniable ecological, social and diet deterioration in America during the last fifty years has had a marked effect on children's health. We see evidence of it in every aspect of their lives — declining educational performance, learning disabilities, mental disorders, obesity, drug and alcohol abuse, hypoglycemia, allergies, chronic illness, delinquency and violent behavior; they're all evidence of declining immunity and poor health.

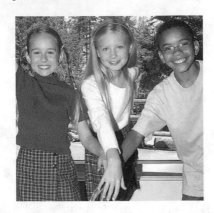

The infiltration of fast food into U.S. schools is insidious. Fast food hamburgers and pizzas are school lunch staples. Soda vending machines with high sugar or aspartame-loaded products are currently readily available on most campuses. (Good news: Increased pressure from the public and legislature means the beverage industry will voluntarily stop selling non-diet sodas to most public schools by 2009.) Still, kids are drinking more soda than ever.... a clear risk factor for osteoporosis and diabetes later in life. In fact, Type 2 diabetes and coronary heart disease, both related to diet and lack of exercise, are on the rise in children. *One-third to one-half* of all new Type 2 diabetes cases are in children between 9 and 19 years old! One-third of all kids have high cholesterol! Autopsies reveal that atherosclerosis begins in childhood. Getting children's obesity under control with a better diet and regular exercise is the best way to solve the degenerative disease problem in children.

Get help from the kids themselves in a health boosting program. Kids don't want to be sick, they aren't stupid, and they don't like going to the doctor any more than you do. They often recognize that natural foods and therapies are good for them. Children have strong natural immunity. A nutritious diet and natural health enhancers like herbs help keep them that way. Evidence shows that giving your child the right nutrients can raise IQ and improve school performance. Kids especially benefit from a high quality multiple vitamin-mineral supplement and the essential fatty acid, DHA (*docosahexaenoic acid*).

Diet Help for Childhood Diseases

Diet is your most important weapon in safeguarding your child's immune defenses. Pathogenic organisms and viruses are everywhere, but they aren't the major factor in causing disease if a child's body is healthy. Well-nourished children handle most infections successfully. They either don't catch the bugs going around, they contract only a mild case, or they develop healthy reactions that get the problem over with quickly. This difference in resistance and immune response is the key to understanding children's diseases.

A wholesome diet can easily restore a child's natural vitality. Healthy foods may take a little more time and attention than ordering a pizza or picking up a "happy meal," but the change in your child's health is worth it. Even children who have eaten a junk food diet for years quickly respond to fresh fruits, vegetables, whole grains, less dairy and sugar. I've seen substantial improvement in as little as one month! A child's hair and skin takes on new luster — they fill out if they are too skinny, lose weight if they are overweight. They sleep more soundly. Their attention spans markedly improve; many learning and behavior problems lessen or disappear.

Keep it simple. Let kids help prepare their own food, even though they might get in the way and it seems more trouble than it's worth. You'll be giving them a better understanding of good food. They're also more likely to eat the things they have a hand in making. Kids learn to appreciate the goodness of whole foods by growing their own food. If possible, plant a vegetable garden that your kids can help out with.

Can't find a recommended product? Call the 800 number in Product Resources for the store nearest you.

Keep only good nutritious foods in the house. Children may be exposed to junk foods and poor foods at school or friend's houses, but you can build a good, natural foundation diet at home. At home, they should be able to choose only from nutritious choices.

Kids have extraordinarily sensitive taste buds. Everything they eat is very vivid to them. The diet program here has lots of variety, so they can experiment and find out where their own preferences lie. There are plenty of snacks, sandwiches, fresh fruits and sweet veggies like carrots — foods children naturally like.

A Short Liquid Detox Cleanse for Childhood Diseases: **24 to 72 hours**

A healing diet for most common childhood diseases, including measles, mumps, chicken pox, strep throat and whooping cough, is fairly simple and basic. It's a therapy that starts with a short liquid elimination fast, followed by a light fresh foods diet in the acute stages.

1: Start cleansing liquids as soon as the disease is diagnosed to clean out harmful bacteria and infection. Give diluted fruit juices like apple, pineapple, grape, cranberry and citrus juices. Take juice of two lemons in a glass of water with maple syrup twice a day to flush the kidneys and normalize body chemistry.

2: Alternate fresh fruit juices throughout the day with fresh carrot juice, bottled water, and clear soups. Give a potassium juice (page 291) or veggie drink once a day. Encourage the child to drink as many healthy cleansing liquids as she or he wants. Light smoothies are favorites with kids. Avoid dairy foods.

3: Offer herb teas throughout the cleanse like a *catnip/lemon balm/echinacea/acerola cherry* blend to rally the body's defense mechanism. Children respond to herb teas quickly, and they like them more than you might think. Make the teas half strength. Add a little maple syrup if the herbs are bitter.

The following teas are effective for many childhood diseases:
- *Elder flowers, boneset (bitter), yarrow* with *peppermint* to induce a cleansing sweat
- *Catnip/chamomile/rosemary* tea to reduce a rash
- *Mullein/lobelia, chamomile, or scullcap* to relax
- *Catnip, fennel, ginger, chamomile* and *peppermint* for upset stomachs
- Herbs for Kids ELDERTUSSIN elderberry syrup for sore throats and for interrupted sleep caused by coughing
- Crystal Star D-CONGEST™ spray to help clear chest congestion
- A *catnip/lemon balm/cinnamon* combo tea for warming against chills
- Herbs for Kids VI PROTECTION BLEND for frequent colds and flu
- *Echinacea* drops in water every 4 hours to clear lymph glands and release infection

4: Acidophilus compounds are exceptional for children. Acidophilus makes a big difference in both recovery time and immune response, especially for getting over the hump of a childhood disease. Acidophilus keeps friendly bacteria in the G.I. tract, especially if the child has taken a course of antibiotics. Bifido-bacteria provides better protection for infants and children than regular acidophilus strains. Nutrition Now CHILDREN'S PB 8 (ages 1-3), DINO ACIDOPHILUS (ages 4 and up), Crystal Star DR. PROBIOTICS™, Jarrow BABY'S JARRO-DOPHILUS, or UAS Labs DDS-JUNIOR work well for children. Use ¼ tsp. at a time in water or juice three to four times daily.

Bodywork therapy for children:
…Give a gentle enema at least once during the detox cleanse to clear the child's colon of impacted wastes that hinder the body's effort to rid itself of diseased bacteria. A *catnip* tea enema is effective and safe.

Can't find a recommended product? Call the 800 number in Product Resources for the store nearest you.

…Oatmeal baths help neutralize rashes coming out on the skin. Herbal baths help induce cleansing perspiration, too, but the child should be watched closely all during the bath to make sure he or she is not getting too hot. Make up a big pot of *calendula* or *comfrey* tea for the bath water. Rub the child's body with *calendula* or *tea tree* oil, or Tiger Balm to loosen congestion after the bath.

…Apply hot *ginger* compresses to affected or sore areas to stimulate circulation and defense response, to rid the body more quickly of infection. Alternate hot compresses with cold, plain water compresses.

…Clear your child's chest congestion with herbal steam inhalations. Use *eucalyptus* or *tea tree* oil in a vaporizer help to keep lungs mucous free and improve oxygen uptake. Planetary ELDERBERRY SYRUP tea for stubborn bronchial infections.

…Dab on with cotton balls, a healing water infusion of *goldenseal, myrrh, yellow dock, black walnut*, and *yarrow*, or Crystal Star ANTI-BIO™ phyto-therapy gel or AloeLife ALOE SKIN GEL to sores and scabs.

Fresh Foods Purification Diet for Children's Diseases: **A 3 day diet.**

Use this diet for initial, acute and chronic symptoms when a liquid detox is not desired, or after a liquid cleanse when the acute stage has passed. A fresh foods diet continues the cleansing activity while the addition of solid foods starts to rebuild strength. Dairy products, except for yogurt should be avoided. This diet should last about three days depending on the strength and condition of the child.

On rising: give citrus juice with a teaspoon of acidophilus liquid, or ¼ tsp. acidophilus powder;
or a glass of lemon juice and water with maple syrup.
Breakfast: offer a choice of favorite fresh fruits. Top with vanilla yogurt, Rice Dream or soy milk.
Mid-morning: Give a vegetable drink, a potassium broth, (page 291) or fresh carrot juice.
Add ¼ tsp. ascorbate vitamin C or Ester C crystals with bioflavonoids.
Lunch: give fresh raw crunchy veggies with a yogurt dip; or a fresh veggie salad with yogurt dressing.
Mid-afternoon: offer a refreshing herb tea, like *licorice root or peppermint* tea,
or Flora KINDERLOVE CHILDREN'S MULTIVITAMIN SYRUP- a warming, good tasting tonic.
or Herbs for Kids MINTY GINGER drops to keep the stomach settled and calm tension;
or another vegetable drink with ¼ tsp. vitamin C added.
Dinner: give a fresh salad with mixed organic, high vitamin A baby greens (a kid favorite), avocados,
carrots, kiwi, romaine; and/or a cup of miso soup or nutritional yeast broth or other clear broth soup.
Before bed: a relaxing herb tea, like *chamomile or scullcap* tea, or Flora Salusan HERBAL REST Syrup.
or a cup of miso broth for strength and B vitamins. Snip 1 tsp. dry sea greens on top if desired.

Note: The cleansing drinks and broths below are full of enzymes critical to a child's health. Use them as a guide for highly nutritive vegetable juices. Your own variations can make them part of a nourishing diet as well. If you have a vegetable juicer, make the juices fresh. See my new book DIETS FOR HEALTHY HEALING for much more.

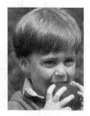

BABY VEGGIE GREEN DRINK FOR KIDS
Kids like baby veggies. Make this in a juicer. Choose fresh veggies that your child likes most.

—Choose green leafy vegetables like baby spinach, sunflower greens and lettuces.
—Add baby bok choy, baby carrots and sprouts.
—Don't forget sweet tasting veggies like cucumbers, celery and tomatoes.

Can't find a recommended product? Call the 800 number in Product Resources for the store nearest you.

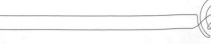

ENERGY SOUP FOR KIDS A liquid salad for kids. Make in the blender.

—Blender blend: ½ cup water, ¼ cup celery, ¼ cup fresh peas, 1 cup salad greens, like baby bok choy, dandelion, lettuces and spinach.
—Add ½ to 1 cup spouts like sunflower greens, alfalfa or mung bean sprouts.
—Add half an avocado for creaminess; add tamari sauce or Bragg's Liquid Aminos for taste.

HEALING FRUIT SMOOTHIE Use fresh fruit for this drink, not canned or frozen.

—Blend 1 banana and 1 peeled orange with some unpasteurized apple juice. Add half a papaya or mango if available, or one-quarter fresh pineapple. Add ¼ tsp. acidophilus powder.

Supplements for a child's fresh foods diet. Give them until the child is symptom free.
• A vitamin/mineral drink, such as 1 tsp. Flora KINDERLOVE CHILDREN'S MULTIVITAMIN syrup in juice, New Chapter EVERYONE'S MULTIPLE or Nutrition Now RHINO CHEWY VITES.

• A good acidophilus. Add vitamin A & D in drops, and ascorbate vitamin C or Ester C crystals in juice.

• Continue the herbal tea choices you found effective during the liquid cleanse, especially *catnip/lemon balm/cinnamon* blends.

• Use a mild herbal laxative, like Nature's Secret ULTIMATE FIBER, in half dosage for regularity. Try Herbs for Kids CATNIP EXTRACT for bouts of colic or stress-related diarrhea.

• Use garlic oil drops or open garlic capsules into juice for natural antibiotic activity; or give Crystal Star ANTI-BIO™ in half dosage; Herbs for Kids SUPER KIDS THROAT SPRAY or Wakunaga KYOLIC liquid

Bodywork is a good choice for children throughout any illness.
• Continue with herbal baths, washes and compresses to cleanse toxins coming out through the skin. Give a soothing massage before bed. Get some early morning sunlight on the body every day possible.

An Optimal Whole Foods Diet for Children:

When the healing crisis passes, and the child is on the mend, begin an optimal nutrition diet, to prevent further problems, and boost energy.

Despite our affluence, many of the basic nutritional needs are not met for U.S. children. Pediatrics Journal 1997 says only a tiny 1% of American kids meet the USDA requirements for all five food groups. Only 36% eat the recommended 2 to 4 servings of vegetables a day; only 30% get 3 to 5 vegetable servings a day. Instead, fats and sugars supply an astounding 40% of American children's daily energy needs! Because much of our agricultural soils are depleted, and most of our foods are sprayed or gassed, micronutrients like vitamins and minerals are no longer sufficiently present in our foods. Today's common childhood nutrient deficiencies, calcium, iron, B-1, and vitamins A, B-complex and C, have a huge impact — slowing down growth, wiping out immune defenses and impairing capacity for learning!

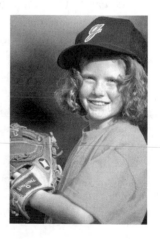

Can't find a recommended product? Call the 800 number in Product Resources for the store nearest you.

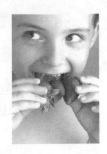

The most health protective diet for children is high in whole grains and green veggies for minerals, vegetable proteins for growth, and complex carbohydrates for energy. Buy organic foods whenever possible. An Environmental Health Perspectives study shows children regularly exposed to pesticides experience serious problems — including low stamina, underdeveloped hand-eye coordination, and significantly poorer short-term memory. Make sure you tell, and graphically *show* your child what junk and synthetic foods are. I find over and over again that because of TV advertising and peer pressure, kids often really don't know what wholesome food is, and think they are eating the right way.

Use superfoods for kids! Superfoods are concentrated nutrients widely popular with adults today (check out the many superfoods listings in this book). They're just as good in healthy diet programs for kids. Mix them in other foods to increase the nutritional content of any meal. Superfood supplements can get some great nutrients into fussy eaters. Crystal Star RESTORE YOUR STRENGTH™ drink is a potent vegetarian blend of sea greens, herbs, and foods like miso, rice protein, and nutritional yeast. Add it to soups, sauces, even salad dressings. Green Foods BERRY BARLEY ESSENCE has natural raspberry and strawberry flavor. Kids like bee pollen, a highly bio-active superfood chock full of nutrients. Sprinkle small amounts on cereals or add it to smoothies.

Diet tips to help keep your child healthier and happier:

I know it's a lot easier said than done to change old dietary patterns to healthier eating… for anybody, but especially for kids. Start by offering something delicious to replace whatever is being taken away.

For example:

…If you want to include more wholesome foods, like fruits and vegetables, start with food forms that children naturally go for—snacks can be dried fruit snacks, and smoothie drinks. Sandwiches, tacos, burritos and pitas can hold vegetables. Most kids like soup… another good place to add vegetables. Let them add sauces or flavors they like.

…If you want to include more whole grains in your child's diet, start by keeping only whole grains in the house. Kids love bagels, for instance…. and pastas, which come in a wide variety of whole grain options. Brown basmati rice is much tastier than white rice if your kid is a "rice kid." Stuffing is a big favorite — make sure it's whole grain with the option they like (nuts and seeds, celery, shrimp and cooked beans are favorites). Popcorn is a healthy snack. Season it with a little soy sauce, or a healthy seasoning blend instead of gobs of butter and salt.

…If you want to add healthy cultured foods to your child's diet, start by keeping a good assortment of yogurt flavors with fruit for snacks in the refrigerator. Offer delicious kefir cheese (available at health food stores) for snack spreads and dips instead of sour cream.

…To reduce the amount of sugar your child is getting, buy delicious, sugar-free snacks. Replace sugar-filled cereals with granola or oatmeal with healthy toppings. Offer dried fruit. Almost every kid likes raisins.

…If you want to reduce the amount of meat and heavy dairy proteins your child is eating, keep good plant protein available. Kids like tofu and grain burgers, especially with their favorite trimmings. Most kids like beans — look for healthy chili blends. Keep peanut butter, and nuts and seeds, like almonds, sunflower seeds and pumpkin seeds around the house for snacks. Recommend them as toppings for everything from soup or salad crunchies to smoothies and desserts. (Seeds and nuts give kids unsaturated oils and essential fatty acids, too.) Eggs are a good protein choice for kids…. one of Nature's perfect foods that's gotten a bad rap. Most kids like deviled eggs, and eggs are great in honey custards, another kid favorite.

…If you want to add more seafood to a child's diet, start with favorites like shrimp, tuna fish or salmon.

…If you want to encourage your child to drink more water instead of carbonated sodas or sweetened drinks, keep plenty of natural fruit juices and flavored waters around the house.

Can't find a recommended product? Call the 800 number in Product Resources for the store nearest you.

Your presence as a loving parental authority is a powerful influence. Gather your family together for a meal at least once a day to establish good eating habits for your kids.

Try this kid-tested healthy diet for your child.

See my book DIETS FOR HEALTHY HEALING for a complete Children's Diet for Disease Control.

On rising: offer a protein drink such as NutriTech ALL-ONE, if the child's energy or school performance level is poor, or if the child seems to be constantly ill, (a child's body must have protein to heal), or 1 teaspoon liquid multi-vitamin in juice, such as Floradix KINDERLOVE MULTI-VITAMIN/MINERAL.

Breakfast: a whole grain cereal with apple juice or a yogurt and fresh fruit;
and/or whole grain toast or muffins, with a little butter, kefir cheese or nut butter;
add eggs, scrambled, baked or soft boiled (no fried eggs);
or have hot oatmeal or puffed kashi cereal with maple syrup or yogurt.

Mid-morning: whole grain crackers with kefir cheese or dip, and fruit juice;
or some fresh or dried fruit, or fruit leathers with yogurt or kefir cheese;
or fresh crunchy veggies with peanut butter or a nut spread;
or a healthy protein bar, or trail mix, stirred into yogurt.

Lunch: a veggie, turkey, chicken or shrimp salad sandwich on whole grain bread, with cheese.
Add trans-fat free corn chips with low fat dip;
or bean soup with whole grain toast, and a small salad, or crunchy veggies with garbanzo spread;
or a vegetarian pizza on a chapati or whole grain crust;
or whole grain spaghetti or pasta with a light sauce and parmesan cheese;
or a Mexican bean and veggie, or rice burrito with fresh salsa.

Mid-afternoon: sparkling juice and a dried fruit candy bar; or fresh fruit or fruit juice, or kefir drink;
or a hard boiled egg and some whole grain chips with a veggie or low fat cheese dip;
or some whole grain toast and peanut butter or other nut butter.

Dinner: pizza on a whole grain, chapati or egg crust, with veggies, shrimp, and low fat cheese topping;
or whole grain or egg pasta with vegetables and a light tomato/cheese sauce;
or a baked Mexican quesadilla with low fat cheese and some steamed veggies or a salad;
or roast turkey with cornbread dressing and salad; or a tuna casserole with rice and peas.

Before bed: a glass of apple juice or a little soy milk, Rice Dream or flavored kefir.

Should your child go veg?

The American Dietetic Association says that a well planned vegetarian diet provides enough nutrients for growing kids. Strict protein combining is not necessary (as was once believed) because a variety of plant protein sources (like beans, nut butters, soy milk and whole grains) provide the proper protein building blocks for children's needs. I'm a believer in the importance of EFA's for a child's developing brain. For strict vegetarians who do not eat seafood (one of the best EFA sources), try a supplement like Flora UDO'S PERFECT OIL BLEND, 1-3 tsp. daily for children 4 to 10, or flax seed oil, 1 tsp. daily, to maximize brain nutrition.

Extra supplements to optimize your child's nutritional health for the long term:

…Acidophilus, liquid or powder: give in juice 2 to 3x daily for good digestion and assimilation. Jarrow BABY JARRO-DOPHILUS, UAS Labs DDS-JUNIOR, American Health ACIDOPHILUS LIQUID, or Solaray BABY LIFE are excellent for children.

…Vitamin C, or Ester C in chewable or powder form with bioflavonoids; in juice, ¼ tsp. at a time 2x daily. For chewable wafers, use 100mg, 250mg, or 500mg potency according to age and weight of the child.

…A sugar-free multi-vitamin and mineral supplement in either liquid or chewable tablet form. Good choices are from Floradix, Natrol, Solaray and Trace Mineral Research.

Can't find a recommended product? Call the 800 number in Product Resources for the store nearest you.

Exercise for kids is a primary nutrient for body and mind. US Public Health studies show a third of American children are unfit. The number of children who are obese has doubled in the last 20 years! Being an overweight child greatly increases the likelihood of being an overweight adult. Exercise is a key to weight control, health, growth and energy. Don't let your kid be a couch potato (the average child watches over 30 hours of TV a week!), or a computer junkie. Encourage outdoor activity, and make sure your child takes P. E. classes in school. Many schools have cut P.E. classes and after school sports due to budget cuts. Statistics show only 29% of kids attend P.E. class every day. Make sure he gets regular exercise outside school, too. Hiking, basketball, swimming, skateboarding and roller-blading are all kid-friendly choices.

About Herbal Remedies for Children's Health

A child's body responds well to herbal medicines. Children are born with naturally well-developed immune systems—a key factor in understanding how to deal with childhood diseases (often, they don't need to be dosed with strong drugs or heroic techniques that are used for adults). Kids often only require the subtle, body strengthening forces that herbs or homeopathic medicines supply. Highly focused allopathic medications can have drastic side effects on a small body. I find that children will drink herbal teas, take herbal drops, syrups and homeopathic medicines much more readily than you might think. The remedies and methods listed in this section are building, strengthening and non-traumatic to a child's system.

Most herbal remedies may be taken as needed. Herbal effects can be quite specific; take the best formula for your particular need at the right time - rather than all the time - for optimum results. Rotating and alternating herbal combinations according to the changing health state of the child allows the body to remain most responsive to herbal effects. Reduce, then discontinue dosage as the problem improves, allowing the body to pick up its own work and bring its own vital forces into action.

Take only one or two herbal combinations at the same time when working with a child's system. Choose the herbal remedy that addresses the worst problem first. Alternate remedies to allow the body to thoroughly use the herbal properties. One of the bonuses of a natural healing program is the frequent discovery that other conditions were really complications of the first problem, and often take care of themselves as the body comes into balance.

Let herbs gently rebuild health. Even when a healing program is working, adding more of the remedy in order to speed healing can aggravate symptoms and bring about worse results!

Herbal remedy dosage goes by body weight. Child dosage is as follows:
½ dose for children 10 - 14 years
⅓ dose for children 6 - 10 years
¼ dose for children 2 - 6 years
⅛ dose for infants and babies

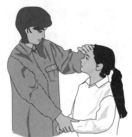

Special Remedies for Children's Problems
Note: Conditions not listed here have their own specific page in the AILMENTS section of this book.

ADD/ADHD: Eliminate refined, chemicalized foods with artificial colorings (the yellow food dye tartrazine has been linked to hyperactivity problems). Reduce sugar intake, esp. sodas (excess phosphorus). Eliminate red meats (nitrates). Add more protein foods (beans, seafood, hormone-free poultry, soy foods, nuts and seeds) to stabilize blood sugar reactions. Natural supplements target symptoms and nourish the brain: Crystal Star Herbs ADD-VANTAGE FOR KIDS™ caps; Metabolic Response Modifiers ATTENTION! softgels with DHA; Homeopathic *Camomilla* (very young children); *Ginkgo biloba* drops (older kids) 60mg daily helps inner ear balance. See ailments section pg.... for a complete ADD healing program. Or see my new book DIETS FOR HEALTHY HEALING for a complete diet to overcome Attention Deficit Disorder.

Can't find a recommended product? Call the 800 number in Product Resources for the store nearest you.

ALLERGIES: (see how to determine specific allergies in the ALLERGIES pages of this book, page 311-316. Consulting with a NAET (Nambudripad Allergy Elimination Technique) practitioner can be useful. For more information, check out www.naet.com.)

General allergy diet guidelines:
• Common allergen foods: dairy, wheat, eggs, chocolate, nuts, seafood and citrus fruits. Try eliminating one at a time for a few weeks and watch to see if there is improvement. Eliminate dairy foods and cooked fats and oils because they thicken mucous and stimulate an increase in mucous production.
• Give lots of water to thin secretions and ease expectoration. Use *fenugreek-thyme-nettles* tea, to help restore breathing and dry out sinuses. *Licorice root* tea helps support adrenals and kids like the taste. An herbal combination of *echinacea, goldenseal and garlic* 2 times daily for 5 to 7 days boosts immunity and clears the lymph system. Use flaxseed oil for essential fatty acids to help regulate the inflammatory response. Mix into foods like salad dressing or in place of butter.

General supplement guidelines: (be sure to give in childhood amounts.)
…Beta-carotene to help heal irritated mucous membranes. One dose per day during allergy season.
…Vitamin C with bioflavonoids acts as an anti-inflammatory. One dose, 3x daily for two weeks.
…Calcium-magnesium for overreactive nerves. Use a ratio of 250mg calcium to 125mg magnesium.
…Herbs for Kids NETTLES & EYEBRIGHT liquid for relief of seasonal and year-round allergies; Nature's Answer NAT-CHOO for runny nose and sneezing.

ASTHMA: Focus on an organic, whole foods diet. Food additives and sulfites are known asthma triggers. Flax oil helps regulate inflammatory response; Gaia OSHA SUPREME drops in water help open bronchials. *Lobelia* tea relaxes wheezing. Bee Pollen granules (1 tbsp.) and B-complex have needed pantothenic acid. Reduce symptoms: Herbs Etc. LUNG TONIC (alcohol free), or Herbs for Kids HOREHOUND BLEND, an expectorant which reduces bronchial inflammation. Use *milk thistle* extract in water daily as a liver cleanser. Vitamin B-12 deficiency is linked to some types of childhood asthma — check with a naturopathic physician and consider adding sea greens to the child's diet. *Astragalus* drops in water help strengthen lungs — use for 2 weeks a month for six months after an asthma attack. Add Vitamin C with bioflavonoids, ½ tsp. in juice 2x daily to lower histamine levels. (Children younger than four should use a vitamin C supplement specially formulated for toddlers.) Magnesium is a natural bronchodilator. Chelated magnesium 100 to 300 mg per day for kids 35 to 115 lbs. Important: Avoid tobacco smoke, wood and gas stoves. Stay away from roach infested areas. (See ASTHMA page 328 for detailed diet recommendations.)

BITES and STINGS: (mosquitoes, fleas, gnats, etc.) Seek immediate medical attention for bites from black widow spiders or other serious bites. Apply B & T STINGSTOP Insect Gel for pain and itch. (Also use as a repellent). Apply *tea tree* oil to the bite, and give vitamin C 100-500mg chewables every 4 hours to neutralize poison. Nature's Path CAL-LYTE helps relieve pain and calm nerves. Crystal Star ANTI-BIO™ gel is an anti-inflammatory or Herbal Answer's ALOE FORCE skin gel. Use vitamin B-1 thiamine, as a natural insect repellent. For prevention, use *neem* oil or Avon SKIN SO SOFT ORIGINAL or BUG GUARD.

BRONCHITIS and CHEST CONGESTION:: go on a mucous cleansing diet to reduce congestion. See the short "Liquid Elimination Cleanse" in this section and the chapter on "Detoxification" for effective juices and broths. After the liquid diet, offer only fresh foods for a day. Avoid dairy foods, sweets and fried foods which continue mucous formation.
…Vitamin C with bioflavs for anti-inflammatory properties; beta-carotene to aid mucous membranes.
…Herbal teas: *thyme, mullein or plantain* tea every 4 hours. *Chamomile-honey* tea for inflammation. Take *peppermint and raspberry* tea 2x daily.

Can't find a recommended product? Call the 800 number in Product Resources for the store nearest you.

…Planetary YIN-CHIAO Bronchitis tabs encourage respiratory tract drainage and stimulates immune response. Herbs for Kids HOREHOUND BLEND is an expectorant; Gaia's Children COUGH SYRUP-WET COUGHS for wet coughs; B & T COUGH & BRONCHIAL SYRUP.

…Zinc to boost immune response; Crystal Star ZINC SOURCE™ throat rescue drops are especially effective.)

…Herbal steam inhalations with *eucalyptus oil, tea tree oil, thyme* or Crystal Star D-CONGEST™ spray help keep lungs mucous free and improve oxygen uptake.

…Hydrotherapy baths with *calendula* flowers or strong *comfrey* tea infusions induce cleansing perspiration. Apply a soothing chest rub with TIGER BALM, WHITE FLOWER or *calendula* oil to loosen congestion.

BRUISES: apply a cold compress (ice inside a towel) immediately. Leave on for 10 minutes — then off for 15 minutes. Repeat cycle 4 times to reduce swelling. Use vitamin C with bioflavonoids to restore integrity of blood vessel walls. Homeopathic *Arnica* 30x eases pain and prevents bruise from becoming larger. BHI TRAUMEEL gel (excellent results!). B & T ALPHA B & B makes black and blue marks go away faster.

BURNS (minor): seek medical assistance for a serious burn. Apply *tea tree* oil or Crystal Star ANTI-BIO GEL™ or Nature's Path BURN-AID or Gaia's Children BURN OIL to promote healing. Give vitamin C and bioflavonoids, beta-carotene, zinc, and B-complex 25 to 50mg to support healing.

COLDS: Crystal Star ANTI-BIO™ drops in water relieve symptoms, often right away. Jarrow GENTLE FIBERS drink helps nasal congestion during the day, and 2 tbsp. *each* lemon juice and maple syrup with 1 tsp. fresh grated ginger at night. Crystal Star ZINC SOURCE™ throat rescue drops boost immunity, soothe a sore throat (take at the first signs). Zand ZINC LOZENGES arrest a nagging cough. Herbs for Kids ECHINACEA-GOLDENROOT is an herbal antibiotic. If using antibiotic drugs, add acidophilus daily. See COLDS page 374-376.

COLIC: if you are nursing, watch your diet carefully. Sometimes mother's milk is acidic from stress or diet. Avoid cow's milk, cabbage, brussels sprouts, onions, garlic, yeast breads, fried and fast foods. If nursing, a weak *fennel seed* tea or Earth Mama Angel Baby MILK MAID tea with added herbs to soothe baby's digestion. Avoid red meat, chocolate, alcohol, sugary foods and caffeine until the child's digestion improves. Use goat's milk instead of cow's milk if the child is drinking milk. Promote healthy gastrointestinal flora: Solaray BABYLIFE for infants, Homeopathic *Colocynthus, Chamomilla* or Hyland's COLIC tabs, or Natren LIFE START ¼ tsp. in water or juice 2-3x daily. Give a dilute B Complex liquid in water once a week. Give papaya or apple juice, or small doses of papaya enzymes for older babies. Give the baby a morning sunbath for vitamin D (also improves digestion). Give a *gentle catnip* enema once a week for gas release. Never give honey to babies less than 1 year old (They love a little maple syrup on your fingertip). Effective weak teas include *chamomile, peppermint and lemon balm* (just use lukewarm dropperfuls) or try Wellements GRIPE WATER with ginger and fennel (highly recommended). Note: Massage is used with excellent results for colic. Check out http://www.em-bry-on-ics.com/wsmassage.html on the web. If symptoms don't resolve after a few months or are accompanied by frequent vomiting, it may be a sign of infant GERD (gastroesophageal reflux disease). Consult with a pediatric gastroenterologist for a professional assessment.

CONSTIPATION: increase the amount of fiber and fluid in the child's diet, with more fresh vegetable salads, fresh fruits, spring water, herbal teas, juices and soups. Soak raisins in senna tea and feed to young children for almost instant relief; use Crystal Star FIBER & HERBS COLON CLEANSE™ for older children. Give weak *licorice* or *mullein* tea and molasses in water, 2 times daily. Herbal Answer's HERBAL ALOE FORCE JUICE to encourage natural detoxification. A gentle *catnip* enema effectively clears the colon of impacted waste. Lactose intolerance is a major cause of childhood constipation. Consider a dairy elimination diet to see if symptoms clear up on their own. See CONSTIPATION, page 381-382.

Can't find a recommended product? Call the 800 number in Product Resources for the store nearest you.

CRADLE CAP: if you're nursing, avoid refined sugar which supports bacteria and yeast. Use Nature's Path FLORA-LYTE, or BABYLIFE by Solaray for infants to foster healthy flora. Massage scalp with vitamin E, olive oil or jojoba oil or Earth Mama Angel Baby BOTTOM BALM for 5 minutes. Leave on 30 minutes, then brush scalp with soft baby brush and shampoo with *tea tree* or *aloe vera* shampoo. Repeat twice weekly. Apply *comfrey root* tea to infant's scalp or dry skin area, and let air dry. Symptoms usually disappear within 10 days. Cradle cap may be a biotin deficiency. Take biotin 1000mcg while nursing; the baby will receive the necessary amount through breast milk.

CUTS: apply *tea tree* oil or Crystal Star ANTI-BIO GEL™ as an antiseptic. Use a *calendula* ointment, or AloeLife ALOE SKIN GEL or B & T CALIFLORA *calendula* gel every 2 or 3 hours. Give 1 Crystal Star DR. ENZYME™ with Protease and Bromelain for inflammation. Apply B & T ARNIFLORA GEL for swelling. Herbs for Kids STINGZZZ™ gel to cool and soothe.

DIAPER and SKIN RASH: give plenty of water to dilute urine acids. Mix *comfrey, goldenseal* and *arrowroot* powders with *aloe vera* gel and apply. Or use *calendula* ointment, liquid lecithin, or a vitamin A, D & E oil. Expose the child's bottom to morning sunlight for 20 minutes for vitamin D. Wash diapers in water with 1 tsp. *tea tree* oil. Motherlove DIAPER RASH RELIEF; Earth Mama Angel BABY BOTTOM BALM; or Jason DIAPER RELIEF ointment. Homeopathic remedies help: *Sulfur, Rhux tox.* Avoid petroleum jelly. Use talc-free powders instead.

DIARRHEA: to prevent dehydration give frequent small sips of water, broths and herbal teas. To give intestines a chance to heal avoid dairy products during diarrhea and for two weeks after a diarrhea bout. Offer easily digested foods — pureed brown rice (B vitamins), bananas, dry cereal, crackers, toast, lightly cooked vegetables, grains and yogurt (friendly intestinal flora). *Lactobacillus* shows good results in clinical research. Use Solaray BABYLIFE or UAS Labs DDS-JUNIOR to help restore healthy flora. Homeopathic remedies like *Arsenicum album and Podophyllum* relieve stress. Offer *slippery elm* tea or *peppermint tea* in juice twice daily. *Red raspberry, chamomile, thyme* teas are also helpful.

EAR INFECTIONS: 80% of kids who take antibiotics for ear infections don't get better any sooner! A new study links kids who constantly suck pacifiers to 30% more ear infections than those who don't. Children exposed to cigarette smoke are more likely to suffer ear infections. Offer water, soups, herbal teas and diluted fruit juices. Avoid dairy foods which make it difficult for ears to drain. Use *mullein* essence, or Motherlove MULLEIN FLOWER ear oil, Crystal Star EAR DEFENSE, Gaia Children EAR DROPS, or *garlic* oil (antibacterial), or warm olive oil ear drops directly in the ear. Or mix vegetable glycerine and *witch hazel*, dip in cotton balls and insert in the ear to draw out infection. Give *lobelia* extract drops in water or juice for pain. Use an *echinacea-goldenseal* combination or Herbs for Kids ECHINACEA-GOLDENROOT to clear infection. Xlear NASAL WASH with xylitol helps flush out bacteria. For babies and toddlers use a small amount of Xlear NASAL WASH as directed during diaper changes. Studies reveals homeopathy reduces pain from ear infections. Consult a qualified homeopath to find out which remedy is right for your child. See EAR INFECTIONS, page 400.

FEVER: a child's moderate fever is usually a cleansing, healing process — a result of the problem, a part of the cure. (See a doctor if fever is high.) Diet should be liquids only - diluted fruit or vegetable juices, herb teas, like peppermint and raspberry, water and broth for at least 24 hours until fever breaks. *Catnip* tea and *catnip* enemas can help moderate a fever. Offer 1-2 cups of the following tea daily as a diaphoretic to help lower fever: grated *ginger rt., peppermint lf., boneset* and a pinch of *cayenne.* Or, try Herbs for Kids TEMP-ASSURE to regulate temperature. Homeopathic remedies for fever, *Aconitum napellus, Camomilla and Bryonia alba* are effective for kids. Use *echinacea-goldenseal* drops, or Gaia's Children COMPOSITION ESSENCE for immune-boosting. Use a cooling spritz with a few drops of peppermint for relief. See FEVER page 414.

Can't find a recommended product? Call the 800 number in Product Resources for the store nearest you.

FLU: during the acute initial stage give only liquid nutrients — fresh vegetable juices and green drinks, hot broths and chicken soup to stimulate mucous release. Refer to the Short Liquid Elimination Fast in this chapter for more detailed information. During the recuperation stage: follow a vegetarian, light diet, such as the Raw Foods Purification Diet For Children's Diseases in this chapter. Anti-viral herbal remedies include: *garlic, echinacea, yarrow, St John's wort, osha root, bee propolis and una de gato. Garlic* is a potent antiviral against influenza. Try KYOLIC LIQUID, ½ tsp. daily. Use Crystal Star VIREX™ in a child's dose to fight the flu virus, ZINC SOURCE™ throat drops for immune boosting zinc, and ANTI-FLAM™ caps along with vitamin C with bioflavonoids to help overcome inflammation. Silver has proven toxic to many viruses as well as bacteria, fungi and parasites. Use Nature's Path SILVER-LYTE liquid in juice. Boiron OSCILLO-COCCINUM may be used for children over two. Dissolve entire contents of one tube in the mouth every 6 hours, up to 3 times a day. See FLU page 417 in this book for more help.

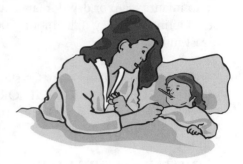

GAS and FLATULENCE: unhealthy food choices, allergies, poor food combinations, eating too fast and not chewing food well are the main reasons for gas in kids. See the Optimal Children's Diet (in this section). Especially eliminate fried foods, excessive sugar and red meat. A plant based digestive enzyme, like Transformation DIGESTZYME or Dr. Green's POWER-PLUS Food Enzymes by Herbal Products Development are helpful. Soak *anise, dill, caraway seed or chamomile* in water or juice and strain off. Give 1 to 2 tbsp. of liquid every 4 hours until digestion rebalances. Use *Catnip* extract, in child dosage, for spasmodic gas pain.

HEADACHES: add stress-busting lavender oil (about 10 drops) to a hot bath in the evening. Calcium and magnesium help calm muscles and relax blood vessels; Nature's Path CAL-LYTE, or Crystal Star ANTI-FLAM™ caps for pain, two at a time for children. *Feverfew drops or valerian-wild lettuce* drops in water help. Herbs for Kids FEVERFEW BLEND, pain-relieving, anti-inflammatory and calming for kids' headaches.

INDIGESTION: give *chamomile or catnip* tea, or a little ground *ginger* and *cinnamon* in water. Use soy milk or rice milk instead of cow's milk. No fruit juice til discomfort passes. One tsp. acidophilus liquid before meals. Herbs for Kids MINTY GINGER and Gaia's Children TUMMY TONIC are high quality herbal blends for kid's tummy aches and indigestion.

JAUNDICE: mainly an infant condition — give a tiny amount of low-dose vitamin E oil on the tip of your finger, or a diluted lemon water with maple syrup. Breastfeed often and expose the child to sunlight regularly. Note: Avoid prescription drugs when breastfeeding. The antibiotic *Azithromycin* has been linked to serious cholestatic jaundice in nursing babies. Ask your physician about the prescriptions you're taking.

MUMPS: the salivary and parotid glands swell and cause pain when chewing or swallowing. Photoluminescence treatments (blood irradiation) are successful for some mumps' cases. To learn more, check out www.natural-healing-centers.com. During acute stage give only liquid nutrients — fresh fruit and vegetable juices, except citrus, green drinks, chicken or vegetable soups. To alleviate pain: heat 1 qt. apple juice with 8-10 cloves. Strain and cool. Anti-viral herbs that work for children include: *garlic, echinacea, yarrow, St John's wort and osha root.* Use Crystal Star VIREX™ caps (half dose) or Herbs for Kids VI PROTECTION BLEND to fight the virus; Crystal Star ANTI-BIO™ extract in water with a little maple syrup, or *burdock* tea every few hours to clear lymph glands, and help overcome infection. Make sure the child gets plenty of rest and sleep.

Supplements for childhood mumps: (give in childhood amounts.)
   …Extra vitamin C with bioflavonoids as an anti-inflammatory. One dose, 3x daily for two weeks.
   …Colloidal or ionized silver helps fight the mumps virus. Use Nature's Path ionized SILVER-LYTE.

Can't find a recommended product? Call the 800 number in Product Resources for the store nearest you.

PARASITES and WORMS: eliminate sugary foods and refined carbohydrates. (See Children's Optimal Whole Foods Diet in this chapter.) High fiber foods like grains, vegetables, especially greens and carrots help both treatment and prevention. Give probiotics like Crystal Star DR. PROBIOTICS™ with FOS, or Solaray BABYLIFE. For very young children, give raisins soaked in senna tea to cleanse the intestines or use Crystal Star PARASITE PURGE™ capsules in child dosage. New Chapter GINGER WONDER syrup, 1-3 tsp. daily. (Research shows 42 components in *ginger* oil kill parasites.) Garlic is a natural antiparasitic; use a garlic enema 2x a week; To prevent reinfection, include garlic as a regular part of the diet or use KYOLIC-LIQUID (½ tsp. daily). Give chlorophyll liquid in water, or epazote herb steeped in juice or yogurt, Nature's Path SILVER-LYTE or herbal pumpkin seed oil tablets by Hain. See PARASITES, page 519.

HEAD LICE: *garlic* and *tea tree* oil fight head lice infestation. Use 25 drops in 1 pint of water. Rub the mixture onto the child's head 3 times daily; rinse hair after third application with strong *goldenseal* tea. Or make a mix of 2 tbsp. olive oil 10 drops <u>each</u> *rosemary and lavender* oil. Massage into damp hair and leave on 1 hour. To shampoo, mix 3 drops <u>only</u> thyme essential oil in a neem shampoo. Let soak 5 minutes, then rinse with water and a white vinegar rinse. Comb hair with a fine-toothed comb to remove lice and eggs. Well in Hand's non-toxic NIT KIT (with oils of *rosemary, thyme, tea tree, peppermint and anise* and Medi-Comb) is an effective alternative to conventional insecticides. Quantum HAIR CLEAN 1-2-3 shows good results in clinical tests with school children.

RINGWORM: apply *tea tree* oil, *black walnut* or *calendula* tinctures, Crystal Star FUNGI FIGHTER™ gel or Nutribiotic SKIN OINTMENT (excellent results usually in 3 to 4 days) on affected area until rash goes away. Use the homeopathic remedy Sulphur 30x or 9c, three times daily, for 3 days. (Use at least one hour before or after using *tea tree* oil because the oil may affect the homeopathic remedy). Boost immune strength with an *echinacea-goldenseal-burdock root* combination 3x a day for ten days. See FUNGAL INFECTIONS pg.420.

SINUS INFECTION: refer to the Short Liquid Elimination Fast in this chapter. See recipes for juices, broths, tonics, etc.in my book, *Detoxification: Recharge, Renew and Rejuvenate Your Body, Mind and Spirit!* A short three day cleansing liquid diet helps clear mucous congestion. Xlear NASAL WASH with xylitol is a specific to help flush out bacteria, Crystal Star ANTI-BIO™ drops or goldenseal liquid drops in the nose to overcome infection and inflammation. Herbs for Kids VI PROTECTION BLEND as a gentle anti-viral. Use Crystal Star D-CONGEST™ drops in warm water to release mucous buildup in the head and chest.

SORE THROAT: give Crystal Star ZINC SOURCE™ throat rescue drops 2 to 3x daily, especially at night for almost immediate relief. Zand ZINC LOZENGES or other zinc lozenges for coughing. Gaia's Children THROAT FORMULA FOR CHILDREN or Herbs for Kids SUPER KIDS THROAT SPRAY to soothe and heal. Give an *echinacea - goldenseal* compound, or Crystal Star ANTI-BIO™ drops to fight infective organisms. Give pineapple juice 2x daily for enzyme therapy. *Licorice sticks* to chew, and *licorice* tea are effective. Give vitamin C lozenges with bioflavonoids to help ease throat inflammation and to fight infection.

SLEEPLESSNESS: avoid stimulants like sugary foods, chocolate or foods containing caffeine. Use Nature's Path CAL-LYTE™ or the calming Homeopathic Hylands CALMS FORTE. Crystal Star RELAX™ caps, 1 before bed, Gaia's Children PASSIONFLOWER-LEMON BALM, Herbs for Kids VALERIAN SUPER CALM, *wild lettuce-valerian* extract drops in water with a little honey, *passionflower, skullcap* and *chamomile teas* are effective.

TEETHING: A cold baby teether can really help. Rub gums with very diluted *peppermint* oil. Give weak *catnip, fennel* or *peppermint* tea to soothe. Add a few daily drops of A, D & E oil to food. Licorice root powder (2 pinches) made into a paste soothes inflamed gums. Use B & T ALPHA TLC, Effective products: Use Noveya BABY TEETHING GEL or Herbs For Kids GUM-OMILE Oil for teething.. (See TEETHING, page 556 for more.)

Can't find a recommended product? Call the 800 number in Product Resources for the store nearest you.

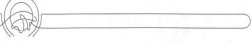

THRUSH FUNGAL INFECTION: Give probiotics like Jarrow BABY'S JARRO-DOPHILUS (also use as a mouthwash). Add vitamin C 100mg or Ester C chewable. Thrush is often caused by antibiotic over use. Give *garlic* extract in water, like Wakunaga KYOLIC, or squirt a pricked *garlic oil* cap in the mouth. Give Nature's Path ionized SILVER-LYTE, or Allergy Research PROLIVE (*Olive leaf* extract) to older kids with thrush.

WEAK SYSTEM: see Optimal Whole Foods Diet For Children in this chapter. Give apple or carrot juice daily. Give Crystal Star RESTORE YOUR STRENGTH™ broth daily. Herbs for Kids ASTRAGALUS extract is a deep immune builder. Add Nature's Path TRACE-LYTE minerals. Add 1 tsp. nutritional yeast for B-complex vitamins and protein. Hyland's BIOPLASMA is a good general homeopathic remedy. Include a daily chewable interferon boosting vitamin C wafer as a preventive.

WHOOPING COUGH: (cases rising almost 85% over the last several years.) A liquid diet during acute stage with juices, broths and water. Add steamed vegetables, brown rice, pineapple and grapes after crisis has passed. Crystal Star STRESS OUT™ muscle relaxer drops in water, or *valerian-wild lettuce* extract, Crystal Star ZINC SOURCE™ throat drops and ANTI-BIO™ capsules as an immune stimulant. Use B & T COUGH & BRONCHIAL syrup to reduce sleeplessness caused by coughing. Give vitamin C with bioflavonoids, ¼ tsp. every hour until stool turns soupy. To soothe respiratory tract, *marshmallow root, slippery elm bark or osha root tea, or lobelia* extract. Apply hot *ginger-garlic* compresses to chest; use a *eucalyptus* steam in a vaporizer at night.

A brief medicine chest for kids:

1: **TEA TREE OIL:** for infections that need antiseptic or antifungal activity, including mouth, teeth, gums, throat, ringworm, fungus, etc. Effective on stings, bites, burns, sunburns, cuts, and scrapes.

2: **RESCUE REMEDY** by Nelson Bach: For respiratory problems, coughing, gas, stomach ache and constipation. A rebalancing calmative for emotional stress and anxiety.

3: **KIDS KIT** from Hylands Homeopathic: A first aid kit with gentle, all-purpose remedies.

4: To help prevent contagious disease after exposure, give 1 *cayenne* capsule 3x a day, 1 chewable vitamin C 500mg wafers 3x a day, and a cup of roasted *dandelion root* tea daily for 3 or 4 days.

5: Gaia Herbs and Herbs for Kids both offer high quality herbal products for children that you can count on for safety and efficacy.

Should you vaccinate your child? *It depends on the vaccination.*

Some, like the flu vaccination, have serious side effects for sensitive people; some can wear off and allow a more serious disease to develop as an adult, like the chicken pox vaccination (a childhood case of chicken pox is a "vaccination" in itself, conferring lifetime immunity). Medical literature from the last 70 years shows a high incidence of vaccination-related injuries and deaths. In just a 39 month period (July 1990-Nov. 1993), over 54,000 adverse reactions as a result of vaccinations were reported to the FDA, including 471 deaths. (The homeopathic remedy *Silicea* is a specific for adverse reactions to vaccinations.) Vaccinated children suffer more colds and ear infections than unvaccinated children. Research shows vaccines may be linked to serious disease like leukemia, Guillain-Barre syndrome, Crohn's disease, meningitis, autism, learning disabilities and encephalitis. My own sense is that most vaccines unnaturally imbalance the immune system, eventually allowing immunological disorders like M.S., lupus, chronic fatigue syndrome, candida and herpes infections to occur later in life.

Can't find a recommended product? Call the 800 number in Product Resources for the store nearest you.

Despite this research, many public schools require all students to be vaccinated. (As of this writing, only 15 states allow parents *not* to vaccinate their children.) Most kids receive 33 doses of viral and bacterial vaccines <u>before</u> they can enter kindergarten. (Some receive 40 or more!)

Are all these inoculations really necessary? A recent study says no. Research published in the Journal of the American Medical Association reveals 20% of U.S. children are given immunizations they don't need. Yet schools threaten lawsuits against parents of unvaccinated children for "putting their child and other children at risk." In one dramatic case, New York state officials threatened to take 77 middle schoolers into custody unless their parents agreed to vaccinate them against Hepatitis B, a disease that kids born to non-infected parents rarely contract! If you choose NOT to have your child vaccinated, consult a health freedom attorney about your rights.

When should you call a doctor?

Herbs are wonderful for most childhood health problems, but sometimes your child may need strong medicine.

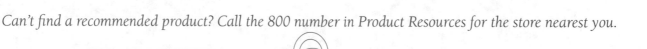

Signs that tell you to call a doctor:
•If your child has chronic stuffy nose and thick discharge that doesn't go away.
•If a fever persists longer than 3 days or returns after 3 days, or is unusually high, or is accompanied by a very stiff neck or headache (signs of meningitis).
•If your child seems lethargic, weak or is hard to wake up.
•If your child has seizures or loses bladder/bowel control.
•If a cold doesn't clear up and a rash or honking cough develops after 7 days.
•If your child shows rapid hard breathing, gasping, wheezing, or pale, bluish skin.
•f your child breaks a bone, gets a deep, blood-gushing gash, or may have ingested a poison.
•If your child shows dehydration signs like no urination, dry lips, sunken eyes, sunken soft spot (baby).
•If your child suffers a blow to the head, experiences dizziness or blurred vision, or becomes disoriented for more than a few minutes (signs of concussion).
•If your child develops severe pain on the right side with vomiting, loss of appetite, fever (appendicitis).
•If your child is recovering from chicken pox or flu virus, and goes into prolonged, vomiting with a fever followed by severe fatigue and confusion, he or she may have Reyes Syndrome, linked to aspirin reaction in children. Symptoms include: agitation, delirium, seizures, double vision, speech impairment, hearing loss and coma. Brain damage and death can result if the child does not get emergency treatment of intravenous glucose and electrolytes within 12 to 24 hours after vomiting starts.

Special notes:
1: Do not use honey (linked to infant botulism) in teas for children less than one year old. Try maple syrup instead.... I've found most kids like it better anyway.
2: Do not use aspirin for children's viral infections. Aspirin given during a viral infection is linked to Reyes syndrome, a dangerous child's liver disease. Aspirin is also linked childhood allergies.
3: Antibiotic drugs can be tough on a small child's system, especially over a long period of time. Question your doctor if an antibiotic prescription seems automatic, especially if your child has a viral infection.

Can't find a recommended product? Call the 800 number in Product Resources for the store nearest you.

Optimum Healing in the Golden Years

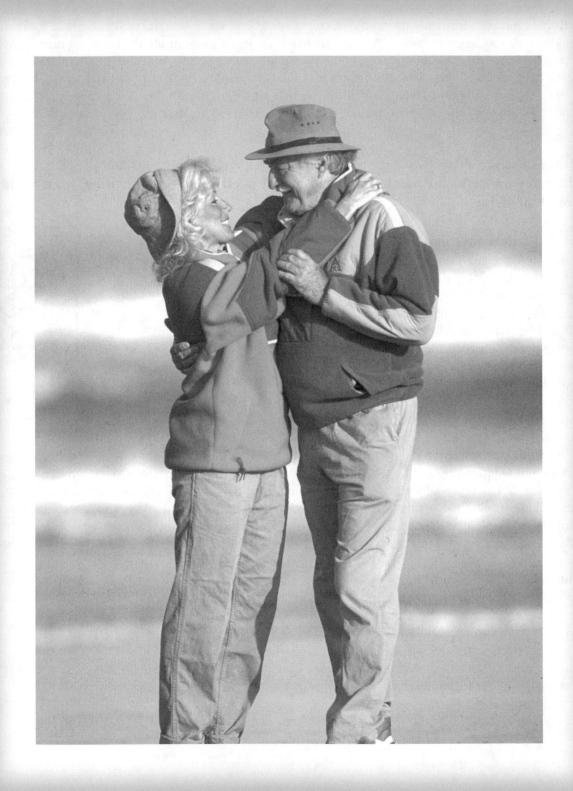

Slow Down Your Aging Clock

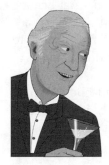

We all have to face it, the aging process we hate is going much faster than we'd like. There are so many interesting things to do and see in the world… without enough time to do them. We all want to extend our life spans with the best health possible.

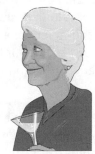

Whenever the gold and silver years begin for you, it's when the fun begins, when hectic family life quiets down, financial strains and needs ease, business retirement is here or not far off, and we can do the things we've always wanted to do but never had time for—travel, art, music, a craft, gardening, writing, quiet walks, picnics, more social life….even starting a new business, just for fun this time. It's doing what we want to do, not what we have to do. We all look forward to these treasure years of life, and picture ourselves on that tennis court, bicycle path or cruise ship, healthy, enjoying ourselves. But, there's a catch—our freedom comes in the latter half of life, and many of us don't age gracefully in today's world.

Yet, science has discovered an amazing paradox. Life expectancy actually lengthens <u>as you age</u>. Youth is not a chronological age. It's good health and an optimistic spirit. The average American child born in 1993 has a life expectancy of 75.4 years. But average life expectancy for someone 85 years is <u>six more years</u>. The longer you live, the longer your total expected life span becomes.

Research also tells us that we are only living two-thirds of the years our bodies are capable of! It's astonishing to realize that human life span is at least 20 to 30 years longer than most of us actually live today. American science is using that goal to increase our life spans at a remarkable rate. In 1928, life expectancy in the U.S. was just 57 years; today, it's 76 years. Researchers anticipate an American woman's life expectancy to rise to between 92.5 and 101.5 by the year 2070. Centenarians, people 100 or over, are the fastest growing segment of the U.S. population. There were 61,000 centenarians living in the U.S. as of the 2000 census. Experts predict that number will grow to 214,000 by 2020!

Age is not the enemy…. illness is.

The hourglass may tell us we're older, but the passage of time isn't what ages us. It's the process that reduces the number of healthy cells in our bodies. Cells themselves don't age; they're sloughed off as their efficiency diminishes, to be replaced by new ones. With the right nutrients, cell restoration may continue for many years past current life expectancy. A long standing diet of chemical-laced foods, pollutants that cause nutrient deficiencies, overuse of prescription drugs and antibiotics, all prevent our seniority dreams from becoming a reality. Eighty percent of the population over 65 years old in industrialized nations today is chronically ill, usually with arthritis, heart disease, diabetes or high blood pressure. If stress is piled on top of poor health, our minds and spirits suffer, too. It's a prescription for aging.

A balanced life is the key to long life.

You can strengthen your lean body mass, boost your metabolism and enhance your immune response. Your cell life is largely genetically controlled, but disease is more often the result of diet, lifestyle or environment. Natural anti-aging techniques are not a magic potion. They are an integrated, hard-core approach to avoiding disease…. the real enemy. In my opinion, they work far better than any of today's "super drugs."

This chapter has clear keys that slow down aging…. how to have a better memory with no senility, better skin tone with fewer wrinkles, a strong heart, bones and immune response, flexible joints and muscles, a youthful metabolic rate and a healthy sex life (good hormone activity keeps your whole body youthful).

Can't find a recommended product? Call the 800 number in Product Resources for the store nearest you.

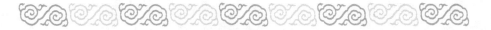

There has never been a better time to grow older. Hundreds of American health organizations focus solely on anti-aging. High tech diagnostic tools now identify diseases early to minimize disease consequences. Newly identified preventive measures keep disease from manifesting symptoms or progressing. In the natural healing world, we're discovering more about the rejuvenating benefits of whole herbs and nutritious foods.

Bodywork techniques like a simple brisk daily walk, increase your lifespan! Stretch out every morning to limber up, oxygenate your tissues, and clear your body of last night's waste and metabolic eliminations. Stretch at night before you retire to insure muscle relaxation and a better night's rest.

Think positive to stay young. Don't worry yourself into old age. Science is validating the mind-body connection in terms of the body's ability to heal. A well-rounded, optimistic life needs friends and family. It's important for you and for them. Doing for, and giving to others at the stage of your life when there is finally enough time to graciously do it, makes a world of difference to your spirit.

Anti-Aging Check-Up:

Are you aging too fast? Don't be overly harsh, but an honest evaluation of the following widely accepted aging signs can identify action areas to slow down some of aging's effects.

…Is your energy level at an all-time low?
…Have you noticed brown spots around your eyes, nose and hands?
…Has your hairline receded? Is your hair showing a lot of gray?
…Do you have some hearing loss or annoying ringing in the ears?
…Are constipation or irregular bowel movements a problem for you?
…Do you have regular insomnia? (especially a sign of adrenal deficiency)
…Do you have joint pain or joint crackling on one side? Do you have knobs on
     your index fingers? Are you stiff when you get up in the morning?
…Does it take longer for you to recover from respiratory infections like colds and flu?
          Do colds frequently become pneumonia for you?
…Is your eyesight worsening? Are you afraid you have macular degeneration, glaucoma or cataracts?
…Is it more difficult for you to lose weight? Have you put on 10-15 pounds that you just can't get rid of?
…Are your eyes usually dry? Do you have trouble tearing? Are your mouth and nasal passages dry?
     If you are a woman, do you have chronic vaginal dryness?
…Is the skin on your hands, arms and neck crepe-y, thinner, bruising easily or getting strawberry marks?
…Have your arms or legs become more flabby? Are your muscles noticeably weaker?
…Are your teeth brittle, with visible chip marks or discoloration? Have you lost teeth to gum disease?
          (Nothing makes you look older than poor teeth. See my "Dental Problems" program on pg. 387-390.)
…Do you experience heartburn, indigestion or gas regularly after eating (a low hydrochloric acid sign)?
…Have you lost some height? Look in the mirror. Is your neck starting to hunch over or at an angle?
…Have you had a recent bone fracture in a fall or accident that wouldn't have meant a break in the past?
…Do you have poor circulation? Are your hands and feet cold even in mild weather?
…Have you noticed a slight but constant trembling of your hands? Are you unsteady when you walk?
…Do you find yourself becoming seriously forgetful? Do you sometimes forget friends' names?
…Have you started to have heart palpitations? or small chest pains?

Start your anti-aging campaign with lifestyle factors that affect aging the most.
—Take a hard look at the prescription drugs you use: Many drugs lead to serious body imbalances by impairing your nutrient uptake, and they can spur a free radical assault that accelerates aging. They also tend to interact, especially drugs that affect hormones, like Viagra, Andro, Propecia or HRT drugs. If you still smoke, you should know smoking greatly increases the body's free radical load, is a clear contributor to premature aging, and is by far the #1 cause of preventable deaths in our country.

Can't find a recommended product? Call the 800 number in Product Resources for the store nearest you.

—Take another look at your diet: You've probably already cut the fat and fried food. But the chemicals in foods like lunch meats, hot dogs and pre-prepared meals are the culprits for early aging. They can create an over-acid condition in the blood, trigger many allergies, and like drugs, deplete the body of antioxidants, setting up a free-radical cascade favorable to disease. Fake fats like olestra (widely popular in snack foods) sabotage body defenses against disease. Research shows fake fats rob the body of vitamins like A, D, E, and K, and carotenoids. *Note: Even if your diet is good, I recommend supplementing with digestive enzymes and HCl with pepsin because digestion normally becomes sluggish with age.*

—Watch your stress levels. A little stress can be good motivation to move you towards a goal. But chronic, excessive stress steals your health and your youth! Over time, high levels of the stress hormone cortisol cause brain cells to age prematurely, or even die off! New research also links high levels of cortisol to middle aged weight gain around the waist.

—Interrupted sleep is a major aging trigger. A recent Lancet study links a lack of sleep to premature aging and serious illness. During sleep, important anti-aging hormones like growth hormone and melatonin are released which help regulate metabolism, heal tissues and boost immune response.

—A sedentary lifestyle paves the way for obesity and chronic disease. But, regular moderate exercise actually reverses the aging process. A recent JAMA study reveals that the bodies of postmenopausal women become up to 20 years more youthful just by lifting weights twice weekly for one year!

—Do you eat sweets or take hard alcohol drinks regularly? A high sugar diet wipes out immunity, reduces tissue elasticity, and interferes with cells' ability to rejuvenate. Sugar is a hidden ingredient in most refined foods. The artificial sweetener aspartame is linked to nerve disorders, dizziness and headaches.

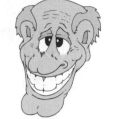

—Take a look at your teeth and gums: Almost nothing shows age faster than discolored teeth, lost teeth or red, receding gums. CoQ-10 helps many gum problems, about 300mg daily at least for the first month; see a good holistic dentist to solve discoloration problems.

—Take a look in the mirror: is your neck at a slight angle? Are your shoulders hunching? You may be losing bone density. Start a strengthening exercise program right away. Make sure it includes elongating, smooth muscle stretches and stick with it. Exercise can rapidly reverse this aging sign.

—Have you moved to a southern climate: 90% of skin cancers and wrinkles are due to sun exposure. Use 40 SPF for your face, up to 26 SPF for your body. Wear a hat.... or face those fine lines in the mirror.

Longevity begins with a good diet

A nutrition rich diet is the center piece of a vibrant long life. Most health experts agree that the food guide pyramid needs modification for better health as we age. Nutritional deficiencies accelerate age-related disorders like dementia and memory loss! Your diet must become even more nourishing and even higher in antioxidants as the years pass. A good diet improves health, provides a high level of energy, maintains harmonious system balance, keeps memory and thinking sharp, staves off disease, and contributes to a youthful appearance. The aging process slows down if you have a good internal environment.

Overeating dramatically hastens the aging process—eating moderately may add as much as ten years to your lifespan. Your body needs fewer calories and burns calories slower as you age. So lower your calories to reduce the signs of aging. A low calorie diet protects DNA molecules from damage, prevents organ and tissue degeneration. Optimum body weight should be 10 to 15 pounds less than in your 20's and 30's. Easily control that annoying slow upward weight gain by composing your diet of 50% fresh foods. Fresh, organically grown foods also protect your skin from the signs of aging. Your skin is a window of your diet. We know the American diet is saturated with chemicals from pesticides, preservatives and additives. Now, over 70% of our foods are genetically altered as well. The brown age spots and rough texture we see on our skin are signs that our bodies are less able to process our foods normally.

Can't find a recommended product? Call the 800 number in Product Resources for the store nearest you.

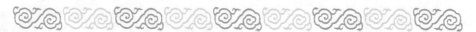

The Best Anti-Aging Foods:

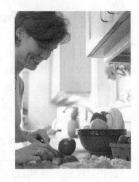

—Fresh fruits and vegetables! Fresh produce gives you the most vitamins, minerals, fiber and enzymes. Plants have the widest array of easy-to-use nutrients for your body. Enzyme-rich fruits and vegetables are the essential link in stamina levels. Organically grown foods insure higher nutrient content and avoid toxic sprays. Have a green salad every day. New research shows the immune cells of vegetarians are twice as effective as meat eaters in killing cancer cells!

…**Fresh fruit and vegetable juices** offer quick antioxidant absorption, which protects the body against aging, heart disease, cancer, and degenerative conditions.

—Sea greens are the ocean's superfoods. They contain all the elements of life and transmit the energies of the sea to us as proteins, complex carbs, vitamins, minerals, trace minerals, chlorophyll, enzymes and fiber. Sea greens and sea foods stand almost alone as potent sources of natural iodine. By regulating thyroid function, they promote higher energy levels and increased metabolism for faster weight loss after 40.

—Whole grains, nuts, seeds and beans for protein, fiber, minerals and essential fatty acids. Sprouted seeds, grains, and legumes are some of the healthiest foods you can eat. They are living nutrients that can go directly to your cells.

—Cultured foods for friendly digestive flora. Yogurt tops the list, but kefir and kefir cheese, miso, tamari, tofu, tempeh, even a glass of wine at the evening meal also promote better nutrient assimilation. Raw sauerkraut is especially good for boosting friendly bacteria. (Avoid sauerkraut processed with alum.) Bonus: Cultured foods act as a mild appetite suppressant for better weight control.

—Fish and fresh seafoods two to three times a week enhance thyroid and metabolic balance, for high quality protein, and for brain nourishing EFA's.

—Plenty of pure water every day keeps your body hydrated. See "Water" on pg. 116 for more info.

—Keep your system alkaline with green drinks, green foods, miso, and grains like rice. I like Green Foods AGELESS ENERGY drink for long term health.

—Healthy, unsaturated fats and oils, 2 to 3 tablespoons a day are enough to keep your body at its best.

—Poultry, other meats, butter, eggs, and dairy in moderation. Avoid fried foods, excess caffeine, red meats, highly seasoned foods, refined and chemically processed foods altogether.

Plant Enzymes are a Key to Anti-Aging

Enzymes are the cornerstone of anti-aging, because they support strong immune response and provide the active food antioxidants which fight free-radicals. Replenishing your enzymes every day builds a body that resists disease, enables healing, and lengthens your life. In fact, Dr. Edward Howell, a founder of enzyme therapy said that "the actual length of life is tied to the increased use of food enzymes because they decrease the rate of your body's enzyme exhaustion."

Enzymes are the workhorses that power our bodies. Millions of enzymes carry out the vital functions that preserve your life. They're called our vital force, because without them we would be a pile of lifeless chemicals.

Can't find a recommended product? Call the 800 number in Product Resources for the store nearest you.

Enzyme depletion and aging go hand in hand. Low enzyme activity is directly related to increased free radical production, abnormal tissue formation (fibrosis) and reduced digestive capacity - all hallmarks of aging. Each of us is born with a battery charge of enzyme energy. The faster you use up this enzyme supply - the shorter your life. Of course enzymes are used up in normal body functions like metabolism and healing. But enzymes are wasted haphazardly throughout life by alcohol, excessive exposure to UV rays, drugs, second-hand smoke and chemical-laced foods. Overcooking food depletes enzymes — they're incredibly heat-sensitive..... the first to be destroyed during cooking above 118 degrees Fahrenheit. Fast food processing, microwaving, and irradiating all seriously deplete enzymes.

Eating food devoid of enzymes forces the pancreas and the liver to use their enzyme stores for digestion. (Critical pancreatic enzyme output may be reduced by as much as 40% in the elderly.) But even this substitute measure doesn't make up for the missing enzymes, because we need the enzymes plants provide to break down our food correctly and deliver nutrients to the blood. Undigested food in the blood forces white blood immune cells to leave their jobs in order to take care of the undigested food, and immune response takes a dive.

You can halt the one-way outflow of enzymes. Enzyme rich foods bring enzymes and antioxidants back into our bodies along with the full array of plant nutrients that keep our immune systems strong. I believe Nature intended us to eat a largely plant-based diet, perhaps to ensure that we received enough enzymes. Cultured foods like yogurt, kefir, soy foods like tofu or tempeh, and raw sauerkraut encourage enzyme activity. If you don't get enough fresh or cultured foods, or if you need extra enzymes for healing, plant based, food enzyme supplements are the next best choice. They're especially useful for anti-aging, digestive and skin disorders (even age spots), inhibiting fibrosis related to atherosclerosis, and fighting free radicals that damage DNA. See "Enzymes and Enzyme Therapy," page 92 for more.

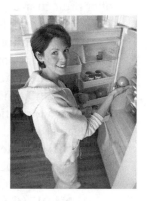

Antioxidants are a Key to Anti-Aging

Free radical production is a normal part of biochemical life. Some free radicals arise normally through metabolism. Your own immune system creates free radicals to neutralize certain viruses and bacteria! When body antioxidants, like the enzymes *superoxide dismutase, catalase* and *glutathione peroxidase* are plentiful and antioxidant intake from foods is high, the body easily handles normal free radical production. But around age 30, the rate of free radical damage begins to outpace the body's production of antioxidants. Even eating the recommended 5-8 serving of fruits and vegetables, may not be enough for free radical protection. A high potency antioxidant supplement can give you an anti-aging boost if your own antioxidants are low.

Important anti-aging antioxidants:
Super green foods are widely popular antioxidants. They should be part of your anti-aging picture. Check out the sections in this book on sea greens, chlorella, spirulina, aloe vera, barley and wheat grass.

...Alpha lipoic acid: may slow or reverse the aging process by increasing metabolic activity and reducing oxidation damage; it increases the free radical quenching power of other antioxidants; significantly boosts body glutathione, a key detoxifying antioxidant.
...Bee pollen: a nutrient source, energy builder and health restorer since ancient times; a full-spectrum rejuvenative food that helps counteract the effects of aging and increases both mental and physical capability.
...CoQ-10: the body's ability to assimilate food source CoQ-10 declines with age. Supplements provide benefits for gum disease, cardiovascular health (CoQ-10 is recommended by many cardiologists), and breast and prostate cancer protection.

Can't find a recommended product? Call the 800 number in Product Resources for the store nearest you.

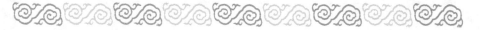

…Carotenes: beta, alpha, lycopene, lutein, astaxanthin, zeaxanthine and others are powerful anti-infectives and antioxidants for immune protection against environmental pollutants, premature aging and allergy control. Lycopene, with twice the antioxidant power of beta carotene, is an anti-cancer carotene, reducing risk for prostate, cervical and pancreatic cancers. *Note: Carotenes work best when used in a combination rather than singly.*

…Vitamin C: an immune-boosting antioxidant, it protects against infections, cancer, heart disease, high blood pressure, arthritis and allergies. Safeguards against radiation, heavy metal toxins and pollutants.

—Bioflavonoids: the anti-inflammatory part of the vitamin C-complex, prevent artery hardening, enhance connective tissue, capillary and vein strength, and control bruising, They also help lower cholesterol and stimulate bile for digestion.

…Vitamin E: an anticoagulant and vasodilator against blood clots and heart disease. Numerous studies show vitamin E reduces risk of a heart attack. It retards cellular and mental aging, works as an anti-aging antioxidant with selenium to quench free radical fires and reduces infections in the elderly. **Tocotrienols:** compounds related to tocopherols, tocotrienols lower cholesterol, and have potent antioxidant and anti-cancer properties. Tocotrienols offer protection against damage to the arterial wall, with a stronger lipid lowering effect. Consider Lane Labs PALM VITEE as an excellent source. Yoanna Vitamin E oil is a wonderful topical choice for skin health and beauty.

…Germanium (organic): a potent antioxidant mineral that detoxifies and boosts natural killer cells. Increases tissue oxygen (poor oxygenation is one of the most common causes of cell injury and disease).

…L-Glutathione: low body levels of glutathione are a biochemical marker for aging, beginning to decline around age 60. An antioxidant amino acid, glutathione works to neutralize drug or radiation toxicity and inhibits free radical formation. It also cleanses the blood from the effects of chemotherapy, X-rays and liver toxins. Protective against age-related eye disorders like cataracts and macular degeneration.

…NAC (N-Acetyl-Cysteine): an antioxidant amino acid and precursor of glutathione. Prevents age-related free radical damage to skin and arteries. Detoxifies from alcohol, heavy metals, smoke, X-rays and radiation. Treats colds and flu. NAC is the acetylated form of cysteine, which provides better absorption.

…NADH (Co-enzyme Nicotinamide Adenine Di-nucleotide): a powerful antioxidant coenzyme involved with the synthesis of ATP (chemical energy) in the body. Used successfully to treat Alzheimer's, Parkinson's, Chronic Fatigue Syndrome and depression. Source Naturals ENADA NADH tablets.

…Oligomeric Proanthocyanidins (OPC's): highly potent antioxidants that strengthen capillaries and connective tissue. OPC's reduce LDL cholesterol that accumulates on arteries causing atherosclerosis.

…Selenium: an antioxidant trace mineral that protects the body from heavy metal toxicity; reduces risk of certain types of cancer (prostate, esophagus, colorectal and lung) and increases body glutathione.

…Royal Jelly: an anti-aging superfood which stimulates the immune system, deep cellular health and longevity, boosts circulation to the skin and supplies key nutrients for energy and mental alertness.

…Zinc: limits the amount of free radicals the body naturally produces, like malondialdehyde (MDA).

Nootropic *(neuroprotective)* brain nutrients are important for anti-aging.

…Choline: one of the lipotropic B vitamins, improves fat metabolism, and it's a memory "vitamin," easily converted to the brain neurotransmitter acetylcholine. Studies show lecithin, a rich source of choline, greatly improves memory. Just eating 2 tbsp. a day for five weeks can do the job!

…GPC (L-alpha glycerylphosphorylcholine) is a precursor to choline which can help repair brain damage caused by aging, Alzheimer's, and stroke. Experts hope it may one day treat brain disorders like Huntington's and Parkinson's diseases which show little or no improvement with conventional therapies. GPC helps preserve and restore important neurons, receptors and membranes that deteriorate with age or illness. It also boosts GABA (gamma-aminobutyric acid), growth hormone and dopamine release, and is well tolerated in human studies.

…Phosphatidylserine: a phospholipid nutrient that helps maintain cell membrane integrity and fluidity. Boosts brain health by increasing neurotransmitter activity and improving glucose metabolism. PS supplements have shown in 25 different human studies to improve or maintain cognition and concentration in older adults. PS can improve quality of life for Alzheimer's patients, and can help reduce depression and mood disorders.

Can't find a recommended product? Call the 800 number in Product Resources for the store nearest you.

...**Acetyl L carnitine (ALC):** An amino acid compound gaining a reputation as a nootropic which reduces age-related mental decline. Available in Italy since 1986, ALC increases alertness and attention span, improves learning and memory, and boosts eye-hand coordination.

...**Vinpocetine:** A derivative of periwinkle, vinpocetine increases cerebral blood flow, brain cell ATP, and utilization of oxygen and glucose. Vinpocetine has been used in Europe for over two decades to treat stroke patients, and has notable effects for enhancing memory. Vinpocetine is added to formulas for eyesight, hearing loss and tinnitus with good results.

Note: A broad spectrum nootropic formula produces best results: Wakunaga of America NEURO•LOGIC has aged garlic extract, lecithin, phosphatidylserine, ginkgo biloba, acetyl-L-carnitine, folic acid, and vitamin B12. Life Extension Foundation COGNITEX combines GPC, vinpocetine, choline and phosphatidylserine.

Herbs Help Slow the Effects of Aging

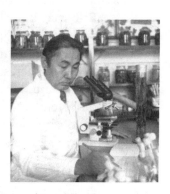

People of every culture since ancient times have searched for the Fountain of Youth. The answer may have been available all along in the youth-extending properties of herbs.

Herbs have wide ranging abilities and far reaching possibilities as rejuvenators. In fact, herbs are at their best in a revitalizing type of role... balancing, toning and normalizing our bodies. Herbs have antioxidant properties that guard against free radical destruction of tissue. Herbs are full of whole essence vitamins, minerals and phytochemicals—potent nutrients that can address aging concerns—better memory, strong gland and metabolic activity, smoother, more elastic skin, energy, and good muscle tone. Herbs have powerful enzymes that make their nutrients easy to absorb.

The three main causes of aging are:
1: cell and tissue damage by free radicals that aren't neutralized because the body lacks antioxidants.
2: reduced immune response that puts the body at risk for disease.
3: enzyme depletion in the body due to lack of enzyme reinforcements from foods or supplements.

Herbal therapy is one of the best defenders your body has for these aging actions.
—Antioxidant herbs scavenge and neutralize free radicals, energize and tone.
—Adaptogen herbs strengthen immunity, and equip your body to handle stress.

Free radicals play a key role in body aging.
They are highly active compounds that spark with an oxidating fire when fat molecules react with oxygen. Although they occur in normal metabolic breakdown, our bodies experience excesses of these cell damagers from air and environmental pollutants. Your body takes 10,000 free radical hits a day just in normal, everyday living!

Free radicals that go unchecked by antioxidants are dangerous — they can actually reprogram your DNA, degrade and deplete your collagen stores (aging your looks), cause premature aging through disease, and break down your natural immune response. Free radicals are the missing link to inflammatory reactions like arthritis, to many diseases including cancer, atherosclerosis, even Alzheimer's disease, and to immune compromised diseases like fibromyalgia and chronic fatigue syndrome.

Lowering the saturated fat in your diet is the single most beneficial step you can take to reduce free radical damage. Heavy, saturated fats depress the body's antioxidant enzyme response to free radical attacks.

Can't find a recommended product? Call the 800 number in Product Resources for the store nearest you.

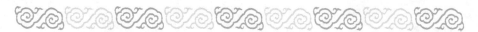

Potent herbal antioxidants for anti-aging:

...Arjuna: an Ayurvedic heart tonic effective for angina pain, arrhythmia and congestive heart failure. High antioxidants in the tannins and flavones prevent oxidative damage linked to heart disease.

...Cat's Claw: a Peruvian rainforest herb known for its benefits for arthritis, irritable bowel syndrome (IBS), immunity, and tumorous growths. Plentiful antioxidants, including proanthocyanidins for anti-aging.

...Pine bark and grapeseed: have powerful proanthocyanidins (OPCs or PCOs), concentrated, highly active bioflavonoids. Fifty times stronger than vitamin E, 20 times stronger than vitamin C, they are one of the few dietary antioxidants that readily cross the blood-brain barrier to protect brain cells and aid memory.

...Ginkgo biloba: is used worldwide to combat the effects of aging. It protects the cells against damage from free radicals, reduces blood cell clumping which leads to congestive heart disease, improves memory and brain activity, restores circulation, helps improve hearing and vision, and fights allergic reactions. Studies show ginkgo extracts stabilize and, in some cases, noticeably improve cognition function and social behavior of severely demented Alzheimer's patients. New studies reveal that ginkgo actually reduces the "stress" hormone cortisol linked to immune suppression, atherosclerosis and brain cell toxicity.

...Bilberry: a bioflavonoid-rich herb that helps keep connective tissues healthy and strengthens small blood vessels and capillaries, factors that keep skin youthful. Bilberry protects against macular degeneration.

...Shiitake mushrooms: promote vitality and are especially valuable as a treatment for systemic conditions related to age-related sexual dysfunction.

...Reishi mushrooms (ganoderma): tonic mushrooms that increase vitality and enhance immunity. They lower cholesterol and high blood pressure, combat bacteria and viruses, may help prevent cancer and aid in the treatment of chronic fatigue syndrome, ulcers and heart disease.

...Astragalus: a strong immune enhancer, adrenal stimulant and gland tonic; a vasodilator that helps lower blood pressure, increase metabolism and improve circulation. It is a specific in liver dysfunction and respiratory problems that involve allergies.

...Hawthorn: bioflavonoid-rich, and adept at counteracting the damaging effects of free radicals on the cardiovascular system. Gentle, but powerful, hawthorn makes the heart a more efficient pump, increasing output of blood from the heart and decreasing resistance from the blood vessels.

...Rosemary: one of nature's finest antioxidants, rosemary is a specific for memory and problems related to aging. Components in rosemary actually prevent the breakdown of acetylcholine in the brain, a key brain chemical for memory. Rosemary is rich in highly absorbable calcium for stress and tension, and shows good results in animal tests for breast cancer. Rosemary in cooking or even steeped in wine is effective for health. Diamond Formulas DIAMOND ETERN-L tabs with rosemary, oregano and anti-aging nutrients are another high quality choice.

...Turmeric: a powerful antioxidant - inhibits oxidative enzymes, chelates and neutralizes the free radical properties of minerals like iron. Animal research shows turmeric reduces brain-damaging plaques linked to Alzheimer's disease. Turmeric also blocks formation of nitrosamines, known cancer-causing carcinogens.

...Garlic: Garlic contains at least 15 different antioxidant compounds. Over 1,000 studies and scientific papers have been published in the last 40 years on garlic. New discoveries show that aged garlic can inhibit platelet adhesion and aggregation, cholesterol synthesis, and arteriosclerosis. Even orthodox medicine acknowledges that garlic reduces the risk of further heart attacks in cardiac patients.

...Ginger: Ginger has at least 12 constituents (maybe more) more powerful than vitamin E.... one compound surpassed vitamin E's antioxidant activity by 40 times! Ginger also works on our eicosanoids.... compounds in our bodies that break down dietary fat that may contribute to sticky blood, atherosclerosis and inflammation. Ginger has at least 5 elements that work on eicosanoids to check inflammatory prostaglandins involved in migraines and arthritis, for instance, and those responsible for sticky blood.

...Wheat germ oil: 1 tablespoon provides the antioxidant equivalent of an oxygen tent for 30 minutes.

Can't find a recommended product? Call the 800 number in Product Resources for the store nearest you.

Potent ginsengs and ginseng-like adaptogens for anti-aging:

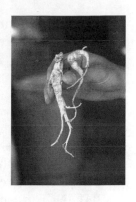

Herbal adaptogens have anti-stress action. They increase resistance to adverse influences by helping the body normalize. Antioxidant herbs like astragalus, shiitake and reishi mushrooms are also adaptogens. Crystal Star Feel Great Now™ with Ginseng is a blend of the best antioxidant, adaptogen herbs.

…Panax Ginseng (red, white and American ginsengs): are the most effective of all adaptogen herbs. Ginseng stimulates both long and short term energy, nourishes reproductive and circulatory systems, has measurable amounts of germanium, energizes the central nervous system, promotes regeneration from stress and fatigue, and rebuilds foundation strength. Red ginseng is particularly beneficial for men since it promotes testosterone production. Asian and American ginsengs both stimulate brain and memory centers.

…Siberian eleuthero: a tonic that supports the adrenal glands, circulation and memory.

…Schizandra: synergistic with eleuthero for stress, weight loss and sports endurance formulas, schizandra supports sugar regulation and liver function, helps keep aging skin healthy through better use of fats.

…Suma: an ancient herb with modern results for overcoming fatigue and hormonal imbalance. Widely used to rebuild the body from the ravages of cancer and diabetes.

…Gotu Kola: a brain and nervous system restorative. Considered an elixir of life and longevity in Chinese medicine, it's a primary nerve and body healer after trauma or illness. Gotu kola has therapeutic applications for the skin, cellulite, wound repair, burns, scars (helps inhibit formation), and varicose veins.

…Fo-Ti (Ho-Shou-Wu): a flavonoid-rich longevity herb. It is a cardiovascular strengthener, increasing blood flow to the heart. Many report hair returns to much of its original color before graying.

…Cordyceps: an adaptogenic, antioxidant mushroom used for centuries in TCM. Gained its fame in 1993 after several Chinese long distance runners won gold medals following a Cordyceps-containing diet. Cordyceps boosts libido in men and women, improves impotence and increases sperm count.

…Jiaogulan: newly popular in America, jiaogulan contains 3 to 4 times as many saponins as Panax Ginseng and some say it has even more powerful regulatory effects on the body. Jiaogulan bolsters immune response, improves fat metabolism, soothes nerves, and enhances endurance. It is becoming well known as an herbal heart protector against high cholesterol and hypertension. Recent studies show that jiaogulan also facilitates natural weight loss by inhibiting the body's tendency to store sugars as fat. I use and recommend Jagulana's line of Jiaogulan products. Visit *www.immortalityherb.com or call 888-465-3686 to learn more.*

Are you considering Anti-Aging Drugs or Hormones?
Read this chapter before you make a decision.

As many as 22 million Americans now use over-the-counter superhormones like melatonin, DHEA, Human Growth Hormone (hGH) and Pregnenolone! Are they really your best choice for anti-aging? We'll explore the benefits and pitfalls.

1: Is Human growth hormone (hGH) really an anti-aging miracle?

hGH, produced by the pituitary gland, promotes bone growth and regulates height. Available only by prescription, <u>daily</u> injections cost up to an astounding $15,000 a year! Older versions of hGH injections, derived from human brain tissue, were banned in 1985 when they were linked to CJD, the human variant of mad cow disease. Children who got the banned hGH version are at higher risk for colon cancer. New, synthetic hGH treatment has some benefits. It helps very, very short children with growth hormone deficiency to grow, and it reduces tissue-wasting caused by advanced AIDS. It accelerates wound healing, and reduces the symptoms of Crohn's disease. It improves skin elasticity and reduces wrinkles, even increases muscle mass and bone density. hGH stimulates a sense of well being in middle aged men, largely because it decreases body fat.

Can't find a recommended product? Call the 800 number in Product Resources for the store nearest you.

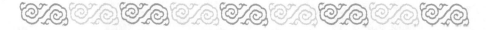

hGH prescriptions have known cautions: hGH increases diabetes risk and is linked to carpal tunnel syndrome and aching joints similar to "growing pains" in youth. Some hGH users develop abnormal bone or tissue growth. One frightening report is the story of a professional athlete who took the hGH to improve his performance and had to have massive skin grafts because his bones literally grew through his skin!

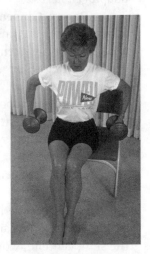

Boost growth hormone levels naturally! Reap the benefits without the drawbacks. Weight training promotes hGH while it increases bone mass and muscle strength. The amino acids arginine (especially when injected), lysine and glutamine taken with niacin boost the release of growth hormone. A 1995 study shows that 2000mg per day of oral glutamine increases hGH release. A full spectrum amino acid complex like Anabol Naturals AMINO BALANCE in conjunction with weight training offers the best results. Note: Very high doses of amino acids may cause stomach discomfort in some people.

Growth hormone microdoses, monitored by a licensed health practitioner, appear to offer the same benefits with fewer health risks! Experts at Allergy Research have developed this new, safer way to supplement the hGH superhormone. Allergy Research Group BIOGEN PRO or Always Young RENEWAL HGH is a microdilution of growth hormone in an easily absorbed oral spray. Preliminary research on several other new oral hGH products also show good results in well being, fat loss, higher energy and skin texture. Native traditionals in Peru claim that the energy herb Maca is a natural source of hGH. Good health food stores have the most advanced versions.

2: Is the highly popular steroid hormone Pregnenolone a good choice for anti-aging?

Pregnenolone, (called PREG), is a steroid hormone made primarily in the adrenal glands from cholesterol. Considered by many the "grandmother of all superhormones," PREG is the precursor to DHEA and progesterone in the body. PREG produces a feeling of well being and increases energy levels; users also report heightened awareness, memory and alertness, primarily because PREG stimulates brain receptors. Pregnenolone also enhances visual and auditory perception - sometimes to hallucinatory levels at higher doses, especially in men. Like DHEA, pregnenolone supplements are synthesized in a lab from wild yam diosgenin.

However, PREG is the most poorly researched of all the superhormones. know its cautions: PREG induces central nervous system excitability and can cause insomnia or shallow sleep; high doses (even 25mg a day) can cause irritability, anger, anxiety or headaches. Special groups of people like pregnant women, people with heart disease or people taking anti-depressant drugs or thyroid medication should avoid PREG. PREG may also convert into excess estrogen or cortisol in the body, resulting in side effects and hormone imbalance. For instance in men, unbalanced estrogen-androgen hormones can increase risk of atherosclerosis and prostate enlargement. For menopausal women, too much cortisol leads to waistline weight gain.

Natural alternatives to PREG? *Gotu kola*, a ginseng-like adaptogen herb boosts mental energy, promotes well being, and heightens sensations without the safety risks of PREG. Try Crystal Star's MENTAL CLARITY™ formula. Meditation and deep breathing also help you sharpen awareness and help you live longer! Studies show that meditating just 20 minutes, twice a day, increases the average lifespan by 65%!

3: Widely publicized for a decade, is melatonin really an anti-aging hormone?

Many people use melatonin as Nature's sleeping pill. Secreted by the pineal gland, melatonin sets our internal biological clock that governs our sleep-wake cycles or rhythms. One of the best benefits of melatonin is its ability to help ward off the effects of jet lag. Melatonin can even help the blind get better sleep, regulating sleep patterns for the sight-impaired by "telling" the person when it's time to sleep. New research shows melatonin can reduce dependence on valium and other benzodiazepine drugs, and improve the symptoms of SAD (Seasonal Affective Disorder). I have met the medical doctor who discovered the hormone melatonin. Besides acknowledging that his

Can't find a recommended product? Call the 800 number in Product Resources for the store nearest you.

work on melatonin revealed that our bodies sense night and day in a deeper way than by sight, he told me that if melatonin hadn't been labeled a hormone first, he would have called it an antioxidant! He showed that as an antioxidant, melatonin helps protect the body from free radical damage. In another hormone effect, melatonin may also reverse the shrinkage of the thymus a little, enabling it to produce more infection-fighting T-cells.

Every hormone has side effects—so does melatonin: Once supplementation begins, the body tends to shut down its own production of melatonin, even impeding regular sleep for good. At high levels, it may temporarily shut down the reproductive system, an effect being used in Europe in a contraceptive called B-Oval, which combines a very high dose of melatonin (75 mg) with progestin. Melatonin can cause nightmares, nausea and stomach cramps, decrease sex drive, even shrink male gonads. There are contraindications. Do not take melatonin with steroid medication, MAO inhibitors or sedative drugs. People with depression, mental illness, epilepsy, women trying to conceive or who are nursing should avoid melatonin.

Note: New Harvard research suggests that production of melatonin may <u>not</u> slow with age, as was previously thought. Low melatonin levels are now believed to be the result of illness or drug use (even aspirin or ibuprofen).

4: DHEA is being promoted for anti-aging for every adult over 45, but is there a downside?

DHEA *(dehydro-epiandrosterone)*, a hormone used by the body to manufacture other hormones, like estrogen, testosterone, progesterone, and corticosterone, is touted as a substance that lowers serum cholesterol, reverses aging symptoms, and promotes energy and libido. DHEA supplements work for post-menopausal women with osteoporosis who are low in DHEA, much the same as estrogen replacement. Other symptoms of menopause are also relieved, and cancer risk associated with estrogen replacement is greatly reduced; it may even be prevented by DHEA's immune potential.

DHEA regulates auto-immune response, stimulating immune defenses to fight infections and monitoring over-reactions that might attack the body. It has proven helpful against lupus and rheumatoid arthritis. Animal research shows the potential of DHEA in preventing cancer, heart disease, and Alzheimer's disease.

DHEA does have side effects: If you take too much, it suppresses your body's ability to make its own. Adult acne is a common side effect, so is excess perspiration, loss of head hair, and increased facial and body hair. DHEA causes irritability, insomnia and mood swings in a significant number of people. It can lead to liver damage, and should not be used by people with ovarian, thyroid or adrenal tumors. It should not be used in combination with blood thinning drugs, aspirin or thyroid medication. Some experts are concerned that high doses of DHEA used longterm may increase risk of prostate cancer by boosting testosterone levels.

Natural alternatives to DHEA? Dioscorea (wild yam), contains diosgenin which some researchers think helps your body produce its own DHEA. Breakthrough technology from Dr. C. Norman Shealy, M.D., Ph.D., uses laminar crystals to restore depleted magnesium, natural progesterone cream, and electrical stimulation of key acupuncture points to boost your own DHEA production naturally. If you're interested, contact Self-Health Systems, 5607 S. 222nd Rd., Fair Grove, MO 65648, 417-267-2900.

My conclusion?

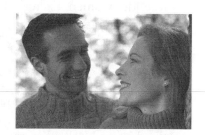

Proper usage of superhormones may lead to improvements in health and quality of life. The technology is advanced and results are promising. But, carelessly taking high dosages of superhormones may be counterproductive, perhaps even dangerous. When you mix hormone-like steroidal substances in the body, you're essentially changing your body chemistry. The wrong mixture may cause side effects or increase your risk of serious disease. A qualified health practitioner can help. Saliva and blood hormone tests are highly recommended. Consider the safe, gentle, natural alternative to superhormones in this chapter.

Note: For more information on these four super hormones, see the LOOK IT UP section in the back of this book.

Can't find a recommended product? Call the 800 number in Product Resources for the store nearest you.

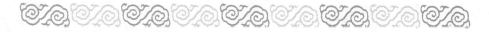

Exercise is an important antioxidant against aging
"Now the evidence is overwhelming that exercise and a long, healthy life go hand in hand,"
Dr. N.P. Napalkov, World Health Organization Assistant Director-General

The newest studies show us that regular exercise extends life-span, reduces cancer risk, and cuts the risk for heart attack in half! Amazingly, exercise boosts immunity even more as you age. Research shows women over 70 who are fit have immune response comparable to women half their age!

Unfortunately, statistics from the National Institutes of Health show that 58% of adult Americans get little or no exercise. Sadly, lack of exercise is responsible for nearly ⅓ of deaths in the U.S.!

Exercise doesn't have to be complicated. Simple stretches every morning oxygenate your tissues, limber your body, and help clear it of the previous night's waste. Stretches at night before bed help insure muscle relaxation and better rest. There are so many ways to bring exercise into your life: yoga, dance (I still like the Twist- great for a tummy bulge), sports like tennis or sailing, aerobic exercise, swimming, walking, jogging, bike riding or hiking. Even deep breathing is a form of exercise.

There are two keys to maintaining regular exercise. Find something that you like, because that's something you'll do on a long term basis; and switch around your exercise activities so you don't get bored. Take an aerobics class one day, swim the next, play tennis on the weekend, etc.

Advantages of regular exercise for a youthful, fit lifestyle:
—Exercise improves blood circulation and our ability to use oxygen for energy.
—Exercise helps reduce the risk for heart attacks and cancer.
—Exercise greatly enhances weight control by fanning the metabolic fires.
—Exercise reduces stress and tension, and encourages relaxation.
—Exercise stimulates hormone production in men and women.
—Exercise helps agility and joint mobility.
—Exercise lowers insulin levels and promotes regular elimination.
—Regular exercise helps manage glaucoma by reducing intraocular pressure.
—Exercise contributes to strength and endurance. Inactivity contributes to fatigue.
—Weight bearing exercise triggers bone mineralization to help deter osteoporosis.
—Exercise releases heavy metals like cadmium, lead and nickel, pesticides and other toxic material through increased perspiration.

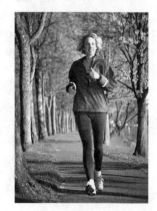

Striking evidence from physical fitness experts shows that regular exercise makes the most difference in the oldest and least fit people! Walking is an "antioxidant nutrient," one of the best exercises for both your body and your brain. Taking a walk every day, especially after your largest meal, boosts circulation, energy, strength, stress reduction and enzyme function. Walking raises your heart rate.... just 20 beats per minute can significantly decrease high blood pressure. Regular exercise also lowers your risk of falls, one of the most serious health threats for older women. Exercise also becomes important to a man as he ages, because it helps maintain his sexual vigor and burns his excess fat.

Deep breathing is a superb anti-aging technique
Deep breathing is a powerful way to decrease stress and increase calm energy. Low body oxygen can cause anxiety, depression, tight muscles, aches and pains, and exacerbate chronic illness. Diaphragmatic breathing is the deepest kind of breathing. Deep diaphragm breathing lowers anxiety levels, relaxes and loosens muscles, and generates an inner feeling of peace and calm. Diaphragm breathing also strengthens heart and lungs, encourages more restful sleep and slows the aging process.

Can't find a recommended product? Call the 800 number in Product Resources for the store nearest you.

Some basic diaphragm breathing steps:

1) Inhale deeply through your nose. Try to fill your lungs.

2) Exhale slowly through your mouth.

3) Breathe deeply for 30 seconds. It takes less than a minute to calm and center yourself during anxious moments. Breathing deeply for just one minute prevents short breaths that negatively affect the oxygen-carbon dioxide content of your blood.

4) Now breathe deeply to fill the lower part of your lungs. Notice the pop-pop feeling in your chest as unused lung pockets open up. Your abdomen extends slightly as you fill it with air. Slowly exhale — your abdomen moves inward.

5) As you breathe in deeply, think of oxygen reaching and recharging all the cells of your body. As you exhale, imagine all the stress and tension leaving your body.

Anti-Aging Techniques for Your Change of Life

The change of life comes to everyone. We recognize menopause as the change of life for women, but, both men and women experience body shape changes and hormonal fluctuations at mid-life. Mid-life change for men, "andropause" is much less discussed, even in the medical community. But it's a real phenomenon and it can cause unusual fatigue, anxiety, loss of muscle, even impotence for a large number of men.

Life changes are natural, and while any change can be difficult, I find a transformation may be just what our bodies need at this phase of our lives. Most people I've talked to adjust, even embrace their changes, especially after they've taken steps in their diet and lifestyle to insure their health for the years to come.

Natural Therapies for a Man's Andropause

Eight in ten family physicians today recognize male andropause as a real change of life for men comparable to female menopause. Symptoms to watch for include: low energy; slowing facial or head hair growth; less muscle mass; lost height or early osteoporosis; enlarged prostate; depression; less strong or less frequent erections; lower than normal sex drive.

1: Reduce fried foods, red meats and fatty dairy foods: they're full of disrupting hormones linked to cancer; reduce caffeine and sugar — all of which deplete the adrenals and drain male energy.

2: Don't go too far: An extremely low fat diet is disastrous for andropausal health. Penn State University studies find it may reduce testosterone levels... almost to preadolescent levels—definitely bad news for an older man! Include healthy fats from seafood and fish, and lean meats such as hormone-free turkey and chicken regularly. Consider flax seed or perilla oil as a healthy oil to use in salad dressings. (Use about 1 tbsp.)

3: Use your diet to prevent prostate cancer: Include cruciferous veggies like broccoli and cauliflower regularly. In one study, men who ate the most cruciferous veggies lowered their prostate cancer risk by 39%. The determining factor may be high 13C (*indole 3 carbinol*) in cruciferous veggies which helps detoxify carcinogens in the body. Diets high in lycopene, a carotenoid high in tomatoes, cut prostate cancer risk by 40%, so include tomatoes and tomato-based products often (cooking boosts the carotene).

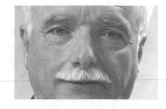

4: Boost your zinc intake to renew sexual potency: Zinc, highly concentrated in semen, is the most important nutrient for male sexual function. Eat zinc-rich foods like liver, oysters, nutritional yeast, nuts and seeds regularly. Add zinc-rich spirulina to your superfood list. Try Ethical Nutrients ZINC STATUS.

Can't find a recommended product? Call the 800 number in Product Resources for the store nearest you.

5: Check your alcohol intake: Heavy drinking can lead to prostate problems and impaired erections. DHT elevation (*di-hydro-testosterone* - a rogue type of testosterone), linked to normal testosterone decline and elevation of female hormones, is definitely undesirable for men.

6: Take care of your prostate: Research documented in the Quarterly Review of Natural Medicine finds *saw palmetto* reduces the symptoms of BPH by blocking DHT (*di-hydro-testosterone*), and inhibiting the enzyme 5-alpha reductase related to prostate enlargement. Consider Crystal Star PROSTATE PROTECTOR™ with *saw palmetto* and *pygeum* to help reduce prostate enlargement and dribbling urine. New Chapter PROSTATE 5LX helps normalize BPH-related symptoms, and also protects against prostate cancer.

7: Revitalize your sexual virility: Try the herb *tribulus terrestris* or *Epimedium* (horny goat weed). An Ayurvedic herb, *tribulus* has been used since ancient times as a treatment for increasing libido and impotence in men. Source Naturals TRIBULUS caps is a good choice. Pinnacle HORNY GOAT WEED caps increase virility and sexual performance, even in cases of impotence. As an alternative, Crystal Star's MALE PERFORMANCE™ caps have a long history of success for strengthening the male system and enhancing the sexual experience.

8: Regular exercise is a vital component of male sexual health: It makes the body stronger, function more efficiently and have greater stamina. In one study, 78 healthy, but sedentary men were studied during nine months of regular exercise. The men exercised for 60 minutes a day, three days a week. Every man in the study reported significantly enhanced sexuality, including increased frequency, performance and satisfaction. Rising sexuality was even correlated with the degree of fitness improvement. The more physical fitness the men were able to attain, the better their sex life!

Natural Therapies for a Woman's Menopause

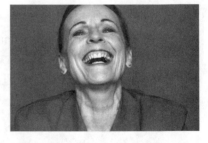

I've worked with women to help their hormone balance during menopause for over 25 years. The best stories come from women who take menopause as an opportunity to embrace the changing needs of their bodies. Gentle herbs are a good choice to regulate hormone fluctuations safely and naturally without the side effects and risks of hormone drugs that overwhelm and disrupt delicate female balance. Most women are highly sensitive to even small fluctuations in hormone levels. In menopause, this sensitivity tends to magnify as hormone shifts become more pronounced. Symptoms to look for: great fatigue, hot flashes and night sweats, mood swings, nighttime panic attacks, slow weight gain, bone loss, vaginal dryness or atrophy (usually pain with intercourse), unusually dry skin and migraine headaches.

1: Reduce the bad fats in your diet: Fats are storage for excess estrogen that lead to many hormone-driven diseases (like breast cancer). Steam and bake foods — never fry. Especially avoid commercial red meats and fatty dairy products (regularly injected with hormones) that disrupt delicate female balance.

2: Add good fats often (plenty of EFA's), like those in seafoods and sea veggies: Women report smoother skin, enhanced mental clarity and increased libido with the hormone balancing Omega 3 essential fatty acids in a high seafood diet. Salmon is particularly beneficial. I try to eat salmon at least once a week. I eat sea veggies every day. I often say if you can keep the EFA's in your diet right, every other nutrient will fall into line.

3: Eat fermented soy foods like tofu, tempeh, miso or soy milk regularly: Recent Italian studies found women who took a soy protein isolate had a 45% reduction in hot flashes! An added perk: Several new studies show that eating just 1.5 oz. of soy foods lowers total cholesterol as much as 9%. LDL, bad cholesterol, drops up to 13%!

Can't find a recommended product? Call the 800 number in Product Resources for the store nearest you.

4: Regulate your estrogen levels: Increase your fiber from whole grains and fresh vegetables. Add boron-containing foods like dark greens (also protects against macular degeneration), fruits, nuts and legumes to strengthen bones against menopausal bone loss.

5. Eat skin nourishing foods to help stave off wrinkles: seafood and sea greens (high in EFAs which nourish and plump the skin); onions and garlic to cleanse the pores; high vitamin C foods like kiwi (boosts collagen production); and plenty of pure water to prevent skin dehydration. I recommend Lane Labs TOKI, a collagen replacement drink mix, in all my anti-aging skin programs.

6: Target menopausal symptoms with herbs. I've used Crystal Star EST-AID™ caps with gentle, phytoestrogen herbs for years as a revitalizer that dramatically reduces hot flashes. The formula has been lab tested in over 200 tests by a third party, non-profit lab. It clearly inhibits breast cancer cell growth in test tubes! Pure Essence Labs TRANSITIONS tabs is another good choice, with black cohosh, isoflavones (soy-free), wild yam, chaste tree and licorice rt., and the nutrients, hesperidin and gamma oryzonal, shown in studies to reduce the frequency and intensity of hot flashes. Use either product with 1500mg of calcium daily.

7: Herbs can come to your rescue if you get panic attacks: Crystal Star WOMEN'S HEART HEALTH™ extract contains *hawthorn, arjuna* and *passionflowers*, herbs that help normalize heart palpitations and reduce stress-related panic attacks during menopause. Gaia VITEX-ALFALFA Supreme is another high quality choice. Ask a knowledgable health professional if an herbal heart stabilizer is right for you.

8: Essential oils reduce menopausal depression: Add a few drops of clary sage, jasmine (also revs up libido), neroli, bergamot or geranium to a diffuser and inhale the aroma for 20 minutes.

9: Naturally lubricate to reduce painful intercourse: During menopause, the vaginal lining may become thin and dry due to reduced circulating estrogen. Painful intercourse increases susceptibility to vaginal infection. Crystal Star WOMAN'S DRYNESS oral extract works almost overnight. Moon Maid VITAL VULVA salve topically relieves dryness and supports the re-thickening of vaginal tissues. Most women only need to use this product for a short period of time because it works so well. Or, apply pure aloe vera gel or natural vitamin E oil. Oral *Panax ginseng* (vials are best delivery system) also helps your body produce more fluid.

Normalizing hormone balance with diet and herbs is a gentle and easy way to sail through menopausal and andropausal body changes. You'll want to... ***keep the change!***

Old age is not determined by the number of years you have lived, but by the ideals you hold, and the enthusiasm of your soul. Youth's beauty is replaced by age's grace.

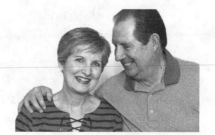

Do not fear death. Dying is one of life's duties... Life is like a play—what is important is not the length of the performance, but how good it is. Round your life off with a good ending.

Can't find a recommended product? Call the 800 number in Product Resources for the store nearest you.

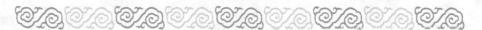

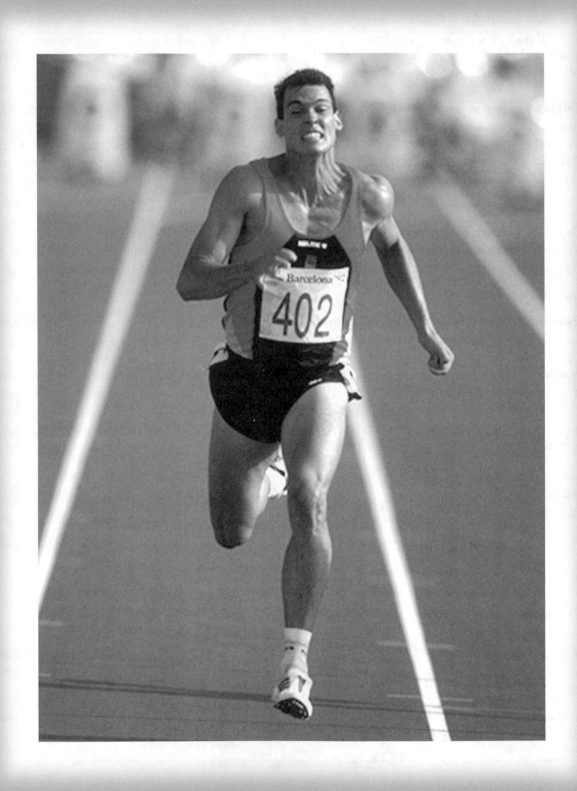

Optimizing Exercise & Sports Performance
Getting the most out of your exercise choices

The latest statistics are shocking! New National Institutes of Health studies reveal that a sedentary lifestyle has the same effect on heart disease risk as smoking a pack of cigarettes a day! Although most Americans know that exercise is critical to good health, that exercise insures weight control and strengthens our hearts, almost 60% of adult Americans get little or no exercise. One in four adults get no exercise at all!

Studies also show that lack of exercise is responsible for nearly one-third of deaths in the U.S. because it increases risk of serious diseases like diabetes, colon cancer and heart disease! The problem has devastating economic consequences too, costing the nation an estimated $1 trillion each year in healthcare services. The problem is so out of control that in June 2002, the White House launched the Healthier US Initiative encouraging all Americans to do some form of physical exercise every day.

Exercise can significantly improve your healing program. It strengthens your whole body — muscles, nerves, blood, glands, lungs, heart, brain, mind and mood. It increases your metabolic rate, muscle mass, oxygen uptake, circulation, and boosts the enzymes that help your body burn fat. Exercise is the key to stress control, low cholesterol and a sharper memory.

Exercise has dramatic anti-aging effects. New aging research shows physically active seniors can turn back the clock 15-20 years! It also stimulates antibody production, enhances immune response, and reduces fatigue. Exercise is the best mood elevator of all! By releasing pain-relieving endorphins, exercise reduces anxiety, relieves depression and extends your lifespan. Today doctors regularly write their patients an "exercise prescription" for relief from disorders like fibromyalgia, addiction, and major depression for which drugs are only moderately helpful.

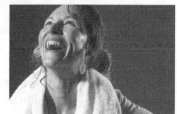

How is exercise tied to brown fat activity and weight control? Brown fat is highly active metabolically, very different from the white fat you see deposited around your body. Brown fat, bound to your skeleton, is filled with tiny, brown-colored mitochondria and cytochromes, chemical powerhouses that produce energy in your cells. Brown fat is thermogenically responsive. When you take in excess calories, your body compensates in part by producing more heat to burn them off instead of storing them as white fat. Brown fat activity explains why some people can overeat and stay slim while other people eat far less but gain weight easily.

For most of us, brown fat becomes less active as we age. Instead of calories being burned off, they get stored as white fat. Keeping your brown fat activated is a big key to weight control as you age. Brown fat activity goes down if your diet is poor and you don't get regular aerobic exercise to increase your lung capacity and elevate your heart rate. Putting on weight and not exercising causes lean muscle tissue to break down, leaving you flabby, with less energy, and ultimately, with even less brown fat activity to burn calories.

We know exercise optimizes metabolism and stimulates calorie burning. Brown fat activity is of enormous interest to exercise coaches and trainers today. The jury is still out on exactly how brown fat and exercise work together, but there's no question that BAT activity and exercise maximize lean muscle and calorie burning. Some experts say using thermogenic foods and supplements before exercise increases energy and helps spare muscle mass. Others say exercise does not maximize brown fat activity, and may interfere with BAT thermogenesis because it raises body temperature. This group recommends exercise 3 to 4 hours after taking a thermogenic formula. They also advise deep breathing and other exercises which don't raise body temperature and don't interfere with BAT thermogenesis (BAT is boosted by exposure to cold).

Exercise-induced thermogenesis (EIT) is different than BAT thermogenesis. EIT is responsible for most body thermogenesis, an automatic response to muscle work that takes place largely in skeletal muscle, not brown fat.

Can't find a recommended product? Call the 800 number in Product Resources for the store nearest you.

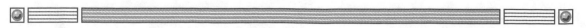

My own sense? Both opinions have merit. People differ widely and dramatically as to how their bodies handle calorie burning and weight loss. Almost everything we are comes into play.... gender, age, ethnicity, environment, background, eating habits, stress reactions and fitness levels. My advice? Eat thermogenic foods and try some of the herbs and supplements that boost calorie-burning. Exercise when it's best for you. Most people see moderate results fairly rapidly in terms of energy, muscle tone and weight loss.

Is exercise difficult for you?

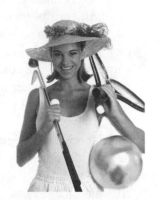

Make it easy. It's as available as your front door. Today we know that you don't have to "feel the burn" to reap the rewards of exercise. Two studies in the Journal of the American Medical Association show moderate exercise is as beneficial for cardiovascular health and overall fitness as high intensity workouts. Pick an exercise that you enjoy and stick to it! A daily, thirty minute walk, breathing deeply, for even a mile a day (½ mile out, ½ mile back) makes a big difference in weight and fat loss. Deep exhalations release metabolic waste along with CO_2; deep inhalations flood your body with fresh oxygen. A walk cleanses your circulatory system, and improves heart strength and muscle tone. It reduces heart attack risk, especially in women. Think of sunlight on your body as heliotherapy adding natural vitamin D for skin and bone health. If you don't exercise, you'll not only lose muscle, you'll lose up to 1% of your bone mass <u>every year</u>.... beginning as early as age 35. Studies show women who exercise regularly after menopause lose 50% less bone than women who don't exercise. Walking, jogging or cycling increases both muscle and bone mass.

Dancing is great aerobic exercise. Legs and lungs both show rapid improvement, not to mention the fun you have. Any kind of dancing is a good workout, and the breathlessness you feel afterward is the best sign of aerobic benefits. Swimming works all parts of your body at once. Noticeable upper arm and thigh definition improvement comes quickly with regular swimming. Just fifteen to twenty steady laps, two or three times a week, and a more streamlined body is yours. (I use water weights when I swim to maximize results.) Cycling gets you somewhere while you exercise. Exercise classes are available, everyday, everywhere at low prices.

If your schedule is so busy that you hardly have time to breathe, let alone exercise, but still want the benefits, there is an all-in-one aerobic exercise. It has gotten resounding enthusiasm and response rates for aerobic activity and muscle tone - all in one minute. The exercise sounds very easy, but is actually very difficult, that's why it works so well. You will be breathless (the sign of an effective aerobic workout) before you know it.

Try this: Simply lie flat on your back on a rug or carpet. Rise to a full standing position any way you can, and lie down flat on your back again. That's the whole exercise. Stand and lie down, stand and lie down — for one minute. Typical repetitions for most people with average body tone are six to ten times in 60 seconds. The record time for an athlete in top competitive condition is 20-24 times in a minute. Be very easy on yourself. Repeat only as many times as you feel comfortable and work up gradually. It is worth a try because it exercises muscles, lung capacity and circulatory system so well.... but don't overdo it.

Watchwords: Choose activities that work for you conveniently and easily. Always make rest a part of it. Work out harder one day, go easy the next; or exercise for several days and take two days off. It's better for body balance, and will increase your energy levels when you exercise the next time. After a regular program is started, exercising four days a week will increase fitness level; exercising three days a week maintains fitness level; exercising two days a week will decrease a high fitness level. But any amount of exercise is better than nothing at all. Vigorous physical exercise is the most efficient way to burn white fat, but every series of stretches and exercises you do tones, elasticizes, shapes and contours your skin, connective tissue and muscles.

Can't find a recommended product? Call the 800 number in Product Resources for the store nearest you.

  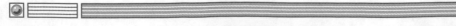

Eating for Energy and Performance

Body building is 85% nutrition. At any level, nutrition is the most important factor for exercise or sports performance. Good nutrition helps eliminate fluctuating energy levels, abnormal fatigue, and susceptibility to injury or illness. Optimal nutrition is the basis for high performance. Protein or carbo-loading before an event can't make up for nutrient short-falls. No anabolic supplement of any kind can give you athletic excellence if you have an inferior diet. When you eat junk foods, you pay the penalty of poor performance.

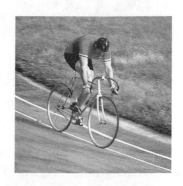

Exercise is integral to good nutrition. In fact, it becomes a nutrient in itself. Most of us notice that when we're exercising we're not hungry. We get thirsty as our bodies call for water and electrolyte replacement... but not hungry. Muscles become toned, heart and lungs become stronger, and fats are lost, but the body doesn't call for calorie replacement right away. Its own glycogens lift blood sugar levels for a feeling of well being. This phenomenon is one of the reasons rapid results are achieved in a body streamlining program. Exercise also promotes an "afterburn" effect, boosting metabolic rate for up to *48 hours* after a workout.

The breakdown of a high performance diet:

—*Sixty to seventy-five percent* should be clean-burning complex carbohydrates—whole grains, pasta, vegetables, rice, beans and fruits. They improve performance, promote muscle fuel storage, and absorb easily without excess fats that slow down weight loss and sap energy.

—*Twenty to twenty-five percent* should be protein—from whole grains, nuts, beans, low fat dairy and soy foods, yogurt, kefir, eggs, and some poultry, fish, and seafood. Vegetable protein is best for mineral absorption and bone density. Strength and muscle mass decline if you get too little protein. But too much protein, especially from red meats (as in the popular "Zone" and "Zone clone" diets) hampers performance. High protein diets can cause dehydration, and can be dangerous even for very fit people. Excess amino acids from too much protein cause toxic ammonia to form in the body. Too much protein may overload your kidneys (you'll feel lower back pain) as your body struggles to eliminate waste by-products from inefficient metabolism. I recommend serious "zoners" drink 10 or 11 glasses a day to make up for water losses. To learn more, see "Protein in a Healing Diet" on pg.98 of this book.

—*Ten to fifteen percent* of an athletic diet should be in energy-producing fats and oils needed for glycogen storage. The best fats are mono-unsaturated oils, a little butter, nuts, low fat cheeses and whole grain snacks.

Other diet fuel: liquid nutrients like fruit juices for natural sugars, mineral waters and electrolyte replacement drinks for potassium, magnesium and sodium. Put superfoods high on your list; they're concentrated, bio-available nutrients that offer an athlete the edge in strength and stamina. Green superfood blends contain concentrates of spirulina, alfalfa, chlorella, sea greens, barley grass, blue-green algae and wheat grass. Bee pollen and royal jelly are rich in essential nutritional elements. Garlic is good for athletes, providing potent antioxidants for anti-fatigue, anti-stress effects.

Surprise! Caffeine sometimes gets a bad rap, but it can boost stamina during your workout by lowering the amount of glycogen your muscles use. It only takes about 2mg to get the effect.

Fluid facts for athletes:

• Two-thirds of your body water is inside your cells (intracellular fluid); the remaining one-third is outside cells (extracellular fluid); only a small portion is in blood plasma.

• Drink plenty of water. Your body needs it to filter and release waste and impurities, and your liver needs it to metabolize stored fats for energy. Six to eight glass of water a day are a must, even if you don't feel thirsty.

Can't find a recommended product? Call the 800 number in Product Resources for the store nearest you.

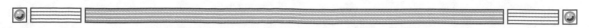

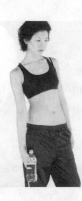

• Dehydration during prolonged exercise causes a drop in blood volume and increases stress on the heart by forcing it to pump harder.

• Water's most important function? For athletes, it's regulating body temperature via sweating. Potassium, magnesium, iron and other minerals are also lost in sweat. Drink at least 16-oz. of high quality water two hours before exercise to avoid exercise-related water-mineral loss. Consider an electrolyte replacement formula like Alacer ELECTROMIX to keep minerals in balance.

• A body water loss of 4-6% reduces muscle endurance and muscle strength. A loss of more than 6% of body weight through sweating causes severe heat cramps, heat exhaustion, heat stroke, coma and in some cases of long distance runners without water, even death.

Three Proven Strength Diets

Strength nutrition enhances endurance, speed and focus. Strength nutrition helps prevent injury, reduces stress, lets you carry more oxygen, replaces ATP, removes lactic acid and improves electrolyte balance. For the serious athlete, strength nutrition can create the edge that makes the difference between winning and losing, especially in the last burst of energy for peak performance.

Athletes' nutrition needs are considerably greater than those of the average person. Normal RDAs are far too low for high performance or competition needs. A training diet should be high in complex carbohydrates for maximum fuel use for muscles, and plenty of amino acids precursors to enhance the body's own growth hormone production. It is vitamin and mineral rich for solid building blocks. Consult a good sports nutritionist, or knowledgable person at a health food store or gym to determine your specific supplement requirements. The important consideration is not body weight, but body composition

Three tried and true strength nutrition diets to choose from:

All three diets are useful for a serious, performing athlete. Competitive training and a training diet alone cannot insure success. Rest time and building energy reserves are also necessary to tune the body for maximum efficiency. When not in competition or pre-event training, extra high nutrient amounts are not needed, and can be hard for the body to handle. A reduced density diet is better for maintaining tone, and can be easily increased for competitive performance.

1: **HIGH ENERGY, ACTIVE LIFESTYLE DIET** - targeted for people who lack consistent daily energy and tire easily, and those who need more endurance and strength for hard physical jobs or long hours. It is also for weekend sports enthusiasts who wish to accomplish more than their present level of nutrition allows.

2: **MODERATE AEROBIC DIET** - for people who work out 3 to 4 times a week. It emphasizes complex carbohydrates for smooth muscle use, and moderate fat and protein amounts. Complex carbohydrates also produce glycogen for the body, resulting in better energy and endurance.

3: **HIGH PERFORMANCE-TRAINING DIET** - focuses on energy for competitive sports action, and long range stamina. For the serious athlete, and for those who are consciously body building for high workout achievement, this diet is a good foundation for significantly improved performance. Sports tests show that adjusting the diet before competition can increase endurance 200% or more — well worth consideration.

Note: See the following 2 pages for a FOOD EXCHANGE LIST and a FOOD AMOUNTS CHART by diet so you can adjust individual needs.

Can't find a recommended product? Call the 800 number in Product Resources for the store nearest you.

  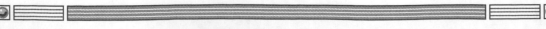

Food Exchange List

Any food in a category may be exchanged one-for-one with any other food in that category. Portion amounts are given for a man weighing 170 pounds, and a woman weighing 130 pounds.

Grains, Breads and Cereals: One serving is approximately one cup of cooked grains, like brown rice, millet, barley, bulgur, kashi, couscous, corn, oats, and whole grain pasta;
   —or one cup of dry cereals, such as bran flakes, Oatios, or Grapenuts;
   —or three slices of wholegrain bread; or three six-inch corn tortillas; or two chapatis or whole wheat pitas;
   —or twelve small wholegrain crackers; or two rice cakes.

Vegetables:
   Group A: One serving is as much as you want of lettuce (all kinds), Chinese greens and peas, raw spinach and carrots, celery, cucumbers, endive, sea greens, watercress, radishes, green onions and chives.
   Group B: One serving is 2 cups cabbage or alfalfa sprouts; or 1½ cups cooked bell peppers or mushrooms;
   —or one cup cooked asparagus, cauliflower, chard, sauerkraut, eggplant, zucchini or summer squash;
   —or ¾ cup cooked broccoli, green beans; onions or mung bean sprouts; or ½ cup vegetable juice cocktail;
   Group C: One serving is approximately 1½ cups cooked carrots;
   —or one cup cooked beets, potatoes, or leeks; or one cup fresh carrot or vegetable juice;
   —or ½ cup cooked peas, corn, artichokes, winter squash or yams.

Fruits: One serving is approximately one apple, nectarine, mango, pineapple, peach or orange;
   —or 4 apricots, medjool dates or figs; or half a honeydew or cantaloupe;
   or 20 to 24 cherries or grapes; or 1½ cups strawberries or other berries.

Dairy: One serving is 1 cup of whole milk, buttermilk or full fat yogurt, for 3gm fat;
   —or one cup of low-fat milk or yogurt, for 2gm of fat;
   —or one cup of skim milk or non-fat yogurt, for less than 1gm of fat;
   —or one ounce of low fat hard cheese, such as swiss or cheddar;
   —or ⅓ cup of non-fat dry milk powder.

Poultry, Fish and Seafood: One serving is 4-oz. of white fish, for 3gm of fat;
   —or four ounces of chicken or turkey, white meat, no skin for 4gm of fat;
   —3 oz. baked tuna (bluefin) for 6.5 gm; 3 oz. baked salmon for 9.5g fat (omega 3's)
   —or one cup of tuna or salmon, shrimp, scallops, oysters, clams or crab for 3 to 4gm of fat.

Note: Beef, veal, lamb, pork, sausage, ham, and bacon are high in saturated fats and cholesterol, and unsound as a use of planetary resources. Many are routinely injected with hormones and antibiotics.

High Protein Meat and Dairy Substitutes: One serving is approximately four ounces of tofu (one block);
   —or ½ cup low fat or dry cottage cheese; or ⅓ cup ricotta, parmesan or mozzarella;
   —or one egg; or ½ cup cooked beans or brown rice.

Fats and Oils: One serving is approximately one teaspoon of butter, ghee (clarified butter) or organic trans-fat free shortening (available from Spectrum Organics' organic palm oil processed at low heat) for 5gm of fat;
   —or 1 tablespoon of salad dressing or mayonnaise for 5gm. of fat; low fat, healthier varieties are available.
   —or 1 tsp. of poly-unsaturated or mono-unsaturated vegetable oil for 5gm. of fat.
   —or 1 tsp. flax seed oil, *perilla* oil or Udo's PERFECTED OIL BLEND for slightly less than 5 gm. of fat (all are ideal, highly usable fat sources).

The following foods are high in fat; amounts are equivalent to 1 fat serving on the diet chart. Use sparingly.
   —2 tablespoons of light cream, half and half, or sour cream; 1 tablespoon of heavy cream;
   —⅙ slice of avocado; ¼ cup of sunflower, sesame, or pumpkin seeds;
   —12 almonds, cashews or peanuts; 20 pistachios or Spanish peanuts; 4 walnut or pecan halves.

Can't find a recommended product? Call the 800 number in Product Resources for the store nearest you.

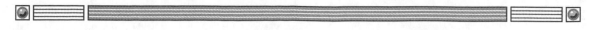

Supplements & Herbs For Bodybuilding & Sports Performance

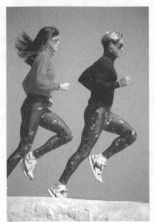

Strength training supplements help both the serious and casual athlete. They help build muscle tissue, maintain low body fat, and improve endurance when the body is under the stress of a workout series. Supplements optimize recuperation time between workouts, enhance muscle growth and speed healing from sports injuries. Antioxidant supplements have become critical for sports performance, because they help maintain the body's defenses against exercise-induced free radicals to combat injury and speed muscle recovery.

The way you take training supplements is as important as what you take. Your program will be more productive if you balance supplements between workout days and rest days. Muscle growth occurs on rest days as your body uses the training you've given it. Increase enhancement by taking vitamins, minerals, and glandulars on rest days. Take proteins, amino acids, anabolics and herbs on workout days, before the workout.

Herbal supplements are good partners in your exercise program. Herbs act as effective food nutrients for body building, offering extra strength for energy and endurance. They have been used since ancient times by athletes. Yarrow and other herbs were used by the gladiators to help heal wounds. Asian warriors and wrestlers used herbs to increase endurance and strength from pre-history. Today, in Russia, Germany, Japan and Korea, herbs are extremely popular with sports enthusiasts and athletes. American athletes are just beginning to see the value of herbs for a winning body.

Herbal supplements work better in combination, and they work best when taken on exercise days, either in the morning with a protein drink, or 30 minutes before exertion.

Herbs you can use for your exercise program:

1: **Antioxidant herbs for aerobic support:** *Siberian eleuthero, ginkgo biloba, barley grass, spirulina, chlorella, panax ginseng, rosemary, white pine bark;* Crystal Star ENERGY GREEN RENEWAL™ drink; Jagulana JIAOGULAN caps; Gaia Herbs ANTIOXIDANT SUPREME.

2: **Adaptogen herbs for body stress:** *Panax ginseng, Chinese astragalus, schizandra, ashwaganda, fo-ti, cordyceps, jiaogulan, Siberian eleuthero, damiana;* Crystal Star ATHLETIC PERFORMANCE™ caps and RESTORE YOUR STRENGTH™ drink, Planetary GINSENG REVITALIZER caps.

3: **Anti-Inflammatory herbs for injuries:** Crystal Star STRESS OUT MUSCLE RELAXER™ drops (often results in 20 minutes), *turmeric extract, St. John's wort oil,* Crystal Star DR. ENZYME™ with Protease and Bromelain. *Lavender* essential oil, mixed with almond oil relieves inflammation; BHI TRAUMEEL *arnica* gel (excellent results); BROMELAIN-PAPAIN 1500mg. for muscle and ligament repair; Transformation PUREZYME helps break down scar build-up, shortens recovery time; Pacific Biologic ORTHOFLEX (herbal analgesic for pain).

4: **Energy Stimulants:** *guarana, ginkgo biloba, damiana, kola nut, gotu kola;* Crystal Star ATHLETIC PERFORMANCE™ caps. Source Naturals TRIBULUS TERRESTRIS caps; Yogi GINSENG NRG tea; Prince of Peace ULTRA GINKGO PLUS ENDURANCE FORMULA vials.

5: **Stamina and endurance herbs:** *Siberian eleuthero, sarsaparilla, wild yam, schizandra, spirulina, American and Chinese panax ginseng, fo-ti;* Crystal Star FEEL GREAT NOW™ with ginseng caps; Jagulana JIAOGULAN PLUS ENERGY FORMULA; Maitake Products SUPER CORDYCEPS; Planetary CORDYCEPS POWER CS-4 (CS-4 shows good results for increasing endurance and exercise performance in clinical trials).

6: **Adrenal tonics:** *licorice, schizandra, ginseng;* Crystal Star ADRENAL ENERGY BOOST™ or Planetary SCHIZANDRA ADRENAL COMPLEX; Herbs Etc. ADRENO-TONIC.

7: **Anabolic stimulants:** *suma, ginseng, Rhaponticum carthamoides(Maral root);* Prince of Peace RED GINSENG-ROYAL JELLY vials; Metabolic Response Modifiers ECDY-20; Always Young HGH WORKOUT FOR MEN.

Can't find a recommended product? Call the 800 number in Product Resources for the store nearest you.

8: **Blood tonics:** *chlorella, spirulina, barley grass, yellow dock, sarsaparilla and goldenseal*; Crystal Star ENERGY GREEN RENEWAL™ and RESTORE YOUR STRENGTH™ drinks; Pure Planet CHLORELLA; Nature's Answer BLOOD SUPPORT.

9: **Circulation activators:** *ginkgo biloba, cayenne, ginger, hawthorn, butcher's broom*; Crystal Star DR. VITALITY™ caps; Zand HAWTHORN FORMULA; Futurebiotics CIRCUPLEX; Natural Balance GREAT LEGS (excellent for varicose veins and feelings of heaviness in the legs).

10: **Metabolic enhancers:** *sarsaparilla, licorice root, bee pollen, royal jelly, panax ginseng, green tea*; Crystal Star ATHLETIC PERFORMANCE ENERGY™ caps and THERMO-THINNER™ caps; Nature's Secret BURN MORE; Gaia Herbs THYROID SUPPORT.

11: **Muscle relaxers for soreness:** *valerian, passionflowers, kava*; Crystal Star STRESS OUT MUSCLE RELAXER™ drops; New Chapter ZYFLAMEND formulas; Natural Balance SUPER FLEX JOINT FORMULA.

12: **Workout recovery - Nerve strength:** *sarsaparilla, suma, carrot*; Crystal Star DR. VITALITY™ tea; and FEEL GREAT NOW!™ with GINSENG caps.

13: **Mineral-rich herbs:** *yellow dock root, barley grass, horsetail, dandelion*; Crystal Star OCEAN MINERALS™ caps; Flora CALCIUM, MAGNESIUM, ZINC AND VITAMIN D liquid; Flora VEGESIL.

Note: Mineral balance is critical for an athlete at any level. Macro and trace minerals are built into every bio-chemical action of athletic movement... energy, digestion, use of protein, nerve transmission, muscle contraction, metabolism, cholesterol levels and blood sugar. Athletes should replace electrolytes lost after workouts. Nature's Path TRACE-LYTE and Alacer ELECTROMIX are both good electrolyte replacement formulas.

Do you really need steroids for high performance?

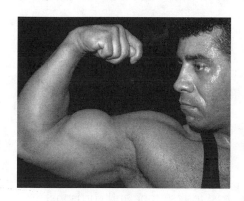

There is enormous pressure on athletes to excel today.... money, national recognition, even international standing all push athletes to ever higher performance. As standards of skill rise in sports competition, the temptation can be almost overwhelming to do whatever is necessary to win. Steroid use, legal and illegal has increased dramatically in response. The downside is, unfortunately, also dramatic. Steroids lead to wholesale destruction of gland tissue, stunted growth from bone closure, male testicle shrinkage, low sperm counts with sterility (noticeable after only a few months of use), male breast enlargement, male pattern baldness, acne, high blood pressure, weakening of connective tissue, jaundice from liver malfunction, poor circulation, and hostile personality behavior and facial changes.

Superhormone steroids like **ANDRO** (*androstenedione*), a by-product of DHEA, are very popular. Studies show ANDRO increases the body's testosterone supply up to three times the normal level! Yet research shows conflicting reports. Studies on one supplement, Norandro, show that ANDRO may not be effective for increasing strength or muscle mass. According to experts at Allergy Research, ANDRO is most effective for accelerating healing from sports injuries. Even though it's synthesized from a natural source, the seeds of the Scotch Pine tree, all reports advise caution, and monitoring under the supervision of a health professional. In some cases, it can boost testosterone levels too much and too fast, causing aggressive behavior and acne. ANDRO may actually convert into estrogen in the body, possibly leading to breast growth or water retention in men. And, the conversion of androstenedione to estrogen can accelerate aging in both men and women! New, cutting edge ANDRO products contains *5, 7-dihydroxyflavone*, a natural flavone which helps block estrogen conversion and reduce androgen side efffects. Don't use ANDRO if you have any hormone-related problems like cancers of the breast, prostate or testes. People with acne, liver disorders, BPH, dysmenorrhea or Cushing's adrenal syndrome should also avoid ANDRO.

Can't find a recommended product? Call the 800 number in Product Resources for the store nearest you.

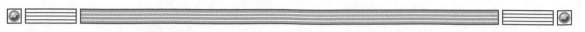

Creatine (*methyl guanidine-acetic acid*), a popular steroid-like supplement, is a booming $100 million business today; in many areas of the country like California and Florida, it is a mainstream supplement. Naturally found in large amounts in the muscles, where it helps provide the energy (ATP) muscles need to move, creatine is formed when the amino acids arginine, methionine and glycine combine in the body. Creatine supplementation is especially useful for the rapid, explosive movements required in many sports, and for increasing muscle mass. But there are risk factors. Creatine forces muscles to retain too much water, leading to muscle strains, dehydration and possible kidney problems. Rod Fleming, a respected colleague and registered physical therapist says, "Dehydration is consistently a problem for people using creatine. I have also personally seen very unusual pectoral muscle tears in people taking creatine supplements. I advise against it." Some users report diarrhea and nausea from creatine loading. Take creatine *only* as directed and drink plenty of fluids. (Don't mix it with fruit juice; creatine can react with fruit juice and transform into creatinine, a metabolic waste product. Don't mix supplemental creatine with caffeine. Caffeine negates creatine benefits.) Creatine food sources are meats and fish.

Ribose is a sports supplement with some advantages over ANDRO and creatine. Ribose is a simple sugar our cells use to convert nutrients into ATP. Supplemental ribose increases energy stores in the heart and muscle cells, especially useful for people with cardiac insufficiency (diminished blood flow to the heart) and athletes who want to recharge muscle endurance and decrease recovery time from workouts. Universal Nutrition's Ribose Caps — maintenance doses equal 3 to 5 grams per day.

HMB (*beta-hydroxy-beta-methylbutyrate*), the latest rage in sports nutrition, found in small amounts in alfalfa and catfish, is a metabolite of the amino acid leucine involved in protein synthesis. HMB promoters say it helps prevent protein breakdown, builds lean muscle tissue, and increases strength gains from resistance training. HMB has gotten mixed reviews for sports enhancement in clinical trials. It is expensive (around $30 for a ten-day supply), but there are no known safety issues as of this writing. 3 grams of HMB per day in combination with resistance training is the recommended dose.

Can herbal steroids do the strength enhancement job?

There are no magic bullets for energy or endurance in sports, but plant-derived steroids called phytosterols do have growth activity similar to that of free form amino acids and anabolic steroids. Amino acids can act as steroid alternatives to help build the body to competitive levels without chemical steroid consequences. They also help release growth hormone, detox ammonia, promote fast recuperation, increase stamina, and support peak performance.

The most well-known of these herbs are:
—*Damiana*, a mild aphrodisiac and nerve stimulant.
—*Sarsaparilla*, *Smilax*, coaxes the body to produce more anabolic hormones, testosterone and cortisone.
—*Saw Palmetto*, a urethral toning herb that increases blood flow to the sex organs; balances testosterone.
—*Siberian and Panax Ginsengs*, adaptogens for balance and energy; increase protein content in muscles.
—*Wild Yam*, an anti-spasmodic that prevents cramping. Contains diosgenin, a precursor to progesterone.
—*Yohimbe*, a testosterone precursor for body building, and potent aphrodisiac for both men and women.
—*Tribulus Terrestris*, an ancient treatment for low libido and impotence; increases strength and stamina.
—*Cordyceps*, a TCM tonic, has testosterone-like effects for stamina and endurance, increases lung capacity and shortens recovery time, excellent for serious athletes.
—*Rhaponticum carthamoides* (*Maral root*)- a non-hormonal anabolic stimulant; contains 20-Hydroxyecdysone (called Ecdy20), which boosts protein production and builds muscle. Russian research shows *Rhaponticum* increases muscle mass and decreases body fat, boosts capacity and endurance, and reduces fatigue. Better than Dianabol without the side effects. Note: Spinach is a good food source of Ecdy 20.

Can't find a recommended product? Call the 800 number in Product Resources for the store nearest you.

Supplementing Your Individual Exercise Requirements

The following pages detail three separate supplement programs:
1) high energy active lifestyle; 2) moderate aerobic workout; 3) high performance and competitive training.

Supplements for a high energy active lifestyle:

Use superfoods to supercharge your diet for energy. Some to try:
—Crystal Star ENERGY GREEN RENEWAL™ drink - a whole green drink with herbs.
—Pure Form POWER GREEN PRO- with certified organic barley grass juice, alfalfa juice and sprouts.
—NutriCology PRO-GREENS with EFA's - green superfoods, herbs, sea greens.
—Nature's Path TRACE-MIN-LYTE - full spectrum minerals from sea greens.
—All One MULTIPLE GREEN (no aspartame, no sugar).
—Esteem SUPER PRO - an ultra-multi plus megaforce nutrients.
—Barleans GREENS- high antioxidants to fight free radicals.
—Universal Nutrition's RIBOSE Caps- for ATP energy.
—Imperial Elixir SIBERIAN GINSENG and SPIRULINA.
—Crystal Star FEEL GREAT NOW™ with ginseng - long range energy and stamina.
—Nature's Secret BEYOND ENDURANCE stamina - energy shake with high protein and amino acids.

Supplements for a moderate aerobics workout:

Superfoods: Boost deep body strength and faster recovery. Some to try:
—Wakunaga KYO GREEN HARVEST BLEND - consists of 44 immune supporting nutrients.
—Green Foods MAGMA PLUS - phytonutrient-rich, 57 ingredients plus prebiotics (FOS) and probiotics.
—Pines MIGHTY GREENS SUPERFOODS - a premium blend of organic greens, superfoods, herbs.
—Esteem GREEN HARVEST- green superfoods plus probiotics, antioxidants and plant enzymes.
—Futurebiotics VITAL GREEN - contains alfalfa leaf juice, barley grass juice, spirulina, and chlorella.
—Nature's Secret ULTIMATE GREEN - 6 superfoods providing protein, vitamins, minerals, and antioxidants.

Minerals: You need minerals to run - for bone density, speed and endurance; as anabolic enhancers.
—Potassium-magnesium-bromelain combo - relieves muscle fatigue/lactic acid buildup.
—Cal-mag-zinc combo with boron - to prevent muscle cramping and maintain bone integrity.
—Chromium picolinate, 200mcg - for sugar regulation and glucose energy use.
—Zinc picolinate, 30-50mg daily for athletes - for immunity, healing of epithelial injuries.
—Crystal Star OCEAN MINERALS™, IRON SOURCE™, CALCIUM MAGNESIUM SOURCE™ caps.
—Herbal Products & Development LAND & SEA high energy mineral tonic.
—Nature's Path CAL-LYTE or HEMA-LYTE iron, electrolytes for strong muscles.
—Eidon MINERAL BALANCING program- hair mineral analysis plus personal supplement program.
—Lane Labs ADVACAL - serious bone builder for active menopausal women and andropausal men.

Vitamins: Metabolize blood and body fats, and enhance muscle growth.
—B-complex, 100mg or more - for nerve health, muscle cramping, carbohydrate metabolism.
—Pure Essence Labs ONE 'N' ONLY- essential nutrients, green superfoods and herbal adaptogens.
—Pure Form LIQUID VITAMIN- ionic minerals, vitamins, amino acids, ginseng, CoQ10, grape seed ext.
—Diamond Formulas HEALTHY HORIZONS- loaded with antioxidants and stress reducers.
—ProLab TRAINING PAKS- provides B-Vitamins to break down carbohydrates, cal/mag for strong bones.

Antioxidants: To increase oxygen use, reduce free radical damage, and to protect against pollutants.
—MICROHYDRIN PLUS caplets- one of the most potent free radical fighters available.

Can't find a recommended product? Call the 800 number in Product Resources for the store nearest you.

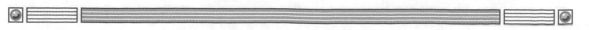

—CoQ-10 - a co-enzyme factor to release energy; excellent for sports enthusiasts with heart conditions.
—Wakunaga KYOLIC SUPER FORMULA 105 - several potent antioxidants.
—NutriCology ANTIOX FORMULA 11- offers a potent mixed antioxidant formulation.

Sports Drinks/Electrolyte Replacements: Use after exertion to replace body minerals.
—Alacer ELECTROMIX, EMERGEN-C and Knudsens RECHARGE drinks.
—Anabol Naturals CARBO SURGE and Nature's Path TRACE-LYTE liquid electrolytes.
—Trace Minerals CONCENTRACE.
—Unipro ENDURA.

Testosterone Support: As part of a natural anabolic program for increased male muscle hardness.
—Crystal Star ATHLETE'S PERFORMANCE ENERGY™ with panax ginseng.
—Muira Puama Bark (potency wood), saw palmetto and sarsaparilla (smilax) herbs (best in combo).
—Anabol Naturals DHEA REJUVAPLEX with L-Glutamine and crystalline vitamine B-12.
—Planetary ANTLER VELVET FULL SPECTRUM: for stamina, sports energy (harvested humanely).
—Unipro TRIBULUS SYNERGY; Source Naturals TRIBULUS TERRESTRIS.

Stimulants: for quick, temporary, energy.
—Universal Nutrition's RIBOSE Caps- for ATP energy.
—Crystal Star ENERGY EXPRESS™ for men and women.
—Imperial Elixir SIBERIAN GINSENG and SPIRULINA.

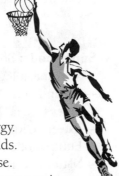

Free Form Amino Acids: Activators to increase body structure and strength.
—Anabol Naturals GH RELEASERS; glutamine 500mg daily with a niacin booster.
—Anabol Naturals AMINO BALANCE - 23 free-form amino acids for tissue repair, energy.
—ProLab AMINO GEL CAPS - complete spectrum essential and nonessential amino acids.
—ProLab LIQUID CARNITINE - strengthen heart and circulatory system during exercise.
—Anabol Naturals MUSCLE OCTANE or AMINO NITRO MAX, BCAAs for ATP energy conversion.
—Glutamine, strong growth hormone release; Unipro BCAA 1000.

Protein/Amino Drinks: Mainstays for muscle building, weight gain, energy, endurance.
—Pure Form WHEY PROTEIN- high branch chain amino acids; chunks of real fruit.
—Metabolic Response Modifiers WHEY PUMPED.
—Unipro PERFECT PROTEIN.
—Bee pollen - complete, natural full spectrum amino acids.
—Unipro PROGAIN- for maximum weight gain and positive nitrogen balance.

Fat Burners: Metabolize blood and body fats, and enhance muscle growth.
—Nature's Path SLIM-LYTE 1200 - chromium to burn fat, not muscle tissue.
—Anabol Naturals GH RELEASERS - metabolic fat burner.
—Pinnacle ALPHA DOPA GROWTH POPPERS- plant based, human growth hormone (HGH).
—Pure Form CALCIUM PYRUVATE- accelerates weight loss; lowers high blood pressure, cholesterol.

Recovery Acceleration: For muscles, joints, ligaments, tendons.
—Proteolytic Enzymes - Transformation PUREZYME for scar tissue build-up, shorter recovery time.
—Crystal Star Dr. ENZYME™ with Protease & Bromelain.
—Bromelain-Papain 500mg - for muscle and ligament repair and strength.
—Universal Nutrition's RIBOSE Caps- for ATP energy.

Can't find a recommended product? Call the 800 number in Product Resources for the store nearest you.

Glandulars: For gland and hormone stimulation.
—Pituitary, 200mg - the master gland, for upper body development.
—Adrenal glandular, Country Life ADRENAL -Tyrosine, Crystal Star ADRENAL ENERGY BOOST™ (herbal).
—Liver, 400mg - for fat metabolism, Enzymatic Therapy LIQUID LIVER EXTRACT w. Siberian Ginseng.
—ProLab PRO PAKS- with orchic extract 1700 mg.

Sports Bars: Rich sources of carbohydrates, protein and fiber. Lots of choices, but many full of sugar, artificial flavors colors, or hidden fat! A small sampling of the best ones available:
—Clif Bars LUNA bars- high protein, low carb with calcium, folic acid, fiber and Omega 3's (women).
—Isagenix ISALEAN bars- high protein with minerals and trace minerals
—Power Foods POWER BARS; SOURCE OF LIFE ENERGY BARS.
—Unipro BURN BAR - low glycemic and supports carbohydrate and protein metabolism.

Supplements for training the serious athlete:
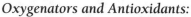

Before you work out:
High Protein Drinks:
—Pure Form WHEY PROTEIN- high branch chain amino acids.
—Unipro MYO SYSTEM XL.
—Metabolic Response Modifiers WHEY PUMPED.
—Garden of Life GOATEIN- goat's milk protein and colostrum with high digestibility.
Unipro PROGAIN- high calories and nutrition for hard gainers.
—All One MULTIPLE VITAMINS & MINERALS GREEN PHYTO BASE (no aspartame, no sugar).

Oxygenators and Antioxidants:
—MICROHYDRIN PLUS caps- the most potent free radical fighter available.
—CoQ-10 120mg daily.
—Unipro AMINO 1000.
—Nature's Path HEMA-LYTE w. electrolytes.
—Nutricology GERMANIUM 150mg to protect the thymus.
—Nature's Secret BEYOND ENDURANCE stamina - energy shake with high protein and amino acids.
—Imperial Elixir SIBERIAN GINSENG and SPIRULINA.

Muscle development and to increase performance:
—Metabolic Response Modifiers BCAA+G - Branched Chain Amino Acids {(BCAAs) and L-Glutamine, essential for building muscle size and strength; Always Young HGH WORKOUT FOR MEN; HGH ADVANCED (women).
—Creatine - 5 to 10gm daily during training (take with plenty of water).
—Arginine-ornithine-lysine to metabolize fats, carnitine to strengthen muscle activity.
—Anabol Naturals AMINO BALANCE, AMINO GH RELEASERS, AMINO NITRO MAX, DIBENCOPLEX.
—Champion MUSCLE-NITROBCAA, ATP energy conversion. Best results: take 10g BCAA's before you train, 3g at night during training. One test finds MUSCLE NITRO improves aerobic capacity by an 300%!

Non-steroidal Anabolic Agents:
—Anabol Naturals DIBENCOPLEX 10000; dibencozide *(coenzyme B-12)* activates protein biosynthesis.
—Universal Nutrition's RIBOSE Caps- for ATP energy.
—Bodyonics ADRENERLIN with Ribose and Mucuna for testosterone help.
—Pure Form SUPER STACK PRO- produces gains in size and strength, and reduces body fat.
—Metabolic Response Modifiers ECDY-20- an extract from Rhaponticum carthamoides *(Maral root-Russian)* shown in studies to be more effective than Dianabol but without side effects.

Can't find a recommended product? Call the 800 number in Product Resources for the store nearest you.

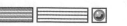

Testosterone Support: To increase muscle hardness.
—Pinnacle METHOXY TEST- natural testosterone production; natural flavones help reduce the amount of testosterone converted in non-anabolic, estrogen hormones.
—Crystal Star ATHLETIC PERFORMANCE ENERGY™ w. panax ginseng; try raw orchic extract, 6 to 10x strength.
—Pure Form TES Sublingual. Use with Pure Form SUPER STACK PRO (substantial increases in strength, energy, endurance; increases muscle size, hardness; blocks estrogen conversion, androgen side effects).
—Unipro TRIBULUS SYNERGY.
—Country Life SUPER STRENGTH YOHIMBE (Use with caution).

Fat Burners:
—Metabolic Response Modifiers META BURN EF (ephedrine-free)- HCA, Green Tea, etc increases fat loss. See a health care provider if taking prescription drugs. Grapefruit compounds can affect drug metabolism.
—Pinnacle MASCULEAN- (men); ESTROLEAN- thermogenics with phytoestrogens (women).
—Anabol Naturals GH RELEASERS; glutamine 500mg daily with a niacin booster.
—Bricker Labs CUT-UP PLUS, Carnitine and Chromium fat-burner.

Herbs:
—Crystal Star FEEL GREAT NOW™ caps with ginseng.
—Crystal Star ATHLETIC PERFORMANCE ENERGY™ caps.
—Futurebiotics MALE POWER: high-potency herb-glandular formula revs your engine.

Recovery Acceleration:
—Metabolic Response Modifiers BCAA+G - Branched Chain Amino Acids (BCAAs) and L-Glutamine for muscle recovery; Always Young HGH ORIGINAL.
—Pure Form POWER JOINT PRO- glucosamine, chondroitin, MSM, and Vitamin C.
—EAS® BETAGEN™- with HMB, Creatine, Grape Powder (take with plenty of water).
—Champion CORTISTAT-PS to reduce cortisol levels and inflammation during a "burning" workout.
—Nature's Path TRACE-LYTE, Knudsen RECHARGE, Alacer ELECTROMIX bring lost minerals.
—Unipro GLUTAGEN & PRO OPTIMIZER (for energy and recovery).
—Eidon SILICA, Now MSM caps help to rebuild and protect joints from injuries.
—NutriCology PHOS-SERINE- reduces muscle breakdown and soreness by lowering cortisol levels.
—Anabol Naturals AMINO BALANCE, AMINO NITRO MAX.

Watchwords for Body Building, Training and Competition:

Cross train. Besides your major sport or activity, supplement it with auxiliary exercise such as bicycling, jogging, walking, swimming or aerobics. This balances muscle use, and keeps heart and lungs strong.

Recuperate. Muscles don't grow during exercise. They grow during rest periods. Alternate muscle workouts with rest days. Exercise different muscle sets on different days, resting each set in between.

Breathe deep. Lung capacity is a prime training factor. Muscles and tissues must have enough oxygen for stamina. Breathe in during exertion, out as you relax for the next rep. Vigorous exhaling is as important as inhaling for the athlete, to expel all carbon dioxide and increase lung capacity for oxygen.

Water. You need good hydration for high performance, cardiovascular activity, overheating and dehydration headaches. An electrolyte replacement drink relieves headaches almost immediately without side effects.

Can't find a recommended product? Call the 800 number in Product Resources for the store nearest you.

   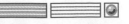

Stretch out. Muscle extensions before and after a workout keep cramping down and muscles loose. Get morning sunlight on the body every day possible for optimal absorption of nutrient fuel.

Weight training. It's good for everybody, no matter what your sport, age or fitness goals. Forty-five minutes of weight bearing exercise three times a week boosts endurance, and strengthens the heart and bones. Women do not get a bulky, masculine physique from lifting weights. They have low levels of testosterone, which influences their type of muscle development. Note: Vitamin E prevents muscle damage from weight training.

Finally.... No pain does not mean no gain. Your exercise doesn't have to hurt to be good for you. Once you work up to a good aerobic level and routine, pushing yourself ever harder won't offer benefits.

How much fat are you burning?

Check your heart rate to see how many fat calories you're burning during your workout. If your heart rate is 70% of maximum, you are burning 20% fat of the total calories per hour/exercise time. If your heart rate is 45% of maximum, you are burning 40% fat of the total calories per hour/exercise time. More fat is burned in low intensity activities because you can take in the extra oxygen needed to burn fat - more than twice as much as carbohydrates per fat gram. (If you reduce maximal effort, you will need to exercise longer to burn the fat.) In addition, there are many high quality diagnostic aids that help you determine your current body fat vs. optimum body fat.

Calorie burning choices:
—**Cross Country Skiing**- 350-1,400 calories per hour
—**Aerobic dancing**- 300-700 calories per hour
—**Calisthenics**- 360 calories per hour
—**Cycling**- 200-850 calories per hour
—**Running**- 400-1,300 calories per hour
—**Stretching**- 60-120 calories per hour
—**Swimming**- 380-850 calories per hour
—**Walking**- 240-430 calories per hour
—**Water Aerobics**- 180-880 calories per hour
—**Weight training**- 260-480 calories per hour

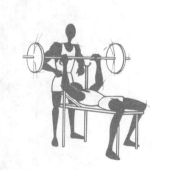
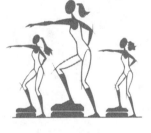
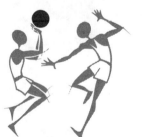
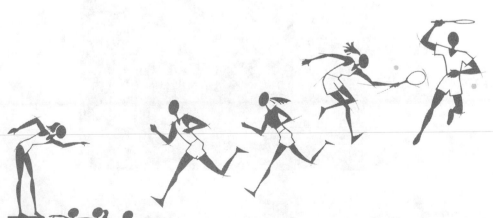

Can't find a recommended product? Call the 800 number in Product Resources for the store nearest you.

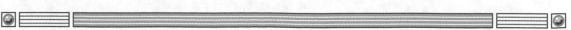

Healing for Pets

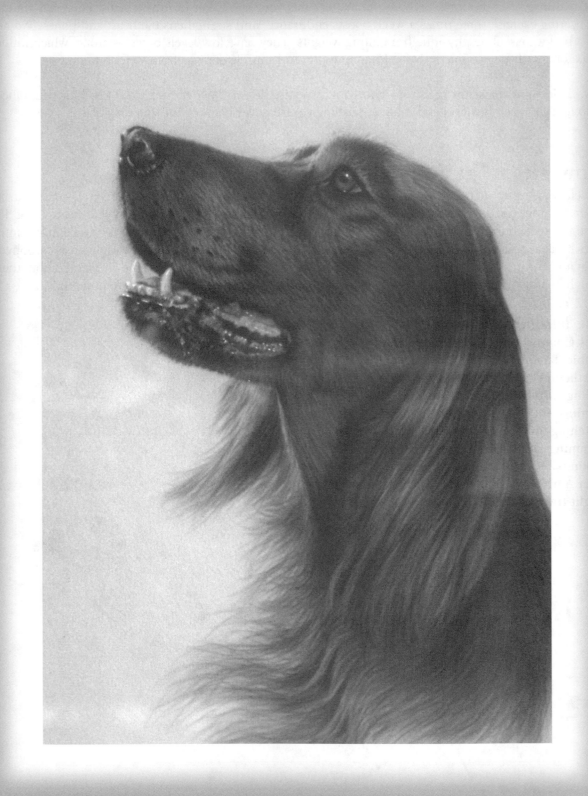

Alternative Healing Options For Pets

Americans are animal lovers. Over 63 million American families have at least one pet. They love us no matter what.... they lower our stress levels, ease our pain and add incredible joy to our lives. Over three-quarters of us feel guilty when we leave our pets at home alone. Having a pet is clearly powerful medicine. The latest research shows pet owners have fewer health problems, visit the doctor less and have less risk for heart disease, high blood pressure and high cholesterol. Today medical doctors even "prescribe pets" to help their depressed patients, the elderly and people dealing with stroke or Alzheimer's. Some evidence shows that animals actually take on the illnesses and stresses of their human counterparts! Clearly, we depend on our pets as they do on us. Strange that somehow, pets have been left behind in good nutrition and health care!

Cats and dogs usually need better nutrition than they get from today's animal foods. Commercial foods often contain low quality ingredients rejected for human consumption, even diseased animal meat laced with high levels of antibiotics. If these foods are the mainstay of your pet's diet, they may destroy its health.

Most brands are saturated with the ingredients we fight to avoid for ourselves...... chemical additives, artificial colors, dyes, preservatives like BHT and BHA — ingredients with known toxicity that are banned for human consumption. Further, much of the meat used in commercial pet food comes from dead, dying, disabled or diseased animals! Did you know that euthanized pets and roadkill are making their way into your pet's food? Cornmeal is a primary ingredient in commercial feed, but many animals, especially cats, cannot tolerate a high carbohydrate diet. Modern pet foods often contain imbalanced essential fatty acids (low Omega 3's and high Omega 6's), leading to skin problems, dull coat or dander. Further, almost all pet food is cooked, pasteurized, canned or microwaved, killing most of the enzymes critical to your pet's healthy body processes.

It's easy to see why so many pets are now victims of the same health problems people face: arthritis, heart disease; thyroid, kidney, adrenal and digestive disorders; chronic infections; diabetes and hypoglycemia; allergies, skin and eye disorders. Like us, animals need the live energy of fresh foods and quality, whole ingredients. Their bodies rely on enzymes even more than ours to protect them from degenerative diseases. It's the reason some animals, even some breeds, tend to eat waste excrement — for the enzymes.

It takes a little more time and effort to feed fresh foods to your pet. I use it as a communication-training time, often with a little by-hand feeding that we both love. Actually, a leftover salad is full of enzyme-rich fresh vegetables, and it makes a big difference to your pet's health. Start them on some veggies young if you can. I remember the day our cat (who recently passed on after living to the ripe old age of 24) turned up her nose at her own cat food and jumped on the kitchen table to eat our dinner salad!

 Healthy Diet for Dogs and Cats

Cats and dogs thrive on the healthy foods that are good for people. A diet with high quality meat or fish, greens and plenty of fresh water is a premium diet for dogs and cats. (Note: Cats need more meat due to their inability to synthesize taurine, and do better with fresh meat. If you have an indoor cat, make up for their inability to catch fresh mice or birds, and offer them uncooked meat.) Most pets need some fresh vegetables every day, too. We've all seen our pets chewing on grass. Mix greens with a little fish, raw liver, kidney or beef, chicken, high quality, low-ash canned or dry food (use meat free of chemicals, and organic vegetables if possible). Most animals like salad greens, pumpkin, sweet potatoes, cucumbers, green peppers, grated carrots (great for birds), parsley, green onions, parsley, celery and vegetable juice. Both dogs and cats like oatmeal, too.

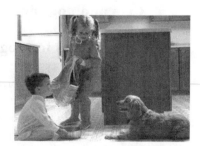

Can't find a recommended product? Call the 800 number in Product Resources for the store nearest you.

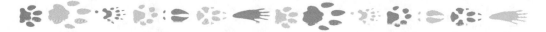

Sadly, most commercial kibble is loaded with preservatives and corn which cause allergies and health problems for many pets. Few commercial animal foods contain any real meat, but rather rely on fillers and "meat by products" with questionable ingredients. Try the <u>chemical-free</u> pet foods found in health food stores. The holistic veterinarians who advise us for this book, feel that many of today's pet ailments are a result of low immune response from chemical-laced foods and environmental pollutants.... just like people.

Note: Animals like people, can become addicted to certain foods if they've eaten them for a long time. Some pets make quick adjustments to diet improvements; others may need new foods introduced gradually. Try a short all-water fast (no more than 24 hours) for an especially finicky pet until it's hungry enough to try the new diet.

Diet watchwords for pets:

1: Try high quality natural pet food instead of commercial brands. Halo-Purely For Pets makes a 100% human grade wet food (SPOT'S STEW) for dogs and cats. Flint River Ranch and Holistic Hounds make good dry dog and cat food that can be mixed with water.

2: Give your pets occasional salmon, shrimp or tuna, and game meats like canned duck or venison for protein-amino acid building blocks, and essential fatty acids for a healthy, shiny coat. These meats, at least (especially if your pet has allergies), haven't been treated with hormones or antibiotics. Uncooked hormone-free beef or turkey from the health food store is a good option. Over the years, I've switched my animals to a largely raw foods diet. As vegetarians, we don't normally keep red meats at our house, but we found that our animals, especially our cats, thrive with raw meat in their daily diet. Note: Avoid raw pork, fish or rabbit meat (high in parasites).

3: Offer occasional dairy foods. Most animals like yogurt, kefir, cottage cheese and eggs. Sprinkle tonic herbs like *nettles, alfalfa or red clover* over food twice a week for extra system strength.

4: A little fruit is OK occasionally to loosen a clogged system, but give sparingly. Dogs and cats like coconut, cantaloupe and apples. Never give a dog raisins or grapes. They've been linked to kidney failure.

5: Give dogs and cats plenty of omega-3 oils from seafood, sea greens, spinach, asparagus and corn. My pets like sea greens so much they eat them dry right from my hand. Add sea veggies (in granular form for ease of use) to your pets food daily to help insure adequate minerals and EFA's in their diet. Sea greens also boost metabolism for overweight pets.

6: Have water always available. Avoid chlorinated water, linked to animal cancer.

7: Feeding time is "together" time for people and animals. Your attention is focused on your pet; they know it and love it. If you're pressed for time, make a meal up all at once and divide it between feedings. For three to four servings: mix, 1 cup quality fish, chicken or turkey (fresh meat is better), 4 tbsp. preservative-free kibble or brown rice, 3 tsp. nutritional yeast, 1 tsp. green superfood powder like barley grass, 1 tsp. flax oil, 1 raw egg, 1 cup chopped vegetables like celery, carrots, zucchini. (If you use broccoli or cauliflower, steam them first so the animal won't get gas). Mix with 1 can chicken-rice soup. Vary dry kibble with brown rice or oatmeal (dogs love oatmeal). I add nutrient-rich sea greens like kelp, dulse or nori to the brown rice.

Cats and dogs need slightly different diets.

—Key foods for dogs:

Include high quality proteins and whole grains for easier digestibility. Dog foods should be low in saturated fat. Contrary to popular advertising, red meat is not a must for their healthy diet. Quality protein can come from eggs, dairy foods, as well as fish or poultry. Dogs tolerate a vegetable diet better than cats because dogs are able to synthesize enough taurine. Make sure your dog's diet doesn't consist of your leftover table scraps (especially spicy foods like cold pizza or anything with onions). Don't feed chocolate of any kind or raisins and grapes to dogs. A little healthy kibble is helpful to deter tartar build-up. PetGuard PREMIUM LIFESPAN dry dog food is one of our favorites (no by products, free of soy, wheat and yeast).

Can't find a recommended product? Call the 800 number in Product Resources for the store nearest you.

Here's a healthy recipe for dog treats I've been using for years. They're a great way to deliver antioxidants, green superfoods, herbs and mushrooms. Mix it to a stiff paste. Spread on a greased cookie sheet to ¼ inch thick. Bake 20-30 minutes at 350° F or until brown. Cut into bite sized snacks. Offer 1-3 cookies daily (adjust to size).

To 1 cup water add:
1 cup smooth peanut butter
1 cup nutritional yeast
1 cup whole wheat flour
3 tbsp. pet powdered supplement of your choice (like Crystal Star Healthy Skin, Coat & Eyes™)
1 tbsp. Green Foods BARLEY DOG
6-10 MICROHYDRIN caps

—Key foods for cats:

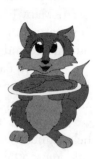

Include raw meat and organ meats like liver, bone meal, sea veggies, whole grains, brown rice and vegetables to provide sustained energy with good ratios of proteins and carbohydrates. Add some wheat bran, corn germ or oatmeal, *borage* or fish oil, and leafy greens three times a week. Taurine, in meat and fish is critical to cats. Without taurine, a cat may develop heart problems or possibly go blind. Too much vitamin A is not good for cats. Excess liver (more than 10% of a cat's diet) may lead to distorted bones, gingivitis, and stiff joints. Raw fish and raw egg whites contain an enzyme, thiaminase which inactivates vitamin B_1, a nutrient animals need to repel fleas and mosquitos. A little healthy kibble is helpful to deter tartar build-up. Old Mother Hubbard WELLNESS dry cat food is one of our favorites (100% Human Grade Ingredients).

Remember:
…Both puppies and kittens need twice the nutrients and calories as adult animals.
…Pregnant and nursing females need more protein, vitamins and minerals.
…Older animals need very digestible foods, less fat and less vitamins, minerals, proteins and sodium.
…Enzymes are essential to health; add in grated veggies to their food.
…Add a small amount of cooked oatmeal to your pets' food once a week to nourish the nervous system.

 Herbs and Supplements for Your Healthy Pet

The same legal battles for access to natural supplements and alternative health care products that were fought (and won) in the 1990's for people, are now being fought for animals. The latest, and ongoing, attack on natural animal health care is the AAFCO (American Assoc. of Feed Control Officials) proposal to ban substances like MSM, glucosamine, chondroitin and herbs from pet foods and supplements. The ban, originally scheduled to go into effect in 2002, would make it impossible for you to purchase many of the healthy pet foods and supplements your animal relies on! As of this writing, many states have chosen to stand behind the safety and efficacy of animal supplements. A few, notably Iowa, have begun issuing notification to companies who sell animal supplements. The National Animal Supplement Council (NASC) has been formed to fight for animal rights to natural supplements and is in ongoing talks with the FDA and AAFCO. To learn more, visit http://nasc.cc.

I continually see that food source supplements are safe, non-invasive medicine for animals. A wholesome diet with a greens supplement needs to be at the base of every healing program. Wheat germ oil, spirulina, kelp, nutritional yeast, bran and lecithin all help keep pets in top condition. Horses, in particular, need the non-toxic joint support that only natural supplements like glucosamine and MSM provide. Herbs and homeopathic remedies are good for animals, too. In fact, humans first learned about herbs from watching animals eat them to cure themselves. Most herbs are effective, gentle, non-toxic, and free of side effects.

For best results, consult your holistic veterinarian or use products specially formulated for pets.

Can't find a recommended product? Call the 800 number in Product Resources for the store nearest you.

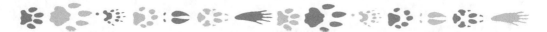

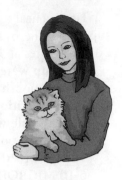

Animal supplement tips:

…Just like us, virtually all pet chronic diseases are directly linked to free radical damage. Consider Ark Naturals, NU-PET GRANULAR GREENS and NU-PET FELINE ANTIOXIDANT for protection against free radicals. PET-LYTE by Nature's Path is a water-based solution of trace minerals for energy and balance.

…In nature, animals consume foods that are whole, raw and fresh. Most domestic animals today eat only processed foods. THE MISSING LINK, by Designing Health is a great all-around nutrient supplement for dogs, cats, birds and horses. It's formulated with natural, human-edible-quality foods and food concentrates. It targets the nutritional gap between what nature provides and what is available in commercial foods.

…Supplement with high omega-3's oils like flax or borage oil to balance the effects of omega-6 overload, common in pet commercial foods. Try Ark Naturals ROYAL COAT and Halo Purely for Pets DREAM COAT.

…Many of today's foods are enzyme deficient, I highly recommend an enzyme supplement for pets. Consider Transformation CAREZYME. Try Green Foods BARLEY DOG and BARLEY CAT, barley grass supplements with garlic, brown rice and nutritional yeast for chlorophyll and enzymes.

…I keep Bach Flower RESCUE REMEDY on hand as a first aid remedy for pet emergencies. RESCUE REMEDY works well for animals that are nervous, scratch compulsively, are depressed or have behavior disorders. It can also help calm an injured or sick animal.

…Animal stress results in widespread behavior problems. Natural therapies can help. WALNUT Flower Remedy helps animals struggling to adapt to a new environment or to a new addition to the family. *Chamomile*, *catnip* and *valerian* soothe acute stress reactions, reduce behavior problems, and are well tolerated by both cats and dogs. Try Ark Naturals HAPPY TRAVELER and Tasha's Herbs EASY DOES IT formulas.

• **Crystal Star Herbal Nutrition has three highly beneficial food supplements for pets.**

—HEALTHY SKIN, COAT & EYES FOR ANIMALS™ offers the benefits of chlorophyll-rich greens to keep their blood strong, their bodies regular and their breath sweet. Rich in carotenes for immune strength, high in antioxidants like vitamin E and life-giving enzymes, HEALTHY SKIN, COAT & EYES FOR ANIMALS™ helps control arthritis and dysplasia symptoms, and protects against damage from rancid fats or poor quality foods. All kinds of animals love it, from hamsters to horses. Some, including our own, won't eat without it!

—AR EASE for ANIMALS™ eases stiffness, boosts mobility in older dogs, especially larger dogs.

—RESTORE YOUR STRENGTH™ drink is an advanced healing combination for pets as well as people. I find this mix to be rapidly restorative for animal systems. Even sick or injured animals seem to know instinctively that it is good for them, and will eagerly take it as a broth from an eye dropper.

Bodywork for a Healthy Pet

• Acupuncture shows excellent results for back pain (horses) and ear infections (dogs).

• Massage therapy and herbal hot packs work for older pets who have dysplasia or arthritis.

• Give your pet plenty of fresh air, exercise and water. Brush and comb your animals often. It keeps their coats shiny, circulation stimulated, and they love the attention. (Brush cats gently; their skin is so sensitive.)

• Avoid chemical-impregnated flea collars. They may have DDT or a nerve gas in them — potentially toxic to your children, your pet, and the environment. Use a mild shampoo with herbal oils like eucalyptus and rosemary instead. The oils interfere with an insect's ability to sense animal's moisture, heat and breath.

• Sprinkle cedar shavings around the animal's bed to keep insects away and to make the area smell nice.

• Halo-Purely For Pets, DERMA-DREAM, Ark Naturals ROYAL COAT and Nature's Path PET-HEAL-AIDE are natural healing skin salves for mange, skin sores and insect bites.

• Finally, pet your pet. Love is always the best medicine. They need it as much as you do.

Can't find a recommended product? Call the 800 number in Product Resources for the store nearest you.

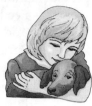

Nutritional Healing For Animals

Special contributions to Animal Healing section come from esteemed experts in holistic animal care.

Except in emergency situations, an optimal diet should be your key concern for natural animal healing. Concerned vets tell me that many animal health problems today are actually caused by poor diets. Health problems are much harder to turn around when highly processed foods are used as the major part of your pet's diet. If possible, use meats without hormones or nitrates and give your pet organically grown veggies.

AMYLOIDOSIS:
—Amyloid, a protein-polysaccharide complex is produced and deposited in tissues during certain pathological states. The liver, spleen and kidney can be affected, as well as any other body tissues.

—Protease product: Transformation PUREZYME or Crystal Star DR. ENZYME™ with protease & bromelain - use as directed 2 to 4 times daily between meals to break down amyloid (glycoprotein).

ANEMIA:
—A diet high in protein, iron, and vitamin B-12. Add land and sea greens (½ tsp. snipped) for iron, minerals and enzymes. Add beef or chicken liver occasionally for protein, B complex, extra B-12 and iron.

—Give 500 to 2,000mg vitamin C, depending on size of animal.

—Sprinkle nutritional yeast flakes on food; or Nature's Path TOTAL-LYTE, an electrolyte yeast mix.

—Pure Planet CHLORELLA - high chlorophyll content helps stimulate production of healthy blood.

ARTHRITIS:
Note: Cats cannot tolerate salicylates from herbs like white willow, drugs like aspirin, or compounds in NSAIDs (Non Steroidal Anti-Inflammatory Drugs). A glucosamine-boswellia blend is best to treat their symptoms.

—Avoid giving refined foods, especially white flour and sugar. Reduce red meat, canned foods and preserved meats like bologna. Add fresh green foods, particularly grated carrots, beets and celery.

—Add ¼ tsp. Green Foods BARLEY CAT or BARLEY DOG in food.

—A 3-month treatment of Winston's JOINT FORMULA shows notable success, especially for older dogs. Winston's Joint Formula is a three part program: 1) lyophilized shark cartilage rebuilds cartilage and bone; 2) synovial fluid lubricates the joints and strengthens the ligaments; 3) bromelain reduces inflammation. In some cases, the improvement is quite rapid and spectacular. For best results, use in conjunction with acupressure massage. For purchasing information, call 1-800-447-2939, or access www.healthyhealing.com.

—Give ¼ tsp. sodium ascorbate or Ester C daily; give 250 to 2,000mg a day (a puppy - 250mg, a great dane - 2000mg). Natural Animal ESTER-C (dog formula and cat formula).

—Crystal Star AR EASE FOR ANIMALS™ ½ tsp. daily.

—Ark Naturals SEA MOBILITY chews, (sea cucumber, MSM, glucosamine, spirulina).

—Green-lipped mussel extract reduces symptoms 30% in arthritic dogs.

—Give shark cartilage (dose by weight); give continually until no evidence of the problem.

—Open 1 capsule MICROHYDRIN, available from royalbodycare.com, dissolve in water; feed one daily.

—Glucosamine-Chondroitin formula, especially with turmeric and boswellia as anti-inflammatories.

—Dancing Paws HI-POTENCY JOINT RECOVERY (therapeutic); JOINT MAINTENANCE (preventive).

—Nature's Path PET-BONE-AIDE (shark cartilage with electrolytes) to aid movement of osteoarthritis.

—Homeopathic *Rhus tox* 12c, one dose per month. Specific anti-inflammatory herbs: *boswellia, turmeric, licorice, devil's claw, alfalfa.*

—Animal chiropractic and acupressure treatments, and magnet therapy reduce pain and improve quality of life.

Can't find a recommended product? Call the 800 number in Product Resources for the store nearest you.

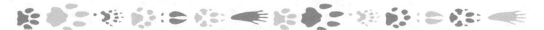

BAD BREATH- BODY ODOR:
—Bad breath can be a sign of disease and dental infections. Consult a holistic veterinarian and schedule regular teeth cleanings.

—Feed more fresh foods, less canned foods. Snip fresh parsley into food at each meal.

—Add a few drops of cider vinegar to water bowl.... for clean teeth against dog breath (and glossy coat).

—Sprinkle a little *spirulina* powder or Green Foods BARLEY DOG or BARLEY CAT on food.

—Pure Planet CHLORELLA: add ¼ to ½ tsp. to food - high chlorophyll deodorizes bad breath. S&M NuTec GREENIES dog bones help freshen breath, clean teeth and improve digestion.

—Life Extension NATURE CALLS drops reduce kitty litter odor, and bedding odors of small animals.

BLADDER INFECTION / FELINE UROLOGICAL SYNDROME (FUS) - INCONTINENCE:
—Put animal on a liquid diet for 24 hours of veggie juices and broths - no solid foods, plenty of water.

—For acute attacks, acidify the urine. Different types of crystal formations can occur in FUS. For struvite crystals <u>only</u> (diagnoses needed by veterinarian), Orthomolecular Specialties CARPON (treats and prevents FUS by acidifying urine and breaking up struvite crystals).

—<u>Avoid dried food entirely during healing</u>. Focus on fresh foods. To make your own healthy cat food: mix together a handful of raw hormone-free meat (cut in small pieces), some grated vegetables (like carrot, zucchini, greens). Add a pinch of parsley to food to help ease urination.

—Add ½ tsp. Transformation CAREZYME, ½ tsp. sea greens flakes, ½ tsp. Pure Planet CHLORELLA, 1 tbsp. flax oil, ½ to 1 cap acidophilus, and 1 tbsp. nutritional yeast. Add in enough water to make a juicy meal. (Low water intake from an all-dry food diet is a primary factor in FUS.) Add 1 tbsp. of brown rice occasionally.

—Open 1 capsule MICROHYDRIN, dissolve in water; feed one daily.

—Enzyme supplements are important. Add a digestive formula like Transformation CAREZYME to all meals. Give a protease product like Enzymedica PURIFY, Transformation PUREZYME or Crystal Star DR. ENZYME™ with Protease & Bromelain, 2 caps, between meals 2 times per day.

—Extra vitamin C daily. Natural Animal ESTER-C for cats - use as directed.

—Vitamin E 100IU daily for a month, then decrease to 400IU once a week.

—Wysong URETIC cat food for bladder infections. Crystal Star TINKLE™ caps for urinary symptom relief. (Adjust dosage to weight of animal. Dosage on the label is for 150 lb. person.)

—Nature's Path PET-LYTE - to flush out gravel. Use as directed.

—Designing Health THE MISSING LINK - use as directed.

—To reduce stress, Natural Labs DEVA FLOWER STRESS/TENSION.

—Avoid "clumping" type kitty litter brands which can contribute to blockage problems. Natural Animal LITTER PLUS - made from 100% organic plant material (peanut shell meal). WORLD'S BEST CAT LITTER is another good choice. Many feed stores have a corn cob mixture that works great as a healthy kitty litter.

—For kidney, liver or bladder disease, protease and digestive enzymes help detoxify fibrosis of affected organs. Use Transformation CAREZYME, (excellent results), mix into meals as directed.

CANCERS - LEUKEMIA - MALIGNANT TUMORS:
—Avoid commercial foods; use as much fresh, unprocessed foods as the animal will accept.

—Animal cancers have shown dramatic improvement with enzyme therapy from plant proteases against tumor growth. Protease enzymes may be used with or without conventional therapy. Use Enzymedica PURIFY or Transformation PUREZYME 3 to 6 times daily (on empty stomach with water, or mixed into a small amount of food if necessary). Add digestive aid Transformation CAREZYME (good results) into meals.

—Lane Labs MGN-3 (*shiitake mushrooms* extract) and Enzymatic Therapy IP-6 (inositol extract) are effective for animal tumors on a case by case basis. Your holistic vet can help you with dosage for your pet.

—Maitake Products, Inc. D-FRACTION EXTRACT (dogs) to help reduce tumor size and for well being.

—Open 1 capsule MICROHYDRIN, dissolve in water; feed one daily.

—Herbal Answers ALOE FORCE juice, 2 to 3 tsp. daily; apply ALOE FORCE gel if tumor is visible.

Can't find a recommended product? Call the 800 number in Product Resources for the store nearest you.

—Natural Energy Plus CAISSE'S tea - 6 to 15-lb animal, use ½ to 1 tsp. dilute tea daily. 16 to 30 lbs- 1 to 2 tsp. dilute tea. Call (941) 363-9770 for more info.

—Give vitamin C as sodium ascorbate powder, ¼ tsp. twice daily for larger animals and cats with leukemia or Alacer EMERGEN-C in water. As tumor shrinks, decrease to a small daily pinch.

—Crystal Star RESTORE YOUR STRENGTH™ broth 2x daily, ¼ cup or as much as animal will take.

—Shark cartilage, give continually until no evidence of the problem.

—Apply Crystal Star ANTI-BIO™ gel to tumorous areas. Some improvement usually in 2 weeks.

—The herb chaparral shows success (check with your holistic vet as to dosage for your pet).

—Preliminary reports suggest the African herb, *Sutherlandia,* can reduce tissue wasting caused by cancer.

—Antioxidants fight cancer-related free radical damage. Ark Naturals NU-PET GRANULAR GREENS.

COAT and SKIN HEALTH:
—Crystal Star HEALTHY SKIN, COAT & EYES FOR ANIMALS™ and acidophilus powder in food daily.

—Add 1-2 tbsp. lecithin granules or Nature's Path LECI-LYTE daily to meals.

—Give vitamin E 100IU daily. Apply E oil or jojoba oil to affected skin areas.

—Add 1 tsp. *spirulina or kelp* powder to food daily. Use PET-SKIN-AID by Nature's Path.

—EFA's are a key. Squeeze 1 black currant oil capsule onto food daily. Add 1 tbsp. flax oil or meal to food.

—Halo-Purely For Pets DREAM COAT (EFA formula) or Ark Naturals ROYAL COAT (fish oil omega 3's).

—Dancing Paws BREWER'S YEAST PLUS (Edible Skin and Coat Conditioner).

—For allergy-related skin/coat problems, try an oatstraw soak (add 4 oz dried oatstraw tops to a hot bath).

CONSTIPATION:
—Add greens and veggies to the diet; mix ½ tsp. to 1 tbsp. bran to each meal; decrease canned food.

—Add Crystal Star HEALTHY SKIN, COAT and EYES FOR PETS™ or fresh dandelion greens for food fiber.

—Mix a little garlic powder with 1 tbsp. olive oil and add to food.

—Natural Animal GENTLE DRAGON INTESTINAL CLEANSER (cat and dog formulas).

—Monas CHLORELLA - ½ tsp. daily in food - chlorella's unique cell walls stimulate the intestine's linings and increase the number of friendly bacteria. LoveMyPet TUMMY EASE for constipation relief.

—Exercise the animal more often. Let it outside more often for relief.

—Give aloe vera juice, 2 tsp. daily; give or open *marshmallow* caps into food.

CUTS, SORES and WOUNDS:
—Apply a goldenseal/myrrh solution, or comfrey salve.

—Arnica tabs or Arnica gel topically to ease pain.

—Apply vitamin E oil. Give vitamin E 100IU daily. Give RESCUE REMEDY for trauma.

—Apply aloe vera gel or Herbal Answer's Herbal ALOE FORCE Gel; give desiccated liver tabs or powder.

—Give vitamin C crystals ¼ to ½ tsp. in water. Apply on sore and give internally during the day.

—Nelson Bach RESCUE REMEDY CREAM.

—1 tsp. unsweetened yogurt, 1 acidophilus cap daily to rebuild friendly flora if using antibiotics.

DEHYDRATION: A major emergency for cats! Check for dehydration by pulling up the scruff of the neck. If skin is slow to return, the animal is dehydrated. Take to a vet as soon as possible. Check for worms, often a cause of dehydration.

—Use *comfrey* tea, or Crystal Star RESTORE YOUR STRENGTH™ broth immediately. Force feed if necessary about 2-oz. an hour. Mix bran, tomato juice and sesame oil. Feed each hour until improvement.

—PET-LYTE by Nature's Path is liquid minerals in electrolyte solution.

—Try to feed green veggies; especially celery, lettuce and carrots for electrolyte replacement. Once the crisis has passed, add *kelp, spirulina* or a green drink to the diet.

Can't find a recommended product? Call the 800 number in Product Resources for the store nearest you.

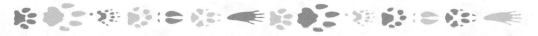

—Give the animal lots of love and attention. Dehydration may be caused by depression. The animal simply curls up and will not eat or drink anything. Bach Flower RESCUE REMEDY is excellent in this case.

DIABETES:
—Strictly avoid sugary foods, especially soft moist animal foods that come in cellophane bags - (very high in sugar, preservatives and artificial colors).

—Lower fat intake. (Use omega-3 oils like flax, ½ tsp. cod liver oil; alternate with a vegetable oil.)

—Beneficial foods for diabetes: Grains - millet, rice, oats, cornmeal, and rye bread. Vegetables - green beans (pods contain hormonal substances closely related to insulin), dandelion greens, alfalfa sprouts, corn, parsley, onion (not for dogs) and garlic reduce blood sugar. Alkalizing foods - grated vegetables, fermented foods like yogurt help counter overacidity due to the disordered metabolism of diabetes.

—Sprinkle nutritional yeast on food; add ½ tsp. to 1 tbsp. lecithin in granular or liquid form.

—Add vitamin C - 500mg to 2000mg daily depending on pet size - divide into 2 or more doses.

DIARRHEA:
—Causes: spoiled food, dairy intolerance, colitis, poisoning, non-food items, worms or harmful bacteria, treats like pig ear. Put animal on a 24 hour liquid diet with diluted aloe vera juice, vegetable juices, broths and lots of water.

—Give plain yogurt, acidophilus liquid and nutritional yeast at every feeding until diarrhea ends.

—Sprinkle crushed activated charcoal tablets on food.

—*Slippery Elm* capsules or tea soothe intestinal lining.

—Dr. Goodpet DIAR-RELIEF homeopathic remedy.

—Transformation PLANTADOPHILUS powder, about ¼ tsp. sprinkled on food.

DISTEMPER:
—If problem is acute, put animal on a short liquid diet with vegetable juices and broths.

—Give vitamin C crystals (sodium ascorbate if possible), ¼ tsp. in water, divided through the day, in an eye dropper if necessary. If vomiting and loss of fluids, give some vitamin C liquid every hour.

—Add brown rice and bran to daily food for B vitamins and system tone.

—Give Dr. Goodpet CALM STRESS homeopathic remedy to calm vomiting.

—Add ½ dropperful B complex liquid and 1 tsp. bonemeal to food daily.

—Give dilute (1 drop extract in 2 tsp. water) *goldenseal-myrrh*, or *echinacea* solution.

—Yogurt or acidophilus rebuild friendly flora; add Green Foods BARLEY DOG to diet.

—Give fresh *garlic*, or a garlic-honey mix daily.; raw liver or liver tablets 3 times a week.

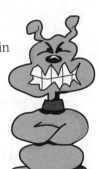

ECZEMA:
—Give zinc 25mg internally, and apply zinc ointment to infected areas.

—Mix cottage cheese, corn or cod liver oil, vitamin E oil, garlic powder, brewer's yeast. Give 1 tbsp. daily.

—Give Green Foods BARLEY DOG daily. Apply solution locally to sores.

—Reduce meat and canned foods. Add fresh veggies and sea greens to the diet.

—Use Nature's Path PET-SKIN-AIDE for healing and rebuilding the skin.

—Add 1 tbsp. flax oil or flax meal to food daily; and give *licorice* tea for cortisone type healing.

EAR MITES:
—Use NATURAL HERBAL EAR WASH by Purely For Pets. Prevents infection, heals abrasions, promotes healthy cell formation and eliminates ear wax and odors. Ark Naturals EARS ALL RIGHT to clean ear canals, and treat ear mite infestation.

—Apply Crystal Star ANTI-BIO GEL™; or make a homemade oil treatment:

Can't find a recommended product? Call the 800 number in Product Resources for the store nearest you.

#1 Combine ½ oz. olive oil and 400IU vitamin E from a capsule in a ½ oz dropper bottle. Put a dropperful in each ear, massage ear canal, let animal shake its head. Gently clean out ear (not deep into ear) with cotton swab. Repeat for 3 days. Let ear rest for 3 days to smother the mites.

#2 Grind 1-oz dried or 2-oz fresh *thyme* and *rosemary* and combine with ½ cup olive oil - let sit in a sunny windowsill or on top of a water heater to rest for 3 days. Shake daily. Strain into a dropper bottle and add 400IU vitamin E. Once a day for 3 days put warmed mixture in each ear. Let ear rest for 10 days. Repeat oil treatment for 3 days to catch egg mites. *Note: Do not use Tea Tree oil on cats - it is toxic to them.*

EYES (CATARACTS) and EAR INFECTION:

—1 tsp. cod liver oil and vitamin E 100IU to the diet. Apply cod liver oil and E oil.

—Try LoveMyPet STINKY EAR OIL for chronic bacterial infections.

—ANITRA'S HERBAL EYEWASH kit by Halo or EYES SO BRIGHT by Ark Naturals for eye infections.

—Ear infection, cider vinegar flush, 2 tbsp. to 1 cup water, twice a week. Macerate 2 cloves of garlic in olive oil. Let sit for 2 weeks. Strain and administer 2-3 drops (warmed) into ears daily until infection clears.

—Homeopathic Nat. Mur, early stages; Sulphuris calc. 12c. every 3 days.

—To arrest cataract development: Homeopathic Phosphorus 2 daily; Silicea, daily; Lutein combo daily.

—Apply an eyebright herb tea or *eyebright-goldenseal-calendula* tea wash to infected area.

—Resource for owners of blind dogs: *Living with Blind Dogs: A Resource Book and Training Guide for the Owners of Blind and Low-Vision Dogs* by Caroline Levin, R.N.

FLEAS - TICKS - MITES:
Give floppy-eared pets a weekly ear inspection for mites and ticks. Severe flea problems cause serious allergic skin reactions.

—Dust ¼ tsp. nutritional yeast and ½ tsp. garlic powder on food 3 times a week.

—Halo-Purely For Pets CLOUD-NINE HERBAL DIP, or Dancing Paws NATURAL FLEA EZE.

—Ark Naturals NEEM PROTECT helps kill fleas and flea larvae, and release them from skin and coat.

—Natural Animal HERBAL FLEA POWDER for dogs and cats with pyrenthrum kills fleas on contact.

—String eucalyptus buds around animal's neck and sleeping area. Stuff a pillow with rosemary, pennyroyal, eucalyptus and mint leaves, and place on animal's bed. Rub *rosemary* oil on coat between shampoos.

—Add a few drops Dawn dishwashing liquid to dog's bath. Often kills fleas instantly.

—Apply *tea tree oil* directly on insect to kill it. Add a few *tea tree oil* drops to pet's shampoo. Leave on 3 to 5 minutes before rinsing. Note: Do not use *Tea Tree oil* with cats - it is toxic to them.

—Apply *jojoba* oil or Aloe Life ANIMAL ALOE on the bitten place to heal it faster.

—Pet Guard HERBAL COLLAR for dogs and cats are a non-toxic alternative to commercial flea collars. The Cancer Prevention Coalition has warned against the use of some commercial flea collars including Sergeant's, Hartz, Zodiac and Longlife brands.

House treatments for fleas, tick and mites:

—Vacuum carpets and bare floors. For carpet infestation, use inorganic salts (sodium borate). Use only 100% pure, non-toxic borates such as TERMINATOR by Canine Care.

—Use carpet and bedding sprays with sea salt, citronella, eucalyptus, tea tree oil, and lemon grass oils.

FOOD ALLERGIES - SEASONAL ALLERGIES:
Finding the right diet can spell relief for your pet, without costly vet visits and harsh steroid drugs. We most often hear about wheat and corn allergies for dogs (especially pasta). If you feed your dog veggies, be careful of all cruciferous veggies which can aggravate gas.

—Transformation CAREZYME; Enzymedica PURIFY or Transformation PUREZYME.

—Consider a HEPA air filter for indoor pets with dust allergies.

—Natural Animal ESTER-C (dog and cat formulas), as directed as an anti-histamine.

—Pet Guard canned cat food offers high quality protein with no allergen preservatives. A cat favorite!

—Natural Balance POTATO & DUCK FORMULA for dogs with allergies. (Highly recommended.)

Can't find a recommended product? Call the 800 number in Product Resources for the store nearest you.

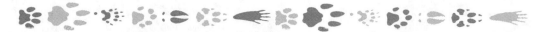

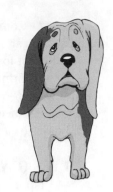

GAS and FLATULENCE:
—Give *alfalfa* or *spirulina* tabs, or Green Foods BARLEY DOG or CAT at each feeding.
—Sprinkle a pinch of *ginger* powder on food at each feeding. Give *peppermint* tea daily.
—Give *comfrey, chamomile, cinnamon, fenugreek* (not during pregnancy).
—Offer them unsweetened yogurt (about 1 tbsp.) with active cultures.

GUM and TOOTH PROBLEMS:
—Apply vitamin E oil, or calendula oil to gums.
—Apply a dilute goldenseal/myrrh or propolis solution to gums.
—Bee balm to help reduce gum inflammation and to fight gingivitis.
—Give a natural fresh foods diet, adding crunchy raw veggies and whole grains.
—Rub vitamin C - a weak solution of ascorbate crystals in water on the gums. Use Natural Animal ESTER-C (dog formula and cat formula), as directed to prevent cavities.
—Open 1 capsule MICROHYDRIN, available from royalbodycare.com, dissolve in water; feed one daily.
—Dancing Paws BREATH-A-LICIOUS dog treats with chlorophyll, peppermint, parsley, dill and fennel help control plaque and tartar. A pet favorite!
—Hepar sulphuris calcareum 12 c. - one dose every 3 days - 3 doses total.

HIP DYSPLASIA and LAMENESS (See also ARTHRITIS):
—Highly recommended: animal acupuncture, acupressure and chiropractic treatments. Some treated animals may be able avoid surgery.
—A natural diet is a key to recovery from joint dysfunction. Add more whole grains like brown rice and oatmeal, and lean meats like turkey and chicken, or organ meats to the diet.
—Mix 1 tsp. sodium ascorbate, or Ester C crystals in water and give throughout the day, every day.
—Natural Animal ESTER-C (dog formula and cat formula), as directed.
—Mix 1 tsp. bonemeal powder in 1 c. tomato juice, with 1 tsp. bran and ½ tsp. sesame oil; give daily.
—Give Crystal Star AR EASE for ANIMALS™ daily, or NU-PET PLUS for pets from Biogenetics.
—WINSTON'S JOINT FORMULA receives excellent reviews from dog owners. Improves quality of life and mobility for most dogs after one month. Sometimes dramatic improvement!
—Give shark cartilage as directed, continually until no evidence of problem. Green-lipped mussel supplements ease pain and stimulate cartilage production.
—Dancing Paws HI-POTENCY JOINT RECOVERY (therapeutic); JOINT MAINTENANCE (preventive).
—Protease enzymes: Transformation PUREZYME or Crystal Star DR. ENZYME™ with Protease and Bromelain 3 times daily.
—Nature's Path CAL-LYTE and PET-LYTE.

HORMONE IMBALANCE: Neutered pets really benefit from herbs that support hormonal systems.
—Herbs for spayed female pets: *wild yam, dong quai, oats, Siberian ginseng.*
—Herbs for neutered male pets: *saw palmetto, damiana* and *Asian ginseng.*

INTESTINAL, DIGESTIVE DISORDER: often caused by spoiled food, non-food items or worms.
—Put the animal on a short 24 hour liquid diet with vegetable juices, broths, and plenty of water.
—Give yogurt, acidophilus liquid or nutritional yeast at every feeding until diarrhea ends.
—Sprinkle crushed activated charcoal tablets on food; use Dr. Goodpet DIAR-RELIEF remedy.
—Give aloe vera juice, 2 to 3 tsp. daily.
—Give Crystal Star HEALTHY SKIN, COAT & EYES FOR PETS™ with ½ tsp. extra *garlic* powder daily.
—Deal with underlying yeast overgrowth. Give *garlic, mullein-myrrh* extract, or *echinacea* extract diluted in water, or *mugwort* tea.
—Give *comfrey* or dilute *cinnamon* tea in the water bowl.

Can't find a recommended product? Call the 800 number in Product Resources for the store nearest you.

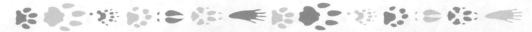

—Ark Natural GENTLE DIGEST with probiotics and *chicory* for animal colitis, occasional constipation.

—Enzyme therapy for inflammatory bowel disease or intestinal disorders: Transformation CAREZYME or Enzymedica DIGEST, mix in meals. Protease: Crystal Star DR. ENZYME™ with Protease and Bromelain, Transformation PUREZYME or Enzymedica PURIFY protease, mixed into a food like cottage cheese.

—Diarrhea: *podophyllum peltatum* 12c. - 1 to 2 doses as needed.

KIDNEY FAILURE (CRF- Chronic Renal Failure):

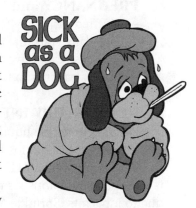

—Conventional vets often recommend a low protein, processed foods' diet for renal failure. Holistic vets tell us that a high protein, raw foods diet can actually help turn around CRF. Protein from raw meat is highly digestible, even when the kidneys aren't functioning well. One report finds a high protein raw meat based diet can produce dramatic reductions in elevated kidney blood tests in just 2 weeks. Make your own animal food with hormone-free organ meats, beef or turkey and pureed vegetables (celery, cucumbers and parsley help kidney problems). Harmony Farms (818-248-3068) and Halshan Foods (888-766-9725) carry high quality raw foods with veggies for pets that you can buy online.

—Learn to administer fluids by injection to help prevent dehydration (it's not very difficult) so you can bring a sense of well being for the animal. Ask your holistic vet.

—N-acetylcysteine (NAC) 50-200mg a day (restores normal filtration) with DHEA 25-100mg a day (supports kidney enzyme activity) has shown good results for some animals. Ask your holistic vet.

LIVER DISORDERS-TOXICITY-MALFUNCTION:

—*Milk thistle seed* or *dandelion rt.* (¼ tsp. per 20 lbs.) support liver recovery from toxic overload, and can sometimes normalize blood tests. Dilute tinctures with warm water for cats.

—If your pet takes several prescriptions, consult a holistic vet and switch to natural remedies if possible.

MANGE & FUNGAL INFECTION:

—Put drops of *tea tree* oil in the animal's shampoo; use every 2 or 3 days. Use *tea tree* oil directly on infected areas by itself or diluted with olive oil. Do not use *Tea Tree* oil with cats - it is toxic to them.

—Apply *pau d' arco* salve, *mahonia* ointment or zinc ointment and fresh lemon juice to relieve area.

—Apply dilute *echinacea* tincture, or *goldenseal-echinacea-myrrh* water solution to affected areas daily.

—Apply Nature's Path PET-SKIN-AIDE for skin healing-rebuilding, or Crystal Star FUNGEX™ gel.

—Apply AZTEC SECRET Indian Healing Clay for deep tissue healing.

—Give daily: 1 tsp. lecithin granules mixed with 2 tsp. cod liver oil, 1 tbsp. nutritional yeast, 2 tsp. desiccated liver powder.

OVERWEIGHT: Pets are following the current obesity trend in humans. New estimates show 60 million dogs and cats (half the pet population!) are overweight. Get a vet check for diabetes and hypothyroidism which exacerbate overweight problems. Add more exercise to your pet's life- 30 minutes daily.

—Reduce canned and fatty foods, and high calorie treats. Increase fresh foods, whole grains and organ meats. Add a vitamin/mineral supplement like Dancing Paws DAILY MULTI VITAMIN & MINERAL to ensure proper nutrition. Open up capsules and sprinkle on foods. Pets love the taste!

—Crystal Star HEALTHY SKIN, COAT and EYES FOR PETS™ for fiber without calories. Lecithin 750mg daily (dogs and cats).

—Sea greens daily to boost metabolism (1 tsp. of snipped sea veggies for dogs and just a pinch for cats.)

—Carnitine boosts fat metabolism (dogs). Ask your holistic vet.

—Apple cider vinegar 1 tsp. (dogs) ⅛ to ¼ tsp. (cats) in water 2x daily.

Can't find a recommended product? Call the 800 number in Product Resources for the store nearest you.

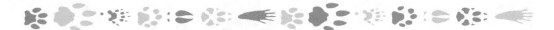

PANCREATIC INSUFFICIENCY:
—Digestive aid product: Enzymedica DIGEST or Transformation CAREZYME - mix into all meals.
—Protease helps clean up and prevent fibrosis- Enzymedica PURIFY or Transformation PUREZYME, mixed into a small treat 3 times daily between meals.

PREGNANCY and BIRTH:
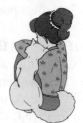
—Give red raspberry tea daily during the last half of gestation for easier birth.
—Give daily spirulina tabs or powder for protein, and sea greens for mineral balance.
—Give desiccated liver tabs (dogs), extra bonemeal, and cod liver oil daily.
—Give extra vitamin C 100mg chewable, and vitamin E 100IU daily.

RESPIRATORY INFECTIONS and IMMUNE STRENGTH:
—Put animal on a liquid diet for 24 hours to cleanse the system, with vegetable juices, broths and water. Offer *comfrey* tea to flush toxins faster. (Nibbling on growing *comfrey* plants is an animal's own natural therapy.)
—Give Crystal Star HEALTHY SKIN, COAT & EYES FOR ANIMALS™ for immune strength. Mild *thyme* tea is an expectorant, antispasmodic and antibacterial for bronchitis. *Mullein* tea is a specific for respiratory irritation due to inhalants. Sprinkle *Mullein* leaves on pet food, too. Horses especially like it.
—Give Crystal Star RESTORE YOUR STRENGTH™ broth 2 times daily, about ¼ cup. Add *astragalus* herb (well tolerated by both dogs and cats) to the broth.
—Add 1 tsp. *bee pollen*, vitamin E 100IU, and ¼ tsp. vitamin C (as sodium ascorbate if possible), dissolved in a cup of water to diet.
—Add 2 to 4 *garlic* tablets and 6 *alfalfa* tablets to the daily diet.
—Colostrum chewables- 1 daily to rev up immune response.
—Atlas IMMUNE BOOSTER- *Agaricus blazei beta glucans* increases effectiveness of natural killer cells.
—PET-LYTE by Nature's Path for foundation strength.
—East Park OLIVE LEAF EXTRACT - (works, but difficult to get cats to take this bitter antibiotic.)

WORMS and PARASITES: *Most parasitic disease treatment must also include medicinal measures.*
—Build up parasite immunity with Crystal Star HEALTHY SKIN, COAT & EYES FOR ANIMALS™ daily.
—Put the animal on a short 24 hour liquid fast with water to weaken the parasites. Then, give Crystal Star PARASITE PURGE™ caps (adjust dosage according to pet's size; dosage on the label is for 150 lb person) with charcoal tabs in water or an electuary for 3 to 7 days. Repeat process in a week to kill newly hatched eggs.
—Mix ½ tsp. *garlic* powder, 1 tsp. pumpkin seed meal, 1 pinch *cloves*; sprinkle on food daily until worms are gone. Give *spirulina* or Green Foods BARLEY DOG or BARLEY CAT for a month after worming.
—Garlic, mullein/myrrh blend; echinacea or black walnut extract diluted in water; or mugwort tea.
—Protease: Transformation PUREZYME or Enzymedica PURIFY, as directed 2x daily between meals.
—Digestion: Transformation CAREZYME or Enzymedica DIGEST - mix into all meals.

Note: Acupuncture is a very successful treatment for animals - especially for arthritis, hip dysplasia, asthma, epilepsy, cervical-disk displacements and chronic infections. To find a certified veterinary acupuncturist, contact International Veterinary Acupuncture Society (IVAS) at (970) 266-0666 or visit them at: www.ivas.org.

Special contributions
to the Animal Healing section come from esteemed experts in holistic animal care.

1)   Dr. Jim R. Smith, DVM, AAVD, does extensive research on enzymes for dietary, therapeutic use with animals. He owns the Animal Allergy Clinics and is a board member of Transformation Enzyme Corporation.

Can't find a recommended product? Call the 800 number in Product Resources for the store nearest you.

2) Special thanks to Dr. Tom Boekbinder of the Carmel Holistic Veterinary Clinic in Carmel, CA for opening the first holistic vet clinic in our community, for his humanitarian efforts in reducing the pet overpopulation problem and for his exceptional care of our own beloved animal companions.

3) Howard Peiper is a nationally recognized expert in the holistic counseling field. He has coauthored 12 books including "Super Nutrition for Animals."

4) Linda A. Mower, D.Hom, is a homeopathic educator, writer and consultant for humans and animals.

5) Special thanks to Dr. Jennifer Wernsing for offering her careful review of this chapter, and for her exceptional care of our own beloved animal companions.

To find a holistic veterinarian in your area, visit the American Holistic Veterinary Medical Association on the web: http://www.ahvma.org or call 410-569-0795.

 ## About Animals & Toxic Substances

There is a wide range of substances that are harmful or lethal to animals. They include pesticides from lawn and garden products, rat poison, commercial flea killers, herbicides like Round-Up, and others. House cleaning products and disinfectants, building and decorating hazards (like paint and outgassing from synthetic carpets) are hazardous when you're only 12 inches off the ground and have to live so close to them.

Use products that are environmentally safe as a general rule. Automobile supplies can be toxic to unsuspecting pets. Antifreeze contains ethylene glycol which possesses a sweet taste animals can't resist. If ingested, it can be fatal, especially to cats.

Many people are unaware of plant poisoning. Laurel, commonly used in dried flower arrangements, Christmas mistletoe, poinsettias, jimson weed, and oleander can cause death in a pet. Dogs who love to dig and chew the bulbs of the hyacinth can experience convulsions.

I recommend the medicine-chest information from The ASPCA's National Animal Poison Control Center, 1717 S. Philo Road, Suite #36, Urbana, IL., 61802. It's a good idea to call them before you have an emergency at 217-337-5030. This organization is the first animal-oriented poison center in the United States. The phones are answered by licensed veterinarians and board-certified veterinary toxicologists. Emergency calls go to 1-888-426-4435 (credit cards, $45 consultation fee).

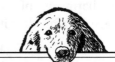

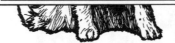

Give more than you get
Leave better than you find
Use less than there is
Smile more than you frown.

Can't find a recommended product? Call the 800 number in Product Resources for the store nearest you.

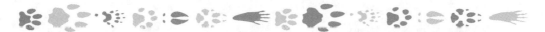

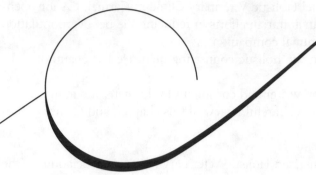

Your Health Care Responsibility

The material on the following pages is intended as an educational tool to offer information about alternative healing and health maintenance options available to the health care consumer today.

I believe we must be respectful of all ways of healing. The crisis intervention measures of drug therapy are sometimes needed to stabilize an emergency or life-threatening situation, but for long term well-being, disease prevention, and many common, self-limiting problems, diet improvement, exercise, and natural medicine choices make good sense. They are gentle, non-invasive, and in almost every case, free of any side effects.

The optional recommendations in this section are not intended as a substitute for the advice and treatment of a physician or other licensed health care professionals. In many cases, the suggestions may be used as adjuncts to professional care, to help shorten the time you may have to use drug treatment, or to help overcome any side effects.

Are there interactions between drugs and herbs? It is important to remember that herbs are foods, remarkably safe in their naturally-occurring state, especially in combinations. They do not normally interact with drugs any more than a food would interact. However, be fair to your doctor and yourself. Discuss your alternative choices with your physician, and always inform your doctor or pharmacist of any other medication you are taking. Pregnant women are especially urged to consult with their health care provider before using any therapy.

I feel that education is the key to making wise health decisions. Part of the job of taking more command of your own health care is using your common sense, intelligence, and adult judgement based on the knowledge of your own body experiences. Ultimately, you must take the full responsibility for your choices and how you use the information presented here.

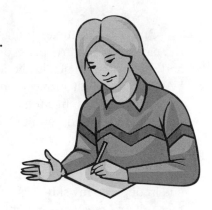

Dear reader, let me tell you a true story about healthy healing...

I embrace things very enthusiastically. When I first heard about a detoxifying diet in the 70's I thought it sounded like just the thing for me. I had fought my weight all my life. I was tired all the time (probably from all the crazy diets I went on to lose weight), and I felt "toxic," constantly getting fever blisters, urinary tract and yeast infections. I had dull hair, poor skin texture, peeling feet and breaking nails. Oh, I remember those days well.

Detoxification seemed like it would solve of lot of health problems. I thought I would be on a cleansing diet all my life.

The trouble was, I had almost no idea how to go about it. The '60s and '70s were the decades that the FDA had what amounted to a "gag order" on all books and information about alternative health methods, healing techniques and products. (You would not be reading this book now if the owner and employees of a very brave health food store in California had not finally challenged this regulation in the early 1980s in the courts and won, after many years and enormous expense.)

But I had a little knowledge and some enthusiastic friends who were detoxing, too, so I started on what was essentially a 5 food diet—cabbage, lettuce with a little salad dressing, apples, oranges, peanut butter (for protein), and a few whole wheat crackers occasionally. I was delighted with my weight loss (I averaged about 90 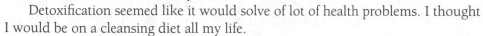 pounds for my 5 foot frame). I rarely ate other things; this went on for several years. I didn't realize it, but my body was going into major malnutrition decline.

Today, with all the information we have about nutrition, most people know this type of diet is not a cleansing diet. It's a prescription for terrible health. All I saw was that I was finally thin.

One week, in the winter of 1981, my energy had dropped so low that I couldn't make it to my job. I had just started working at the town's small health food store, and I loved my work, so this was very unusual.

I didn't realize it but I had already slipped into shock—the hours and days were slipping by like a dream. I lived alone with my dogs and cats, but my colleagues from work wondered why I wasn't there. Thankfully, one of them came to check up on me. He saved my life.

I had already collapsed, and was lying by my front screen door. He scooped me up and got me to the nearest emergency room. It was eight-thirty in the morning, at a very small Seventh Day Adventist hospital in a small California town. There were 12 people in the building. Everyone worked feverishly to save me, but my blood pressure dropped rapidly. The staff saw me slip into a coma—they thought they had lost me.

All I knew was that I was floating—above my body, the operating table and the doctors who were working on me. It was all very interesting. I saw all the frantic emergency room procedures—like a TV show.

And then… I can see as clearly as when it happened, I floated to a top corner of the room. A million colors were swirling around me. I saw a dark tunnel with a white pinpoint of light miles away at the end. I turned to go to it… then everything when black, and I don't remember any more.

I was in a coma, and even though I didn't know it, I had made it.

Eventually I regained consciousness, and woke up full of tubes and needles on a breathing machine. My blood was so toxic, the hospital had to have plasma flown in every 5 hours to give me a slow but complete transfusion. It kept me alive, but I wasn't regaining health, slipping back and forth into unconsciousness. The doctors wanted to MED-Evac me to Stanford University for specialized treatment, but I knew that I would just become a number, so I wouldn't go.

One of the fortunate things about a Seventh Day Adventist hospital in those days was that they listened to the patient. I couldn't speak, of course, but I could write. So, I asked for green drinks from the health food store and the hospital staff allowed a small refrigerator to be brought in for them. It was then that a miracle began. Within hours I felt stronger; within days, they removed the respirator; within a few more, they removed all the tubes and needles. In a total of twelve days after I regained consciousness, I left the hospital, very very weak, weighing 69 pounds, and unable to walk because my legs would not support my weight.

I knew I had been given another chance at life and a tremendous challenge to regain my health. My hair had either fallen out or turned white; some of my veins has collapsed from the needles. I had pulled retinal tissue in one eye; my skin was peeling off at my fingertips. The hospital thought they might have to amputate my toes unless I regained circulation in my feet fast.

I started reading everything I could get my hands on about natural healing and herbal remedies. I started formulating herbal formulas to bring each part of my body back to health. It began to happen. I could see a new me emerging, with curly hair, and a better skin tone and texture (no wrinkles) than I had before the illness. My circulation came back (no toe amputations); my energy returned stronger than it had been in many years.

The experience and the healing changed my life. I saw that herbs are far more than remedies for colds and flu. They can bring your health back from serious illness… literally from death's door. I was enormously impressed. I decided to devote my life to reaching out to others—to talk about the power of herbs, to write about their healing abilities, to return some of the essential universal knowledge that we've lost. I gained my degrees from Clayton College of Natural Health over the next several years.

That early attempt at cleansing was almost fatally misguided. One of the reasons I wanted to write this Healthy Healing book was to pass along all I've learned about healthy healing. Hundreds of thousands of people have been helped by this information. I hope you will too. Pass it along!

To your best health,

Linda Page

PS: What others have said...

"In the holistic health field, no one has written as comprehensively as Dr. Page in her book *Healthy Healing*. I highly recommend this book and personally use Dr. Page's knowledge and applications in my practice. It is a must-read for everyone, health practitioner and lay person alike." -Howard Peiper, N.D. *Author of numerous books on nutrition including two best sellers on ADD/ADHD. His latest book is "Kiss Your Life Hello."*

"I have used your book, *Healthy Healing*, as a reference, actually almost a bible, for the past few years after my yoga instructor suggested it for infertility advice. Your book, and some of your products have made a profound difference in the quality of my life!" -Kathleen D.

"There is no way for me to express appreciation to you for saving and improving my life. You are not just selling books.... you are helping people to help themselves." -Mal H.

A message to interested readers...

The Ailment Healing section of this book recommends many fine natural health products that I and my staff have used and reviewed for effectiveness and safety under label dosage and conditions.

There are special recommendations for Crystal Star Herbal Nutrition products in the Herb and Supplement heading. I formulated these products and have been involved in healing experiences with them for over 25 years. The suggested uses for them in this book are for conditions I have either personally witnessed or heard directly from the first hand knowledge of people who used the products successfully for their health problems.

This book is all about furthering real knowledge about what really works for human health - not just laboratory results or even animal studies, but what works for us. I consider first person knowledge to be incredibly valuable in this effort.

My goal is to pass on to you all the information I have gained in the health field with products I have used and worked with. You can have every confidence that the products suggested under the health conditions in this book have had success for their recommendation.

Linda Page

Linda Page, PhD. and Traditional Naturopath

Access is important.
If you are interested in knowing more about the Crystal Star herbal formulas, call Crystal Star Herbs directly at 1-800-736-6015.

Crystal Star is carried nationwide. If you know the product you want, go to your natural food store. If they don't have it, they can easily order it for you.

If you prefer the convenience of internet ordering, you can get product information from www.healthyhealing.com.

If you wish to contact the Healthy Healing offices, you can call 831-583-9372.

How to use the "pink pages" therapy charts...

Each ailment chart includes two therapy categories:
—Diet and Lifestyle Support Therapy
—Herb, Superfood and Supplement Therapy

Alternative medicine is all about you.... your individual problem, and your individual solution.
It's easy to put together the best healing program for yourself. There are many effective remedies to choose from. Each remedy in this book has been carefully chosen and personally tested.

You can have every confidence that the recommended remedies have been used and found to be effective, in some cases by thousands of people. I develop and work with the healing programs over many years; they are constantly updated with new information.

Here's a good way to start:
First: Follow all the diet and nutrition recommendations. No matter what your health problem is, your diet is your "first responder" healing tool.

Second: 1) Choose one recommendation from <u>each healing target</u> (numbered, boldface, underlined) under the interceptive therapy plan. Use these choices together for a complete healing program.

or

2) Identify your symptoms using the healing targets (numbered, boldface, underlined) under the interceptive therapy plan. Then choose remedies to target those symptoms.
(All given doses are daily amounts unless otherwise specified. Dosage listed is for the major time of healing, and is not to be considered as maintenance or long term. The rule of thumb for natural healing is one month for every year you have had the problem.)

Healthy Healing addresses many serious diseases with expanded therapy recommendations. The step-by-step, full scale diets I suggest for these problems are "real people" diets. People with specific health conditions have used them and have related their experiences to me. Over the years, I've seen that diseases change—through mutation, environment, or treatment—a person's immune response to them changes. Healthy Healing's diet programs are continually modified to meet new, changing health needs.

Every edition of Healthy Healing offers you the latest knowledge from a wide network of natural healing professionals - nutrition consultants, holistic practitioners, naturopaths, nurses, world health studies and traditional physicians in America and around the world.

The most significant information is the evidence of people who have tried the natural healing methods for themselves, experienced real improvement in their health, and wish to share their success with others. Pick the suggestions that you feel instinctively strong about. They are invariably the best for you, and will be the easiest to incorporate into your lifestyle.

Refer to "Look It Up," on page 570 for more information about any recommended healing agent.

No prescription is as valuable as knowledge.

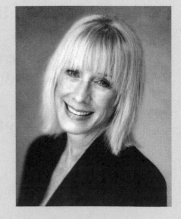

Abscesses

Boils, Carbuncles, Furuncles

Abscesses are a manifestation of low immune resistance to pathogenic organisms. They often follow a staph, viral or bacterial infection, and represent part of your body's toxin cleansing mechanism. Most abscess sufferers experience accompanying swelling of nearby lymph glands. Abscesses of all kinds are a result of toxin overload in the colon, liver and blood, usually from an acid-forming diet high in chocolate, trans fats and sweets, and too many fats from red meat and dairy foods.

Boils, inflamed, pus-filled sores, often attended by chills, malaise and fever, exhibit weeping, white (rather than clear), drainage.

Along with **furuncles,** they have common sites on gums, buttocks, the back of the neck and armpits. Both are usually staph infections of sebaceous glands, especially around hair follicles (often caused by a rough or contaminated razor blade).

Carbuncles are groups of boils where the staph infection extends out into the subcutaneous layers of the skin.

Recurrent attacks of boils and abscesses indicate a depressed immune system. Extreme cases may require medical treatment. Diabetics are at special risk for abscesses as are people who lack vegetable protein and essential fatty acids. (For Dental Abscesses see page 389.)

Diet and Lifestyle Support Therapy

Nutritional therapy plan:

1—Start with a short cleanse: 1 to 3 days of fresh juices (pg. 172) followed by a fresh foods diet for 1 to 2 weeks to balance body chemistry pH.

2—Eat cultured foods: yogurt, kefir, etc. for friendly intestinal flora. Add acidophilus to your diet, sprinkled over food or as a supplement, especially if taking high dose courses of antibiotics for an abscess infection. Consider UAS DDS-PLUS™.

3—Drink 6 glasses of water daily.

4—To prevent recurring boils: try daily *dandelion root tea* to keep liver clear.

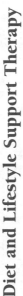

—Medicinal food applications: Apply tomato paste to bring boil to a head, and soothe the pain too. •Simmer flax and fenugreek seeds together until soft. Mash pulp. Apply to abscess as a compress. •Mix and apply fresh grated garlic mixed with lemon juice.

—Bodywork: *Warning:* Squeezing a boil or abscess can force infectious bacteria into the bloodstream. Hot compresses bring boils to a head instead - 3 compresses, 3x daily. •*Burdock root* Dab with *tea tree* oil.

1—Take a *catnip, aloe vera juice,* or *wheat grass juice* enema at least once during healing to clean out toxins.

2—Expose abscess to morning sunlight 15 minutes a day.

—Apply effective skin healers: Choose 1 recommendation.
•AloeLife ALOE SKIN GEL, or Herbal Answers HERBAL ALOE FORCE gel.
•*Tea tree* oil, *manuka* oil or Thursday Plantation TEA TREE ANTISEPTIC CREAM.
•Hot epsom salts compress - 2 tbsp. salts to 1 cup hot water, apply to bring to a head. *Fenugreek* compresses help soften boils.
•AZTEC SECRET Indian Healing Clay- Mix with apple cider vinegar and use as a poultice to draw out toxins.

Herbal, Superfood and Supplement Therapy

Interceptive therapy: Choose 2 to 3 recommendations.

1—Flush out infection: •Crystal Star ANTI-BIO™ caps, 6 daily for 1 week; with •CLEANSING & PURIFYING™ Tea for 1 week, or •*Aloe vera* juice, 2 tbsp. in juice morning and evening; or •*Myrrh* tincture. •*Garlic* or *nettles* extract caps, 2 caps 3x daily to purify the blood. •*Echinacea* extract- take internally to flush out infected lymph glands, apply directly to abscess (good results). •Apply Crystal Star ANTI-BIO™ gel 3x daily.

2—Take down swelling and pain: •Crystal Star ANTI-FLAM™ caps 6 as needed. •Transformation PUREZYME protease, or •Crystal Star DR. ENZYME™ with protease and bromelain, a detoxifying anti-inflammatory, 6 caps daily. •*Cleavers* tea, 3 times daily.

3—Neutralize toxins: Apply •Nutribiotic GRAPEFRUIT SEED SKIN SPRAY or •COLLOIDAL SILVER SPRAY. Add •Nutribiotic GRAPEFRUIT SEED extract capsules, too.

4—Skin healing: •Diamond HERPANACINE capsules, 6 daily. •Enzymedica PURIFY all proteas, 4 daily. •*Burdock root* tea 2 cups daily, a blood purifier to restore sebaceous gland function. •Earth's Bounty O₂ spray, a skin biocleanser

5—Preventive measures: •Planetary YELLOW DOCK SKIN CLEANSE tabs prevent recurrence. •UAS DDS-PLUS™ with FOS caps or other probiotics 3x daily. •*Burdock* root tea 2 cups daily, to restore sebaceous gland function. •Beta carotene 100,000IU daily; vitamin E 800IU daily, zinc 50mg daily, vitamin C with bioflavs. 3 to 5 grams daily for 1 month (may also apply a C solution).

—Superfood therapy: Choose 1 or 2 recommendations.
•Crystal Star ENERGY GREEN RENEWAL™ drink for EFA's, 1 heaping tsp. in 8-oz. ALOE VERA JUICE each morning.
•Nutricology PROGREENS w. EFA's.
•Liquid chlorophyll - apply on gauze pad, then to abscess as a poultice (see pg. 76). Take chlor-phyll liquid internally, 3 tsp. daily in water to purify blood.
•Propolis tincture: apply directly, take internally, twice daily.
•AloeLife FIBERMATE drink daily to cleanse intestinal tract.

Can't find a recommended product? Call the 800 number listed in Product Resources for the store nearest you.

Acidity, Acidosis

Restoring Body Chemistry Balance

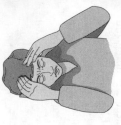

Balanced body chemistry pH is vital to health and immune response. Your body has alkaline parts (like blood) and acid parts (like the inside of the stomach), but if over-all body chemistry is too acidic, you open yourself up for arthritis-type diseases. Duodenal ulcers wait in the wings if your body is continually over acid. A healthy body keeps large alkaline reserves to meet the demands of excess acid-producing foods. When these are depleted beyond a 3:1 ratio, health can be seriously threatened.

Modern medicine solves the overacidity problem by prescribing antacids or ever stronger acid blocking drugs like *Tagamet* or *Prevacid*. These techniques may make sense short term by providing relief, but over the long term, they further disrupt pH levels, and may even lead to antacid dependency. (Most of us know someone who swallows mouthfuls of antacids daily. For them, one day without antacids leads to a roaring case of heartburn, even when diet choices are good!) New acid blocking drugs have worrisome side effects. In some studies, diarrhea, abdominal pain and nausea occur more in *Prevacid* users than in a placebo group. One user I spoke to feels his recent hair loss is due to the drug.

Here's the problem: When antacids are taken regularly, the GI tract and entire body fluctuates between too alkaline or too acidic. Abnormal pH, too acidic (below 7.3) or too alkaline (higher than 7.5), leads to health problems like diarrhea or constipation, malnutrition (from the inability to use nutrients in the GI tract), gallbladder problems, hiatal hernia and indigestion. pH disruption alters the ecology of the bowel environment, too, potentially causing a dramatic overgrowth of harmful microorganisms. Diet therapy is the key to recovery from acidity and acidosis. Add alkalizing drinks and fresh foods (rich in enzymes), and reduce those trigger "acid stress" foods to help turn around the majority of acidosis cases.

What signs indicate an over-acid condition? GERD (gastroesophagael reflux); frequent skin eruptions that don't go away; sunken eyes, dark-circles under eyes; rheumatoid arthritis or fibromyalgia; gastritis; burning, foul-smelling stools and anal itching; poor digestion; ulcer flare-ups; bad breath and body odor; alternating constipation and diarrhea; insomnia; bloating; kidney or gallstones; gum disease; very low blood pressure; frequent migraine headaches.

What causes an over-acid condition? Poor diet tops the list.... generally, excess acid-forming foods like caffeine, fried foods, tobacco, and sugary foods, leading to poor kidney, lung, liver or adrenal function , and mineral imbalances. Mental stress and tension are usually involved. Excessive exercise which causes lactic acid to build up in the muscles and tissues may be a factor. Acidosis itself is often related to or caused by arthritis, diabetes or borderline diabetes. (Refer to those pages in this book.)

Home pH Testing

Acidity or alkalinity are stated in pH values. The neutral point, where a solution is neither acid or alkaline, is pH 7. Water has a pH of 7.0. A pH above 7.0 is alkaline; maximum alkalinity is pH 14. A pH below 7.0 is acid; maximum acidity is pH 0. Ideal pH range for saliva and urine is between 6.0 and 6.8. The body is naturally slightly acidic. Values below pH 6.3 are considered too acidic; values above pH 6.8 are too alkaline. Measure saliva and urine pH on litmus paper. Normal saliva pH is 6.4. If saliva pH is above 6.8, it may indicate digestive problems; below 6.0 may mean liver and blood toxicity. Urine pH cycles between 4.5 and 5.8 in the morning, to a high of 7.0 during the day, averaging 6.4 in a 24 hr. period. If urine is too acid, below 6.0, it may indicate dehydration or kidney stress. Too alkaline (over 8), may be a sign of liver, kidney or pancreas dysfunction.

Colon pH is critically important to your health. It should be in a narrow range of 6.8 to 7.0. If it is too alkaline (above 7.0), yeasts and pathogenic bacteria grow. To lower the pH of the colon, implant a good L. bifidus colon culture. Most of the bacteria in the colon is bifidus.

You can determine whether your body fluids are either too acidic or too alkaline. Purchase nitrazine paper, at a drugstore, or Trimedica ALKAMAX pH papers, and test your saliva or urine. For accuracy, take the test either before eating or one hour after eating. The color of the paper changes to show if your system is too acidic or alkaline. If your results show an imbalance, eliminate either acid-or alkaline-forming foods (see next page) from your diet until you achieve proper homeostasis.

Can't find a recommended product? Call the 800 number listed in Product Resources for the store nearest you.

Acidity, Acidosis

Diet and Lifestyle Support Therapy

Nutritional therapy plan:

1—Go on a short 24 hour (pg. 173) liquid diet to cleanse excess acid wastes. Drink an alkalizing juice: 8-oz.tomato juice, 1 tsp. each wheat germ, nutritional yeast and lecithin daily. Use lemon juice if tomato aggravates your acidity. Drink 1 to 2 glasses of unsweetened cranberry juice daily, or Knudsen JUST CRANBERRY juice.

2—For the next 3 days, eat only fresh foods to complete the alkalizing process. Eat (Cooked foods tend to increase acidity.) Eat chlorophyll-rich green foods daily.

3—Then eat a diet of 75% alkalizing foods..... fresh and steamed vegetables (especially asparagus), sprouts, fruits and fruit juices, miso soups, brown rice, sea vegetables, green drinks, ume plums, honey, etc. Have a Potassium Drink twice a week (below).

4—For the next 2 weeks, acid-forming foods should be no more than 25% of your diet. Avoid foods like coffee and caffeine-containing foods, meats, dairy foods (except yogurt or kefir), poultry, eggs, beans or lentils, peanuts and legumes, cheeses, yeasted breads, most pre-prepared foods and most condiments.

5—Have a glass of wine or Crystal Star STRESS ARREST™ tea at dinner to relax your body and nerves.

POTASSIUM JUICE

This is the single most effective juice for cleansing, neutralizing acids and rebuilding the body. It is a blood and body tonic that provides rapid energy and system balance.
For one 12-oz. glass: Juice in a juicer 3 Carrots, 3 Stalks Celery ½ Bunch Spinach, 1 tbsp. snipped, dry Sea Greens, ½ Bunch Parsley. Add 1 tsp. Bragg's LIQUID AMINOS if desired.

POTASSIUM ESSENCE BROTH

If you don't have a juicer, make a potassium broth in a soup pot. While not as concentrated or pure, it is still an excellent source of energy, minerals and electrolytes.
For a 2 day supply: Cover with water in a soup pot 3 to 4 Carrots, 3 Stalks Celery, ½ Bunch Parsley, 2 Potatoes with skins, ½ Head Cabbage, 1 Onion, and ½ Bunch Broccoli, 2 tbsp. snipped, dry Sea Greens. Simmer covered 30 minutes. Strain and discard solids. Add 2 tsp. Bragg's LIQUID AMINOS or 1 tsp. Miso. Store in the fridge, covered.

—Lifestyle bodywork:
•Get some mild exercise every day for body oxygen. A daily walk is a good choice, with deep breathing exercises (deep breathing naturally alkalizes the body). Take another walk before you go to bed to relax and settle your system for the night.
•Metabolic factors influence pH balance. Learn about your personal metabolic type; visit *www.bloodph.com* on the web. It provides a list of Metabolic Typing practitioners.

—Herbal healing application:
•Crystal Star HOT SEAWEED BATH™ twice a week to rebalance your body's pH.

Herbal, Superfood and Supplement Therapy

Interceptive therapy: Choose 1 or 2 recommendations.
1—For biochemistry balance: •Crystal Star FIBER & HERBS COLON CLEANSE™ caps, or •Planetary Formulas TRIPHALA for 1 month (highly recommended); add •Crystal Star OCEAN MINERALS™ caps or 2 tbsp. snipped dry sea veggies daily. •Trimedica ALKAMAX powder (electrolytic alkaline buffers). Or take • Arise & Shine THE ALKALIZER, and add • one tsp. cider vinegar and 1 tsp. maple syrup in a glass of water each morning for a month (highly recommended)

2—Increase elimination of toxins: •Ginger compresses on the kidneys, and take •two ginger caps with each meal; or •Crystal Star DR. ENZYME™ with Protease and Bromelain (as directed between meals), or •Prevail ACID EASE tabs; •HCL Pepsin tabs after meals (contraindicated for peptic ulcers).

—Effective herbal healing:
• *Chamomile* tea or *Fennel seed* tea
• Homeopathic *Berberis vulgaris*
• Wisdom of the Ancients YERBA MATÉ tea

—Superfood therapy: Choose one recommendation.
•AloeLife ALOE GOLD concentrate.
•Nature's Answer SEACENTIALS GOLD (excellent).
•Green Foods CARROT ESSENCE.
•Nutricology PRO GREENS w. EFA's.
•Crystal Star RESTORE YOUR STRENGTH™ drink or caps.
•Pure Form WHEY PROTEIN - no artificial sweeteners, real chunks of fruit.

—Preventives: Choose 1 or 2 recommendations.
•Alkalizing enzymes, like Transformation GASTROZYME formula.
•B-complex 100mg with extra pantothenic acid 500mg daily.
•Ascorbate vitamin C crystals with bioflavonoids, 3000mg daily for 4 weeks.
•Futurebiotics VITAL K, 2 tsp. daily.
•Probiotics: Jarrow Formulas JARRO-DOPHILUS™, or UAS DDS-PLUS + FOS for better pH balance.

—Supplements for kids: Choose 1 recommendation.
•Prevail VITASE for kids.
•Green Foods BARLEY ESSENCE (berry flavor).
•*Catnip* or *horsetail* tea.
•Probiotics: Natren LIFE START or Nutrition Now RHINO ACIDOPHILUS.

Can't find a recommended product? Call the 800 number listed in Product Resources for the store nearest you.

Acne

Pimples, Blemishes

Teenage acne has been common since at least Greek and Roman times. Four out of five teenagers develop it as hormones rage and try to adjust to new roles. But today's adults see another bump raise its ugly head! Adult acne is prevalent, and rising, a clear sign of today's chronic stress, continuing body imbalance and poor diets.

Whiteheads (comedones) are plugs of oil and dead skin cells under the surface of the skin that block oil from flowing to the skin surface. They may turn into blackheads (open comedones) when they reach the skin surface, or spread under the skin, rupture and irritate (the more you try to pop them out the deeper they seem to go and the more they inflame). Mega-doses of vitamins may aggravate acne because too much iodine and vitamin E can stimulate sebaceous glands to produce too much oil. Adult acne along the jawline along with irregular periods and excessive hair on face and abdomen, can be a sign of polycystic ovarian syndrome.

Media reports tell us that acne is not triggered by food choices, but new studies show our Western diet of sugary, over processed foods is at least partly to blame. Too much sugar raises insulin and IGF-1 (Insulin Growth Factor) levels, triggering the production of excess testosterone and sebum which clog pores and cause breakouts. Sugar-saturated skin is susceptible to acne, because a rise in blood sugar is multiplied by 5 by the time it gets to the skin. Note: Tetracycline and other antibiotics prescribed for acne often don't help much, and they may lead to antibiotic-resistance when used long term. Accutane, a prescription drug for severe acne, has been linked to birth defects, bone loss, depression, even higher suicide risk.

Blood cleansing herbs are a proven traditional herbalist's tool to help acne heal from the inside out. The newest thinking incorporates blood cleansing formulas, and also targets acne inflammation. Reducing the inflammatory response minimizes acne severity and prevents breakouts. Crystal Star BEAUTIFUL SKIN™ caps, tea and gel (soak in cotton balls and apply, often works overnight for breakouts) are premier anti-inflammatory compounds, especially formulated for good results for acne sufferers. Follow the initial acne diet, (see next page), then adopt a low glycemic diet like the one on pg.463 to help regulate your body's sugar use for long term acne relief.

Do you have acne? Not all pimples are acne. Acne blemishes are not only inflamed but infected and often occur on the face, chest and back, too, with rough textured, flaking, red skin patches. Some experts think acne is in fact a type of eczema-like dermatitis. Cystic Acne (fluid-filled cysts) are the ones that cause itching and scarring.

What causes acne? Gland imbalance (particularly related to the pituitary), and hormone imbalance (particularly related to male testosterone activity) during teenage years. For adult acne: stress is the biggest cause for men (confirmed in studies); for women, it's hormone imbalances around menstrual periods, some oral contraceptives, polycystic ovarian syndrome (PCOS), and pregnancy. Both teenage and adult acne are aggravated by poor digestion of fatty foods, lack of green veggies and essential fatty acid deficiency. Poor liver function, constipation, genetic predisposition and illicit drug abuse are related to acne development.

What about *Acne Rosacea?*

Rosacea is the hyperactive, inflammatory response of skin capillaries to stress, heat, foods and some cosmetic chemicals like *salicylic acid* and *alpha hydroxy acids*. Its hallmarks are red, acne-like bumps, white heads, broken capillaries and redness over the facial T-zone. People of Celtic descent and menopausal women seem to be most affected. The medical approach to rosacea is antibiotic treatment along with *metronidzole* (Metrogel), an antiparasitic agent. Both treatments seem to provide only temporary results and can actually worsen rosacea over the long term.

Avoid rosacea triggers. Menopausal women can fight back triggering hot flashes with phytohormone-rich herbs like Crystal Star EST-AID™ or Pure Essence Labs TRANSITIONS. Both reduce hot flashes and night sweats triggers. Limit: spicy foods, hot drinks, vinegar, meat marinades, alcohol, tomatoes, red peppers, caffeine, chocolate and excess salt. Include betaine HCl 600mg with extra pancreatin 1400mg. Avoid: prolonged sun or heat exposure (i.e. from a heater or dry sauna), or intense exercise (only during flare-ups). Soothe your skin: Crystal Star RED SKIN RELIEF™, Dreamous Corp. BIOPATHIC THERAPY serum and Dr. Diamond HERPANACINE caps (all show excellent results). Crystal Star ANTI-BIO™ caps work (highly recommended, start with 6 daily) if there is accompanying *H. pylori* infection (many roasacea sufferers). Use either formula with *Evening Primrose Oil* for best results.

Can't find a recommended product? Call the 800 number listed in Product Resources for the store nearest you.

Acne

Diet and Lifestyle Support Therapy

Nutritional therapy plan:

1—Go on a short 3 day liquid cleanse (pg. 172) to clean out acid wastes. Use apple, carrot, pineapple, papaya juices, and 6 glasses of water daily.

2—Add more fiber - especially from fresh foods. Have a salad every day. Add often to the diet: whole grains, green veggies, brown rice, sprouts and apples.

3—Choose turkey, chicken, vegetable protein (beans, tofu, sprouts); avoid red meat.

4—Drink green tea each morning or Crystal Star GREEN TEA CLEANSER™ or Green Foods SHOGUN IMPERIAL green tea tabs. **For adult acne prevention: Boost skin cell immune function with a daily cup of white tea (highly recommended for skin).

5—Eliminate acne trigger foods: white flour foods, sugary and fried foods, soft drinks, caffeine, chocolate, fatty dairy, hard cheeses, nightshade plants - eggplant, peppers, tobacco, tomatoes, peanut butter, additive-laden foods. Limit: wheat germ, shellfish, high iodine foods like kelp (some cases), cheese, citrus, eggs, salt.

6—Add acidophilus and vitamin C if taking antibiotics for acne. Mix ¼ tsp. vitamin C crystals with 1 tbsp. acidophilus liquid, take 4x daily.

—Medicinal food applications for acne scars:

• Place fresh pineapple on scars for enzyme therapy.
• *Stevia* extract drops - apply directly.
• Take Omega-3 oils for extra EFAs.
• Mix a little tomato paste with a little non-fat powdered milk. Apply to pimple and leave on 10 minutes to greatly reduce spot.
• Apply cider vinegar or fresh lemon juice. Dab on sores at night for 2 to 3 weeks. Sometimes amazing results.

—Lifestyle measures:

• Sleep an extra hour. Hormone and sebum levels increase when sleep is disrupted.
• Get fresh air and exercise daily.
• Ice it. As soon as you feel a pimple coming on, wrap an ice cube in saran wrap and hold it on the pimple for a few minutes. (Doesn't work for existing zits, though.)
• Get early morning sun on the face. Sunlight acts as a natural antibiotic, boosting porphyrins chemicals which attack bacterial infections in the skin.
Note: Sunlight aggravates acne rosacea, a different skin problem, common in adults.

—Preventive measures:

• Touching sores spreads breakouts. Squeezing pimples or blackheads causes inflammation and scarring. Apply Earth's Bounty O₂ SPRAY. Do not squeeze. Whiteheads will come to the surface for elimination. Apply Mychelle CLEAR SKIN serum to trouble areas.

Herbal, Superfood and Supplement Therapy

Interceptive therapy: Choose 2 or 3 recommendations.

1—Relieve inflammation and infection first: • Crystal Star ANTI-BIO™ caps, 2, 4x daily for 1 week. Use • Diamond HERPANACINE caps (good reliable results).

2—Rapid improvement: • Crystal Star BEAUTIFUL SKIN™ tea. Drink and dab on with cotton balls. • Crystal Star BEAUTIFUL SKIN™ caps and gel take down inflammation fast; • Planetary YELLOW DOCK SKIN CLEANSE (skin detox).

3—Tissue healers: Take bromelain 1500mg to relieve inflammation. • Anabol Naturals AMINO BALANCE; Vitamin A 50,000 IU daily for one month only; • Pancreatin to digest oils. • Vitamin E with selenium to normalize glutathione. • B-complex 100mg daily for stress-caused acne (around chin). • Add 100mg zinc daily with beta carotene 100,000IU (very effective). Homeopathic *Ledum palustre* for adult acne, *Hepar sulphuris* for youth acne.

4—Add EFAs and enzymes: • *Evening primrose* oil 4-6 daily, • flaxseed oil, 1TB daily; or *lemon grass,* or *ginger tea* daily. Boost enzyme development for better fat and protein metabolism. Try Transformation LIPOZYME.

—Superfood therapy: Choose two recommendations.

• AloeLife FIBER-MATE drink, ½ tsp.
• Barlean GREENS (high chlorophyll, high antioxidants)
• Green Foods CARROT ESSENCE or Wakunaga KYO-GREEN drink.
• Crystal Star ZINC SOURCE™ extract. Critical enzymes for detoxing from alcohol (and acne causing sulfites) are zinc dependent.

—For adult acne: Choose 2 or more recommendations.

• Diamond HERPANACINE capsules 3 to 6 daily (excellent results).
• Prince of Peace RED GINSENG-ROYAL JELLY vials, one daily, especially for adult acne.
• Take *saw palmetto* extract, 30 drops 2x daily, to reduce excess testosterone.
• For acne related to menstrual cycle: Take *Burdock* and *Vitex* extract under the tongue 3x daily til clear with B₆ 50mg daily. Mix aloe vera skin gel with 1 pinch each *burdock rt.* and *vitex* powder and 1 tsp. gentle clay mask powder. Apply, dry and rinse.
• Apply Nutribiotic FIRST AID skin spray to stop infections (highly recommended).

—Acne scar healing applications: Choose one recommendation to pat on.

• For infection: *Goldenseal-myrrh* tea, or • Jason NEW CELL ACNE THERAPY.
• Pat on essential oils: *chamomile, tea tree, rosemary, lavender.*
• Steam face with Swiss Kriss Herbs, or a red *clover-elder-eucalyptus* steam. • Wash with *tea tree* or *calendula* soap. Yoanna ALOE CAMOMILE EXFOLIATOR for scar reduction.
• Zia Cosmetics HERBAL MOISTURE GEL (adult acne, rosacea). • Crystal Star SCAR REDUCER™ roll-on. • Camocare CAMOCARE GOLD clear solution.
• Herbal Answers ALOE FORCE SKIN gel, or AHAs, like Noni of Beverly Hills AHAs.

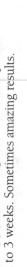

Can't find a recommended product? Call the 800 number listed in Product Resources for the store nearest you.

Addictions

Alcohol Abuse

Fully one-third of Americans are heavy drinkers; over half of us consume over 14 drinks a week. Alcohol abuse is brought on and marked by stress, depression, a no-confidence vote about one's self, and nutritional deficiencies. It also runs in families; three-quarters of alcoholics have a genetic disorder metabolizing alcohol. Alcohol dependence is a disease, not a character flaw, and it leads to other problems. (Over-the-counter pain relievers now carry a liver damage warning for anyone who drinks 3 or more drinks a day.) Cirrhosis of the liver means premature death for over 26,000 alcoholic people every year. Up to 35% of alcoholics develop hepatitis, also life threatening. Complementary therapies are ideal because they can address the devastating consequences of chronic alcoholism: nutrient (especially mineral) deficiencies, cognitive impairment, immune suppression, liver disease, even diabetes and pancreatitis. **Do you think you might be alcoholic?** Do you use alcohol for daily calories instead of food? Do you experience frequent short term memory loss (dementia may occur at late stages). Has nervousness and poor coordination become noticeable? Do you lack emotional control? Are you aggressive and abusive towards friends and family? **Note to men:** The liver controls hormone balance. Excessive alcohol especially affects men and their estrogen levels through liver damage. Abuse means enlarged breasts, reduced sex drive and beard growth, shrunken testes.

Diet and Lifestyle Support Therapy

Nutritional therapy plan:

1—No alcohol detox program will work without liver regeneration. A liver detox removes alcohol residues and shortens withdrawal significantly. **Use the LIVER DETOX program on pg. 199.**

2—Then follow the HYPOGLYCEMIA DIET (pg. 463) for 3 months. Take a daily protein drink, like •Solgar WHEY TO GO to balance body chemistry and replace electrolytes quickly. Add 1 tbsp. flax oil to control fatty liver.

3—Think B-vitamins, EFA's, protein and minerals for a solid nutrition base. Especially add magnesium-rich foods like wheat germ, sea veggies, nutritional yeast, whole grains, brown rice, leafy greens, sweet potatoes, low-fat dairy, eggs and fish. Add flax seed to help metabolize excess estrogen.

4—Avoid fried foods, sugary or heavily spiced foods and caffeine. They aggravate alcohol craving. Sodas speed up alcohol release in the blood.

5—Red Star nutritional yeast broth or miso soup every night for B vitamins and to curb craving.

6—Dehydration is a hallmark of alcohol abuse. Drink lots of water daily, and plenty of green or white tea to eliminate alcohol toxins.

—**Lifestyle measures and bodywork:**

•Making major lifestyle reform may be your best medicine for changing body chemistry. It may seem overwhelmingly difficult at times, but this step works at the cause of the problem to curb the craving for alcohol's effects. It almost always begins the road to lasting success and is often the only way.

•Although it states the obvious, avoid places, people and situations that sharpen your desire to escape via alcohol.

•Acupuncture (especially ear and head) and massage therapy realignment help curb craving for alcohol.

•Aerobic exercise, like a daily walk for system oxygen.

•Epsom salt baths for faster detox and mineral therapy.

Herbal, Superfood and Supplement Therapy

Interceptive therapy: Choose 2 to 3 recommendations.

1—**Support your detox:** Crystal Star •ADDICTION WITHDRAWAL™ caps for 3 months, or •Maitake Products MUSHROOM EMPERORS. Try •Crystal Star DR. VITALITY™ caps and tea with white and green tea, ginger and cayenne (rapid results).

2—**Improve brain communication:** •Crystal Star CALCIUM-MAGNESIUM SOURCE™ caps, a rapid calmer; •5-HTP 50-100mg. •Spirulina 500mg daily; add EFA's from High Lignan Flax Oil 2 tbsp. daily (men) or *Evening Primrose Oil* 2000mg (women) also helps mood swings.

3—**Curb alcohol craving:** • Pacific BioLogic's RECOVERY AMERICA is first line defense; • Planetary KUDZU RECOVERY, or •Glutamine, 2000mg with •Tyrosine 1000mg. *•St. John's wort* balances serotonin levels, reduces cravings. *Passionflower-hops* tea controls craving, regulates blood sugar. •Acetyl-Carnitine 1000mg daily reduces liver damage; •Time Release Niacin 500mg 2x daily; Country Life DMG, 125mg boosts energy.

4—**Calm, soothe anxiety reactions and nerves:** •Taurine 500mg; *•Scullcap-black cohosh* tea. •*Kava kava* calms nerves (but also magnifies intoxification levels).

5—**Supplements help overcome critical nutrient deficiencies:** •Vitamin C, up to 10,000mg daily during an alcohol detox (very good results). •B-complex, 100mg 2x daily. B-vitamin deficiency increases alcohol craving. •Zinc 50mg 2x daily. Critical enzymes for alcohol detox are zinc dependent.

6—**Preventive measures:** •DLPA 750mg with magnesium 500mg daily. •Solaray CHROMIACIN regulates blood sugar. •Lithium orotate 5mg for 6 weeks, especially if there is bipolar disorder, too.

—**Superfood therapy:** Choose 1 or 2 recommendations.
•Crystal Star ENERGY GREEN RENEWAL™.
•Unipro PERFECT PROTEIN drink.
•Nutricology PRO GREENS w. EFA's.
•Wakunaga HARVEST BLEND shores up deficiencies.

Can't find a recommended product? Call the 800 number listed in Product Resources for the store nearest you.

Addictions

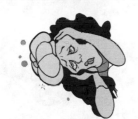

Alcohol Poisoning and Toxicity Reactions, Hangover

A high-stress, fast-paced, jet-lag lifestyle overloads your body's biochemical detox systems (especially your liver) so that too much alcohol the night before gets you a steamroller effect the "morning after." Hangovers take an economic toll, too. Poor job performance and work absenteeism caused by hangovers cost the economy $148 billion every year! A hangover should be gone by five o'clock the next day. If it isn't, you probably have alcohol poisoning... a severe type of hangover with dehydration thrown in. Your body can't work adequately unless you give yourself a break. There are effective natural means of reducing alcohol's damage to your body and brain, but the real idea is to reduce alcohol consumption below the toxicity level.

Do you have a toxic hangover? It's more than just mental dullness, sensitivity to light, a headache or a bad taste in your mouth. A toxic hangover means muscle cramps, all over body shakiness and weakness, and usually vomiting. Initial withdrawal symptoms include high anxiety, rapid pulse with tremors, hot flashes and drenching perspiration, dehydration, insomnia and sometimes hallucinations. A cleanse can help. See page 168 for more information and my book DETOXIFICATION for a complete alcohol cleanse.

Diet and Lifestyle Support Therapy

Nutritional therapy plan:

1—Restabilize your body with vitamin B-rich, high fiber foods like brown rice and vegetables to soak up alcohol.
•If your hangover doesn't go away, you may have alcohol poisoning. Take a catnip, chlorophyll or coffee enema, and the following liver tonic.
Quick liver tonic for alcohol poisoning: Steep 20 minutes - *hibiscus, cloves, allspice,* juice of 2 lemons and *Milk Thistle Seed* 120mg extract in grape or orange juice. Drink slowly. •2 pinches Red Star NUTRITIONAL YEAST in water alleviates nausea

2—Cranberry juice protects the liver. Drink O.J. and tomato juice too, or Knudsen VERY VEGGIE SPICY juice. Their fructose helps the body burn alcohol. Rapid results.

3—NO "hair of the dog" drinks; they drag out a hangover. Crackers and honey, or dates at bedtime burn up and soak up alcohol. 16-oz. water at bedtime and in the morning stave off a killer headache. •Homeopathic *Kali phosphoricum* helps morning breath caused by dehydration.

4—Drink white instead of red wines. They have less congeners by-products to make hangovers worse.

5—Knudsen's RECHARGE electrolyte replacement. (Rapid energy results).

Lifestyle support:
•Get outside in the fresh air - the more oxygen in the lungs and tissues, the better.
•Take a sauna for 20 minutes to help release toxins through the skin. Scrub skin with a dry skin brush. *Kava kava* calms nerves, (but also magnifies intoxification levels) If you take kava for depression or tension, don't drink alcohol for at least 6 hours after taking it. You'll get highly intoxicated. In addition, don't use kava at all if you drink a lot of alcohol cr take medications that affect the liver. The combination may adversely affect liver health.
•If alcohol poisoning is severe, you may need a stomach pump at an urgent care center.
•Apply cold compresses to the head before and after a long hot shower to neutralize and wash off toxins coming out via the skin.

Herbal, Superfood and Supplement Therapy

Interceptive therapy: Choose 2 to 3 recommendations.

1—**Before drinking, minimize brain toxicity:** •N-Acetyl Cysteine (NAC) 600mg with •Evening Primrose oil 1000mg caps, and •Prince of Peace GINSENG-ROYAL JELLY vials or •B-complex 100mg before drinking and before retiring to boost glutathione (excellent results). •Living Essentials CHASER caps reduce shakiness. •Kudzu caps, or •Planetary KUDZU HERBAL suppress ethanol.

–**For liver support:** •Floradix GALLEXIER liquid, •Crystal Star LIVER CLEANSE FLUSHING™ tea.

2—**After you drink:** •Crystal Star ANTI-FLAM™ or New Chapter ZYFLAMEND PM caps (excellent results for hangover prevention). –**For withdrawal:** •Alacer EMERGEN-C with bioflavs ½ tsp. in water, with •B-complex 100mg. • Homeopathic *Nux vomica* for sour stomach. •*Scullcap* tea soothes nerves and oxygenates, and •5-HTP - 50mg.

–**Curb cravings:** *Siberian eleuthero* extract drops in *angelica root* tea.
–**For energy:** •Crystal Star FEEL GREAT NOW!™ with Ginseng caps, or •Planetary GINSENG REVITALIZER tabs.

3—**Antioxidants end the misery:** Take 1 each: EVENING PRIMROSE oil 1300mg. Country Life B-12 sublingual, 2500mcg; Country Life DMG, 125mg tablet, Glutamine 1000mg, L-carnitine 1500mg for better mental performance.

4—**Nervines and enzyme therapy:** •*Sweet Violet* tea, 3 cups daily. •*Cayenne-ginger* capsules settle stomach, relieve headache. •*Dandelion-burdock-ginger* tea with honey quells nausea. •UAS Labs DDS-PLUS or •Jarrow JARRO-DOPHILUS with FOS remove acetylaldehyde, linked to hangovers.

—Antioxidant hangover chasers:
•Mix tomato juice, green and yellow onions, celery, parsley, hot pepper sauce, rosemary, fennel seeds, basil, water and Bragg's LIQUID AMINOS. Drink straight down.
•Herbal Answers ALOE FORCE drink.
•Jarrow GENTLE FIBERS.

Can't find a recommended product? Call the 800 number listed in Product Resources for the store nearest you.

Addictions

Drug Abuse, Rehabilitation

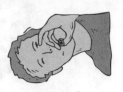

Caffeine Addiction

One of the most widely used stimulants in the world, caffeine is in coffee, tea, cocoa, chocolate and herbs like *cola* nuts and *yerba maté* tea. It is in medicines like Excedrin, Anacin, Vanquish and Bromo-seltzer. It is an ingredient of almost every weight loss drug and many soft drinks. Over 80% of American adults drink coffee; almost everybody else gets caffeine in some form. Clearly caffeine is a quick energy pick-me-up, and a memory stimulant, but just as clearly, excessive use of caffeine (over 5 cups of coffee a day) can lead to anxiety, sleeplessness, high blood sugar levels, rapid heartbeat, exhausted adrenals and increased tolerance – all signs of addiction.

Good ideas for successfully cutting down on caffeine without the agony of withdrawal:

1: Have a cup of energizing herb tea instead of coffee. Try •DR. VITALITY™ tea (slower, longer energy), or •Prince of Peace RED GINSENG-ROYAL JELLY vials, or GINKGO with TIBETAN RHODIOLA vials (almost immediately noticeable results).

2: Strengthen adrenal glands with herbal formulas: •Crystal Star FEM SUPPORT CFS STAMINA™ drops for women, or •ADRENAL ENERGY BOOST™ caps for men or Planetary SCHIZANDRA ADRENAL COMPLEX.

3: Normalize body chemistry with *Siberian eleuthero* or *panax ginseng, ashwagandha, gotu kola, jiaogulan, reishi mushroom.*

4: Take •Natra-Bio homeopathic *CAFFEINE WITHDRAWAL RELIEF,* zinc 30mg daily (caffeine leaches out body zinc stores), and add a B-Complex 100mg daily.

5: For withdrawal headaches: •Crystal Star ANTI-FLAM™ caps, 2–4 at a time; or •Gaia Herbs MIGRA-PROFEN.

6: For constipation, try triphala caps, longterm; •Zand CLEANSING LAXATIVE, short term.

7: Consider aromatherapy: oils of *peppermint, rosemary,* and *lemon balm* gently help awaken the mind.

Prescription Drug Dependence

Widespread dependence on prescription drugs is serious today – especially mood altering tranquilizers, pain killers, anti-depressants, and anti-psychotics. Addiction to benzodiazepines is especially insidious. Some people report severe withdrawal symptoms which persist over years! Others, like amphetamines, create an addictive high in a metabolic process similar to that of body endorphins. A 1998 study shows that 17% of Americans over 60 are addicted, and that many seniors mix alcohol with their prescription drugs for even more risk.

—**Signs that addiction is occurring:** 1) The body builds up a tolerance to the drug, so that the user increases dosage regularly. 2) There is decreased desire to work, with inattentiveness, mood swings, restlessness, temper tantrums, crying spells, etc. 3) There is unusual susceptibility to illness because the immune system and the liver are weakened. 4) Withdrawal headaches, insomnia, light sensitivity, hot flashes, diarrhea and disorientation occur when the user stops taking the drug. 5) Drug-seeking behavior like juggling prescriptions from different doctors and frequent trips to emergency rooms are signs that a prescription drug addiction is out of control. Some tranquilizers can be replaced with herbal remedies to avoid dependence, but specific prescription information is necessary to make withdrawal straightforward and safe. For many prescription drug addicts, a liver detox can be of great benefit. Always seek guidance from a practicing naturopath or holistic doctor for the best results.

Three types of herbs are needed to wean yourself from addictive prescription drugs.

—Nervines, like *scullcap* and *passionflower,* relax and rebuild your nerves. Try •Crystal Star RELAX™ caps.

—Tonic adaptogens, such as *ginseng, astragalus,* or *chlorella* strengthen and normalize the body.

—Liver detox herbs, like *milk thistle seed, dandelion rt.* or *turmeric* (curcumin), help rebalance your system.

About Marijuana Use

Marijuana use is rising again in the U.S., this time with propagation techniques that make THC content over 200% greater than 20 or 30 years ago! Marijuana is no longer the mild, euphoric 3 or 4 hour high of the 60's and 70's. It is addictive. Those dependent on it are either constantly thinking about it, intoxicated, or recovering from its influence. Both mental and physical health are affected - blood sugar balance, muscle coordination, reaction time and emotional deterioration. Work habits suffer from low ambition, family life and relationships suffer from apathy and non-communication.

Can't find a recommended product? Call the 800 number listed in Product Resources for the store nearest you.

Casual marijuana users are generally not aware of new research about this drug. Its newly increased strength means many more people are experiencing exaggerated effects.... acute anxiety, paranoia, incoherent speech, extreme disorientation and hallucinations lasting up to 12 hours. Marijuana also impairs the reproductive system, especially in terms of reduced male sperm count; reduces short and long term memory; and depresses immune response.... by as much as 40%. Tests show that risk of a heart attack increases up to five-fold in the first hour after smoking marijuana! Even smoking medicinal marijuana may be unwise for patients with heart disease. Further, marijuana smoke today contains the same health-damaging carcinogens as tobacco smoke, *only now in much higher concentrations.* Its smoke is inhaled more deeply and held in the lungs longer than tobacco, leading to severe lung damage. The diseases of nicotine smokers now beset marijuana smokers - especially chronic bronchitis, emphysema and lung cancer. Marijuana withdrawal is characterized by anxiety, sleeplessness, tremors and chills.

Simple nutrition and lifestyle changes go a long way toward minimizing discomfort and craving.

—Marijuana leaches B vitamins: make brown rice and broccoli mainstays of your diet during the withdrawal period. Follow a Hypoglycemia Diet (pg. 463) to control sugar cravings.

—Take a protein drink each morning: •ALL ONE MULTIPLE green plant base, •Unipro PERFECT PROTEIN, •Crystal Star RESTORE YOUR STRENGTH™ drink with sea greens.

—Take antioxidants like tyrosine 500mg daily, plenty of •vitamin C with bioflavonoids or Alacer EMERGEN-C (2 packets a day, good results), •B-complex, and herbal nerve relaxers like *rosemary aromatherapy,* or •Crystal Star RELAX CAPS™ (results in about 25 minutes).

—Exercise re-oxygenates your tissues to help you kick the craving. Marijuana makes for flabby bodies.

Does your body need to clean out drug or alcohol toxins?

Americans have an expensive river of chemicals coursing through our national veins. We take $140.6 billion worth of prescription drugs each year. Fourteen million Americans—1 in every 13 adults—are alcoholic or abuse alcohol. At a cost to taxpayers of nearly $300 billion dollars a year in health care costs, extra law enforcement, automobile accidents, crime, and lost productivity, addiction may be the nation's number one health problem. Nicotine addiction alone costs the U.S. economy a price tag of $138 billion. Society's use of "hard" or "pleasure" drugs is also prevalent. Still, experts believe the most serious addictions are those to prescription drugs. More than one million people a year (3 to 5 percent of admissions) end up in hospitals as a result of negative reactions to prescription drugs.

Clearly, modern drugs play lifesaving roles in emergency situations and they can help numerous health problems, especially short term, but most people begin taking drugs to alleviate boredom and fatigue, or to relieve pain. A detox program helps enormously to release drugs and alcohol from your system, but withdrawing after long time use can produce harsh effects. Detox spas and clinics are everywhere today, staffed by health professionals that can help you with a dependency cleanse, especially if addiction has been long term.

Drugs and alcohol not only add to poisons in your body but can aggravate an original health problem. You must fortify your body enough to be able to resist returning to the addictive substance. A drug detox releases stored residues, at the same time changing lifestyle habits so that you are no longer dependent on them. A well-nourished body can offer enough of a sense of well being and strength to melt the relapse urges and desires.

Do you think you might be addicted?

—Do you only feel happy and relaxed after having a drink or taking an antidepressant or mood elevating drug? Does a day without alcohol or drugs lead you to overwhelming emotional or physical pain?

—Do you relieve stress with a drink or a drug? Do you get severe headaches that feel like a continual hangover?

—Are the whites of your eyes dingy? Is the lower lid yellow? Is your skin slightly yellow? Do you sweat a lot? *Signs of liver exhaustion.*

—Does your stomach protrude but you are thin everywhere else? *It's a sign of liver inflammation.*

—Have you lost your appetite? Have you gotten unusually thin? Do you have an intolerance for fatty foods? *Signs that drugs are replacing your body's normal call for food.*

—Is your digestion always bad? Do you have a metallic taste in your mouth? Are you drowsy after meals? *Habitual drug and alcohol users suffer from chronic sublclinical malnutrition, and multiple depletions of critical nutrients. Vitamins, minerals, amino acids, fatty acids and enzymes are all depleted, some by 50 to 60 percent. See following page for more.*

Can't find a recommended product? Call the 800 number listed in Product Resources for the store nearest you.

—Do you have short term memory loss? It's one of the first signs of alcohol abuse; brain damage is another, signalled by lack of motor coordination.
—Do you have esophagus impairment, reflux after eating, high blood pressure, or pancreatitis? Are your stools a pale color? All signs of low enzymes and impaired nutrient use.
—Are you always tired? Extreme fatigue usually means poor liver health, adrenal exhaustion or low thyroid.
—Are you foggy mentally? Intolerant to certain foods? Overly sensitive to chemicals?
—Do you crave sweets? Is your blood sugar low? Do you get dizzy or black out? Signs of rampant hypoglycemia from alcohol or drug overload.
—Do you feel shaky and sweaty? Do you often get a "wired," nervous feeling, sometimes with heart palpitations? Central nervous system overload is a sign of addiction.
—Are you unusually anxious, even paranoid? Do you lose your temper or get in a bad mood easily? Do you feel depressed and cry a lot? Typically late symptoms of alcohol abuse.
—Is your immune response low? Have a cold or flu all the time? Drugs weaken the immune system over time.
—Do you avoid spending time with friends and family? Withdrawal from normal social and family contacts is often a clear sign of dependency.
—Are you missing more and more work or school days? Late stage addicts focus on only one goal, getting more of the addictive substance and using it.
—Do you blame others or circumstances for your drug use? Do you deny that you have a problem? Denial and blame run deep in addictions. An addict feels he is victim of life's injustices, rather than chemically dependant

What does it feel like to withdraw from drugs or alcohol?

Withdrawal symptoms are the same as addiction symptoms, only worse and more frequent. Breaking destructive habits is hard. Your body, mind and spirit all react in concert when a substance you think you depend on is removed. The initial withdrawal phase is usually the most difficult part of an addiction detox and can last from two or three days, to a week, a month or more. You'll get chronic headaches, usually with diarrhea as your body tries to release toxins faster, and a lot of irritability and anxiety. Some people experience hallucinations, disorientation or irrational thinking. Some people go into depression or unexplained crying episodes. You'll probably sleep poorly, and your sleep will be interrupted during the night. Most people in withdrawal are sensitive to light and noise, hot and cold flashes, and they sweat profusely. Without the addictive substance, most people lack the energy or motivation to get out of bed in the morning.

But every day gets easier. I encourage people to look at each episode of discomfort as a little victory on the road to recovery. One of the laws of the universe is that we don't have to fight the same battle twice. As your body dislodges and removes more toxins day by day, you have the satisfaction of knowing they can be gone for good. Natural mood enhancers, like St. John's Wort and Kava Kava, that our bodies are equipped to handle, help in the weaning process from addictive substances. Ginkgo biloba extract for a month speeds up your brain and circulation processes so you're better able to face the world. Panax Ginseng is a good choice to rebalance both body and brain chemistry.

Is your brain chemistry to blame for your addiction?

Many experts believe disordered brain chemistry plays a key role in proneness to addiction, theorizing that addiction may be a symptom of a deeper imbalance within the limbic system that predisposes an addictive response. In the limbic system, the center of the brain which controls emotional response, there are two basic pathways, excitatory and sedative. A wide range of feelings (from deep sleep to euphoria) begins in these pathways through neurotransmitters like dopamine, epinephrine, norepinephrine, serotonin and gamma amino butyric acid (GABA). Drugs and alcohol disrupt the limbic system, causing severe depletions of these neurotransmitters– it's why addicts and alcoholics are so prone to mood swings and depression!

Curtis Harned, formerly of Pacific BioLogic, an herbal company making great strides in finding effective, natural therapies for addiction, recommends an orthomolecular approach focusing on normalizing brain neurotramitters and limbic system health. Harned says, "Individuals who suffer low baseline populations of excitatory neurotransmitters are subject to depression states, and vulnerable to dependency on stimulant drugs. Low baseline populations of sedative neurotransmitters result in people suffering anxiety disorders. They are vulnerable to dependency on depressant drugs.... Of premier value is the nutrient therapy using neurotransmitter precursor amino acids, vitamins and minerals, and beneficial "orthomolecular" compounds."

Pacific BioLogic's NUTRITION IN RECOVERY HANDBOOK and RECOVERY AMERICA morning and evening formulas are used with excellent results in treatment facilities all over the country today. Call 800-869-8783 for ordering information and their complete program.

Can't find a recommended product? Call the 800 number listed in Product Resources for the store nearest you.

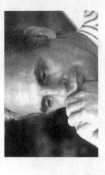

Addictions
Drug Abuse, Rehabilitation

The origins of addictions range from inherited genetics, childhood behavior patterns, allergies to certain foods (especially the inability to metabolize carbohydrates properly), brain neurotransmitter deficits, even estrogen dominance. But most people begin taking drugs to alleviate boredom, to relieve pain, or to cope with depression. Club drugs like Ecstasy, GHB and ketamine are the latest rage, for enhancing euphoria, sexuality and stamina. Don't be fooled.... all street drugs, whether chemical or so-called herbal are very strong and usually adulterated. Multiple depletions of critical nutrients set off addictive chain reactions, seriously affect brain chemistry, or much worse. Just one botched concoction can cause sudden death, coma, even a persistent vegetative state! At the least, nutritional health is severely compromised, often taking the form of metabolic disorders like low blood sugar, hypothyroidism, liver malfunction, poor food absorption or diarrhea even when meals are good. It takes a year or more to detoxify the blood of drugs. **Do you think you might be addicted to drugs?** Watch yourself for constant financial problems (all of your money goes to drugs); unusual irritability, shakiness; bouts of nerves and anxiety, memory loss; irregular heartbeat with sweating and cramps; headaches, hallucinations (both auditory and visual). Natural lifestyle therapies help treat addictions by minimizing the discomfort and maximizing the healing process.

Diet and Lifestyle Support Therapy

Nutritional therapy plan:
A cleanse can help get rid of drug residues quickly. See page 168 for more information and my book DETOXIFICATION for a complete cleanse.

1—Most addictive drugs create malnutrition. Improve your diet to overcome nutrient deficiencies caused by substance abuse. Include plenty of slow-burning complex carbohydrates from whole grains and fresh vegetables, and vegetable protein from soy, grains and sprouts. Good choice: a HYPOGLYCEMIA DIET, page 463.

2—The brain is dependent on glucose for energy. Drug withdrawals often mean blood glucose levels drop. Sweating, tremors, palpitations, anxiety and cravings result. Eliminate sugars, alcohol and caffeine. They aggravate the craving for drugs.

3—Enzymes restabilize body chemistry: fresh plant enzymes, especially leafy greens and sea greens for antioxidant carotenoids, minerals and EFAs; or •Enzymedica DIGEST.

Lifestyle support:
•Biofeedback, chiropractic, massage therapy, yoga and acupuncture techniques have a high success rate in overcoming drug addictions.

•Heal ulcers in the nose: apply *tea tree oil*, or B&T CALI-FLORA GEL.

—**Help for specific drugs:** Strong drugs, from LSD to hard alcohol to nicotine to heroin. can put you at higher risk for Alzheimer's disease due to microvascular blockage and cerebral dementia. Nicotine increases craving for drugs by stripping the body of stabilizing nutrients.

Nutrients to try: Methionine for heroine; Tyrosine, NADH and Siberian eleuthero for cocaine and Ecstasy; CoQ-10 up to 300mg for prescription drugs; LITHIUM orotate 5mg for uppers and depressants; Pacific BioLogic S.T.O.P. for opiates (very good clinical results); B-complex 150mg for LSD. Melatonin is a specific for Valium withdrawal- 2mg 30 minutes before bedtime nightly for 6 weeks.

Herbal, Superfood and Supplement Therapy

Interceptive therapy 7-step plan: Choose one recommendation under each category.

1—Normalize body chemistry: •Crystal Star ADDICTION WITHDRAWAL™ caps, and •DR. VITALITY™ tea, for 3 months. •Prince of Peace GINSENG-ROYAL JELLY vials. •Lobelic extract drops under the tongue every half hour can sometimes normalize an overdose situation.

2—Clean out drug residues: •Crystal Star TOXIN DETOX™ or •DETOX™ caps 4 daily; •Sun CHLORELLA tabs; •Yogi DETOX tea; • Herbal Clean QUICK TABS (results temporary). •Highly recommended: Pacific BioLogic RECOVERY AMERICA, morning and evening formulas show excellent results in treatment facilities.

3—Detoxify the liver: •Crystal Star LIVER CLEANSE FLUSHING™ tea or •GREEN TEA CLEANSER™, or •Flora BILIV tea with •*Milk Thistle Seed* extract for 2 months, and •B-complex 150mg daily.

4—Lessen withdrawal discomfort: •Crystal Star RELAX™ caps (fast acting), *Valerian-wild lettuce* extract for sleepless anxiety; •Natural Balance HTP:Calm; *gotu kola* caps: glutamine 1000mg; •DLPA 750mg for cravings and depression. Try *Chamomile* for stress, *scullcap* for nerves, *ginkgo biloba* for memory loss, chromium to rebalance sugar levels.

6—Increase energy: •Crystal Star FEEL GREAT NOW!™ with Ginseng caps, or •MENTAL CLARITY™ caps; •*Siberian eleuthero*; •*astragalus* extract.

7—Replenish neurotransmitters: •Enzymatic Therapy THYROID/TYROSINE caps (fast results.) •NADH 10 mg daily; •Country Life RELAXER (GABA with taurine). •Vitamin C crystals, up to 10,000mg daily, with niacin 1000mgdaily.

—**Superfood therapy:** Choose 1 or 2 recommendations.
•All One MULTIPLE GREENS or Body Ecology VITALITY SUPER GREEN.
•Crystal Star RESTORE YOUR STRENGTH™ drink and caps (especially for overcoming prescription drug dependency).
•Nutricology PRO GREENS.
•Pure Essence FLORALIVE helps replace friendly G.I. flora.

Can't find a recommended product? Call the 800 number listed in Product Resources for the store nearest you.

Adrenal Gland Health

Adrenal Exhaustion

Stress in America has skyrocketed, especially since the September 11th attacks. The passage of time has not lessened it; collectively, our health toll has been enormous. Many experts say it's getting worse. Over 1 million Americans miss work every day because of stress-related disorders. Adrenal burn-out is called "America's invisible epidemic," with up to 80% of U.S. adults suffering adrenal fatigue at some point in their lives. It's the primary cause of today's exhaustion illnesses like chronic fatigue syndrome, mononucleosis and EBV. It's involved in candidiasis and fibromyalgia syndromes. Low blood sugar attacks and increased allergies are often the result of exhausted adrenals.

Type A personalities, competitive people who push themselves to their limits in every endeavor, appear to be the most often affected. But, truth be told, more and more Americans are shouldering more responsibility in their families, working harder and longer hours than ever just to get by, getting less sleep that they need.... so adrenal burn-out is affecting more people.

When functioning well, our adrenal glands are Mother Nature's wonderful tools for dealing with stress. Two tiny, walnut sized glands that rest on top of our kidneys, and weigh no more than a grape, the adrenals are our body's major steroid factories, producing almost 150 vital hormones that keep us healthy. Comprised of the medulla, which secretes adrenaline and norepinephrine to help the body cope with stress by increasing metabolism, and the cortex, which maintains our body balance by regulating sugar metabolism as well as a complex array of steroid hormones, including cortisone, DHEA, aldosterone, progesterone, estrogen, and testosterone.

Medical doctors often ignore adrenal dysfunction unless it is severe or part of illnesses like Addison's disease or Cushing's syndrome (see next page). However, a skilled naturopath can assess your adrenal health and offer support therapies that help the body resist stress, and really make a difference in your well being. Menopausal complaints, like hot flashes and panic attacks, may be completely relieved with a natural adrenal program.

Adrenal dysfunction is almost entirely caused by a poor diet and a high stress lifestyle.

If you're using steroid drugs extensively for arthritis, asthma, allergies, skin problems or M.S., these drugs can cause the adrenals to shrink in size. If your diet is overloaded with sugar, fried foods, salty snacks and caffeine; if you're overusing alcohol or nicotine, your adrenals are more than likely on stress overload. Note for menopausal women: Adrenal health is critical after menopause because these glands shore up hormone production to keep a woman healthy, active, and beautiful after estrogen production is reduced by the ovaries. Stress depletes B and C vitamins, too. Menopausal women should be aware of their levels of these vitamins for adrenal health.

Are your adrenals exhausted? **Three or more yes answers should alert you.**

—Are your energy and alertness chronically low for no discernible reason? Is even mild exercise of any kind a burden?

—Do you have frequent unexplained moodiness, unusual crying spells, unfounded guilt?

—Do you have severely cracked, painful heels? Do you have nervous moistness of hands and soles of feet?

—Do you have brittle, peeling nails or extremely dry skin?

—Do you get heart palpitations, anxiety spells or panic attacks... usually followed by great fatigue?

—Do you have chronic heartburn and poor digestion? Do you constantly crave salty foods or sweets?

—Do you have frequent yeast or fungal infections? Do you have severe reactions to odors or certain foods?

—Do you have chronic lower back pain (adrenal swelling)? If you press your adrenals in the small of your back, do they hurt?

Test yourself for adrenal dysfunction: Ragland's Test is a common diagnostic procedure used by chiropractors, massage therapists and naturopaths with a home blood pressure testing kit:

1. Lie down, rest for 5 minutes. Take a blood pressure reading. Systolic blood pressure should be below 120, diastolic blood pressure below 80.

2. In one minute, stand up, take another reading. Systolic blood presure should rise by about 5 points. If it drops, your adrenals are probably working poorly. The amount of drop is in ratio to the amount of adrenal dysfunction.

Can't find a recommended product? Call the 800 number listed in Product Resources for the store nearest you.

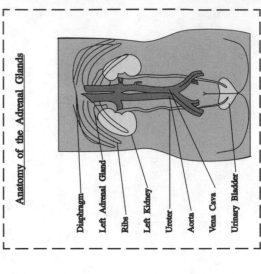

Anatomy of the Adrenal Glands

Diaphragm
Left Adrenal Gland
Ribs
Left Kidney
Ureter
Aorta
Vena Cava
Urinary Bladder

Do you have Addison's Disease?

Addison's disease is an autoimmune disorder which destroys the adrenal cortex. The adrenal glands become completely unable to secrete steroid hormones. Immune response decreases, energy levels fall rapidly; even small stresses lead to serious health collapse. Addison's disease may be lifelong and life threatening. Medical doctors strongly recommend corticosteroid hormone replacement to regulate blood sugar levels, blood pressure and electrolyte levels. Medical therapy now allows most people with Addison's disease to live a full life today.

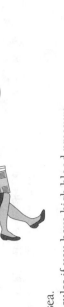

Warning signs to watch for:

—unexplained weight loss usually accompanied by severe nausea and/or vomiting

—chronic fatigue (especially muscular weakness); unusual irritability and depression

—changes in pigmentation (skin darkening)

—light-headedness and dizziness upon standing from low blood pressure

—cravings for salty foods (loss of body salt from electrolyte imbalance is common in Addison's disease)

Watchwords:

• A good diet is critical. Alcohol, caffeine, tobacco, and highly processed foods must be avoided.

• Stimulate and balance ACTH with organic Nutricology ADRENAL CORTEX and PITUITARY concentrate.

• Take Red Star Nutritional Yeast, 2 tbsp. daily; with extra B Complex 100mg and pantothenic acid 100mg.

• Rebalance electrolytes: Use sea veggies for their chelated minerals and/or Nature's Path TRACE-LYTE minerals from the sea.

• Take Licorice root tea or extract drops to reduce the hydrocortisone broken down by the liver; use deglycyrrhizinated capsules if you have high blood pressure.

• Take royal jelly, up to 100,000mg daily; or Prince of Peace AMERICAN GINSENG-ROYAL JELLY vials or GINKGO-ROYAL JELLY with Rhodiola vials (highly recommended).

Do you have Cushing's Syndrome?

Cushing's is a rare, dysfunctional disease caused by an overactive adrenal cortex. Cushing's syndrome is allowed by immune suppression, and sometimes brought on by an overdose of steroid drugs, (particularly those used for rheumatoid arthritis), or a benign pituitary gland tumor. It is a metabolic disease that causes kidney stones to form. It is characterized by a fat stomach, face and buttocks, but severe thinness in the limbs. There is muscle wasting and weakness, poor wound healing, thinning of the skin leading to stretch marks and bruising. Peptic ulcers, high blood pressure, mental instability, and diabetes accompany Cushing's. The face may get acne-like sores and the eyelids are often swollen. Cushing's appears in women five times more than men; there is scalp balding, excess body and facial hair (hirsutism), brittle bones, along with a wide variety of menstrual disorders.

Our experience with Cushing's has been limited, but the following protocols are helpful:

—A vegetarian diet, low in fat, salt, sugar, with high potassium foods - bananas, broccoli, sea greens, etc.

—Add green drinks, like Nutricology PRO-GREENS, chlorella, germanium and protein for healing, or Crystal Star ENERGY GREEN RENEWAL™ drink regularly.

—Take potassium supplementally - daily sea greens, 2 tbsp. snipped sea veggies, any kind, over rice, salad greens or soup, herbal potassium drinks (see page 291, like Futurbiotics VITAL K, or Crystal Star RESTORE YOUR STRENGTH™ drink, or capsules like Crystal Star OCEAN MINERALS™, sea plant iodine and potassium source capsules, or New Chapter OCEAN HERBS iodine and potassium.

Note: If you're worried about your adrenal health, a hormone saliva test can be very telling. Contact ZRT Laboratories (503-466-2445) or visit www.salivatest.com for more information.

Can't find a recommended product? Call the 800 number listed in Product Resources for the store nearest you.

Adrenal Gland Health

Diet and Lifestyle Support Therapy

Nutritional therapy plan:

SEE DIET FOR HYPOGLYCEMIA page 463 for specifics.

A good diet and plenty of rest are essential. Potassium is the principal mineral lost when adrenal health is compromised. Potassium-rich foods like sea veggies, bananas, kiwis, potatoes, broccoli and fish help recharge adrenal energy.

Other key nutrients: B vitamins (royal jelly shows excellent results); vitamin C (helps convert cholesterol to adrenal hormones); zinc foods, like brown rice, grains, sunflower seeds, pumpkin seeds, nutritional yeast, bran, eggs, oysters, etc.; magnesium foods like green leafy vegetables, almonds, apricots, avocado, carrots, citrus fruits, lentils, salmon, flounder; and the amino acid tyrosine. I use about 500mg daily.

1—Eat small, instead of large meals, low in sugar and fats. Eat lots of fresh foods, cold water fish, brown rice, legumes, dark greens and whole grains.

2—Put sea greens at the top of your list of adrenal enhancing foods. Add potassium-rich foods like potatoes, salmon, seafood and avocados to your diet.... about 3 to 5 grams daily. Cut down on high sodium foods.

3—Avoid hard liquor, tobacco and excess caffeine during healing.

4—Avoid fats, fried, salty foods, red meats, sugary foods and fast foods.

5—Each morning, make a fresh mix of 2 teaspoons each flax seed, bran, nutritional yeast, toasted wheat germ, and maple syrup and add to your favorite cereal or yogurt. Or, have a cup of miso broth every evening, adding 2 teaspoons each nutritional yeast and toasted wheat germ to boost benefits.

Lifestyle bodywork:

•Massage therapy is effective in improving adrenal function. Therapists use muscle testing to determine the degree of dysfunction, and then work to clear the adrenal pathways through cranial and nerve massage treatment.

•Take a Crystal Star HOT SEAWEED BATH™ for a noticeable adrenal energy boost.

•Take an arm-swinging walk every day for adrenal health

•Don't smoke. Nicotine encourages adrenal surges.

Herbal, Superfood and Supplement Therapy

Interceptive therapy: Choose 2 to 3 recommendations.

1—Stimulate hormone and adrenal rebalance: •Crystal Star ADRENAL ENERGY BOOST™ caps 2x daily, with FEEL GREAT NOW™ caps; (rebuilding energy for both men and women over 40); •Planetary SCHIZANDRA ADRENAL COMPLEX; •CC Pollen High Desert ROYAL JELLY with ginseng, 2 tsp. daily; •Nutricology GERMANIUM 150mg daily.

—**For women:** Add •Allergy Research Group ADRENAL CORTEX or •Crystal Star OCEAN MINERALS™ sea plant iodine-potassium caps. • For severe adrenal insufficiency, DHEA 5mg (short term). •Jiaogulan caps or tea (highly recommended).

—**For men:** Add •Prince of Peace American GINSENG-ROYAL JELLY with Rhodiola vials, 1 daily; or Planetary GINSENG ELIXIR tabs; •Panax ginseng root, or Siberian eleuthero-astragalus capsules, 4 daily. •Rhodiola rosea caps or tea (highly recommended).

—**Adrenal support from herbs:**

•Evening primrose oil 4-6 daily.

•Siberian eleuthero and panax ginsengs directly support the medulla.

•Licorice root tea (reduces the hydrocortisone broken down by the liver; use deglycyrrhizinated capsules if you have high blood pressure).

•Hawthorn extract - 1 dropperful as needed for a feeling of well-being.

•Gotu kola extract caps 6 daily, also help rebuild nerves.

—**Superfood therapy:** Choose 1 or 2 recommendations.

•Crystal Star RESTORE YOUR STRENGTH™ drink or caps with sea veggies.

•Wakunaga KYO-GREEN drink.

•Green Kamut JUST BARLEY drink.

•Nutricology PRO-GREENS with EFAs.

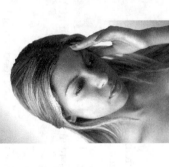

—**Preventives:** A good multiple works for adrenal exhaustion. Try •Diamond Formulas HEALTHY HORIZONS (highly recommended).

•Adrenal glandular - Country Life ADRENAL with TYROSINE or organic Nutricology ADRENAL CORTEX.

•Enzymatic Therapy LIQUID LIVER with Siberian eleuthero.

•Pantothenic acid 1000mg daily, with B-complex 100mg and Tyrosine 500mg.

•Ascorbate vitamin C 3000mg or Ester C 1500mg blocks excess cortisol.

•Enzymes: CoQ-10 100mg daily, Enzymedica DIGEST, Crystal Star DR. ENZYME™ with protease and bromelain, or Prevail VITASE boost adrenal cortex.

Can't find a recommended product? Call the 800 number listed in Product Resources for the store nearest you.

AIDS and HIV Infection

AIDS Related Syndromes

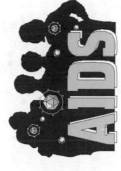

Despite the advances of modern medicine, serious, incurable diseases are spreading around the world at an astonishing rate. HIV infection has gone beyond the gay community, to heterosexuals and to babies from infected parents. AIDS has become a global epidemic in just twenty short years. At this writing, nearly 40 million people worldwide now live with HIV-AIDS. Over 70% of them live in Africa where AIDS suppressing drugs are not widely obtainable, and safe sex practices are not culturally accepted. So far, a staggering 23 million have died.

In the U.S., nearly 1 million people are living with HIV. One-quarter of them don't even know it! Sadly, after almost a decade of decline, this number is again rising, with heterosexual women now the fastest growing group of people infected with HIV. New AIDS drugs in America have offered a false sense of protection, and risky sex practices have risen as a result.

AIDS and its cousin diseases are the result of immune system breakdown. The body becomes unable to defend itself. Long believed to be caused by the HIV (human immunodeficiency virus), a retro-virus that affects DNA and T-cells, there is a growing body of evidence that severe AIDS is influenced by nutritional factors.

AIDS occurs in stages: 1) an asymptomatic state when HIV is most often passed; 2) a mononucleosis-like stage with one or more AIDS-related complexes; 3) "full blown" AIDS. The protocols in this section are for those who have been diagnosed with HIV but are asymptomatic, for those who have decided to reject orthodox AIDS treatment for alternative methods, and for those who have tried orthodox treatment, but showed no improvement and want to use alternative techniques (even new highly acclaimed drugs are failing, especially in advanced cases).

Advanced HIV-AIDS drug cocktails offer new hope, but they are not free of side effects or serious risks. In fact, researchers estimate that 50% of deaths attributed to AIDS are actually the *result* of the toxic side effects of antiviral drugs! More concerns: Drug-resistant HIV strains can emerge and the viral load may skyrocket if the drugs are discontinued.

Other severe drawbacks: • Diarrhea due to digestive difficulty (HIV itself compromises digestive function); • Adult-onset Diabetes; • Birth defects in children born to infected mothers; • Lipodystrophy syndrome- fatty growths on the neck and back; • Anemia and resulting chronic fatigue; • Liver toxicity; • Bone marrow toxicity (AZT).

If you decide to use a combination of orthodox and alternative treatments, seek out a knowledgeable naturopath. There are over 122 HIV-AIDS drugs in development, and mixing natural products with the powerful drugs used for AIDS can be dangerous. A qualified holistic physician offers the best results.

Are new HIV home tests a good choice?

Pharmacies now carry HIV tests, costing $40 to $50 that you can perform privately in your home. If you're reluctant to get HIV screening from a doctor, home tests can be a good choice. There are some drawbacks: 1) You must send in your sample to a lab; 2) Your results will be communicated to you over the phone a few weeks later; 3) Brands without FDA approval may provide unreliable results. Most communities now offer free, confidential HIV screening. Look under AIDS-HIV in the yellow pages to find a clinic. Regardless of your chosen screening method, knowing your HIV status is critical to your health and to your sexual responsibility in the modern world.

Is there hope if you are HIV positive?

Testing "anti-body positive" does not mean that you have AIDS, only that you have been exposed to the HIV virus. Being HIV positive does not even mean that you will develop AIDS. It is a warning, not a sentence. At least 5% of people diagnosed HIV positive never develop full-blown AIDS. Most infected people co-exist with HIV. The face of AIDS has changed dramatically since the late 90's. Protease inhibitor "cocktails" and genetic modifying drugs, coupled with a healthy diet, elimination of recreational drugs and responsible sexual behavior has improved HIV status.

HIV positive people are recognizing that the destructive lifestyle factors leading to their diagnosis can be changed to prevent re-infection, and that lifestyle therapies can greatly improve their health condition and help keep them symptom free. Often, if the infection is caught early, if lifestyle and nutritional healing measures are embraced, HIV infection can be managed and a patient can live a full, productive life.

Can't find a recommended product? Call the 800 number listed in Product Resources for the store nearest you.

What does it take to survive AIDS?

Although new drug treatment options have already changed the face of HIV-AIDS, researchers still find that even when 99% of the virus appears to be destroyed, resistant strains can appear within days. Thousands of long term AIDS survivors are free of HIV symptoms. In every case I know, the survivor consciously decided to take charge of his or her own life and healing. All energies were channeled into the therapies each thought were right for them. They faced reality, knew there was no silver bullet, realized that the process would be long and hard, that the battle would take great courage. Almost universally, AIDS survivors believe that they grew in their humanity, compassion and maturity by taking responsibility for their enormous task. They felt that they gained strength, confidence and control of their lives - and indeed, became the kind of person they always wanted to be.

A phenomenon of AIDS survival is the intense desire to reach out to other sufferers with courage and hope.

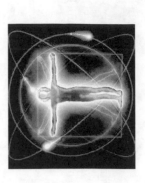

Here are their survival watchwords:

1: **Don't think or behave like a victim - you must fight for your life.** Expect favorable results from your courageous lifestyle steps. There is no invariably fatal diagnosis - no mortal can decide when or if someone will die.

2: **Take charge of your own healing.** Educate yourself about alternative approaches and treatment. Seek life re-inforcing modalities. Lifestyle therapy must be part of recovery. Destructive life patterns must be stopped.

3: **Avoid stress,** learn to laugh, exercise, eliminate harmful drugs and alcohol, reduce red meat and sugar.

4: **Seek the healing power of God and of Love.** You are not alone - seek people and relationships that support your great effort.

Have no fear of death - look forward to your life.

AIDS risks and symptoms you may not know

—**It is fairly easy to transfer HIV virus through anal intercourse, more difficult through vaginal or oral sex.** Powerful proteins in tears, saliva and pregnant women's urine, friendly flora in the intestinal tract, and HCl in the stomach produce a hostile environment that destroys HIV. There is no such protection in the colon. Suppression of the immune system is believed to occur when the HIV virus slips through the intestinal wall and into the bloodstream. Normal immune response is to attack the virus with macrophages that then die and are removed through the lymphatic system. These toxic wastes are finally dumped into the colon on its last leg of clearance from the body, but in an unprotected colon without friendly bacteria or good defensive pH environment, new HIV viruses hatch from the dead macrophages and multiply in the feces, repeating the cycle again and again. The immune system cannot detect the virus in the colon and does not marshal its forces until the infection is in the bloodstream; ...often too late if immune defenses are already exhausted.

—**HIV is never the only culprit in AIDS.** Immune suppression, often related to unhealthy lifestyle activities, comes before HIV. Syphilis is usually present in AIDS victims, as are parasites and other viruses that set the stage for AIDS and related complexes.

—**Parasites are a co-factor in AIDS.** An immune-suppressing lifestyle allows parasites to easily take hold. If you have frequent bacterial infections and use antibiotics that don't help, have your stool tested for parasites. Amoebic parasites allow the virus to spread by rupturing your immune defense cells that try to engulf and destroy it. Parasites also worsen drug side effects, and reduce the body's capacity to benefit from HIV drugs. Some physicians report that when parasite infections are curbed, the HIV viral load goes down to undetectable levels.

—**You can continually re-infect yourself!** Destructive lifestyle actions like continual exposure to HIV and STD's through sexual excess and multiple sex partners, excessive use of alcohol, sharing needles or "snort straws" for drugs expose you to the virus by putting you in direct contact with infected blood.

—**Hepatitis predisposes you to HIV infection, because the liver is so weakened it cannot play its part in resisting infection.** By the same token, HIV also predisposes you to hepatitis by grinding down liver defenses.

—**Symptoms can appear anywhere from 6 months to 3 years after infection. If you feel you are at risk, here are early symptoms to watch out for:** 1) diarrhea that lasts longer than a week; 2) swollen glands and lymph nodes in the neck area, armpits and groin; 3) inability to heal even minor ailments like a small cut, bruise or cold; 4) unusual fatigue; 5) white patches in the mouth and trouble swallowing (thrush); 6) nail ringworm fungus.

—**These further symptoms mean that AIDS is undeniable:** 1) purplish blotches that look like hard bruises occurring on or under the skin, inside the mouth, nose, eyelids or rectum that do not go away (Kaposi's Sarcoma); 2) pneumonia; 3) swollen glands that never go down; 4) persistent dry, hacking cough (unrelated to smoking); 5) fevers and night sweats that last for days or weeks; 6) severe, unexplained, debilitating fatigue; 7) persistent diarrhea that doesn't go away; 8) unexplained, rapid weight loss; 9) visual disturbances; 10) personality changes; 11) dementia or memory loss, confusion and depression.

Can't find a recommended product? Call the 800 number listed in Product Resources for the store nearest you.

Addressing AIDS Related Syndromes

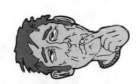

Serious diseases accompany AIDS and play a major role in susceptibility to it. Studies show many of these side-effect syndromes can be addressed with natural, lifestyle therapies. Several observational studies of AIDS infected adults in the U.S. show a 30% reduction in the rate of disease progression when a multivitamin is used. The goal of the suggestions in this therapy section is to increase underlying body system support. System strength is the key to reducing the chances of succumbing to full-blown AIDS or to one of these related infections.

• PNEUMOCYSTIS CARINII (PCP):

A rare form of pneumonia, affects over 70% of all AIDS cases and is the leading cause of AIDS-related death. PCP is thought to be caused by a fungal parasite. Even though new cases of PCP have diminished, as a result of anti-retroviral therapy and new anti-Pneumocystis drugs, PCP is still the most common life threatening infection in people with AIDS whose T-cell counts are below 200.

—**Alternative healing protocols for PCP:** •Black Carrot (*Lomatium dissectum*) extract, (an anti-viral, anti-fungal, anti-bacterial immune stimulant), 30 drops 4x daily, and •Crystal Star RESTORE YOUR STRENGTH™ broth with • VIREX™ caps to guard the respiratory tract; •Pacific BioLogic RESIST 2 (a potent anti-fungal, anti-viral, antibiotic complex). •Earth's Bounty O₂ caps, and O₂ skin spray rubbed on the feet morning and evening; •Nutricology GERMANIUM 150mg daily for interferon production; •Crystal Star D-CONGEST™ extract ventilates the lungs and stimulates the liver to produce anti-histamines; •Potassium broth (page 291) and *milk thistle seed extract* strengthen the liver; •American Biologics DIOXYCHLOR boosts oxygenation; •Enzymatic Therapy MEGA-ZYME and LIVA-TOX stimulate the pancreas to attack foreign proteins in the blood; •Ester C 5000mg for collagen production and healing of infected tissue; •Nutricology SYMBIOTICS powder (rinse mouth 3x daily); •Bromelain 1500mg twice daily; •highest potency ROYAL JELLY, a prime source of pantothenic acid; •Herbal Answers ALOE FORCE or •Aloe Life ALOE GOLD drink rebuilds immunity. *Note:* eat vegetables lightly steamed rather than eaten raw – the protozoan parasite thought to cause pneumocystis lives in the soil and is destroyed by heat. Deep breathing exercises morning and evening help recovery from pneumocystis.

• KAPOSI'S SARCOMA (KS):

Human herpes virus 8 (HHV-8) is widely thought to be the cause of Kaposi's sarcoma in people. Research suggests HHV-8 is spread through deep kissing. Experts suspect this only poses a problem for people with HIV or transplant patients. KS appears as benign skin tumors, but when they accompany AIDS drugs, KS lesions become a serious tissue cancer. (When the drugs are stopped, the lesions often regress.)

—**Alternative healing protocols for KS:** •Curcumin (*turmeric*) extract 10 capsules daily (or more) inhibits tumor necrosis factor (TNF); •Beta Glucan 1500mg stimulates white blood cells; •Crystal Star ANTI-BIO™ gel with *una da gato* and *ginseng* to control infection; •CoQ₁₀ 300mg daily; •PCOs 100mg 3x daily, from *white pine* or *grape seed* oil help restore interleukin; •Grifron MAITAKE MUSHROOM extract or D-fraction Maitake Mushroom extract boosts macrophages and T-cell production (good clinical results); note: mix •D-fraction extract with DMSO and apply to lesions 4x daily, or add Maitake mushrooms to food; •Olive leaf extract, 1 capsule 4x daily to reduce lesions. •Herbal Answers HERBAL ALOE FORCE gel applied directly to lesions; •*Black Carrot* extract (see a clinical naturopath); •Nutribiotic GRAPEFRUIT SEED EXTRACT and SKIN SPRAY are important for healing with the macrobiotic diet page 348. broth (page 291) and •Green Foods CARROT ESSENCE, are important for healing with the macrobiotic diet page 348.

• EPSTEIN-BARR VIRUS (EBV):

A herpes family, chronic fatigue disease, Epstein-Barr is a cause of mononucleosis. EBV lives and hides in B-cells of the immune system, producing antibodies that react against tissue cells to affect immune response. Symptoms are swollen lymph nodes, fever, chills, severe fatigue, chronic sore throat, usually pneumonia. Around 20% of people with HIV develop B-cell lymphoma, linked to Epstein-Barr virus (EBV)

—**Alternative healing protocols for HIV-related Epstein Barr:** •garlic suppositories and Crystal Star VIREX™ caps help kill the virus; •American Biologics DIOXYCHLOR; •UAS DDS-PLUS +FOS or Jarrow Formulas JARRO-DOPHILUS for all-important micro-flora; •AloeLife ALOE GOLD juice each morning; •ECHINACEA EXTRACT or *maitake mushroom* extract to stimulate interferon, and •PANAX GINSENG extract helps mobilize anti-bodies, try •Prince of Peace GINSENG ROYAL JELLY VIALS, 1 daily; •Earth's Bounty O₂ CAPS or O₂ SPRAY rubbed on the feet twice daily; •Crystal Star ENERGY GREEN RENEWAL™ or •Nutricology PRO GREENS drinks with EFAs help rebuild immune strength; •Enzymatic LIQUID LIVER, or •Crystal Star LIVER RENEW™ caps with extra *milk thistle seed* extract, •Alpha Lipoic acid 300mg daily, and •MICROHYDRIN PLUS for 3 to 6 months; •Crystal Star DETOX: FAT & SUGAR RELEASE™ caps, •Enzymatic Therapy LYMPHO-CLEAR or •Herbs, Etc. LYMPHATONIC help relieve lymph node swelling

Can't find a recommended product? Call the 800 number listed in Product Resources for the store nearest you.

• MUSCLE WASTING:

Malabsorption and metabolism irregularity (fat is spared while protein is burned), characterized by severe, unhealthy weight loss and muscle loss can be helped with superfoods. Normalizing body fluid levels, calories and protein is a critical step in fighting infections. Many drugs for AIDS leach valuable nutrients from already weak bodies, making superfoods like •Pure Planet CHLORELLA, •Crystal Star RESTORE YOUR STRENGTH™ drink, or •Life Extension WHEY ISOLATE protein drink even more important.

—**Alternative healing protocols for HIV-related wasting syndrome:** •Liddell VITAL hGH or Nutricology BIOGEN PRO, oral growth hormone products fight tissue wasting (recommended, milder therapy than drug HgH injections). •Consider the South African herb *Sutherlandia* (some patients show weight increases within 6 weeks), available through African Red Tea Imports: *www.africanredtea.com.* •Nature's Path CAL-LYTE, taken with food to fortify against malabsorption, food allergies, degraded gastric membranes, leaky gut, and toxic lymph glands; •Herb Care Chinese bitter melon (*Charantia*) tea and caps, inhibits the virus and treats gastrointestinal infection; •a *panax ginseng- licorice root* tea helps sugar balance, while inhibiting virus replication; •CoQ-10 300mg daily works for stronger blood; •Metabolic Response Modifiers BCAA+G (Branched Chain Amino Acids plus Glutamine), are essential for building muscle size and strength. Or, •Arginine 2000mg and •Glutamine 3000mg 2x daily help defeat muscle loss. Focus your diet on metabolic care, with large amounts of vegetable juices, especially potassium broth (page 291), and •Pines MIGHTY GREENS drink. •Eat complex carbohydrate foods first, protein foods last, and plenty of high fiber foods. Include yogurt, kefir and kefir cheese, and high sulphur foods like garlic and onions. •Essential fatty acids inhibit TNF (tumor necrosis factor), linked to catabolic muscle wasting. Consider •Udo's PERFECTED OIL BLEND, 2 tbsp. per day and daily sea veggies sprinkled over your brown rice and daily salad. Avoid absolutely: caffeine, (drink herbal teas, like green or white tea instead, or try •Crystal Star DR. VITALITY™, green and white tea blend with ginger, for best digestion), all pork and other fatty meats, enzyme-inhibiting foods like unfermented soy products and peanuts, table salt and sugary foods. Cook all beans VERY well. They're great protein, but tend to inhibit enzyme activity unless thoroughly cooked. If enzymes are hard for your body to make, try •Crystal Star DR. ENZYME™ caps with protease and bromelain to help.

• CYTOMEGALOVIRUS (CMV):

A salivary, herpes-type virus, associated with Epstein Barr infection, CMV produces retinitis (lesions on the retinas which can lead to blindness), fever, low white blood cell count and fungal infections of the gastro-intestinal tract. Risk of CMV is highest when CD4 cell counts are below 100.

—**Alternative healing protocols for HIV-related Cytomegalovirus:** •*nettles* extract; •*tea tree oil* mouthwash; •Earth's Bounty OXY CAPS or O₂ SPRAY rubbed on the feet twice daily; •Enzymatic Therapy MEGA-ZYME to digest foreign proteins and •PHYTO-BIOTIC 816 for parasitic infestation. •Acupuncture treatments taken along with *shiitake* and *maitake mushroom* and *astragalus* extracts (or Health Concerns ASTRA-8) have shown good results against symptoms. •*Feverfew* to reduce severe headaches; •Nutricology ADRENAL CORTEX organic glandular caps; •*black carrot* extract (from a clinical naturopath) or •Crystal Star VIREX™ caps along with •*Milk Thistle Seed* extract and •MICROHYDRIN PLUS, and •Alpha Lipoic acid 300mg daily.

• HERPES SIMPLEX VIRUS:

Some experts theorize that HIV only progresses to actual AIDS in the presence of the herpes virus HHV-6A. Ongoing herpes outbreaks are a co-factor in HIV/AIDS progression because they overburden the immune system. If you have HIV, get herpes outbreaks under control for your ongoing health. AIDS-related herpes is aggravated by UV sunlight; antioxidants have protective effects. Merix Health Products RELEEV caps have profound anti-herpes activity. See HERPES pg.535 in this book for the newest products and protocols to consider.

• CANDIDA-THRUSH:

Candida overgrowth is a major cause of reduced digestive capacity in HIV. Chronic thrush mouth infections increase risk for PCP (Pneumocystis Carinii). Melaleuca, Inc. BREATH AWAY *tea tree* oil mouthwash significantly reduces AIDS related thrush. (AIDS 1998;12:1033-7) For candida, use dairy free •UAS DDS-PLUS +FOS or Pure Essence FLORALIVE for all-important micro-flora and see pg.359 for my anti-candida diet with a healing program.

• PARASITES:

Drug therapy may be necessary for severe parasite infestations. Herbal antiparasitic therapy can help: Crystal Star PARASITE PURGE™ caps; or Nature's Secret PARA-STROY. See PARASITES pg.519 for more information.

Can't find a recommended product? Call the 800 number listed in Product Resources for the store nearest you.

A Holistic Approach to Overcoming HIV and AIDS

Holistic therapies show more promise than ever for AIDS and its related syndromes. Alternative treatment programs are enormous factors in showing that HIV and AIDS are no longer inevitably fatal as they once were. Holistic treatments are often seen as the key to abating symptoms, slowing the advance of the virus itself, and improving quality of life. Success is bringing in more expertise to the field of AIDS therapy... holistic physicians, homeopaths, naturopaths, chiropractors, therapists, nutritional counselors and more. The following protocol is a holistic therapy program that has achieved measurable success with AIDS and its attendant conditions. Doses are generally quite high in the beginning. They may be reduced as improvement is observed. Treatments may be used together or separately as desired, along with the recommendations of a competent professional who has your personal case knowledge. Note: Address allergies and malabsorption problems before beginning alternative HIV treatment.

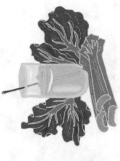

DETOXIFY: choose 2 or 3 products and protocols especially to cleanse lymph and liver tissue, particular HIV targets.

...*Lymph and liver cleansing is the key:* American Biologics DIOXYCHLOR, Enzymatic Therapy LIVA-TOX; or Crystal Star LIVER RENEW™ caps with GREEN TEA CLEANSER™.

...*Flush and detoxify the tissues:* Calcium ascorbate vitamin C crystals, or a mixed mineral ascorbate with bioflavonoids. Take orally 10-20 tsp. daily for 2 to 3 weeks, then reduce to 10 grams twice a week. Mega-doses may be resumed as necessary. Intravenous dose, 100-150 grams daily for 2-3 weeks, reducing to 30 grams a week.

...*Clean out toxic waste, normalize organs:* If not too weak, detoxify with a weekly wheat grass colonic.

...*Thermo-therapy:* both a sauna and an overheating bath (pages 182-183) severely attenuate virus and tumor cells by the sudden raising of body temperature. In vitro tests show an amazing reduction of infected cells by as much as 40%. (Karl Kroyer, France 1998.)

DIET: choose 2 or 3 products and protocols to normalize your body chemistry.

...*Rebalance body pH with micro-flora:* acidophilus complex with bifidus, like Nutricology SYMBIOTICS, 3 tsp. daily or UAS DDS-PLUS™ with FOS 6 daily. Sprinkle acidophilus on food for an extra probiotics boost.

...*Take carrot juice, fresh vegetable juices daily:* a good juicer is critical to potency. Take a potassium juice (page 291) 2x daily with garlic extract or Wakunaga AGED GARLIC extract and flax oil for needed fatty acids.

...*Get concentrated green foods daily:* Sun CHLORELLA, 20 tablets or 2 pkts granules daily, Green Foods GREEN ESSENCE or CARROT ESSENCE; Crystal Star ENERGY GREEN RENEWAL™ drink. Wakunaga KYO-GREEN, or Nutricology PRO-GREENS for brain performance.

...*Add egg lipids from egg yolk lecithin, a specific for HIV:* highest potency, Source Naturals EGGS ACT liquid. Chew DGL tablets to neutralize acids.

...*Whey protein helps inhibit HIV at every meal:* or use Life Extension WHEY ISOLATE protein drink for highly absorbable protein and digestive enzymes to deter HIV deterioration.

PHYTOBIOTIC HERBAL THERAPY: choose 2 or 3 products to reduce viral load and boost immune response.

...*Block viral replication, boost immune response:* St. John's wort extract (*recently seen in tests to inhibit the HIV virus*), and Cat's Claw extract 2x daily, proven against retro-virus replication; Crystal Star VIREX™ (with *lomatium, St. John's wort, protease, usnea and andrographis*); and ANTI-BIO™ caps with *echinacea, goldenseal* and *myrrh.* Echinacea stimulates interferon against HIV virus that hides in memory T-cells. *Note: Avoid standardized St. John's wort if you're taking indinavir. It may reduce levels. Cat's Claw is incompatible with AZT and DDI. Antacids may also reduce the effectiveness of AIDS drugs.*

...*Fight infection:* Aged aloe vera juice, 2-3 glasses daily, blocks the virus spread, and reduces herpes lesions (good results on slowing replication). Take with black carrot (*lomatium dissectum*) extract 30 drops 4x daily to fight HIV infection.

...*Protect the liver:* Milk thistle seed boosts immune response too, long term.

...*Enhance your immune forces:* Essiac tea 3x daily, Flora FLOR-ESSENCE tea, or *panax ginseng;* also Crystal Star FEEL GREAT NOW!™ with *panax ginseng* and *Siberian eleuthero.*

...*Restore homeostasis:* Drink 4-6 cups daily of the following restorative tea: *prince ginseng roots, dry shiitake mushrooms* and their soaking water, *echinacea angustifolia root, schizandra berries, astragalus, pau d'arco bark, St. John's wort.* Steep 30 minutes.

Can't find a recommended product? Call the 800 number listed in Product Resources for the store nearest you.

ANTIOXIDANT -ENZYME THERAPY: The natural products below can boost white blood cell and T-cell activity.

...*Increase leukocytes and white blood cell activity:* American Biologics SHARKILAGE 740mg - 1 cap per 12 pounds of body weight for 3 weeks before meals then 4-6 caps daily.

...*For neuropathy from AIDS drugs:* Acetyl-Carnitine 1000mg for 3 days. Rest 7 days, then 2000mg for 3 days. Rest 7 days. Take with *evening primrose oil* 4000mg daily.

...*Optimum liver detoxification:* LIPOIC ACID 150mg 3x daily.

...*Germanium:* highest potency 200mg 6x daily, or 150mg sublingually, 4x daily, with astragalus extract.

...*Healing enzymes:* Transformation PUREZYME, anti-viral protease enzyme therapy- 370,000 HUT daily.

...*Antioxidants:* CoQ₁₀ 300mg, Pycnogenol or grape seed PCO's, 200mg daily, Planetary REISHI SUPREME or Maitake Products MUSHROOM EMPERORS.

...*Respiratory improvement:* Solaray QUERCETIN PLUS 500mg 3x daily.

...*Overcome the side effects and nerve damage from AZT:* Glutathione 50mg 2x daily.

...*Help deactivate HIV:* NAC - a stable form of L-cysteine, with glutathione 50mg 2x daily.

...*MICROHYDRIN PLUS:* a superior antioxidant, 2 caps daily.

...*Change the cell environment with Bio-oxidation therapy:* The body produces H_2O_2 naturally as part of its immune defenses. Use catalytic H_2O_2 with shark cartilage by injection, (qualified practitioner only), or rub Earth's Bounty O_2 SPRAY on the feet twice daily. Alternate H_2O_2 use, 4 days on and one week off for best results.

BODY NORMALIZING MEASURES: choose 2 health maintenance products.

...Vitamin C with bioflavonoids, 10-30g daily, injection (ask your holistic physician) or orally.

...300,000IU mixed carotenes to stimulate T-cell activity.

...NAC (N-acetyl-cysteine), high potency as directed.

...Acetyl L-carnitine 500 milligrams daily to normalize energy production in the cells. Works well against peripheral neuropathy and lipodystrophy caused by AIDS drugs.

...Nutricology GERMANIUM 150-200mg daily for interferon production.

...CoQ₁₀ 300mg daily, with GLUTATHIONE 100mg 2 daily.

...UAS DDS-PLUS with FOS (5 billion viable *Bifidobacterium longum, Lactobacillus acidophilus, and 100 grams FOS*).

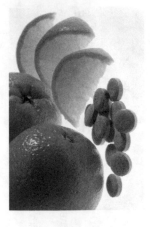

Diet Defense Against HIV and AIDS

HIV itself isn't deadly. It simply weakens the immune system to the point where its T4 reserves are exhausted and can't fight. Thousands of research papers show that AIDS' immune system failure directly correlates to specific vitamin, mineral and amino acid deficiencies. Malnutrition is the number one reason for low immune response. A high resistance, immune-building diet is the key to health. Your intestinal environment must be changed to create a hostile site for the HIV virus. AIDS victims need about 4000 calories a day, double the normal amount, to sustain body weight.

The liquid and fresh foods diet on the next page represents the first "crash course" stage of the change from cooked to living foods. It is for the ill person who needs dramatic measures - concentrated defense in a short time. It has been very helpful in keeping an HIV positive person symptom free, even in symptom recession during full-blown AIDS. The diet also helps prevent other attendant diseases associated with low immunity.

The suggested step-by-step program on the next page is a modified, enhanced macrobiotic diet, emphasizing more fresh than cooked foods, and mixing in acidophilus powder with foods that *are* cooked to convert them to living nourishment with friendly flora. As with other immune-suppressing viral diseases, HIV lives on dead and waste matter. (AIDS experts theorize that HIV feeds off undigested proteins in the colon.) For several months at least, eat a vegetarian diet, low in dairy, yeasted breads and saturated fats. Meats, fried foods, dairy products except yogurt and kefir, coffee, alcohol, salty, sugary foods, and all refined foods must be eliminated. Recreational drugs should be eliminated, as well as unnecessary prescription drugs. The ultra purity of this diet controls multiple allergies and sensitivities that occur in the auto-immune state, yet still supplies the needs of a body that is suffering great nutrient deprivation. For most people, this way of eating is a radical change, with major limitations, but the health improvement rate against HIV is excellent.

Remember: This diet is only a "jump start." Working with nutritionist is highly recommended over the long-term. See also the Blood Cleansing Detox Diet in this book (pg. 203).

Can't find a recommended product? Call the 800 number listed in Product Resources for the store nearest you.

The Diet:

On rising: take 3 tbsp. cranberry concentrate in 8-oz. of water with ½ tsp. ascorbate vitamin C crystals with bioflavonoids and ½ tsp. Nutricology SYMBIOTICS with FOS; or a Jarrow FERMENTED SOY ESSENCE protein drink.

Take a brisk walk for exercise and morning sunlight.

Breakfast: have a glass of fresh carrot juice with 1 tsp. Bragg's LIQUID AMINOS, and whole grain muffins or rice cakes with kefir cheese; or a cup of plain yogurt blended with a cup of fresh fruit, sesame seeds, walnuts; or oatmeal, amaranth or buckwheat pancakes with yogurt and fresh fruit; and ½ tsp. Nutricology SYMBIOTICS with FOS, or Transformation PUREZYME powder mixed in 8-oz. of aloe vera juice or AloeLife ALOE GOLD drink.

Midmorning: take a weekly colonic. On non-colonic days, take potassium essence (page 291), with 1 tsp. Bragg's LIQUID AMINOS and ½ tsp. ascorbate vitamin C crystals with bioflavs; and have another fresh carrot juice, or pau d'arco tea, with ½ tsp. Nutricology SYMBIOTICS with FOS added.

Lunch: a green salad with lemon-flax oil dressing, plenty of avocado, nuts, seeds and alfalfa or broccoli sprouts; or an open-faced sandwich on rice cakes, or a chapati with fresh veggies and kefir cheese; or a cup of miso soup with rice noodles or brown rice, and some steamed veggies, shiitake mushrooms and tofu with millet or brown rice; and take a cup of pau d' arco tea or 8-oz. aloe vera juice with ½ tsp. ascorbate vit. C, and ½ tsp. Nutricology SYMBIOTICS with FOS added.

Midafternoon: have 2 drinks: another carrot juice with Bragg's LIQUID AMINOS and ½ tsp. Nutricology SYMBIOTICS with FOS added; then a green drink like Pure Planet CHLORELLA, Barleans GREENS, or Crystal Star ENERGY GREEN RENEWAL™, with ½ tsp. ascorbate vitamin C crystals added.

Dinner: have a baked potato with Bragg's LIQUID AMINOS, yogurt or kefir cheese and a green salad, and black bean or lentil soup; or a fresh spinach or artichoke pasta with steamed veggies and lemon-flax oil dressing; or a Chinese steam stir-fry with shiitake mushrooms, brown rice and vegetables.

Sprinkle on ½ tsp. Nutricology SYMBIOTICS with FOS over any cooked food at this meal.

Before Bed: have 2 drinks: a glass of aloe vera juice with ½ tsp. ascorbate vitamin C crystals and ½ tsp. Nutricology SYMBIOTICS with FOS added; then a fresh carrot or papaya juice, or body chemistry balancing drink like Crystal Star RESTORE YOUR STRENGTH™ broth.

Note 1: Unsweetened herb teas and bottled water through the day offer additional toxin cleansing and system alkalizing.
Note 2: Add ½ tsp. ascorbate vitamin C powder with bioflavs to any drink throughout the day until the stool turns soupy.
Note 3: Because nutrient absorption is so degraded in HIV infection, supplemental probiotics are recommended throughout the day to normalize friendly flora and keep the GI environment as healthy as possible. This, in turn, keeps body resistance high to bacterial, viral and fungal invaders (especially Candida yeast). If you are regularly using antibiotics drugs or eating antibiotic laced foods, probiotics help correct this imbalance and resolve the resulting yeast infection.

To Your Health

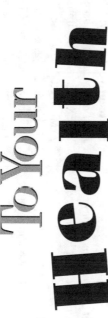

You must stay strong.... you must be able to survive while research for answers against the HIV virus goes on.

Often, a strong person is able to develop resistance to the virus symptoms that lasts for many years.

Can't find a recommended product? Call the 800 number listed in Product Resources for the store nearest you.

AIDS and HIV Infection

Diet and Lifestyle Support Therapy

Nutritional therapy plan:

Low immune response is clearly tied to compromised nutrition. Diet improvement is the key to keeping HIV infection from becoming AIDS. Intestinal pH environment must be changed for disease protection.

1—Extreme toxicity, fatigue and AIDS malabsorption forestalls a liquid detox plan (too harsh for a weakened system). Three glasses of fresh carrot juice and a potassium broth (pg. 291) daily keeps a detox ongoing. A good juicer is necessary.

2—Your diet should have the best possible nutrition. A modified macrobiotic diet is ideal for resistance and immune strength. Produce should be fresh and organically grown when possible. See diet suggestions page 308-309.

3—No fried, fatty foods (they aggravate diarrhea). A low sugar, low fat diet is best if you have fatty accumulations related to drug therapy. Coconut oil is easily digested with anti HIV activity. Avoid concentrated sweeteners and chemicalized foods of all kinds. Avoid protein from dairy and red meat, esp. fried meat, quite difficult to digest for people with HIV. Limit high gluten foods: wheat bread, barley, rye, commercial pastas and cereals, and bakery goods.

4—Anti-parasite enzyme foods: cranberry, pineapple, papaya.

5—Flush with fresh lemon juice (a specific for HIV), or 6 cups mild herb teas and pure water daily. Add ½ tsp. ascorbate vitamin C and ¼ tsp. Nutricology SYMBIOTICS to each daily drink (good results). Invest in a yogurt maker for highly potent friendly flora.

—Lifestyle practices and bodywork to avoid HIV:

•Acupuncture, meditation, massage therapy, visualization help normalize symptoms.
•Get fresh air and sunlight on the body every day. Get mild exercise daily, and plenty of rest. Do deep diaphragmatic breathing exercises morning and evening (page 250).
•Earth's Bounty O₂ spray- Use 2x a day on soles of the feet.
•Overheating therapy inhibits HIV growth. See pg. 182. Hydrotherapy is effective in re-stimulating circulation. Take a sauna or overheating bath (see page 183).
•Hormonal imbalance and depletion contribute to AIDS' progression. Consider a hormone blood panel or saliva test to assess your levels.
•Shaman Pharm. Sangre de Drago, NORMAL STOOL FORMULA reduces excess GI water without constipation. Simple GOLDENSEAL root extract drops are also effective.
•**Practice safe sex.** Use condoms even for oral sex. Latex condoms are 98-100% effective in preventing transmission if used correctly. •Avoid anal intercourse.
•Avoid needle-injected pleasure drugs and snortable drugs. (HIV can be spread with shared "snort straws.")
•Make sure any blood transfusion plasma has been tested for HIV virus (a regular practice in the U.S.)

Herbal, Superfood and Supplement Therapy

Interceptive therapy: Choose 4 or 5 recommendations.

Plant anti-virals have been among the most effective treatments against HIV. •Crystal Star VIREX™ caps fortify immune response, fight the virus. •Transformation Enzyme PURE-ZYME 370,000 HUT, (see directions). •East Park OLIVE LEAF EXTRACT 4x daily helps drop viral loads, acts as a natural protease inhibitor. •Arkopharma FLU GUARD, anti-retroviral boxwood extract, keeps CD4 levels high (good results in new trials). •CARNIVORA® Immune Enhancer caps, help eliminate HIV from blood (highly recommended). •Turmeric (curcumin) inhibits TNF, a cytokine that increases HIV in T-cells.

•*Garlic*, a measurable selenium plant source inhibits TNF. Garlic suppositories at night help kill HIV in the colon. •Planetary TRI-CLEANSE removes toxins from the colon. *Pau d'arco*

•*Una da gato - St. John's wort* extract (proven effective against retro-viruses). *Pau d'arco* boosts immune response; *Siberian eleuthero* extract, T-cell helpers.

•Chinese antivirals: *Panax ginseng, Astragalus, Reishi, Turkey Tail, Shiitake mushrooms*; Grifron PRO MAITAKE D-FRACTION extract, *Atractylodes, Schizandra, Ligustrum.*

•*Evening primrose oil*, infected cells crack up when bombarded with GLA.

•PSP Marketing VITAL PSP PLUS to raise immune T-cells. Use with PSP Marketing VIRAMAX (humic acid) for help in reducing viral load (highly recommended).

•Quercetin 1000mg (blocks HIV same way as AZT) with BROMELAIN 1500mg.

•Melatonin - clinically -shown to increase T-helper cells, natural killer cells, and lymphocyte production. Reduces AZT toxicity, 3-30mg. daily.

—Superfood therapy: Choose 1 or 2 recommendations.

•Sun Chlorella WAKASA GOLD chlorella drink.
•Crystal Star GREEN TEA CLEANSER™ to help inhibit HIV.
•Alacer EMERGEN-C, 93% of patients note improvement (highly recommended).
•American Health ACIDOPHILUS liquid (fermented soy).

—Detox, purifying supplements:

•Egg yolk lecithin. Active lipids help make cell walls virally resistant. •Herbal Answers ALOE FORCE JUICE, 4 tbsp. daily to curb virus spread with *echinacea* extract to stimulate interleukin; *turmeric* to inhibit TNF. •Nutricology GERMANIUM 150mg daily for interferon production. •Glutamine up to 20g twice daily.

—Detoxification bodywork:

•You must detoxify the liver for holistic healing to be effective. See LIVER CLEANSING, page 199 in this book.

•Remove infected feces from intestinal tract. Take both a colonic and an enema implant with *aloe vera, wheat grass* or *spirulina* once a week until recovery is well underway. Follow up with one treatment a month. •Use implant-enemas with supergreens like *chlorella* or *spirulina*, or micro-flora like •UAS DDS-PLUS FOS, or •Enzymatic Therapy PHYTO-BIOTIC HERBAL FORMULA.

Can't find a recommended product? Call the 800 number listed in Product Resources for the store nearest you.

Allergies–Chemical

Multiple Chemical Sensitivity (MCS), Environmental Illness, Drug-Contaminant Reactions

Allergic reactions to chemicals are multiplying. We're exposed every day to more chemicals than any generation in history. One-third of Americans have sensitivities to chemicals! Multiple Chemical Sensitivity (MCS), now called a "silent epidemic," alone affects at least 15 million Americans, most of them women and children. Over 4½ billion pounds of pesticides are used in America every year! (76 million pounds in our homes.) Irritants range from petrochemicals and estrogenic chemicals, to combustion residues from household appliances, to paints and household cleaners. Benzene, fluoride, formaldehyde, and carcinogens from carpeting and dry cleaning affect our brains. Other culprits include: gas stoves, asbestos from older buildings, chlorine bleach, laundry detergent (for less chemicals, try T-Wave Cleaning Capsules), fabric softener, nail polish remover, synthetic perfumes, moth balls and insect repellents.

Repeated chemical exposures set off rampant free radical reactions, as well as allergic responses. (Free radical damage to liver function from environmental pollutants also lowers histamine levels.) Environmental illness, sick buildings, Gulf War syndrome, nerve damage, attention deficit disorder in children, latex and insecticide allergies, are only the latest in a growing list. People with severe environmental illness may even become "dispossessed," living a nomadic life in the attempt to find a safe haven.

Worse, our bodies use up enormous amounts of nutrients trying to detoxify us from these chemicals, nutrients that could have been used to keep us happy and healthy. Research shows 60% of people with chemical sensitivity have a vitamin B6 deficiency; 30% have a vitamin C deficiency; and 30% are deficient in vitamins B1, B2, B3, and B5. While many physicians do not recognize MCS as an official disorder, natural health practitioners regularly treat it with encouraging results.

Allergies to chemicals and contaminant allergens are called Type 2 allergies. Reactions to chemicals are frequently a defense mechanism, the body's attempt to isolate an offending substance by storing it in fatty tissue. An allergic reaction of this type only occurs after the second exposure to the irritant when your body's histamine response is alerted. Repeated exposures set off massive free radical reactions as the body's contaminant toleration levels are reached; toxic overload results and a severe allergic reaction sets in. Not only does the toxic overload from chemicals in the environment cause allergic reactions, it also impairs the body's immune response to them. Worse, chemical sensitivities initiate other allergy reactions, so that the sufferer becomes allergic to nearly everything else. Drug reactions mimic allergy reactions but usually don't involve the immune system (IgE antibodies).

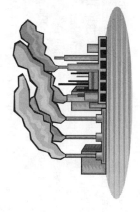

Signs that you may have a Type 2 allergy to chemicals and contaminants:

- Unexplained migraine headaches? Usually with nausea or diarrhea?
- Frequent skin rashes for no explained reason?
- Feel "under the weather" no matter how much sleep you get? Are your ears ringing, especially at night?
- Frequent colds and flu, or chronic respiratory inflammations and low immune response to them?
- Frequently moody and depressed for no reason?
- Gained or lost weight recently for no reason? (Chemical allergies may cause abnormal metabolism.)
- Do you have chronic musculoskeletal pain or fibromyalgia?
- Do you have an autoimmune condition like M.S., rheumatoid arthritis, Hashimoto's thyroiditis, lupus?
- Do you use pesticides in your house or yard?
- Are you regularly exposed to toxic metals, chemicals or minerals at work?
- Have you ever had breast implants?
- Do friends and family tell you that your personality changes?
- Are you often spacey? Is your brain foggy; your mind sluggish? Is your memory unusually bad?
- Do you have a child that's chronically hyperactive or who has difficulty learning?

Want to find an MD who practices environmental medicine? Check out www.aaem.com or call 316-684-5500.

Can't find a recommended product? Call the 800 number listed in Product Resources for the store nearest you.

Allergies-Chemical

Diet and Lifestyle Support Therapy

Nutritional therapy plan:

1—Go on a short blood purifying cleanse (pg. 203) to begin toxin release. Have one each daily:
- a glass of fresh carrot juice
- a carrot-beet-cucumber juice
- a cup of miso soup with sea greens
- a bowl of high fiber cereal to bind and eliminate toxins in the G.I. tract. Sprinkle on nutritional yeast, toasted wheat germ and lecithin granules.

2—Eat organically grown foods when possible. Avoid canned foods. Avoid caffeine, which inhibits liver filtering, and foods sprayed with colorants, waxes or ripening agents.

3—Eat legumes and sea greens to excrete lead. Cruciferous veggies like broccoli and cauliflower help metabolize excess estrogen from hormone mimicking chemicals. Eat a daily apple if you're in a polluted area. Apple pectin removes metal toxins.

4—Lower bad saturated and trans fats; omega-3 fats with essential fatty acids: sea greens, flax, grape seed and olive oils build resistance.

5—Avoid food contaminants like artificial sweeteners, MSG and fake fats like Olestra. Use bottled water for cooking and drinking. Consider fluoride free toothpaste, like Nature's Gate SPEARMINT or Weleda PINK TOOTHPASTE with Myrrh.

Lifestyle Bodywork:

- Use Coca's Pulse Test or muscle testing to identify allergens. (See page 316.)
- Acupuncture, chiropractic, massage therapy are most effective against chemical allergies.
- Take a sauna once a week to accelerate toxin release.
- Removing amalgam fillings eliminates symptoms for some MCS sufferers.
- Nambudripad's Allergy Elimination Techniques (NAET) show success.

Ideas to avoid contaminants:

- Seek out trees to live around. Trees produce oxygen and remove many air pollutants. • Invest in an air filter. Pay attention to unhealthy air alerts; stay indoors if you have chemical sensitivities.
- Avoid antacids; they interfere with enzymes, and your body's ability to carry off chemical residues.
- Avoid as much as possible: smoking and secondary smoke, pesticides and herbicides, phosphorus fertilizers, fluorescent lights, aluminum cookware and deodorants, electric blankets; microwave ovens.
- Wear natural fiber, like silk or cotton.

Herbal, Superfood and Supplement Therapy

Interceptive therapy: Choose 2 to 3 recommendations.

1—**Detoxify your blood:** for 6 weeks, •Crystal Star TOXIN DETOX™ caps (*with amla fruit, seaweed, apple pectin*), or •Crystal Star DETOX BLOOD PURIFIER™ caps with CLEANSING & PURIFYING™ TEA; •Glutathione 150mg daily; •Tyrosine 500mg daily; use •magnesium 800mg if you have TIA episodes.

2—**Support your liver:** •Crystal Star LIVER RENEW™ caps along with LIVER CLEANSE FLUSHING™ tea for 1 month to restore the liver. Then •FIBER & HERBS COLON CLEANSE™ caps with *milk thistle seed* extract; or •Planetary TRIPHALA INTERNAL CLEANSER caps; •B-complex 100mg daily with extra B$_6$ and pantothenic acid.

3—**Neutralize histamine reactions:** •Crystal Star fast acting D-CONGEST™ spray (good results). •Bilberry extract (natural quercetin), or •Quercetin 1000mg with bromelain 500mg take down swelling. •Biotec Foods CELL GUARD with SOD.

4—**Neutralize allergen response:** •MSM 400mg 2x daily, •Nutricology ADRENAL CORTEX GLANDULAR; •*Evening primrose oil* 3000mg daily, •Kelp 10 tabs daily, or •Crystal Star OCEAN MINERALS™ (sea plant iodine and potassium) caps, or •New Chapter OCEAN HERBS, or •Crystal Star IODINE, POTASSIUM, SILICA drops 3x daily.

—**Superfood therapy:** Choose 1 or 2 recommendations.
Blood detox helps, chemical exposure sets off rampant free radicals.
- Crystal Star ENERGY GREEN RENEWAL™ or GREEN TEA CLEANSER™
- Sun Wellness CHLORELLA
- Green Foods GREEN MAGMA
- AloeLife ALOE GOLD juice
- Green Foods CARROT ESSENCE blend
- Pines MIGHTY GREENS drink

—**Effective herbal healing resources:** •*Garlic* oil caps, 2-4 daily. •*Dandelion-nettles* caps, 6 daily. •*Pau d'arco* tea 4x daily. •Nutribiotic GRAPEFRUIT SEED EXTRACT caps. •*Licorice* rt. tea or •Crystal Star ADRENAL ENERGY BOOST™ caps.

Preventives:

—**Antioxidants fight chemical assault and boost immunity:**
1) Vitamin C with bioflavonoids, up to 5000mg boosts immunity against MCS. 2) Vitamin E 400IU w/selenium 200mcg. 3) CoQ-10, 120mg. 4) Grapeseed PCO's 100mg. 5) Quercetin 1000mg. 6) Vitamin B-12 2000mcg. 7) Beta or marine carotene 150,000IU.

—**Glandulars reinforce the body at its deepest level:**
•Nutricology ADRENAL CORTEX ORGANIC GLANDULAR, THYMUS ORGANIC GLANDULAR caps.

Can't find a recommended product? Call the 800 number listed in Product Resources for the store nearest you.

Allergies-Seasonal

Seasonal Hayfever, Allergic Rhinitis, Respiratory Allergies

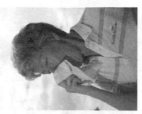

Allergies are an epidemic as civilization's 21st century begins. Over 60 million Americans suffer from allergies - more than 20% of the population! Respiratory allergies affect between 35 and 50 million people. Allergies used to be defined as inappropriate immune responses to substances like cat hair, dust or wheat, and seasonal conditions, like dust, pollen or spores that weren't normally harmful. Today, the dramatic rise in allergies is due to substances that are harmful, like environmental pollutants, asbestos and smoke exhaust fumes. Stress and adrenal exhaustion, common problems in western societies (see page 300), set the stage. Enzyme imbalance and essential fatty acid deficiency are also usually involved.

In response to all the sniffing and sneezing, the FDA recently approved over-the-counter sales of (*loratadine*) Claritin, an anti-allergy medication linked to animal liver tumors in high doses! Most drugstore medications for environmental allergies only mask symptoms, often cause drowsiness and have a rebound effect. ***The more you use them, the more you need them.*** The newest ones are strong side effects like rapid heartbeat. Even older antihistamines can be dangerous. Diphenhydramine (Benadryl) impairs driving performance more than alcohol. Steroid drugs for hayfever allergies, if taken for long periods, do not cure and often make the situation worse by depressing immune defenses, and impeding allergen elimination. On top of all this, environmental allergens frequently interact in the bodies of allergy sufferers, activating and aggravating other irritants. Then, even the most powerful drugs do not relieve symptoms.

Do you have seasonal allergies?

Substances that cause allergy reactions are called allergens. Respiratory allergies to environmental allergens like air pollutants, asbestos or heavy metals, and seasonal allergens to dust, pollen, spores and mold, are called Type 1 allergies. This type of allergy develops more easily if your body has excess mucous accumulation to harbor the allergen irritants.

Spore and pollen allergens produce congestion as the body tries to seal them off from its regular processes, or tries to work around them. Your body forms a mucous shield around the offending substances, making you start to feel the allergy symptoms of sinus clog, stuffiness, headaches and puffy eyes. Sometimes your body throws this excess off through the skin, and you get skin irritations or a sore throat. An allergic response to spores and pollen may cause a histamine release that swells nasal passages and membranes, producing symptoms like runny, itchy nose and eyes, sneezing, coughing attacks, bronchial and sinus infections, skin rashes, asthma, insomnia, menstrual disorders and hypoglycemia.

Signs that you have a Type 1 allergy to environmental or seasonal allergens:

- Do you have chronic lung, bronchial and sinus infections with itchy, watery nose and eyes?
- Do you get frontal headaches with sneezing, coughing attacks and sore, scratchy throat?
- Does your face swell up, with itchy, rashy skin?
- Do you have a skin rash on your arms or torso?
- Do you have trouble sleeping ?
- Do you have dark circles under your eyes that don't go away with sleep?
- Do you have unusual menstrual pain and congestion?
- Do you have hypoglycemia? candida albicans yeast overgrowth? or learning disabilities?

A strong immune system is critical to preventing the allergic reaction symptomology of opportunistic diseases like herpes, candida albicans or chronic fatigue syndrome (CFIDS). Allergy-prone people produce an overabundance of complex proteins known as antibodies—which trigger special cells known as mast cells—which release inflammation-causing chemicals called histamines and leukotrienes throughout the body. A "histamine reaction" occurs when your body tries to neutralize the chemicals through a severe allergic reaction.

Medical treatment for most allergies consists of antihistamines, steroids and desensitization shots. Laser surgery can now vaporize mucous-forming nasal tissue. People with allergies know that these treatments seldom work for very long because they don't get to the cause of the problem. At best, they provide temporary relief of symptoms; at worst, they create side effects which may be worse than the allergy itself.

Can't find a recommended product? Call the 800 number listed in Product Resources for the store nearest you.

Allergies-Seasonal

Diet and Lifestyle Support Therapy

Nutritional therapy plan:

Note: Use Coca's Pulse Test or muscle testing to identify allergens. (See page 316, 378)

Diet change and cleansing your internal environment is the most beneficial thing you can do to control allergic rhinitis reactions. For a complete program to overcome allergies, see my book COOKING FOR HEALTHY HEALING for diet and recipes.

1—Focus on a plant-based diet. Animal fats produce inflammatory leukotrienes linked to allergies.

2—Begin with a 3 to 7 day cleanse (pg. 202) to get rid of mucous build-up, and release allergens. Drink lots of water during your cleanse, take Yogi BREATHE DEEP tea for lung cleansing, Crystal Star GREEN TEA CLEANSER™ to relax breathing.

3—Have a cup of green tea each morning (and at bedtime) to thin mucous. Take hot miso or chicken soup to release mucous. Celery juice daily helps flush allergens.

4—Eat non-mucous-forming foods: fresh veggies and fruits (high antioxidants and anti-inflammatory activity reduce reactions), cultured foods like yogurt, high vitamin C foods like citrus and berries, seafoods, and fundamental sulphur from cabbage, onions and garlic. Get plenty of essential fatty acids from Omega-3 oils like flax, and EFA's from sea greens, arugula and spinach.

5—Avoid preserved and canned foods, sugary foods, caffeine, and fatty, mucous-forming foods during healing. This means dairy products and high gluten foods.

Lifestyle measures:

Avoid allergens. Stay indoors, esp. in the a.m. and exercise indoors on dry, windy days. Invest in an air filter or run an air ionizer to reduce indoor allergens. Stop smoking and avoid secondary smoke. It magnifies allergies reactions.

—Acupressure points for relief:

Note: Acupuncture and chiropractic are also both effective.

1—During an attack, press tip of nose hard as needed.

2—Press hollow above the center of upper lip as needed.

3—Press underneath cheekbones beside nose, angling pressure upwards.

Bodywork: •Take 1 tsp. fresh grated horseradish in a spoon with lemon juice. Hang over a sink to release great quantities of mucous fast.

•*Eucalyptus* steams ease breathing. Add 2 pinches *eucalyptus leaves* to a lot of hot water. Use a towel to cover your head; hang over the pot; inhale the steam for 5 to 10 minutes.

•Exercise is important to increase oxygen uptake. Take a daily walk with deep breaths.

•Use relaxation techniques. Stress depresses immunity and aggravates allergies.

Herbal, Superfood and Supplement Therapy

Interceptive therapy: Choose 2 to 3 recommendations.

Natural therapies build resistance and offer symptom relief without side effects.

1—Natural antihistamines: •Crystal Star ANTI-HST™ caps (very fast acting, usually within 25 minutes); or •Pure Essence ALLER-FREE with protease and amylase enzymes (digests foreign proteins in the blood and breaks down histamine). Try •Trimedica MSM 500mg 2x daily to counter IgE anti-body response; •Ascorbate Vitamin C or Ester C with bioflavonoids 5000mg daily during high risk seasons acts as a natural antihistamine. •Grapeseed PCO's 100mg or •Baywood Dr. Harris Original ALLERGY FORMULA; •Quercetin 1000-2000mg daily, with •Bromelain 1000mg; •*Cat's Claw* or *Ginkgo Biloba* extract; •CoQ$_{10}$ 200mg daily; •NAC (n-acetyl cysteine) 200mg at bedtime (effectively thins mucous).

2—Liver support: *Dandelion-nettles* tea, morning and evening (very effective), or •freeze-dried *nettles* caps for allergic rhinitis.

3—For mucous congestion: •Crystal Star ANTI-BIO™ 4 caps at a time, or XLEAR nasal wash with xylitol flushes out allergens, take •Crystal Star D-CONGEST™ spray for clearer breathing at night; •Zand DECONGEST HERBAL; •Apply *cayenne-ginger* chest compresses. •Apply BREATHE RIGHT post nasal strips. •Chew Altoids strong peppermints to clear up a stuffy nose (very effective).

4—Reinforce defenses against allergens: •B-complex with extra pantothenic acid 500mg; •Crystal Star ADRENAL ENERGY BOOST™ formulas; •raw thymus and adrenal daily. •Mixed carotenes 150,000IU daily; •Nutricology GERMANIUM 150mg.

5—Stabilize a bad reaction: •Tyrosine 1000mg daily; •Maitake Products REISHI caps or Planetary REISHI SUPREME drops. •Quercetin 2000mg with bromelain 1000mg; •Studies say *butterbur herb* is as effective as *cetirizine* (Zyrtec) for hay fever. •Apply MSM gel topically to allergy-related skin rashes.

6—Homeopathic remedies help acute attacks without side effects: •LifeSpan Nutrition SNEEZE-EZE as needed (highly recommended); •*Euphrasia*; •*Zincum Gluconicum* nasal gel; •BioForce POLLINOSAN tabs; •BioForce SINUSAN tabs;•Bio-Allers POLLEN-HAYFEVER; •Similasan ALLERGY EYES drops (excellent results) to relieve eye itching and NASAL SPRAY to relieve drippy nose.

—Superfood therapy: Choose 1 or 2 recommendations.

•NutriCology PRO GREENS with EFA's.

•Herbs, Etc. ALLER-TONIC.

•CC Pollen 24-HOUR ROYAL JELLY for pantothenic acid or •CC Pollen ALLER BEE-GONE (not if you are allergic to bees). Take with •*Evening primrose oil* 4000mg daily for 3 months.

•AloeLife FIBER-MATE dink.

Can't find a recommended product? Call the 800 number listed in Product Resources for the store nearest you.

Allergies-Food

Food Sensitivities and Intolerances, Celiac Disease

Food intolerances are often confused with food allergies. A food allergy is an antibody reaction — an immune system response to a food your body sees as a pathogen or parasite. A food intolerance is a non-immune reaction, usually an enzyme deficiency to digest a certain food. For example, people with a lactose intolerance experience the bloating, cramping and diarrhea of an allergy reaction, but the symptoms are really due to a deficiency of the enzyme lactase, which helps digest milk sugar. Lactose intolerance affects between 30-50 million North Americans, a full 75% of African Americans and over 90% of Asian Americans. Celiac disease is a sensitivity to gluten, a wheat protein (celiac disease affects about 20% of Americans).

Food sensitivities of all kinds are growing as people are more exposed to chemically altered, genetically-modified, enzyme-depleted foods. Low enzyme activity means food assimilation is only partial, leaving large amounts of undigested fats and proteins that the immune system treats as potentially toxic. Prostaglandins, leukotrienes, and histamines enter the bloodstream in an immune response and allergy reactions occur.

You're highly likely to experience allergic reactions if you eat a lot of fast foods. Fast foods are often loaded with food additives - nitrites, aspartame, MSG and sulfites. Chemically altered, sprayed, or injected foods also put your body under a lot of stress - resulting in low gastric pH, leaky gut syndrome or candida albicans yeast overgrowth. Watch your diet closely if you're a frequent traveler. Jet lag stress, insufficient sleep, unusual or unfamiliar foods, chemically sprayed or adulterated foods all lay the groundwork for allergic reactions.

Do you have a food allergy or intolerance?

Food allergies may be hereditary; a child is twice as likely to develop food allergies if one parent has them, or four times as likely if both parents have them. Food allergies are common in children; many result from feeding babies meats and commercial dairy foods before 10-12 months. Babies do not have the right enzymes to digest these foods. Feed mother's milk (by far the best choice), soy milk or goat's milk for 10 months to avoid food allergies. Ninety percent of food reactions are caused by certain proteins in cow's milk, peanuts, eggs, corn, wheat, coffee, mushrooms and soybeans. These foods may be healthy in themselves, but they are often heavily sprayed or treated; in the case of animal products, also injected with antibiotics and hormones.

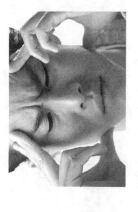

Signs that you have a Type 2 food allergy or intolerance:

• Are you unable to eat normal amounts of a food? Are you nauseated after eating?
• Do you get cyclical headaches with blurred vision or mental fuzziness after eating?
• Do you get a runny nose; itchy, watery eyes, sweating, heart palpitations, or hives after eating?
• Do you have chronic fatigue syndrome (CFIDS)?
• Do you get heart palpitations, with sweating, rashes or puffiness around the eyes after eating?
• Does your abdomen swell excessively after eating with heartburn or stomach cramps and gas?
• Have you gained significant weight even though your diet hasn't changed?
• Do you have Crohn's disease, irritable bowel syndrome or alternating chronic diarrhea and constipation?
• Do you have hypothyroidism or hypoglycemia? or osteoarthritis?
• Is your child irritable, flushed (especially earlobes) or hyperactive after eating? Does he wet the bed?
• Does your child have chronic ear infections and congestion… if an infant, does he get colic?

If your answers are largely yes to these questions, you may have an allergy or sensitivity to certain foods or food additives. Americans consume 8 to 10 pounds of food additives each year! Regardless of the food, the reaction symptoms are similar. Inflammation occurs from histamine release into tissue mast cells, walling off the affected body area until immune response agents can restore health. But this process takes time. If the body is re-exposed before health is renewed, inflammation and symptoms, especially mucous congestion, become chronic. For more, see also CANDIDA ALBICANS Page 358.

Can't find a recommended product? Call the 800 number listed in Product Resources for the store nearest you.

Allergies-Food

Diet and Lifestyle Support Therapy

Nutritional therapy plan:

1—A short colon cleansing diet (page 196) clears the system of allergens. The best ongoing diet? Enzyme-rich, organic fresh foods.

2—Food elimination diet: helps eliminate allergen foods, especially if you are overweight, have candida, sluggish thyroid or hypoglycemia.

• Find out what foods you're allergic to by following an elimination diet. For one week, eat foods like brown rice, sweet potatoes, all cooked vegetables, and non-acidic fruits - foods that are less likely to cause reactions. When symptoms improve, add other foods one at a time to see if they aggravate symptoms. For best results, eat each new food three times a day for 2 days. Foods that trigger symptoms are likely allergens.

3—Take 2 tbsp. cider vinegar with maple syrup at each meal.

4—Eat cultured foods, like yogurt and kefir to add G.I. friendly flora.

5—Problem foods: wheat, sugar (esp. if you have skin problems), dairy foods (except yogurt or kefir), fruits, yeast, mushrooms, peanuts, eggs, soy, coffee, corn, beer.

6—Safer food choices: rice milk, goat's milk, almond milk, sweet potatoes, winter squash, rice flour, puffed rice, flat breads, brown or wild rice, millet, buckwheat, amaranth, quinoa, non-citrus fruits, date sugar, maple syrup, almond or sesame butter, egg replacer made from flax or arrowroot.

Note 1: One of the most insidious effects of food allergy is weight gain. Eliminate wheat from your diet to stop allergy-related weight gain. (Wheat keeps you from absorbing EFAs, the good fats that help control weight.)

Note 2: For severe lactose intolerance, watch for hidden lactose in foods like bread, cereals, deli meats, salad dressings, breakfast drinks, instant soup, even some prescription and over-the-counter drugs.

Coca's Pulse Test: can help you find and eliminate foods that harm.

Dr. Arthur Coca, an immunologist, discovered that when people eat foods to which they are allergic, there is a dramatic increase in heartbeat — 20 or more beats a minute above normal. Pulse rate is normally remarkably stable, unaffected by digestion, ordinary physical activities or normal emotions. Unless a person is ill or under great stress, pulse rate deviation is probably due to an allergy.

COCA'S PULSE TEST

1. Take your pulse when you wake in the morning. Using a watch with a second hand, count the number of beats in a 60-second period. A normal pulse is 60-100 beats per minute.

2. Take your pulse again after eating a suspected allergy food. Wait 15 to 20 minutes and take your pulse again. If your pulse rate has increased more than 10 beats per minute, omit that food from your diet.

Herbal, Superfood and Supplement Therapy

Interceptive therapy: Choose 2 to 3 recommendations.

• Use Coca's Pulse Test (opposite), or muscle testing (page 378) to identify allergens. The skin-prick and RAST tests used by many allergists often misdiagnose food allergies unless a rotation-reintroduction diet is also used.

• NAET (Nambudripad Allergy Elimination) combines muscle testing, acupuncture and chiropractic techniques to help eliminate allergies and sensitivities. Many allergy sufferers report good results.

1—Help your body produce antihistamines: •Pure Essence ALLER-FREE caps; •CoQ-10, 200mg daily.

2—Reduce allergic reactions: •MSM 1000mg daily; •LifeSpan Nutrition SNEEZE-EZE as needed (highly recommended); •Reishi mushroom extract; •Omega-3 flax oil for EFAs; •Liquid chlorophyll 1 tsp. in water 3x daily before meals.

3—Cleanse the GI tract: Crystal Star BITTERS & LEMON CLEANSE™ extract helps stimulate - normalize bile activity; green tea (or •Crystal Star DR. VITALITY™ green and white tea); aloe vera juice each morning. •A *garlic-catnip* enema balances colon pH.

4—Add proteolytic enzymes: •Quercetin 1500mg daily with bromelain 1500mg daily for antioxidants plus enzymes. A full spectrum enzyme like Herbal Products POWER PLUS ENZYMES, or Enzymedica DIGEST. To reduce inflammation reactions, use •Enzymedica PURIFY, •Crystal Star DR. ENZYME™ with protease and bromelain, or •Transformation PUREZYME for protease.

5—Add probiotics: • American Health ACIDOPHILUS liquid or •Nutricology SYMBI-OTICS acidophilus, take ¼ tsp. in liquid before meals;

6—Support adrenals: •Crystal Star DR. VITALITY™ tea or caps.; •Ester C up to 5000mg daily with bioflavonoids.

7—Herbal enzymes boost immunity, normalize digestion: (choose 1) •*Milk thistle seed* extract; •*Dandelion root-nettles* tea; •*Echinacea-goldenseal root* caps; •Gaia SWEET-ISH BITTERS.

—**For gluten intolerance:** •Bio-Allers FOOD ALLERGY GRAIN. •Crystal Star CANDIDA YEAST DETOX™ caps especially if you have unexplained weight gain.

—**For celiac disease:** shore up related deficiencies: • Nature's Secret ULTIMATE B, •Crystal Star CALCIUM SOURCE™, •Crystal Star IRON SOURCE BLOOD BUILDER™ extract.

—**For lactose intolerance:** •Lactaid drops or tablets; • Nature's Plus SAY YES TO DAIRY; •Country Life DAIRY-ZYME; •Transformation powder DIGESTZYME for children and adults.

—**Superfood therapy:** Choose 1 or 2 recommendations.
•Jarrow GENTLE FIBERS drink mix cleanses the bowel.
•New Chapter GINGER WONDER syrup- 1 tbsp. in 8-oz. water 2x daily.

Can't find a recommended product? Call the 800 number listed in Product Resources for the store nearest you.

Alzheimer's Disease

Senile Dementia, Cerebral Atherosclerosis, Loss of Memory, Korsakoff's Syndrome

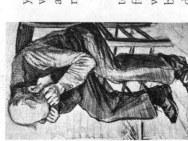

The number one fear of older Americans (and their families) isn't heart disease or cancer.... it's Alzheimer's. As more people live into their 80s, 90s, and beyond, cases of Alzheimer's and dementia are rising fast. Alzheimer's disease now affects 4 million Americans at a cost of over $100 billion in nursing care and lost wages of family members. As many as 10% of all seniors over 65 have Alzheimer's; 50% of those over 85 are affected. By 2050, as many as 14 million Americans are expected to fall victim to the disease! Alzheimer's disease progresses slowly, but inexorably, with increasing rapidity to the final devastating stages where communication is almost non-existent, feeding and elimination functions uncontrolled.

Alzheimer's disease is a progressive, degenerative condition that attacks the brain forming neurofiber tangles and plaques believed to result in dementia symptoms. Memory loss and disorientation are the first symptoms as the brain shrinks and nerves degenerate, but eventually there is almost complete loss of physical function, the body breaks down and reverts to childhood in terms of care. It's a devastating, relentless assault that's rising at a rapid rate in industrialized countries worldwide. A substantial number of those diagnosed with Alzheimer's appear to really be victims of too many drugs, or have nutritional deficiencies that can be reversed. Although orthodox medicine has been unable to make a difference in this relentless disease, natural therapies have been successful in slowing brain deterioration. Ask a holistic physician about chelation therapy to reduce heavy metal toxicity.

Do we know what causes Alzheimer's?

Medical science does not know entirely, but increased oxidative damage from free-radicals plays a prominent role in Alzheimer's development. Low body-brain oxygen (perhaps because of lack of exercise) and anemia are common, probably caused by free radical damage. Genetic factors may also be involved, too, but environmental exposure to harmful chemicals, aluminum or inorganic silicon are thought to be a key. Estrogen disrupters like those in pesticides have been found in Alzheimer's sufferers.

Other markers are acetylcholine deficiency in the brain along with arteriosclerosis. Poor or obstructed circulation throughout the body is an accompanying factor. Lipofuscin, a brown fluid forming on brain neurons means overactive immune response causing chronic inflammation and destruction of neurons. Other regularly seen conditions - thyroid malfunction, high homocysteine levels, aluminum toxicity, possible mercury toxicity, and bad reactions to drugs like oxybutynin chloride for incontinence or some antihistamines.

Note: Once touted as preventive medicine against Alzheimer's, new studies conclude that HRT (Hormone Replacement Therapy) may not provide protection for women if taken less than 10 years. In fact, a recent Journal of the American Medical Association study (2000) showed women with mild to moderate Alzheimer's who were taking estrogen actually had a higher level of dementia than those who weren't!

On a more positive note, however, studies reveal the lion's mane mushroom *Hericium erinaceus* stimulates the growth of neurons, and may play a role in inhibiting brain dysfunction caused by Alzheimer's disease, senility, or traumatic injury. Consider Maitake Products SUPER LION'S MANE caps.

Does one of your family members have signs of Alzheimer's?

•A noticeable loss of ability to think clearly or remember familiar names, places or events?
•Loss of touch with reality? confusion about events? constantly repeating oneself?
•Difficulty in finishing thoughts or following directions? inability to learn new information?
•Clear, unexplained personality or behavior changes with confusion, paranoia or poor judgement?
•Poor coordination with shuffling movements instead of normal steps?   •Problems speaking, understanding, reading, or writing?
•Unexplained depression or sleep disturbance? (Supplementation may offer dramatic improvement.)
•Does the person often wander away from home? or get lost in familiar places?
•Frequent incontinence, reduced ability to bathe or dress without help?

Can't find a recommended product? Call the 800 number listed in Product Resources for the store nearest you.

Alzheimer's Disease

Diet and Lifestyle Support Therapy

Nutritional therapy plan:

1—Good nutrition deters Alzheimer's onset. Red meats and sugar are big culprits. Avoid food chemicals linked to brain dysfunction like trans fats in fried foods, bakery goods and snack foods; chemical sweeteners; and MSG. Add high fiber foods and brain nourishing EFAs from seafood and sea greens, flax oil, and olive oil. —A good brain mix: wheat germ, lecithin granules, nutritional yeast, oat bran, flax oil and molasses. Two tbsp. mornings with cereal or juice.

2—Eat a largely vegetarian diet: avoid red meats, linked to amyloid neuro-fiber tangle build-up. Alzheimer's is also linked to synthetic estrogens injected into some red meats and in pesticides. Eat curry (anti-inflammatory) and sea greens (binds to heavy metals) often for brain protection. •Magnesium-rich foods like greens and sea veggies reduce brain activity and deter Alzheimer's. •Moderate wine drinking may boost brain activity and deter Alzheimer's.

3—Eat B vitamin foods that deter aluminum toxicity: brown rice, whole grains, nutritional yeast, molasses, liver, fish and wheat germ.

4—Eat vitamin C foods like oranges, broccoli, kiwi fruit and tomatoes; and vitamin E foods like nuts, seeds and leafy vegetables to reduce your risk as much as 70%. In a recent JAMA study (2002), people with the highest intakes of vitamin C and E were the least likely to develop Alzheimer's.

5—Eat tryptophan-rich foods: Low tryptophan is linked to Alzheimer's. Add poultry, low-fat dairy, and avocados to the diet.

6—Drink unfluoridated water. Beware of fluoridated water. It increases absorption of aluminum from deodorants, pots and pans, etc. by over 600%! Avoid aluminum and alum containing products: cookware, deodorants, dandruff shampoos, anti-diarrhea compounds, canned foods, salt, buffered aspirin / analgesics, antacids, refined, fast foods, relishes, pickles, tobacco, etc. Read labels!

Lifestyle watchwords:

•Consider removing silver amalgam dental fillings. Mercury toxicity releases into the brain and affects brain health.

•Decrease prescription diuretics if possible. They leach potassium and nutrients needed by the brain.

•Use pain killers or sleeping pills sparingly; they can leach acetylcholine from brain tissue.

Bodywork:

•Daily exercise in fresh air is medicine against Alzheimer's. •Hot and cold hydrotherapy showers boost brain and circulation. •Deep breathing exercises oxygenate the brain, for energy and well being.

Herbal, Superfood and Supplement Therapy

Interceptive therapy: Choose 2 to 4 recommendations.

1—Reduce glyco-protein amyloid strings, overcome brain damage: •Transformation PUREZYME, protease 3 to 5 capsules; •Ethical Nutrients MAGNESIUM-MALIC ACID. •Phosphatidyl Choline 5000-10,000mg. •COLOSTRUM fights E. coli which produces fibers similar to Alzheimer's.

2—Slow brain deterioration: •Alpha Lipoic Acid 600mg daily (good results in halting Alzheimer's progression in one study); •NADH, 10mg in the morning before eating (highly recommended). •Phosphatidyl serine 100mg 3x daily for 3 months, or GPC (glyceryl-phoshorylcholine) or DHA for 3 months (Nature's calcium channel blocker, good results) . •Lion's mane mushroom Hericium erinaceus extract (see previous page). •Lysine 1000mg daily; •Acetyl-Carnitine 2000mg; •CoQ-10, 200mg. Vitamin E 2000 IU daily (use under a doctor's supervision).

3—Fight inflammation: or Crystal Star DR. ENZYME™ with protease and bromelain; •New Chapter ZYFLAMEND caps; •Nexrutine caps® (proprietary extract of Phellodendron amurense); •Life Extension SUPER CURCUMIN w. Bioperene.

4—Normalize body chemistry: Panax ginseng or reishi mushroom drops; •Kyolic FORMULA 108 for high homocysteine (common in Alzheimer's); Siberian eleuthero drops; •B-complex for mental power also lowers homocysteine levels; •MICROHYDRIN PLUS; •Transformation EXCELL-ZYME; •Nutricology ANTI-OX II. •Donq quai-peony formula for menopausal women. A ginseng formula like •Crystal Star FEEL GREAT NOW!™ caps with ginseng helps balance testosterone levels for men.

5—Enhance memory retention: •Huperzine-A, 200mcg, 2 daily (all natural best). Herbs like panax ginseng and royal jelly; •Crystal Star MENTAL INNER ENERGY™ drops in water. Chelation therapy cleans arterial pathways - Metabolic Response Modifiers CARDIO CHELATE. •Ginseng–Gotu Kola, •Rosemary tea daily. or •Planetary BRAIN STRENGTH BACOPA-GINKGO stabilize symptoms. •Crystal Star IRON SOURCE™ caps may improve conversation ability.

6—Nourish the brain: •IODINE, POTASSIUM, SILICA drops in water, or •Flora VEGE-SIL to prevent aluminum build-up; •Vitamin Research VINPOCETINE 30mg daily enhances memory; •Brain EFAs: Evening primrose 3000mg daily, vitamin E 800IU daily, and DHA.

—**Superfood therapy:** Choose 1 or 2 recommendations.
•Crystal Star RESTORE YOUR STRENGTH™ drink, or caps.
•Nutricology PRO-GREENS.
•Pines MIGHTY GREENS superfood
•Prince of Peace GINSENG–ROYAL JELLY vials.

Can't find a recommended product? Call the 800 number listed in Product Resources for the store nearest you.

Anemia

Hemolytic, Iron-Deficiency, Folic Acid, Aplastic, Pernicious, Thalassemia, Sickle Cell

Iron-Deficiency: chronically low hemoglobin caused by a lack of iron, or poor absorption of iron. Twenty percent of American women suffer from iron-deficiency anemia. *Hemolytic or megaloblastic*: vitamin B-12 and/or folic acid deficiency (your body may be unable to absorb them) which means interference in the production of red blood cells in bone marrow. Red blood cells are destroyed more quickly than they are replaced. *Thalassemia*: an inherited defect, usually affecting people of Mediterranean origin. *Sickle Cell*: an inherited defect, common among blacks, with severe pain caused by blood clots. *Pernicious*: an auto-immune disease affecting nerve and digestive systems, caused by failure of the digestive tract to absorb vitamin B-12, common among the elderly. *Folic acid*: low folic acid interferes with red blood cells. *Aplastic*: progressive bone marrow failure, often caused by toxic exposure. **Anemia symptoms are wide ranging**: great fatigue, characterized by apathy, dizziness and fainting; shortness of breath, usually with heart palpitations; bleeding gastric ulcers; heavy menstruation; low libido; slow healing, headaches which engender violent mood swings and irritability, spots before the eyes, brittle nails, hair loss, dark urine and yellowish skin pallor. Anemia is linked to recurring infections and underlying immune compromised diseases like Crohn's, Lupus, Candidiasis. See those pages in this book for more.

Diet and Lifestyle Support Therapy

Nutritional therapy plan:

1—Anemia is almost always linked to low leafy greens intake. Eating patterns show that vegetarians eat more iron than meat eaters. Vegans eat the most iron of all! Vegetable and herbal iron sources are best for absorbability. Make a B-12/folic acid mix: nutritional yeast, molasses, wheat germ, bee pollen granules, sesame seeds, dulse flakes; sprinkle 2 tbsp. daily over food (noticeable activity; highly recommended for at least 2 months). Cultured foods like yogurt, kefir, miso and tofu help friendly flora and vitamin B-12.

2—Iron-rich foods: liver, organ meats, figs and raisins, seafood, molasses, beets, tofu. brown rice, dark greens, whole grains, poultry, eggs, grapes, yams, almonds and beans.

3—Manganese and vitamin C foods help iron uptake: whole grains, green vegetables, nuts, pineapple, eggs, citrus, cruciferous veggies, tomatoes and peppers.

4—Potassium rich foods improve red blood cell count: broccoli, bananas, sunflower seeds, artichokes, vegetables, whole grains, kiwi, dried fruits or a potassium broth (pg. 291).

5—Avoid iron-depleting sodas, caffeine, chocolate, red meat, milk, excess alcohol.

—Lifestyle measures:

•Avoid pesticides, sprays and fluorescent lighting that cause body mineral leaching.
•Mild exercise daily enhances oxygen uptake. Morning sunlight boosts vitamin D.
•Poor food combining accounts for an amazing amount of low iron. Check out a food combining chart at your health food store.
•Parasite infestations cause anemia. It's worth it to get a check
•Ethical Nutrients ZINC STATUS checks for zinc deficiency (linked to pregnancy-related anemia) and is a supplement.

—Watchwords:

•If your baby is pale, lacks energy and drinks cow's milk instead of breast milk, he or she may be anemic. Cow's milk may promote loss of iron in stools.
•Chemotherapy methotrexate drugs may cause anemia by interfering with folic acid.
•Limit NSAIDS drugs linked to gastrointestinal bleeding

Herbal, Superfood and Supplement Therapy

Interceptive therapy: Choose 2 to 3 recommendations.

1—**Improve red blood cell count:** •Crystal Star IRON SOURCE™ caps with dandelion and dulse; •Nutricology PRO-GREENS w. EFAs, or Pure Planet SPIRULINA can increase iron levels over 300%! • Pure Planet CHLORELLA; •Floradix LIQUID IRON.

2—**Improve iron absorption:** •Crystal Star ENERGY GREEN RENEWAL™ drink for extra iron and zinc needed for iron absorption; •Planetary TRIPHALA COMPLEX; •Nutricology LAKTOFERRIN enhances iron absorption (decreases nausea and constipation of iron supplements); •Pure Planet AMLA C PLUS; •Iron-enhancing herbs: *yellow dock, red raspberry, dandelion, dulse, amla berry, kelp* (esp. during pregnancy).

3—**B vitamins boost absorption:** •Nature's Secret ULTIMATE B; Transformation SUPER-CELLZYME; •for B-12: Spirulina-bee pollen caps, •Prince of Peace American GINSENG-EOYAL JELLY vials; or Sublingual B-12, 5000mcg; •B-complex 10Cmg w. extra B₆ 10Cmg daily. •Crystal Star DR. PROBIOTICS with FOS™ or UAS DDS-PLUS boost B-12. •Solaray ALFA-JUICE stimulates bone marrow production.

4—**Iron-enhancing resources:** •Crystal Star OCEAN MINERALS™ caps and ZINC SOURCE™ spray. •*Siberian eleuthero,* or •Nature's Secret ULTIMATE IRON, Betaine HCl or manganese at meals. •Zinc 50mg daily, or •Source Naturals OPTI-ZINC caps.

Special anemia types:

—**Folic acid anemia:** Folic acid 800mcg with B-12 and zinc 50mg (regains menstrual periods) ; and Sun Wellness CHLORELLA tabs, 15 daily.

—**Sickle cell anemia:** add antioxidants daily: zinc 50mg (helps children grow normally), vitamin E 800IU, folic acid 800mcg, vit. B-6 200mg, vitamin C 5000mg, garlic.

—**Thalassemia:** vitamin E 800IU with CoQ₁₀ 120mg daily.
—**Pernicious anemia:** Folic acid 800mcg daily.

Red Blood Cell

Can't find a recommended product? Call the 800 number listed in Product Resources for the store nearest you.

Anxiety Reactions

Panic Attacks, Phobias, Obsessive-Compulsive Disorder

Anxiety disorder is the most common mental illness in the U.S! Over 19 million Americans suffer from clinical anxiety and panic disorders, and phobias (extreme fear). Another 35 million suffer mild to moderate anxiety symptoms. Women are twice as likely to suffer from anxiety as men. Further, the shock of the September 11th tragedy, the repeating of the experience in our minds and the new fears that the vulnerability to our freedom has revealed, add more layers of anxiety that affects our health. A survey by the Pew Institute finds 1 in 3 Americans have frequent insomnia and interrupted sleep since September 11th…. even now, years after the attack! The health toll after Worl War II was much the same.

What causes anxiety reactions?

Anxiety and phobias are more than just frightening. A Harvard study shows that people who react to stress this way are 4 times more likely to have high blood pressure, heart spasms, heart disease and hypoglycemia than those who don't. During a panic attack, terror is so great that one loses all sense of reality. Severe, long term financial problems and economic insecurity can generate this kind of fear. Some people even feel that they are going to die. Anxiety is tied to emotional stress encountered in daily life - relationship difficulties, job demands, food allergies, B-vitamin, calcium and magnesium nutrient deficiencies, even our increasingly crowded, noisy environment. Drugs can provide good short term results in anxiety reduction, but over the long term, they pose serious drawbacks like addiction and oversedation. Anti-depressant drugs like Prozac, besides their side effects, change body chemistry, making you more at risk for a panic attack, and abnormal behavior. Some people report withdrawal symptoms worse than heroin, lasting for years! In contrast, a natural approach with nervine herbs and lifestyle support works well to help reduce crippling symptoms and help regain control over your life.

What does an anxiety attack look like?

Most people shiver or tremble. Heartbeat becomes rapid, concentration and focus are difficult, thoughts race, sleep is elusive. Most suffer indigestion, ulcer or colitis attacks. Irritability, high blood pressure, head and neck aches, dizziness, excessive perspiration, dry mouth and shortness of breath all abound.

Are you having a panic attack or a heart attack?

Many women confuse panic attacks with heart attacks during menopause because their symptoms seem so severe. Menopausal heart palpitations and nighttime anxiety attacks are extremely common. When I first went into menopause, I remember waking up terrified that I was having a heart attack, but found out later that it was a panic attack.

Panic attack signs to look for:

If you have the following symptoms, you're probably suffering from a panic attack. It will more than likely pass quickly. If symptoms persist, seek out a health practitioner. Herbs offer relief from nighttime panic attacks. I keep Crystal Star HEART PROTECTOR FOR WOMEN™ for panic attacks extract (*hawthorn, arjuna, ashwagandha* and *passionflowers*), by my bed for immediate relief.

- hyperventilating or feeling short of breath especially at night.
- racing heartbeat, dizziness or feeling faint.
- bolting upright out of bed in the early morning hours.
- feeling like you're "going crazy" or losing control; being full of fear that has no basis in reality.

Heart attack warning signs: Seek medical attention immediately! Ignoring symptoms could mean risking your life.

- Pressure or pain in the center of the chest lasting more than a few minutes.
- Numbness spreading to the face, neck or arms, usually on one side.
- Chest pain and severe headache with light-headedness, sweating, nausea or shortness of breath.
- Dimness or loss of vision, especially in one eye. Trouble talking or understanding speech.
- Unexplained sudden fatigue or back pain.

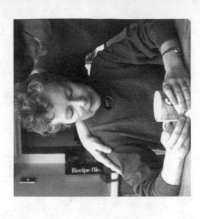

Can't find a recommended product? Call the 800 number listed in Product Resources for the store nearest you.

Anxiety Reactions

Diet and Lifestyle Support Therapy

Nutritional therapy plan:

1—To deter panic attacks, avoid alcohol, caffeine, nicotine. They deplete B vitamins, your body's natural tranquilizers.

2—Avoid trigger foods: sugar, aspartame loaded foods, coffee, alcohol, nitrate-preserved meats, MSG, fast foods, salty, fried foods, cola drinks.

3—Eat simple, calming, comfort foods during the day to prevent a panic attack at night...brown rice, mashed potatoes, creamy yogurt, oatmeal, steamed vegetables, etc. Consider rice milk or goat's milk (rich in B-vitamins) instead of cow's milk.

—Good nutrients for your diet:

• Foods rich in calcium for both stress and immune response: sesame seeds, almonds, soy foods, low fat dairy products, and leafy greens.

• Foods rich in magnesium protect nerves: sea greens, wheat germ, bran, most nuts.

• Foods rich in B vitamins support the adrenals and fuel the nerves: nutritional yeast, whole grains and brans, nuts, beans.

• Foods rich in vitamin C help control a stress response: peppers, greens, broccoli, kiwi, acerola cherries.

Bodywork diet support:

• Hypnotherapy is extremely successful for panic attacks and anxiety.

• Relax. Take an epsom salts bath, get a massage therapy treatment, do yoga or meditate. A sleep pillow filled with flax seeds and lavender shows good results.

• Regular exercise reduces symptoms. Do aerobic exercise, or take a hike or run every day possible.

• Deep breathing is a natural tranquilizer: 1) exhale with a whoosh. 2) inhale through your nose slowly. 3) hold your breath for a count of six. 4) exhale with a whoosh. Repeat four more times.

—Lifestyle measures:

• Most panic attacks take place in the early morning hours.

Next time, put the 5 a.m. willys into perspective:

1: Get out of bed, turn on a TV show, take a shower; see the sun rising and life going on. Get dressed and walk outside.

2: Stretch, exercise a little, or walk your dog. There is a body chemical basis for fear, released in hormone secretions. Exercise oxygenates the body, replacing that function.

3: Think positive. Review a recent success, remind yourself of talents and abilities.

4: You are not alone, no matter what situation you are in. Don't let stress make you violent toward those you love, or against yourself, for instance, through a heart attack.

5: No matter what it is, it will pass.

Herbal, Superfood and Supplement Therapy

Interceptive therapy: Choose 2 to 3 recommendations.

1—**Herbal calmers help, often in 20 minutes:** Relora, 750mg as needed; New Life TRYPTOZEN helps lower cortisol (effective as benzo-diazepines); •Nelson Bach RESCUE REMEDY drops (highly recommended); •*Kava kava* (see contra-indications), •*Ashwagandha* or •*Siberian eleuthero* extracts; •Crystal Star RELAX CAPS™ as needed (usually helps within 25 minutes), or STRESS ARREST™ Tea; or Pinnacle's RHODAX, a rhodiola extract capsule we find very helpful, especially for men.

2—**Rebuild nerves-relieve anxiety:** •*Gotu kola, scullcap* or *passionflower* extracts. •*St. John's wort* extract, or •*Valerian–Wild Lettuce* extract drops in water with a little honey (works well for kid's stress reactions); •Jarrow THEANINE relaxes and improves concentration; •B-complex 100mg with extra B_6 50mg, niacinimide 500mg, thiamine 500mg and taurine 500mg, 3x daily.

3—**Adrenal tonics help the body handle stress:** •Crystal Star MUSCLE RELAXER™ drops (works very fast to calm), and •ADRENAL ENERGY BOOST™ caps; •*Evening Primrose* oil 3000mg daily, also adds EFAs. •Ayurvedic *Shankhpushpi* to regulate adrenaline and cortisol production

4—**Aromatherapy can often help right away:** •*Lavender* or *ylang-ylang* oil on the temples; •*Chamomile* or *Rose* oil; •aromas of apples and cinnamon.

5—**Tonic adaptogens rebalance body chemistry:** •Crystal Star FEEL GREAT NOW!™ caps with Ginseng. •Pure Essence ENERGY PLUS tabs (good results) or *Dong Quai-Damiana* extract. •Enzymatic Therapy ANTI-ANXIETY. •*Hawthorn-Arjuna-Passionflowers* drops for panic attacks or *Hawthorn* extract as needed for heart palpitations.

6—**Vitamin C helps prevent an anxiety response:** •Pure Planet AMLA C PLUS (take for 2 months at least); •Ester C with high bioflavonoids 1500mg daily.

—**Anti-stress amino acids and minerals are calmers and balancers:** •GABA 750-1000mg, during an attack mimics valium effects without sedation. •Natural Balance HTP: CALM, at night before bed. •Magnesium: critical support for heart stability and calcium balance. •Tyrosine 1000mg, between meals. •Enzymatic Therapy ANTI-ANXIETY. •Homeopathic *Ignatia* tablets.

—**Superfood therapy:** Choose 1 or 2 recommendations.

•Crystal Star RESTORE YOUR STRENGTH™ drink with sea veggies and EFAs..

•Nutritional yeast broth or miso broth before bed.

•Green Foods CARROT ESSENCE.

Can't find a recommended product? Call the 800 number listed in Product Resources for the store nearest you.

Appendicitis
Chronic Appendix Inflammation

Your appendix and tonsils are lymph organs that make white blood cells. Appendicitis is the inflammation of the small 2 inch appendix tube opening into the beginning of the large intestine. It's the most common reason a child requires emergency abdominal surgery. It is usually caused by blockage from a small, hard lump of fecal matter, which itself results from a fiber-deficient diet. Appendicitis is rare in countries where people eat a high fiber diet. The blockage stops the natural flow of fluids, unfriendly bacteria swarm in – inflammation and infection result. Some doctors believe appendicitis serves as a lightening rod for the body, attracting infections and localizing them in an unimportant spot in the body to be dealt with more easily.

__Early Symptoms:__ It starts with constipation, the inability to pass gas and a low grade fever… it's followed by central abdominal pain, nausea and vomiting, pain which then shifts to the right lower abdomen as the inflammation spreads - then sharp intense, stabbing pain on the lower right side at the waist. Important: Do not take enemas or laxatives (even herbal) during an attack because they may cause your appendix to burst. Perforation and rupture of the organ is a major medical emergency, and you need emergency treatment. DON'T DELAY!

Diet and Lifestyle Support Therapy

__Nutritional therapy plan:__ *Reduce the risk of developing appendicitis by avoiding chemicalized and fried foods and making sure your diet is high in fiber.*

__1__—Go on a short spring cleanse (pg. 172) to gently clear and clean the intestine. Take one potassium drink (pg. 291) daily during your cleanse.

__Appendix specific teas: (choose 1)__
#1) 2 tbsp. *agrimony*, 2 tbsp. *echinacea rt.*, 1 tbsp. *chamomile*, 1 tbsp. *wild yam root.*
#2) 2 tbsp. *agrimony*, 2 tbsp. *calendula.*

__2__—Eat sweet fruits for a day to encourage healing. Then, resume a simply cooked, mild foods diet. Include a glass of carrot juice daily for 2 weeks.

__3__—Add a fiber-rich drink to your diet. Fiber is critical in preventing fecal blockages that result in appendicitis. Try AloeLife FIBERMATE gentle fiber or Jarrow GENTLE FIBERS drink mix.

—__Warning:__ Take no solid food or laxatives during an appendix flare-up.
—Keep the colon clean. Constipation is usually at the heart of an attack. __After an attack subsides, gently clean the colon of infection: (choose 1)__ •Solaray TETRA CLEANSE or •Planetary TRIPHALA caps. •Yerba Prima COLON CARE. •Crystal Star FIBER & HERBS COLON CLEANSE™ caps. Use a mild catnip enema if needed.

—__Lifestyle measures:__ *The suggestions here are for chronic, recurring appendicitis.*
•Chronic or grumbling appendicitis can be treated herbally with some success. Any hint of complications or deterioration of your condition must be taken seriously. Get emergency help!
• *Note:* it's a vicious circle, using too many laxatives to make up for fiber deficiency results in low peristalsis, which then causes toxic build-up; many people end up using excessive antibiotics which then causes poor bowel flora and poor immune response. Do not take enemas or colonics during an attack.
•Use alternating hot (*cayenne/ginger*) and cold (plain) compresses on affected region and along spinal area to stimulate healing circulation.

Herbal, Superfood and Supplement Therapy

__Interceptive therapy: Choose 2 to 3 recommendations.__
Take liquid supplements when possible - they're easier on your system.
__1__—__Reduce infection:__ •Crystal Star ANTI-BIO™ drops every 2 hours.
__2__—__Reduce inflammation:__•Crystal Star ANTI-FLAM™ caps.
__3__—__Reduce spasms:__ •Crystal Star MUSCLE RELAXER™ caps or STRESS OUT™ drops. (Drops usually help within 20 minutes.)
__4__—__Flush lymph toxins:__ •*Echinacea* extract 4x daily for a month after an attack to keep lymph glands flushed. •Herbs Etc. LYMPHA-TONIC softgels with *echinacea* and *red root.*
__5__—__Preventive measures:__ Choose 1 or 2 recommendations.
•__Daily vitamins:__ •Transformation SUPER-CELL-ZYME. •Beta carotene 100,000IU; •vitamin E 800IU daily; •zinc picolinate 30mg; •Ester C powder ¼ tsp. in water 4x.
•__Plant enzymes:__ •Liquid chlorophyll in water 3 tsp. daily; •Rainbow Light AD-VANCED ENZYME SYSTEM tablets at meals or Herbal Products and Development POWER PLUS enzymes, or •Crystal Star DR. ENZYME™ with protease and bromelain to help reduce inflammation.
•__Probiotics:__ •Nutricology SYMBIOTICS powder, ¼ tsp. in water 3x daily; •Natren LIFE START powder for friendly flora, •UAS DDS-PLUS with FOS, for better intestinal peristalsis.

—__Superfood therapy:__
•Crystal Star RESTORE YOUR STRENGTH™ drink, very alkalizing.
•Nutricology PROGREENS w. EFAs.
•Green Foods CARROT ESSENCE.

__The Appendix__
Large Intestine
Small Intestine
Appendix

Can't find a recommended product? Call the 800 number listed in Product Resources for the store nearest you.

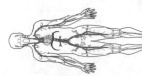

Arteriosclerosis - Atherosclerosis
Clogging and Hardening of the Arteries

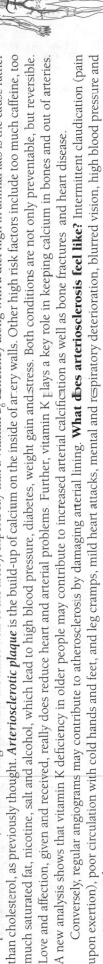

Both arteriosclerosis and atherosclerosis block the flow of blood from the arteries to the heart, and damage the circulatory system. **Atherosclerotic plaque** is largely composed of cholesterol, but since it begins under the inner wall of the artery, experts say that a vitamin B_6 deficiency along with a diet high in animal fats is the cause rather than cholesterol, as previously thought. **Arteriosclerotic plaque** is the build-up of calcium on the inside of artery walls. Other high risk factors include too much caffeine, too much saturated fat, nicotine, salt and alcohol, which lead to high blood pressure, diabetes, weight gain and stress. Both conditions are not only preventable, but reversible. Love and affection, given and received, really does reduce heart and arterial problems. Further, vitamin K plays a key role in keeping calcium in bones and out of arteries. A new analysis shows that vitamin K deficiency in older people may contribute to increased arterial calcification as well as bone fractures and heart disease.

Conversely, regular angiograms may contribute to atherosclerosis by damaging arterial lining. **What does arteriosclerosis feel like?** Intermittent claudication (pain upon exertion), poor circulation with cold hands and feet, and leg cramps, mild heart attacks, mental and respiratory deterioration, blurred vision, high blood pressure and sometimes sexual impotence.

Diet and Lifestyle Support Therapy

Nutritional therapy plan:

1—Reduce coffee to 1 cup daily. Instead, drink green tea especially, and have ½ a grapefruit for artery clearing flavonoids each morning. Eat high fiber whole grain cereals.

2—Reduce your cholesterol. Avoid fatty foods like red meats, dairy foods, especially fried fast foods, often fried in re-used, rancid oil, the worst for your arteries!

3—Reduce high phosphorus foods: sodas, beef, pork, poultry. They promote negative calcium balance. Eat sea veggies - loaded with vitamin K which keeps calcium in bones.

4—Eat antioxidant-rich vegetables like fresh greens. In tests, vegetarians have healthier hearts and arteries. Stroke risk from clogged arteries decreases by 35% for each increase of 3 fruit or vegetable servings a day.

5—Reduce homocysteine: 1) B Complex 100mg daily. Add 50mg extra of B_6 and 400mcg extra of folic acid; 2) Four garlic capsules (about 1200mg a day) maintain aortic elasticity; 3) Daily ginger prevents blood "stickiness;" 4) Red wine, one glass with dinner. (*See complete program on page 440*).

6—For arteriosclerotic retinopathy: reduce fats, especially saturated fats from meats in your diet. Reduce sugar intake to help normalize blood sugar balance.

Lifestyle measures:

The American Heart Association says people over 50 have twice as much arterial calcification as younger people. Still, atherosclerosis can begin in early childhood! Autopsies reveal fatty deposits in the arteries of children just 5 years old today!

•Stop smoking - it accelerates arteriosclerosis by making blood platelets sticky and more likely to form arterial clots. Relax. Meditation proves to be good for your arteries.

•Avoid chlorinated water. Chlorine may promote atherosclerosis by oxidizing LDL in artery walls.

•Exercise… a brisk daily walk keeps arteries young. Aerobic exercise helps raise HDL levels. Then, use a dry skin brush over the body to stimulate circulation.

•Take an alternating hot and cold shower to increase blood circulation.

Herbal, Superfood and Supplement Therapy

Interceptive therapy: Choose 2 to 3 recommendations.

1—**Normalize blood circulation:** •Crystal Star HEART PROTECTOR FOR MEN or HEART PROTECTOR FOR WOMEN™ caps; •Planetary HAWTHORN HEART tabs.

—**Silica returns circulation:** •Flora VEGESIL, •Eidon SILICA. •Aortic *Glycosaminoglycans* improve circulation and artery health- Enzymatic Therapy AORTA-GLYCAN.

•Daily *Garlic* capsules help normalize blood pressure levels.

2—**Oral chelation - good results:** •Metabolic Resp. Modifiers CARDIO-CHELATE oral chelation with EDTA (highly recommended).

3—**Inhibit atherosclerosis forming:** •Lane Labs PALM VITEE w. toco-trienols (excellent results); Nutricology NATTOZYME (breaks down fibrin, a blood clotting protein, which builds up on arteries) •*Ginkgo biloba* extract and chromium picolinate 200mcg relieve claudication pain; •Health from the Sun FRENCH PARADOX with resveratrol.

4—**Antioxidants are front line defense:** Their negatively charged electrons prevent and remove positively charged plaque build-up. •MICROHYDRIN PLUS caps 3 daily; •PCO's from *grapeseed* or *white pine* 100mg daily; •CoQ-10, 100mg daily, and •Zinc picolinate, 30mg daily. •Futurebiotics CIRCU A.V. tabs.

5—**Liver support balances fats:** •*Milk thistle* seed extract, 3 to 6 months; •Crystal Star GREEN TEA CLEANSER; •Acetyl-Carnitine 1000mg; •Niacin 500mg daily (flush free OK). •Sun Force CoQ₁₀ in flax oil, or *evening primrose* oil caps 4000mg daily.

—**Superfood therapy:** Choose 1 or 2 recommendations.

•Nature's Secret ULTIMATE FIBER (very good feedback from users).
•Crystal Star CHO-LO-FIBER TONE™ drink or caps
•All One TOTAL FIBER COMPLEX.
•Jarrow GENTLE FIBERS.
•New Chapter GINGER WONDER syrup- 1 tbsp. in 8-oz. water 2x daily.

Can't find a recommended product? Call the 800 number listed in Product Resources for the store nearest you.

Arthritis

Joint and Connective Tissue Diseases

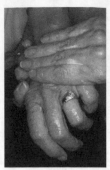

The term arthritis (joint inflammation), refers to over 100 diseases that attack joints and connective tissue. Degenerative joint and rheumatic diseases include gout, lupus, ankylosing spondylitis (arthritic spine), psoriatic arthritis (skin and nail arthritis), infective arthritis (bacterial joint infection), fibromyalgia and rheumatism. Today more than 40 million Americans are afflicted by one or more of these crippling conditions, now the leading cause of disability in the U.S. Arthritis is the country's number one crippling disease, affecting up to 80% of people over 50. Estimates say arthritis cases are rising... over 60 million people in the U.S. will be afflicted in the next two decades. Add to that, people suffering from arthritis-like diseases—gout, bursitis, tendonitis and lupus, and the figure becomes staggering.

Arthritis isn't a simple disease. It affects not only bones and joints, but also blood vessels, kidneys, skin, eyes, brain and immune response. Conventional medicine has not been able to address arthritis very well. NSAIDs (*non-steroidal anti-inflammatory drugs*), commonly used to relieve its pain, send 76,000 people to the hospital and kill 7,600 people each year! Research shows even the new COX 2 inhibiting drug, Vioxx, prescribed for arthritis may increase risk of blood clots, heart attacks and stroke. Natural therapies based in lifestyle changes, however, work extremely well, addressing the causes of arthritis while reducing pain and discomfort without the devastating consequences of long term drug therapy. Some, like glucosamine sulfate actually help rebuild joints and prevent further destruction.

Does your body need an arthritis detox?
Start your program with a detox to jumpstart the healing process for joints, connective and immune response.

Is your body showing signs that it needs an arthritis detox?
See the highly recommended Arthritis Sweat, page 187. It works.

—Are you stiff when you get up in the morning? Do you have marked redness and swelling in your fingers, shoulders or neck when it's cold and damp?
—Are your joints starting to crack and pop? Do you experience back or joint pain when you move? Does it get worse with prolonged activity?
—Are you noticing bony bumps on your index fingers? Or bony spurs on other joints?
—Are you anemic? Is your complexion unusually pale? Have you recently lost weight but weren't on a diet?
—Are you more than 20 pounds overweight and starting to feel the extra weight in your knees and hips?
—Is your digestion poor? Do you have food allergies? Do you have long-standing lung and bronchial congestion?
—Are you usually constipated? Do you suffer from ulcerative colitis?
—Do you take more than 6 aspirin a day? Are you on a long-term prescription of corticosteroid drugs? (Either of these may eventually impair the body's own healing powers.)

Try this 3 day nutritional arthritis detox:
Include at least six glasses of cool fresh water daily in your arthritis healing diet.
—*On rising:* take a glass of lemon juice and water; or a glass of fresh grapefruit juice. (Acidic citrus fruits help enzymes alkalize the body); or Crystal Star GREEN TEA CLEANSER™.
—*Breakfast:* take a potassium broth or essence (pg. 291); or a glass of carrot/beet/cucumber juice.
—*Mid-morning:* have apple or black cherry juice; or a green drink, like Green Foods BARLEY ESSENCE, or Crystal Star ENERGY GREEN RENEWAL™ drink.
—*Lunch:* have a cup of miso soup with sea greens snipped on top, and a glass of fresh carrot juice with 1 tsp. Bragg's LIQUID AMINOS.
—*Mid-afternoon:* have another green drink, or alfalfa/mint tea, or Crystal Star CLEANSING & PURIFYING™ tea.
—*Dinner:* have a glass of cranberry/apple, or papaya juice, or another glass of black cherry juice.
—*Before Bed:* take a glass of celery juice, or a cup of miso soup with 1 tbsp. of nutritional yeast.

Follow your detox with a fresh foods diet for 1 month. 1) Fresh fruits and vegetables, with lots of green leafy greens, rich in enzymes. 2) Low sulfur and arthritis are linked. Eat sulfur-containing foods like broccoli, onions, cabbage and garlic. 3) Fiber keeps crystalline wastes flushed. Eat whole grains like rice and oats. 4) Bioflavonoids strengthen connective tissue. Eat (and drink) cranberries, grapes, papayas and citrus fruits, or try Jarrow GENTLE FIBERS drink. 5) Have cold water fish like salmon for high omega-3 oils twice a week.

Drink more water to relieve pain and stiffness. Water helps restore healthy cartilage as it relieves osteoarthritis symptoms. Chondroitin sulfate, a specific nutrient for arthritis, is the molecule in cartilage that attracts and holds water. Healthy joints are 85 to 90% water, but since cartilage doesn't have its own blood supply, chondroitin sulfate aids the chondroitin "molecular sponge" in providing joint nourishment, waste removal and lubrication. Limit alcoholic beverages since they are especially dehydrating.

Can't find a recommended product? Call the 800 number listed in Product Resources for the store nearest you.

The Different Faces of Arthritis

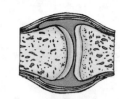

Synovial Joint

OSTEOARTHRITIS: degenerative joint disease, is the most common form of arthritis. OA is characterized by significant cartilage destruction and hardening, followed by the formation of large bone spurs (osteophytes) on weight-bearing joints like the knees, hips, spine, and hands. At its most severe, small bone chips break off, causing great pain and inflammation. The first signs of OA show up as morning stiffness especially in damp weather, then pain as the joints move, worsening with prolonged activity. Osteoarthritis is considered an aging condition, because decades of use lead to degenerative creaking and cracking of joints, and the body has less ability to repair itself. Osteoarthritis affects more women than men, but a man 20 pounds overweight doubles his risk of knee and hip arthritis. Osteoarthritis is repairable, especially with body chemistry improvement. Food allergies almost always contribute to osteoarthritis symptoms, so a good detox followed by a diet with plenty of fresh vegetables is the first place to start (see previous page). Standard drug therapy with aspirin or NSAIDS drugs like MOTRIN suppress inflammation, but may promote OA progression by damaging cartilage and inhibiting maintenance of normal collagen structures. Numerous studies show that glucosamine sulfate, a natural body substance, stimulates the production of cartilage components even better than NSAIDS drugs.

—**Natural therapies for osteoarthritis:** •For women: Crystal Star PRO-EST BALANCE™ roll-on gel, Maitake Products REISHI caps, and •Crystal Star ADRENAL ENERGY BOOST™ caps for adrenal exhaustion; •SAMe reduces pain and improves mobility, 600mg daily. •Vitamin B-12 2500mcg daily. •For men: Ayurvedic BOSWELLIA with zinc 50mg (excellent results) . •For both: cherries and cherry juice take the "bumps" out of knuckles by helping eliminate acids. Flush acids out with a diuretic like •Crystal Star TINKLE™ caps or •TINKLE™ tea as needed. Bitters herbs like •Crystal Star BITTERS & LEMON™ extract stimulate better digestion: Pain relievers: •Home Health CELADRIN joint cream; •Biochemics PAIN RELIEF; •W.F. Young ABSORBINE CHRONIC arthritis strength. Outdoor exercise for extra vitamin D helps osteoarthritis. *See also general recommendations for arthritis.*

RHEUMATOID ARTHRITIS: affects more than 6 million Americans, the vast majority of them women. RA is a chronic, auto-immune, inflammatory disease in which rogue immune cells attack the synovial membrane that cushions joints. When this connective membrane becomes inflamed, it invades and damages nearby bone and cartilage, resulting in pain, loss of movement, and eventually destruction of joints. Damage goes further, because RA also inflames blood vessels and the outer lining of the heart and lungs. People with RA often feel sick and feverish all over, and suffer severe fatigue. Most have food allergies, amoeba infestation, anemia, ulcerative colitis, chronic lung and bronchial congestion, and liver malfunction. Common causes include calcium depletion, adrenal exhaustion, prolonged use of aspirin or steroid drugs, that eventually impair the body's immune response; low fresh vegetable intake, and high intake of mucous-forming foods, auto-toxemia from constipation, resentments and a negative attitude toward life that locks up the body's healing ability.

...**PSORIATIC ARTHRITIS:** an easily aggravated rheumatoid-like arthritis, affects 1 out of 10 patients with psoriasis. •*Burdock* tea, 2 cups daily and daily applications of wild yam cream are two specifics for this type of arthritis. Immune support is essential. Try •Biotec Foods ANTI-STRESS ENZYMES, 6 daily for several months. Crystal Star •LIVER RENEW™ caps or LIVER CLEANSE FLUSHING™ tea and •BLADDER KIDNEY COMFORT caps or tea support liver function and kidney elimination of toxins.

—*Natural therapies for rheumatoid arthritis:* Eat fresh salmon or tuna twice a week. Use olive oil frequently. Focus on "live" foods with plenty of fresh vegetables and salads. Consider Betaine HCl if you have low stomach acid (common in RA). Take •Phoenix Biologics BOVINE TRACHEAL CARTILAGE (natural chondroitan sulfates), •*Evening Primrose Oil* 4000mg daily, •Nutricology PRO-GREENS drink with EFAs; •vitamin E 800IU along with *ginger* caps daily; •Natural Balance MODUCARE plant sterols decrease cytokine secretions linked to RA inflammation. •Reduce inflammation significantly with New Chapter Zyflamend, or Crystal Star ANTI-FLAM™ caps (4 at a time), or PCO's from grape seed oil, 300mg daily. •CAPSAICIN and Tiger Balm rub-on cremes help, as do hot sulphur and mud baths at a spa. Enzyme therapy alleviates pain and swelling: Transformation PUREZYME 6 caps 3x daily; •bromelain 1500mg, or try •Crystal Star DR. ENZYME™ with protease and bromelain. •B-complex 100mg with pantothenic acid 500mg and folic acid 400mcg reduce stiffness •Thymus extract boosts immune response; •Japanese research shows "sand baths" (where the sufferer buries arthritic joints in the sand for at least 15 minutes) reduces swelling (good results).

RHEUMATISM: rheumatism myalgia, referred to today as Fibromyalgia (see page 416 for more specific recommendations): characterized by pain, muscle stiffness, and tenderness in soft-tissue, where excess acid settles in the joints causing inflammation, and inhibiting production of natural cortisone. (Cortisone feeds adrenals and helps metabolize proteins.)

—**Improve body chemistry to relieve rheumatism:** Start with •Crystal Star CLEANSING & PURIFYING™ tea, cider vinegar and water each morning, or a diuretic like •Crystal Star TINKLE™ caps to release congestive sediments.. Build your healing diet around acid-absorbing and anti-inflammatory foods like potatoes, turnips, green beans and carrots; white grape juice and apples stimulate digestion. Alfalfa has a long history of success for rheumatism - eat alfalfa sprouts often, take alfalfa tablets or •Solaray ALFA-JUICE caps, or •Crystal Star ENERGY GREEN RENEWAL™ drink with alfalfa. Anti-rheumatics: •New Chapter ZYFLAMEND AM & PM highly recommended), or anti-inflammatories like a glucosamine-chondroitin supplement, or • ginger, both as compress and supplement 2-4 capsules daily, works for rheumatism. For long term musculo-skeletal support, try •Crystal Star RESTORE YOUR STRENGTH™ drink with circulatory stimulants, like *cayenne/ginger* caps and •Capsaicin rub on cream. For immune health, Tri-Medica COLOSTRUM shows good results for rheumatic myalgia. •Crystal Star RELAX CAPS™ relieve arthritic muscles. •*Wintergreen* oil and •Wakunaga GLUCOSAMINE GLUCOSAMINE SOOTHING cream are good rub-ons for pain relief.

Can't find a recommended product? Call the 800 number listed in Product Resources for the store nearest you.

325

Arthritis

Diet and Lifestyle Support Therapy

Nutritional therapy plan: See previous page for an arthritis cleansing diet.

1—Change to a low-fat, mostly vegetarian diet - the single most beneficial thing you can do to control any kind of arthritis, even in long-standing cases.

2—Avoid arthritis trigger foods: corn, wheat, rye breads, bacon and pork, beef, eggs, coffee, oranges and milk. Nightshade foods like peppers, eggplant, tomatoes and potatoes; mustard, colas, chocolate. Diets high in hydrogenated oils and refined sugar aggravate flare-ups.

3—Cut down on: alcohol, fried foods, dairy foods, black tea, salty, highly spiced foods.

4—Add body balancing foods: green tea, artichokes, cherries, cabbages, brown rice, oats (not for rheumatoid arthritis), shiitake mushrooms, cold water fish, sea greens, fresh fruits, vegetables, leafy greens, garlic, onions, olive oil, flax seed oil, sweet potatoes, squashes, ginger and parsley.

5—Arthritis V-8 Special: add to a bottle of Knudsen's VERY VEGGIE JUICE, 4 tbsp. each: wheat germ, lecithin granules and nutritional yeast flakes. Take 8-oz. twice daily.

•Add New Chapter GINGER WONDER syrup (a COX2 inhibitor) with 1 pinch cayenne pepper, 1 pinch turmeric powder to any healing drink. (Highly recommended.)

Things to know:

•High doses of aspirin, NSAIDS and cortisone for arthritic pain can hamper your body's ability to maintain bone strength.

•Nightshade plants may trigger arthritis: Tobacco is a nightshade plant. MOTRIN is also a nightshade derivative, and should not be used by nightshade-sensitive people.

—Bodywork:

•To relieve pain, press the highest spot of the muscle between thumb and index finger. Press in the webbing between the two fingers, closer toward the bone that attaches to the index finger. Press into the web muscle, angling the pressure toward the bone of the index finger. Press for 10 seconds at a time.

•Massage therapy, acupuncture, hot and cold hydrotherapy (page 185), epsom salts baths, chiropractic treatments and overheating therapy (page 182) are all effective.

•Regular exercise is a key. Strong muscles act as shock absorbers against arthritis pain.

•Get sun on your body for vitamin D.

—Healing applications:

•Home Health CELADRIN cream for stiffness; •BHI TRAUMEEL healing gel; •*Arnica* gel for soreness; •*Boswellin* creme; •Biochemics PAIN RELIEF lotion. •Capsaicin creme, *cayenne-ginger* compresses; Home Health CELADRIN cream (use in the AM for stiffness relief). •Emu oil. •Soak hands in oatmeal for 15 minutes for relief.

—**Desert healers are some of the best:** *Yucca* extract, *Jojoba* oil to apply, *Aloe vera* gel and juice, •*devils claw* extract (clinically tested activity).

Herbal, Superfood and Supplement Therapy

Interceptive therapy: Choose 2 to 3 recommendations.

1—**Repair joints, reduce pain:** •Crystal Star ANTI-FLAM™ caps with natural COX-2 inhibitors; •GLUCOSAMINE-CHONDROITIN 4 daily jumpstarts healing; (Some evidence says men with a high risk for prostate cancer shouldn't use chondroitin sulfate.) Shark cartilage has natural chondroitin sulfates. Try •Lane Labs ADVACAL (noticeable results). Use with •CMO (*cetyl-myristoleate*) 500mg, like Jarrow TRUE CMO, •Omega-3 flax or fish oil 3x daily. Expect pain to lessen in 2 to 4 months. •Dreamous FULL SPECTRUM HGH. •Solanova NEXRUTINE up to 9 caps a day for severe pain relief.

2—**Reduce inflammation:** •Transformation PUREZYME protease: •MSM 750 to 1000mg. •Quercetin 1000mg w/Bromelain 1500mg; •Niacinamide inhibits pro-inflammatory interleukin-1, 3000mg daily; •DLPA 1000mg for pain. • Herbal anti-inflammatories: •New Chapter ZYFLAMEND COX-2 inhibitors, or Crystal Star ANTI-FLAM™ (excellent results for both). Ocean anti-inflammatories: •Green-lipped mussel and sea cucumber caps 1500-2000mg for 2 months. •Wakunaga GLUCOSAMINE rub-on cream.

—*Nettles therapy: nettles extract suppresses pro inflammatory proteins - their sting on affected joints can dramatically reduce symptoms. Use with guidance of an herbalist or holistic professional.*

3—**Antioxidants help regenerate cartilage - immunity:** •SAMe protects synovial fluid that degrade cartilage (as effective as ibuprofen). •CoQ$_{10}$ 300mg daily; •Carnitine 2000mg daily; •Grapeseed PCO's 300mg daily; •Vitamin E 800IU daily.

4—**Boost collagen synthesis:** •Lane Labs TOKI, collagen replacement drink (highly recommended, noticeable results in hands and fingers) - add Hyalogic Synthovial Seven drops for an even better one-two punch. •Ester C 500mg with bioflavs, up to 10 daily.

5—**Normalize body pH:** •Rainbow Light ADVANCED ENZYME system; •Transformation REPAIRZYME; •Crystal Star DR. ENZYME™ w. protease / bromelain (good results).

6—**Enhance adrenal activity:** •Prince of Peace ROYAL JELLY/GINSENG vials daily. •Nutricology ADRENAL CORTEX organic glandular caps; •Crystal Star ADRENAL ENERGY BOOST™ caps with *Evening Primrose oil* 3000mg daily.

—**Superfood therapy:** Choose 1 or 2 recommendations.

•Take cortisone for arthritis? You may be zinc deficient. Crystal Star ENERGY GREEN RENEWAL™ drink or caps and ZINC SOURCE™ spray extract.

Stimulate natural cortisone: •Alfalfa tabs 10 daily; •Solaray ALFA-JUICE caps; •Sun Wellness, or Pure Planet CHLORELLA 1 tsp. daily.

•Green Foods MAGMA PLUS barley grass.

•Wakunaga KYO-GREEN - take with glucosamine for 1 month. Continue with KYO-GREEN for 3 months.

•Aloe Life ALOE GOLD drink.

•Pure Planet TART CHERRY CONCENTRATE (esp. for gouty arthritis).

Can't find a recommended product? Call the 800 number listed in Product Resources for the store nearest you.

Asthma
Allergic Breathing Disorder

Asthma, inflammation of the bronchial tubes, is a severe respiratory allergy reaction. Since 1980, asthma has increased by 75% in America, with a 50% rise in the last decade, mainly due to more environmental pollutants. It now affects 4 percent of the U.S. population. about 18 million people, 2.5 million of whom have needed emergency treatment. More alarming, a new study by The Pew Environmental Health Commission concludes that 29 million people will have asthma by 2020! Asthma is the leading serious, chronic illness in children under ten, (2:1 ratio of boys to girls), with a death rate of about 5,000 kids a year. Some scientists believe that America's high rates of asthma are a result of a marked decrease in vitamin C anti-oxidants. Unlike other mammals, humans can't manufacture vitamin C on their own; we must obtain it from eating vitamin C rich foods or taking vitamin C supplements. An asthmatic's difficult breathing, choking, wheezing, coughing is actually a failure to exhale, not inhale. In asthma, the lung airways become red, swollen and full of thick mucous. Bronchial spasms constrict airways. The inflamed, constricted airways react, often progressively, to asthma triggers (see below). Drug-free natural therapies can help reduce the need for medication. Still, emergency medical measures may be necessary to arrest severe asthma attacks which can be life threatening.

What triggers asthma?

Food allergies to sugar, dairy foods and wheat often trigger asthma attacks. Most asthma sufferers are sensitive to food additives, sprayed produce, animal dander and molds, too. Beware of aspirin if you are at risk for asthma. Asthma in kids can be aggravated by a chronic fungal or parasite infection. Adult asthma is aggravated by adrenal exhaustion, hypoglycemia and GERD (gastroesophageal reflux disease). Pollutant irritants like smoke, chemical toxins and factory emissions, cold, flu or pneumonia infections can bring on an attack. Emotional stress like anxiety can triple your asthma risk! It makes sense to know your triggers. Asthma sufferers report relief when the trigger is eliminated from their diet or environment.

Note 1: Steroid drugs for asthma help *temporarily* by opening restricted airways. Over the long term, they can impair immune response and severely weaken the bones. Many pred-nisone users end up needing joint replacements to correct bone loss! Studies show even regular use of bronchodilating inhalers like albuterol may lead to frequent, more severe attacks.

Note 2: Acetaminophen (Tylenol) used weekly may increase asthma attacks up to 79%! Why? Acetaminophen depletes levels of glutathione, an antioxidant that protects the lungs.

Signs you might need an asthma chest congestion cleanse: Is your body full of mucous congestion?

Your body needs some mucous. We're taught that mucous is a bad thing because it obstructs our breathing during a sinus infection, asthma or a cold. But mucous is also a needed lubricant and an important body safeguard. We take about 22,000 breaths a day. Mucous gathers up irritants like dirt, pollen, smoke and pollutants we take in along with our oxygen to protect mucous membranes in the respiratory system. Foods that putrefy quickly inside your body are the ones most likely to produce excess mucous like meat, fish, eggs and dairy products. These foods also slow down transit time through your gastrointestinal tract. Allergies and asthma mean extra mucous in the respiratory system and colon. Chronic bronchitis means excess mucous in the bronchi. Some of us carry around as much as 10 to 15 pounds of excess mucous!

You probably have too much clogging mucous if..... 1) your breathing is labored, you wheeze, cough or choke when you exhale. 2) you have chronic sinus congestion, a runny nose and sneezing. 3) you find yourself using a lot of over-the-counter drugs for allergy or asthma to clear your chest 4) you catch every infection that goes around (remember excess mucous is a breeding ground for infectious pathogens that cause colds and flu). See pg. 175 for my best recommendations for a mucous cleansing diet.

—**You may have asthma, the most serious Type 1 allergy reaction if:** 1) you have difficulty breathing, especially after mild exertion. 2) you have chronic sinus congestion with itchy, watery nose and eyes. 3) you get headaches with sneezing, coughing and scratchy throat. Asthmatic colds are often accompanied by ear infections, and a croupy cough. 4) your face swells up, with itchy, rashy skin. 5) you are unusually tired with trouble sleeping at night.

—**You may have a Type 2 allergy to chemicals and contaminants if:** 1) you get unexplained migraines. 2) you are frequently moody and depressed for no reason 3) your friends and family tell you that your personality changes, that you are often space-y or that your memory is getting unusually bad. 4) you have a child that is chronically hyperactive.

—**You may have a Type 2 food allergy if:** 1) you get cyclical headaches with mental fuzziness after eating. 2) you get heart palpitations, with sweating, rashes or puffiness around the eyes after eating, usually also accompanied by high blood pressure. 3) your abdomen becomes excessively swollen after eating with heartburn or stomach cramps. 4) you've gained significant weight even though your diet hasn't changed. 5) you have a child that's irritable, flushed and hyperactive after eating. (Regardless of the food, most food allergy symptoms are similar. Inflammation is started by a release of histamines into tissue mast cells, walling off the affected body area until immune response agents can restore health. But this process takes time. If the body is *re*-exposed before health is renewed, inflammation and mucous congestion become chronic.)

Can't find a recommended product? Call the 800 number listed in Product Resources for the store nearest you.

Asthma

Diet and Lifestyle Support Therapy

Nutritional therapy plan:

1—Food sensitivities play a major role in asthma attacks. During an attack, eat only fresh foods. Include fresh apple or carrot juice daily. Add plenty of water to thin mucous secretions.

2—See pg.175 for a complete lung mucous congestion cleanse. To control asthma nutritionally, reduce salt and starchy foods. Asthma is common when salt intake is high.

3—A largely vegetarian diet offers significant improvement. Leukotrienes that contribute to asthma reactions are derived from arachidonic acid found in animal foods.

4—Avoid dairy products: they generate the most mucous. Avoid foods with sulfites (esp. commercial wine), preservatives or MSG, high gluten breads, oily and fried foods and sugary foods. Avoid soft drinks and caffeine. (Pancreatin, 1400mg before meals helps digest fats.)

5—Magnesium foods relax bronchial muscles: green leafy veggies, seafood, nuts, poultry, whole grains. Relax constricted breathing: Green tea or Crystal Star GREEN TEA CLEANSER™. Eat fresh fish for anti-inflammatory EFAs to reduce asthma.

6—Get more B-vitamin foods: fish, brown rice, nutritional yeast, sea veggies, sunflower seeds, soy foods and fish. Vitamin B-6 deficiency is common in asthma sufferers today because some asthma medications deplete B-6 stores.

•Make a syrup of pressed garlic juice, cayenne, olive oil and honey. Take 1 tsp. daily as a liver cleanser.

Home and lifestyle measures:

•Avoid tobacco smoke, wood and gas stoves.
•Keep home temperature less than 70 degrees, humidity less than 55%. •Use *eucalyptus* oil in a vaporizer at night. Launder with perfume/dye-free detergents. Vacuum often.
•Keep indoor plants in your home as natural air filters.
•Deep breathing exercises bring asthmatic wheezing under control. Expel toxins by taking a walk, a day at the beach, (helps 85% of asthmatics), or bicycle ride. Try to stay away from cortisone compounds that eventually weaken the immune system, and over-the-counter drugs that often drive congestion deeper.

—Bodywork:

•First: stay active to keep breathing strong. Stay physically fit. Extra weight makes breathing difficult.
•A twenty minute oxygen bath helps right away. See page 186 for instructions.
•Take a *catnip-garlic* enema once a week.
•Acupuncture, biofeedback, guided imagery, yoga and massage therapy are effective.
•Gently scratch the lung meridian from top of shoulder to end of thumb to clear chest of mucous. Massage between the shoulder blades.

Herbal, Superfood and Supplement Therapy

Interceptive therapy: Choose 2 to 3 recommendations.

1—Clear mucous, control spasms: •Crystal Star STRESS OUT™ muscle relaxer drops (works fast, sometimes within 25 minutes to ease spasms) or •CoQ₁₀ 200mg; •Crystal Star MUSCLE RELAXER™ caps. •Oshadi FRANKINCENSE aromatherapy.

2—Antihistamines for asthmatics: Crystal Star •ANTI-HST™ caps. •Quercetin 2000mg daily, with Bromelain 1000mg; •Vitamin C up to 8000mg daily with bioflavs.; •Vitamin E 400IU with selenium 200mcg or Eidon SELENIUM liquid; •Sublingual DMG (100mg) before exercise; NAC (n-acetyl cysteine) 600mg 2x a day.

—For acute attacks: •*Lobelia* extract under the tongue relaxes chest constriction (highly recommended, dilute for kids); or sniff an anti-spasmodic oil like *lavender, rosemary, or anise.*

—Bronchodilators: •*Ginkgo Biloba* extract 50mg 3x daily; •magnesium 400-800mg daily eases breathing. Ayurvedic: •*Coleus Forskholii;* •*Sida cordifolia;* •*Cordyceps sinensis; Note:* Bronchodilating drugs deplete B6; a high quality B-complex daily like Nature's Secret ULTIMATE B works well.

—Bronchodilators for kids: •Calcium 500mg, •Magnesium 250mg, or •Floradix MAGNESIUM liquid for bronchodilating help. •B₁₂ 2000mcg every other day, •Vitamin C 1000mg, •B-complex 50mg.

3—Minimize allergic reactions: •Futurebiotics MSM 400mg 2x daily, with •MICRO-HYDRIN PLUS. Ease stress, the most common asthma trigger for children, with *Reishi mushroom* drops in water. •Multiple reactions: *una da gato* drops.

4—Ease cough, release mucous: •Herbs Etc. LUNG TONIC; •Crystal Star D-CONGEST™ drops; •Yogi BREATHE DEEP tea; •Zand DECONGEST herbal; •*Wild cherry* syrup; •*Echinacea-goldenseal* extract. •Apply a hot *ginger* compress to the chest, then use light percussion on the back to release mucous faster.

5—Reduce inflammation: Add EFAs: •*Evening Primrose oil* 500mg (kids), 2000mg (adults). •Omega Nutrition ESSENTIAL BALANCE.

6—Normalize adrenal and immune response: •Crystal Star ADRENAL ENERGY BOOST™ caps; •*Astragalus-echinacea* extract; •Transformation PUREZYME protease.

—Superfood therapy: Choose 1 or 2 recommendations.
•AloeLife ALOE GOLD drink relieves inflammation.
•3 tbsp. of flax seed daily.
•Jarrow GENTLE FIBERS for extra vitamin C and bioflavs. Good preventive help.
•Klamath BLUE GREEN SUPREME.
•Barleans GREENS for high antioxidants.
•Prince of Peace ROYAL JELLY vials for active B-vitamins.

Can't find a recommended product? Call the 800 number listed in Product Resources for the store nearest you.

Attention Deficit Hyperactivity Disorder

Learning Disabilities, Autism, Tourette's Syndrome

Hyperactive behavior and learning disorders are serious — affecting up to 2 to 3 million children today.... at least one child in every classroom in the U.S! A Mayo Clinical study shows children now have a 7.5% chance of being diagnosed with ADHD between the ages of 5-18. Worse, statistics say that 3 to 7% of all U.S. *adults* may be afflicted with ADHD. *ADD (Attention Deficit Disorder)* is ADD accompanied by hyperactivity. ADHD exhibits extreme emotional instability, with aggressive destructive behavior including self-mutilation. Victims may be chronic liars and have difficulty listening, following directions or completing tasks. Most exhibit stress syndromes like chronic thirst, chronic colds, sneezing, and coughing. *Autism* is almost a "mind-blind" condition diagnosed in the first 30 months of a child's life. It is characterized by withdrawn behavior, lack of emotion and speech, extreme sensitivity to sound and touch. Autistic children have a brain malfunction (related to abnormal serotonin metabolism in the brain) that creates a barrier between them and the rest of the world. Children at greatest risk are male with low birth weight, and a family history of diabetes or alcoholism. *Tourette's Syndrome* is an involuntary movement and vocal disorder, often socially disabling. Tourettes is amazingly common, affecting 1 out of every 2,000 people.

Is ADHD over-diagnosed?

Researchers say it may be, because so many other lifestyle conditions are involved. For example, **Americans consume 8-10 lbs. of additives and 150 lbs. of sugar a year, both of which play a huge role in ADHD.** People with ADHD have sensitivities to food chemicals and sugars which worsen their symptoms. The Journal of Pediatric Research reveals children with ADHD are less able to compensate for the stressful effects sugar has on the brain than other children. A diet high in trans fats and saturated fats is another known brain offender. Hyperactivity may be a sign of either hypoglycemia or food allergies or both. Post-traumatic stress disorder anxiety and depression mimic Attention Deficit Disorder signs. Many experts say the multiple, wide-ranging vaccines now given to children before they enter kindergarten play a role in autism development. Autism also has allergy, parasite, yeast infection or fungal links. Heavy metal poisoning (especially lead) causes excess ammonia waste in the brain, affecting its stability.

The Ritalin craze: make an informed choice! Are we drugging a whole generation with Ritalin with no thought to long term effects?

Drug therapy with Ritalin, (*Methylphenidate*) a central nervous system stimulant used to improve concentration and reduce impulsive behavior is the conventional approach for dealing with ADHD. Ritalin's popularity is growing. DEA figures show that since 1990, the production of Ritalin type drugs has risen 741%! Prescriptions in the U.S. have doubled in the last 10 years. In some schools, 6 out of 100 children take Ritalin every day! Still, the media reports that the drug is underused! School officials and medical professionals alike push Ritalin on kids in an effort to curb school disturbances. A number of dramatic cases have judges ordering kids put back on Ritalin after their parents tried to take them off the drug. I believe Ritalin is all too often used as a "band-aid" to deal with a problem that could respond to less invasive therapies. Ritalin does not cure ADHD, and it can have serious side effects. Sleeplessness, facial tics, headache, stomachache, depression, decreased appetite, high blood pressure, seizures and heart palpitations have all been linked to Ritalin. It shouldn't be used if a child is severely depressed, has hypertension or epilepsy. More worries: Canadian research reveals that more than 9% of children who take Ritalin develop symptoms of psychosis like hallucinations or paranoia! Some information shows that Ritalin may even affect a child's growth.

Ritalin may interact with other drugs. There are 21 reported drug-drug interactions with Ritalin, including some over-the-counter cold medicines. Like other amphetamines, Ritalin may cause small vessel damage in the heart. In one disturbing report, a 14 year-old boy died of a heart attack related to long term Ritalin use. Ritalin is chemically similar to cocaine, and is often sold and snorted for a "quick high" on school campuses. In fact, "Ritty" is one of the top ten abused prescription drugs on the street today!

New ADHD Drugs on the Radar. Parents clearly want an alternative to Ritalin, but new ADHD drugs, like Adderral and Concerta are not much better, disrupting normal sleep patterns and seriously depressing appetite, bad news for a developing body! Like Ritalin, they are habit-forming and produce side effects like dizziness, anxiety, headaches, stomach aches and para-noia. One million prescriptions were written for Strattera, a non-stimulant medicine for ADHD, just between November 2002 and June 2003. But mood swings, reduced appetite, nausea and fatigue top the list of Strattera's side effects. Reports include increased anxiety and hot flashes, a major problem for women in the throes of menopause who may be using the drug.

The Bottom Line on ADHD Drugs. ADHD drugs are all too often used as "skill enhancers" to help children get good scores on tests and receive teacher approval. There are even reports of parents stealing their children's ADHD drugs for their own cognitive enhancement. I believe the drug overload of today's society is a sad testament to the enormous pres-sure our children (and adults) are on to perform and produce at any cost, even at the cost of resorting to mind altering drugs. While there are cases where drug therapy may be necessary to stabilize ADHD symptoms, most experts agree that nutritional therapy should be your primary focus for long term relief.

Can't find a recommended product? Call the 800 number listed in Product Resources for the store nearest you.

Attention Deficit Hyperactivity Disorder

Diet and Lifestyle Support Therapy

Nutritional therapy plan: Your child might not need a Ritalin prescription for ADHD relief. Food allergies and hypoglycemia play a huge role in ADD symptoms. Short term fixes like sugar, caffeine or stimulant drugs to improve focus in fact worsen the disorder.

1—Diet improvement is the key to changing ADD behavior. Simple diet changes can make a big difference. Results are almost immediately evident, generally within 1 to 3 weeks. When behavior normalizes, maintain the improved diet to prevent reversion.

2—Food sensitivities play a major part in attention disorders. Reduce sugar intake (always involved in ADHD). Use stevia instead of sugar to sweeten drinks or baked foods. Reduce carbonated drinks (Excess phosphorus). Eliminate red meats (nitrates).

3—Use muscle kinesiology (page 378) to determine allergens, or test foods like milk, wheat, corn, chocolate, citrus with an elimination diet. •UAS DDS-JUNIOR probiotics.

4—Ongoing diet: green salads, high vegetable proteins (beans, soy foods, nuts, seeds), whole grains, plenty of fresh fruits and vegetables.... no junk or fast foods. Use organically grown foods when possible. Miso soup before bed.

5—Include calming tryptophan-rich foods like turkey, tuna, wheat germ, yogurt and eggs. Add lecithin granules to whole grain cereal or yogurt for brain boosting phosphatides. Lewis Labs high phosphatide lecithin, or Red Star nutritional yeast.

6—Add EFA-rich foods: sea foods and sea greens, spinach, canteloupe, soy foods. Stay away from trans fats in fried food, baked goods and snack foods which disrupt brain function. •I like Maine Coast Sea Vegetables daily for stabilizing minerals and EFAs.

Lifestyle support:

•Homeopathic remedies have proven valuable for behavior and social problems. But diagnosis and remedy are very individual. See a qualified homeopath for best results.

•Avoid aspirin and amphetamines if your child has ADHD.

•Use full-spectrum lighting when possible for better mood.

•Read food labels carefully. 70% of kids with ADD react to chemical additives. **ADD-ADHD triggers:** artificial flavors and colors, artificial sweeteners, preservatives like BHA (*butylated hydroxyanisole*) and BHT (*butylated hydroxytoluene*). Yellow food dye tartrazine is clearly implicated in hyperactivity. Other culprits: sulfiting agents, casein, citric acid, chocolate, high fructose corn syrup, hydrogenated oils, MSG (*monosodium glutamate*), sodium nitrates, caffeine, smoke flavoring and yeast. Consider an elimination diet (see pg. 316 to help you find out exactly which foods are a problem for you).

The A.D.D. Nutrition Solution, by Marcia Zimmerman C.N., is an excellent resource for information on nutritional approaches.

—**Bodywork:** •Massage therapy, acupressure and hypnosis have shown some success. Biofeedback treatments reduce ADD symptoms for 85% of sufferers. •Consider Cranio-Sacral therapy if there was birth trauma. •Warm baking soda-sea salt baths.

Herbal, Superfood and Supplement Therapy

Interceptive therapy: Choose 2 to 3 recommendations.

1—**Improve behavior problems:** •DMAE, 100 to 500mg daily in divided doses; •Crystal Star RELAX CAPS™ (fast acting), and ADD-VANTAGE FOR KIDS™ caps •Herbs Etc. KIDALIN, •Metabolic Response Modifiers ATTENTION! gels with DMAE and phos. serine, or •Planetary Formulas CALM CHILD. •Homeopathic *Camomilla* -young kids.

2—**Focus attention:** •NADH 2.5mg daily. •*Rosemary* tea or aromatherapy oil rubber on temples; •*Gotu Kola* or *Siberian eleuthero* extract 20 drops in water. •Diamond DIAMOND MIND for adult ADD (good results). Some prescription drugs block EFA conversion in the brain. EFA's are over 60% of the brain, critical to its balance. EFA's like DHA (*docosahexaenoic acid*) improve focus (good results).

3—**Calming herbs:** •Crystal Star CALCIUM SOURCE™ drops in water, a rapid calmative. •Crystal Star *valerian-wild lettuce* extract, *lemon balm* or *catnip* tea; •Hylands CALMS or CALMS FORTE; •Crystal Star STRESS ARREST™ tea (rapid); •*St. John's wort* (not if child is on prescription drugs); •Nature's Way RESTLESS CHILD; •Taurine 500mg.

4—**Enhance neurotransmitters - brain serotonin:** •Stress B Complex with extra pantothenic acid 100mg and B₆ 100mg; •PSP Marketing VITAL PSP PLUS (excellent results); nervines like *gotu kola* and *scullcap* calm hyperactivity safely. •*Ginkgo biloba* drops - older kids (60mg 3x daily also helps inner ear balance). Maitake Products REISHI caps (adults); Practitioners use •GABA 100mg and •Phos. Serine with good results, 100mg daily (300mg daily for children over 50 lbs). Results take up to 4 months.

5—**Add electrolyte minerals:** •Nature's Path TRACE-LYTE minerals or Alacer ELEC-TROMIX; •Add magnesium 400mg and •Premier Lithium .5mg. Check the child's iron-deficiency may result in learning disability. •Klamath CALM KID with blue green algae.

6—**For allergic reactions:** •Chromium 150mcg 3x daily with •Vanadium 150mg.

7—**Balance prostaglandins:** •New Chapter SUPER-CRITICAL DHA 100; •Source Naturals FOCUS DHA 100mg. Udo's PERFECT OIL BLEND, 1 tsp. daily; also •*Black currant oil* •*Evening Primrose oil*, 500mg for kids; •Omega-3 flax oil.

—**Natural Autism therapy:** Magnesium 400mg; B-complex with extra B₆ 100mg (UAS DDS-JUNIOR for synthesis of B vitamins); •Black walnut, an anti-fungal. Ask a qualified practitioner for dose. •Vitamin C with bioflavonoids, 2000mg daily -best in powder; ¼ tsp. every 2 hours in juice; •Eidon ZINC liquid if high copper levels, common in autism. •A gluten and casein free diet can produce improvements in social behavior, cognitive skills and communication for some autistics.

Can't find a recommended product? Call the 800 number listed in Product Resources for the store nearest you.

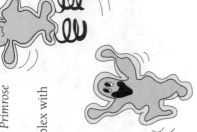

Back Pain

Lumbago, Herniated Disc, Scoliosis, Sciatica

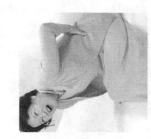

Friend and fellow author Dr. Art Brownstein (*Healing Back Pain Naturally*) says "back pain...can drive a person to thoughts of suicide." The spine is the seat of human nerve structure, so it manifests much of your body's stress. 80% of Americans suffer back pain sometime in their lives - almost 40% wind up with crippling back pain. Back pain is the leading cause of disability for Americans 18-45 years old! *Lumbago* is any pain in the lower back. *Sciatica* pain radiates along the sciatic nerve, buttocks and back of the leg. A *herniated disc* occurs when the outer disc covering ruptures and the soft filling bulges into the spot. Major back surgery, like removing discs, may do more harm than good. Surgery works for only 1% of patients, and should be considered as a last resort. Diet improvement, supplements, a chiropractor or massage therapist who treats more than just the physical problem is often the best path to relief. • *Note:* Experts say poor posture is the #1 cause of back pain. Slouching and slumping heavily stress your back and neck muscles. **What else causes back pain?** High heels, artery blockage, emotional stress, poor posture, improper lifting, even financial woes. Risk is increased if you're overweight, if you don't eat leafy greens, if you're dehydrated, if you have arthritis or osteoporosis, if your protein and calcium are low, or if you sleep on a too-soft mattress.

Diet and Lifestyle Support Therapy

Nutritional therapy plan:

1—Your diet should be high in minerals and vegetable proteins. Vegetarians have stronger bone density. Add high protein foods from the sea - seafoods, fish, sea greens.

2—Drink at least 6 glasses of water daily. Much back and rheumatoid pain is due to chronic dehydration. You need to keep acid particles flushed to keep kidneys functioning well. Uric acid aggravates back pain.

3—Avoid sugar, red meats, dairy foods (except for yogurt and kefir) and caffeine. Add alkalizing foods: fresh or steamed veggies and veggie juices, green drinks, sprouted whole grains, miso soups, brown rice, sea veggies, lemons and limes, ume plums.

4—Reduce the fat in your diet. The greater the deposits of fatty plaque, the greater the degeneration of spinal discs.

Which pain relievers for back pain? The Amer. Pharmaceutical Assoc. says, "..... studies over the last few years show that low dose (60-300mg per day) aspirin and over the counter NSAIDs (non-steroidal anti-inflammatory drugs) like ibuprofen are associated with a significant risk of GI bleeding and upper GI hemorrhage. NSAIDs users are at approximately three times greater risk of developing serious GI events which include gastric ulceration, bleeding and DEATH than nonusers." Incredibly, new statistics show NSAIDs send 76,000 people to the hospital and kill 7,600 people annually in the U.S.! Heat wraps are up to 50% MORE effective than over-the-counter pills at relieving back pain. Herbal heating pads may be the best choice for your back.

—**Effective herbal compresses and topicals:** •Apply ice packs if pain lasts over 48 hours.
•Home Health CASTOR OIL PACKS.
•Biochemics PAIN RELIEF lotion.
•DMSO with ALOE GEL.
•New Chapter *Arnica-Ginger* gel, or •B &T TRIFLORA GEL.
•Tiger Balm PAIN RELIEF PATCHES, or WHITE FLOWER oil.

Herbal, Superfood and Supplement Therapy

Interceptive therapy: Choose 2 to 3 recommendations.

1—**Relieve pain:** •Crystal Star STRESS OUT™ muscle relaxer drops under the tongue (highly recommended, can help within 20 minutes). •Apply *cayenne-ginger* heat packs -work wonders (page 76). •Crystal Star MUSCLE RELAXER™ caps 4 at a time, for back spasm control. •Natural Balance SUPER FLEX BACK FORMULA with natural COX-2 inhibitors; •DLPA 1000mg; •MSM 1000mg.

2—**Build strong cartilage:** •Lane Labs ADVACAL; •Crystal Star CALCIUM-MAGNE-SIUM SOURCE™ caps; Jarrow BIOSIL (orthosilicic acid); •Country Life LIGATEND 6 daily. •Bovine tracheal cartilage 1000mg daily; •Rainforest Remedies BACK SUPPORT.

3—**Reduce inflammation:** •Quercetin 1000mg with Bromelain 1500mg daily; or Transformation REPAIRZYME caps •Glucosamine-chondroitin, 1500/1200mg daily with vitamin C 5000mg and boron 3mg daily for better uptake. •Crystal Star ANTI-FLAM™ caps for longer term pain control with DR. ENZYME™ with protease and bromelain; •Homeopathic *Horse Chestnut* - results in about 3 to 6 days.

—**Sciatica:** Extra potassium, 500mg daily, and CoQ-10, 200mg daily. •Crystal Star RELAX™ caps ease nerve pain.

—**Scoliosis: arthritis-like back pain:** •Glucosamine-chondroitin; •Vitamin B$_{12}$ 5000mcg. •*Evening primrose oil* 3300mg; •Calcium 1500mg-magnesium 750mg; •*devil's claw* compound; *lavender-chamomile* aromatherapy oils help control spasms.

—**Superfood therapy:** Choose 1 or 2 recommendations.
•AloeLife ALOE GOLD, an anti-inflammatory.
•Nutricology PRO-GREENS WITH EFAs.
•Crystal Star ENERGY GREEN RENEWAL™ or RESTORE YOUR STRENGTH™ drinks, for absorbable potassium, and chlorophyll strength.
•Fit for You MIRACLE GREENS with barley grass.
•Unipro PERFECT PROTEIN or Solgar WHEY TO GO.
•A potassium drink (pg. 291) as a kidney cleanse.

Can't find a recommended product? Call the 800 number listed in Product Resources for the store nearest you.

Bad Breath and Body Odor

Halitosis, Bromidrosis

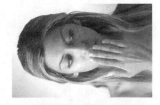

Bad breath and body odor are the most common problems people have, over 50% of Americans complain about bad taste in the mouth and foul smelling perspiration. Both are really manifestations of the same problems - poor diet or poor food digestion causing rotting food and bacteria formation that the body throws off through the skin and breath. Four hundred types of bacteria can survive in the mouth alone - over 80 cause smelly sulphur-rich gasses. **Are bad breath and body odor more serious than just poor digestion or poor hygiene?** Sometimes they are... a raging candida yeast infection, post-nasal drip from a chronic sinus infection, smoking (usually along with heavy caffeine intake), and gum disease are regularly involved. Up to 35% of Americans have full-blown gum disease; another 40 million Americans have chronic sinus infections. Nevertheless a high enzyme, fresh foods, green vegetable diet can't be stressed enough in controlling these problems. In addition, popular weight loss diets that propound an extraordinarily high protein, low carb regimen, often lead to inadequate protein digestion, dry mouth, dehydration and sluggish digestion. Stress, anxiety, food intolerances, low HCl and liver malfunction may be implicated. *A TCM analysis can help determine the cause of bad breath or body odor. Call the American Association of Oriental Medicine at 888-500-7999.*

Diet and Lifestyle Support Therapy

Nutritional therapy plan:

1—Keep your internal environment clean. Try •Crystal Star DR. VITALITY™ tea (with lightly detoxing green and white tea), to keep your body feeling fresh.

2—Diet improvement is the single most beneficial thing you can do to get rid of bad breath and body odor. Start with a 24 hour liquid diet (pg.173) with apple juice and 1 tbsp. psyllium husks, or Planetary TRICLEANSE to cleanse the bowel.

3—Deodorize your digestive tract. For 7 days, add 1 tsp. liquid chlorophyll to apple juice to cleanse digestive tract. Try Alfalfa-Mint tea, or green tea after meals (more effective than mint, parsley or chewing gum against bad breath). Eat smaller meals, and chew well for best enzyme activity.

4—Make sure your diet has crunchy, cleansing, fiber-rich foods like fresh fruits and veggies. Eat high chlorophyll foods: parsley, greens, sprouts.

5—Eat cultured foods like yogurt or kefir for intestinal flora.

6—Drink 6 glasses of water daily to flush your GI tract. When your body is dehydrated, mouth secretions become concentrated and odorous.

7—Eat light, less concentrated foods - esp. heavy animal protein (avoid red meats), and heavy sweets, caffeine, dairy foods, fried foods - especially onions, curry, garlic.

—Expressly for body odor: •Think zinc. Take 15-50mg daily, or Ethical Nutrients ZINC STATUS; •Dilute essential oils of *lavender, thyme, juniper, rosemary or myrrh* - put a few drops on a cotton pad; apply to your underarms.

Natural body deodorants:
•Dab underarms and feet with vinegar or aloe vera gel.
•Avalon LAVENDER deodorant with rosemary (good results).
•Natural mineral crystal deodorants.

•When you shower: Use a dry skin body brush or loofah to remove toxins coming out on the skin. Then use an oatmeal/honey scrub soap; or take a mineral bath like Para Labs BATH THERAPY.

Herbal, Superfood and Supplement Therapy

Interceptive therapy: Choose 2 to 3 recommendations.
Do you have bad breath? Lick the back of your hand. Let dry a few seconds, then sniff. A metallic, sour or fishy odor should alert you.

Expressly for morning breath: Floss well before bedtime. Brush the back of tongue and teeth with baking soda rather than toothpaste. Use a tongue cleaner. Don't use mouthwash. Morning breath should be eliminated.

Breath fresheners: Try •Nature's Answer PERIOWASH; •Melaleuca, Inc. BREATH AWAY; •BioForce DENTA-FORCE breath spray.

1—**Bitters herbs stimulate better digestion:** (Take extracts, bitters don't work unless you can taste them.) •Crystal Star BITTERS & LEMON CLEANSE™ drops each morning;
•Gaia GOLDENROD flower extract.

2—**Spices are natural antacids, break up gas:** Put pinches in water of *cloves, ginger, cinnamon, nutmeg* or *anise-* drink down. Chew on *anise* or *fennel seeds*; they contain cineole, an antiseptic that destroys bacteria.

3—**Intestinal cleansers:** •Crystal Star GREEN TEA CLEANSER™ each morning; •American Health HERBAL-TONE gentle laxative tabs at night; •Nature's Secret SUPER CLEANSE; or •AloeLife FIBER-MATE.

4—**Control mouth, gum infections:** •Nature's Answer PERIOWASH w. oregano oil; •Home Health PERI-DENT gum massage. •Nature's Gate Green Tea with Ester C Toothpaste; •propolis lozenges; •*myrrh* extract, *tea tree* or *eucalyptus* oil rubbed on gums.

5—**Probiotics and enzymes:** •Acidophilus caps 4-6x daily. Try •American Health ACIDOPHILUS liquid. •1 tbsp. cider vinegar in water before each meal; •Betaine HCl with papain before each meal (especially before meat protein); •Schiff ENZYMALL tabs with ox bile or •Crystal Star DR. ENZYME™ with Protease and Bromelain between meals.

—Superfood therapy: Choose 1... •Crystal Star ENERGY GREEN RENEWAL™ drink or caps. •Fit for You MIRACLE GREENS. •Pure Planet CHLORELLA.

Can't find a recommended product? Call the 800 number listed in Product Resources for the store nearest you.

Bedwetting
Child and Adult Enuresis

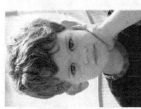

Bedwetting, involuntary urination during the night beyond the normal age of 3 to 7 years old, affects about 5 million, or 10% of children, mostly male. Some boys continue to have a bedwetting problem into their teens. Amazingly, bedwetting also affects over 150,000 adults, a rising number. **Most experts acknowledge that the problem stems from three bases:**

•**Physical** - very deep sleep patterns with decreased REM sleep, a bladder infection, a blood sugar imbalance like hypoglycemia or diabetes, and most commonly, food allergies, especially to excess sugar, salt, spices or dairy foods.

•**Psychological** - emotional anxiety and behavioral disturbances; bad dreams or dreams about using the restroom. New theories point to deeply hidden stress reactions from sexual abuse, both in adults and children.

•**Mechanical** - including an immature or poorly formed bladder, inherited organ weakness, a compressed nerve or congenital obstruction in the bladder region.

In addition, since nutritional therapies have such notable success in helping bedwetting, I believe that nutritional deficiencies are also a part of the problem.

Diet and Lifestyle Support Therapy

Nutritional therapy plan:

1—Avoid oxalic acid-forming foods, such as cooked spinach, sodas, rhubarb, caffeine, cocoa, chocolate, etc.

2—Getting rid of junk foods is a key. Irritants like high sugar foods, salty or extra spicy foods always seem to be involved.

3—Avoid food colorings, additives, preservatives and cow's milk as possible allergens.

4—Take a small glass of cranberry/apple juice each morning to clean the kidneys.

5—No liquids before bed. Eat a little celery instead to balance organic salts.

6—A spoonful of honey before bed.

Lifestyle measures:

•See a chiropractor or massage therapist if a compressed nerve or obstruction is the suspected cause. (Excellent success for adult sufferers.)

•Muscle testing (applied kinesiology) is effective here in determining what allergies may be the cause. See pg. 378.

•Guided imagery techniques have some success. Within the first few hours of sleep, give the child reassuring messages without waking him.

•Good circulation is a key. Good daily exercise is an answer; especially bicycle riding.

—Lifestyle TLC:

•Leave a night light on so child feels free to get up at night.

•Give a relaxing massage before bed to ease muscles and fears. Try *lavender* essential oil mixed in almond oil.

•Decrease your child's stress about bedwetting by giving encouragement rather than punishment. Praise him for not wetting the bed. Sometimes a reward system helps.

•Make sure home emotional environment is supportive. Divorce proceedings, and recently, abuse activity are notably involved in bed wetting.

•Make bedtime regular and stress-free. Consider a happy bedtime story and a lullaby.

Herbal, Superfood and Supplement Therapy

Interceptive therapy: Choose 2 to 3 recommendations.

1—Preventives: •Crystal Star BLADDER-KIDNEY CONTROL™ caps before dinner, half strength for kids; or •BLADDER-KIDNEY COMFORT™ tea (daytime) or •*Thyme* tea midafternoon. •Give the child *cinnamon* sticks to chew on before bed, or make *cinnamon* tea from *cinnamon* extract drops in water. •*Cornsilk* or *plantain* extract drops in water. •*Ginkgo biloba* extract drops in water, mixed with a little honey before bed for better circulation. •For an elderly wetting problem, try *century* tea.

2—Relax stress before bed: •Crystal Star RELAX CAPS™ or •*valerian/wild lettuce* extract in water; *scullcap* extract drops in water; *lemon balm* tea.

3—Minerals strengthen tissues: •Crystal Star CALCIUM SOURCE™ extract drops in water; •*Parsley-oatstraw-juniper-uva ursi* tea daily (not at bedtime). •Twin Lab Chondroitan sulfate A 250mg daily; •Mezotrace SEA MINERAL COMPLEX chewable (good results); •Flora FLORADIX children's multivitamin; •Magnesium 100mg daily; •*Horsetail* herb extract in water; rub on abdomen; •Body Essentials SILICA GEL.

—Highly effective homeopathics:

•Hyland's BEDWETTING tabs before bed. •BSI Equisetum for bedwetting during dreams or nightmares. •Standard Homeopathics Enuraid (adults).

—Superfood therapy: Choose 1 recommendation.

•Twin Lab LIQUID K PLUS to strengthen tissues.
•Futurebiotics VITAL K.
•AloeLife FIBER-MATE drink, ½ tsp.
•Country Life CAL SNACK, milk-free chewable calcium (kids like it).
•Green Foods CARROT ESSENCE blend drink or BERRY BARLEY ESSENCE.

Can't find a recommended product? Call the 800 number listed in Product Resources for the store nearest you.

Bladder, Urinary Tract Infections

Bacterial Cystitis, Incontinence

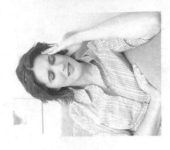

Bladder infections are very common in women; less common in men (largely tied to prostate problems). A UTI is the most frequent reason a woman seeks medical attention; any woman who's had one knows the pain can be all-consuming during the acute stage. One in 5 American women will have at least one urinary tract infection in her life; of those 20% will have another, 30% will have a third. An astounding 80% of women who have had 3 bladder infections will have a 4th. Simultaneous staph and strep infections, or diabetes may affect the kidneys, making the problem more serious - an alarming number result in kidney failure. Some women go on to develop a condition called "chronic UTI" where they relapse into a full blown bladder infection every few weeks. Treat a UTI at the first sign of infection. Untreated, recurrent bladder infections can ultimately result in serious kidney problems. Some STD's mimic UTI symptoms. Natural therapies help clear the infection and strengthen the urinary system. Get checked and consult a holistic clinic if there is no improvement within 5 days. Beware long courses of antibiotics for a UTI. This can really backfire and may leads to infections like bacterial vaginosis and chronic yeast infections. Vaginal pH can become so imbalanced from antibiotics that another UTI is almost inevitable! UTI medications can have some awful side effects, too: Nausea, vomiting, diarrhea, even visual changes or eye pain may occur.

What puts you at risk for a bladder infection? What triggers them?

Bladder infections develop when bacteria like E. coli (often from contaminated meat or water), or chlamydia ascend the urethra and enter the bladder where they reproduce and infect. Long courses antibiotics for a staph, strep, bronchitis, or a cold may fuel resistant organisms because normal immune response becomes depressed. Sexual intercourse is a trigger for some women because it can cause E. coli bacteria to migrate up the urethra. ("Honeymoon" cystitis is related to frequent sexual activity or rough sex.) Experts believe that the active chemical in spermicidal creams and foams, nonoxynol-9, causes recurring cystitis and yeast infections. Kidney malfunction or kidney stones (usually from lack of adequate fluids), diabetes, food allergies (especially to high fructose corn syrup), and excessive caffeine can be factors. Tampons or diaphragms pinching the neck of the bladder, hampering waste elimination may be involved.

Do you have the symptoms of a bladder infection?

—Do you have urgent, burning, painful, overly frequent urination, especially at night?

—Is your urine smell is strong, foul-smelling, cloudy or bloody; is there a urethral discharge?

—Is urination pain attended by lower back and abdominal pain? Is the pain is accompanied by chills and fever as the body tries to throw off infection?

(If you have pain above the waist, it may be a kidney infection or kidney stones instead of a bladder infection.)

Home Bladder Infection Tests:

90% of bladder infections are caused by overgrowth of E.coli bacteria which ascends the urine tube (urethra) and enters the bladder to reproduce and infect. The infection increases the concentration of nitrites in urine. A home test available at pharmacies can detect the nitrites with dip strips that change color when urine comes in contact with the impregnated chemicals. If you are at frequent risk for bladder infections, check yourself weekly so you can nip the infection at the beginning with natural remedies.

Note: Some women develop symptoms of a bladder infection, but don't show the expected amounts of bacteria or nitrites in their urine. If your test results conflict with symptoms of infection, know that a diagnosis by an alternative practitioner gives more weight to your symptoms than to the test. You should too. If you experience symptoms of bladder infection, but your home test turns out negative or marginally positive, call your practitioner. Treatment is usually recommended regardless of test results, because of the risk of kidney infection.

Are you suffering from urinary incontinence?

People may not want to talk about it, but the numbers don't lie. *Nineteen million Americans suffer from bladder control problems.* Eighty percent are women! In the U.S. we spend nearly $30 billion on adult diapers and medical treatments for incontinence every year! Stress incontinence and urge incontinence are the most common types of bladder control problems.

Do you fit these incontinence profiles? 1) —Do you regularly experience the sudden, but uncontrollable urge to urinate? (urge incontinence). 2) —Do you experience urine leakage when you exercise, laugh, cough or sneeze? (stress incontinence). 3) —Do you experience dribbling after urination? (a sign of weakened or damaged *pubococcygeus* (PCG) muscles). Natural therapies help rebuild and strengthen the urinary system for long lasting results, not just symptom relief. *See the following page for specific recommendations.*

Can't find a recommended product? Call the 800 number listed in Product Resources for the store nearest you.

Bladder, Urinary Tract Infections

Diet and Lifestyle Support Therapy

Nutritional therapy plan:

1—Change body pH: Eat a yeast-free diet - no baked breads during healing. Cut out coffee! A new study shows women who drink more than 4 cups a day more than double their urinary incontinence risk. Drink *Schizandra* tea or *Fennel seed* tea daily instead.

2—Flush the bladder: Water is a key to any bladder/kidney cleanse. The biggest problem for most UTIs is bacteria getting out. I use concentrated, organic cranberry juice with no added sweeteners in bottled water (cranberries have substantial D-Mannose against *E. coli* infection), 6 to 8 glasses daily.

3—Purify bladder and urethra: watermelon seed tea (very good results) or carrot/beet/cucumber juice reduces infection. Watermelon juice or chlorophyll-rich superfood drinks are another option. For some, drinking 2 Alka-Seltzer tabs in water begins eliminating UTI infection almost immediately.

4—Increase urine flow: Drink 10 glasses of water, diluted, unsweetened fruit juices and herbal teas daily to flush out bacteria. A tip: Add 1 tsp. VITAMIN C crystals to your drinks to acidify urine. Vitamin C chewables every 4 hours also works well. Increasing urine acidity reduces bacterial overgrowth since bacteria thrive in alkaline environments.

5—Acute stage: take 2 tbsp. cider vinegar and honey in water at morning, yogurt at noon, a glass of white wine at night.

6—Avoid acid-forming foods: caffeine, tomatoes, cooked spinach, chocolate. Avoid sugary foods, sodas; fried, salty and fatty foods; and dairy foods. Reduce meat protein.

7—Add alkalizing foods: celery, watermelon, ume plum, blueberries, green drinks and potassium drinks (pg. 291), garlic and onions. Use antibacterial spices like *oregano, thyme, rosemary, lemon balm* and *sage*. Add sea greens to your diet. They are valuable tissue toners and an easily available plant source of vitamin B-12.

—Lifestyle tips for incontinence:

• Biofeedback and acupuncture are successful for incontinence, regardless of cause. Medicare coverage for biofeedback for incontinence is now mandated by the Health Care Financing Administration (HCFA). For a biofeedback practitioner visit go to the website *www.aapb.org.* Association for Applied Psychophysiology and Biofeedback.

• Kegel exercises help incontinence. Losing excess weight offers significant help.

Bodywork:

• Acupuncture sometimes relieves pain almost immediately.

• Apply wet heat, or hot *comfrey* compresses on lower back and kidneys.

• Massage abdomen with a blend of 1-oz. *almond oil*, 3 drops *sandalwood oil*, 2 drops each *cedarwood oil, cypress oil* and *lavender*, 1 drop *frankincense oil*.

• Use a mild *catnip* or liquid *chlorophyll* enema to clear wastes.

• Wipe from front to back, and wash rectum with gentle soap and water after bowel movements.

• Avoid scented bubble baths and soaps. Consider tea tree oil soap.

Herbal, Superfood and Supplement Therapy

Interceptive therapy: Choose 2 to 3 recommendations.

1—Control infection, bacterial adhesion: •Crystal Star BLADDER-KIDNEY COMFORT™ caps, 2 every 3 hours at the first hint of infection (highly recommended), and/or •BLADDER-KIDNEY COMFORT™ cranberry compound tea (with 2 •ANTI-BIO™ caps each cup if problem is severe). Add •Crystal Star DR ENZYME™ with protease and bromelain to reduce inflammation. •D-Mannose by Biotech Pharmacal, Ark. is a miracle remedy for chronic UTIs. It prevents *E. coli* from adhering to urinary walls (1 tsp. in water every 3 hours, and works almost immediately with excellent reports; or take •cranberry caps every 3 hours. Cranberry and Cat's claw are powerful anti-microbials and anti-inflammatories. •Nutribiotic GRAPEFRUIT SEED EXTRACT caps 2 daily, and a glass of water with 1 tsp. baking soda. •Homeopathic *cantharis* can sometimes stop a UTI immediately.

—For intercourse-related UTIs: Rinse vagina with •*goldenseal-echinacea* tea. •Homeopathic *Staphysagria-* is a specific for intercourse-related UTIs. •D-Mannose, 1 tsp. daily as a preventative. Do not use a diaphragm if you are prone to bladder infections. Urinate before intercourse and after intercourse.

2—Curb pain and inflammation: •*Goldenseal-echinacea* extract and *kava* extract drops in water. For chronic infections take •Futurebiotics VITAL K and *uva ursi* caps for 14 days to disinfect. On the tenth day, begin Solaray CRAN-ACTIN caps, then •*cat's claw* extract for 10 days. Take •Ayurvedic *Crataeva nurvala*, if there are also bladder stones.

—Reduce painful spasms: Use an herbal muscle relaxer like Crystal Star MUSCLE RELAXER™ to stop those bladder spasms. •Hot sitz baths 2x daily for ½ hour relieve pain and ease urination. Add 3 drops *tea tree oil*, 2 drops each *bergamot oil, juniper oil,* and *thyme oil,* drop *eucalyptus oil.* •If there's also hemorrhaging, take 1 oz. *marshmallow rt.,* steep in 1 pt. hot milk. Take every ½ hr. to staunch bleeding.

3—Re-establish vaginal flora to reduce recurrence: High potency probiotic supplements with extra FOS (*fructo-oligosaccharides*) crowd out harmful bacteria and normalize the urinary system. Take •UAS DDS-PLUS or Jarrow JARRO-DOPHILUS, 6 daily with garlic caps 6 daily; •add vitamin C 1000mg and Lysine 1000mg every 2 to 3 hours.

• Use a lactobacillus suppository, or 1 tbsp. acidophilus powder in warm water as a douche for 4 days after treating a UTI with antibiotics.

4—Incontinence, men and women: add vitamin C 3000mg daily. •Crystal Star BLADDER-KIDNEY CONTROL™ caps. •Crystal Star PROSTATE PROTECTOR™ caps. For BPH results within 48 hours. • B12 deficiency is linked to incontinence in the elderly. Use a high potency sublingual B-12, up to 2500-10,000mcg.

—Superfood therapy: Choose 1 recommendation.

• Green Foods GREEN MAGMA.

• Genesis Today 4 KIDNEY, BLADDER & URINARY HEALTH juice.

• Herbalist & Alchemist BLUEBERRY extract, rich in antioxidant tannins

Can't find a recommended product? Call the 800 number listed in Product Resources for the store nearest you.

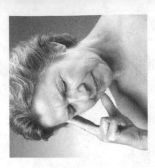

Bladder, Urinary Tract Infections

Interstitial Cystitis, Chronic Urethritis

Chronic UTI's may not be due to infection, but to an auto-immune reaction. Interstitial cystitis (IC), a non-bacterial form affecting 700,000 Americans (90% of them women over 40 with a history of bladder infections), has been called "migraine of the bladder," because many of the same things that either trigger or benefit migraine headaches affect interstitial cystitis the same way. In IC, the space between the bladder lining and the bladder muscle is chronically, painfully inflamed. Leaks in the bladder wall allow urine to irritate bladder tissue, even to destroy the bladder lining. The bladder becomes tough and atrophied, in severe cases shrinking to a size where it will only hold 1 or 2 ounces. Normal urination becomes impossible; urine is cloudy, with a foul odor. Endometriosis frequently accompanies IC, magnifying already great pain in the lower abdomen and perineum. Attend to healing immediately. A natural approach may be best because IC does not respond to antibiotics and may be aggravated by drug treatment. Some antibiotics actually attack the bladder lining when there is no infection to attack. The active chemical in spermicidal creams and foams, nonoxynol-9, increases risk of all types of cystitis. Experts theorize that environmental and food allergies are IC triggers. Pelvic congestion from heavy menstrual periods, constipation, or dehydration are also involved.

Diet and Lifestyle Support Therapy

Nutritional therapy plan:

1—Cranberry juice doesn't help interstitial cystitis. Add cilantro to veggie drinks and carrot juice instead in acute stages and for prevention.

2—Drink extra water all day as soon as you feel a UTI coming. For some, adding 2 Alka-Seltzer tabs to the water begins eliminating pain almost immediately.

3—Cleanse bladder and kidneys with watermelon juice or watermelon seed tea. Strengthen them with well-cooked beans (esp. adzuki) and sea greens. Increase leafy greens and high fiber foods.

4—Avoid IC triggers: Aged protein foods like yogurt, pickled herring, vinegar, preserved or smoked meats, cheeses, yeasted breads, sauerkraut, citrus fruits or juices and red wine until condition normalizes.

Avoid acid-forming foods - like coffee, alcohol, black tea, colas, chocolate, citrus fruits, tomatoes, spicy foods, soy sauce, and foods with additives like NutraSweet.

Quick tip: AkPharma Prelief® helps to reduce the symptoms of IC by reducing the acids in foods (very good results for this difficult type of infection).

Lifestyle bodywork:

•Do not wear tampons. Wash anal area with mild soap and water after bowel movements. •Chiropractic treatments help correct nerve compression problems linked to chronic bladder infections. •Acupuncture works well for pain and symptom relief.

•Hot sitz baths bring cleansing circulation to area. See sitz baths page 188. Press hard with alternating hot and cold compresses on pubic bone and clitoris.

—**Pain relieving:** drink as teas, use as hot abdominal compresses. •*Cornsilk-Horsetail* tea or a •Six day tea blend: 1 handful each- *uva ursi or buchu leaves, echinacea root, cut, nettle or dandelion leaves.*

—**For chronic urethritis:** •*Cat's claw* tea 3 cups daily, 2 weeks (results within 3 days). •*Ginkgo Biloba* extract (more effective than tetracycline). —**For urinary stones:** Eat cilantro and take *Tribulus/Cilantro* caps; or try a *Gravel root* combination tea.

Herbal, Superfood and Supplement Therapy

Interceptive therapy: Choose 2 to 3 recommendations.

1—**Control pain/swelling:** •Crystal Star BLADDER-KIDNEY COMFORT™ caps every 3 hours at first twinges of pain, and/or •BLADDER-KIDNEY COMFORT™ tea with 2 •ANTI-BIO™ caps each cup. •Add Crystal Star DR. ENZYME™ with protease & bromelain for inflammation or •*cat's claw* tea 3 cups daily, with •6 *goldenseal-echinacea* caps, or •Crystal Star ANTI-BIO™ caps, 6 a day during acute periods. *Note:* if multiple sensitivities are involved, try a simple uva ursi tea.

—**For chronic infections:** •Solaray CORNSILK BLEND caps daily for 10 days, then •*cat's claw* extract for 10 days. •Crystal Star MUSCLE RELAXER™ caps for spasmodic cramping, 4 at a time or •STRESS OUT™ muscle relaxer drops under the tongue (for almost immediate temporary relief), or •*scullcap* drops every 2 hours for pain.

—**Reduce interstitial scarring:** •Transformation PUREZYME protease restores immunity, reduces scarring. •Solaray *Centella Asiatica* extract caps help heal ulcers.

2—**Control inflammation:** •At first signs of infection, take 1 tsp. baking soda in 8-oz. water to alkalize urine before it reaches the bladder (excellent). •Then, take a calcium carbonate capsule or •Enzymatic Therapy ACID-A-CAL cap every 12 hours until pain is reduced; then •Nutribiotic GRAPEFRUIT SEED extract drops in water for 1 month.

3—**Combat auto-immune reaction:** D-Mannose may be helpful in some cases. Experts say that women with IC may have an abnormal autoimmune response to even normal levels of bacteria, so flushing regularly with D-mannose can offer relief from painful bladder spasms and abdominal pressure. Add •six days of *Echinacea-Goldenseal-Astragalus* extract; •Vitamin C therapy: ascorbate or Ester C powder, ¼ tsp. every 2 hours during acute stages, then •Lysine 1000mg with bromelain 1500mg daily.

—**Superfood therapy:** Choose 1 or 2 recommendations.
•Esteem GREEN HARVEST with eight strains of probiotics.
•Crystal Star ENERGY GREEN RENEWAL™ - critical minerals.
•Herbal Aloe ALOE FORCE juice, ot •Solaray ALFAJUICE, very potent..

Can't find a recommended product? Call the 800 number listed in Product Resources for the store nearest you.

Bone Health

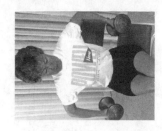

Healing Bone Breaks, Preventing Brittle Bones, Regrowing Strong Cartilage

Your bones are alive! Bone is far more complex than we ever thought.... bone needs far more nutrition than we ever think about giving it. We don't think much about our bones until we age, but nearly 87% of teenage girls and 64% of teenage boys aren't getting enough calcium, let alone other bone-building nutrients. If we extend those low nutrient numbers through life, over 50% of America's future women and one in eight men will develop osteoporosis fractures. Most research shows mineral deficiency or poor assimilation from low enzymes, and a poor diet high in refined foods, meat protein and soda, causing phosphorus imbalance are at the root of bone problems. French research shows a significant correlation with increased hip fracture in drinking water. Most of America's tap water (64%) is already fluoridated, with pending legislation for the rest of the country. *You mineral bone mass may have decreased if you have one or more of the following signs:* 1) prematurely gray hair (before 40) along with thinning skin; 2) easy bone breaks and poor bone healing; 3) shifting teeth, gum disease, lots of plaque on the teeth; 4) brittle nails that break too easily; 5) joint and tendon soreness along with unusual muscle weakness (especially chronic lower back pain); 6) you take frequent courses of steroid drugs. Smoking inhibits bone growth and increases bone brittleness.

Diet and Lifestyle Support Therapy

Nutritional therapy plan:

1—There is much more to strong bones than just calcium. Without the proper balance of other minerals as well as vitamin D, you won't absorb the calcium. Vegetarians have denser, better formed bones, stronger immunity.

—Soda warning: USDA research finds that men who drink 5 cans of cola a day for 3 months absorb less calcium, increasing risk for bone deterioration!

2—Feed your bones. Focus on mineral-rich vegetable proteins: sesame seeds, almonds, Red Star or Lewis Labs NUTRITIONAL YEAST extract drink, MISO broth, sea greens (vitamin K, too). •Daily sunlight on the body for vitamin D

3—Key nutrients: *Calcium and silica*: green and sea veggies, fish, seafood, whole grains, soy protein, yogurt. *Boron*: dried fruits, nuts, seeds, honey, wine. *Vitamin C*: papayas, kiwi, strawberries, bell peppers, broccoli, cantaloupe. *Manganese* (helps make collagen): pineapple, sea veggies.

4—Bone leaching foods: red meats, fried and fast foods and sodas. Sugar and caffeine inhibit calcium absorption. Excess salt decreases bone density.

Lifestyle support: •Some medicines put bone health at risk: L-thyroxine, a thyroid stimulant; steroid drugs like hydrocortisone, cortisone and prednisone (prescribed for rheumatic conditions and respiratory diseases); phenytoin and phenobarbital (anti-seizure drugs); heparin, a blood thinner; furosemide, a diuretic; and No-DOZ, a stimulant.

•These drugs may hamper your bone repair ability: Ibuprofen, NSAIDS like Naproxen, Fenclofenac, Indomethacin, Sulindac, Keto-profen, Diclofenac, Aspirin, Piroxicam, Flur-biprofen, Asopro-pazone. (British LANCET.)

•Aerobic exercise and light weight training are key bone builders and strengtheners. Exercise significantly increases bone mass even after you've stopped growing! •Take an ocean swim or walk for extra minerals.

•Aluminum pots, deodorants, aluminum-containing antacids may increase risk of hip fractures, leaching calcium from the body.

Herbal, Superfood and Supplement Therapy

Interceptive therapy: Choose 2 to 3 recommendations.

1—Build bones with more bone nutrients from herbs: •Silica: Crystal Star OCEAN MINERALS™ iodine, potassium, silica caps, •Body Essentials SILICA GEL, or Jarrow BIOSIL for collagen formation. •Calcium: Crystal Star CALCIUM-MAGNESIUM SOURCE™ caps or drops; •Flora CALCIUM liquid; or •Eidon MINERAL BALANCING PROGRAM.

2—Improve daily assimilation of bone nutrients: •Magnesium, 400mg; •Vitamin D 400IU; •B-complex 100mg, extra B-6 100mg and folic acid 400mcg. •Manganese 5mg; •Betaine HCl 650mg. •Enzymedica DIGEST; or •Transformation Enzyme PURE-ZYME - provides amino acids that help calcium uptake. (Very good results.)

3—Healthy glands for good bones: Estrogen/progesterone balancers: •Crystal Star FEM-SUPPORT™ CFS Stamina drops. •Bilberry extract (herbal bioflavs have estrogen-like activity); •Crystal Star PRO-EST BALANCE, plant progesterone roll-on; •DHEA 25mg daily; •Pure Essence Labs FEM CREME; •INDIUM-EASE (indium) -up to 694% higher gland mineral uptake.

4—Help remodel your bones: •Lane Labs ADVACAL FAST RELEASE ULTRA (highly recommended, good clinical results); Natural Balance IPRI-FLAVONE (menopausal women). •Nature's Path TRACE-MIN-LYTE; •CoQ10 200mg daily; •Jarrow HYDROXYAPATITE; •Evening Primrose Oil 4000mg. Note: Love your liver -vital to forming bone marrow.

5—Bone knitters and healers: •Apply B & T ARNIFLORA gel. •Tape on a Comfrey poultice for 3 days. Change daily to start healing faster. •Suspected bone cancer - yarrow tea, or •Natural Energy Plus CAISSE'S TEA or Flora FLOR-ESSENCE® tea.

—Superfood therapy: Choose 1 or 2 recommendations.
•Prince of Peace GINSENG ROYAL JELLY vials or •royal jelly-ginseng caps.
•Green Foods CARROT ESSENCE.
•Solaray ALFAJUICE, vitamin K.
•AloeLife ALOE GOLD for HCl.

Can't find a recommended product? Call the 800 number listed in Product Resources for the store nearest you.

Brain Power and Health

Better Memory, More Mental Activity, Less Mental Exhaustion

With tens of billions of neurons and more than 100 billion cells, our brains are a million times more powerful than any computer! In fact some scientists say the human brain is the most complex computer in the universe, with a database big enough to record and store over 10 million books! NEWSFLASH! It has long been speculated that brain cells do not regenerate, but new research reveals people actually do produce new brain cells well into adulthood. The brain makes up less than 3% of our body weight, but uses over 25% of our oxygen, more than 25% of glucose and 20% of our blood supply! Research shows high levels of stress hormones stunt new brain cell development, while ample levels of serotonin, the "feel good" hormone, enhance it. The brain is our primary health managing organ, and it's incredibly sensitive. Even damage to just a small part of the brain has devastating consequences; We see clear evidence of this in strokes and Parkinson's disease.

Do you really only use just 10% of your brain? We all hear this myth from childhood (especially when we do something stupid). We do use all of our brain, but clearly, we still have much to learn about how the brain works and how to heal the brain from serious disorders. We know that brain health is intertwined with immune response (it's especially sensitive to free radical damage), with glandular function (especially sexual response), and via the hypothalamus, with the cardiovascular system. A tiny, but important limbic system organ, the hypothalamus regulates production and release of insulin, as well as thyroid, stress, sex and growth hormones. Imbalances in the limbic system have wide ranging effects from hormone disruption to serious mental disorders. The hippocampus is the brain's memory center, sorting and storing working memory, and short term and long term memory. The size of the hippocampus is markedly reduced in advanced Alzheimer's disease.

Clearly, the best brain activity comes from feeding it and using it. Your brain is hungry… nutrient fluctuations and deficiencies can send the brain into a major decline! In contrast, brain nutrients have a rapid, noticeable effect on brain performance. Long term brain nourishment can straighten out even grave mental, emotional or coordination problems. For better or worse, the brain responds rapidly to stimulants of all kinds, to tranquilizers and antidepressants, even to drugs, like beta blockers, calcium channel blockers and antihistamines… usually at the expense of memory and alertness. Take a look at your brain's "diet" if you have trouble concentrating, if you're gloomy or depressed for no real reason, if you always feel stressed and burned out, or if your memory has noticeably deteriorated. You may need more brain nutrition. *Note:* Exercise is a key brain nutrient, increasing oxygen and blood supply which the brain depends on for well being. Studies show physically active seniors demonstrate much better thinking and memory skills than their sedentary counterparts.

Does your brain power need a boost?

…Do you feel mentally foggy, spacy or slow? Have you lost the ability to concentrate?

…Do you frequently have unexplained depression, gloominess or bad moods?

…Have you lost the ability to remember well or for a reasonable length of time?

…Do your muscles respond more slowly than usual? Is your muscle coordination poor?

…Do you feel anxious or paranoid?

…Do your nerves feel raw and on edge no matter how much sleep you get?

…Are you often tired for no physical reason?

…Do you cry unexpectedly and often for no explained reason?

Science divides memory into three different classifications:

1) **working memory** (the ability to remember a phone number or address in the moment to complete a task);
2) **short-term memory** (the ability to remember what you had for dinner last night or where you left your car keys);
3) **long-term memory** (the ability to remember to significant events, names of family members and friends, and important birthdays).

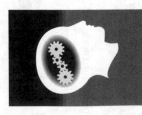

Memory is dependent on how effectively brain cells communicate with each other through neurotransmitter activity. It is also intimately connected with emotional response, a reason why your wedding day may be crystal clear in your memory but last week's dinner is a big blur. Or why love songs instantly recall a time in our lives, but the latest rap music doesn't make a memory connection. Optimism and relaxation assure better memory, too. Studies show classical music is especially good for brain function. The vagus nerve, which extends from the brainstem to the body's internal organs, acts a messenger between the brain and body. The vagus nerve keeps your brain informed on everything from your heartbeat to how full your

Can't find a recommended product? Call the 800 number listed in Product Resources for the store nearest you.

stomach is. The vagus nerve is also believed to be involved with how emotional response affects memory. Scientists still have more to learn about how this communication works, but animal studies suggest arousal hormones like adrenaline use the vagus nerve to tell the brain to "hang on" to important memories.

Is memory loss *inevitable* as you age?

Aging is not synonymous with mental decline. We have all known seniors who are just as sharp (if not sharper) as younger people. Check these factors that may be affecting your memory and see the corresponding pages in this book for natural recommendations.

Memory loss is linked to....

...chemo and high blood pressure drugs; or alcohol or drug abuse

...depression, lack of sleep or low neurotransmitter levels

...chronic stress causing elevated cortisol (shrinks the hippocampus); post traumatic stress disorder

...poor circulation (reduced blood flow and oxygen to the brain); narrow blood vessels (arteriosclerosis)

...TIAs (transient ischemic attacks- mini strokes) or brain disease (Alzheimer's, brain tumors)

...heavy metal toxicity; free radical damage

...nutrient deficiency or malabsorption (common in the elderly); adrenal or thyroid dysfunction

The brain is one of those things in life that passes our understanding. Physiologically, a memory is just a few thousand chemicals firing in a set pattern. But our memory is much more. Our brain chemicals rise and fall as we experience emotions and feelings that are "attached" to a memory. Your brain may call your heart, endocrine, immune and gastrointestinal systems to attention. We see evidence of this in people suffering from post traumatic stress disorder who experience heart palpitations, cold sweats and nausea when they recall the traumatic event. We also see evidence of this in our experience of sexuality and love. We can remember our romantic encounters with the same euphoria, ecstasy and fondness of the original event.

The spirit is intertwined with the mind. In fact, the body fails without the harmonious working support of the mind and spirit. (In contrast, if the body fails, most people believe the spirit is set free.) The brain is the perfect example of the mind-body connection at work. When mind and spirit are in balance, you really are your own best healer- no matter how serious your disease may be. But how do we rally the mind and spirit for healing? Some practitioners use guided imagery which has been shown to help bolster cancer patients' immune systems, and reduce fear and pain. Massage therapy, biofeedback, and meditation are also widely used to bring together the mind, body and spirit with good results.

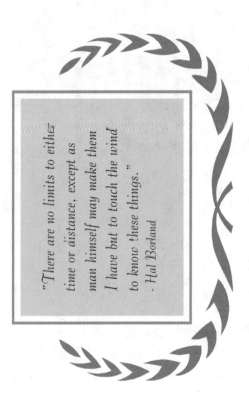

"There are no limits to either time or distance, except as man himself may make them I have but to touch the wind to know these things."
- Hal Borland

Can't find a recommended product? Call the 800 number listed in Product Resources for the store nearest you.

Brain Power

Diet and Lifestyle Support Therapy

Nutritional therapy plan:

1—Brain cells are almost 60% EFAs. Keep your brain well oiled with omega-3 oils for EFAs: Sea greens, spinach, arugula, other leafy greens, fish, shellfish have plenty of DHA and EPA oils; sprouts, fertile eggs, olive, perilla and flax oils, avocado, nuts and seeds, cantaloupe, wheat germ and beans are other good food sources of EFAs.

• Drink plenty of water for brain health. An Italian study shows that even a 2% loss of body fluid affects short term memory! Try PENTA water for a noticeable difference.

• Avoid saturated fats and trans fats. High saturated fat meals cut off glucose, your brain's main energy supply. (Avoid sugary foods though; they lower blood sugar that nourishes the brain.) Trans fat chemicals replace natural DHA in brain cell membranes and disrupt neuron communication.

2—Add glutathione enhancing foods for neurotransmitter energy: eggs, spinach, parsley, watermelon and cruciferous veggies.

3—Lack of protein, potassium or other minerals cause mental burnout. Make a brain booster: mix 2 tbsp. each: lecithin for phosphatides and memory lapses, nutritional yeast for myelin formation. Take 1-2 tbsp. of the mix daily in juice.

4—Increase antioxidants to boost brain activity: 1 cup green or white tea each morning (or try Crystal Star DR. VITALITY™ green and white tea.) 1 to 2 glasses of wine at dinner; eggplant often (its antioxidant *nasunin* protects against free radicals).

Lifestyle support:

• Get your sleep! We all need rejuvenating downtime. Even a few hours of sleep loss causes memory problems.

• Build more brain circuits by reading and playing mental games. Do a Sunday crossword puzzle. Boost brain circulation by an arm-swinging ½ hour walk.

• Deep breathing works wonders. (See page 250, and Paul Bragg's book on SUPER POWER BREATHING, a good health investment.)

• If you're dieting, remember that a low fat diet can rob your body of critical Omega-3 fats, especially DHA, the primary building blocks for your brain, heart tissue and eyes. Your memory, attention span, focus and learning ability will suffer. So will your vision and cardiovascular performance.

• Chronic stress causes elevated cortisol which damages the hippocampus. Transcendental meditation lowers cortisol and raises DHEA to combat stress, helping you reach a state of restful alertness that enhances mental ability.

• Hyperbaric oxygen therapy shows promise for treating traumatic brain injury, cerebral palsy, stroke and more.

• Alcohol, tobacco and marijuana inhibit brain release of vasopressin, impairing memory, attention and concentration, and increase the need for neurotransmitter replenishment.

Herbal, Superfood and Supplement Therapy

Interceptive therapy: Choose 2 to 3 recommendations.

1—**Boost neurotransmitter connections:** •Crystal Star MENTAL CLARITY™ caps (noticeable rapid activity); •Wakunaga NEURO-LOGIC, or •Life Extension Foundation COGNITEX with GPC (Glycero-PhosphoCholine); •Phosphatidyl Serine (PS) 1000mg, GABA or Choline 600mg. (If choline levels are low, Huperzine A 50mg allows levels to rise.) •Tyrosine 3 grams daily aids dopamine, norepinephrine, epinephrine production;
•*Evening primrose oil* 3-4 daily; •For bad moods, add 5-HTP, 50mg at night.

2—**Enhance brain blood flow:** •*Ginkgo Biloba* extract 3x daily; •*ginger-cayenne* caps 4 daily; •Vitamin Research VINPOCETINE 30mg daily. •Magnesium 800mg.

3—**Sustain your brain with herbs and EFAs:** Ginseng curtails release of stress hormone cortisol to boost brain activity. •Crystal Star FEEL GREAT NOW!™ with ginseng caps, or •MENTAL INNER ENERGY™ drops; •Planetary BACOPA-GINKGO BRAIN STRENGTH tabs; •Source Naturals NEUROMINS DHA. •Brain tonics *Ginseng-Gotu Kola, Ashwagandha* and *Fo-Ti root.*

4—**Sharpen your memory:** •Acetyl-Carnitine, 2500mg daily; •Crystal Star MENTAL CLARITY™ caps; •Dr. Diamond DIAMOND MIND; •New Chapter NEUROZYME with DHA and *Chinese Club moss;* •DHEA, with pregnenolone boosts memory. Try aromatherapy oils for the brain: *peppermint, rosemary* (apply to temples), *frankincense, vanilla.*

5—**B's are for brain power:** •B-complex 150mg with extra niacin and B-6 250mg.
•Nature's Secret ULTIMATE B; •Sublingual active B-12, 2500mcg.

6—**Antioxidants boost brain energy, target inflammation:** •Glutathione 100mg daily;
•Transformation PURE-ZYME and •Alpha Lipoic Acid neutralize toxins and recycle glutathione; Vitamin C 4000mg daily reduces cortisol; •Acetyl-L-carnitine 1000-2000mg a day to repair and energize the brain. •CoQ$_{10}$, 200mg; with vitamin E 400IU for best results. •Source Naturals ENADA NADH tabs for brain energy.

—Superfood therapy: Choose 1 or 2 recommendations.

•Nutricology PRO-GREENS with EFAs.
•Health from the Sun TOTAL EFA.
•Crystal Star RESTORE YOUR STRENGTH™ drink or caps.
•Prince of Peace GINKGO BILOBA-RED PANAX GINSENG vials, 1-2 daily, and ROYAL JELLY-PANAX GINSENG vials, 1 daily. (fast-acting)
•Futurebiotics VITAL K drink to help reduce damage to brain neurons.
•MICROHYDRIN PLUS antioxidant therapy.

Can't find a recommended product? Call the 800 number listed in Product Resources for the store nearest you.

Bronchitis
Acute and Chronic

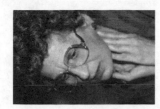

Chronic bronchitis is an infectious inflammation of the bronchi, largely a direct result of prolonged exposure to irritants like cigarette smoke, air pollutants and environmental chemicals, a rising problem in today's world. The typical victim is forty or older, with lowered immunity from prolonged stress, fatigue or smoking. The disease usually develops slowly over a course of years, but will not go away on its own. The person becomes increasingly susceptible to respiratory infections which suppressive cold preparations and lack of exercise aggravate. The recent type of viral bronchitis, which affects women, is very hard to treat, and lasts from 3 weeks to 5 months.

There are two types of bronchitis. **Chronic bronchitis** can be incapacitating, and lead to serious, even potentially fatal lung disease. Bronchial walls thicken, bronchial tissue becomes inflamed, and mucous becomes thicker and more profuse. Breathing is difficult with shortness of breath from clogged airways. A mucous-producing cough and wheezing lasts for 3 months or more. Most sufferers are constantly tired and weak from this constant low grade lung infection, and lose weight. **Acute bronchitis**, inflammation of the bronchial tree, is generally self-limiting, like a bad chest cold, with eventual complete healing. Symptoms feel like a deep chest cold, there's a slight fever; inflammation; headache, nausea, lung and body aches and a hacking, mucous-y cough.

Diet and Lifestyle Support Therapy

Nutritional therapy plan:

1—Go on a short mucous cleansing liquid diet to get rid of the thick chest mucous. Then follow a largely vegetarian, cleansing diet for 3 weeks. Avoid sugars, dairy, starchy and fatty foods during healing to reduce congestion. See pg. 202 for my Mucous Congestion Cleansing Diet.

2—Take cleansing soups, broths, hot tonics, high vitamin C juices, vegetable juices and green drinks. •Liquid chlorophyll, 1 tsp. in water before each meal.

3—Take lemon juice in water each morning and flax seed tea each night during acute stages to alkalize the blood and keep bowels clean to better eliminate excess mucous.

4—Make an onion-honey syrup: Put 5 to 6 chopped onions and ½ cup honey in a pot and cook over very low heat for two hours. Strain and take 1 tbsp. every two hours.

—**Superfood therapy:** Choose 1 or 2 recommendations.
•Crystal Star RESTORE YOUR STRENGTH™ drink daily for 1 month.
•AloeLife ALOE GOLD 2 tbsp. daily.
•Barleans GREENS for antioxidants.
•Alacer EMERGEN-C replaces electrolytes, anti-viral action.

Lifestyle bodywork support:
•Take a hot sauna; follow with a brisk rubdown, and chest-back percussion to loosen mucous. Rub on the chest: *tea tree* oil, or Earth's Bounty O₂ OXY-SPRAY (fast results).
•Avoid commercial cough suppressants. Coughing gets rid of mucous. Apply alternating hot and cold witch hazel compresses to the chest. •Use *eucalyptus* oil in a vaporizer for anti-inflammatory properties.
•Deep breathing exercises morning and before bed help clear lungs. Get fresh air and sunshine every day.
•Cover mouth and nose with a scarf or mask so that infectious micro-organisms are not sucked into the lungs.

Herbal, Superfood and Supplement Therapy

Interceptive therapy: Choose 2 to 4 recommendations.

1—**Reduce inflammation, infection:** •*Oregano* oil caps as directed. •Crystal Star ANTI-BIO™ extract 1 dropperful twice daily, with ANTI-FLAM caps™ 4 at a time. New Chapter ZYFLAMEND caps or extract 2x daily. •Add *reishi mushroom* extract, Maitake Products REISHI caps, for T-cell immune defenses. •Protease 175,000 to 375, 000 HUT daily. •Bromelain 2000mg daily, or •Crystal Star Dr. ENZYME™ with protease and bromelain.

2—**Expectorants get rid of thick, irritating mucous:** •*Lobelia* extract drops during acute stage; •*cayenne-ginger* capsules and also apply *cayenne-ginger* compresses to the chest. •NAC caps (N-acetyl-cysteine), 2 daily; •Crystal Star D-CONGEST™ drops.

3—**Soothe the hacking cough:** •Han HONEY LOQUAT syrup (excellent activity); •*marshmallow root* tea - gargle twice daily and at night; •Zinc lozenges or •Crystal Star MUSCLE RELAXER™ caps 4 at a time (rapid results).

4—**Antioxidants re-establish lung capacity:** •Bayberry-Ginger caps, 4 to 6 daily, a powerful antioxidant relieves acute conditions. •Vitamin A 10,000IU with vitamin C with bioflavonoids up to 5000mg, and magnesium 800mg daily. •LYCOPENE 10-25mg. •Nutricology organic THYMUS and COLOSTRUM help restabilize immunity.

—**For chronic bronchitis:** Astragalus extract or Planetary Jade Screen extracts (excellent results). •CoQ₁₀ 200mg daily; •*mullein* tea 2 cups daily; •*cayenne-garlic* or *elecampane* caps 6 daily; •*Cordyceps* extract, or •Metabolic Response Modifiers CORDYCEPS 750mg; or •*echinacea-goldenseal* extract for 1 month; •Gaia Herbs LOMATIUM OSHA SUPREME. •Bromelain caps 2000mg a day improves lung capacity, reduces coughing (clinical tests), or •Crystal Star DR. ENZYME™ caps with bromelain and protease to reduce inflammation. Crystal Star VIREX™ caps to reduce hanging-on infection.

—**For acute bronchitis:** Make a tonic tea: Steep 1TB each in 4 cups hot water for 25 minutes - *Licorice rt., horehound, lemon grass, osha, coltsfoot, lobelia, pleurisy rt., mullein.* Try olive leaf extract, or use homeopathic B&T Bronchitis-Asthma Aid.

Can't find a recommended product? Call the 800 number listed in Product Resources for the store nearest you.

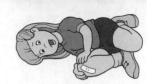

Bruises, Cuts, Abrasions

Easy Bruising, Blisters, Black Eyes, Hard to Heal Wounds

Bruising is a normal body reaction to a minor trauma, occurring when capillaries rupture from an injury, causing blood to leak out, discoloring adjacent tissue. Easy bruising usually means you have thin capillaries and weak vein walls. Its root cause, and the cause of hard to heal wounds, is almost always a flavonoid deficiency, nutrients that strengthen vein and capillary walls. Although the elderly are most affected, it's common for people who are overweight, or who take anti-clotting drugs. Poor circulation, anemia and liver malfunction are other reasons for easy bruising, and can be a clear sign that the body needs foundation nutrient support. Easy bruising is easy to correct through diet changes (add minerals and collagen boosters) and supplements (vitamin K). For frequent, excessive bruising, see a physician for a clotting time blood test... it may also be an early warning sign of cancer. *Note: Do not take aspirin if you bruise easily. It allows blood seepage that leads to discoloration.* Healing from a bruise gets worse with age, because underlying skin layers become weaker and thinner; coarser, more random collagen fibers offer less support for capillaries. For some, the slightest bump causes bruising. Large, dark purple bruises may appear spontaneously and can take weeks or months to go away.

Diet and Lifestyle Support Therapy

Nutritional therapy for bruises:

1—Keep diet light, low fat, mineral-rich to build skin infrastructure. Avoid clogging dairy foods during healing. Eat fresh greens daily to replenish cell rebuilding nutrients.

2—Give yourself more protein to heal: seafood, soy foods like tempeh and tofu, green superfoods like spirulina and chlorella. Eat enzyme rich foods like sprouts, papayas and pineapple to encourage enzyme healing.

3—Eat vitamin K rich foods - alfalfa sprouts, sea greens, leafy greens, peppers, citrus fruits. Eat vitamin C and bioflavonoid-rich foods like citrus, strawberries and other berries, grapes, peppers and broccoli.

4—Apply pineapple or white vinegar directly to a bruise to remove blueness; orange to a black eye; milk to a blister.

—**Bodywork applications for bruising:**

•Apply ice cubes wrapped in a cloth for 15 minutes just after a bruise occurs. Remove for 10 minutes, then repeat ice pack. Then 10 minutes each -hot and cold washcloths.

•Take a bruise bath: make strong *rosemary-thyme* tea. Strain; add to a hot bath. Soak for 30 minutes.

•Apply *calendula* or *plantain* salve for bruises and blisters.

•For stubborn bruises, massage in a few drops of *rosemary, fennel, tea tree or lavender* oil to 1-oz. *jojoba* oil.

Nutritional therapy for cuts:

•Take a green veggie drink for hard-to-heal wounds. •Apply wheat germ oil-honey mix. •Apply a thick honey (or sugar) coat, natural antibiotics, to the cut and wrap.

—**Bodywork applications for cuts or abrasions:**

•Apply hot and cold *witch hazel* or *lavender* compresses, or clean with H_2O_2 and apply *tea tree* oil drops every 3 hours. •Apply weak C solution directly. •Apply *Echinacea-Arnica-Calendula* compresses, or B & T CALIFLORA. Note: For a deep cut, apply *calendula* salve only after the inside begins to heal. It heals so fast that the outside closes up before the inside is healed.

Herbal, Superfood and Supplement Therapy

Interceptive therapy for bruises: Choose 2 to 4 recommendations.

1—**Reduce bruises:** •*Horse Chestnut Seed* extract can take down a bruise as you watch; so can •BHI TRAUMEEL gel daily. (*Amazingly fast*). •Homeopathic *Arnica* 30C or B & T ARNIFLORA gel; Ledum for a severe bruise. •*Rosemary* essential oil, •*Ginkgo biloba* extract, or •*cayenne-ginger* disperse bruising by raising circulation. •Crystal Star's VARI-VAIN™ has active herbal anti-inflammatories. •Apply DMSO a.m.- p.m. for 3 days.

2—**Rebuild skin, capillary strength:** •*Bilberry* extract or •Crystal Star IODINE, POTAS-SIUM, SILICA drops or Eidon SILICA minerals for collagen; *gotu kola* caps 6 daily. •Vitamin C with bioflavs 1000mg every 2 hrs. •Vitamin K 100mcg daily for a month.

3—**Enzyme therapy:** •Crystal Star DR. ENZYME™ with protease and bromelain; •Transformation PUREZYME protease; •Bromelain 1500mg daily, or •Nature's Plus ULTRA BROMELAIN 1500mg. •Apply until swelling goes, *bromelain/papain* powder paste.

4—**Rebuild connective tissue:** •Lane Labs TOKI, collagen replacement promotes new cell growth, reduces discolorations. •B-complex with extra pantothenic acid 500mg.

Interceptive therapy for cuts:

1—**Encourage healing:** •*Evening Primrose* oil with bromelain 1500mg for hard to heal wounds. •Ethical Nutrients ZINC STATUS for slow healers. •*Gotu kola* caps 6 daily. •Take Ester C with bioflavonoids, 5 grams daily. •Nutricology GERMANIUM 150mg.

2—**Reduce infection:** •Apply *cayenne* tincture to stop bleeding; •Apply Crystal Star ANTI-BIO™ gel (with *una da gato*), and •take Crystal Star ANTI-BIO™ for a week. •Apply Nutribiotic GRAPEFRUIT SEED SKIN SPRAY (excellent activity).

—**Superfood therapy for bruises and cuts:** Choose 1 or 2 recommendations.

•Crystal Star BIOFLAV. FIBER & C™ drink (highly recommended).

•Herbal Answers HERBAL ALOE FORCE (polysaccharides directly stimulate tissue regeneration). Drink and apply.

•Alacer EMERGEN-C drink mix.

•Solaray ALFAJUICE with high vitamin K.

Can't find a recommended product? Call the 800 number listed in Product Resources for the store nearest you.

Burns

1st and 2nd Degree Burns, Sunstroke, Heatstroke

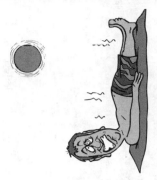

Burns are identified as 1st, 2nd, or 3rd degree according to the severity of damage and the number of skin layers affected. **First degree burns**, usually from sunburn, exhibit minor blistering and pain, affecting only the surface layer of the skin (the epidermis). **Second degree burns** damage the next lower layer (the dermis), with blistering, scarring, hair follicles burned off, even gland structure damage. **Third degree burns** are the most serious, with extensive tissue damage to all skin layers, often injuring muscles and other tissue as well, oozing, charring, severe loss of body fluids and shock. Get medical help fast for anything other than a first degree or small second degree burn. Don't use drugstore burn medications over large body areas or for serious burns. They are for minor burns only. If there is severe itching, redness or swelling, if fever, chills or great fatigue appear, get to a medical clinic. The suggestions on this page are for 1st degree or small 2nd degree burns only. If the burn is 3rd degree, treat for shock until help arrives. **Heatstroke and sunstroke** are an over-reaction to heat and sun exposure. Symptoms are evident first by thirst, severe headache and fatigue, then rapid pulse and dizziness, often vomiting, and a "shock-y" condition of decreased alertness, can even lead to brain damage or death. *See Shock page 538, Sunburn and Skin page 543.*

Diet and Lifestyle Support Therapy

Nutritional therapy plan:

1—Apply ice water, then vinegar soaked compresses.

2—Drink lots of fluids like potassium broth (pg. 291) and veggie drinks. Eat plenty of protein and mineral-rich foods for tissue repair.

3—For immediate relief with no blistering or irritation, dip cotton balls in fresh *ginger juice* or strong black tea or green tea and apply. Colgate toothpaste is a good burn salve.

4—Give electrolyte drinks or a little salty water. No alcoholic or caffeinated drinks- they dehydrate. Electrolyte replacements: Alacer EMERGEN-C, 2 pkts. Lemonade, limeade, mineral water. PENTA bottled water offers rapid rehydration.

—**Effective kitchen compresses:**

• *Peppermint oil* drops mixed with *wheat germ oil* and honey. *(Rosemary Gladstar)*

• Fresh ginger juice or inside of a banana peel for swelling.

• Egg whites or raw potato for scalds

• Baking soda or vinegar in water for acid/chemical burns.

—**Soothing applications:**

• Earth's Bounty OXY-SPRAY. • Body Essentials SILICA GEL.

• Burn applications: *elder flower, red clover, yarrow, goldenseal rt.* tea. • *Calendula* gel or St. Johns *wort-Comfrey-Calendula* salve reduces pain. or • New Chapter ARNICA-GINGER gel. • *Thyme oil* or *Tea tree oil.*

Immediate procedures: • Flush with cold water if skin is not charred; then apply ice packs until pain is relieved. Cut away loose clothing. If skin is charred, apply cloths dipped in aloe vera gel or juice, or a fresh *comfrey leaf* or *plantain herb* poultice. • Make a water solution of Vitamin C crystals and apply. • Take **Cayenne** for shock: ¼ tsp. tincture, or 2 opened caps in 1 tsp. warm water.

—**For sunstroke or heatstroke:** • To prevent: drink plenty of fluids and don't over-exert when it's hot. Dress in loose, light clothes. Get out of the sun immediately. • Apply ice packs, wrap the person in a cold wet sheet. Get medical help for shock immediately.

Herbal, Superfood and Supplement Therapy

Interceptive therapy: Choose 2 to 3 recommendations.

1—**Reduce pain and swelling:** • Apply Aloe Life ALOE SKIN GEL, or • Blender blend your own burn gel: to every ¼ cup aloe vera gel, add ¼ tsp. vitamin E oil, ¼ tsp. vitamin C powder and ½ tsp. *lavender* or *chamomile* essential oil; then apply. • Apply Crystal Star ANTI-BIO™ GEL, or • *St. John's wort* oil. Use • Crystal Star ANTI-FLAM™ caps; • NutriBiotic grapefruit seed extract SKIN SPRAY. • Take vitamin C, 3-5000mg daily.

2—**Reduce risk of shock:** • Nelson Bach RESCUE REMEDY (medicine chest necessity). • For fluid loss: B-complex 100mg, calcium-magnesium-potassium w. vitamin D.

3—**Accelerate healing:** • Make a skin healer tea to help new collagen form, apply 3x times daily: *Comfrey, nettles, marshmallow, horsetail, scullcap, red clover.* • Take Flora VEGE-SIL caps, • Crystal Star IODINE, POTASSIUM & SILICA™ drops; • *Green tea-gotu kola* caps and tea. • Take Nutricology GERMANIUM 150mg.

4—**Normalize your skin tissue:** • Chi's Enterprise WHOLE SKIN OINTMENT (excellent for burns- Call 800-457-5708 to order); • New Chapter TRUE TAMANU oil (speeds healing and healthy skin growth); • Proteolytic enzymes, bromelain 1500mg and papain for healing; • American Biologics SUB-ADRENE for cortex formation, 3x daily. • Guard with beta carotene 25,000IU and vitamin C 1000mg daily.

—**Homeopathic burn remedies:**

• Use *Arnica* for bad burns, followed by *Hypericum* tincture; • *Apis* for a stinging burn; • *Phosphorus* for electrical burns; • *Urtica Urens* for 2nd degree burns that itch and sting.

—**Superfood therapy:**

• Nutribiotic PRO GREENS with EFAs.

• Crystal Star ENERGY GREEN RENEWAL™ drink or caps.

• Crystal Star BIOFLAVONOID, FIBER & C SUPPORT™ drink.

• Futurebiotics VITAL K.

Can't find a recommended product? Call the 800 number listed in Product Resources for the store nearest you.

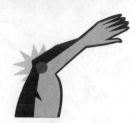

Bursitis

Acute or Chronic Tendonitis, Tennis Elbow

Bursitis is either the acute or chronic inflammation of a bursa, the sac-like membrane of connective tissue that contains joint protecting fluids. (The **tennis elbow** form of bursitis is a result of a direct blow or repetitive pressure to a bursa area.) *Tendonitis* is inflammation of the lining of the tendon sheath and its enclosed tendon, especially where tendons pass near bones. Both tendonitis and bursitis may develop calcified deposits (thought by most experts to be a result of poor nutrient absorption) in the shoulder, elbow, hip or knee. Both can result from strain, a blow to the affected area, or in the case of bursitis, as a secondary symptom of arthritis or rheumatism. Naturopaths believe an acid-forming diet, which causes chronic metabolic imbalance, opens the door to both tendonitis and bursitis, (and to rheumatoid arthritis or gout). Smoking produces excess acid; stress, toxemia and infection may also be involved. **When is it bursitis?** Both tendonitis and bursitis mean inflammation and tenderness where tendons affix to bones, causing limited motion in the affected body part. Shooting pains are severe, with swelling and redness, especially in the morning and damp weather. Intense pain occurs when lifting or backward rotating the arm. *See Arthritis, page 324 for more information.*

Diet and Lifestyle Support Therapy

Nutritional therapy plan:

1—Avoid acid-forming foods, like caffeine, salts, fried highly processed foods, red meats, nightshade plants like tomatoes, potatoes and eggplant.

—Cleanse acids: take 2 tbsp. cider vinegar and 2 tbsp. maple syrup in water each morning for 2 weeks.

2—Best: Vegetarian and alkaline foods like celery, avocado, potato, wheat germ, sweet fruits, sprouts, leafy and sea greens, nutritional yeast, oats.

3—High magnesium foods: Greens, green and yellow veggies, sea veggies.

—**For calcium-magnesium uptake:** Salmon, sea foods, sea veggies. Leafy greens, spinach, watercress, broccoli, cauliflower. Cultured foods: yogurt, tofu, miso, kefir, sauerkraut.

4—Have a carrot-beet-cucumber juice with extra celery juice twice a week to "scour" out sediment residues.

5—Take high Omega-3 flax oil, or cold water fish oil, ½ to 1 tsp. 3x daily. Improvement usually in 2 – 6 weeks.

Lifestyle bodywork support:

•Acupuncture and reflexology treatment excellent for bursitis.

•Apply ice packs to inflamed area during acute stages. Apply wet warm compresses in later stages for fast healing.

•Hot castor oil packs or •Hot *comfrey-olive oil* compresses.

•Take an epsom salts bath once a week with several drops of rosemary essential oil.

•Magnet therapy has now been proven effective for bursitis.

•Regular mild aerobic and stretching exercises keep your joint system flexible.

•Use affected area gently. No intense athletic activity until trauma is relieved.

—**Soothing, healing applications:** •Baywood TOPICAL SUPER COOL RELIEF; •DMSO liquid with aloe vera gel 2x daily. •Wakunaga GLUCOSAMINE soothing cream. •Nature's Way CAYENNE HERBAL ointment. •A *burdock-lobelia* tea poultice.

Herbal, Superfood and Supplement Therapy

Interceptive therapy: Choose 2 to 3 recommendations.

1—**Reduce inflammation:** •Source Naturals sublingual B$_{12}$ daily for 2 weeks, then every 2 days for two weeks. (Injections for a week highly recommended.) •Country Life LIGA-TEND 4 daily; •Crystal Star ANTI-FLAM™ caps, 4 at a time for intense pain or •Solaray TURMERIC capsules 500mg; •Enzymatic Therapy ACID-A-CAL to dissolve sediment. Apply to reduce inflammation: •B&T TRI-FLORA analgesic gel, •Chinese WHITE FLOWER oil, •Biochemics PAIN RELEAF, or •DMSO roll-on as needed (works within a day).

2—**Improve body pH for arthritis-like symptoms:** Herbal Products and Development POWER PLUS ENZYMES; •Betaine HCl 650mg; •Biotec EXTRA ENERGY ENZYMES with SOD; •Quercetin 3000mg daily with bromelain 1500mg; •Trimedica ALKAMAX caps. •Crystal Star CLEANSING & PURIFYING TEA™ flushes kidneys. •Echinacea extract or Herbs, Etc. LYMPHATONIC flushes lymph system. •UAS -DDS PLUS with FOS caps, or Jarrow JARRO-DOPHILUS.

3—**Reduce spasms and pain:** •Crystal Star STRESS OUT™ muscle relaxer extract drops for fast relief (sometimes less than 20 minutes). •Take DLPA 1000mg as needed. •Use *Lobelia-mullein* or *crampbark* tincture as an antispasmodic rub.

4—**Rebuild connective tissue:** •Crystal Star ADRENAL ENERGY BOOST™ caps, or •American Biologic SUB-ADRENE extract for essential cortex formation. Apply •Body Essentials SILICA GEL to joints, take •Eidon SILICA MINERAL supplement or •Eidon ZINC liquid daily (good results in our tests). •Vitamin C or Ester C with bioflavs 3000mg daily for collagen formation.

—**Superfood therapy:** Choose 1 or 2 recommendations.
•Planetary TRICLEANSE drink.
•Edge Labs JOINT FLEX drink with MSM.
•Solaray ALFAJUICE.
•New Chapter GINGER WONDER syrup- 1 tbsp. in 8-oz. water 2x daily to boost circulation to the painful area.

Can't find a recommended product? Call the 800 number listed in Product Resources for the store nearest you.

Cancer
A New Look at an Old Foe

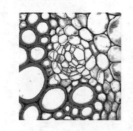

Cancer is reaching epidemic proportions in the U.S. New sad statistics show that more than one in three Americans will get cancer. More than 3 million Americans are being treated for cancer. 1.3 million are newly diagnosed each year. The numbers are even higher for lung and advanced breast cancer, and cancers of the pancreas, liver, bone, ovary and colon.

Recent research shows that conventional therapies still fail <u>50% of the time</u>, even though new drugs and technologies in medical cancer treatment are aimed at killing cancer, but not patients. The medical community recognizes the downsides and limitations of these treatments. Clearly, chasing each of the more than 200 different diseases now classified as cancer with a drug for the different needs and complexities of each one is futile. Still, the best research shows that if we spent more time on <u>cancer prevention</u> rather than treatment, the number of cancer deaths in the U.S. could drop by nearly a third. That translates into 100,000 fewer cancer cases and 60,000 prevented cancer deaths by 2015!

Information about cancer is changing fast. New knowledge offers more choices that really help.

By age 30, millions of your cells have already taken one step towards becoming cancerous. Molecular research has most scientists convinced that cancer is a result of DNA "gone bad." Cancer cells are normal cells that have been altered by a chemical or other enabler that allows the cell to survive, but without the safety controls of normal cells. Cancer-filled cells can no longer do their assigned job for your body. Instead, cancer cells have only one job....to survive. Cancers attack when immune defenses and blood health are low. Boost your immune response to reduce your risk for cancer (and to treat cancer successfully). Promote an internal environment where your immune system can stay effective, and cancer and degenerative disease can't live. Cancers don't seem to take hold where oxygen and minerals (especially potassium) are high in vital body fluids. Love your liver! It's a powerful chemical plant that keeps immunity strong. Love your thymus! It is the seat of the immune system.

Natural therapies are making great strides in the cancer battle. The most promising therapies:

Diet improvement is a key because up to 40-60% of cancer risk is determined by your diet choices! Percentages like these mean that good food choices could have helped prevent 385,000 to 700,000 new cancer cases. Nutrition deficiencies accumulate over a long period of time - years of too much over processed food, trans fats and red meats, entrenched habits of too little fresh fruits and vegetables.... eventually leaves our bodies with very little to protect us. Hormone-driven cancers like ovarian, breast, uterine, kidney, bladder, prostate and colon cancers are closely related to the kind of protein and fat we eat, especially oxidized fats from meats, and oxidized fats from meats, and oxidized fats from junk foods and fried foods. Alcohol abuse, too much sugar and barbecued meat can also be traced back to cancer development. Poor nutrition ultimately changes body chemistry. The immune system can't defend your body properly when biochemistry is altered. It can't tell its own cells from invading toxic cells, and in confusion may attack everything or nothing.

Cancer fighting food nutrients. Your diet is the place to start.

Your diet is your major weapon against cancer. Whole food nutrition allows the body to use its built-in restorative and repair abilities. A healthy diet can intervene in the cancer process at many stages, from its conception to its growth and spread. Even if your genetics and lifestyle are against you, your diet may still make a tremendous difference in your cancer odds. For example, certain body chemicals must be "activated" before they can initiate cancer. Food can block the activation process. Antioxidant foods can snuff out carcinogens, nip free radical cascades in the bud, and even repair some cellular damage.

Certain foods accelerate body detoxification, and prevent the genetic ruin of cells, a prelude to cancer (one of the reasons I emphasize a detoxification diet as part of cancer control). Healthy food chemicals in cells can determine whether a cancer-causing virus, or a cancer promoter like too much estrogen will turn tissue cancerous. Even after cells have massed into structures that may grow into tumors, food compounds can intervene to stop more growth. Some actually shrink the patches of precancerous cells.

Although far less powerful at later stages, diet can still influence the spread of cancer. Wandering cancer cells need the right conditions to attach and grow. Foods can foster a hostile or a favorable environment. So even after cancer is diagnosed, the right foods may help prolong your life. Even if your genetics and lifestyle are against you, your diet may still make a tremendous difference in your cancer odds. Massive new research is validating what naturopaths like myself have known for decades. The more fruits and vegetables you eat, the less your cancer risk, from colon and stomach cancer, to breast and even lung cancer. People who eat plenty of fruits and vegetables have half the risk of people who eat few fruits and vegetables. Studies show that even small to moderate amounts of fruits and vegetables make a big difference. Two fruits and three vegetable servings a day show amazing anti-cancer results. Eating fruit twice a day, instead of twice a week, can cut the risk of lung cancer by 75% even in smokers. One National Cancer Institute spokesman said it is almost mind-boggling, that ordinary fruits and vegetables could be so effective against such a potent carcinogen as cigarette smoke. The evidence is so overwhelming that researchers are beginning to view fruits and vegetables as powerful preventives that could substantially wipe out the scourge of cancer. What an about-face this is for cancer study!

Can't find a recommended product? Call the 800 number listed in Product Resources for the store nearest you.

Foods that provide prime cancer-fighting nutrition:

1) *Vitamin C rich fruits and vegetables:* citrus, tomatoes, peppers, broccoli offer anti-oxidant protection and neutralize cancer-causing free radicals.

2) *Yogurt and active culture foods:* help neutralize carcinogens and de-activate enzymes that allow body substances to turn into cancer.

3) *Antioxidant foods:* green and white tea, wheat germ, soy foods, yellow, orange and green vegetables, citrus fruits, and olive oil help normalize pre-cancerous cells.

4) *Fiber-rich foods:* whole grains, fruits and vegetables absorb excess bile and improve intestinal bacteria.

5) *Phyto-chemical foods:* especially broccoli, cabbage and cauliflower help break down carcinogens and remove them from the body. These same vegetable compounds also break down excess estrogens that are responsible for some types of breast cancer.

6) *Folic acid foods:* wheat germ, greens, beets, asparagus, fish, sunflower seeds, citrus fruits are potent. Folic acid is critical to DNA synthesis so normal cells don't turn cancerous.

Enzyme Therapy: **Enzyme activity maintains the delicate balance between cancer cell production and cancer cell destruction.**

I'm a big believer in the power of enzymes to keep cancer cells in check. I've seen first hand that taking effective enzyme supplements can boost immune response, with powerful anti-inflammatory effects (protease), highly beneficial in cancer treatment. Enzyme therapy improves immune response, chemically alters tumor by-products to lessen cancer's side effects, and changes the tumor's surface to make it vulnerable to immune system response. Re-establishing metabolic balance is the key to nutritional therapy for cancer. Pancreatic enzyme and plant proteases show special promise with specific anti-cancer activity that can help shrink tumors and rally the immune system. *Note:* Avoid antacids. They interfere with enzyme production, and the body's ability to carry off heavy metal toxins.

Two examples of enzyme therapy's amazing results for cancer treatment:

...*Pancreatic Enzymes:* Pancreatic enzymes (derived from animals) are used therapeutically in the famous Gonzales-Isaacs Cancer Program. Their theory submits that a low pancreatic enzyme supply is involved in all types of cancer development. Their program replenishes pancreatic enzymes to significantly reduce active tumors and prevent additional cancer cell growth. Pancreatic cancer responded with particularly good results, even in normally fatal cases of advanced pancreatic cancer. In their pilot study, 36% of patients lived three years on the treatment (even the newest cancer drug trials show only a 19 month survival rate). The National Cancer Institute has funded $1.4 million for a large-scale, controlled clinical trial of the Gonzales-Isaacs approach to treating pancreatic cancer. Additional case studies now document patients with other types of terminal cancer who enjoyed longer survival time and/or tumor regression while on pancreatic enzyme therapy. The Gonzales-Isaacs protocols incorporate individualized diet programs, supplement programs and detoxification treatment like coffee enemas. *For information on Gonzales-Isaacs study, call Cancer Information Service at 1-800-4-CANCER (1-800-422-6237) or visit http://www.dr-gonzalez.com/.*

...*Plant Proteases:* Plant enzyme proteases, enzymes that digest protein, are powerful medicine. Taken on an empty stomach, protease goes directly to the bloodstream to reach body tissues for healing action. Protease helps dissolve the fibrin coating on cancer cells which prevents them from being detected. Without their fibrin "cloak," cancer cells are easy prey to a strong immune system. Proteases helps shrink tumors by stimulating removal of dead or abnormal tissue while enabling healthy tissue. Practitioners regularly use plant protease to accelerate recovery after cancer surgery. Consider Crystal Star DR. ENZYME™ with Protease and Bromelain or Transformation Enzyme PUREZYME, both high potency protease formulas.

Medicinal Mushrooms: **They can intervene in cancer progression at most stages and improve a patient's ability to fight the cancer.**

Today many natural health practitioners use mushrooms to help prevent and treat cancers, and improve a patient's immune health and well-being.

Maitake D-Fraction: maitake D-fraction helps stimulate programmed cell death (apoptosis) of prostate cancer cells, and can improve results of chemo and radiation, and reduce side effects. New tests reveal maitake D-fraction is highly effective even with metastatic prostate cancer by inducing 90% cell death.

    Royal Agaricus: the highest known content of immune boosting beta glucan of all mushrooms, stimulates interferon and natural killer cells, boosts cancer recovery.

    Shiitake: contains lentinan and LEM for strong anti-tumor power (clinical studies). Shiitake do not directly attack cancer tumors, but instead bolster the body's own natural ability to eliminate tumors. Japanese studies find that chemotherapy patients who also receive lentinan injections survive significantly longer with less tumor growth, than patients who receive chemotherapy alone. Shiitake are currently the source of two mushroom-based cancer drugs used in Japan.

    Reishi: detoxify and disperse toxins. Reishi are successful in protecting against bacterial and viral infections caused by poor immune response or chemo/radiation.

    Turkey Tail: New research shows turkey tail mushrooms can improve cancer survival rate, and boost recovery from chemo and radiation.

    Cordyceps: an excellent endocrine rebuilding tonic, I've personally known cancer patients whose strength significantly improved with cordyceps supplements.

Need a good source of medicinal mushrooms? Contact Maitake Products, Inc. at 800-747-7418.

Can't find a recommended product? Call the 800 number listed in Product Resources for the store nearest you.

Anti-Neoplaston Therapy: Anti-Neoplastons may be a "miracle" for some cancers.

They've been controversial since they were first discovered by Dr. Stanislaw Burzynski in 1967. Thankfully, legal problems, office raids, and both personal and professional harassment didn't stop him from getting his therapy to cancer patients who needed it. Anti-neoplastons are non-toxic chemicals synthesized from peptides (protein-like substances) and amino acids in human blood and urine. Intrigued by anti-neoplastons when he discovered them in abundance in healthy patients, but almost completely absent in advanced cancer patients, Dr. Burzynski theorizes that anti-neoplastons function as a kind of secondary defense system, separate from the immune system, which help reprogram defective cells. Brain, prostate, ovarian, pancreatic, and bladder cancer, some types of lung and breast cancer, even lymphoma have all had notable improvement with anti-neoplaston therapy. In some cases, tumors have shrunk or disappeared after just a few weeks of the therapy. Anti-neoplastons can be administered by injection, orally or through a catheter. Treatment can range from $36,000 to $60,000 per year. Reported side effects include: gas, rashes, fever, chills or changes in sodium levels. But compared to the devastating side effects of chemo drugs and radiation therapy, anti-neoplaston therapy may be a viable, less toxic alternative for many cancer patients. *Find out about this potentially life-saving therapy, contact Burzynski Research Institute at 713-335-5697 or visit http://www.cancermed.com on the web.*

Regular exercise: Just 30 minutes a day can make all the difference.

Exercising 3 times a week can almost be considered a "cancer defense" in itself. While one out of three Americans falls victim to cancer, only one out of seven active Americans does. The American College of Sports Medicine reports that unfit men (determined in treadmill tests) are 80% more likely to die of cancer than fit men. Exercise acts as an antioxidant to enhance body oxygen use, altering the way body chemistry controls fat retention, and accelerating passage of waste out of the body. Exercise may reduce breast cancer risk in older women by reducing the amount of estrogen produced by fat cells, and converting more fat into muscle. The Journal of the National Cancer Institute says regular exercise cuts breast cancer risk by 40%! Other tests find active people have 50% less risk of colon cancer than inactive people. Even smokers can reduce their lung cancer risk by exercising regularly. Along with a low fat, high fiber diet, exercise is now a big part of a lifestyle plan to prevent prostate cancer progression. Pick exercises that are fun. Rotate your routine often to reduce boredom. People-pleasing favorites are long walks or beach runs, bicycling, yoga and dancing.

Knowing the early detection signs: You can bring in risk reducers early if you know early tell-tale signs:

1) a change in bowel or bladder habits, especially blood in the stool. 2) chronic indigestion, bloating and heartburn, especially difficulty swallowing. 3) unusual bleeding or discharge of the vagina. 4) lumps or thickening of breasts or testicles. 5) chronic cough or constant voice hoarseness; bloody sputum. 6) growth or changes in warts or moles, or scaly skin patches that never go away, especially if they become inflamed or ulcerate. 7) unusual weight loss. 8) long, unexplained anemia or fatigue.

Cutting the Risk: How can we take more control of our health and lives to prevent cancer?

It's easy to get the idea that anything and everything can cause cancer. It seems like we're assaulted from all sides by cancer activators that we can't control. That's because cancer is not a single disease with a single cause, but a multi-dimensional disease with many factors. Yet, most cancer is preventable. Ninety percent of all types of cancer relate to diet, lifestyle habits (especially smoking), and environmental pollutants and chemicals. At least 20,000 of the 70,000 chemicals people come in contact with regularly are toxic. Hereditary factors account for 5% of cancer cases, but even these are largely influenced by diet and environment. The fact that most cancers *are* related to lifestyle causes means that we can positively affect their source factors ourselves – both to prevent cancer from occurring and helping ourselves when it has.

Watchwords for cutting your risk:

...**Improve your diet:** #1) *Reduce intake of fats and sugars.* Environmental toxins become lodged in the fatty tissue of animals in our food chain, then in our tissues when we eat them. Fat from cancer tissue regularly tests almost double the safe amount of chlorinated pesticides. And, sugar is a major cancer feeder. In a 21 country study, breast cancer incidence rose in areas of high sugar consumption. #2) *Reduce intake of red meats.* Cancer is closely related to the protein and fat in red meats, fast foods and fried foods. #3) *Eat vegetables every day.* The best chance for cancer isn't drugs or surgery - it's diet and lifestyle choices you can make yourself. Fresh foods, superfoods and herbs (and the phyto-chemicals they contain), are powerful cancer fighters. The more fruits and vegetables you eat, the less your cancer risk, regardless of the type of cancer.

...**Keep your immune system strong:** U.S. industries alone generate 88 billion pounds of toxic waste per year. Environmental toxins can damage cell DNA, which leads to cell mutation and tumor development. A daily green drink like Barleans GREENS or Crystal Star ENERGY GREEN RENEWAL™ drink means high antioxidants for immunity.

...**Use enzyme therapy:** #1) Have a fresh green salad every day as a source of hydrolytic enzymes to stimulate immune response. #2) Take CoQ$_{10}$ 100mg daily to boost immunity.

...**Detoxify and cleanse your body at least twice a year:** Superfoods and juices accelerate natural body detox activity and prevent the genetic ruin of cells, a prelude to cancer.

Can't find a recommended product? Call the 800 number listed in Product Resources for the store nearest you.

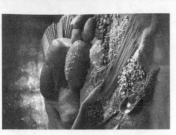

A Macrobiotic Cleansing and Balancing Diet for Cancer

Cancer used to be extremely rare. The devastating disease we know as cancer today emerged gradually, but then began to rise at extraordinary rates as industrial societies became more dependent on technology instead of nature. The dramatic increase is only minimally due to new diagnostic tests, or to calling old diseases, like consumption, cancers. Has our lifestyle over the last 25 years really been that bad? Smoking alone is expected to cause more than 180,000 cancer deaths in 2003; synthetic estrogen hormones seem to permeate our lives; and experts note the parallel of our society's huge rise in chemicals to the expansion of organ cancers. On the plus side, rising evidence from cancer survivors shows that a good chance of success comes from improving our lifestyle to normalize cells out of control. **⅓ of cancer deaths are related to nutrition. Dramatic diet changes can mean dramatic results.** Cancer cells seem to crave dead de-mineralized foods. They find it easy to live and grow in the unreleased waste and mucous deposits in the body. A macrobiotic diet is an effective tool against cancer. It helps rebuild healthy blood and cells, and prevents diseased tissue from continuing to grow. Macrobiotic eating is high in vegetable fiber and protein, low in fatty foods that can alter body chemistry and enhance cancer potential in cells. It is stimulating to the heart and circulatory system through its emphasis on Asian foods like miso, green tea and shiitake mushrooms. It is alkalizing with umeboshi plums, sea veggies and soy foods. It is high in potassium, natural iodine and other minerals. Its greatest benefit is that it is cleansing and strengthening at the same time, and offers truly balanced eating, easily individualized for one's environment, the seasons, and the health of the person using it. The strict form given here for an intensive healing program may be followed for three to six months.

Before each meal, and before bed: take 2 to 4 tbsp. aloe juice concentrate in water (detoxifies and eases nausea if you are undergoing chemotherapy or radiation).

—**On rising:** take a potassium broth or essence (page 291); or carrot-beet-cucumber juice to clean liver and kidneys; or cranberry concentrate (2 tsp. in water) or red grape juice; or a ginseng restorative tea; or Crystal Star RESTORE YOUR STRENGTH™; or a superfood drink like Green Foods CARROT ESSENCE. Consider Arise & Shine CLEANSE THYSELF PROGRAM - a specific for cancer patients, with many reports of success.

—**Breakfast:** have Pulsating Parsley Juice: 6 carrots, 1 beet, 8 spinach leaves, handful fresh parsley; then, make a mix of 2 tbsp. each: nutritional yeast, wheat germ, lecithin, bee pollen granules. Sprinkle some on a whole grain cereal or granola, or mix with yogurt and dried fruit; use on fresh fruit, like strawberries or apples with kefir or kefir cheese; add a whole grain breakfast pilaf like Kashi, bulgur or millet, with apple juice or kefir cheese topping.

—**Mid-morning:** take a cup of Crystal Star CLEANSING & PURIFYING™ TEA, or fresh wheat grass juice or a potassium drink (pg. 291); Pure Planet CHLORELLA, Green Foods GREEN MAGMA; Crystal Star ENERGY GREEN RENEWAL™. Or an herb tea, like pau d'arco, Essiac tea, or Flora FLORESSENCE tea; or a glass of fresh carrot juice; or a cup of miso soup with fresh ginger and sea greens snipped on top. (Have 2 tbsp. dry sea greens daily.)

—**Lunch:** have a Super V-7 veggie juice: 2 carrots, 2 tomatoes, handful each of spinach and parsley, 2 celery ribs, ½ cucumber, ½ green bell pepper. Add 1 tbsp. of a green superfood powder: Crystal Star ENERGY GREEN RENEWAL™; NutriCology PRO-GREENS, Green Kamut GREEN KAMUT, Vibrant Health VITALITY SUPERGREEN. Or, have steamed broccoli or cauliflower with brown rice, or an oriental stir fry with brown rice and miso sauce; or a fresh green salad with whole grain pitas; or a black bean, onion or lentil soup, or a 3 bean salad.

—**Mid-afternoon:** green tea, Crystal Star GREEN TEA CLEANSER™, and whole grain bread sticks or crackers with kefir cheese or a soy spread; or raw veggies dipped in sesame salt.

—**Dinner:** have brown rice and steamed vegetables with maitake or shiitake mushrooms. Snip on 2 tbsp. dry sea veggies (like dulse, arame or nori), 1 tbsp. flax or olive oil, and nutritional yeast; or have a brown rice, millet, bulgur, or kasha casserole with tofu, or tempeh and some steamed vegetables, or a hearty dinner salad with sea greens, nuts and seeds, and whole grain bread or chapatis, or baked, broiled or steamed fish or seafood with rice and peas or other veggies, or stuffed cabbage rolls with rice, and baked carrots with tamari and a little honey.

—**Before bed:** have a cup of shiitake mushroom or ginger broth; green tea exhibits anticancer and cancer chemoprotective effects; or a glass of organic apple juice.

See my book COOKING FOR HEALTHY HEALING *for a complete diet program for cancer control.*

To help macrobiotic balance work correctly with your body, avoid the following foods: —Red meat, poultry, preserved, smoked or cured meats of all kinds, and dairy foods. —Coffee, black teas and carbonated drinks of all kinds (even juices). —All frozen, canned and processed foods; white vinegar, and table salt. —Sugars, corn syrup and artificial sweeteners; and tropical and sweet fruits. —Limit hot spices and nightshade plants like tomatoes, potatoes, peppers and eggplant if you also have rheumatoid arthritis. —Artificially colored foods, chemical-laced and microwaved foods. These foods clog the system so that the vital organs cannot clean out enough waste to maintain health. If you like junk foods, you'll find it difficult to starve out cancer cells; but as healthy cells rebuild, your cravings for these chemical-laced foods will subside.

See the next page for recommended supplements and herbal aids for an intensive macrobiotic cleanse.

Can't find a recommended product? Call the 800 number listed in Product Resources for the store nearest you.

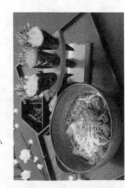

Cancer

Diet and Lifestyle Support Therapy

Nutritional therapy plan for prevention:

1—Juices and teas are key anti-cancer protocols: veggie juices, citrus juices, green or white tea, pau d'arco, roobios red bush tea (key antioxidants). A daily glass of red wine (not breast cancer) and a daily glass of aloe vera juice. •AloeLife ALOE GOLD juice or Herbal Answers HERBAL ALOE FORCE are highly recommended.

2—Have miso, shiitake mushrooms, sea veggies and nutritional yeast 5 times a week.

3—Reduce meat proteins, and saturated and trans fats. Have fresh fish instead.

4—Probiotics, like UAS DDS-PLUS or •Jarrow JARRO-DOPHILUS with FOS to retard cancer cell growth. Sprinkle on food daily.

5—Cook with garlic, rosemary, turmeric, sage and oregano.

—**The best cancer-fighting foods** –organically grown: •*carotene-rich foods*: all red, orange, yellow fruits and veggies; tomatoes; green vegetables. Have a fresh green or sea-weed salad every day! •*antioxidant foods soak up free radicals*: garlic, onions, broccoli, sea veggies (kombu is a high fucoidan source–a substance found to cause cancer cells to self-destruct), leafy veggies, chiles, grapes, berries, carrots, turmeric, green tea, white tea, citrus. •*steamed cruciferous vegetables*: broccoli, broccoli sprouts, cabbage, brussels sprouts, cauliflower, kale and all dark greens. •*protease inhibitors*: beans (esp. soy), potatoes, corn, hibiscus tea, brown rice. •*high fiber foods*: whole grains, especially brown rice, apples, fruits and vegetables. •*enzyme-rich foods and herbs*: pineapple, papaya, mangoes, miso, sprouts, ginger, all fresh fruits and vegetables. •*lignan foods*: fish, flax oil, walnuts, berries.

Lifestyle bodywork support:

•Morning sunlight and regular exercise every day possible accelerate the passage of toxins (esp. for organ cancers). Yoga is especially good. No healing program will make it without some exercise. Avoid barbecued, blackened meat (has carcinogenic hydrocarbons).

•Guided imagery effectively helps the immune system work better, encourages the hormone system to stop making abnormal cells. See a good practitioner for real help.

•Enemas clean out purefaction: A coffee enema once a week for a month (1 cup strong brewed in 1 qt. water), castor oil enema, chlorella implants or a wheat grass retention enema.

—**Poultices for external growths:** •AloeLife ALOE SKIN GEL, or •Green clay poultice. •Garlic/onion or comfrey leaf poultice. •Dr. Christopher's BLACK DRAWING ointment (very strong); •Lane Labs SUN SPOT ES (highly recommended); •Crystal Star ANTI-BIO™ gel with una da gato.

—**Reduce side effects of chemotherapy or radiation:** •Reishi or turkey tail mushroom or Maitake D-fraction extract; Natural Balance MODUCARE plant sterols reduce nausea, hair loss, mouth sores. New Chapter GINGER WONDER syrup for nausea. •Apply kukui nut or sea buckthorn oil for chemo or radiation burns. •Nettles tea can dissolve adhesions.

Herbal, Superfood and Supplement Therapy

Interceptive therapy plan: Choose 2 to 3 recommendations.

1—**Detoxify:** •Crystal Star DETOX BLOOD PURIFIER™ caps, •GREEN TEA CLEANS-ER™ or •Flora FLORESSENCE tea each morning. Give yourself a weekly •vitamin C flush (also relieves pain) - up to 10g daily (until stool turns soupy). •Una da gato, if liver fluke parasites are involved–many cancers; •Calcium D-Glucarate 400mg daily, promotes glucuronidation to help eliminate toxins. •DAILY DETOX by M.D

2—**Discourage tumor growth:** ; •Dr. Rath's VITACOR PLUS and •Nutricology MODIFIED CITRUS PECTIN help stop cancer cell replication and metastasis; •Carnivora Research CARNIVORA® Immune Enhancer; •American Biosciences IMMPOWER; •Ginger extract, the world's best herbal inhibitor of 5-LO enzyme; •European mistletoe helps repair damaged DNA; •Enzymatic Therapy IP-6 (inositol); 800mg daily.

3—**Mushroom therapy (pg. 346) improves ability to fight cancer:** •Maitake mushroom extract or •Grifron MAITAKE D-FRACTION extract stimulate cancer cell death. •Agaricus mushroom stimulates interferon. •*Shiitake mushroom*, or Lane Labs NOXYLANE 4 from shiitake mushroom (triples natural killer cell activity.) •*Reishi* or •Maitake Products REISHI caps detox-fy, disperse toxins. •*Cordyceps* especially for breast cancer.

4—**Protect against free radical damage:** •Glutathione 150mg daily; •Lipoic acid, or •Jarrow ALPHA LIPOIC ACID 600mg daily; •Rosemary essential oil; •Astragalus extract. •Allergy Research GLUTATHIONE with vitamin C; •NutriCology LAKTOFERRIN with colostrum and TOTAL IMMUNE formula; •Flora VEGESIL or •Eidon SILICA MINERAL SUPPLEMENT; •Esteem IMMUNE LIFE with thymus; •INDIUMEASE (indium).

5—**Anti-angiogenesis blocks tumor support:** •Lane Labs SHARK CARTILAGE, or •Phoenix Biologics BOVINE TRACHEAL cartilage. Lane Labs ANGIOPM, 6 caps daily for one month (highly recommended fresh bindweed leaf extract. Not during pregnancy, surgery, heart disease or a healing wound).

6—**Natural anti-neoplastons reduce tumors:** •Green or white tea: •folic acid 800mcg; •vitamin E 800IU. •EFA's and Omega-3 oils: Evening Primrose oil 4000mg daily; fish or flaxseed oil, 1-oz daily for cancer. •NutriCology PRO-GREENS with EFA's.

7—**Enzyme therapy:** •Transformation Enzyme PUREZYME or Enzymedica PURIFY protease therapy between meals dissolves fibrin coating on cancer cells allowing immune defenses to work. Purifies the blood by breaking down protein invaders. •CoQ₁₀ 600mg daily or •Enzymatic Therapy VITALINE® COENZYME Q₁₀ 100mg with Vitamin E.

8—**Cancer fighters:** •Germanium 150mg and MODIFIED CITRUS PECTIN inhibit tumor metastasis; •grapeseed PCO's 300mg daily; •Beta-carotene 200,000IU daily, or •PHYCOTENE MICRO-CLUSTERS; •Eidon liquid SELENIUM (can cut cancer risk in half!); •Ester C with bioflavs 3000mg daily; •MICROHYDRIN PLUS.

9—**Superfood therapy:** •Pure Planet CHLORELLA or SPIRULINA. •Fit for You MIRACLE GREENS with barley grass. •Vibrant Health GREEN VIBRANCE

Can't find a recommended product? Call the 800 number listed in Product Resources for the store nearest you.

Recommendations for Specific Cancer Sites

Cancer is not one disease, but many. There are four types of cancerous growths: 1) *carcinomas*- affecting the skin, glands, organs and mucous membranes; 2) *leukemias*- blood cancers; 3) *sarcomas*- affecting connective tissue, bones and muscles; 4) *lymphomas*- affecting the lymph system. There can be more than one type of cancer in a location. The link between all cancers is this: certain cells become de-sensitized to normal growth constraints, then the damaged cells grow uncontrolled and may move (metastasize) to other sites in the body. Cancer is complex. There is no simple solution. Vigorous treatment is necessary on all fronts. But, more people are overcoming this devastating disease every day. Use the specific site recommendations along with the general cancer healing recommendations on preceeding page. Working with a natural health practitioner is advised.

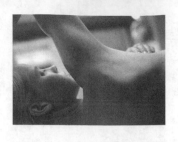

Breast Cancer
American Cancer Society statistics tell us that over 211,000 women fell victim to invasive breast cancer in 2003.

Of those, almost 40, 000 are expected to die of it, *up 50%* from a generation ago. 75% of all cases occur in women over 40, with post-menopausal, overweight women at highest risk. If you're more than 25% above your ideal weight, your risk rises because fat cells are the storage depots for environmental estrogens, pesticides, organo-chlorine residues and other chemical toxins. Weight gain around age 30 increases the long-term risk of breast cancer, too. A 10-pound increase raises the risk by 23%, a 15-pound increase by 37%, and a 20-pound increase by 52%. Women who have overly high, or imbalanced estrogen secretions and higher breast density are at high risk. Examples: women who had their first period before age 12, those who did not go through menopause until after age 55, those who did not have a child before age 30, those who did not carry a pregnancy full-term, and those who smoke. Women whose diet is high in meats and dairy foods have a higher risk. Many food animals are injected with hormones that add to the environmental estrogens circulating in a woman's body. Women who eat soy foods have lower levels of circulating estrogen. Vegetarians have fewer instances of breast cancer because they process estrogen differently.... and they are less exposed to hormone-injected animals like beef and pork. Long term synthetic estrogen and/or oral contraceptive use, and estrogen-containing pesticides are also risk factors for breast cancer. Indeed, there is a veritable assault on female hormone balance from man-made estrogens. Regular exercise is a key to fighting breast cancer, because it favorably alters body chemistry to control fat deposits which store excess estrogen, and increases fat metabolism, which helps flush out excess estrogens. Try to limit your exposure to environmental estrogens.

Are you at risk of developing breast cancer? Synthetic estrogens can stack the deck against women by increasing their estrogen levels hundreds of times.

Studies released in the last few years draw a clear connection between HRT (hormone replacement therapy) and breast cancer. A 2000 study shows women taking HRT for just five years have a 40 percent greater risk of developing breast cancer. Another study finds that long-term HRT may boost the odds of one of the most dangerous types of breast cancer as much as 85 percent! (Thankfully, some research shows that this higher risk for breast cancer greatly diminishes when a woman has been off HRT treatment for five years.) Five percent of breast cancer cases appear in women who inherit the BRCA 1 or BRCA 2 gene. These women have up to 85% chance of developing the disease. (Many women with these genes are having prophylactic (preventive) surgery to remove both breasts and their ovaries before there are even signs of cancer!) The greatest breast cancer rise is in women born after World War II, an era that ushered in massive amounts of new chemicals, processed foods, and drugs like super strong antibiotics and hormone therapy into American life. Estrogen imitators like many pesticides, household chemicals and common plastics developed during the war then found their way into agriculture and household products without the normal years of testing for long term health effects. Only in the last five years have we realized how common synthetic estrogens are. Breast or prostate cancer in a woman's father's family doubles her risk. Chemotherapy does not seem to improve a woman's chances for survival, especially if the cancer has spread to the lymph nodes.

The mammogram debate: Early detection can mean less radical medical intervention, but it is not prevention. A healthy lifestyle should be the primary goal.

Studies from the 1970's and 80's showing that mammograms reduced death rates are now seen to be seriously flawed. Mammograms have improved in the last 20 years, but I still hear enough horror stories about swift fibroid onset to feel that mammograms should not be done without suspected cause. The scientific community itself is debating whether death rates from breast cancer are reduced at all by mammograms in women under 50. Younger women's breasts are dense, so mammograms only detect dangerous lesions in young women about 50% of the time. Further, low-dose radiation can cause breast fibroids, so mammograms in younger women should only be needed if there are abnormal lumps or nipple infections. A major problem is that mammograms can't distinguish between slow growing tumors and aggressive ones. Thus, some non-invasive, non life threatening cancers may be treated more aggressively than necessary. Even in women over 50, mammograms should be undertaken with care. A recent study in the National Cancer Institute Journal shows radiologists report false positives 16% of the time! Women who have annual mammograms after fifty may receive up to three false positives in their lifetime causing unbelievable emotional trauma. Research also shows mammograms miss cancer 15% of the time! By the time a tumor reaches detectable size, it has probably been growing for 10 years or more and may even have spread.

Can't find a recommended product? Call the 800 number listed in Product Resources for the store nearest you.

Is Thermography an effective alternative to mammograms? FDA approved in 1982, thermography is a highly advanced health scanning technique that offers the benefits of breast cancer screening without the drawbacks of mammogram radiation. Over 12,000 articles worldwide detail its success. Angiogenesis (new blood vessel growth produced by tumors) generates abnormal heat in the area of a tumor. Thermography takes measurements of skin surface temperature to determine cancer risk. Thermography is very precise, and may be a better tool than mammograms for detecting breast cancer, finding abnormalities in breast tissue 8-10 years before mammogram detection. It can also reveal the state of body organs, determine if imbalances are present and what might be causing them. Experts say it can show if an organ or system is susceptible to tumors before there are even signs on an X-ray or CT scan. Thermography can help you determine whether supplements you're taking are helping or hurting you. Some doctors recommend using thermography in conjunction with traditional breast cancer detection mammograms. But, for women who refuse mammograms because of their high rate of false positives and false negatives, their link to fibroids and X-ray-harmed breast tissue, thermography offers a non-invasive technique to keep them better informed of their breast health. To find a skilled thermography practitioner, visit *www.thermography.net* on the web to learn more.

What signs should alert you to possible breast cancer? Nipple discharge, or scaly skin patches around nipples or nipple retraction are common. Breast lumps, especially firm lumps with poorly defined edges that don't move when touched or don't change during your cycle, often along with breast skin irritation or dimpling and change in breast texture or color are serious alert signs. Also, watch for unusual enlargement of lymph nodes in the armpit. Any breast changes not related to your regular menstrual cycle should be watched. Chronic swollen sores around your mouth, gums or jaw, severe unexplained morning nausea and hypothyroidism linked to low iodine can be early warning factors.

—Alternative healing protocols: Reduce animal fats in your diet to cut your breast cancer risk by 33%. Especially avoid fats and trans fats from sugary foods, snack foods, fried foods, dairy foods and high sugar alcoholic drinks. Increase your fiber and antioxidants from fruits, vegetables, whole grains and soy. Add vegetables like broccoli and cauliflower with estrogen-reducing effects. Foods rich in carotenoids (esp. lutein), like dark greens, tomatoes and watermelon can improve breast cancer prognosis, or take mixed carotene PHYCOTENE MICROCLUSTERS from sea greens available at royalbodycare.com. British research shows frequent water consumption may reduce breast cancer risk by 79%! Drink plenty of bottled water, or consider a high quality water filtration system like AQUASANA. Find an organic supply of chicken and turkey with no hormone injections. Fish, especially wild salmon, provides protective EFAs. Sea greens provide EFAs and protective plant minerals, like copper, zinc, chromium, manganese and magnesium, critical to detoxification pathways, and reduce the cancer-promoting effects of chemical overload. **Hypothyroidism is regularly involved in breast cancer.** Sea greens are a natural iodine source that balances thyroid activity. Use 2 tbsp. daily of dry sea greens, or take •Crystal Star OCEAN MINERALS™ iodine, potassium, silica caps or drops.

Crystal Star EST-AID™ is a lab-tested, proven cancer inhibiting formula. Add •Lane Labs NOXYLANE from *shiitake mushroom* (increases natural killer cell activity.) for 6 months. *Cordyceps mushroom tests* have been especially effective for fighting breast cancer. *Carnivora juice* treatment shows good results (Dr. Helmut Keller). •Vitamin C, up to 10,000mg with bioflavonoids (a proven cancer deterrent); Lane Labs PALM VITEE tocotrienols help inhibit cancer growth. •COX II inhibitors work: •New Chapter ZYFLAMEND and •CoQ-10, 300mg daily. •*Milk thistle* seed extract inhibits cancer cell replication; •PCO's, 300mg daily (from *white pine bark or grape seeds*) are some of the most potent antioxidants and free radical scavengers known - 50% more potent than vitamins E or C. **Stimulate glutathione:** •New Life hormone-free COLOSTRUM and Nutricology MCP show great promise for breast cancer. •GLUCOSAMINE-CHONDROITIN 4 daily helps reduce bone pain. **Protective measures:** Low body levels of the hormone melatonin may raise breast cancer risk; •melatonin, .1 to .3mg at night. •Nature's Way DIM-Plus (*Diindolylmethane*) helps balance estrogen for breast cancer prevention; •Royal jelly, ¼ tsp. daily, with *pcnax ginseng, Evening Primrose Oil,* 3000mg daily boost EFAs and boost adrenal activity. •Vitamin E 400IU, selenium 200mcg daily, and folic acid 400mcg. •Calcium D-Glucarate 2000mg help detoxify carcinogens.

Prostate Cancer

Prostate cancer afflicts one in nine men over age seventy in the U.S. and it's striking at an ever earlier age (25% of cases occur in men under 65). This year over 220,000 new prostate cancer cases will be diagnosed… around 30,000 men die each year. Death rates for prostate cancer have been declining since the early 1990's. But hard hit African American men have a much higher prostate cancer incidence, and death rates twice as high as white men. Their prostate cancer incidence went up an astounding 300% just from 1985 to 1996!

Prostate cancer is clearly associated with the conversion of normal testosterone to di-hydro-testosterone by the enzyme 5-alpha reductase, (one consequence of a high fat, high sugar, low fiber, high cholesterol diet). A vegetarian diet is a proven weapon against prostate cancer, since high fiber, low-fat foods excrete hormones linked to its onset. The 50% drop in American male sperm counts along with the doubling of prostate cancer in the last 50 years, has focused research on environmental estrogens, androgens and pollutants that may put men at risk. Abnormally high ratios of estradiol to testosterone may be a big factor in prostate cancer development. A monthly self-exam should be a part of your prevention plan if you are over fifty. Men with osteoporosis are at higher risk. *Note: The supplement chondroitin sulfate used in natural arthritis treatment may accelerate prostate cancer growth. Consider other natural options like glucosamine sulfate, and anti-inflammatory enzymes and herbs instead.*

Can't find a recommended product? Call the 800 number listed in Product Resources for the store nearest you.

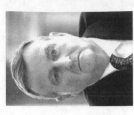

The PSA Test:

The Prostate Specific Antigen (PSA) blood test has meant better diagnosing of prostate cancer. Unfortunately, the PSA test has also produced an epidemic of prostate radiation and surgery, procedures that can be as devastating as the disease. Studies show that surgery often only extends life a few months. Almost 2% of men die within 90 days of prostate cancer surgery, and 8% experience severe heart and lung complications. Because surgery and radiation damage nerves that lead to the penis and rectum, both treatments regularly cause incontinence (over 12%) and impotence (over 10%). Radiation treatments frequently initiate a free radical cascade that reduces immune response. *Get a second opinion if you are diagnosed with prostate cancer.* Two out of three men with border-line high PSA levels don't have prostate cancer. In fact, as you age, the acceptable level for a PSA goes up, since most elderly men have *some* prostate cancer cells. PSA's under 4.0 are accepted for low risk, but a 60-year old man can have a PSA of 6.0 without having cancer. Most men with prostate cancer do not die of it. Life expectancy with surgery and radiation is almost the same as with no treatment for this localized, non-invasive cancer. Unless surgery is absolutely necessary, monitored "watchful waiting" may be a better choice for avoiding the enormous pain and disability.

You should be concerned, however, about invasive prostate cancer, which rapidly engulfs the organ and spreads through the body. This deadly form of prostate cancer is increasing among men in their 40's and 50's in all western countries. Dr. Burzynski's Antineoplaston Therapy really takes down PSA numbers, for some men to a normal 1.3, even after metastasis.

What signs alert you to prostate cancer? lumps in prostate or testicles; thickening and fluid retention in the scrotum; persistent, unexplained back pain or pain in the pelvis or upper thighs; frequent, straining or difficult urination, similar to benign prostatitis. If the cancer outgrows the small prostate gland, it often eats its way into the bladder or rectum, even the pelvis and back, causing severe damage. Note: if you're considering the new testosterone therapy for better sex drive, consider that testosterone therapy may stimulate prostate cancer.

—**Alternative healing protocols:** Improve your diet: •Add soy foods. Soy has at least five proven anti-cancer agents, with anti-estrogenic activity that can retard development of prostate cancer. •Add quercetin foods like green tea, garlic, onions, apples, leafy greens and red wine to your daily diet. Quercetin guards against cancer cell proliferation. •Reduce animal fats to 15% or less of your calorie intake. Barbequed red meat is linked to metastatic prostate cancers. •Add more fish and seafood instead. Recent research shows eating fish and seafood more than three times a week reduces prostate cancer metastasis risk. •Reduce sugars and refined carbohydrates which increase insulin production and raise prostate cancer risk. •Reduce dairy foods like cow's milk, ice cream, and cheese. Eliminate caffeine or sodas. •Add 4 to 6 grams of fiber daily from whole grains, flax seeds, vegetables and fresh or dried fruits. •Include carotene-rich foods like broccoli, and green and orange vegetables. Just one serving a day of lycopene-rich foods like tomatoes, grapefruit or watermelon juice reduces the risk of developing prostate cancer by 82%! Or take 10mg lycopene supplement. •Add cruciferous veggies to help detoxify hormone-disrupting pollutants. Consider Nature's Way DIM-PLUS, 200mg daily, if you are at high risk.

—New research shows that **ginger** is the world's greatest herbal inhibitor of 5-LO enzyme, a food source for prostate cancer cells. Without their only food source, prostate cancer cells die in 1 to 2 hours. I recommend daily *ginger* for every man at risk for, or currently in the grip of, prostate cancer. •New Chapter PROSTATE 5lx is a premier prostate support formula rich in herbal 5-LO inhibitors, like *ginger rt.* and *saw palmetto berry.* New Chapter ZYFLAMEND shows good results in prostate cancer inhibition, and cancer cell apoptosis (programmed cell death) in new Columbia University in vitro tests. •Phyto-hormone-rich •Crystal Star PROSTATE PROTECTOR™ caps with *saw palmetto, pygeum,* and *potency wood* for help in inhibiting the DHT form of testosterone linked to prostate cancer. •Raintree Nutrition N-TENSE with antimicrobial, anti-tumor herbs like *graviola* (I have personally seen positive effects). Use as directed. **Antioxidants retard cancer cell growth:** •CoQ₁₀, 300mg daily, •Wakunaga AGED GARLIC EXTRACT or *garlic* capsules 8 daily inhibit cancer growth. •calcium D-Glucarate 2000mg daily, •Zinc 50mg daily and •EVENING PRIMROSE oil 4000mg daily. •A three month course of •*milk thistle seed extract* or *nettles extract* helps your liver metabolize excess fats. Include •vitamin C 10,000mg daily (see page 193). **Protective measures:** Rich antioxidants like glutathione 100mg daily, •vitamin E 400IU with mixed tocopherols 400IU and selenium 400mcg daily; •PCO's from *grapeseed* or *white pine,* 200mg daily, especially against invasive cancer. •Nutricology MCP (modified citrus pectin), helps prevent cancer metastasis. •Melatonin .1 to .3mg. at night may act as a prostate cancer deterrent. **Exercise is a must** for men dealing with prostate cancer (new research shows exercise slows prostate cancer growth by 30%!), as is 15 minutes a day of early morning sunlight on the genitals for vitamin D. African-American men have a 40% higher rate of prostate cancer than white men because they synthesize less vitamin D. Black men should add 400IU vitamin D daily. Cautions: 1) If you have prostate cancer, avoid DHEA supplements. DHEA can be converted to testosterone which may stimulate the cancer.

Testicular Cancer

Today about 7,400 men a year are diagnosed with testicular cancer. That's twice the number of cases from 30 years ago! Testicular cancer is highly curable when caught early. Even stage 3 testicular cancer (the most advanced) has an 80% cure rate. American cyclist Lance Armstrong won the Tour de France in 1999 after surviving *advanced* testicular cancer! Unlike prostate cancer, it's a younger man's disease, usually striking men under 35. It's much more common among sedentary men than active men (over 70% higher for men who sit more than 10 hours a day than those who sit less than 2 hours a day). Many experts believe exposure to xenoestrogens in the womb or the environment may be linked to testicular cancer risk.

Can't find a recommended product? Call the 800 number listed in Product Resources for the store nearest you.

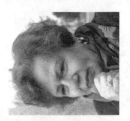

What signs alert you to testicular cancer? Testicular cancer spreads quickly - it can move to lymph nodes in a few months. Early detection means less impotence, higher survival rates. Roll each testicle between thumb and forefinger to check for lumps, tenderness or swelling. A history of undescended testicles is linked to testicular cancer.

—**Alternative healing protocols:** most recommendations for prostate cancer apply to testicular cancer. •Especially reduce saturated and trans fats. •Add green tea to your morning diet. •Add EFAs from *Evening primrose oil* and sea greens to your diet. •Add Vitamin C, 5000mg daily, along with selenium 200mcg and mixed carotenes 100,000IU daily.

Cervical, Uterine *(Endometrial)* Cancer Even after dysplasia surgery, recurrence is common if lifestyle changes aren't made.

Women who take estrogen replacement therapy for menopausal symptoms are especially at risk (symptoms are clearly aggravated by excess estrogen). Over-weight women, especially if they smoke, are at significant risk (smoking secretes toxins into cervical mucous). Women, between the ages of 55 and 75, especially those who have never been pregnant, (or conversely, have had more than five births), are vulnerable. Using oral contraceptives for 5 or more years in a row, a history of frequent abortions or sexually transmitted disease like chlamydia and cervical dysplasia are linked. Virtually all cases of cervical cancer are triggered by HPV the *human papilloma virus*. A new gene test to check for HPV (human papilloma virus) may one day replace the PAP. Untreated cervical cancer usually spreads to un-derlying connective tissue, lymph glands, the uterus and urinary tract. Serious vaginal infections like trichomonas, exposure to heavy metals, asbestos and herbicides increase risk The drug tamoxifen may also increase the risk of endometrial cancer.

What signs alert you to cervical or uterine cancer? Infertility or difficulty getting pregnant should alert you. Symptoms advance steadily.... unusual bleeding after menopause; discharge between menstrual periods; painful, heavy periods; vaginal bleeding during intercourse indicate the presence of polyps. A class 4 PAP smear is a clear pre-cancerous sign.

—**Alternative healing protocols:** •**Reduce fatty meats and dairy foods** in your diet immediately. These animal crops receive hormone and antibiotic injections. The excess estrogen correlation between these foods and uterine cancer is undeniable. **Add food protectors:** Fresh fruits and vegetables, especially cruciferous vegetables (a vital food medicine against this cancer), oranges, tomatoes, carrots and artichokes. Add •soy foods 3 times a week and •2 tsp. high potency royal jelly daily (tested effective). •Add sea greens for carotenes or take a carotene supplement like sea greens PHYCOTENE MICROCLUSTERS from Healthy House daily. •Crystal Star CALCIUM-MAGNESIUM SOURCE™ or an herbal calcium with *nettles* to prevent pre-cancerous lesions from becoming cancerous. •Take *Evening Primrose Oil*, or high Omega-3 flax oil and COQ10 300mg daily. •Ester C, up to 10,000mg daily and •vitamin E 800IU daily with selenium 200mcg daily. **Natural progesterone protection:** •Pure Essence Labs FEM CREME. *Note:* the American Cancer Society has dropped its recommendation that women have a PAP test every year - advising it only if the woman is at high risk. Women over 30 at low risk are now advised to get a PAP test every 2 to 3 years If you have a Type II PAP smear, take •green drinks daily, use •Crystal Star WOMAN'S BEST FRIEND™ for 3 to 6 months; Nature's Way DIM-PLUS *(diindolylmethane)*, 400mg daily; and •folic acid 800mcg daily.

Ovarian Cancer Investigate unusual symptoms with your doctor right away. Long term estrogen replacement therapy increases ovarian cancer risk.

Women at risk seem to be those who have never had children, didn't breastfeed, are past menopause or are overweight from a high fat diet. Excess ovulation, especially from fertil-ity drug treatment, adds to the risk. NutraSweet is implicated in ovarian cancer. Avoid it, especially in hot drinks. Check the dates on products that contain NutraSweet. Old NutraSweet breaks down into DKP, a tumor-causing substance. Use a talc-free condom during intercourse; do not dust your perineum with talcum. Asbestos exposure is also implicated, as well as some anti-inflammatory drugs (salicylates, non-steroidals, and cortico-steroids). Some reports show that the risk of developing leukemia from platinum-based chemotherapy (with cisplatin or carboplatin) for ovarian cancer is high enough to outweigh the benefits.

What signs alert you to ovarian cancer? In early stages, ovarian cancer has no symptoms, except abdominal bloating and pain, chronic, unexplained indigestion, weight loss, abnormal bleeding, frequent urination. There may be no signs until the cancer has metastasized. If caught early, ovarian cancer can often be stopped with surgery and lifestyle changes.

—**Alternative healing protocols:** •Add EFAs: Omega-3 rich flax oil, or *Evening Primrose Oil* 300mg daily. Boost your fresh fruits and vegetables, especially cruciferous veg-etables. Keep fats low, and include soy foods for protein instead of meats or dairy foods. •Add sea greens, 2 tbsp. daily as a source of iodine therapy and carotenes, especially if a thyroid disorder is involved. Avoid fried foods and commercial eggs. **If you are at a high risk,** •drink green tea or Crystal Star GREEN TEA CLEANSER™ every morning. (Green tea shows dramatic reduction in ovarian cancer risk.) •A recent in vitro National Cancer Institute study shows indole-3-carbinol (I3C) and DIM (diindolylmethane) inhibit ovarian cancer cells and enhance chemo effectiveness. Try •Nature's Way DIM-PLUS 400mg daily. Take high potency •Prince of Peace ROYAL JELLY-GINSENG vials daily. **Add anti-oxidant supplements:** •mixed carotenes 150,000IU daily, like Royal Bodycare PHYCOTENE MICROCLUSTERS from sea plants; •Ester C, up to 10,000mg with bioflavonoids daily, vitamin E 800IU daily with selenium 200mcg. Take •milk thistle seed extract and green superfoods like •Green Foods GREEN MAGMA, or •Crystal Star ENERGY GREEN RENEWAL™ drink for 3 months. Use •Pure Essence Labs FEM CREME for natural progesterone protection. The Gonzales-Isaacs Program has shown good results in some cases (page 346).

Can't find a recommended product? Call the 800 number listed in Product Resources for the store nearest you.

Bladder-Kidney Cancer (Renal Cell Carcinoma)

America adds more than 50,000 new cases of bladder and kidney cancer every year. Smoking is implicated as a main cause in both bladder and kidney cancers. Chlorine from drinking water is linked to 4,200 cases of bladder cancers a year! A history of cystitis and polycystic kidney disease add to the risk. Men have a 4 times higher risk for bladder cancer than women. Men working in dye, rubber or leather industries also have a higher bladder cancer risk. High use of diuretic drugs increases risk of renal cell cancer.

What signs alert you to bladder-kidney cancer? Bloody or difficult urine; sometimes side or loin pain.

—**Alternative healing protocols:** Increase your fresh vegetables, especially carrots, or •Green Foods CARROT ESSENCE. Have steamed cruciferous veggies daily to help detoxify carcinogens. Drink up to ten 8-oz glasses of water a day. I recommend PENTA bottled water. Have fruit twice a day. Have cold water fish twice a week. Take •garlic 10 tablets daily. Take •una da gato extract twice daily. Take high potency lactobacillus, or •UAS DDS-PLUS with FOS or •American Health ACIDOPHILUS LIQUID and add antioxidants: vitamin A 40,000IU (short term), B-6 250mg, vitamin C 3000mg, vitamin E 400IU with selenium 200mcg, and zinc 50mg to help prevent bladder cancer recurrence. Take •Nutricology MODIFIED CITRUS PECTIN (MCP) to inhibit growth into other sites. Add •sea greens to your diet for further antioxidants and iodine therapy; 2 tbsp. daily.

Colon / Colo-Rectal Cancer

Over the long term, experts say that 90% of colon cancer may be avoidable through diet improvement for colon protection.

Because America's diet is still loaded with fat, red meat and refined carbohydrates and still low in protective fiber, colon cancer has become the number two cause of cancer death in the U.S. 50,000 people die every year from it. New studies show overweight men and women (especially those who smoke) are particularly at risk. Don't be fooled by studies which failed to show a low fat, high fiber diet provided colon cancer protection. Experts now say those tests were flawed because they only measured short-term benefits while colon cancer takes decades to develop. Long standing family diet habits which lead to a family history of colon cancer, colitis and diabetes are regularly involved. A low fat, high fiber diet can dramatically reduce development of benign polyps that usually lead to colon cancer. A seasonal colon cleanse (see page 196) and regular exercise may be your best defense against colon cancer. Numerous studies show that daily exercise and sunshine lower the risk of colon cancer.

What signs alert you to colon cancer? persistent diarrhea, changing to persistent constipation for no apparent reason, blood in the bowel movement, and a change in shape of the stool to a thin, flattened appearance. Often pain and gas in the lower right abdomen, as well as unusual weight loss and fatigue. Colon cancer begins as polyps on the colon walls. For pre-cancerous polyps, •take vitamin C with bioflavonoids 5000mg daily and a daily green drink like Green Foods GREEN MAGMA.

—**Alternative healing protocols:** high fiber foods, like an apple, banana, 1 cup raspberries and a green salad every day, as part of a low fat, low meat diet are still the keys for colon cancer protection. Add whole grain cereals, especially wheat bran that moves through the colon quickly, fresh vegetables, especially cruciferous vegetables, moderate amounts of olive oil, soy foods (protease inhibitors), legumes and high fiber foods like dried fruits. Include carotene-rich, antioxidant foods like tomatoes, watermelon and fresh greens. Add calcium rich foods like broccoli and dark greens (also a good source of lutein, a protective phytonutrient against colon cancer). Especially avoid fatty red meats, alcohol and sugary foods.

—**Inhibitory vitamins:** the strongest inhibitory is •vitamin E 800IU with selenium 200mcg. **Calcium offers colon cancer protection:** Lane Labs ADVACAL FAST RELEASE 4 daily; vitamin C 5000mg daily with bioflavonoids (can dramatically lower risk); beta carotene 100,000IU; •MSM, 1000mg is a chemo-preventive for colon cancer. •Boost EFAs like GLA such as in •EVENING PRIMROSE oil 3000mg daily and Omega-3 rich flax seed oil to reverse pre-cancerous changes in the rectum; take flax seed tea for fiber. Drink • green tea or Crystal Star GREEN TEA CLEANSER™ each morning. •Nutricology MCP (Modified Citrus Pectin) helps prevent tumor spread. Normalize colon environment: •B-complex 100mg daily; •folic acid 800mcg daily. •CoQ$_{10}$, 300mg daily. •Carnitine 2000mg daily, •acidophilus daily with meals; •New Chapter ZYFLAMEND caps inhibits inflammatory Cox-2 enzyme.

—**Inhibitory herbs:** •Garlic is a proven colon cancer inhibitor; 10 capsules daily may reduce tumors by 75%. •Cat's claw extract (una da gato), •Ginkgo biloba and astragalus extracts reduce tumor development. •Research shows Turmeric extract capsules help inhibit colon tumors; •Shark cartilage (try Lane Labs SHARK CARTILAGE), or bovine trachael cartilage, inhibit tumors from forming new blood vessels. Tumors also shrink from lack of nutrients as the blood vessels shrivel. Shark cartilage is rich in calcium, a specific preventive for colon cancer. **Ginseng-based herbal combinations speed healing and normalize cell structure.** Ginseng enhances antibody response, strengthens the immune properties of cellular connective tissues, normalizes blood cells according to need, normalizes cell structure and has a distinct activity against radiation. •GINSENG/REISHI extract has shown in vitro results against colon cancer cells. •Drink ginseng tea if you've had polyps surgically removed to recover faster. Try ginseng tea during healing. •Shiitake mushrooms contain the polysaccharide, lentinan, an anti-cancer agent and immune cell stimulant. •Turkey tail mushrooms help reduce tumor development. •Green drinks like Pure Planet CHLORELLA with easily absorbed calcium, help prevent colorectal tumors. •Jarrow JARRO-DOPHILUS with FOS encourages a healthy gut environment.

Note: The traditional herbal formula •ESSIAC has been effective for colon cancer. In my experience, it isn't complex enough to address cancer as it exists today. Including pau d'arco for immune response, and panax ginseng for reverse transformation on malignant cells with Essiac formulas may be able to address today's more complex cancers. Contact Syracuse Cancer Research Institute at 315-472-6616 to see if treatment with hydrazine sulfate is right for you.

Can't find a recommended product? Call the 800 number listed in Product Resources for the store nearest you.

Home Colorectal Cancer Screening Tests: Available through medical supplies stores and some pharmacies.

You can test for possible colon cancer yourself, but all colorectal cancers cannot be detected by this test. False positives are not uncommon. Other factors besides cancer can introduce small amounts of blood into the stool. Aspirin, hemorrhoids, gastrointestinal problems, and some foods like popcorn may cause blood in the stool. To reduce risk of false results, follow directions scrupulously. Early-stage colorectal tumors release a tiny amount of blood, which becomes incorporated into the stool and can be detected. Some tests rely on chemically impregnated toilet paper to detect the blood. If the toilet paper changes color after use, it indicates a positive result. Others require the user to place a sheet of test paper in the toilet bowl following a bowel movement. If a color change appears on the paper, blood is present in the stool.

Stomach and Esophageal Cancer

In the last 25 years, esophageal cancer has increased 350%, faster than any other cancer!

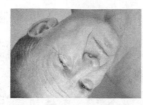

Esophageal cancer is linked to the high rates of GERD (gastroesophageal reflux disease) in America. (See pg.425 of this book for recommendations to reduce GERD.) A high fat, low fiber diet is always linked to stomach cancer and stomach polyps. The elderly are especially at risk, because of low stomach acid (HCl) production and less dietary fiber; many have pernicious anemia. Smoking is a high risk factor. Dietary habits contribute to onset - high intake of red meat and nitrates, heavy alcohol use; low intake of fresh fruits, vegetables, and the vitamins C and E in them which significantly inhibit the formation of nitrosamines. Research reveals eating 1½ cups of berries a day may cut the risk for esophageal cancer in half! The gastric pathogen *H. pylori* is strongly linked to stomach cancer, another result of nitrite metabolism.

What signs alert you to stomach cancer? Stomach cancer takes a long time to develop, sometimes as much as fifteen years. Do you have pain after eating? Do you take large amounts of antacids regularly? Chronic indigestion, heartburn or GERD (gastroesophageal reflux disease) and gastritis, all contribute.

—Alternative healing protocols: Eat 3 servings of fresh vegetables at every meal. especially crucifers like broccoli for antioxidants and vitamin C. (Eating Chinese white cabbage just once a week may cut risk for gastric cancer in half.) Eat small frequent meals - no large meals. Take probiotics like •Nutricology SYMBIOTICS with FOS with meals. Limit alcohol to a small drink a day. Limit salt to less than 2500mg a day. Avoid cured meats and smoked foods like bacon, ham or hot dogs, and hot peppers. **Reduce caffeine:** •Drink green tea, •Crystal Star DR. VITALITY™ green and white tea, or •Crystal Star GREEN TEA CLEANSER™. •Add soy foods 3 times a week. Add whole wheat and wheat bran. Add garlic 8 caps daily or Wakunaga KYOLIC AGED GARLIC extract. **Add glutathione-rich foods:** avocados, asparagus, grapefruit, oranges and tomatoes, or take glutathione 100mg daily. **Take green superfoods:** •Pines MIGHTY GREENS or Crystal Star ENERGY GREEN RENEWAL™. •Take CoQ₁₀ 300mg daily. **Take proteolytic enzymes:** •Transformation Enzyme PURE-ZYME high protease formula) or •Crystal Star DR. ENZYME™ with protease and bromelain or •bromelain 1500mg daily. **Inhibitory vitamins:** •all carotenes, vitamin C and E 800IU with selenium 200mcg. •Cat's claw extract (*una da gato*) and turkey tail mushroom reduce tumor development. •*Siberian eleuthero*, a specific to stomach cancer, extends life for some by as much as 5 years

Lung Cancer

Lung cancer is still the leading cause of cancer deaths worldwide. •Have an apple every day, it's a prime lung protector.

Lung cancer is still rising in the U.S. as well, with around 172,000 new cases annually and the astounding rate of 157,200 deaths per year! Women who smoke are especially vulnerable - twice as likely to develop lung cancer as male smokers. 85% percent of lung cancer cases are attributable to cigarette smoke, (including potentized marijuana strains, 100 times more likely to cause lung cancer than tobacco). The remaining 15% is attributed to heavy metals, radioactive exposure, radon gas which leaches into tap water, toxic chemicals like pesticides and herbicides, chronic bronchitis and T.B. •Chinese herbal medicine is a vanguard in broncho-pulmonary cancers. Seek out a Traditional Chinese Medicine specialist.

What signs alert you to lung cancer? a persistent cough and chest pain, hoarseness, sore throat, increasingly, blood in the sputum. The cough changes and worsens, chest pain, pneumonia and bronchitis recur and increase as the cancer grows. There is unusual sweating, poor circulation, feverishness and unhealthy weight loss as the disease progresses.

—Alternative healing protocols: Carotenes hold the key to deterring lung cancer. There are over 600 carotenes in orange, red and yellow fruits and vegetables. Lung cancer risk has been reduced by 75% with the nutritional therapy of lycopene-rich tomatoes, broccoli, and watermelon.... eat at least 3 servings 3x a day during healing. •PHYCOTENE MICROCLUSTERS (mixed carotenes) from marine plants. •Crystal Star OCEAN MINERALS™ caps contain rich carotenes. •Reduce dairy foods in your diet. Improving your vegetable intake supplies more absorbable calcium for healing. A *Nutrition and Cancer* study shows an herb and vegetable soup can more than triple survival time for advanced lung cancer patients (one of the deadliest cancers), far surpassing the success of chemotherapy treatment. (*Soup ingredients were soybeans, mung beans, shitake mushrooms, red dates, scallions, garlic, lentils, leeks, hawthorn fruit, onions, ginseng, angelica root, licorice, dandelion root, senegal root, ginger, olives, sesame seeds and parsley. Note: The commercial product is available on www.sunfarmcorp.com.*) •Add sulphur-rich garlic tabs 6-10 daily. •Add lentinan-rich shiitake mushrooms and soyfoods 3 times a week.... good protease inhibitors to block lung cancer. **Risk protectors:** •Vitamin C is a critical protective nutrient against lung cancer - 5000mg or more daily. •Vitamin E 1000IU with selenium 200mcg. •Calcium D-Glucarate 2000mg daily, •Nutricology GERMANIUM 200mg, and •Nutricology LACTOFERRIN with colustrum. •Drink green tea daily or take Crystal Star GREEN TEA CLEANSER™ each morning. •Cat's claw (*una da gato*) helps reduce tumors, for some even after metastasis. •Reishi mushrooms boost interferon. Apply •Earth's Bounty O₂ SPRAY to the chest for more tissue oxygen.

Can't find a recommended product? Call the 800 number listed in Product Resources for the store nearest you.

Liver and Pancreatic Cancers

Organ cancers are some of the most difficult to deal with.

Organ cancers are so deep in the body, their influence on all body systems is widespread, and they metastasize quickly. A high fat diet, smoking, pancreatitis, diabetes, cirrhosis, being overweight and lack of exercise increases your risk.

What signs alert you to liver and pancreatic cancer? Extreme tiredness is usually first. If cancer develops near the bile duct, jaundice may also occur.

—**Alternative healing protocols:** A macrobiotic diet has led to a long remission in one documented case. See pg. 348. Fresh vegetables are the key, especially cruciferous vegetables, like broccoli and cabbage, at least 3 servings per meal for antioxidants and vitamin C. Several studies show that high vitamin C intake reduces the risk of pancreatic cancer. •Take up to 10,000mg daily with bioflavonoids. •**Carotenes are critical**, especially lycopene-rich foods like tomatoes and watermelon. •Watercress and arugula with almost 500 different carotenes are liver cancer specifics, or take •PHYCOTENE MICROCLUSTERS with mixed carotenes from sea greens. **Green drinks are essential:** try •Crystal Star ENERGY GREEN RENEWAL™, or •AloeLife ALOE GOLD, or •Sun Wellness Chlorella WAKASA GOLD. Add 2 tsp. high Omega-3 flax oil to any drink. •Lane Labs NOXYLANE 4 improves natural anti-tumor defenses. •Alpha Lipoic Acid 600mg daily. •Allergy Research LAKTOFERRIN with colostrum boosts immune strength. **Herbal medicines have a proven record.** Mega-doses are important at first. •Include: *schizandra, milk thistle seed, shiitake and maitake mushrooms, dandelion, ginkgo biloba, pau d'arco, echinacea, and saw palmetto.* **Enzyme therapy is critical in organ cancers.** •Enzymedica PURIFY (protease) •Crystal Star DR. ENZYME™ with protease and bromelain or •bromelain 1500mg daily. **Significant to any program:** •CoQ-10 300mg daily, L-Carnitine 3000mg daily, Chromium picolinate 250mcg daily, Glutathione 100mg daily. •Avoid alcohol. Reduce fats and add soy foods to your diet at least three times a week as a protease inhibitor. The Gonzales-Isaacs Program shows excellent results in many cases. A ten-year study shows *European Mistletoe* extract may prolong life for pancreatic cancer patients. Visit *www.iscador.com* to learn more. Beware of the drug *loratadine* (Claritin), an antihistamine. It causes liver tumors in animal tests.

Brain Cancer

Most brain tumors grow slowly for years, but when they become large, progressive problems develop quite rapidly. The use of pesticides in pest strips have been linked to brain cancer, especially in children. Excessive intake of Nutrasweet has produced a high incidence link with brain tumors. The brain is also often a site for the metastasis of other tumors, usually from the lungs, ovaries and breast. Question closely the call for a brain biopsy; it could set the cancer cells free to roam the rest of the body.

What signs alert you to brain cancer? recent onset of cluster headaches, and neurological symptoms like sudden numbness, twitching or seizures; weakness, lethargy, night sweats and unexplained nausea; personality change usually with mental decline; double vision and poor motor coordination; unusual weight loss.

—**Alternative healing protocols:** Find an acupuncturist with a track record in treating brain tumors. Add prayer and meditation to your life. Qi Gong and deep tissue massage reduce stress that impairs healing. Keep your immune system strong with •plenty of fresh vegetable juices and aloe vera juice. **Use superfoods:** •Chlorella, •Green Foods GREEN ESSENCE, or WHEAT GERM extract. •Use a fresh grape juice poultice on the nape of the neck. Leave on until dry; continue treatment until tumor regresses. Supplement with •Grifron MAITAKE D-FRACTION or Nutricology ARTEMESIA caps, (cross the blood-brain barrier). Take • Nutricology Germanium 150mg; and •vitamin E 800IU with selenium 200mcg. •GINKGO BILOBA extract for brain circulation. •Use Lane Labs BENE-FIN shark cartilage for glioblastoma multiform tumors, or Phoenix Biologics Vita Carte as directed. **New research:** Squalamine from shark liver oil slows brain cancer in animal tests; it's being evaluated in Phase II studies for brain cancer. Nu-Gen Nutrition SQUALAMAX is a good choice. —**For brain tumors:** Phosphatidyl choline (PC 55) 4 daily; carnitine 2000mg daily; Vitamin C therapy: 5,000mg daily; B Complex 150mg daily, with extra pantothenic acid 500mg, and folic acid 400mcg for neuroblastoma to help deter spread. Check out *www.cancermed.com* or call 713.335.5697 to find out more about Antineoplaston therapy, used with good results on brain tumor patients.

Lymphoma

Rates of non-Hodgkin's lymphoma have doubled since the 1970's.

Lymphomas are lymphatic system cancers, including Hodgkin's and non-Hodgkin's lymphomas, and lymphatic leukemia. Lymphomas may be related to mercury fillings in the mouth. Check to see if you should have them removed. Exposure to herbicides, solvents and vinyl chloride petro-chemicals is implicated in both Hodgkin's and non-Hodgkin's diseases, especially when immunity is already compromised because of long term conditions like hypoglycemia, viral triggers (HIV, Epstein-Barr) or prescription drug addiction.

Early signs include: swollen sore lymph nodes, especially in the neck. If the lymph nodes stay swollen for more than 3 weeks, get a medical diagnosis. Frequent and often painful, burning urination, blood in the urine, extreme lethargy, unexplained weight loss, night sweats, an intermittent fever, itchy skin, genital herpes, and frequent cold sores.

—**Alternative healing protocols:** A low sodium, vegetarian diet produces good results. Start with a liver cleansing diet, (page 199) Superfoods show the most promise for detoxification, especially •Sun Wellness Chlorella WAKASA GOLD, and •AloeLife ALOE GOLD drinks. Use •American Biologics DIOXYCHLOR as directed, reishi or maitake mushroom

Can't find a recommended product? Call the 800 number listed in Product Resources for the store nearest you.

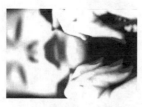

extracts, or •REISHI-CHLORELLA extract; •Nutricology GERMANIUM 200mg daily, •high potency royal jelly, ½ tsp. 4x daily, and •Crystal Star ANTI-BIO™ extract 6 daily to clear the lymph nodes of poisons. •Enzymatic Therapy VITALINE chewables CoQ10, 100mg. 3 daily; •Flora FLOR-ESSENCE tea for immune boosting. Add carotenes, especially lycopene from tomatoes and watermelon, to your diet. Add soy foods and cruciferous veggies like cabbage to block tumor nourishment. •Coffee enemas can help relieve pain. •Tests show St. John's wort can inhibit leukemia cell growth. *Contact Syracuse Cancer Research Institute at 315-472-6616 to find out if treatment with hydrazine sulfate may be right for you.*

Skin Cancer Skin cancer is an undeclared epidemic of our time.

Of all cancers, it is the most common (1 in every 3 cancers is skin cancer), and the fastest rising (800,000 new cases each year), claiming about 10,000 deaths a year. Over 90% of skin cancers are caused by over-exposure to ultra-violet radiation from the sun, increasing in toxicity as the earth's protective ozone layer is depleted. Some evidence shows that a genetic predisposition to certain reactions to the sun's UV rays and diet overabundance of fried foods and trans fats is also involved. Exposure to coal tar, pitch, creosote, and radium all show up in skin cancers. Age (usually 55 or over) and gender (50% more males get skin cancer) are factors. One in 75 people (largely white people with fair skin) will be diagnosed with melanoma in their lifetime. Use water-proof sun screen, and let it soak in before going out in the sun. I like MyChelle SUN SHIELD and Lane Labs ANTI-AGING PHYSICIAN SPF skin protector. (Apply sunscreen before insect repellent or the sunscreen won't work). Apply olive oil to skin after sunbathing to protect the skin from UV damage. Fair skins... avoid tanning salons and sunlamps. Early morning sunlight on the skin every day for 15 minutes can help heal ulcerations. Midday sun aggravates them.

There are 3 kinds of skin cancer: 1) *squamous cell carcinoma*, fast growing, looks like a red papule or a psoriasis-type patch with scaly crusted surface, appearing on sun-exposed areas. Later, it becomes hard and nodular; may become a lesion on the face, lips or ears. Curable with appropriate treatment. 2) *basal cell carcinoma*, least dangerous, but most common. Characterized by small, shiny, firm nodules, or crusty lesions that look like local dermatitis - does not metastasize. A shiny, pearly border develops after 3 or 4 months with a center ulcer. 3) *malignant melanoma*, a deeply rooted cancer that arises from the type of cells found in moles. It is serious, can be fatal, because it can metastasize to other organs, especially lymph nodes. Severe sunburns as a child boost melanoma risk. Early signs look like a freckle or mole, but melanomas have an irregular border, and are dark brown or black. Warning signs include itchiness, tenderness, hardening, or any visible change in size or color. Early stage melanomas are 95 to 100% curable.

—Alternative healing protocols: Reduce the fat and sugary foods in your diet immediately. Stop smoking; it's linked to recurring skin cancers. Eliminate hard alcohol drinks; reduce wine intake to 2 drinks a day or less. Add soyfoods to your diet. Soy saponins slow the growth of some skin cancers. Eat leafy greens daily for carotenes like lutein. Eat orange and yellow vegetables 3 times a week for more carotenes. Eat cold water fish like salmon twice a week. Take 1 tsp. each, wheat germ oil and nutritional yeast in •Aloe vera juice 2x daily.

•Drink green tea, or take Crystal Star GREEN TEA CLEANSER™, apply Lane Labs SKIN ANSWER gel to lesions (excellent results). •Take high potency Prince of Peace ROYAL JELLY-GINENG vials and 2 cups of *burdock* tea daily to normalize skin cells. **Normalize the epidermis:** •Alpha hydroxy acids, like Noni of Beverly Hills AHA's. •CoQ10 300mg daily, and EVENING PRIMROSE OIL caps 3000mg daily. Take •Flora VEGE-SIL for connective tissue. Take proteolytic enzymes like •Enzymedica PURIFY, 10 daily and •bromelain 1500mg with turmeric extract caps to reduce swelling. •Nutricology GERMANIUM 150mg is an immune stimulant. **Skin cancer healing applications:** •apply a Germanium solution in water; •hot comfrey compresses, •tea tree oil, •green clay poultices, •B & T CALIFLORA gel, •Earth's Bounty O₂ spray on affected areas, and on soles of feet. (Usually noticeable change in 3 weeks.)

For basal cell carcinomas: Apply and take MSM 1000mg daily. **Skin application 2x daily:** •Open a Lane Labs SHARK CARTILAGE capsule and mix with ¼ tsp. vitamin C crystals and DMSO. •Aloe Life ALOE SKIN GEL for 3 months. Results usually in 3 to 4 weeks. •Massage sandlewood essential oil into skin papillomas. Take •ascorbate or Ester C powder, ½ tsp. hourly to bowel tolerance during healing, for collagen production and connective tissue growth. **Protection:** •NAC (N-acetyl cysteine) 400mg daily during summer months; Selenium 200mcg and vitamin C 1000mg daily.

For squamous cell carcinoma: Preliminary evidence shows caffeine may act as preventive. Drink green tea daily if you are high risk. **Apply an escharotic salve** through which tumor cells can exit: •equal parts *garlic* powder, *goldenseal* rt. powder, zinc powder - mix into *calendula* ointment. Apply daily until tumor is destroyed, usually 4 weeks. The commercial product is called •HERBAL VEIL 8 by Viable Herbal Solutions (770-579-6323). •Consider Lane Labs SUN SPOT™ ES gel, rich in glycoalkaloids- (excellent results in clinical trials). Take •mixed carotenes (best), or •beta carotene 150,000IU; drink carrot juice daily. •Apply a combination of vitamin A and vitamin E oil to reverse skin cancers in early stages and prevent recurrence. •Add vitamin E 400IU and selenium 200mcg to your daily diet. Apply a Germanium solution in water.

For malignant melanomas: •Histidine, 1000mg 3x daily. Take •Milk Thistle Seed extract drops 3x daily in red clover tea (a specific for melanoma) or •Planetary Formulas PAU D'ARCO DEEP CLEANSING tabs. Take •pycnogenol 300mg daily, and apply Earth's Bounty O₂ SPRAY. Apply Crystal Star ANTI-BIO™ gel, *calendula* gel, *birch bark* extract or a *goldenseal/myrrh* solution. **Applications:** •Open a Lane Labs SHARK CARTILAGE capsule and mix with ¼ tsp. vitamin C/*garlic* paste, or a *turmeric* paste. A 1995 study in Alternative Therapies shows the 5-year survival rates of melanoma patients following the Gerson diet were considerably higher than those reported elsewhere. Find out more on the Gerson diet, check out *www.gerson.org* on the web.

Can't find a recommended product? Call the 800 number listed in Product Resources for the store nearest you.

Candida

Candidiasis, Leaky Gut Syndrome, Thrush

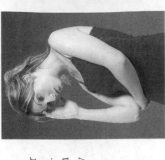

Candidiasis is a state of inner imbalance, not a disease. It is a stress-related condition marked by a seriously compromised immune response and it's extremely hard to overcome. Today, over 40 million Americans of all ages suffer from it. *Candida albicans* yeast itself is common, normally living harmlessly in the gastrointestinal tract and genito-urinary areas. But when immune response is reduced from repeated rounds of antibiotics, birth control pills or steroid drugs, a high sugar or refined carbohydrate rich diet, and a lifestyle short on rest, the body loses its intestinal balance and candida yeasts multiply too rapidly, voraciously feeding on excess carbohydrates in the digestive tract.

Even more worrisome, Candida is *dimorphic*, meaning it can change from a yeast into a fungus. In its fungal form, candida is invasive, with root-like tendrils that penetrate the intestinal tract, paving the way for Leaky Gut Syndrome and multiple food sensitivities to take hold. Candida may infect any part of the body. The most common sites are nail beds, skin folds, feet, mouth, sinuses, ear canal, belly button, esophagus, vaginal tract, urethra, even intestines. Assist your weakened defenses or candida colonies will flourish throughout the body and keep releasing toxins into the bloodstream.

Do you have a Candida infection?

Most of the orthodox medical community still chooses not to recognize, diagnose or treat Candidiasis seriously. It's no wonder since three out of the four main contributors - overuse of antibiotics, excess consumption of sugar, mercury dental fillings and birth control pills come from conventional medical practice. Instead, alternative professionals like Naturopaths, Homeopaths, Chiropractors and massage therapists see and deal with most cases. Their energy and dedication have dramatically advanced our knowledge of the symptoms and etiology of Candidiasis to better pin-point symptoms and treatment, to investigate its many companion diseases, to shorten healing time, to lessen overkill, and to understand the overriding psychological aspect of the disease.

Watch out for lifestyle factors that promote Candida infection:

1) *Poor diet* - especially excessive intake of sugar, starchy foods, yeasted breads and chemicalized foods.
2) *Repeated use of antibiotics* - long term use of antibiotics kill protective bacteria that keep candida under control, as well as harmful bacteria.
3) *Hormone medications* like corticosteroid drugs and birth control pills.
4) *A high stress life*, too much alcohol, little rest.

Signs that you may have a candida infection:

...Do you have recurrent digestive problems, severe bloating or flatulence?
...Do you have rectal itching, or chronic constipation alternating to diarrhea?
...Do you have a white coating on your tongue (thrush)? Do you crave sugar, bread, or alcoholic beverages?
   (Be forewarned. People with severe candida who eat a lot of sugar can actually become drunk because candida yeast can ferment sugar and carbohydrates and produce alcohol!)
...Have you been unusually irritable or depressed? Do you catch frequent colds that take weeks to go away?
...Are you bothered by unexplained frequent headaches, muscle aches and joint pain?
...Do you feel sick, yet the cause cannot be found? Do your symptoms worsen on muggy days?
...Has your memory been noticeably poor? Do you have a space-y feeling, find it hard to focus your thoughts?
...If you are a woman, do you have serious PMS, menstrual problems or endometriosis? or chronic vaginal yeast infections or frequent bladder infections?
...If you are a man, do you have abdominal pains, prostatitis, or loss of sexual interest?
...Do you have chronic fungal infections like ringworm, jock itch, nail fungus or athlete's foot?
...Do you have hives, psoriasis, eczema or chronic dermatitis?
...Are you bothered by erratic vision or spots before the eyes?
...Are you oversensitive to chemicals, tobacco, perfume or insecticides?
...Have you recently taken repeated rounds for 1 month or longer, of antibiotics or steroid drugs, like Symycin, Panmycin, Decadron or Prednisone, or acne drugs?

Can't find a recommended product? Call the 800 number listed in Product Resources for the store nearest you.

Symptoms for candida albicans overgrowth occur in fairly defined stages:

1st symptoms: Heartburn; chronic indigestion with gas and bloating; recurring cystitis or vaginitis; chronic fungal dermatitis skin rashes like eczema or acne, and nail infections.

2nd symptoms: Allergy reactions: chronic bronchitis, hives, sinusitis, hayfever, chronic headaches or migraines, muscle pain, sensitivity to odors. Ear infections are signs in children that candida is out of control.

3rd symptoms: Nervous system reactions: extreme irritability; confusion, a "spacey" feeling; night time panic attacks; memory lapses and trouble concentrating; fatigue and lethargy, often followed by acute depression.

4th symptoms: Gland and organ dysfunctions: hypothyroidism, adrenal failure, and hypoglycemia; ovarian problems, frigidity and infertility, male impotence, low sex drive.

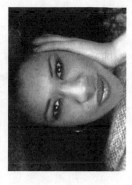

It may be difficult to detect *Candida albicans* overgrowth. Candida can mimic symptoms of over 140 different disorders. For instance, chronic fatigue syndrome, *salmonella*, intestinal parasites and mononucleosis have similar symptoms, but require very different treatment. Get a candida test before starting a healing program. *Call Antibody Assay Labs (1-800-522-2611), for a blood test for candida immune complexes and candida antibodies. For information on electrodermal candida screening, call Harmony Health Systems (770-345-6614).*

Is your Candida aggravated by food allergies? Check yourself with Coca's Pulse Test:

Dr. Arthur Coca, an immunologist, discovered that when people eat foods to which they are allergic, there is a dramatic increase in their heartbeat — 20 or more beats a minute above normal. Pulse rate is normally very stable, not affected by digestion, ordinary physical activities or normal emotions. Unless a person is ill or under great stress, pulse rate deviation is probably due to a food allergy. This test can help you can find foods that harm.

1. Take your pulse when you wake in the morning. Using a watch with a second hand, count the number of beats in a 60-second period. A normal pulse rate reading is 60 to 100 beats per minute.

2. Take your pulse again after eating a suspected allergy food. Wait 15 to 20 minutes and take your pulse again. If your pulse rate has increased more than 10 beats per minute, omit the food from your diet.

A successful protocol for overcoming candida includes the following stages:

Stage 1: Kill the yeasts through diet change and enzyme supplement therapy. Avoid antibiotics, steroid drugs and birth control pills, unless there is absolute medical need.

Stage 2: Cleanse the dead yeasts and waste cells from the body with a soluble fiber cleanser or bentonite. Colonic irrigation and herbal implants are effective here.

Stage 3: Strengthen your digestive system by enhancing its nutrient assimilation. Fortify afflicted organs and glands, especially the liver. Restore normal metabolism and promote friendly bacteria in the G.I. tract.

Stage 4: Rebuild immune response and stimulate immune well-being throughout the healing process.

Candida Cleansing Diet for the First Two Months of Healing

Diet therapy is the best way to rebuild strength and immunity from candida overgrowth. Your initial cleansing diet should focus on releasing dead and diseased yeast cells from the body... a phase that may require 2-3 months for complete cleansing. Also use this diet as the basis for a "rotation diet," in which you slowly add back individual foods during healing that cause an allergic reaction to candida. As you start to see improvement, and symptoms decrease (usually after two months), start to add back some whole grains, fruits, juices, a little white wine, some fresh cheeses, nuts and beans. Go slowly, add gradually. Test for food sensitivity all along the way until it is gone. Don't forget that sugars and refined foods will allow candida to grow again.

I have been working with candidiasis since 1984 and find repeatedly that a too-rigid diet does not work over the long term. The sufferer cannot stick to it (except in a restricted, isolated environment), and the body becomes imbalanced in other ways. The recommended diets in this book, and my book "DETOXIFICATION" are real people diets, used by people suffering from candida who have shared their experience with us. The healing diets and detoxes are continually modified to meet the changing needs of the disease and to benefit from the network of new information.

Can't find a recommended product? Call the 800 number listed in Product Resources for the store nearest you.

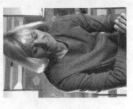

Note 1: **Superfood therapy is critical:** (Choose one or two and add to your diet any time) •Crystal Star ENERGY GREEN RENEWAL™ drink; •Fit for You MIRACLE GREENS; •Nutricology PROGREENS with EFAs; •Futurebiotics VITAL K; •Vibrant Health GREEN VIBRANCE; •AloeLife ALOE GOLD.

Note 2: **Probiotics are critical to restore a healthy internal environment:** (Choose one and add to your diet either sprinkled on food or taken with water throughout the day).
•Garden of Life FUNGAL DEFENSE; •American Health ACIDOPHILUS liquid; •UAS DDS-PLUS.

Note 3: **Enzyme therapy is critical to recovery:** Enzyme therapy along with diet therapy and anti fungal herbs speeds up recovery time. Some people feel better within 2 days!
•Pure Essence CANDEX; •Crystal Star DR. ENZYME™ with protease and bromelain; •Enzyme PUREZYME, high protease formula.

—*On rising:* two tsp. cranberry concentrate, or 2 tsp. lemon juice in water, or a fiber cleanser like AloeLife FIBERMATE or Crystal Star FIBER & HERBS COLON CLEANSE™ to clean the colon; or a cup of Crystal Star GREEN TEA CLEANSER™; if you have gas, take 1 tsp. unfiltered apple cider vinegar with 1 tsp. maple syrup.

—*Breakfast:* NutriTech ALL 1 vitamin/mineral drink in water; then take 1 or 2 poached or hard boiled eggs on rice cakes with a little butter or flax oil; or almond butter on rice cakes or wheat free bread; or oatmeal with 1 tbsp. Bragg's LIQUID AMINOS; or amaranth or buckwheat pancakes with a little butter and vanilla; or a vegetable omelette with broccoli; or scrambled eggs with onion, shiitake mushrooms and red pepper; or brown rice with onions and carrots; or oatmeal or cream of buckwheat.

—*Mid-morning:* take a strengthening potassium drink (page 291) or Sun Wellness CHLORELLA or Green Foods GREEN MAGMA, or Crystal Star DR. VITALITY™ green and white tea blend; or a cup of miso soup with sea greens snipped on top; or a cup of *pau d' arco* tea, *echinacea* or *chamomile* tea, or a small bottle of plain mineral water.

—*Lunch:* fresh greens, seafood, chicken or turkey with lemon/coconut, olive or flax oil dressing; or vegetable or miso soup with sea veggies snipped on top and buttered cornbread; Rejuvenative Foods VEGI DELITE cultured veggies; or steamed veggies with brown rice; or wheat free bread sandwiches, with mayonnaise or butter, some veggies, seafood, chicken or turkey; or tuna or wheat-free pasta salad, with mayonnaise or lemon/oil sauce.

—*Mid-afternoon:* have some rice crackers, or baked corn chips, with a little kefir cheese or butter; or some raw veggies dipped in lemon/oil dressing or spiced mayonnaise; or a small mineral water and hard boiled or deviled egg with sesame salt or sea vegetable seasoning.

—*Dinner:* baked, broiled or poached fish or chicken with brown rice or millet with flax oil and veggies; or a tofu and veggie casserole with sea greens; or a baked potato with Bragg's LIQUID AMINOS, Rejuvenative Foods VEGI DELITE (health food store refrigerator case) cultured veggies; or a vegetable stir fry with brown rice, sea veggies and a miso or light broth soup; or a vegetarian pizza with snipped sea veggies, on a chapati or pita crust; or a hot wheat-free, veggie pasta salad.

—*Before bed:* have a cup of herb tea such as *chamomile, peppermint,* or Crystal Star STRESS ARREST™ tea or a cup of miso soup.

Note: Unless you have a food sensitivity (see Coca's Pulse test on the previous page), nutritional yeast *does not* cause or aggravate candida albicans yeast overgrowth. It is one of the best immune-enhancing foods available. Candida yeasts need minerals to thrive, and they deplete the minerals from our bodies. Supplement minerals to shore up mineral deficiencies caused by the yeast. •Restricting sugar in your permanent diet is essential.

Golden Rules *for controlling candida overgrowth:*

Candida albicans yeast takes advantage of lowered immunity to overrun the body. A healthy liver and a strong immune system are the keys to lasting control of candida. The whole healing-rebuilding process may take 6 months or more, and is not easy. The changes in diet, habits and lifestyle are often radical. Some people feel better right away; others go through a rough "healing crisis." (Yeasts are living organisms - a part of the body. Killing them off is traumatic.) But most people with candida are feeling so bad anyway, the knowledge that they are getting better pulls them through the hard times. Be as gentle with your body as you can. Give yourself at least 3 to 6 months. I know you want to get better quickly, but multiple therapies all at once can be self-defeating, psychologically upsetting, and traumatic on your system. Just stick to it and go at your own pace.

Can't find a recommended product? Call the 800 number listed in Product Resources for the store nearest you.

Candida

Diet and Lifestyle Support Therapy

Detoxification bodywork:

Applied kinesiology works well to test for candida food and product sensitivities. Avoid antibiotics, birth control pills and steroids unless absolutely necessary.

•**Enema:** Take the night before your cleanse to flush the colon and jump start detoxification; it allows a more expedient release of dead yeast cells and toxins from the body.

•**Stop candida transmission:** Use a cleansing vaginal douche and penis soak, or *pau, d' arco* tea, or 1 tsp. tea tree oil in 2 cups water as a douche or soak.

•**Irrigate for best results:** At least one colonic during a candida detox.

•**Exercise:** A brisk walk for more body oxygen, a positive mind and outlook….essential to overcome candida body stress.

•**Rest:** A key to overcoming yeast-induced fatigue.

•**Flower remedies:** Nelson Bach Rescue Remedy; or Natural Labs Deva Flower Cleansing Remedy or Fearfulness (dread is a primary emotion of candida and CFIDS victims).

•**Microcurrent therapy:** New patents show that microcurrents neutralize pathogens, fungi, viruses, bacteria and parasites. *Call Sota Instruments for more info: 800-224-0242.*

Nutritional therapy plan:

1—*Food recommendations for the initial diet*… a long, restrictive list, but for the first critical weeks, when energy-sapping yeasts must be deprived of nutrients and killed off, it is the only way. Candida yeasts grow on sugars, carbohydrates, preserved, over-processed foods, molds and gluten breads.

2—*Don't eat the following foods for 4 to 6 weeks:* Sugar or sweeteners of any kind (use stevia instead: gymnema sylvestre extract helps handle sugar cravings); gluten bread or yeasted baked goods, fried foods, dairy products (except plain kefir or kefir cheese, yogurt or yogurt cheese), smoked, dried, pickled or cured meats, sweet potatoes or regular potatoes, mushrooms, nuts or nut butters (except almonds or almond butter), most fruits and fruit juices, dried or candied fruits, coffee, black tea, carbonated drinks (phosphoric acid binds up calcium and magnesium), alcohol or foods with vinegar. Avoid antibiotics, steroid drugs, birth control pills and tobacco.

3—*Acceptable foods during the first stage*…a short list, but diet restriction is the best way to stop candida yeast overgrowth: Fresh and steamed veggies (especially onions, garlic, ginger, cabbage, and broccoli), vegetable juices, raw cultured sauerkraut, poultry, seafoods and sea greens, olive or coconut oil, ghee, eggs, mayonnaise, brown rice, mochi rice bread, amaranth, buckwheat, barley, millet, miso soup and tofu, vegetable pastas, plain or vanilla yogurt, rice cakes-crackers, some citrus fruit and herb teas, especially white tea and pau d' arco tea. Have a green drink, green tea and miso soup every day.

4—**Probiotics re-establish internal balance:** •Garden of Life FUNGAL DEFENSE; •UAS DDS-PLUS; •Rejuvenative Foods VEGI-DELITE.

Herbal, Superfood and Supplement Therapy

Interceptive therapy: Choose 1 suggestion in each category.

Rotate anti-yeast and anti-fungal products, so yeast strains don't build up resistance to any one formula. Herbs normalize and balance.

1—Kill the yeasts: •*Pau d' Arco* tea, 4 cups daily (soak nails for nail fungus, or use as a douche for vaginal fungus); •*Echinacea* extract or *echinacea-barberry* extract (if there is diarrhea), 4× daily; •Crystal Star CANDIDA YEAST DETOX™ caps, 6 daily with GREEN TEA CLEANSER™ (helps leaky gut). Add •*Black Walnut* extract and •KYOLIC AGED GARLIC extract; •Nature's Secret CANDISTROYER or Gaia Herbs CANDIDA SUPREME. •Nutribiotic GRAPEFRUIT SEED extract; •Olive leaf extract eats candida, try •East Park *Olive Leaf* extract (good results); •Nutricology PROLIVE 1500mg daily; •New Zealand *Psuedowintera Colorata* (Horopito), clinically tested effective against candida.

—**Enzyme therapy is highly recommended:** Enzyme therapy in conjunction with diet therapy and anti fungal herbs speeds up recovery time. Some people feel better within 2 days. •Bromelain 1500mg daily; •Pancreatin 1400mg w. HCL; •Transformation Enzyme PUREZYME or •Enzymedica PURIFY; •Pure Essence CANDEX caps or Enzymedica CANDIDASE help digest candida's cell walls and excess sugar.

2—Cleanse dead yeasts and wastes: •AloeLife FIBER-MATE drink; •Crystal Star BWL-TONE IBS™ caps. •Gaia CANDIDA SUPREME VITAL CLEANSE; •Crystal Star DR. VITALITY™ tea or •Yogi GREEN TEA SUPER ANTI-OXIDANT with Grapeseed extract; •Nutricology PERMAVITE for leaky gut syndrome.

3—Detoxify the liver: •Crystal Star LIVER RENEW™ caps also helps enhance immune status; •Vibrant Health RED MARINE ALGAE, •Oceanic carotenes 200,000IU; or 2 tbsp. snipped sea greens daily; SAMe (*S-adenosylmethionine*) 800mg daily; •*Milk Thistle Seed* extract Alpha Lipoic Acid up to 400mg daily.

—**Shift internal ecology from unhealthy to healthy:** •Lane Labs NATURE'S LINING restores, strengthens the stomach wall (very good activity). •Planetary Formulas TRIPHALA; •Glutamine increases IgA levels; NAG (*N-acetyl-glucosamine*) deters candida adherence.

4—Enhance adrenal and thyroid activity: •Crystal Star RESTORE YOUR STRENGTH™ and ADRENAL ENERGY BOOST™ caps or •Nutricology ADRENAL organic glandular caps; •Biotin 1000mcg with Nature's Secret ULTIMATE B; •taurine 500mg.

5—EFA's fight fungal action, inhibit yeast overgrowth: •*Evening Primrose Oil* caps, 1000mg 4 daily; •Solaray CAPRYL, or Solgar caprylic acid tabs up to 1200mg; •Coconut oil is a rich source of caprylic acid with 50% lauric acid, a disease-fighting fatty acid. •Body Ecology COCONUT OIL, 3 TBSP. daily. •Allergy Research Group *oregano* oil caps, or Oshadi *oregano* oil, 1 drop 2x daily in 1 tsp. flax oil (also helps leaky gut).

6—Antioxidants, minerals prevent further infection: •Nutricology Germanium 150mg; •Trid Earth's Bounty O_2 SPRAY on abdomen; Kal COLOSTRUM 1 daily; •Grapeseed PCO's 100mg 3x daily; •Nature's Path TRACE-MIN-LYTE.

Can't find a recommended product? Call the 800 number listed in Product Resources for the store nearest you.

Addressing Candida Related Syndromes

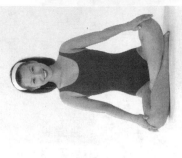

Candida may infect virtually any part of the body.... so a wide range of related problems can accompany a candida infection. The most common sites are nail beds, skin folds, feet, mouth, sinuses, ear canal, navel, esophagus, intestine, vaginal tract and urethra. Candida also infects deep internal organs, which sometimes results in serious disease. Likely sites of infection include the thyroid and adrenal glands, kidneys, bladder, bowel, esophagus, uterus, lungs and bone marrow.

LEAKY GUT SYNDROME: a bowel disorder symptoms similar to Crohn's disease, connected to candida through compromised allergy-immune response. Breaches in the gut wall and flaccid gut tissue mean too much gut permeability, which allows foreign food and toxin molecules into the bloodstream where they are attacked by the immune system. Wide nutrient deficiencies occur because the inflamed gut tissues can't absorb them. Fatigue and bloating set in. Food sensitivities get worse. New food allergies usually appear.
—**Natural treatment recommendations (use several):** Reestablish normal gut permeability with •vitamin C and bioflavonoids (an ascorbic acid flush once a week, page 193, and up to 5000mg daily); •Kal COLOSTRUM, 1-3 daily, or •Nutricology PERMAVITE help heal damaged gut wall, a specific for leaky gut; •Omega-3 fatty acids from flax oil and sea greens, or •Trimedica SEAGEST inhibit inflammatory chemicals; L-Glutamine 500mg 3x daily normalizes the gut barrier; probiotics like •Pure Essence FLORALIVE, or •UAS DDS-PLUS with FOS reseed colonic flora; •NAG (*N-acetyl-glucosamine*) rich in mucopolysaccharides, restabilizes connective tissue. Daily •*ginger* tea helps take down inflammation; •*Marshmallow, slippery elm* and *cat's claw* also reduce inflammation and help normalize gut mucous membranes. Add •Zinc 50mg for 30 days and bromelain 1500mg daily for enzyme therapy.

THRUSH (oral candidiasis): usually a childhood candida condition, thrush appears as creamy white patches or sores on the tongue or mucous membranes of the mouth. Corners of the mouth may also be red and cracked. The primary cause of thrush is widespread antibiotic use.
—**Natural treatment recommendations: (use several):** •Probiotics are a key: •UAS DDS-JUNIOR or •Natren LIFESTART by mouth, and use as a rectal suppository. •Add vitamin C 100mg or Ester C chewable. •Give garlic extract drops in water, or squirt a pricked garlic oil cap in the mouth or give KYOLIC by Wakunaga. •COLLOIDAL SILVER drops or Nature's Path SILVER-LYTE are effective. Use •Melaleuca, Inc. BREATH AWAY tea tree oil mouthwash; tea tree oil; homeopathic Thuja, •*Black Walnut* extract. •Disinfect toothbrush with 3% hydrogen peroxide frequently.

VAGINAL CANDIDA (Vulvovaginitis): a thick, white, leukorrhea vaginal discharge with itching and redness all around the genitalia.
—**Natural treatment recommendations (use one or more):** •Pure Essence Labs CANDEX caps (highly recommended), use as directed; •Natren GY-NA-TREN caps and inserts; •Nutricology SYMBIOTICS powder as a vaginal application (apply powder to a tampon and insert or open a capsule and apply); garlic capsules 6 daily or •insert a peeled *garlic clove* and leave in overnight. Use •*Cat's Claw* extract 30 drops and *goldenseal* extract 30 drops in 2 cups water as a douche 2x daily. •GRAPEFRUIT SEED EXTRACT liquid or capsules may also be used as a vaginal douche or enema. •Beta-carotene 100,000IU daily, or 2 tbsp. dry snipped sea greens daily (a key diet source of mixed carotenes). •Soak a washcloth in a dilute tea tree oil solution and apply to infected areas. Use •Thursday Plantation TEA TREE OIL to inhibit candida growth. Follow directions, or 1 tsp. tea tree oil in 2 cups water as a douche. Consider •*pau d' arco* tea as a douche. Make your own highly effective herbal douche: •brew a strong tea of *garlic cloves, echinacea root, myrrh, calendula flowers* and *thyme*. Fill a squirt bottle - wash perenium after defecating to keep from re-infecting; may also douche the vagina. Apply un-sweetened plain yogurt topically to relieve discomfort. Wear 100% cotton underwear. Synthetic fibers trap in moisture and heat, an environment where candida flourishes. Note: Be sure to follow the treatment recommendations for intestinal candida on page 361. Vaginal candida is dependent on intestinal candida. Cure is not likely if you only address the vaginal infection. See pg. 561 for my complete healing program for vaginal yeast infections.

PARASITE INFESTATION: parasites encourage candida growth by reducing normal immune response. Some naturopaths say that up to ⅔ of people suffering from candida also have a parasite infestation.
—**Natural treatment recommendations:** High dosage of probiotics is effective. May be sprinkled on food or taken as a capsule 6-10 daily. Choose and use a broad spectrum, multi flora supplement for 12 weeks- •UAS DDS-PLUS with FOS, •Nutricology SYMBIOTICS. •Nature's Secret PARASTROY, a two-part anti parasite formula. *Garlic* is a natural antiparasitic; use a garlic enema 2x a week. •COLLOIDAL SILVER or Nature's Path SILVER-LYTE are effective.

Can't find a recommended product? Call the 800 number listed in Product Resources for the store nearest you.

NAIL FUNGUS: usually begins as painful swelling of finger or toe tips, with pus that later develops around the nails. If the infection occurs under the nails, it may cause loss of the nail.

—**Natural treatment recommendations (use one or more):** •apply *tea tree oil* on affected areas several times daily. • Soak nails in *Pau d'Arco tea* or Nutribiotic GRAPEFRUIT SEED EXTRACT. See pg. 504 for more information. • *Evening Primrose Oil* caps, 1000mg 4 daily; Solaray CAPRY_, or Solgar caprylic acid tabs up to 1200mg. •Coconut oil is a rich source of caprylic acid with 50% lauric acid, a disease-fighting fatty acid. •Body Ecology COCONUT OIL, 3 TBSP. daily. •Allergy Research Group *oregano* oil caps, or Oshadi *oregano* oil, 1 drop 2x daily in 1 tsp. flax oil (also helps leaky gut).

CANDIDA PENIS INFECTION: Infects the tip (glans penis); almost always a result of a ping-pong effect, where a man has a sexual partner who has candida vaginitis, and the infection bounces back and forth between them. Men most at risk are those who have diabetes.

—**Natural treatment recommendations:** In most cases, the same treatment protocols effective for vaginitis are also effective for penile candidiasis. Sexual partners should use a cleansing vaginal douche or penis soak or *pau d'arco tea*; or 1 tsp. tea tree oil in 2 cups water as a douche or soak to prevent re-infection.

CANDIDA SKIN INFECTION: characterized by itchy, scaly skin patches, candida fungus lesions are red-looking pustules that appear in moist places like the groin, underarms, navel, anus, buttocks or webbing of fingers and toes. Crusts that form on the scalp usually cause hair loss.

—**Natural treatment recommendations:** Apply tea tree or manuka oil; or •Crystal Star FUNGEX™ skin gel, or Nutribiotic GRAPEFRUIT SEED SKIN OINTMENT, or East Park TOPICAL CLEANSING BAR (*olive leaf extract*).

Use Muscle Testing to see which foods and supplements will work for you.

Muscle kinesiology testing is a personal technique to use when buying a healing food or product. You can estimate a product's effectiveness for your own body needs and make-up.

You'll need a partner to help. Here's how:

1: Hold your arm out straight from your side, parallel to the ground. Have a partner take hold of the arm with one hand just below the shoulder, and one hand on the forearm. Your partner should then try to force down towards your side, while you exert all your strength to hold it level. Unless you are in ill health, you should easily be able to withstand this pressure and keep your arm level.

2: Then, simply hold the item that you desire to test against your diaphragm (under the breastbone) or thyroid (the point where the collarbone comes together below the neck). The item may be in or out of normal packaging, or in its raw state, like a fresh food.

3: Holding the item as above, put your arm out straight from your side as before and have your partner try to press it down again. If the item is beneficial for you, your arm will retain its strength; your partner won't be able to force it down. If the item is not beneficial, or would worsen your condition, your arm can be easily pushed down by your partner.

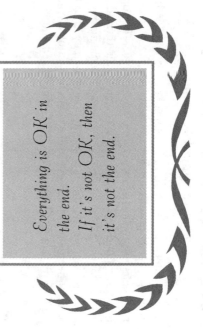

Everything is OK in the end.
If it's not OK, then it's not the end.

Can't find a recommended product? Call the 800 number listed in Product Resources for the store nearest you.

Carpal Tunnel Syndrome

Repetitive Strain Wrist Injury

Carpal tunnel syndrome is the most common ailment of the computer age. Far more widely spread than originally thought, 2.5 million *new* carpal tunnel cases are diagnosed each year! Today, one in five workers suffer from tingling, pain and swelling, poor grip, and intense numbness in the wrist and hand that often involves shoulder nerves as well. Women are greater victims because they have narrower carpal tunnels and smaller muscles than men. Continued, repetitive stress on the wrist, hand and arm nerves from knitting or needlework, or assembly-line task work are the most common causes, but diseases like arthritis, diabetes, even thyroid disease, also cause the same type of nerve inflammation pain and numbness. Vitamin B$_6$ deficiency, and/or birth control pills creating a B$_6$ deficiency lead to carpal tunnel. Nerve pressure and fluid retention from obesity or during pregnancy increase your risk. (See weight loss programs on pp. 564-569 of this book.) Standard medical treatment is usually cortisone shots to control swelling, or in severe cases, surgery to enlarge the carpal tunnel opening. Natural therapies can both relieve pain and help prevent development of CTS. Left untreated, muscle atrophy of the wrist and hand is likely to develop.

Diet and Lifestyle Support Therapy

Nutritional therapy plan for prevention:

1—Vitamin B$_6$ helps CTS. Eat a diet rich in vitamin B$_6$ foods: leafy greens, whole grains, liver, beans and legumes.

2—Eat 1 green salad, 2 tbsp. sea greens, 1 cup miso soup daily.

3—Add fluid-balancing foods to keep from retaining excess fluid: hormone-free chicken and turkey, fish, beans, wheat germ, whole grains. Add celery for good cell salt activity.

4—Avoid foods like caffeine, hard liquor and soft drinks that bind magnesium. Reduce refined carbohydrates, trans fatty acids, and dairy foods that aggravate symptoms.

5—Take a glass of lemon juice and water each morning. Make a mix with 2 tsp. each: lecithin granules, nutritional yeast, molasses, toasted wheat germ; take 1 tbsp. daily.

Lifestyle bodywork support:

—*Self Test for CTS:* Hold out your right hand, bend your left index finger and tap the middle of your right wrist where the wrist joins your hand. A tingling sensation or shooting pains down your fingers mean possible carpal tunnel problems.

•Take short work breaks during the day, stretch frequently.

•Chiropractic, massage, yoga, hypnosis are effective for CTS injuries. 70% of carpal tunnel patients have pinched neck nerves; treatment can eliminate a need for surgery.

•Try a CATS PAW ergonomic hand exerciser. Work up to 10 minutes of exercise each night to relieve pain and numbness. Visit www.catspaw.com for more information.

Bodywork exercises for relief:

1) Effective hand exercise: With palms down, spread fingers apart as far as you can. Count to five. Relax. Repeat.

2) Stand with arms at your side. Lift arm in front to shoulder level, palm up. Spread fingers and point them to the floor. Bring fingers up into a fist and flex wrist toward you. Pull fist to your face.... slowly. Make a muscle with your arm and fist. Turn your head toward the fist, straighten arm, open your fist. Spread fingers again and point them to the floor. Turn your head to your other shoulder and repeat the exercise.

Herbal, Superfood and Supplement Therapy

Interceptive therapy: Choose 2 to 3 recommendations.

1—Relax tingling nerves: •Crystal Star STRESS OUT™ muscle relaxer extract (relief usually felt within 25 minutes). •Planetary MYELIN SHEATH FORMULA or •Country Life LIGA-TEND caps. Relax nerves with extracts of •*scullcap, passionflower* or *lobelia*.

•Massage area with Earth's Bounty O$_2$ SPRAY.

2—Control pain - inflammation: Vitamin B$_6$ 250mg daily, with B-complex 100mg and Bromelain 1500mg for 3 months (highly effective for many). •Cyanotech BIOASTIN (*astaxanthin*); clinical tests reduce pain severity and duration. •Crystal Star ANTI-FLAM™ caps 4x daily, or •Solaray QBC-PLEX or *turmeric* extract caps. •New Chapter ZYFLAMEND (effective herbal Cox-2 inhibitor); •GLUCOSAMINE-CHONDROITIN 4 daily. •DLPA 500mg as needed. Massage area frequently with •*cajeput* oil or •Chinese WHITE FLOWER oil.

3—Restore nerve health: •Crystal Star RELAX CAPS™ as needed (usually relief felt within 30 minutes); Anabol Naturals AMINO BALANCE; •Evening Primrose Oil 500mg, 4 daily; •Choline 600mg daily, with manganese 10mg.

•**Homeopathic:** Hylands NERVE TONIC or *Arsenicum* as needed. B & T ARNI-FLORA if you do computer work.

4—Strengthen wrist tissue: •Crystal Star CALCIUM SOURCE™ caps; •Nutrapathic CALCIUM/COLLAGEN caps. • Lane Labs TOKI, collagen replacement drink.•Crystal Star IODINE, POTASSIUM SILICA extract or •Flora VEGE-SIL 2x daily, rebuild collagen. •Vitamin C with bioflavs 5000mg daily for connective tissue. •Country Life GABA w. Taurine.

5—Boost circulation to painful area: •*Ginkgo Biloba* extract 3x daily; niacin (flush-free OK) 500mg daily; •Capsaicin cream. • New Chapter GINGER WONDER syrup.

—Superfood therapy: (Choose one or two recommendations)

•Green veggie drinks or a Potassium Juice pg. 291.

•Fresh carrot juice or Green Foods CARROT ESSENCE.

•Pure Planet TART CHERRY CONCENTRATE.

•Jarrow GENTLE FIBERS drink.

Can't find a recommended product? Call the 800 number listed in Product Resources for the store nearest you.

Cataracts and Macular Degeneration

Lens Opacity

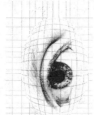

Cataracts block light entering the eye. The eye lens which focuses light, hardens and becomes cloudy or opaque. Over 4 million people (80% of people 75 and older), feel like they're looking through a piece of smoked glass, with blurry or double vision, or glare. Smokers are 63% more likely to develop cataracts. Cataracts are related to free radical damage, diabetes (page 394), steroid drugs and steroid inhalers for asthma, radiation and excessive exposure to UV light. Too much dietary fat may boost risk as much as 80%! Cataract surgery is the most common operation for people over 65, performed over 1 million times a year at a cost of $3.5 billion dollars! Most operations are repeated in 2 to 5 years; complications like detached retina, glaucoma, corneal edema, and infections affect 28,000 people every year. Natural therapies can arrest, even reverse early cataracts. **Age-related macular degeneration (AMD)**, affects 13 million Americans and is the leading cause of blindness in people over 60. It affects the center part of the eye, characterized by accumulated oxidized fat (lipofuscin) and thinning macular pigment. AMD means blurry, distorted vision, trouble reading even large type, and seeing faded colors. Glasses don't help. Driving is difficult because of blind spots. People with light eyes are more at risk. AMD is linked to smoking, low carotene intake, UV sunlight, but can be aided or reversed with nutritional therapy.

Diet and Lifestyle Support Therapy

Nutritional therapy plan for prevention:

1—Reduce trans fat foods (esp. salty snacks). Avoid sugary foods, red meat, caffeine.

2—Add magnesium foods: seafoods, whole grains, green veggies, molasses, nuts, eggs (full of zeaxanthin). Add berries of all kinds for anthocyanins. High vitamin A and C foods reduce your risk by 40%.

—**"See" foods prevent cataracts:** •Stabilize blood sugar: green or white tea each morning. •Take a daily cataract herb tea: 2 tbsp. each: *ginkgo leaf, catnip, rosemary, shredded ginger, lemon balm.* Blender blend with 2 cups blueberries. Or try Herbalist & Alchemist BLUEBERRY extract (excellent). •Dehydration is implicated in cataracts. Try PENTA water, microclustered for rapid hydration. •Photosensitivity from standardized *St. John's wort* may increase cataracts risk.

—**"See" foods for macular degeneration:** A high fat diet, smoking, too much alcohol and over-exposure to ultra-violet light increase risk. Carotenoids, (specifically lutein and zeaxanthin) in dark greens can cut risk up to 50%! •Consider Hain Pure Foods VEG-GIE JUICE fortified with FloraGLO lutein. Eat lutein-rich foods like kale, collard greens, spinach, mangoes (for cataracts, too). •Eat zinc-rich foods: all sea foods and sea veggies (tests show eating fish 3 times a week reduces risk of AMD blindness up to 50%), whole grains, beans, pumpkin seeds. •2 to 4 glasses of wine a month cuts risk of AMD 20%!

—**Bodywork:**

•Don't smoke. Smoking causes massive free radical damage to the eyes and is now linked to Age-Related Macular Degeneration (AMD). See page 413.

•Acupressure and massage therapy stimulate energy flow to your eyes. Important.

•Avoid long exposure to the sun. Get outdoor exercise early in the day. Wear wrap around sunglasses for protection. Wear amber or blue-blocking sunglasses. Dark sunglasses with no UV filter dilate pupils, allow destructive UV rays in.

•Avoid aspirin, drugstore antihistamines and cortisone as detrimental to eye health. •Hyperbaric oxygen therapy boosts oxygen, really improves vision. *Check out www.drcranton.com.*

Herbal, Superfood and Supplement Therapy

Interceptive therapy: Choose 2 to 3 recommendations.

1—**Strengthen eye tissue and nerves:** •Allergy Research Group OCUDYNE with Lutein; •Quercetin 2000mg with bromelain 1500mg daily. •Homeopathic *Silicea* tabs; (full of zeaxanthin). Add berries of all kinds for anthocyanins. High vitamin A and C foods •Solaray VIZION, •Esteem Products BRIGHT EYES or •Nature's Life I-SIGHT; •High potency *royal jelly* 2 tsp. with •*spirulina* tabs 8 daily; •Vitamin C 3000mg daily (long term vitamin C intake can prevent cataracts in women under 60. *AJCN 2002*); •Betaine HCl 600mg. (People with AMD have low hydrochloric acid levels.) Try •American Health APPLE CIDER VINEGAR tabs.

2—**Strengthen eyes with super bioflavonoids:** •Take *bilberry* or *elderberry* extract for PCO activity, or •PCO's 100mg 3x daily from *grapeseed* or *white pine*, or *ginkgo biloba* extract, or •Herbalist & Alchemist BLUEBERRY extract. •Take Crystal Star EYES RIGHT™ drops with Taurine 500mg and NAC (*N-acetyl-cysteine*) improves visual acuity (good results). •Good eye-washes: •Aloe vera juice, *rose hips* tea, or •Life Extension BRITE EYES.

3—**Boost antioxidants against free radical damage:** Antioxidants in C, E and carotenoids lower the common cataract risk of oxidative stressors like ultraviolet light, boost glutathione, and de-activate heavy metals and pollutants: Similisan CATARACT drops (excellent results). •New Chapter SUPERCRITICAL DHA to support cell membranes; •MICROHYDRIN PLUS from royalbodycare.com. •Glutathione 100mg daily w. Vitamin E 400IU; •Vitamin C with bioflavonoids 5000mg daily; •Alpha lipoic acid, 300mg daily (good results); •Barleans GREENS; •CoQ-10 100mg 3x daily.

4—**Eye vitamins for more macular pigment:** high intake of carotenes lowers risk of macular degeneration- •Green Foods CARROT ESSENCE; •Beta carotene 150,000IU daily, or •PHYCOTENE MICRO-CLUSTERS, mixed sea greens carotenes at Healthy House; •B-complex 100mg daily; •Vitamin E 800IU with selenium 200mcg daily, •Taurine, 2000mg daily, •Zinc 50mg 2x daily or Eidon ZINC liquid slow onset.

5—**Balance your blood sugar to see better:** •Crystal Star SUGAR CONTROL HIGH™ caps; •*Bilberry* extract decreases sorbitol accumulation, helps remove chemicals from the eyes.

Can't find a recommended product? Call the 800 number listed in Product Resources for the store nearest you.

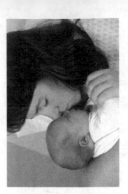

Cerebral Palsy

Muscle-Nerve Dysfunction

Cerebral palsy is a broad term for brain-centered motor disorders, almost always occurring as a birth defect in premature, very low birth weight babies (less than 3½ pounds). Damage to the cerebrum causes a paralysis (palsy) in one or more parts of the body. It's a crippling disease and the damage never heals. There are about 9,000 new cases in the U.S. each year. The highest risk factor today is for tiny premature infants whose mother has AIDS, or has been addicted to drugs (causing low oxygen supply to the brain). Also implicated, measles infection in early pregnancy, clogged motor control centers in the fetus' brain, infant diseases like encephalitis, meningitis, herpes simplex and heavy metal poisoning. It's an unusually harsh disease; victims have almost no control over voluntary muscles, which results in abrupt, jerking, muscle contractions and spastic, convulsive seizures. Typically, children with CP have above average intelligence, but they don't appear so, because their muscles often appear atrophy, which can result in drooling and speech impairment. Some experts argue for intravenous magnesium during pregnancy to strengthen muscle development and prevent cerebral palsy in premature births.

Diet and Lifestyle Support Therapy

Nutritional therapy plan:

1—A modified macrobiotic diet is effective. See pg. 348 in this book.

2—Provide organically grown foods as much as possible. Include plenty of leafy greens and a fresh salad every day.

3—Go on a gentle juice cleanse one day a week until symptoms improve (usually noticed in 3 to 4 months). Take a potassium broth (pg. 291) every other day during the cleanse.

4—Avoid chemicalized foods, trans fats, concentrated proteins from red meats, fried foods, caffeine and canned foods.

5—Boost magnesium intake during pregnancy: dark green vegetables, seafood and sea greens, whole grains, cultured foods like yogurt, cottage cheese and kefir, beans and almonds.

6—Boost B vitamins and choline: Make a mix with 2 tbsp. each: nutritional yeast (high in riboflavin, a specific for CP), lecithin, toasted wheat germ. Sprinkle daily over cereal or mix in juice.

—Lifestyle measures:

•Stay away from all pesticides and agricultural sprays. Many affect the nervous system, especially if that system is fragile and sensitive.

—Bodywork:

•Use hot and cold hydrotherapy to stimulate nerve circulation.

•Schedule regular massage therapy for the muscles; it's a key deterrent to atrophy. Massaged babies with cerebral palsy also may show more organized motor activity.

•Physical therapy is a key tool for preventing muscle deterioration and contracture.

•Apply Earth's Bounty O₂ SPRAY applied to affected muscle areas.

Herbal, Superfood and Supplement Therapy

Interceptive therapy: Choose 2 to 3 recommendations.

1—Relax and repair nerves: Crystal Star RELAX CAPS™ 2-4 daily (improvement results reported), Crystal Star STRESS ARREST™ tea, as needed for tension, with •Evening Primrose Oil caps 6 daily. Or •Gotu Kola (*Centella asiatica*), with •*Ginkgo Biloba* extract for brain - nerve stability. •An effective nerve strengthening tea: one part each: *gotu kola, bilberry, ginger, butcher's broom, scullcap*. •*Hawthorn* extract 4x daily for circulation and a feeling of well-being. •Country Life RELAXER caps (GABA with Taurine); •Metabolic Response Modifiers Glucosamine-Chondroitin complex 3 to 4 caps daily for spinal - nerve pain; •Tyrosine 500mg daily for L-Dopa formation.

2—Strengthen muscles to help control spasms: •Crystal Star MUSCLE RELAXER™ capsules. •Crystal Star BLADDER-KIDNEY CONTROL™ caps in water for urinary incontinence.

3—Boost magnesium for better muscle coordination: •Magnesium 800mg; •Crystal Star OCEAN MINERALS™ for stability. •Pregnant women at risk for premature birth and toxemia from drugs, should take magnesium 400mg during pregnancy to reduce risk of brain injury from birth asphyxia.

4—Choline therapy: •Twin Lab CHOLINE/INOSITOL caps; •Source Naturals PHOS-PHATIDYL CHOLINE in lecithin, 3 softgels daily; •Jarrow MEGA PC-35, up to 12 daily.

5—Boost your B's for calm and tension relief: •B-complex 150mg daily; •REAL LIFE TOTAL B, sublingual (contains 250% of B-12 RDA) to reduce muscle atrophy.

—Effective antioxidants: •*Rosemary* tea; •Natural vitamin E 400IU 3x daily. •CoQ-10 200mg daily; •Octacosanol 1000mg 4 daily.

—Effective superfoods: Choose 1 or 2 recommendations.

•Crystal Star RESTORE YOUR STRENGTH™ drink.

•Red Star NUTRITIONAL YEAST broth or MISO, 1 tbsp. in water before bed.

•Prince of Peace GINSENG-ROYAL JELLY vials or GINKGO with RHODIOLA vials. (excellent).

Can't find a recommended product? Call the 800 number listed in Product Resources for the store nearest you.

Chicken Pox

Varicella Zoster Virus

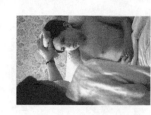

Chicken pox is a herpes-type viral disease, usually a childhood ailment, lasting from 7 to 10 days. One out of chicken pox provides immunity against recurrence for the rest of your life. Adults are vulnerable if they didn't have chicken pox as children. It can be life-threatening (12,000 hospitalizations, about 100 deaths a year) if the child has a compromised immune system (such as undergoing chemotherapy treatment). Commonly caused by an airborne virus, chicken pox preys more on kids whose immune response is low from a diet with few green vegetables, too many sugars and mucous-forming foods. Widespread chicken pox vaccination has meant fewer cases per year, but the chicken pox vaccine itself may imbalance the immune system, eventually allowing more immunological disorders to take hold, even into adulthood. In rare cases, problems including serious brain reactions and low blood count have occurred after the chicken pox vaccine. **For more on child-hood vaccinations, see pg. 236.** For most children, symptoms include a mild fever and headache, with small, flat, pink blisters all over the body that erupt, crust and leave a small scar. Both blisters and scabs are highly infective and extremely itchy. Keep the child isolated from other kids, frail elderly people, or those who haven't had chicken pox. Complications may include chronic ear infections and secondary skin infections.

Diet and Lifestyle Support Therapy

Nutritional therapy plan:

1—Take 2 lemons in water with a little maple syrup every 4 hours to flush the system of toxins and clean the kidneys.

2—Stay on a liquid diet with plenty of fruit and vegetable juices for the first 3 days of infection. Then eat mostly fresh foods for the rest of the week, with apples, bananas, yogurt, avocados and a daily green salad. Try •Knudsen's organic VERY VEGGIE JUICE.

3—Avoid all dairy foods except a little yogurt or kefir cheese. Make a morning blender drink for kids: 8 strawberries, ½ cup vanilla yogurt, 1 tbsp. toasted wheat germ.

4—Get plenty of vitamin C in your diet: strawberries, pineapple, papaya, kiwi, cruciferous veggies like broccoli.

—Watchwords:

•Do not give aspirin to your child. It has been linked to Reye's syndrome, a rare but deadly disease that can afflict children after bouts of chicken pox or some types of flu. It also tends to aggravate sores. Early Reye's syndrome warning symptoms include persistent vomiting and combative behavior.

—Bodywork: •Use a *catnip* enema during acute stage to clean out toxins.

•**Baths and compresses control itching, help healing:** 1 handful of each dried herb to 1 qt. hot water. Steep 10 minutes, strain. Add to a bath, or apply as a wet compress to control itching. —*Rosemary-calendula blend; Peppermint-ginger root blend; Pleurisy root or Witch Hazel.* —Oatmeal or cider vinegar-sea salt baths soothe itches.

•**Effective topical applications:** —To prevent scarring: •Crystal Star SCAR RE-DUCER™ gel, •Thursday Plantation ANTISEPTIC CREAM or •New Chapter MANUKA OIL, or •*Lemon Balm* cream. •Earth's Bounty O₂ SPRAY to reduce scarring.
— Aloe vera gel, or AloeLife SKIN GEL.
—B & T CALIFLORA gel.
—St. John's wort oil or salve. Or pat on *licorice root* tea.

Herbal, Superfood and Supplement Therapy

Interceptive therapy: Choose 2 to 3 recommendations.

1—**Mineral-rich herbs offer key bio-chemical ingredients for neurotransmission:** •*cayenne-lobelia* caps every 4 hours; •Herbs Etc. EARLY ALERT with *echinacea angustifolia, echinacea purpurea* and *pallida;* Klamath POWER 3 caps 4 daily.

2—**Antihistamine herbs reduce itching, redness:** •Crystal Star ANTI-HST™ caps (very fast activity), •Crystal Star ANTI-FLAM™ caps reduce inflammation; •Nutribiotic GRAPEFRUIT SEED skin spray for infection.

 —**Effective homeopathics:** •*Rhus Tox;* •*Pulsatilla.*

3—**Nervine herbs help calm and relax:** •Crystal Star VALERIAN-WILD LETTUCE extract drops in water. •SHINGLE-EEZE by Merix (apply topically for nerve pain), or RELEEV topical by Merix to help dry up sores quickly (excellent results).

4—**Help heal sores:** Apply Crystal Star HERPEX™ LYSINE/LICORICE gel to sores, or Crystal Star ANTI-BIO™ gel; or a *goldenseal-myrrh* solution if sores are infected; or a strong tea of *yellow dock, burdock* and *goldenseal roots* every 4 hours.

5—**Vitamins for chicken pox:** •Extra vitamin C is essential. Begin taking vitamin C when diagnosis is made: Vitamin C or Ester C crystals, ¼ tsp. every 3 hours to bowel tolerance, to relieve itching and neutralize viral activity. Also important: •Vitamin A 10,000IU or Beta carotene 25,000IU; natural vitamin E 400IU daily. •Apply vitamin A and E oil to scabs; zinc 30mg 2x daily for a month to re-establish immunity. •Nutricology THYMUS ORGANIC GLANDULAR for production of T-lymphocytes.

 —**Effective superfoods:** Choose 1 or 2 recommendations.
•Crystal Star RESTORE YOUR STRENGTH™ for minerals.
•Pure Planet CHLORELLA drink as an antiviral.
•Beehive Botanicals fresh royal jelly in honey. Take internally and apply to sores.
•Green Foods BERRY BARLEY.
•New Chapter GINGER WONDER syrup– 1 tbsp. in 8-oz. water 2x daily- swish as a mouthwash.

Can't find a recommended product? Call the 800 number listed in Product Resources for the store nearest you.

Cholesterol

Hyperlipidemias, High Serum LDL or VLDL, High Triglycerides

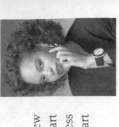

We hear about cholesterol almost daily. High cholesterol affects up to 60 million Americans, yet there are probably more misconceptions about it than any other body element. High cholesterol by itself is a major factor for coronary heart disease. But it's also linked to stress. People under stress *with* cholesterol levels over 240 are 3 times as likely to die of heart trouble. New research links high cholesterol to greater risk of early Alzheimer's disease. An English study shows, however, that progression may be inhibited, even prevented from occurring by taking PCO's like those found in grapeseed oil, white pine bark or flax seed. Cholesterol itself is a fat-related substance essential to every body function, and also is affected by everything you eat. Over-indulgence in artery clogging foods like trans or saturated fats and sugars (especially if your metabolism is also sluggish) leads to serious deposits in arterial linings. If your diet lacks good fiber, cholesterol becomes implicated in gallstones.

There are two kinds of cholesterol found in your blood. (Dietary cholesterol comes from dairy products and meat, and, like saturated and trans fats, can be a factor in high cholesterol.) HDL, high density lipo-protein, or good cholesterol, LDL/VLDL, low density and very low density lipo-proteins, or bad cholesterol are found in the blood stream. Oxidized LDL-cholesterol poses a particular health hazard to the heart, because it significantly contributes to arterial plaque accumulation and to high blood pressure. Strangely however, high cholesterol levels do not seem to increase heart disease risk in people 70 and older. Triglycerides are sugar-related blood fats that usually appear on your thighs and hips. High triglycerides cause blood cells to stick together, impairing circulation and leading to heart attack. If your triglyceride level is above 250, your heart attack risk is twice as high.

What level should your cholesterol be?

Cholesterol screening results can be complicated. Pay close attention to your test results and beware. Some cholesterol-lowering drugs are actually harmful. New research on statin drugs, widely touted for cholesterol reduction, shows that if you take them without making healthy lifestyle changes, death rates, heart attacks or heart disease are NOT reduced. Side effects of cholesterol-lowering drugs like Zocor, Mevacor and Pravachol include liver toxicity, kidney failure, impotence, stomach distress and vision impairment. A study in Journal of Clinical Pharmacology, says these drugs also deplete CoQ_{10} up to 50%, an essential co-enzyme that strengthens the heart and arteries. Here's what's tested in today's cholesterol screening.

...LDL (low density lipoprotein), the "bad" cholesterol, carries cholesterol through the bloodstream for cell-building, but leaves the excess behind on artery walls. Signs that this has happened are poor circulation with cold hands and feet, leg cramps, difficult asthmatic breathing, dry skin and hair. Ideal LDL levels are less than 130 mg/dL. Levels of 130 mg/dL to 159 mg/dL are borderline high. Over 160 mg/dL is high. High LDL cholesterol accumulated on arteries walls can eventually block the flow of blood to your heart or brain, resulting in a heart attack or stroke. The first signs you see may be uncomfortable heart palpitations and dizziness.

New research shows that almost half of all heart diseases patients have pattern-B LDLs, smaller and denser than normal LDLs. Pattern-B LDLs make their way into blood vessels 40% faster than normal LDLs, so fat is deposited on artery walls faster than it can be removed. Studies show people with more than 25% of pattern-B LDL cholesterol have three times the normal risk of heart diseases — even when their total LDL count is normal! Future cholesterol screening may have more precise tests which show the level of pattern-B LDL cholesterol.

...HDL (high density lipoprotein), the "good" cholesterol helps prevent narrowing of the artery walls by transporting excess LDL cholesterol to the liver for excretion as bile. Ideal HDL cholesterol levels should be 60 mg/dL and above. Levels below 35 mg/dL are too low.

...Triglycerides increase the density of LDL cholesterol molecules. Ideal triglyceride levels are less than 200 mg/dL. 200 to 399 mg/dL is considered borderline. Levels 400 mg/dL and above are too high and dangerous to health. Every ounce of triglycerides you eat adds 250 calories (the weight of a raisin).

...Total cholesterol levels should be less than 200 mg/dL. Levels 200 to 239 mg/dL are borderline high. Over 240 mg/dL is high and puts you at an increased risk for heart disease. Low cholesterol levels (below 180) affect 10% of Americans and can be dangerous, a risk factor for hemorrhagic stroke! If your cholesterol levels are high, the cholesterol reduction program on the next page of this book has been successful for hundreds of people.

Can't find a recommended product? Call the 800 number listed in Product Resources for the store nearest you.

Cholesterol

Diet and Lifestyle Support Therapy

Nutritional therapy plan:

1—Cholesterol in foods like eggs isn't a culprit. Research from Kansas State U. shows eating eggs in moderation has little impact on blood cholesterol levels. Eggs are a whole food, with phosphatides to balance the cholesterol. The big contributor to high blood cholesterol levels is saturated fat and over-eating. Focus instead on plant foods like red yeast rice (good results). Vegetarians who occasionally eat eggs and small amounts of low fat dairy are at the lowest risk for arterial or heart disease.

2—Still the key to lower cholesterol: reduce bad fats and add daily dietary fiber. Reduce sugar to lower triglycerides.

3—Foods that lower bad cholesterol: soy foods (*isoflavones*), olive oil (research shows adults who consume 2 tbsp. of extra virgin olive oil a day for just one week have less LDL oxidation!), walnuts, avocados, yams, whole grains like oats, high fiber fresh fruits and vegetables, garlic, onions, green tea, beans, yogurt and cultured foods. Best: Shiitake mushrooms.

4—Substantially reduce or avoid animal fats, red meats, fried foods, fatty dairy foods, salty foods, refined foods. Reduce or eliminate refined sugar and carbohydrates which elevate insulin levels, another high cholesterol culprit.

5—Eat smaller meals, especially at night. A little wine with dinner reduces stress and raises HDL's.

Lifestyle bodywork support:

• Reduce your body weight. Many overweight people have abnormal metabolism. If you are 10 lbs. overweight, your body produces an *extra* 100mg of cholesterol every day.
• Exercise is preventive medicine for cholesterol. Even if you cut your fat, you need to exercise to lower your LDL's. Take a brisk daily walk or other regular aerobic exercise of your choice to enhance circulation and boost HDL.
• Eliminate tobacco use of all kinds. Nicotine raises cholesterol levels.
• Practice a favorite stress reduction technique at least once a day. There is a correlation between high cholesterol and aggression. Men who are the most emotionally repressive have the highest cholesterol levels.

Note: If you're taking statin drugs to lower your cholesterol, know that they may interact with antioxidant supplements (like vitamin C and E). In one recent test, the combination of antioxidant supplements and statin drugs caused protective HDL levels to drop by 22%!

Herbal, Superfood and Supplement Therapy

Interceptive therapy: Choose 2 to 3 recommendations.

1—**Balance your LDL to HDL levels (the real secret):** • Wakunaga FORMULA 104 lecithin, cholesterol; • *Reishi* extract drops; • Red yeast rice; • Policosanol (Nature's statin) 5-30mg daily to inhibit LDL oxidation without reducing good HDL levels.

2—**Support your cardiovascular health:** • Hawthorn extract 3x daily. • Metabolic Response Modifiers CARDIO-CHELATE oral chelation. • Vitamin E 400IU daily and TOCOTRIENOLS 48mg. or • Lane Labs PALM VITEE tocotrienols (very good results).

3—**Boost your antioxidant intake:** • CoQ$_{10}$ 100mg daily (especially if taking cholesterol-lowering drugs). • Grapeseed PCO's 100mg daily; • BILBERRY, ELDERBERRY or HAWTHORN extract 2x daily for PCOs; • Carnitine 1000mg. daily.

4—**Lower LDL's bad fats:** • Udo's PERFECTED OIL BLEND; • *Evening Primrose Oil* 4000mg daily for 2 months; • Omega-3 rich flax oil caps 3 daily; • Magnesium 800mg daily or • Flora MAGNESIUM liquid.

5—**Raise your HDL's:** • *Panax ginseng* (also protects the liver); • *Suma root*; • Solaray ALFA JUICE caps; • Herbs Etc. CHOLES-TERO-TONIC.

6—**Lower your LDL, VLDL, triglyceride levels:** • Grifron MAITAKE mushroom caps; • Heart from the Sun BASIKOL with phytosterols (Mayo clinic tests) or • Jagulana JIAOGULAN (Chinese clinical tests). • *Cayenne-Ginger* capsules 2 daily; • AGED GARLIC EXTRACT (Kyolic), or • *Garlic-Fenugreek* caps 6 daily (decreases bad cholesterol 10%). • Nutricology NAC (*N-acetyl-cysteine*) 1000mg daily, or • Nutricology GUGGUL LIPIDS (guggulipic lowers blood fats over all). • Chromium 200mcg helps triglycerides.

7—**Help your liver metabolize cholesterol:** • Green tea or Crystal Star GREEN TEA CLEANSER™ each morning; • *Milk Thistle Seed* extract for 3 months; • *Dandelion root* tea; • Schiff ENZYMALL with ox bile daily. • Solaray LIPOTROPIC 1000. • Esteem CARDIO-LIFE; • Planetary TRIPHALA as directed.

Note: If dietary changes haven't helped you, use niacin therapy to reduce harmful blood fats. (Do not use if you are glucose intolerant, or have liver disease or a peptic ulcer.) Flush free niacin is OK. Men's effective dose: 1500mg daily; women's dose: 1000mg daily. Take Nature's Way NIACIN 100mg with glycine 500mg if sugar sensitive. • Futurebiotics CHOLESTA-LO with garlic and niacin.

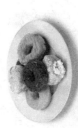

—**Effective superfoods:** Choose 1 or 2 recommendations.
• Jarrow GENTLE FIBERS.
• Red Star NUTRITIONAL YEAST.
• Jagulana JIAOGULAN tea.
• Green Foods BERRY BARLEY ESSENCE.
• GINSENG-LICORICE drops.

Can't find a recommended product? Call the 800 number listed in Product Resources for the store nearest you.

Chronic Fatigue Immune Dysfunction Syndrome

Epstein Barr Virus, Hypoadrenalism

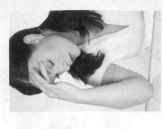

Chronic fatigue and immune dysfunction syndrome (CFIDS) is sometimes referred to as a condition without a cause. Today, as the number of sufferers approaches one million Americans, we know the opposite is true. There are a wealth of causative factors. Many experts say CFIDS is a result of mixed infections with a wide group of viruses involved.... Epstein-Barr virus (EBV), herpes simplex viruses (genital, oral and herpes virus 6, which causes childhood roseola), and cytomegalovirus (CMV) are clearly implicated. CFIDS association with hypoglycemia is well-known. *Candida albicans* yeast (caused by antibiotic overload and excessive sugar intake) and parasite infestations are highly suspect.

Incredibly, new research shows that the polio virus, long considered conquered, may be resurfacing 20 to 30 years after childhood vaccinations against it, as Post-Polio Syndrome, now seen as CFIDS. Environmental contaminants contribute by lowering immune response, allowing CFIDS a path to develop through exhausted adrenal glands. Growing evidence points to high stress lifestyles, overwork and a degenerative imbalance in the endocrine/metabolic systems (particularly the hypothalamic-pituitary-adrenal HPA axis). In fact as our immunity drops lower, almost anything can be the final trigger for CFIDS. Onset is abrupt in almost 90% of cases.

The number of people suffering from medically incurable viral conditions is increasing at an alarming rate. No conventional medical treatment or drug on the market today can help fatigue syndromes; most hinder immune response and recovery. Thankfully, natural healers and therapists have been working with these difficult to diagnose and treat fatigue syndromes since the early eighties. *Call CFIDS Hotline (800) 442-3437, and see MONONUCLEOSIS, page 499 for more info.*

Do you have Chronic Fatigue Syndrome?

Latest estimates reveal that between 800,000 to 2 million Americans are struggling with chronic fatigue syndrome right now. Although anyone (even children) can be affected by CFS, it strikes women more often and much harder. Over 85% of CFS victims are women, usually between 30 and 50, most are outgoing, productive, independent, active, overachievers. Women *under 45* are at the highest risk. Clearly it seems, today's overworked, overstressed "superwomen" are paying the price of their hectic lifestyles in terms of health.

Variations of CFS have been known since the 1800s. Chronic Fatigue Syndrome is most prevalent in the Western industrialized countries where a 40-60 hour work week, single parent households and raising children is the norm. At the root of CFS development is immune system malfunction (often from a highly toxic environment), a lifestyle that dramatically outruns personal energy reserves and the presence of a virus or group of viruses.

Symptomology for Chronic Fatigue Syndromes - A CFIDS Profile

The outward symptoms for chronic fatigue conditions are similar to mononucleosis, HIV infection, candidiasis, cytomegalovirus, M.S., lupus, Lyme disease and fibromyalgia. There are many AIDS-like reactions, but CFIDS does not kill, is not sexually transmitted as once thought, and can go into remission. Get tested for viral titers that measure your body's reaction to the virus, or to elevated levels of EBV anti-bodies for correct treatment.

—**First symptoms**: unusually persistent (for at least 6 months), debilitating fatigue and lethargy, where there has been no previous history of fatigue. It's tiredness that does not resolve with bed rest, and is severe enough to reduce average daily activity below 50% percent of normal. The CFIDS victim experiences classic flu or mononucleosis symptoms - chronic low grade fever and throat infections, headaches, unexplained muscle weakness, gastrointestinal disturbances, and sore lymph nodes in the armpit and neck.

—**Second symptoms:** ringing in the ears, chronic exhaustion, interrupted sleep, long term depression and self-doubt, moodiness, irritability, mental fogginess and muddled thinking, continuing low grade infections and fevers, worsening allergies, diarrhea, sharper muscle aches and weakness, numbness and tingling in the hands and feet, disorientation and vertigo.

—**Third symptoms:** extreme fatigue, isolation, herpes infections, aching ears and eyes, night sweats, blackouts, extremely low immune response resulting in almost constant infections, paranoia, chronic exhaustion, loss of appetite which usually results in extreme weight loss, an MS-like nerve disorder with heart palpitations.

Can't find a recommended product? Call the 800 number listed in Product Resources for the store nearest you.

Knowledge is part of the cure for CFIDS. Some things to recognize:

...CFIDS develops from opportunistic retroviruses that attack a weak immune system. **But it is main ained through other agents:** 1) mononucleosis or yeast related problems; 2) food allergies that are either a related cause or a result; 3) long standing emotional stress or grief, or low levels of cortisol, an immune-stimulating hormone secreted in response to stress; 4) environmental pollutants that cause chemical sensitivities; 5) CFIDS sufferers are far more likely to be smokers, and they suffer more; 6) widespread, long-term use of antibiotic or steroid drugs; 7) a low nutrition diet. The best way to begin is to schedule several tests for conditions that mimic CFIDS. I suggest tests for candida albicans yeast, parasite infestation, food allergies, mononucleosis, and herpes virus so they can be ruled out first.

...Chronic fatigue syndromes act like recurring systemic viral infections, viruses that often go undetected because their symptoms mimic simple illnesses like colds, flu, or acute, but less debilitating, mononucleosis. Following the acute stages, these retro-viruses penetrate the nuclei of immune system T-cells where they can survive and replicate indefinitely. Multiplication of the virus and recurring symptoms appear with the organism ruptures and releases into the bloodstream. This can occur at any time, but almost always arises when a person is under stress or has reduced immune response due to a simpler illness like a cold.

...CFIDS and EBV take longer to overcome than Candida or Herpes virus. The symptoms are similar, but CFIDS viral activity is more virulent and debilitating to the immune system. Entrenchment in the glands (especially the adrenals), organs (especially the liver) and circulatory system (hypotensive) is more deep-seated. It takes two to four weeks to notice consistent improvement, and six months or longer to feel energetic and normal. Most people do respond to natural therapies in three to six months. Many achieve near normal functioning in two years even though the virus may persist in the body.

...CFIDS symptoms are greatly reduced by aerobic exercise. Even light stretching, shiatzu exercises, yoga or short walks are noticeably effective when done regularly every day (a good idea for preventing recurrence, too).

...Good diet and lifestyle habits are paramount in keeping the body clear of toxic wastes and balancing the lymphatic system. Drink plenty of fresh liquids, and clear the bowels daily. High doses of aspirin, NSAIDs or cortisone for arthritic type pain can hamper your body's ability to maintain bone strength and adrenal health.

...Mind and attitude play a critical role in the status of the immune system and energy levels for overcoming CFS. Be gentle with yourself. Don't get so wound up in the strictness of your program that it further depresses you and takes over your life. The people who learn to identify and manage mental, emotional and physical stress in their lives recover fastest. Laughter is still the best medicine.

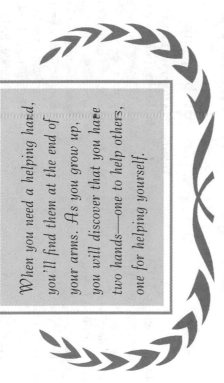

When you need a helping hand, you'll find them at the end of your arms. As you grow up, you will discover that you have two hands—one to help others, one for helping yourself.

Can't find a recommended product? Call the 800 number listed in Product Resources for the store nearest you.

371

Chronic Fatigue Immune Dysfunction Syndrome

Diet and Lifestyle Support Therapy

Nutritional therapy plan for prevention:

1—Keep the diet at least 50% fresh foods during intensive healing. Emphasize foods that build immunity. Include often: **Defense foods:** white and green tea, cruciferous vegetables; **Antibody forming foods:** shiitake mushrooms, onions and garlic; **Oxygenating foods:** wheat germ, spirulina, sea greens; **Mineral-rich, B-complex foods:** sea greens, brown rice, dark greens; **High fiber foods:** prunes and brans; **Cultured foods:** yogurt and miso; **Protein foods:** seafoods, nuts, seeds and whole grains.

2—See the *Diet for Hypoglycemia* on page 463. *Licorice tea* helps balance blood sugar and is specific for CFIDS. Avoid allergen-prone, body-stressing foods: junk and fast foods, caffeine, refined sugars, alcohol, dairy, gluten and chemicals.

3—Immune defense cells are created in bone marrow. Take a protein drink every morning to keep new cell development strong: Lactose-free Solgar WHEY TO GO.

4—**Add green superfoods to your daily diet.** •Crystal Star RESTORE YOUR STRENGTH™ drink (also combats hypothyroidism), and GREEN TEA CLEANSER™ promotes detoxification. Try •Nutricology PRO-GREENS with EFAs, or Pines MIGHTY GREENS with EFAs, or •Fit for You, Intl. MIRACLE GREENS- high stamina, pH balance.

—Lower your homocysteine levels:
— 4 garlic caps (1200mg a day) maintain aortic elasticity.
— B₆, 50mg and folic 800mcg help reduce homocysteine.
— red wine, 1 glass with dinner (unless alcohol intolerant).

Lifestyle bodywork support:
•Avoid all tobacco. Nicotine destroys immunity. It takes 3 months to rebuild immune response even after you quit.

•Take a daily deep-breathing walk for oxygen uptake. Walk for a half hour to stimulate lymphatic system and cerebral circulation. Highly recommended: Yoga and swimming.

•Get 20 minutes early morning sunlight on your body every day possible for vitamin D.

•Apply Matrix Health OXY-SPRAY onto soles of the feet for body oxygen. Alternate use, one week on and one week off. Too much reactivates symptoms. A little is great; a lot is not.

•Relax. An optimistic mental attitude and frame of mind play a major role in releasing body stress, a big factor in lowered immunity. Remember that immune stimulation itself has an anti-viral effect.

•Stretching exercises and massage will cleanse the lymph system and enhance oxygenation. Use hot and cold alternating hydrotherapy to stimulate circulation.

•Overheating therapy helps control retro-viruses. See page 183 for at-home technique.

Herbal, Superfood and Supplement Therapy

Interceptive therapy: Choose several recommendations.

1—Fight the viral infection: •*St. John's wort* (also an antidepressant); •Crystal Star VIREX™ caps (with *St. John's wort*); •Nutricology PROLIVE *olive leaf* extract caps; •*Usnea* extract 30 drops 2x daily or Crystal Star VIREX™ caps; •Pure Planet RED MARINE ALGAE 1000mg for 3 to 6 months. •Garlic caps 8 daily; •Nutribiotic GRAPEFRUIT SEED extract caps. •Vitamin C or Ester C crystals w. bioflavonoids, ¼ tsp. every half hour to bowel tolerance for 10 days - to flush the tissues with anti-viral action. Then reduce to 3-5000mg daily.

2—Take non-depleting energizers: •Acetyl-Carnitine 2000mg daily (often dramatic improvement); •Sublingual B-12, 2500mcg; •Ethical Nutrients MALIC-MAGNESIUM; •Imperial Elixir SIBERIAN ELEUTHERO; •*Dong quai-damiana-ashwagandha* extract; with •Crystal Star ADRENAL ENERGY BOOST™ caps.

3—Enzyme therapy enhances digestion, reduces inflammation: •NADH 10mg or Kal NADA each morning; •CoQ-10 Chewables, 100mg 2x daily; •Nature's Plus Bromelain 1500mg daily; •Futurebiotics VITAL K; •Natren BIFIDO FACTORS; UAS-DDS PLUS with FOS; •Crystal Star DR. ENZYME™ with protease and bromelain.

4—Balance body chemistry to boost healing: take 1 dropperful in water of any of these extracts: •*Suma* or *Siberian eleuthero* extract, •*Ginseng-Reishi mushroom* extract, •*Hawthorn* extract, •Rainbow Light ADAPTO-GEM. •Crystal Star PRO-EST BALANCE™ roll-on, with •*maitake mushroom* caps.

6—Detoxify, repair your liver: •Crystal Star LIVER CLEANSE FLUSHING™ tea for 2 weeks, then LIVER RENEW™ caps with extra *Milk thistle seed* extract for 2 months; •A wheat grass enema, once a week, to help detoxification.

7—Strengthen your nervous system: •SAMe (*S-adenosyl methionine*) to boost serotonin, dopamine and phos. serine levels, 800mg daily. •L-theanine for less stress and better focus, 100-300mg. daily *Ginkgo Biloba* extract or •Prince of Peace GINKGO-RHODIOLA vials as needed; •Herbal Magic GINKGO-GINSENG caps; •*Evening Primrose oil* 4 daily or Udo's PERFECTED OIL BLEND, 1-2 tbsp. daily.

8—Relieve muscle pain, improve sleep: Crystal Star NIGHT CAPS™. •Herbs Etc. DEEP SLEEP softgels (highly effective); •Flora Calcium-Magnesium liquid or Crystal Star CALCIUM MAGNESIUM SOURCE™ caps before bed. •5-HTP 300mg. before bed if there is also depression (not for bipolar). •*Chamomile* tea before bed.

9—Rebuild immune strength: •GINSENG-LICORICE extract (a specific for CFIDS); Astragalus extract 1 large dropperful; •Crystal Star DR. VITALITY™ green and white tea; •Echinacea extract if swollen lymph glands; •Vitamin E 400IU with selenium 200mcg; •PCOs: pine bark or grapeseed, 200mg daily. •Longevity Science PROBOOST (thymic protein A)- good results for CFS; •Nutricology ORGANIC THYMUS; •Tyrosine 1000mg daily.

Can't find a recommended product? Call the 800 number listed in Product Resources for the store nearest you.

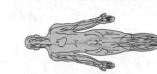

Circulation Problems

Sluggish Blood Flow, Intermittent Claudication, Chillblains, Raynaud's Disease

It isn't hard to see why circulatory health is so important. It delivers our river of life throughout the body. It transports heat from the body interior to the skin. It carries antibodies to infections. It helps move waste products to elimination channels. **Sluggish blood flow** is a first sign of serious disorders. High blood pressure, high cholesterol, arteriosclerosis, varicose veins, phlebitis, and heart disease are all dependent on circulatory health. **Claudication** is a peripheral artery disease, characterized by pain in the legs due to obstructed blood flow (aggravated by lack of exercise, a low fiber diet and constipation). **Raynaud's disease,** often the result of underlying atherosclerosis from using a jackhammer or chain saw over many years, is marked by numb, cold, white hands and feet even in warm weather because small arteries contract and cut off blood flow. **Chillblains** are painful, itchy patches on the hands and feet. Boost your circulation if you have cold hands and feet, chronic migraines, ringing in the ears, leg cramps or prickling swollen ankles (usually accompanied by varicose veins), dizziness, shortness of breath or irregular heartbeat when standing quickly, high triglyceride and cholesterol levels, poor memory, or frequent nosebleeds. *See HIGH BLOOD PRESSURE page 452 and HEART DISEASE page 440.*

Diet and Lifestyle Support Therapy

Nutritional therapy plan for prevention:

1—Keep your colon clear and cholesterol low with a high fiber diet; at least 60% fresh foods. Avoid large or heavy meals. Eat smaller meals more often, instead. Avoid red meat, fried, fatty foods (especially trans fats in snacks), low fiber foods, sugary foods. Limit your caffeine and salt. Have soy milk instead of dairy.

2—Eat citrus fruits, juices and dried fruits - good bioflavonoid content to strengthen vein and tissue walls. Try •Jarrow GENTLE FIBERS drink.

3—Add circulation boosting spices: *cayenne, mustard, garlic, ginger, turmeric, rosemary*.

4—Raynaud's disease: Drink lots of liquids. follow a hypoglycemic diet. Green or white tea daily or DR.VITALITY™ tea with *green* and *white tea, ginger, hawthorn*.

5—Make a circulation drink: take daily for almost immediate improvement: Mix ½ cup tomato juice, ½ cup lemon juice, 6 tsp. wheat germ oil, 1 tsp. nutritional yeast.

—Lifestyle and bodywork measures:
•Biofeedback is notably successful for cold hands and feet.
•Avoid smoking and excess alcohol that restrict blood flow.
•Apply alternating hot and cold *cayenne-ginger* compresses to areas in need of stimulation. Or wrap feet in towels soaked in *cayenne-ginger* solution.
•Use a dry skin brush before your daily shower.
•See a massage therapist for a structure work-out to clear obstructions.
•Take a brisk walk every day to get your blood moving.

—For chillblains: •Nature's Way CAYENNE PAIN RELIEVING ointment or *cayenne-ginger* capsules, 2 daily.

—For claudication: sit with legs elevated on an ottoman when possible. No knee high hosiery. Massage legs each morning with •CAPSAICIN cream. Apply evening hot sea salt compresses to the legs. •Clinical tests show a daily morning walk with •Ginkgo biloba extract, 10-15 drops 4x a day, or •Pacific BioLogic ADAPTRIN for significant improvement in walking and reduced pain (excellent results).

Herbal, Superfood and Supplement Therapy

Interceptive therapy: Choose 2 to 3 recommendations.

1—Boost your circulation nutrients: •Crystal Star HEART PROTECTOR™ caps for MEN and WOMEN; •*Hawthorn, Bilberry* or *Ginkgo Biloba* extracts; •Pacific BioLogic ADAPTRIN (highly recommended) •Country Life sublingual B-12, 2500mcg.

—For claudication: •*Ginkgo biloba* extract 120mg daily; •Solaray CENTELLA VEIN (to decrease leg swelling and heaviness) or •Crystal Star HEARTSEASE CIRCU-CLEANSE™ tea daily; •Enzymedica PURIFY with protease enzyme. •Flora MAGNESIUM liquid helps combat deficiency—common in claudication.

—For Raynaud's Disease: •*Cayenne/ginger* caps 4 daily; •Crystal Star OCEAN MINERALS– iodine and potassium caps. •New Chapter GINGER WONDER syrup and •Magnesium 800mg daily. •Crystal Star GREEN TEA CLEANSER™

2—Stimulate sluggish circulation: •Crystal Star HEARTSEASE CIRCU-CLEANSE™ tea, or a *Chinese Wolfberry-Ginger* combo; •*Ginger* tea daily. •Niacin therapy: 250mg 3x daily (flush-free OK). •Natural Balance GREAT LEGS; •*Butcher's broom* caps tea or Nutricology NATTOZYME, natural blood thinners. •Effective massage oils: *Juniper oil; Rosemary oil.*

3—Strengthen-elasticize veins: •Carnitine 500mg 2x daily for poor leg circulation; •Esteem Products BEYOND RELIEF caps; •Solaray CENTELLA ASIATICA caps; •Vitamin E 400IU with selenium 200mcg daily; •Ester C with bioflavonoids 3000mg daily; •Metabolic Response Modifiers CARDIO CHELATE w. EDTA; •Golden Pride HEART HEALTH PAK. •*Garlic* keeps blood pressure normal and HDL levels down; •*Horse chestnut* extract (not if on anti-coagulant drugs).

4—Flavonoids tone circulation: •*Bilberry* and *Siberian eleuthero* extracts; •Quercetin 1000mg with bromelain 1500mg.

5—Balance prostaglandins to smooth out circulation: •*Omega-3 flax oil* 3x daily; •*Evening Primrose oil* 2000mg daily.

6—Antioxidants boost long-term circulatory health: •*Panax ginseng*; •CoQ-10, 200mg daily; •Pine or grapeseed PCO's 100mg.

Can't find a recommended product? Call the 800 number listed in Product Resources for the store nearest you.

Cols

Upper Respiratory Infections

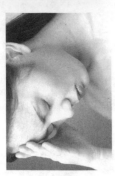

The common cold is quite common.... Americans catch about 66 million colds a year, costing the U.S. economy a whopping $40 billion a year! In any two week period during high risk seasons, almost one-third of the U.S. suffers from a cold. Children in daycare are especially susceptible; they experience up to one dozen colds every year! Your body is talking to you when you get a cold. A cold is usually your body's attempt to cleanse itself of wastes, toxins and bacterial overgrowth that build up to a point where natural immunity can't overcome them. The glands are always affected, and as the endocrine system is on a 6 day cycle, a normal cold usually runs for about a week as your body works through all of its detoxification processes. Work with your body, not against it, to get over a cold. Natural remedies are effective in speeding recovery and reducing discomfort. In my experience, most drug store cold remedies halt the body cleansing/balancing processes, and generally make the cold last longer. **See Flu page 417 for what to do for flu.**

Do you have Chronic Colds?

Over 200 different viruses cause colds. Although we hear most often about rhino-viruses and their involvement in the misery we know as a cold, we are constantly exposed to cold-causing organisms without them actually causing a cold. Your immune system health is the deciding factor in whether you "catch" a cold or not. The medical world is well aware of this, so today there seem to be almost as many drugstore cold remedies, as there are colds.... most of them symptom-suppressing with side effects. A cold is usually a cleansing condition, so it may be better to just let it happen, let your body start fresh, with a stronger immune system. Still, without a doubt, it's hard to work, sleep, and be around other people with miserable cold symptoms. Traditional herbal wisdom is effective for minimizing misery while your body gets on with its job of cleaning house.

Twelve Steps to Better Cold Care

1) A daily walk revs up immune response and gives you some fresh air. A walk puts cleansing oxygen into your lungs, and stops you from feeling sorry for yourself. It works wonders!
2) Take ascorbate vitamin C or Ester C, 1000mg every hour, preferably in powder form with juice, throughout the day. Take zinc lozenges as needed, or propolis throat spray.
3) Don't smoke or drink alcohol (other than a little brandy and lemon). They suppress immunity. Avoid sugary foods, fried foods, and dairy foods. They increase production of thick mucous.
4) Eat lightly but with good nutrition. Nutrient absorption is less efficient during a cold. A vegetarian diet is best at this time so the body won't have to work so hard at digestion.
5) Drink plenty of liquids; 6-8 glasses daily of fresh fruit and vegetable juices, herb teas and water to help flush toxins through and out of your system.
6) Keep warm. Increase room humidity so your mucous membranes will remain active against the virus or bacteria. Don't worry about a fever unless it is prolonged or high. (See fevers as cleansers and healers, page 414.)
7) Take a long hot bath, spa or sauna. Lots of toxins will pass out though the skin. For prevention, take daily alternating hot and cold showers at the beginning of cold season to stimulate immune response. Repeat any time you feel the first signs of discomfort.
8) Stay relaxed. Let your body concentrate energy on cleaning out infection. Go to bed early, get plenty of sleep. Most cell regeneration occurs between midnight and 4 a.m.
9) Use XLEAR nasal wash every day to help keep any bacteria that enters your breathing passages from multiplying.
10) Think positively about becoming well. Optimism is often a self-fulfilling prophecy.
11) Wash hands and clean countertops frequently to prevent virus spread.
12) Rest is important. Light exercise is better than vigorous exercise during a cold.

Can't find a recommended product? Call the 800 number listed in Product Resources for the store nearest you.

Do you have a Cold or the Flu? Here's How to Tell.

Colds and flu are distinct and separate upper respiratory infections, triggered by different viruses. (Outdoor environment - drafts, wetness, temperature changes, etc. do not cause either a cold or the flu.) The flu is more serious, because it can spread to the lungs, and cause severe bronchitis or pneumonia. In the beginning stages, the symptoms of colds and flu can be similar. Both conditions begin when one or more of the over 200 hundred viruses that cause a cold or flu penetrate the body's protective barriers. Viruses don't breathe, digest food or eliminate, but they do replicate themselves with a vengeance. Nose, eyes and mouth are usually the sites of invasion from cold viruses. The most likely target for the flu virus is the respiratory tract. Colds and flu respond to different treatments. The following symptomatic chart can help identify your particular condition and allow you to deal with it better.

A Cold Profile Looks Like This:

—Slow onset. No prostration.
—Body aches - largely due to the release of interferon (an immune stimulator).
—Rarely accompanied by fever and headache.
—Localized symptoms like sore throat, sinus congestion, listlessness, runny nose, sneezing.
—Mild fatigue and weakness as a result of body cleansing.
—Mild to moderate chest discomfort, usually with a hacking cough.
—Sore or burning throat common.

A Flu Profile Looks Like This:

—Swift and severe onset.
—Early and prominent prostration with flushed, hot, moist skin.
—General symptoms like chills, depression and body aches.
—Extreme fatigue, sometimes lasting 2-3 weeks.
—Acute chest discomfort, with severe hacking cough.
—Sore throat occasionally.
—Accompanied by high (102°-104°) fever, headache, sore eyes, achy muscles.

Note: Seek medical attention immediately if you have symptoms like difficulty breathing, unrelenting fever, severe fatigue, nausea, and vomiting- signs of inhalation anthrax.

If you have a hanging on cold, that just won't let you get well:
Here's a tried and true method used by thousands for over 2 decades…

—For 3 days:
Drink 3 cups of Crystal Star Cleansing and Purifying Tea™ or *Dandelion Root* **tea to release congestion. Take 6 capsules daily of Crystal Star Fiber and Herbs Colon Cleanse™ caps to eliminate the excess mucous that keeps harboring the infection.** This method removes the bacteria that keep seeping back into your body from your colon and bowel, and reinfecting you.

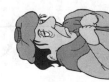
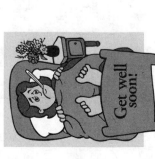
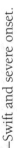

An ascorbic acid flush - a great tool to fight colds and flu:

An ascorbic acid flush accelerates a detoxification program, improves body chemistry to neutralize allergens and fight cold and flu infections. It promotes more rapid healing, and protects against further illness.

1: Use ascorbate vitamin C or Ester C powder with bioflavonoids for best results.

2: Take ½ tsp. every 20 minutes until a soupy stool results. Note: Use ¼ tsp. every hour for a very young child; ½ tsp. every hour for a child six to ten years old.

3: Then reduce the vitamin C dosage slightly so that you have a mealy, loose stool, but not diarrhea. Your body will continue to cleanse. You will be taking approximately 8-10,000mg daily depending on your body weight. Continue for one to two days for a thorough flush.

Can't find a recommended product? Call the 800 number listed in Product Resources for the store nearest you.

Colds

Diet and Lifestyle Support Therapy

Nutritional therapy plan:

1—For a cold: Go on a liquid diet during acute stage, with green or potassium drink -pg. 291 to clean out infected mucous. Take Alacer EMERGEN-C drink mix (*very effective*).

2—Take 2 tbsp. cider vinegar, and 2 tsp. honey in water, or *garlic/ginger* tea morning, and *garlic/miso* soup night. Or 2 tbsp. each lemon juice and honey, and 1 tsp. fresh grated *ginger* at night, or •Planetary formulas OLD INDIAN syrup.

3—When fever and acute stage has passed, eat light meals - fresh and steamed vegetables, fresh fruits and juices, brown rice, mushrooms (esp. shiitake), and cultured foods for friendly intestinal flora.

4—Avoid dairy products of all kinds, red meats, caffeine, sugary, fried or fatty foods during a cold. Chicken soup with pinches of *garlic* and *cayenne* increases mucous release and reduce inflammation.

5—Drink eight glasses of liquids daily, especially green tea, peppermint tea, white tea, and tangerine juice. Crystal Star GREEN TEA CLEANSER™ combats infection.

6—To release quantities of mucous all at once if you have a streaming cold: take fresh grated horseradish in a spoon with lemon juice, and hang over the sink; or use onion-garlic syrup for gentler mucous release.

7—Boost immunity with glutathione foods: brussels sprouts, avocado, asparagus, watermelon, oranges, peaches and green superfoods like chlorella and barley grass.

—Bodywork:

•Open all channels of elimination with hot baths; take ginger caps or tea, hot broths and tonics, brandy and lemon, and catnip enemas.

•Apply hot ginger compresses to the chest.

•Massage therapy opens up blocked body meridians.

—Acupressure press points:

1) For a scratchy, hoarse throat: press just behind the nail and the first joint of the thumb, on the outside.

2) To unclog a stuffy nose: press on the cheek, at the flare of the nostrils where they join the cheek.

•Aromatherapy steams, with or without a vaporizer are effective:

—*Eucalyptus* opens sinus passages.

—*Frankincense* boosts immune response and speeds recovery.

—*Wintergreen* relieves nasal congestion.

—*Mint* or *chamomile* relieve headaches.

—*Tea tree* oil combats infection.

Herbal, Superfood and Supplement Therapy

Interceptive therapy: Choose 2 to 3 recommendations.

1—During initial stage: •Merix Viramedix C & F caps with viracea® can stop a cold in its tracks if used when symptoms start (highly recommended); •Crystal Star ANTI-BIO™ caps 6 daily; Life Rising YIN CHIAO tabs (excellent results) •Vitamin C crystals, ¼ tsp. every half hour to bowel tolerance to flush, neutralize toxins; COLLOIDAL SILVER drops every 3 hours.

2—During acute phase: •*Ginger/Bayberry* caps every hour to promote sweating, eliminate toxins (strong for adults only). •Zand HERBAL LOZENGES, •Crystal Star ZINC SOURCE™ throat rescue spray; •XLEAR (Clear) nasal wash flushes out infection (excellent results); •Beehive Botanical PROPOLIS THROAT spray.

 —Fight the infection: •Crystal Star ANTI-BIO™ caps or extract to lush lymph glands for 6 days. •*Elderberry-mint-yarrow* tea is a good throat coat. •A nasal salt irrigation removes pathogens from mucous membranes and clears breathing quickly: add ½ tsp. sea salt to a cup of warm water. Fill a dropper with liquid, tilt your head and fill each nostril; then blow your nose.

 —Deactivate the cold: Mix in a glass of aloe vera juice: ¼ tsp. vitamin C crystals, 2 tsp. SAMBUCOL elderberry syrup, ½ tsp. turmeric powder (or open a *curcumin* capsule), 1 opened capsule *echinacea*, ½ tsp. *propolis* extract.

 —Cleanse congestion: •*Cayenne-ginger* or •*Cayenne-garlic caps; •Echinacea-goldenseal* caps or Herbs Etc. ECHINACEA-GOLDENSEAL; •*Dandelion root tea; •Crystal Star* D-CONGEST™ spray; •Zand DECONGEST extract; XLEAR nasal wash (good results); •Nutribiotic GRAPEFRUIT SEED extract spray, or gargle (3 drops in 5-oz. water).

 ...Homeopathics: •B&T ALPHA CF; •*Aconite*-fever, sneezing; •*Eupatorium Perfoliatum*-sweating; •Hylands C-PLUS.

3—During recovery phase: •*Usnea* extract; glutamine 1000mg daily; •Nutribiotic NASAL SPRAY & EAR drops; •Zinc lozenges kill throat bacteria-one study reports 50% improvement!

4—Re-establish immune health: •Immudyne MACROFORCE w. beta glucan; •Vitamin C, 5000mg daily decreases cold's severity; •Nutricology NAC (N-acetyl-cysteine) boosts glutathione; •*panax ginseng, astragalus* extract or *Siberian eleuthero* extract boost lymphocytes and interferon; •Enzyme therapy: •Planetary ANDROGRAPHIS the "king of bitters;" or •Flora FLORADIX GALLEXIER.

5—High risk season preventives: •Nutricology PERMA VITE or Solgar WHEY TO GO balance intestinal structure, or •Acidophilus liquid 3 tsp. daily; •Garlic caps; •Beta carotene 100,000IU, or mixed carotene PHYCOTENE MICROCLUSTERS from Royal Bodycare. •Nutricology LACTOFERRIN w. colostrum. •Zinc 30mg daily; •Ethical Nutrients ZINC STATUS, tests for deficiency and is a supplement.

Can't find a recommended product? Call the 800 number listed in Product Resources for the store nearest you.

Cold Sores, Canker Sores, Fever Blisters
Mouth Sores (HSV-1)

Mouth sores caused by the *Herpes Simplex 1 (HSV-1)* virus are highly contagious - you can get them from kissing, sharing eating utensils, drinking glasses, even a towel. According to the American Social Health Association, 80% of American adults are carriers of HSV-1! One in five of them will experience outbreaks. Mouth herpes sores crop up about 20 days after exposure, as a series of red, painful, pus-filled bumps on lips, nose or chin. Inside of the mouth is usually also sore. Accompanying flu like symptoms or a fever aren't unusual. Symptoms last about 2 weeks, a week of great pain and oozing, followed by a week where a scab forms and finally drops off. Note: Almond oil in skin and lip care products can be a trigger.

Fever blisters or **canker sores** occur after a fever or illness, sometimes triggered by a food allergy, such as to high arginine foods or gluten sensitivity, even to Sodium lauryl sulfate toothpaste, or by B-vitamin or iron deficiencies. They are yellowish or grayish and occur on the tongue, inside the cheeks or on the gums. Canker sores occur most often in women, generally because of hormone imbalances, especially PMS. They can also be caused by Crohn's disease (related to great nutrient losses) or emotional stress.

Diet and Lifestyle Support Therapy

Nutritional therapy plan for prevention:

1—Body pH balance is important. Add more cultured foods for prevention: yogurt, kefir, raw sauerkraut, etc. Add sea greens (2 tbsp. snipped, dried) daily for a month.

2—Eat a mineral-rich diet: lots of salads, raw and cooked vegetables, whole grains; baked potatoes and steamed broccoli are especially good. Fresh carrot juice once a week.

3—Avoid high arginine foods, such as coffee, chocolate, peanut butter, nuts, seeds, etc. Avoid nightshade plants like eggplant and peppers.

4—Avoid red meats, caffeine, fried foods, and especially sugary foods and sweet fruits.

—**Tannins and bioflavonoids from food help. Apply:**
• Red wine residues; • Black or green tea, cold tea bags; • Grapes and grape juice; • Apples, apple juice • Strawberries.

—**Rinses normalize mouth pH:** Swish these in the mouth every half hour. • *echinacea*, *lemon balm* or *chamomile* tea; • *goldenseal-myrrh* tea; • Aloe vera juice; • Salty water.

—Effective topical applications:

• During the acute stage: Apply Nutribiotic GRAPEFRUIT SEED SKIN SPRAY or Merix RELEEV topical solution or propolis extract - powerful anti-infectives.

• Then apply any of the following: *Calendula* ointment; • *Witch hazel*; • *Black walnut* hulls tincture; • *Tea tree oil*; • Aloe vera gel; • *Comfrey-aloe* salve; • *Lemon balm* cream; • *Geranium* essential oil; • B & T SSSTING STOP; • Mychelle LOVE YOUR LIPS as a preventative.

• Apply ice packs frequently to stop movement of virus from nerves to the skin. Follow with vitamin E oil.

• Relax more. Get plenty of sleep and rest. Use sunblock more often, and avoid sun exposure during outbreaks.

• For chronic canker sores, switch to a sodium lauryl sulfate-free toothpaste like Nature's Gate SPEARMINT.

Herbal, Superfood and Supplement Therapy

Interceptive therapy: Choose 2 to 3 recommendations.

1—**Reduce pain and inflammation:** Apply RELEEV by Merix- works in 24 hours to heal lesions, (stops pain almost immediately, 75% of people get relief in 24 hours or less). Or • take Crystal Star HERPEX™ capsules 6 daily (both highly recommended); take
• Crystal Star ANTI-FLAM™ or DR. ENZYME™ with protease and bromelain to reduce pain and inflammation long term. Take daily and apply • *Echinacea-goldenseal* extract. Take
• Ester C crystals with bioflavonoids, ¼ tsp. every 2-3 hours in juice, and make a strong C solution in water, apply directly to sores until they subside. • Niacinamide 500mg 4x daily for canker sores. • Apply *Licorice Root* or *Cat's Claw* extract drops every hour.

2—**Fight the virus:** • Merix Health RELEEV caps and • Pure Planet RED ALGAE help prevent and arrest virus replication. • Take L-lysine 500mg 4x daily; apply • Crystal Star HERPEX™ lysine-licorice gel or SUPER LYSINE PLUS cream on blisters. • Take St. John's wort caps, or apply St. John's wort salve. Take • Crystal Star VIREX caps 6 daily.

—*Homeopathics:* Hylands Hylavir; *Rhus Tox.*

3—**Rebalance your body:** • Crystal Star RELAX CAPS™ as needed to calm; • *Burdock* tea
2 cups daily to balance hormones. • *Licorice* extract, or a mouthwash made from • Deglycyrrhizinated Licorice chewable tablets (apply directly, take internally). • Propolis ointment (heals lesions faster than acyclovir); • B Complex 100mg daily with extra B_6 250mg, and pantothenic acid 100mg, or • Nutritional Yeast 2TB daily. • UAS Labs DDS Plus + FOS, or Natren LIFE BIFIDO-FACTORS, ¼ tsp. in water 4x daily to rinse mouth.

—**Proteolytic enzymes for better body pH:** • Bromelain 1500mg, 7 days; • Enzymatic Therapy DGL tabs 4 daily.

4—**Heal your skin:** • Diamond HERPANACINE tablets. • Enzymatic Therapy HERPILYN cream. • Red clover tea.

—**Superfood therapy:** • Crystal Star RESTORE YOUR STRENGTH™ alkalizes the body. Take Jarrow GENTLE FIBERS drink for extra flavonoids.

Can't find a recommended product? Call the 800 number listed in Product Resources for the store nearest you.

Colitis, Irritable Bowel Syndrome

Ulcerative Colitis, Spastic Colon Ilietis

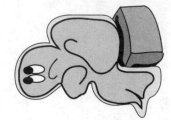

Over 70 million Americans suffer from a digestive disorder. Irritable Bowel Syndrome affects as many as one in five U.S. adults! A chronically inflamed, painful colon, IBS is often a result of food allergies (65%), usually a gluten reaction to wheat, or cheese, corn or eggs. Lactose intolerance symptoms mimic those of IBS and colitis. Most victims are women between 20 and 40 with stressful jobs or lifestyles. Colon membranes become irritated and inflamed, and the body forms pouchy pockets in reaction. In severe cases, ulcerous lesions line the sides of the colon (ulcerative colitis).

If there is also appendicitis-like sharp pain, seek medical help immediately. Conventional medicine hasn't been able to address IBS or colitis very effectively. The IBS drug, Lotronex, taken off the market in November 2000 and re-approved with restrictions, has been linked to severe intestinal problems and several deaths! Natural therapies are effective and reduce the need for drugs. Diet changes are a must. Healing herbs and supplements will not work without diet changes.

What causes IBS and colitis? The most notable culprit is our modern diet with excessively processed foods and sugar loaded foods, accompanied by a lack of fresh foods that supply natural dietary fiber and enzymes. Food allergies to this type of diet play a part; so do yeast diseases like *candida albicans*, and parasites, which may infest up to one in 6 Americans today. Dutch tests show up to 20% of IBS sufferers have a lactose sensitivity. (A lactose free diet reduced IBS hospital stays by 75%!) Other research shows 78% of Irritable Bowel Syndrome (IBS) patients have overgrowth of abnormal bacteria in the small intestine which is aggravated by too many antibiotics which reduce immune response. Too many non-steroidal anti-inflammatory drugs that damage the gut lining are another major factor. Heavy smokers and coffee drinkers are at higher risk, as are tense and anxious people under long emotional stress or depression. A small number of cases are genetically prone.

Colitis symptoms appear in stages: First symptoms include weakness, lethargy and fatigue; the second stage proceeds to abdominal cramps, distention and pain, which is relieved by bowel movements; the third stage involves recurrent constipation, usually alternating with bloody diarrhea and mucous in the stool; the next stage sees the onset of rectal hemorrhoids, fistulas and abscesses, and unusual urgency to defecate, followed by dehydration, mineral loss and unhealthy weight loss with abdominal distention. •An electrolyte replacement drink can help a great deal to control the painful diarrhea. Butyrate has shown success (by prescription for ulcerative colitis). See also CROHN'S DISEASE page 384 for more information.

You can use muscle kinesiology to determine I.B.S. diet triggers:

Muscle testing is a personal technique to help determine your response to a food or substance. Used before buying a healing product, it lets you estimate the product's effectiveness for your own body needs and make-up. You will need a partner for the procedure.

1: Hold your arm out straight from your side, parallel to the ground. Have a partner hold the arm with one hand just below the shoulder, and one hand on the forearm. Your partner should then try to force down towards your side, while you exert all your strength to hold it level. Unless you are in ill health, you should easily be able to withstand this pressure and keep your arm level.

2: Then, simply hold the item that you want to test against your diaphragm (under the breastbone) or thyroid (the point where the collarbone comes together below the neck). The item may be in or out of its packaging, or in its raw state, like a fresh food.

3: While holding the item as above, put your arm out straight from your side as before and have your partner try to press it down again. If the substance or product is beneficial for you, your arm will retain its strength, and your partner will be unable to force it down. If the substance or product is not beneficial, or would worsen your condition, your arm can be easily pushed down by your partner.

Can't find a recommended product? Call the 800 number listed in Product Resources for the store nearest you.

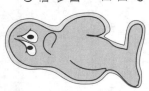

Use your stool as a tool to tell your body state:

Few of us are comfortable talking about what goes on (or doesn't go on) in our private moments in the bathroom — even with our own physician. That's too bad because your stool can be surprisingly revealing about your health status. Elimination varies from person to person, but for optimum health, you should eliminate 2-3 times a day (one time for each meal). Healthy bowel movements should be brown to light brown, light brown to float, bulky (not compacted), and easy to pass. While it's normal for stool to have some odor, it shouldn't be strong or pungent (signs of longer bowel transit time and a diet too high in animal proteins and saturated fat). If you don't fit this model, you're not alone. Most Americans have some degree of colon toxicity, largely as a result of our diets high in fast foods, chemicalized foods and low in fiber-rich whole grains, and fruits and vegetables.

Your stool can be an important tool to help you assess your digestive health.
A few things to watch for:

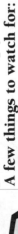

—Bloody or mucous-covered stools can be a sign of Crohn's disease, ulcerative colitis, even colon cancer. It can also be a sign of inflamed, irritated hemorrhoids. Report symptoms like these to your physician right away.

—Thin, ribbonlike or flattened stools are usually the sign of an obstruction like a polyp that narrows the elimination pathway. It can also be a sign of Irritable Bowel Syndrome or spastic colon.

—Stools that are large, messy and leave a film in toilet water signal malabsorption. If the problem is chronic, consider consulting a qualified health professional. Malabsorption problems lead to nutritional deficiencies.

—Abnormally fatty stools may signal pancreatitis, inflammation of the pancreas that can lead to diabetes.

—Extremely foul-smelling stools may mean you have a deficiency of "friendly bacteria" that inhabit your intestines, a diet too high in red meat protein, or Candida yeast overgrowth.

—Greenish stools may mean you should cut down on sugar. If you are a vegetarian who doesn't consume a lot of sugar, it may mean you need more whole grains in your diet.

—Pale, greyish stools can be a sign of liver or gallbladder problems.

—Black, tar-like stools may mean you have bleeding in your upper digestive tract. Report these symptoms to your physician right away.

—Reddish stools are usually the result of eating a lot red foods. Beets are the frequent cause here.

—Dark brown stools can be the result of too much salt in the diet.

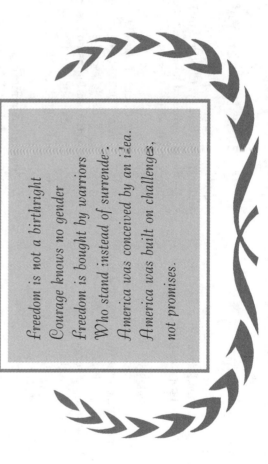

freedom is not a birthright
Courage knows no gender
freedom is bought by warriors
Who stand instead of surrender.
America was conceived by an idea.
America was built on challenge,
not promises.

Can't find a recommended product? Call the 800 number listed in Product Resources for the store nearest you.

Colitis, Irritable Bowel Syndrome

Diet and Lifestyle Support Therapy

Nutritional therapy plan:

1—During the acute stage of an attack: Go on a mono diet for 2 days with apples and apple juice. (A short vegetable juice-brown rice cleanse helps people who are sensitive to sorbitol in apples.)

2—Then eat a low fat diet with plenty of fiber, but low roughage, like white rice to start. Lightly cook foods, never fry; add few salts.

3—Include fresh fruits, fruit fiber from prunes, apples and raisins (not if fructose intolerant- many people with IBS), green salads with olive oil and lemon dressing, whole grain cereals like oatmeal or brown rice (not wheat), and steamed veggies.

4—Have a glass of mixed vegetable juice daily for the first two weeks. Have fresh carrot juice 3 times a week. •WHEAT GRASS juice, shows good results for ulcerative colitis. Keep your body well-hydrated - 6 to 8 glasses of water a day, or try •Herbal Answers ALOE FORCE juice.

5—Eat cultured foods, like yogurt and kefir for friendly intestinal flora.

6—Eat small, frequent meals. No large meals. Eat fruits alone, on an empty stomach.

7—Clean up your diet: Avoid coffee and caffeine foods, sodas, nuts, seeds, dairy and citrus while healing. Cut back on saturated fat (high quality coconut oil is OK). Eliminate sugary foods, fried foods, sorbitol, dairy foods. (Lactose intolerance affects 30% of people with IBS. Statistics show symptoms resolve for up to 40% of those who eliminate dairy completely from their diets.) Eliminate wheat foods (another major irritant) of all kinds. Highly spiced foods are an irritant.

—Watchwords:

•Do not take aspirin. Use an herbal analgesic, or non-aspirin pain killer.

•Avoid antacids. They often do more harm than good by neutralizing body HCl.

•Consciously practice relaxation techniques like meditation and deep breathing to reduce stress.

—Bodywork:

—Effective gentle enemas to rid the colon of fermenting wastes and relieve pain. Tip: Add 1 cup of sesame oil to your choice of below to loosen and release impacted wastes.

—Peppermint tea

—White oak bark

—Slippery elm

—Chamomile

—Lobelia

•Reduce stress: Biofeedback and hypnotherapy are especially helpful for IBS.

•Acupressure helps: Stroke abdomen up, across and down.

•For trapped gas, try the Child Yoga pose.

Herbal, Superfood and Supplement Therapy

Liquid and chewable supplements are best for colitis irritation.

Interceptive therapy: Choose 2 to 3 recommendations.

1—Relieve pain and inflammation: •Take cat's claw (*una da gato*) extract, 3 capsules or 3 droppers daily -usually results in 5 days; or Nature's Way CELL MEND with *cat's claw* and IP-6; •*peppermint* oil is a specific for colitis and IBS, 2 capsules 3x daily, or 5 drops in tea. I like •Crystal Star GREEN TEA CLEANSER™ 2 cups daily with 5 peppermint oil drops 2x daily. •Glutamine 500mg 4x daily. •Take Planetary Formulas TRIPHALA caps, or •Crystal Star BWL-TONE IBS™ (results in 3 days). •High Omega-3 flax oil 3 capsules daily.

—Effective anti-spasmodics: •Crystal Star •MUSCLE RELAXER™ caps 4 at a time, or •Heather's •STRESS OUT™ drops (fast relief). •*Peppermint/ginger* tea reduces griping, gas or Tummy Tamers PEPPERMINT OIL capsules. •Apply warm ginger compresses to spine and stomach.

2—Neutralize, remove allergens: •Gaia TUMERIC-CATECHU SUPREME; •Crystal Star BITTERS & LEMON CLEANSE™ drops, or •*Milk Thistle Seed* drops in water each morning. •QUERCETIN reduces histamine reaction. •*Yellow dock* extract (rapid relief).

3—Soothe the intestines: Nutricology PERM A VITE intestinal permeability powder (with *slippery elm*, L-glutamine, MSM, intestinal glandular complex, N-acetyl-d-glucosamine, *stevia*); or Trimedica SEAGEST with anti-inflammatory white fish. Or try •Nature's Answer SEACENTIALS GOLD at bedtime. Take •*chamomile* tea 4 cups daily; •*slippery elm* or *pau d'arco* tea as needed; •Try VITEX extract for premenstrual I.B.S.

4—Calm tension: •Crystal Star *Valerian-Wild Lettuce* drops in water; •scullcap tea; •Natural Balance 5HTP. Calm.

5—Enzyme therapy normalizes digestive system: •Crystal Star DR. ENZYME™ with protease and bromelain, or •Bromelain 1500mg daily; •American Health papaya enzyme chews; •Biotec BIO-GESTIN; •pancreatin 1400mg before meals. •Alta Health CANGEST powder (especially for wheat allergy reactions); •Enzymatic Therapy DGL chew tabs before meals, PEPPERMINT PLUS (enteric-coated *peppermint oil*) between meals, GUGGUL-PLUS each A.M. •*Caraway-Peppermint Oil* combo, (good results).

6—Immune system support is crucial: •Lane Labs NATURE'S LINING helps re-build gastric tissue (excellent results). •Allergy Research Group NAG 500mg, or •Source Naturals Glucosamine sulfate for mucous membrane health. •Prince of Peace Royal Jelly -Ginseng vials daily. •Sun Wellness CHLORELLA powder in water or •chlorophyll liquid 3 tsp. daily in water before meals; •Beta carotene 150,000IU daily for colitis ulcers; •Eidon ZINC liquid; •Kal COLOSTRUM to rebuild gut lining.

—Superfood therapy: (choose 1 or 2 recommendations.)

•Wakunaga KYO-GREEN drink.

•AloeLife FIBER MATE drink.

Can't find a recommended product? Call the 800 number listed in Product Resources for the store nearest you.

Constipation & Waste Management
Colon and Bowel Health

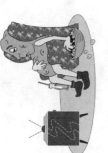

Most poor health conditions stem from poor elimination in some way. Naturopaths believe that old, infected material in bowel pockets causes as much as 90% of all disease. It's understandable, the colon and bowel are the depository for all waste material after food nutrients are extracted and processed into the bloodstream. Decaying food ferments and forms gases, then 2nd, even 3rd generation toxins which often reabsorb into the body and nearby organs. The colon becomes a breeding ground for putrefactive bacteria, viruses, parasites, yeasts and more. This is especially dangerous for your health because healthy intestines act as your body's second immune system. Ideally, we should eliminate after each meal (bowel transit time should be about 12 hours), but some experts say the average American is 50,000 bowel movements *short* over a lifetime because our bowels are so sluggish. Chronic constipation is the #1 gastrointestinal complaint in the U.S., affecting almost 5 million people and responsible for 100,000 hospitalizations every year! The accompanying signs of infrequent bowel elimination are almost as bad as the problems it causes — fatigue, irritability, headaches and mental dullness, gas, nausea and depression, coated tongue and bad breath, body odor and sallow skin.

What causes constipation?

It's more than just a poor diet, although there's no question that too little fiber, too many fried, sugary foods and too much red meat, caffeine and alcohol are the biggest culprits. Allergies to cheese and dairy foods play a big role, especially in kids. Most of us don't drink enough water, especially when we travel, so the first day or so of any trip is spent renormalizing bowel regularity. The enormous rise in the use of antidepressant or opiate drugs along with increasing hypothyroidism are big reasons for constipation in western cultures. Lack of exercise around the world is a major factor.

Specific elements causing constipation and colon toxicity come from three basic areas:

1) *Chemical-laced foods, and pollutants in the environment*, ranging from relatively harmless to very dangerous. Your body can tolerate a certain level of contamination. But when that level is reached, and immune defenses are low, toxic overload causes illness. A strong system can metabolize and excrete many of these toxins, but a constipated body harbors them. As more and different chemicals enter and build up in your system, they tend to interact with those that are already there, forming mutant, second generation chemicals more harmful than the originals. Evidence in recent years suggests that much bowel cancer is caused by environmental agents.

2) *Accumulation of body wastes and metabolic byproducts* that are not excreted properly. Unreleased wastes can also become a breeding ground for parasite infestation. Recent medical research says that 3 out of 5 Americans will be infected by parasites, at some point in their lives! An astounding figure.

3) *Slowed elimination time*, allowing waste materials to ferment, become rancid, and then recirculate through the body tissues as toxic substances, usually resulting in sluggish organ and glandular functions, poor digestion and assimilation, lowered immunity, faulty circulation, and tissue degeneration.

Step-By-Step Diet Change for Colon Health

The rewards of a regular, energetic life are worth it. A high fiber, low fat diet, with lots of fresh foods both cures and prevents waste elimination causes. Even a gentle, gradual improvement from low fiber foods helps almost immediately. In fact, a graduated change is better than a drastic about-face, especially if the colon, bowel or bladder are painfully inflamed. Progress can be felt fairly quickly, but if constipation is a chronic problem, it may take three to six months to rebuild tissue elasticity with good systol/diastol action. After an initial colon juice diet, (page 196), rebuild healthy colon tissue and energy for 1 to 2 months. Emphasize high fiber from fresh vegetables and fruits, cultured foods to increase enzyme production, and alkalizing foods to prevent irritation while healing. Drink 6-8 glasses of healthy liquids every day; avoid dairy drinks (a major cause of constipation).

Could a bentonite clay cleanse help you?

Bentonite clay is a mineral substance with powerful absorption qualities that can pull out suspended impurities in the body. It helps prevent proliferation of pathogenic organisms and parasites, and sets up an environment for rebuilding healthy tissue. Used short term only, it is effective for lymph congestion, blood cleansing and reducing toxicity from environmental pollutants. It may be used orally, anally, or vaginally for acute problems. It works like an internal poultice, drawing out toxic materials, then draining and eliminating them through evacuation. For best results, especially avoid white sugar and flour, and dairy products during this cleanse. 1. To take as an enema, mix ½ cup clay to an enema bag of water. Use 5 to 6 bags for each enema set. Follow the normal enema procedure on page 189, or the directions with your enema apparatus. 2. Massage across the abdomen while expelling toxic waste into the toilet. Note: Bentonite clay packs are also effective applied to varicose veins and arthritic areas.

Can't find a recommended product? Call the 800 number listed in Product Resources for the store nearest you.

Constipation and Waste Management

Diet and Lifestyle Support Therapy

Nutritional therapy plan for prevention: Chew food well, and eat smaller meals.

1—*On rising*: take a glass of lemon juice and water, or Herbal Answers HERBAL ALOE FORCE JUICE with herbs, with 1 tsp. liquid acidophilus added.

2—*Breakfast*: Fiber foods are a key, experts recommend 40-45 grams daily: fiber isn't digested; it simply moves through your system, moving other foods with it. Soak prunes, figs and raisins overnight; take 4 tbsp. with 1 tbsp. blackstrap molasses, or mix with yogurt. •Or mix flax seed, oat bran, raisins and pumpkin seeds with yogurt, apple juice, or a light miso broth. Add 2 tsp. nutritional yeast or Lewis Labs FIBER YEAST; or have oatmeal with yogurt or apple juice; or a bowl of fresh fruits with apple juice or yogurt.

3—*Mid-morning*: take a green drink like Esteem GREEN HARVEST, or Crystal Star ENERGY GREEN RENEWAL™, or green tea or Crystal Star GREEN TEA CLEANSER™, or carrot juice.

4—*Lunch*: Add plenty of intestinal brooms: a fresh green salad with lemon/olive oil dressing, or yogurt or kefir cheese; or steamed veggies and a baked potato with soy or kefir cheese; or a fresh fruit salad with yogurt or cottage cheese topping.

5—*Mid-afternoon*: have green tea or raw crunchy veggies with a low fat soy spread.

6—*Dinner*: have a dinner salad with black bean or lentil soup; or a stir fry and miso soup with sea veggies snipped on top; or a baked vegetable casserole with yogurt sauce; or a vegetable or whole grain pasta with a light lemon sauce.

7—*Bedtime*: have apple or papaya juice, or aloe vera juice.

—Bodywork:

•Think twice about taking antibiotics, drugstore antacids and milk of magnesia. They kill friendly intestinal flora.

•A protective level of fiber in your diet can be measured:
1) the stool should be light enough to float.
2) bowel movements should be regular, daily and effortless.
3) the stool should be almost odorless, signalling less transit time in the bowel. There should be no gas or flatulence.

•Start your program with a colonic irrigation. (Page 189 for how.) A grapefruit seed extract colonic is very effective; a wheat grass retention enema helps if there is colon toxicity along with constipation. (Dilute to 15 to 20 drops per gallon of water.)

•A catnip enema once a week keeps cleansing going. (Page 189 for how.) Enemas may be given to children - small amounts according to size and age. Allow water to enter very slowly; let them expel when they wish.

•Take a daily walk to stimulate regularity. •Have a regular daily time for elimination. •Massage lower back to ease passage of waste. •Don't ignore the urge to defecate. Bowel movement suppression contributes to chronic constipation.

Herbal, Superfood and Supplement Therapy

Interceptive therapy: Choose 2 to 3 recommendations.

1—Cleanse the body of old wastes: •Crystal Star FIBER & HERBS COLON CLEANSE™ caps 2, 3x daily for one to three months. •Nature's Secret A.M./P.M. ULTIMATE CLEANSE or SUPERCLEANSE tabs. •Earth's Bounty OXY-CLEANSE removes old hardened wastes.

—For a quick occasional cleanse: take 3000 to 5000mg vitamin C with bioflavonoids over a two hour period; or an herbal laxative tea to flush wastes gently over a 24-hour period; or Zand CLEANSING LAXATIVE tabs.

2—Prevent constipation: •Omega-3 flax oil caps; •1 tbsp. sesame oil before bed (overnight relief). •magnesium 400mg, or •Rejuvenative foods VEGI DELITE raw sauerkraut.

—Probiotics prevent constipation, and overcome antibiotic residues: •UAS - DDS PLUS with FOS; •Nutricology SYMBIOTICS; •Transformation PLANTA-DOPHI-LUS powder (also helps liver function); •Prevail INNER ECOLOGY; •Jarrow Formulas JARRO-DOPHILUS.

3—Normalize digestion and intestinal functions: •Solaray TETRA CLEANSE or •Nature's Way 5 SYSTEM CLEANSE; •Herbasway LIVER ENHANCER tea; •*Fennel-ginger* caps or *Garlic* caps, 4 daily; •caps, 4 daily; •*Turmeric* or *goldenseal-myrrh* extract drops in water enhance bile flow.

4—Promote a healthy, odor-free stool: •Planetary Formulas TRIPHALA 4 daily; •*Milk thistle seed*, or *dandelion* extract enhance bile output and soften stool.

5—Natural laxatives and regulators: •Bee pollen 2 tsp. daily; •*Senna leaf/pods* (sparingly, a little goes a long way); •*cat's claw* caps 6 daily; •*Cascara* caps increase peristalsis; •Aloe vera juice. •Lane Labs H₂ GO tabs as needed.

6—Enzyme therapy re-establishes body pH balance: •Transformation RELEA-SEZYME daily; •Papaya enzymes 1000mg daily to digest milk proteins and sugars. •*Peppermint* or *ginger* tea provide plant enzymes that specifically balance digestion.

7—Add food-source fiber: A food source multi-vitamin controls initial gas and stomach rumbling as your added dietary fiber combines with the minerals in the G.I. tract. •AloeLife FIBER-MATE drink; or •Jarrow GENTLE FIBERS drink. •Apple pectin tabs; •Maitake mushroom holds moisture in bowel-increases peristalsis.

—Superfood therapy: (choose 1 or 2 recommendations.)
•All One TOTALLY FIBER complex.
•New Chapter GINGER WONDER syrup- 1 tbsp. in 8-oz. water 2x daily.
•Nutricology PRO GREENS with flax.
•Planetary TRI-CLEANSE drink mix.
•Futurebiotics COLON GREEN for gentle regularity.

Can't find a recommended product? Call the 800 number listed in Product Resources for the store nearest you.

Cough

Chronic Cough, Dry, Hacking Cough, Smoker's Cough

A coughs signals an inflamed respiratory tract infection. It's a body defense mechanism, a protective reflex for cleansing the trachea and bronchial tree of excess mucous and toxic material. A chronic cough, however (one that lasts more than two or three weeks), is usually not the result of an infection in itself. It may be evidence of a low grade, chronic infection of throat and sinuses, which commonly occurs from a hanging-on cold or flu. More often, it's evidence of long term throat irritation from smoking, environmental irritants like pollens or chemical pollutants, sometimes a drug side effect or the result of GERD (Gastro-Esophageal Reflux Disorder). This kind of cough is rough, dry (no phlegm or mucous) and hacking, like a smoker's-throat cough from constant irritation. Regard this kind of cough as a sign of low immune response; treat it topically, and with an immune-stimulating program. Eliminate smoking and secondary smoke as much as possible from your environment. *Note:* Avoid drugstore over-the-counter cough suppressants, which can make the problem worse. Suppression can force the infection deeper into tissues. *See Sore Throat, Colds and Flu pages for more information.*

Diet and Lifestyle Support Therapy

Nutritional therapy plan:

1—Start with a short colon cleansing juice diet (pg. 196) to rid the bowel of current wastes. Avoid all dairy foods during acute stages.

2—Take 2 tbsp. honey and 2 tbsp. lemon juice in water or cider vinegar to stop the tickle; or take a cup of hot black tea with the juice of 1 lemon and 1 tsp. honey.

3—Take a cup of hot water with 2 tbsp. brandy and 2 tbsp. lemon juice to help stop a cough at night.

4—Drink cleansing fruit juices. Eat high vitamin C foods: sprouts, green peppers, broccoli, citrus and cherries.

5—Help expel mucous if your cough is from a cold: hot, pungent foods like chilies and garlic bring up phlegm.

6—*Make your own honey/onion cough syrup:* Slice a large onion into rings and place in a bowl. Cover with honey and let stand 24 hours. Strain off liquid mixture and you have a powerful anti-microbial cough elixir.

•*Make the popular thyme-honey cough syrup for kids:* put 3 tbsp. *thyme* leaves in a quart jar. Add 2 cups boiling water. Close lid and let steep til cool. Strain off liquid; add 1 cup honey, a 1" piece *ginger* or a piece of orange peel. Refrigerate. Take 1 tsp. every hour as needed.

Lifestyle bodywork support:

•Steam *eucalyptus, peppermint* or tincture of benzoin in a vaporizer at night to clear respiratory passages.

—**Use topicals directly on the throat:** (choose 1 recommendation.)
•*Ginseng-licorice* drops; •*slippery elm* lozenges; •*Zinc gluconate* lozenges, or •*Zand HERBAL* lozenges; •*horehound, licorice* or *wild cherry* drops or syrups; •Olbas Cough Syrup and pastilles.

—**Effective gargles:** •*Tea tree* drops in water or New Chapter TEA TREE gargle; •*Slippery elm* tea or lozenges for dry coughs; •*Aloe vera* juice; •*Echinacea-goldenseal* solution.

Herbal, Superfood and Supplement Therapy

Interceptive therapy: Choose 2 to 3 recommendations.

1—**Soothe and control the cough:** •Herbs, Etc. OSHA ROOT COMPLEX syrup. For smoker's cough, take vitamin C 3000mg and Alpha Lipoic acid 300mg daily.

2—**Get rid of excess mucous:** •New Chapter ECHINACEA GINGER TONIC; •Herbs Etc. RESPIRATONIC; •*Echinacea extract* to release mucous.

3—**Reduce throat inflammation:** •Crystal Star MUSCLE RELAXER™ capsules, 4 at a time reduces spasmodic coughing (highly recommended), or STRESS OUT™ muscle relaxer drops (very fast acting). •Nature's Way homeopathic SORE THROAT formula. •Crystal Star ZINC SOURCE™ throat rescue (fast relief drops for throat tickles); •Herbs, Etc. ECHINACEA-GOLDENSEAL complex soothes mucous membranes.

4—**Overcome the infection:** •Planetary OLD INDIAN WILD CHERRY BARK SYRUP, hourly as needed; •Propolis extract or lozenges as desired, or •Beehive Botanicals PROPOLIS THROAT SPRAY; •*Garlic* capsules 6 daily.

5—**Strengthen immune response:** •Beta or mixed carotenes 50,000IU daily. •Ascorbate vitamin C or Ester C powder: ¼ tsp. every half hour to bowel tolerance. •Esteem Products IMMUNE LIFE with thymus gland and CoQ10.

—**Cough teas** (choose 1): •*Wild cherry* to suppress a cough (good for kids); •*Clove* tea for spasmodic cough; •*Marshmallow* with honey for dry cough; •*Coltsfoot* for cough with mucous (small amounts only); •*Sage-rosehips* tea with lemon juice, honey and ginger.

—**Effective homeopathic remedies** (choose 1): •BioForce *Biotussin* drops and tabs; •Hylands Cough Syrup; •B&T Cough Syrup; •Standard *Hylavir* tablets.

—**Effective superfood therapy:** (choose 1 or 2 recommendations.)
•Pure Planet AMLA C PLUS.
•*Aloe vera* juice with herbs.
•Prince of Peace GINSENG-ROYAL JELLY vials, 1 daily.

Can't find a recommended product? Call the 800 number listed in Product Resources for the store nearest you.

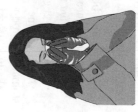

Crohn's Disease
Regional Enteritis

Crohn's disease, chronic inflammation of the digestive tract, strikes 30,000 Americans each year. It affects 400,000 Americans today and is rising. It's characterized by painful ulcers that form along the length of the gastrointestinal lining from rectum to mouth. Alert signs are diarrhea with a low grade fever, abdominal pain and distention from food residue and gas. While ulcerative colitis affects only the mucosa layers of the bowel, Crohn's disease inflames the whole muscle layer of the bowel and the connective tissue below that. In severe cases, Crohn's ulcers (which often bleed) may drill holes right through the gut and require emergency surgery. The ulcers leave thick scar tissue that narrows and hardens the tract, hindering elimination. 50% of Crohn's sufferers have food allergies. Wheat intolerance (celiac disease) is common. A poor diet with low fiber, too much sugar and fried foods is always involved. Smoking and a diet high in animal protein are risk factors. Many Crohn's sufferers follow a candida pattern with abnormal weight loss, depression, anemia and joint pain. A strict, highly nutritious, mild foods diet is an effective, non-toxic alternative to steroid drugs. See also DIVERTICULITIS page 398 and COLITIS page 378. •*Need a Crohn's-friendly practitioner? Call the California Naturopathic Assn. (530) 676-4842.*

Diet and Lifestyle Support Therapy

Nutritional therapy plan for prevention:
Crohn's disease sufferers can react to almost anything, no matter how mild or soothing. Start slowly, noting your reactions carefully.

1—Nutrition spells relief for Crohn's: Start with an alkalizing liquid diet for 3 days: carrot and apple juice, grape juice, pineapple and green vegetable drinks.

2—Add mild fruits and vegetables for a week: carrots, lettuce, potatoes, yams, apples, papayas, bananas and sea greens. Add steamed and raw vegetables, brans, cultured foods for 2 weeks: yogurt, kefir, miso, etc., and especially fresh salads.

3—Add rice, whole grains, wheat germ, tofu, hormone-free turkey, fish and seafood for healing protein and EFAs.

4—Your continuing diet should be high in gentle fiber sources and fresh veggies, low in fats. (Avoid too much fiber during flare-ups.) Most people experience relief with a disaccharide-free diet - mainly avoid table sugars, milk sugars, refined carbs.

6—Avoid foods like popcorn, nuts, seeds, and citrus while healing. Eliminate fatty meats, high fat dairy and fried foods, and chemicalized foods.

7—Drink bottled water. Over-treated tap water can wreak havoc on an inflamed bowel. Note: Consider the Specific Carbohydrate Diet if your Crohn's disease is not responding. This diet has helped many Crohn's sufferers to remain drug-free and in remission. Read *Breaking the Vicious Cycle* by Elaine Gotschall for diet details.

—**Lifestyle and bodywork measures:**
•Eat smaller meals, more frequently.
•Use *peppermint tea* enemas once a week for 1 month.
•Apply hot wet *ginger* compresses to stomach, lower back.
•Avoid commercial antacids. They can make the inflammation worse by causing the stomach to produce more acid.
•Reduce stress in your life. Acupuncture, yoga and meditation have all been successful with Crohn's.

Herbal, Superfood and Supplement Therapy

Interceptive therapy plan: Choose 2 to 3 recommendations.
Use liquid or powdered supplements for less irritation during flare-ups.

1—**Ease the pain:** •Crystal Star ANTI-FLAM™ caps (4 at a time) to ease pain without aspirin. •*Cat's Claw* extract drops in water for 1 month; •Enzymatic Therapy IBS caps, chewable DGL tabs as needed.

2—**Essential fatty acids (EFAs) reduce inflammation:** Nature's Way FISOL enteric coated fish oil caps help reduce relapse rate; •*Evening primrose oil* caps 2000mg daily; •Omega-3 flax oil 2 tbsp. daily, or •Barleans FLAX oil caps 3 daily.

3—**Normalize bowel functions:** •Crystal Star BWL-TONE IBS™ caps 4 daily, with GREEN TEA CLEANSER™ for 3 months. •Mix 1 tsp. bee pollen in 1 cup of *chamomile* tea - 2x daily. •*Garlic* capsules 4-6 daily. •Enzymatic Therapy LIQUID LIVER with *Siberian eleuthero*. —**Plant enzyme therapy normalizes quickly:** •Quercetin with bromelain 1500mg; or •chewable bromelain, or papaya enzymes after meals, or •Solaray QBC complex; •Planetary TRIPHALA caps (very helpful). •Consider Betaine HCl with pepsin if your hydrochloric acid level is low.

4—**Heal tissue damage:** •Crystal Star DR. ENZYME™ with protease and bromelain; •Ethical Nutrients ZINC STATUS test and supplement; •Flora FLORADIX MULTI-VI-TAMIN; •Pure Essence Labs ONE 'N' ONLY multiple; •Country Life sublingual B-12; •Dreamous FULL SPECTRUM growth hormone spray.

5—**Antioxidants re-establish immune response:** •Glutamine 500mg - as effective as prednisone in controlling Crohn's. •Ascorbate vitamin C with bioflavs- pwdr. ¼ tsp. 4 to 6x daily. •OPCs from grapeseed, 150mg daily.

5—**Reculture friendly flora:** •American Health LIQUID ACIDOPHILUS; •Nutricology SYMBIOTICS; •Transformation PLANTADOPHILUS powder.

—**Superfood therapy:** •Garden of Life PRIMAL DEFENSE (homeostatic soil organisms); •AloeLife ALOE GOLD JUICE; •Lewis Labs FIBER YEAST each A.M. •Solgar WHEY TO GO.

Can't find a recommended product? Call the 800 number listed in Product Resources for the store nearest you.

Cysts and Polyps

Benign Tumors, Lipomas, Wens, Skin Tags

Benign lumps or bulges just under the skin can arise from excessive growth of fat cells, internal, unreleased toxins or infections. They are commonly found anywhere on the skin, but also internally, on the intestinal, urethral, genital passage linings. They can be annoying, unsightly, and in some cases lead to cancer. **Cysts** or **polyps** in the colon, bladder or cervix, may lead to rectal, urethral or vaginal bleeding. Some **vaginal cysts** can become painfully inflamed and infected, and bleed during intercourse. **Sebaceous cysts** under the skin result from gland outflow blocked with sebum deposits and accumulation of dead skin cells. **Wens** usually form over nerve ganglia. **Skin tags** (*acrochordons*) are small outgrowths of skin tissue connected to a soft stalk. They usually appear after age 45 or 50, are soft and can be bent easily (unlike a tumor lump). The can be removed with a scalpel or scissors, burned off or frozen off with liquid nitrogen. (See Skin Tags, page 562).

Most benign growths are responsive to the body's growth-regulating mechanisms and receptive to natural therapies. A low fat diet plays a major role in preventing new growths. Homeopathic remedies work to reduce cysts and polyps. A good homeopath can recommend the correct treatment for your type of growth. The remedies here have been successful in reducing cyst size and inflammation. Don't smoke. Nicotine aggravates gland imbalances that allow deposits to form.

Diet and Lifestyle Support Therapy

Nutritional therapy plan:

1—Go on a short 1 to 3 day liquid diet (page 172) to set up a healing environment, stimulate the liver and clean the blood. Follow with a fresh foods diet the rest of the week. •Add 1 tbsp. wheat bran to any morning juice daily for 3 months to prevent colon polyps.

2—Avoid red meats, caffeine, fatty dairy foods.

3—Keep your diet low in animal fats, high in fish, seafoods, sea vegetables, and EFA oils like flax and olive oil. Eliminate fried foods, chocolate, margarine, shortening and trans fats. Add red peppers with plenty of capsaicin to your diet.

4—Have plenty of miso soup with garlic and onions, brown rice, shiitake mushrooms, dark leafy greens and cruciferous vegetables like broccoli.

Bodywork therapy:

—*If the growth is increasing in size:* •Apply Nutribiotic GRAPEFRUIT SEED extract directly, 2x daily. Make and apply an •escharotic salve through which tumor cells can exit: **equal parts:** *garlic powder, goldenseal powder, comfrey or cayenne powder* - mix into *calendula* ointment. Apply daily until tumor is destroyed, usually 4 weeks. •Take and apply *Cat's Claw* extract daily for 3 months, or •*Pau d' arco* tea, 3 cups daily.
•Apply Crystal Star ANTI-BIO™ gel (with pau d'arco and vit. C) for several weeks.
•Apply Herbal Answers ALOE FORCE SKIN gel directly.
•Apply liquid garlic directly with a cotton swab. Or •Use a *garlic powder, lobelia, cayenne* poultice to draw out infection.

•Apply *tea tree oil* for 4 to 6 weeks.
•Apply fresh comfrey compresses until cysts shrinks. Hot compresses bring cyst closer to the skin surface.

•Exfoliate regularly with a loofah or dry skin brush to keep sebaceous glands open.
•Massage into affected area daily, Earth's Bounty O₂ SPRAY for 3 weeks, for noticeable reduction without pain.
•Use only hypoallergenic cosmetics to avoid irritants.

Herbal, Superfood and Supplement Therapy

Interceptive therapy plan: Choose 2 to 3 recommendations.

1—Program to dissolve cyst: Take •Transformation Enzyme PUREZYME, 15 daily (375,000 HUT protease), •Source Naturals WELLNESS RESPONSE Transfer Factors 5 daily, •Crystal Star ANTI-BIO™ extract as an anti-infective, and apply ANTI-BIO™ gel directly, •Grifron MAITAKE D-FRACTION extract 6 drops 3x daily, or •Lane Labs NOX-YLANE 4, 8 capsules daily until growth decreases in size (highly recommended). Add •Solaray CENTELLA ASIATICA caps 4 daily for cytotoxic effects.

2—Clear the lymph system, regulate liver metabolism: For 2 months: •*Echinacea* extract 2x daily; •*Chaparral* caps 6 daily; •*Milk Thistle Seed* extract 4x daily; •Herbs, Etc. LYMPHATONIC softgels. •Crystal Star DR. ENZYME™ with protease and bromelain; •Diamond HERPANACINE caps, 4 daily. •*Evening primrose oil* 3000mg daily.

3—Shield your immune warriors from toxins that aggravate tumor cells: For 1 month: •Mixed carotenes 100,000IU daily, •Ascorbate vitamin C crystals with bioflavs ¼ tsp. 4x daily; •CoQ-10 300mg daily, •Zinc picolinate 50mg 2x daily, then 30mg daily for another month.

—**Improve fat metabolism with EFA's for lipomas and wens:** •Lane Labs BENE-FIN shark cartilage caps, 9 daily for 4 months; •Acetyl-Carnitine 500mg 2x daily; •Omega-3 rich flax oil 2 tbsp. daily. *Note:* I have used a version of Michael Tierra's PAU D'ARCO DEEP CLEANSING capsule formula, 4 daily for 2 months with success for lipomas: Combine *pau d' arco, echinacea root, chaparral, red clover, poria mushroom, gotu kola, kelp and panax ginseng.*

—**For colon polyps:** •1500mg daily calcium with Nature's Secret ULTIMATE A.M./P.M. CLEANSE (good results); •Nutricology GERMANIUM 150mg daily; •Folic acid 400mcg; •Vitamin E 800IU with selenium 200mcg daily until condition clears.

—**Superfood therapy:** •Crystal Star RESTORE YOUR STRENGTH™ drink; •Pure Planet CHLORELLA - tested anti-tumor properties; •Aloe Life ALOE GOLD juice with herbs for 3 months; •Fit for You, International MIRACLE GREENS for detox help.

Can't find a recommended product? Call the 800 number listed in Product Resources for the store nearest you.

Dandruff

Seborrheic Dermatitis, Pityriasis

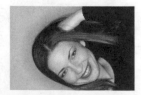

50 million people in the U.S. have it. $300 million is spent every year on products to control it. **Pityriasis** (simple dandruff) is a dry scalp problem, and can usually be controlled with a better diet, cleansing and brushing. **Seborrheic dandruff** appears as dry, scaling flakes in the hair, eyebrows and around ears, nose or forehead. More severe cases show a red, weeping, itching, burning scalp, even unsightly crusts. It looks like a dry skin condition, but seborrheic dandruff is actually the opposite - too much oil is produced, clogging highly active sebaceous glands. Seborrhea appears when skin cells turn over at a faster rate than normal and break away in large flakes into the hair, mostly in the winter months. Dandruff causes range from a scalp imbalance caused by lack of essential fatty acids, yeast overgrowth, or an allergic reaction to excessively strong or harsh hair dyes. Commercial dandruff preparations are suspect because some contain coal tar, and some contain selenium sulfide, a chemical that reduces the production of skin tissue and has been linked to hair loss (because it dries hair out even more) and nerve damage. Diet improvement with more green vegetables and less fat, sugar and alcohol is the key to long term dandruff control for either kind of dandruff. *See Eczema-Psoriasis page 403 for more.*

Diet and Lifestyle Support Therapy

Nutritional therapy plan for prevention:

1—Boost vegetable proteins to keep metabolically active scalp cells working right: soy, nutritional yeast and wheat germ, plenty of fresh fruits and vegetables.

2—Eliminate fried foods. They clog the body so it can't eliminate wastes properly. Try Crystal Star GREEN TEA CLEANSER™ to keep the system metabolically active.

3—Avoid allergy foods: dairy foods, white flour, chocolate, nuts, shellfish -sometimes involved with dandruff. Reduce sugars. Sugar depletes the body of B vitamins.

4—Add sulphur-rich foods: lettuce, oats, red peppers, onions, cucumber, eggs, fish, cabbage, wheat germ.

5—Eat cultured foods: yogurt and miso for healthy intestinal flora, better digestion.

Lifestyle bodywork support:

• Drugstore ointments may do more harm than good by clogging sebaceous glands.

• Massage head with both hands and all the fingers, for 5 minutes to stimulate circulation and slough dead skin cells.

• *Make your own disinfecting dandruff treatment:* 1) Add to a glass bowl, 1 small handful each: *nettle, witch hazel and rosemary leaves.* Add enough boiling water to cover and let steep one hour. Strain. Add ½ tsp. *tea tree oil.* Pour mixture into a mild, unscented shampoo and use twice weekly. OR 2) Add drops of *tea tree oil, rosemary, cedarwood or burdock* oil to your shampoo; massage in - use daily.

• **Dandruff controlling rinses:**

—Oily scalp: apply 1 cup white vinegar. Leave on 15 min.

—Dry scalp: Mix 2 drops vanilla extract with 2 tbsp. mayonnaise. Massage into scalp. Put on a shower cap. Leave on 20 minutes. Or, for one week, apply water-honey (excellent results) to scalp at night to moisturize. Rinse in the morning.

—Itchy scalp: rinse hair 3 times a week with *ginger* tea. Or, try •Organix South NEEM OIL shampoo.

—Leave in rinse: Make hot *thyme-rosemary-yarrow* tea with 1 tbsp. thyme, 1 tbsp. yarrow, 1 tbsp. rosemary to 1 cup water. Cool, strain, massage in. (smells like a country garden).

Herbal, Superfood and Supplement Therapy

Interceptive therapy plan: Choose 2 to 3 recommendations.

1—**Control the causes of flaking:** Add a few drops •Nutribiotic GRAPEFRUIT SEED EXTRACT to shampoo and use daily; or use •Crystal Star ANTI-BIO™ extract or capsules. •Jason TEA TREE OIL SCALP THERAPY or NATURAL JOJOBA SHAMPOO; •Home Health EVERCLEAN dandruff shampoo (very good results). •Rinse hair with cider vinegar after every wash to keep sebum deposits from clogging pores.

2—**Restore scalp's natural balance with EFA's:** •Evening Primrose Oil 3000mg. •Ecco Bella NEEM shampoo; •Omega-3 flax oil 3 tbsp. daily; •Hemp seed oil 1 tbsp. daily.

—**Oil balancing herbal conditioning treatments:** 1) Mix the juice from fresh grated *ginger* with an equal amount of *sesame oil.* Rub on scalp at night. Rinse in the morning. Use for 1 week. 2) Steep *bay* leaves in *olive oil* until fragrant. Rub on scalp before shampoo. Leave on 30 minutes, shampoo out. 3) Massage *jojoba* or *rosemary oil* into scalp. Leave on 1 hour. Shampoo out.

3—**Lubricate and balance with oil-based vitamins:** •Take vitamin E 400IU with selenium 200mcg; •Schiff emulsified A & D; •Choline/inositol caps; •PHYCOTENE MICROCLUSTERS; •Nature's Secret ULTIMATE OIL.

4—**Nourish with minerals:** •Futurebiotics HAIR, SKIN, NAILS tabs 2 daily; •Green Foods IONKELP tabs; •Flora VEGE-SIL. •Borlind of Germany Dado Sens EXTRA DERM shampoo with dead sea salts for extra body; •Eidon SELENIUM liquid; •Zinc picolinate 50mg daily; •B-Complex 100mg daily with extra B$_6$ 100mg, PABA 1000mg, niacin 500mg for circulation; or •Nature's Secret ULTIMATE B. •Biotin 600mcg daily.

—**Superfood therapy:** (choose one recommendation.)

•Crystal Star RESTORE YOUR STRENGTH™, highly absorbable minerals.

•Prince of Peace GINSENG-ROYAL JELLY vials for B-vitamins.

•Green Foods VEGGIE MAGMA, extra vegetable protein.

•Nutricology PRO-GREENS with EFA's.

Can't find a recommended product? Call the 800 number listed in Product Resources for the store nearest you.

Dental Problems

Tooth Tartar and Plaque, Tooth Decay, Bruxism, Salivary Stones, Mercury Amalgams

An astonishing 90% of Americans today have some form of gum disease or tooth decay. Almost 15 million Americans have lost all their teeth! (Keeping your own teeth healthy can keep you younger longer. Studies show that the more natural teeth you are missing, the quicker you will age.) Although the American public has been led to believe that fluoride is the best solution (fluoride has been in city water supplies since World War II), clearly fluoride isn't a "magic bullet" for dental health. In fact, a University of Arizona study finds that the more fluoride a child drinks, the more cavities appear in the teeth. Evidence shows highly fluoridated water is even linked to cancer, neurological impairment, bone pathology and low IQ scores in children. Note: studies show breast fed children have straighter teeth.

Do you have dental problems?

If you have bad breath, a bad taste in your mouth, a noticeable sticky film on your teeth, you probably have **plaque**, the film in which harmful mouth bacteria live. It can begin to damage teeth and gums within 12 hours after a meal. Brush at least twice a day and floss at least once before going to bed. Relax more. Stress reduces salivary flow allowing bacteria to flourish. **Salivary stones** cause swelling and jaw pain just in front of the ear, and a stone-like growth that blocks saliva. They're also tied to too much red meat and caffeine that cause constipation and acid in the system. Take your vitamins and eat more fresh foods to keep cavities down.

Are mercury amalgam fillings safe? Although not all people with amalgam fillings are sensitive to the mercury release, there seems to be no doubt that there are definite immuno-toxic effects for people who are. Mercury is a heavy metal that kills beneficial bacteria and allows resistant strains, which are also antibiotic-resistant, to flourish. The best choice is still to have the fillings gradually removed and replaced. After removal, go on a 2 to 3 month detox program to re-ease the mercury from your bloodstream.

Need to find a holistic dentist? Visit the Holistic Dental Association's website; do an online search, http://www.holisticdental.org.

Is the fluoride in your water and toothpaste poisoning you?

I was shocked when I read the new studies on fluoride toxicity and its deadly effects on health, especially for postmenopausal women, young children and developing babies. I was even more shocked to find out that big business is still dumping this hazardous waste, into the public water supply. Europe paid attention to those studies and is now 98% fluoridation-free. Many U.S. cities are beginning to reject fluoride legislation. **(See Water page 119.)**

Most of us have been brought up to believe fluoride was good for teeth. Fluoride has been added to the water supply and toothpastes for decades, because studies conducted by our Public Health Services showed fluoride had health benefits for teeth. Newer large-scale studies show no difference in decay rates of permanent teeth in fluoridated and non-fluoridated areas. In addition, fluoride sources were different decades ago. They weren't a by-product of the phosphate fertilizer industry as they are today; they were a product of the aluminum industry, sodium fluoride. Today, the type of fluoride that's added to almost 70% of our water supply is hydrofluosilicic acid... much more problematic than the sodium fluoride of years ago. Hydrofluosilicic acid is only 40-50% fluoride. The rest is heavy metals, like arsenic, lead, aluminum, and uranium-238. It's full of waste pollutants, sludges and chemicals that are virtually untreated by the scrub system used to process it before it is dumped into our water.

Signs and symptoms of fluoride toxicity:

• bone damage — early signs of osteoporosis, too-easy bone fractures
• unusual thyroid problems and immune weakening
• higher than normal birth defects or cancer in an area
• signs of early Alzheimer's disease
• dental fluorosis, a first sign of fluoride poisoning is marked by pitted or white specked teeth
• nervous system malfunctions; a tendency to kidney problems, cardiovascular problems like arrhythmias
• learning disabilities; lower than normal IQ scores in children (fluoride is more toxic than lead)

The dedicated people from Citizens for Safe Drinking Water work hard to protect the water supply from mandatory water fluoridation. For more information, you can contact them at 1-800-728-3833.

Can't find a recommended product? Call the 800 number listed in Product Resources for the store nearest you.

Diet and Lifestyle Support Therapy

Nutritional therapy plan for prevention:

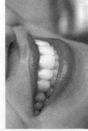

1—Eat crunchy teeth-cleaning foods: fresh vegetables, celery, carrots, broccoli, cauliflower, apples, etc. Chew well. Avoid soft, gooey foods and dairy foods like ice cream that leave a film on teeth.

2—Eat high mineral foods for strong teeth: green leafy vegetables, broccoli, cabbage, and high fiber whole grains. Have a fresh salad every day.

3—Focus on cranberries, cashews, cardamom seeds, especially green tea. All have anti-adhesion properties to keep plaque from adhering to teeth. Strawberries are a good tooth cleanser. Rub strawberry halves on teeth. Add yogurt as a viable source of calcium.

4—Reduce fats, sugars and carbs (which turn into sugar). A high fat diet means high lipid levels in saliva and a higher risk of tooth decay. Sugars significantly increase plaque accumulation. Mouth bacteria feed off sugar, reproduce and eliminate acid wastes simultaneously. Within 5-10 minutes of eating sugar, acid production begins and lasts for 20-30 minutes. The more acid produced, the more chance it has to penetrate through tooth enamel and begin the cycle of tooth decay! (Note: Nibbling low fat cheese after eating sugar neutralizes cavity-causing acids.)

5—Potato chips are the worst. They turn into sugar and stick to your teeth. Drink water after eating them and all sugary foods and carbs to flush out plaque acids.

6—Add hot foods that make your eyes water: wasabi (Asian horseradish), chili peppers (also good sources of C). They inhibit bacteria growth that cause cavities.

Lifestyle bodywork support:

• To remove tartar: Dry brush first to loosen tartar. Then mix equal parts cream of tartar and sea salt, or baking soda and sea salt and scrub teeth.

• Floss daily. Nothing makes you look older than bad teeth.

• Electric toothbrushes can make home cleanings more efficient. High quality electric toothbrush bristles can rotate up to 4,200 times a minute, removing much more plaque from tooth surfaces, in between teeth and even under the gum line that regular toothbrushes can't touch. The Interplak and Rotadent models come highly recommended.

—Natural oral care:

• Excellent home cleaning kit: Nature's Answer ORAL HEALTH PROGRAM.

• Anti-bacterial, anti-fungal for almost every mouth problem: *Tea tree oil* products.

• To whiten: •Peelu has natural chlorine that whitens, removes tarter and controls plaque; it also has natural vitamin C. •Or, apply a pinch of baking soda and 3% hydrogen peroxide on your toothbrush. Brush for 3 minutes, rinse thoroughly.

Herbal, Superfood and Supplement Therapy

Interceptive therapy plan: Choose 2 to 3 recommendations.

1—**Boost antibacterial mouth activity:** •*Ginseng-licorice* extract drops in water as a mouthwash to inhibit bacteria and harmful sugars. •MICROBRITE, whitening powder available on Royal-Health.Com to remove and prevent tartar build-up; •Nature's Answer PERIOBRITE for deep cleaning; •Beehive Botanical PROPOLIS & HERBS THROAT SPRAY as needed. •*Eucalyptus* extract to prevent cavities; •Neem toothpaste to remove tarter; •Bloodroot (*sanguinaria*) helps remove plaque.

2—**Build tooth enamel:** •Crystal Star IODINE, POTASSIUM SILICA™ extract drops in water as a mouthwash; or take •Flora VEGE-SIL caps daily. •Apply baking soda mixed with water drops in a paste to teeth. Leave on 5 minutes to remineralize. To remineralize teeth, with antiseptic activity. •MICROBRITE Powder; •Thursday Plantation Tea Tree paste or •Eco-Dent tooth powder supports remineralization.

3—**Strengthen teeth and gums:** •Ester C crystals with bioflavs. and rutin, 1/4 tsp. 3x daily in water. Swish and hold in mouth before swallowing for best results. Or, use •Ester C chewables as needed. •Solaray ALFAJUICE capsules 4 daily; •Spirulina tabs 6 daily; or •Klamath POWER 3 capsules. Massage gums with •vitamin E oil; take internally 400IU daily.

4—**Control mouth infections:** •CoQ-10, 200mg daily, or Douglas Labs CoQMELT chewables daily; •*Myrrh* drops as needed; •B complex 100mg daily; •Beehive Botanicals PROPOLIS TINCTURE. •Papain chewables; •Omega-3 fatty acids like *flax* oil control inflammation. •Nutribiotic GRAPEFRUIT SEED EXTRACT in water as a natural mouthwash. •Add 3 drops *tea tree* oil to water as a mouthwash.

—**For salivary duct stones:** •Rinse mouth with equal parts *goldenseal root* and *white oak bark* tea to reduce swelling and bleeding. •Rinse mouth with *ginger root* tea; apply *ginger* compresses to area. •Rinse mouth with Crystal Star IODINE, POTASSIUM, SILICA extract in water, take *kelp* tabs 6 daily. •Alacer EMERGEN-C daily.

—**For bruxism:** take a calcium-manesium-zinc combination daily to reduce stress.

—**Mercury Amalgam Detox:** After having fillings removed, try this 5-point program for two months to protect against mercury exposure. •MICROHYDRIN PLUS, 2 daily. •Pure Planet CHLORELLA. •L-glutathione 100mg daily; •N-acetyl-cysteine 600mg with extra vitamin C, 3000mg daily. • 4 *garlic* capsules, 1200mg daily.

—**Superfood therapy:**

•Crystal Star GREEN TEA CLEANSER™ or •Crystal Star DR.VITALITY™ tea - green and white tea for immune function and detoxification (good preventive). •C'est Si Bon CHLORENERGY, 1 packet daily.

Can't find a recommended product? Call the 800 number listed in Product Resources for the store nearest you.

Dental Problems

Toothaches, Dental Abscesses, TMJ (Temperomandibular Joint Syndrome)

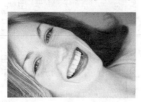

Pay attention to your teeth. Ignore them and you'll lose them. Many dentists now realize that you need to see a nutritionist as well as a dentist if you have chronic toothaches and infections. The number one way to keep your mouth clean is to eat a natural diet. Natural wisdom about wisdom teeth?.... check to see that they're growing in straight and have enough room; eat right so they don't decay; clean them well. Healthy teeth help your mouth's immune system to work. *TMJ* is a painful, arthritis-like syndrome that links various dental and other health problems to jaw misalignment (usually only on one side, sometimes caused by tooth grinding at night or a neck injury that doesn't heal). Approximately 10 million people suffer from TMJ, three times as many women as men. TMJ symptoms include painful jaw movement and jaw clicking, headaches, ringing in the ears, sinus pain, hearing loss, depression, dizziness and facial neuralgia. Natural therapies are an excellent choice to manage TMJ. Research in the Journal of the American Dental Association shows 60 to 90% of people with TMJ improve when they use holistic therapies like jaw exercises, massage, acupuncture, cranial manipulation and relaxation techniques. Stress is more involved in tooth and jaw pain than once thought. Relax.

Diet and Lifestyle Support Therapy

Nutritional therapy plan for prevention:

1—Eat primarily fresh foods during acute stages to speed healing, with plenty of leafy greens and vegetable drinks. Try Crystal Star DR. VITALITY™, a green and white tea blend for tooth and gum health each morning.

2—To prevent recurring tooth problems, eat lots of crunchy, crisp foods, such as celery, and other raw vegetables, nuts and seeds, and whole grain crackers. Chew food very well.

3—Eat calcium-rich foods: greens and shellfish. Eat salmon twice a week for anti-inflammatory EFAs.

4—Reduce citrus juices if you have weak teeth. They're great for your insides, but not for your teeth. Avoid soft, gooey foods. Sweets and sodas especially damage weak teeth.

Apply directly to area for pain:

1) Ice the jaw; take a little wine or brandy and hold on the aching area as long as possible. Hot and cold packs increase circulation and reduce pain.

2) Mix 20 drops of clove oil with 1-oz. brandy. Apply with a cotton swab to toothache area. Up to 90 minutes relief!

3) Hot *Ginger* or *Comfrey root* are effective jaw compresses.

—**Use a cotton swab to apply these:** •Chinese WHITE FLOWER oil. •Propolis tincture (Beehive Botanicals). •1 tsp. acidophilus dissolved in water. •Black walnut extract (anti-infective). •Vanilla extract. •Apply *Bilberry* or *Hawthorn* extract drops for on-the-spot bioflavonoids.

Lifestyle bodywork support:

•For TMJ: Massage therapy, biofeedback and chiropractic adjustments.
•Acupressure technique: Squeeze the sides of each index finger at the end. Hold hard for 30 seconds.

•For dental abscesses: Rinse mouth with a solution of equal parts *goldenseal root* and *white oak bark tea* to take down pain and swelling.

Herbal, Superfood and Supplement Therapy

Interceptive therapy plan: Choose 2 to 3 recommendations.

1—**Control infection:** •Crystal Star ANTI-BIO™ caps, or apply ANTI-BIO™ extract with a cotton swab directly on inflamed area - a good disinfectant after a root canal. •Pacific BioLogic TOOTHACHE caps, fast pain relief; •*Echinacea-myrrh* extract. •Twin Labs PROPOLIS extract. •MICROBRITE, available on royalbodycare.com, reduces plaque that causes infection.

2—**Reduce inflammation:** •Apply *clove oil* directly to painful tooth, or chew whole cloves; •Apply *lobelia* tincture; •Take Solaray TURMERIC caps, or •Crystal Star ANTI-FLAM™ caps, 4 as needed for pain; or •BROMELAIN 1500mg. or Crystal Star DR. ENZYME™ with protease and bromelain; •*Evening Primrose Oil*, 1300mg 2x daily.

3—**Rebuild strong teeth:** •CAL-MAG-ZINC, 4 daily, with boron 3mg. •Crystal Star CALCIUM MAGNESIUM PLANT SOURCE™ and •Crystal Star IODINE, POTASSIUM SILICA™ drops in water as a mouthwash; or take •Flora VEGE-SIL caps daily.

4—**Rebalance mouth pH:** •Reculture your mouth with American Health CHEWABLE ACIDOPHILUS with bifidus, especially for wisdom teeth. •Swish and hold De Souza liquid chlorophyll (in a small amount of water) daily for one month.

—**Remedies for dental abscesses:** Colloidal Silver - take internally, apply directly. Myrrh extract - apply directly. For dry socket abscesses - *sage tea.* **Homeopathics:** •*Chamomilla* - neuralgic aches; •*Belladonna* - throbbing pain; *Mercurius* - foul breath; •*Silicea* - pus drainage; •*Bryonia* - acute pain.

—**For TMJ:** Take •B-complex 100mg with extra B₆ 100mg, niacin 100mg. •Take DLPA 1000mg as needed. •*Cayenne-ginger* caps take down inflammation. Take •CoQ-10, 200mg daily, or Douglas Labs COQMELT chewables daily; as a preventive. •Fight free radical damage-MICROHYDRIN PLUS; •Nerve and pain relaxing herbs: *Kava Kava* caps, or *Valerian-Wild Lettuce* extract, •Homeopathic remedies for TMJ: *Cal. Phos., Mag. Phos., Chamomilla, Rhus Tox.*

—**Superfood therapy:** •Wakunaga KYO-GREEN for jaw arthritis; •Nutricology PRO-GREENS + flax; •Crystal Star ENERGY GREEN RENEWAL™; •Pure Planet SPIRULINA.

Can't find a recommended product? Call the 800 number listed in Product Resources for the store nearest you.

Dental Problems - Gum Disease

Periodontal Disease, Gingivitis, Pyorrhea

75% of the U.S. population over 35 has some form of gum disease. Even many children show signs of gingivitis today. Periodontal disease is a progressive disorder that affects both gums and bone structure around teeth. Plaque on gums hardens into tartar, forming deep pockets between gums and teeth roots, leading to loosened teeth and eventual bone damage. Gum disease is a sign of nutrient deficiencies like vitamins A, C, D and calcium, and of body chemistry out of balance. Left untreated, it can lead to periodontitis (chronic infection and bone degeneration), the most common cause of tooth loss in America. Experts say there is high correspondence between periodontitis and disorders like arthritis, diabetes and cadiovas-cular diseases. Some anti-depressant drugs can cause saliva reduction followed by gum disease. Advanced cases of periodontitis are extremely difficult to treat successfully. Still, holistic therapies that rebalance body chemistry through diet improvement, supplements and irrigation, are sometimes good alternatives to surgery. Start now to protect your mouth if you have red, swollen, tender gums that bleed when you brush, chronic bad breath that no amount of mouthwash helps, loose shifting teeth, pus between teeth and gums, receding gums that leave the root surface of teeth exposed, or the loss of even cavity-free teeth.

Diet and Lifestyle Support Therapy

Nutritional therapy plan for prevention:

1—Focus on whole foods. Dental disease was extremely rare before the 1930s, when people ate whole, seasonal, fresh foods. The same high fat, low fiber, fast food diet implicated in heart disease, cancer, diabetes and osteoporosis is also involved in dental disease.

2—Cranberries, cashews, cardamom seeds, wasabi and green tea have anti-adhesion properties to arrest plaque acid, and keep plaque from adhering to teeth - a major cause of gum disease. Clean, soothe, rebalance gums with fresh strawberry halves, baking soda, honey or lemon juice. Use stevia, a good-for-your-gums sweetener.

3—Eat raw, crunchy, high fiber foods to stimulate gums: apples, celery, Grape Nuts cereal, seeds, chewy grains. Have a green salad every day. Chew well.

4—Eat high vitamin C foods like broccoli, green peppers, sea greens, kiwi, papaya, cantaloupe, and citrus fruits.

5—Eat vitamin A, carotene-rich foods like dark leafy greens, yellow and orange veg-etables and fruits, fish, sea vegetables.

6—Avoid caffeine, sugary foods and carbonated drinks that form plaque acids. Sodas are a major dental problem with high phosphorous levels that leach calcium from teeth and the jaw bone and erode protective enamel that prevents tooth decay.

Lifestyle bodywork support: Regular professional cleanings are imperative to recovery from gingivitis and periodontitis. •Chlorophyll liquid 3 tsp. daily before meals; or dilute with water and apply directly to gums.
•Nature's Answer ORAL HEALTH program, for dental disease. Good results!
•Rub *Goldenseal-Myrrh* powder mixed with aloe vera gel on gums. Great after dental surgery to heal, reduce swelling.
•Chew propolis lozenges. Use propolis toothpaste.
•Thursday Plantation TEA TREE toothpaste.
•Rinse with salt water or olive leaf extract solution at first signs of gum infection.
•Use a rubber tipped stimulator to massage the gum area daily.

Herbal, Superfood and Supplement Therapy

Interceptive therapy plan: Choose 2 to 3 recommendations.

1—**Control the infection:** •Take Crystal Star ANTI-BIO™ caps, and rub ANTI-BIO™ extract, or *myrrh* extract, *Lobelia* extract, or *Tea Tree Oil* drops directly on gums. For immediate relief and prevention: •CoQ$_{10}$ 200mg daily, or •Enzymatic Therapy VITALINE chewable CoQ$_{10}$. •Make up a vitamin C solution with water and ascorbate C powder with bioflavonoids, rub directly on gums. Take vitamin C 5000mg daily. •MICROBRITE, avail-able on royalbodycare.com, reduces plaque that causes gum infection. •Durafresh ORAL RINSE (great for bad breath and dental infection); •*Licorice* extract is anti-bacterial.

2—**Reduce inflammation, stop bleeding, relieve pain:** Rub •*Clove oil or Calendula* tincture on gums to relieve pain. Mix 6 drops *Myrrh-goldenseal* extract in wa-ter, rinse mouth to stop bleeding. •Put 6 drops *tea tree oil*, or Nutribiotic GRAPEFRUIT SEED extract or Nature's Answer PERIOWASH in a water pik, use daily for recurring gum infections (excellent reports). •Take three anti-inflammatories 2x daily: Quercetin 1000mg, Bromelain 1500mg, Lysine 500mg; •Crystal Star ANTI-FLAM™ caps for gin-givitis and abscesses. or •Body Essentials SILICA GEL, 1 tbsp. in 3-oz. water 3x daily - or rub directly on gums. •Rub American Biologics DIOXYCHLOR gel directly on gums.
•Enzymatic Therapy ORA BASICS with WILLOCIN caps for pain.

3—**Heal and strengthen gums:** •*Gotu Kola* extract or *St. John's wort* tea promotes heal-ing; •*Ginkgo Biloba* extract for healing circulation and flavonoids; •Crystal Star OCEAN MINERALS™ caps strengthen gums (takes about 3 weeks). •Quantum GUM THERAPY; •prick vitamin A & E emulsion caps, rub oil on gums. •Lane Labs ADVACAL Ultra or Flora Cal/Mag/Zinc liquid with Vitamin D to reduce alveolar bone loss.

4—**Add EFAs to rebalance body chemistry:** •*Evening Primrose Oil* caps 1000mg daily; •Omega-3 flax oil 2 tbsp. daily; •Pure Essence Labs ONE 'N' ONLY multivitamin helps prevent gum disease.

—**Superfood therapy:** •Pure Planet AMLA C PLUS tabs. •AloeLife ALOE GOLD drink with *myrrh.*

Can't find a recommended product? Call the 800 number listed in Product Resources for the store nearest you.

Depression

Bi-Polar Disorder, Paranoia, Mood Affective Disorder

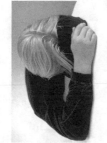

Depression is the most common adult psychiatric disorder, and it's on the rise worldwide. Today, the World Health Organization recognizes depression as one of the top four disabling diseases in the world! Mood disorders affect 30 million Americans (women more than men) and we spend over $20 billion on treatment. Over 20 million prescriptions for Prozac alone, a so-called "wonder" antidepressant drug, have been filled since its debut in 1987. Clever marketers now even push mood elevating drugs for shyness or ordinary sadness! Yet Prozac has been linked to 23,067 adverse drug reactions, 1,436 suicide attempts, and up to 1,313 deaths! Clinical depression is much more than a case of the blues. Depression is both a mental and emotional state, a feeling of being in a box that you can't escape. It's closely tied to disease; over 80% of terminal cancer patients have a history of chronic depression.

Depression today is identified in two parts — underlying circumstances, as well as more incidental traits.

Underlying origins for depression: 1) The great loss of a spouse or child, and the inability to express grief; 2) Bottled-up anger and aggression turned inward; 3) Negative emotional behavior often learned as a child; 4) Biochemical imbalance (such as copper) involved with neurotransmitter, amino acid and other nutrient deficiencies; 5) Hypothyroidism, often misdiagnosed as depression; 6) Drug-induced depression.

Incidental markers for depression: 1) Hypoglycemia or sugar or alcohol dependency; 2) prescription drug addiction or intolerance; 3) chemical or food allergies; 4) hormonal imbalances related to childbirth, PMS or menopause; 5) negative emotions as a result of the inability to cope with prolonged, intense stress. 6) Research from the Journal of Orthomolecular Medicine links mercury fillings to manic depression. *See Anxiety and Chronic Fatigue Syndrome pages for more information.*

Are you depressed?

At some point in their lives, one in five Americans will experience a depression episode. The elderly, the lonely and drug abusers used to be the prime depression candidates, but no longer.... Baby Boomers (men and women), city residents, teens, even children now have identifiable depression. Over twenty-eight million Americans take anti-depressant drugs or anxiety medications to control depression symptoms. While many of these drugs do seem to relieve symptoms at least temporarily, they can have disturbing side effects. Low libido, dry mouth and eyes, dizziness, nausea, headaches and insomnia are only some of Prozac's side effects. Even more frightening, in a 1990 study in Journal of American Psychiatry, Prozac led to "intense, violent suicidal preoccupation!" Numerous other studies link popular anti-depressants like *imipramine* and *amitriptyline* to increased aggression and suicidal ideas NOT present before the drug was used! *If you are on anti-depressant drug therapy, ask your physician before adjusting or stopping your medication.*

Major depression may be indicated if you answer yes to two or more of the following signs:

— Have you lost your appetite with marked weight loss, or do you eat a lot with new weight gain?
— Do you sleep excessively, and feel lethargic, sad, pessimistic and worthless when you're awake?
— Do you often feel like you're going a mile a minute one moment and totally tired the next?
— Have you lost interest or pleasure in regular activities you used to like? Has your sex drive decreased?
— Has you energy been exceptionally low, to the point of doing almost nothing all day?
— Do you drink more alcohol than you used to? Do you feel self-reproach or constant guilt?
— Do you have trouble thinking or concentrating? Do you forget things more easily than you used to?
— Have you had paranoia attacks or hallucinations usually with headaches, sweating, heart palpitations?
— Are you often irritable, with recurring problems with friends and family members?
— Have you started taking more and more mood altering drugs or antidepressants?
— Do you feel isolated from others with recurrent thoughts of death or suicide?

Depression is a serious disorder that needs serious attention. We all get the blues from time to time, but major depression is different. The lifestyle program on the next page is effective for a wide range of people. Consult with a healthcare professional to find out what natural therapies are right for you.

Can't find a recommended product? Call the 800 number listed in Product Resources for the store nearest you.

Depression

Diet and Lifestyle Support Therapy

Nutritional therapy plan: Nutrition is a key to brain behavior.

1—Many prescription drugs create nutrient deficiencies. If you are taking MAO inhibitor drugs, control your diet with care: Avoid alcohol, cheese, red meat, yeast extract and broad beans - foods rich in tyrosine. Eliminate preserved foods, fast foods and junk foods. Avoid sugary foods, refined carbohydrates and caffeine - they wreak havoc on blood sugar levels. Trans fatty acids in fried foods, baked goods and commercial snack foods further disrupt brain chemistry.

2—Make vegetable protein about 15% of calorie intake. Include proven depression fighters: fish, seafoods, sea greens, spinach, avocados, olive oil; tryptophan foods like turkey, potatoes and bananas.

3—Eat foods rich in calcium, magnesium and B vitamins. Have a glass of carrot juice twice a week with a pinch of sage and 1 tsp. Bragg's LIQUID AMINOS for adrenal stress.

4—Drink plenty of pure, bottled water. Some common water treatments can cause neurotransmitter imbalances.

5—Make a brain mix of lecithin granules, nutritional yeast, wheat germ, pumpkin seeds; take 2 tbsp. daily. and take New Chapter GINGER WONDER SYRUP, 1 tbsp. daily.

Lifestyle watchwords:

•67% of people with no apparent cause for their depression *benefit* from sleep deprivation. A single sleepless night can wash away depressive symptoms. *Amazing.*

•Before you try PROZAC, (it has had more side effect complaints than any other drug) ask your doctor about hypnotherapy, biofeedback or acupuncture... relaxation techniques with success in overcoming chronic depression.

•*The two major classes of antidepressant drugs seem to block the effect of herbal nervines. Don't take St. John's wort if you take PROZAC. While St. John's wort has been maligned as useless in the media for depression, research shows it is more effective than placebo in treating mild to moderate depression. In some cases, even severe depression has responded to St. John's wort therapy.*

Bodywork support:

•Exercise anxiety away. Give your body plenty of oxygen. Exercise is an anti-depressant nutrient in itself. Deep brain breathing exercises work, too. (See Paul Bragg's BRAIN BREATHING book).

•Depression increases risk of osteoporosis. Get some daily sunlight on the body for vitamin D, a natural serotonin boost.

•Yoga stretches and regular massage help clear the mind.

•Acupuncture banishes the blues in 90% of women by increasing their brain endorphins.

•Aromatherapy helps: Try essential oils of jasmine, geranium, rosemary and basil.

Herbal, Superfood and Supplement Therapy

Interceptive therapy plan: Choose 2 to 3 recommendations.

1—Relieve depression, improve your mood: •Crystal Star DEPRESS-EX™ extract or caps for mental calm; •New Chapter ST. JOHN'S SC27; Pacific BioLogic EMOTIONAL RESCUE formulas; •NADH 10mg daily with *St. John's Wort*, a natural MAO inhibitor. If hypothyroid related, take *St John's wort* with sea veggies or other thyroid support. •*Ginkgo Biloba* (not with blood thinners) or *Hawthorn* extract for a feeling of well-being. •MACA tabs 1000mg daily and •*Rhodiola Rosea*, an herbal serotonin booster, are both very effective mood lifters (try Pinnacle RHODAX for men). •*Kava-Kava* caps 2 daily (not with alcohol); •Gaia Herbs PHYTOPROZ SUPREME caps.

2—Fight depression with essential fatty acids: •*Evening Primrose oil* 3000mg daily; •Omega-3 flax oil 2 tbsp. daily; Health from the Sun TOTAL EFAs; •New Chapter DHA 100; •Nature's Secret ULTIMATE OIL; Spectrum Norwegian fish oil for bipolar disorder.

3—Amino acids boost your brain energy: •SAMe 400-1600mg daily helps rebuild the brain's stockpile of mood elevating hormones. Research shows SAMe banishes depression in 1 month for 70% of women -as effective as Prozac without the side effects; •Dr. Diamond DIAMOND MIND for mental stamina and alertness; •Glutamine 1000mg daily; •Country Life Maxi-B with taurine, or MOOD FACTORS caps as needed; •Tyrosine 500mg or •DLPA 1500mg as needed; •GABA 1000mg, mimics valium without sedative effects.

4—Nerve tonics and relaxers: •Crystal Star RELAX™ caps for nerve repair; •Gotu Kola for nerve support; •Sublingual B-12, 2500mcg every other day for 2 months; •5-HTP 50-100mg at bedtime for 2 months. •Vitamin C with bioflavonoids, 3000mg daily helps withdrawal from chemical dependencies. •B-complex 150mg. •Take *black cohosh*, Natrol SAF capsules, or melatonin .3mg at bedtime for 3 months if depression is hormone related. •Eidon SELENIUM liquid and •Magnesium 1000mg daily, for mood swings.

—Before retiring, drink •*chamomile-spearmint-scullcap* tea; or make an •anti-depression pillow with fresh-dried mugwort leaves, rosemary, California poppies, lemon balm and mint. Stuff a pillow for sweet sleep.

5—Adaptogen herbs help normalize body chemistry: •*Panax ginseng, Siberian eleuthero* extract or *suma* or Prince of Peace GINSENG vials; •Maitake Products REISHI tabs for inner calm, nerve restoration; •Planetary GINSENG ELIXIR or Reishi Supreme tabs; •Nelson Bach RESCUE REMEDY for stress reactions; •Homeopathic *Ignatia* for grief due to loss of a loved one or relationship breakup.

—Superfood therapy: (Choose one or two recommendations.)
•Crystal Star RESTORE YOUR STRENGTH™.
•Pure Planet 100% PURE SPIRULINA.
•Prince of Peace American Ginseng - Royal Jelly vials, or Ginkgo-Siberian Ginseng-Rhodiola vials (highly recommended, fast acting).

Can't find a recommended product? Call the 800 number listed in Product Resources for the store nearest you.

Diabetes

High Blood Sugar, Type 1 (Insulin Dependent), Type 2 (Largely non-insulin Dependent)

The Centers for Disease Control show diabetes reaching epidemic proportions, *doubling* between 1999 to 2000! Today, 17 million people have diabetes. One million more are diagnosed each year. Another 6 million people have it, but don't yet know it. WHO expects 300 million cases worldwide by 2025. With its complications (stroke, heart attack, blindness), diabetes is now the 7th leading cause of death in the U.S. Alert: Type 2 diabetes is increasingly being diagnosed in overweight children and adolescents who get little exercise and live on fast foods.

Health care costs of diabetes: $132 billion a year. Diabetes is a degenerative disease, strongly linked to long-term diet overload of highly processed carbohydrates and sugar, and lack of fiber. It's a vicious circle disease, in which poor fat and sugar metabolism lead to obesity.... which then leads to diabetes. The cycle keeps going. Diabetes makes you want to eat more, so symptoms are aggravated, as well as brought on by eating too much fat, too many sugary foods and too much fast food (especially caffeine and alcohol). This type of diet overworks, then damages the pancreas, so your body loses the ability to produce or use insulin correctly, the hormone that helps convert food into energy. As simple carbohydrates and sugars cease to be metabolized, they accumulate in the body and are stored as fat. Excess body fat and lack of exercise bring on insulin resistance, so less energy is moved into the cells. Type 2 diabetics produce insulin, but it isn't used properly (insulin resistance). Type 1 diabetes, a juvenile condition, is more severe and almost entirely dependent on insulin to sustain life.

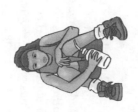

Do you know the signs of diabetes?

Type 2: Largely Non-Insulin Dependent

—Are you always thirsty? Do you urinate too often?
—Do cuts and bruises heal slowly? Get frequent infections?
—Have you lost weight? Constantly tired? or drowsy?
—Is your vision blurry? mental acuteness foggy?
—Do you get leg cramps, or prickling in fingers or toes?
—Have you experienced episodes of impotence?

Type 1: Insulin Dependent

—Is the person unusually thirsty? Urinate too often?
—Is the person extremely hungry? unusually wanting to eat?
—Is the person unusually tired, lethargic drowsy, irritable?
—Does the person having unusual trouble learning?
—Has the person lost weight lately for no reason?
—Do cuts and bruises heal slowly?

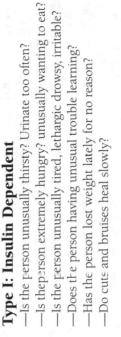

Blood sugar balancing diet for diabetes control

Diet improvement is absolutely necessary to overcoming diabetes. Although some Type 2 diabetics must take insulin to regulate blood sugar levels, others can balance their blood sugar without drugs by following a controlled diet along with regular exercise. The diet below, in addition to balancing blood sugar use, has the nice "side effect" of healthy weight loss. (Since high blood sugar is also an indication of high triglycerides, the diet also generally reduces triglycerides.)

—**On rising:** take the juice of two lemons in a glass of water with 2 tsp. Pure Planet CHLORELLA powder.

—**Breakfast:** take a glass of aloe vera juice, or All One TOTALLY FIBER COMPLEX drink mix in apple juice or water to regulate sugar curve; or make a mix of 2 tbsp. each: nutritional yeast, wheat germ, lecithin granules, rice or oat bran. Sprinkle some daily on breakfast foods, or mix into yogurt with fresh fruit; or have 1) poached egg on whole grain toast; 2) muesli, whole grain or granola cereal with apple juice or vanilla rice milk; 3) buckwheat or whole grain pancakes with apple juice or molasses.

—**Mid-morning:** have a green drink like Crystal Star ENERGY GREEN RENEWAL™ or Green Foods GREEN MAGMA; or a sugar balancing herb tea, like *licorice* or *dandelion* tea.

—**Lunch:** have a green salad, with marinated tofu, and mushroom soup; or baked tofu, tofu burgers or turkey with steamed veggies and rice or cornbread; or a baked potato with yogurt or kefir cheese, or soy cheese and miso soup with sea vegetables; or a whole grain sandwich, with avocado, low fat or soy cheese, a low fat sandwich spread and watercress.

—**Mid-afternoon:** have a glass of carrot juice, and/or fruit juice sweetened cookies with a bottled water or herb tea; or watercress/cucumber sandwiches with a low fat sandwich spread; or a hard boiled egg with a veggie dip, and bottled water.

—**Dinner:** Keep it light! Have a baked or broiled seafood dish with brown rice and peas; or a stir-fry with rice, veggies and miso soup; or a beans and rice dish with onions and peppers; or whole grain or veggie pasta salad; or a mushroom quiche with whole grain crust and yogurt/wine sauce, and a small green salad. A little white wine is fine with dinner for relaxation and has surprisingly high chromium content. Beware! Overconsuming any alcohol can cause blood sugar to soar.

—**Before bed:** take Jarrow GENTLE FIBERS drink mix with apple juice; or MISO, 1 tsp. in warm water.

Can't find a recommended product? Call the 800 number listed in Product Resources for the store nearest you.

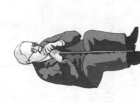

Controlling Complications Associated with Diabetes

Diabetes frequently leads to other health problems. Use the recommendations as needed for specific diabetic complications. Don't stop or reduce insulin without monitoring by your physician.

...DIABETIC CATARACTS, GLAUCOMA, RETINOPATHY (damaged retina), RETINITIS: the leading cause of new blindness in the U.S., is a disorder of the light sensitive retina caused by diabetes. **—Alternative healing protocols:** •Bilberry extract 2x daily for effective flavonoids; •Ginkgo biloba extract 3x daily for blood vessel circulation to the eyes; •PCO's from *grapeseed* or *white pine bark*, 100mg 3 times daily to reduce vascular fragility; •Quercetin 1000mg with bromelain 750mg 2x daily; •Lane Labs BENE-FIN shark cartilage caps 1200mg for blood vessel, capillary support; •magnesium 1200mg daily; •Ester C powder with bioflavonoids, ¼ tsp. at a time, 4 to 6x daily; •vitamin E 400IU 3x daily, especially for retinitis; •Planetary TRIPHALA caps as directed; •Solaray CENTELLA ASIATICA for optic nerve support; •B-complex 100mg daily with taurine 500mg.; MICROHYDRIN PLUS, royalbodycare. com, an antioxidant for the eyes. Note: Avoid foods sweetened with the additive aspartame. A diabetic retinopathy diagnosis may often really be aspartame toxicity in the eye.

...DIABETIC CARDIOVASCULAR COMPLICATIONS: People with diabetes are twice as likely as non-diabetics to suffer from coronary heart disease and stroke, five times as likely to suffer from arterial disease. **—Alternative healing protocols:** Use ginger in cooking often. Soy foods (esp. good for menopausal women at risk for diabetes-related heart disease), •Ginkgo biloba or •Bilberry extracts 120mg daily; •PCOs from *grapeseed* or *white pine bark*, 200mg daily; •gymnema sylvestre extract to lower blood lipids; •taurine to reverse blood clotting; •CoQ-10 100mg daily with vitamin E 400IU 2x daily to increase blood flow, decrease platelet aggregation; or •Golden Pride HEART HEALTH PAK daily, or •Metabolic Response Modifers CARDIOCHELATE. •Omega-3 flax oil, 2 tsp. daily helps keep arteries free of fats. Take •Country Life vitamin B-12 sublingual 2500mcg with carnitine 1000mg. To help lower cholesterol: •MICROHYDRIN PLUS (rapid results) available from royal-health.com; •niacinamide 500mg 2x daily, and •chromium picolinate 200mcg daily, or •Solaray CHROMIACIN.

...DIABETIC CIRCULATORY PROBLEMS AND ULCERS: —Alternative healing protocols: consider chelation therapy. Today, it is an easy clinic procedure... and it works. Or try •Metabolic Response Modifers CARDIOCHELATE as directed. Take •American Biologics emulsified vitamin A & D 25,000/1,000 IU (beta-carotene is not effective for diabetics, who cannot convert it to A). Drink aloe vera juice each morning. Take •zinc/methionine 30mg 2x daily to improve zinc status without affecting copper levels. Clean ulcers of necrotic tissue and apply a comfrey poultice, or •Country Comfort GOLDENSEAL/MYRRH salve. •AloeLife SKIN GEL (excellent results), •B & T CALIFLORA gel, or •tea tree oil/olive oil compresses.

...DIABETIC OBESITY: Weight control problems and heart disease run in a vicious circle. Obesity is a risk factor for heart disease; obesity is a risk factor for diabetes. Thus, diabetes is a risk factor for heart disease. Excess body fat plays a key role in Type II diabetes by contributing to insulin resistance - the inability of the body to deliver glucose to the cells for energy. Good diabetic meals are small, frequent (up to 6 mini meals a day), largely vegetarian, and low in fats. Slow-burning complex carbohydrates, like whole grains, beans and vegetables reduce insulin requirements. In fact, a diet like this allows some people to reduce, even stop their prescription medications. (Check with your doctor.) **—Alternative healing protocols:** You must lower your sugar and fat intake. Get help from •stevia herb, or •gymnema sylvestre herb before each meal to help normalize pancreas activity and increase insulin output; •Lewis Labs FIBER YEAST in the morning helps, or •Edge Labs CARB OUT drink with chromium picolinate and white kidney bean extract; or •chromium picolinate 200mcg daily. •Source Naturals RELORA caps reduce stress-eating; •Acetyl-carnitine 1000mg, •Magnesium 800mg, and •Vitamin E 400IU daily help overcome insulin resistance. Most diabetics suffer from essential atty acid deficiency. My favorite sources: •Evening Primrose oil 4000mg daily, flax oil 2 tbsp. daily, and sea greens (any kind works. I like Maine Coast delicious roasted seaweed, available at healthyhealing.com), 2 tbsp. daily snipped on soup, salad or rice. A weekly dry sauna helps regulate sugar and control cravings.

...DIABETIC NEPHROPATHY: Kidney disease resulting from diabetic small blood vessel malfunction. **—Alternative healing protocols:** Avoid red meats - eat fish or chicken instead - especially salmon; take •gymnema sylvestre water soluble extract before meals; •alpha lipoic acid 600mg daily; •Acetyl-carnitine 500mg daily; Lane Labs BENE-FIN shark cartilage caps for blood vessel and capillary support.

...FOOD ALLERGIES: When testing for glucose tolerance, be sure to take food tolerance tests to determine food allergies. Avoid foods like red meats and hard cheeses, refined carbohydrates like white breads, and preserved foods. Eating a lot of processed meats like salami, bologna and hot dogs increases diabetes risk by 46%. Choose sea foods or hormone-free poultry protein instead. Avoid cow's milk especially and all fatty dairy foods. There is a definite link between cow's milk and Type 1 Juvenile Diabetes. Keep your diet high in fresh fruits and vegetables for fiber. Aspartame (in sweeteners like NutraSweet, Sweet 'N' Low and Equal) deplete insulin reserves. **—Alternative healing protocols:** •HCL 600mg with meals, digestive enzymes after meals, like •Transformation DIGESTZYME with PUREZYME, or •Prevail DAIRY ENZYME formula for lactose intolerance. Regular coffee can decrease insulin sensitivity by as much as 15%. Avoid it if you have diabetes. Green tea may be a better choice. USDA research shows green tea's catechins enhance insulin activity.

Can't find a recommended product? Call the 800 number listed in Product Resources for the store nearest you.

...DIABETIC NEUROPATHY: Damage to peripheral nerves characterized by numbness, tingling, pain, cramping in hands and feet. —**Alternative healing protocols:** Follow a vegetarian diet; take •Alpha lipoic acid 600mg daily to lower blood sugar and reduce severity and frequency of symptoms; take •Quercetin with Bromelain 2x daily, or Solaray QBC COMPLEX; Take •MSM 800mg daily to strengthen nerves; •PCO's from *grapeseed* or *white pine bark*, 300mg daily reduce vascular fragility; •*gotu kola* capsules 6 daily provide nerve support. •*Ginkgo Biloba, Hawthorn* or *Bilberry extracts* enhance circulation; •*Evening Primrose Oil caps* 4000mg, or •choline 600mg help nerve damage; •biotin 1000mcg 6x daily; •Apply capsaicin cream or Nature's Way CAYENNE PAIN RELIEVING ointment to affected areas for pain relief. •Magnetic foot pads produce good results; •Nature's Secret ULTIMATE B shores up deficiencies, add vitamin B-12 sublingual 2500mcg, every other day for a month; •Vitamin C 3000mg, •Acetyl-L-Carnitine (ALC) 2000mg •Magnesium 800mg daily.

Is Syndrome X the future of Diabetes?   Are you on the path to Syndrome X?   New research says you may be.

Syndrome X is estimated to affect up to 95 *million Americans* - one of the most serious health threats facing the modern world! Syndrome X is a very complex condition, but the common denominator is insulin resistance (diabetes). Insulin fluctuations overwhelm the body, and the cells become resistant to insulin. Blood sugar levels soar out of control, setting off a damaging free radical cascade, inflammation and metabolic problems. The condition often goes undetected by doctors for years, because Syndrome X complications are so varied. Gland problems like infertility, polycystic ovary syndrome and irregular menstruation are often involved, so are increased risk of colon and breast cancer, lupus, and liver disease. Any one of these problems is a threat - combined in the Syndrome X pattern, even lethal. Insulin resistance causes great damage to the cardiovascular system and blood vessels. High blood pressure is common, and people with Syndrome X have very high risk of heart attack, stroke and coronary heart disease. Excess insulin also provokes the liver to make more cholesterol, dump more fats into the bloodstream, and allow more fat storage, reasons why people with Syndrome X have such a hard time losing weight. Excess fat around your waist is a primary sign. The medical approach to Syndrome X relies on using a different drug "patch" for each problem, so the typical patient is juggling 4 or 5 different prescriptions, (and possibly adverse drug reactions and side effects). For example, statin drugs used to control high cholesterol are highly toxic to the liver. Using them long term can compound Syndrome X complications like fatty liver disease and obesity. Natural therapies, in contrast, are well suited to treat Syndrome X, helping to rebalance blood sugar levels, and get high blood pressure and cholesterol back under control without side effects or toxicity. Ask a holistic practitioner if natural treatments are a good option for you.

What's causing the Syndrome X epidemic? Our lifestyle bears much of the responsibility. The main triggers of Syndrome X are lack of exercise, and diet overloads of sugar, refined carbs, saturated and trans fats. Smoking, chronic stress and alcohol abuse accelerate it. Heredity may play a role. African American women, Hispanics, Native Americans and Pacific Islanders who have adopted a western lifestyle (and eating patterns) are the hardest hit by this syndrome, but the epidemic is growing in all of America's middle aged baby boomer population.

Are you at risk for Syndrome X?   *Three or more of these symptoms may be a sign.*

• Obesity, especially if you have an apple shaped body (excess weight around the middle) or a protruding stomach (a sign of liver enlargement).
• Diagnosed high cholesterol or triglycerides. Fasting blood glucose higher than 110. Cholesterol deposits on the skin (xanthelasma).
• Poor circulation or arteriosclerosis. Blood pressure greater than 140/85 mmHg.
• Poor immune response with frequents colds, flu or candida yeast infections. Retinal changes, cataracts.
• Polycystic ovaries (signs include irregular menstruation, hirsutism, acne and obesity).

Natural therapies for Syndrome X: *Key natural recommendations that you can easily implement.* Choose several recommendations.

1) Get diet triggers under control. Never fry! Avoid excess caffeine, saturated and trans fats, alcohol, salt, sugary foods and refined carbohydrates. Focus on healthy proteins from seafood or hormone-free turkey, non-starchy vegetables, and whole grains (oats and oatmeal especially good). Eat fruits in moderation until balance is achieved. 2) Low essential fatty acids worsen Syndrome X by triggering inflammation. Eat seafood (especially salmon) 3 times a week for Omega 3 fatty acids. Add regularly: sea veggies, olive oil and dark greens like spinach are good sources of EFA's. Consider EVENING PRIMROSE OIL 3000mg daily. 3) Drink green tea or Crystal Star GREEN TEA CLEANSER™ daily to maximize metabolism and block starch absorption. Consider a cholesterol-balancing drink like Jarrow GENTLE FIBERS. 4) Maitake Products MAITAKE SX FRACTION helps reduce blood glucose and insulin resistance (clinical tests). 5) Alpha lipoic acid 250-600mg daily improves insulin sensitivity, and is an antioxidant, liver and nerve protector (check with your physician if you are also on drug therapy). 6) Milk thistle seed extract, 15 drops daily for 1-3 months strengthens the liver and reduces insulin resistance. 7) Chromium 200mcg daily helps rebalance blood sugar levels (check with your physician if you are on drugs). 8) If you have high homocysteine (common in Syndrome X), use my 3 point program to lower it on pp 440. 9) Very important! Strive for 30 minutes of aerobic exercise daily. No program for Syndrome X will work for long without regular exercise.

Can't find a recommended product? Call the 800 number listed in Product Resources for the store nearest you.

Diabetes

Diet and Lifestyle Support Therapy

Nutritional therapy plan:

Start with diet improvements. Don't skip meals. Most diabetics should eat 6 mini meals a day, especially if they're on insulin therapy.

Your ongoing diet should be low in fats and total calories, largely vegetarian, rich in good fats like olive oil and proteins from sea greens, unroasted nuts, green superfoods like barley grass, spirulina and chlorella, and vegetable sources like soy foods and whole grains, for lecithin and chromium. Vegetables especially supply slow-burning complex carbohydrates that don't need much insulin for metabolism, preventing rapid blood sugar spikes. 50 to 60% of the diet should consist of fresh or simply cooked vegetables.

1—Eliminate sugars, alcohol, fried, fatty, refined carbohydrates and high cholesterol foods. Avoid cow's milk especially and all fatty dairy foods.

2— Avoid caffeine and caffeine foods (except green or white tea), hard liquor, food coloring and sodas. Even "diet" sodas have phenylalanine that can affect blood sugar levels.

3—Sweeten with stevia herb, or Trimedica SLIM SWEET instead of sugar. Stevia doesn't have sugar's insulin requirements and reduces food cravings. One of my staff knows a diabetic who required a foot amputation as a result of chronic high blood sugar reactions.

4—High fiber foods are a key, and in mild cases, can lead to discontinuation of insulin therapy. Fiber improves control of glucose metabolism, lowers cholesterol and triglyceride levels, and promotes weight loss. Poor bio-chemistry often results from being overweight. Use a fiber weight loss drink, like All One TOTALLY FIBER COMPLEX or Jarrow GENTLE FIBERS.

5—Chromium-rich foods are key: whole grains, nutritional yeast, string beans, eggs, cucumbers, liver, onions, garlic, fruits, cheese, shiitake mushrooms, wheat germ, etc.

6—A daily green salad with Omega-3 flax oil dressing for EFAs. Eat salmon twice a week.

—Bodywork and lifestyle measures:

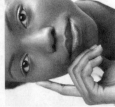

•Don't smoke; nicotine increases desire for sugary foods.

•Exercise! Insulin resistance drops by nearly 2% for every 200 calories burned through exercise. Walking is the best exercise for diabetics, to increase metabolism and reduce need for insulin. A daily 3mph walk decreases risk by 50% !

•Alternating hot and cold hydrotherapy boosts circulation.

•Hot tub therapy: A study reported in the New England Journal of Medicine shows soaking in a hot tub for 30 minutes a day for three weeks lowers blood sugar levels 13%!

•Deep therapy massage helps regulate blood sugar use.

•Avoid phenylalanine. No Nutra-Sweet or Aspartame products. Check labels on colas, diet drinks, they may trigger diabetes.

•Get eight hours of sleep a night. Sleep deprivation increases diabetes complications.

Herbal, Superfood and Supplement Therapy

Interceptive therapy plan: Choose 2 to 3 recommendations.

1—Stabilize blood sugar: •Crystal Star SUGAR CONTROL HIGH™ helps insulin balance; •Pacific BioLogic BITTER MELON caps help both high and low blood sugar attacks; •Nutricology GLUCOSOL with *banaba*, clinically proven to activate cellular glucose transport. (Ask a practitioner if you're on insulin). •Adapters like GTF Chromium or chromium picolinate 200mcg. •VANADIUM 25mcg daily (diabetics usually make enough insulin, chromium and vanadium help them use it.) •Siberian eleuthero extract or •Imperial Elixir SIBERIAN ELEUTHERO or •Grifron MAITAKE SX FRACTION (enhances insulin sensitivity) •vitamin E, 800IU daily; •*Bilberry* extract or *rosemary* tea balance blood sugar. •*Neem* and *turmeric* powder, ¼ tsp. each in 1 tsp. honey before meals.

2—Lower blood sugar levels: •Lipoic acid 600mg daily (lowers glucose levels up to 30%); •Crystal Star FEEL GREAT NOW!™ (with ginseng, a proven aid to blood sugar control); or •*Olive Leaf* extract or •Nutricology PRO-LIVE; •Biotin 3000mcg daily. •PSP Marketing VITAL PSP PLUS improves glucose absorption; •*Fenugreek seed* tea daily, •Vitamin C 3000mg helps blood sugar levels in non-insulin dependent diabetics. •Magnesium 400mg combats insulin resistance. •*Devil's club* infusion to lower blood sugar levels in type 2 diabetics.

3—Normalize pancreas / insulin activity: •*Gymnema sylvestre* extract before meals helps repair the pancreas, and damage to liver and kidneys. •Ester C 3000mg daily increases insulin tolerance, normalizes pancreatic activity. •Glutamine 1000mg with acetyl-carnitine 1000mg; •DHEA 25mg increases cell sensitivity to insulin. •*Burdock, Pau d'arco* or *Astragalus* tea, for 3 months; •*garlic* capsules 6 daily.

4—Help prevent nerve damage with EFAs: •*Evening Primrose Oil* capsules 1000mg daily, •Omega-3 flax or fish oil (for DHA) 3000mg daily; Planetary REISHI SUPREME.

5—Raise your antioxidant defenses: •Alpha lipoic acid 300mg daily; NAC (N-acetyl-cysteine) 150mg, Pycnogenol or grape seed PCO's 200mg daily; CoQ10 120mg per day.

6—Boost energy: •Crystal Star ADRENAL ENERGY BOOST™ caps for cortex support with ENERGY GREEN RENEWAL™ for stable energy. •Spirulina tablets 6 daily to elevate mood. —**A vitamin regimen solves many diabetes problems:** Solaray B-12 2500mcg. B-complex 100mg, with pantothenic acid 500mg daily for adrenal activity, niacin 250mg stimulates circulation, zinc 50mg for more immune strength. Magnesium/potassium/bromelain helps control blood pressure. Nature Made DIABETES HEALTH PACK (replenishes nutrients drained by the disease).

—Superfood therapy: Choose one or two recommendations.
•Herbal Answers ALOE FORCE JUICE.
•Futurebiotics VITAL K.
•All One TOTALLY FIBER COMPLEX.
•Green Kamut JUST BARLEY.

Can't find a recommended product? Call the 800 number listed in Product Resources for the store nearest you.

Diarrhea

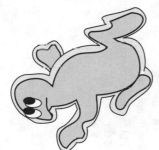

Chronic Diarrhea, Traveler's Diarrhea, Poor Nutrient Absorption

Diarrhea, uncomfortably frequent, fluid and excessive bowel movements, is your body's way of ridding itself of something disagreeable or harmful. Diarrhea is one of the body's best methods of rapidly throwing off toxins. While the abdominal cramps, low fever and general fatigue are unpleasant, unless diarrhea is chronic, it may be best to let it run its cleansing course. If it continues for more than two to three days, dehydration may ensue, (dangerous for the elderly and very young children). Take steps to ensure adequate fluid intake and to replace vital electrolyte minerals. Note: No drugstore remedy I have found is as effective as diet correction with herbs or natural supplements.

What causes diarrhea? Besides a body cleansing reaction to bad food, chemicals in food or water, or a viral bug like flu, intestinal parasites may be the biggest culprit. (Some estimates say 1 in 6 Americans now have them.) Food allergies often play a role, especially allergies to lactose, fructose or gluten foods. Today, poor food absorption because of lack of enzymes may be a leading cause (if you use a microwave for most of your meals this may be the case); low enzymes are also implicated in liver or gallbladder disease. *Note:* hemorrhoids are linked to diarrhea and obesity - not just constipation as one might think.

Diet and Lifestyle Support Therapy

Nutritional therapy plan: *An apple a day is an excellent preventive.*

1—For chronic diarrhea: Go on a juice diet for 24 hours (pg. 173) to clean out harmful bacteria. Add 2 tbsp. cider vinegar in hot water with honey 2x daily, and 2 tsp. roasted carob powder in apple sauce with 1 tsp. of cinnamon morning and evening. Then, take for 3 days: Miso soup or vegetable broth with snipped sea veggies, papaya juice, a green salad, toast, and brown rice with steamed veggies. Add pectin foods like apples or bananas.

2—Avoid dairy products, and fatty and fried foods during healing. Eat small meals and chew food well. Add fiber to your continuing diet with whole grain brans, amaranth cereal (an astringent), brown rice and fresh vegetables. Add yogurt, kefir and cultured foods for friendly flora. Drink plenty of liquids to keep from getting dehydrated.

3—Mix 1 tbsp. each: *psyllium husk, flax seed, chia seed,* and *slippery elm* in water. Let the mix soak for 30 minutes. Take 2 tbsp. at night for 2 days before bed.

4—**For kid's diarrhea:** Catnip, nettles, sage or thyme tea. •Red Raspberry tea

—To curb symptoms:

•Apply ice packs to the middle and lower back.
•If no inflammation is present, use mild *catnip* or *fenugreek seed* tea enemas to soothe and rid the body of toxic matter.
•For babies: give finely grated apples followed by oatmeal.
•For older children: give oat flakes; let them chew and wet them with saliva; don't give any other food for at least 2 hours.

—For travel diarrhea and irregularity: 1) Eat only ripe bananas and yogurt for 24 hours - especially if in a 3rd world country to help your body retain water and absorb salt. Eat high fiber foods on your trip.... brown rice, salads, vegetables. 2) Drink black orange pekoe tea w. lemon, pinch of cloves. 3) Have a glass of wine with meals - 6 times more effective in killing bacteria than Pepto Bismol.

Herbal, Superfood and Supplement Therapy

Interceptive therapy plan: Choose 2 to 3 recommendations.

—For chronic diarrhea:

1—Control the infection: •Crystal Star ANTI-BIO™ caps or extract •Nutribiotics GRAPEFRUIT SEED extract caps counter gastrointestinal infection. •Sangre de Drago extract (esp. useful for E. coli infections)• BLACK WALNUT HULLS extract, 2x daily.

2—Soothe discomfort and cramping: *Peppermint-Slippery Elm* or *chamomile* tea; *Blackberry-elderberry-cinnamon* tea; •New Chapter GINGER WONDER syrup as needed.

3—Help dry up diarrhea: •Activated charcoal tabs with Cal/Mag/Zinc at night (temporary); •Herbalist & Alchemist *Yellow dock* extract; •Body Essentials SILICA gel.

4—Rebalance bowel functions: •BWL TONE-IBS™ for gentle rebalance. •Pure Planet CHLORELLA. •Vitamin A 10,000IU daily; •Garlic caps 6 daily; •Bayberry-barberry tea; •Pancreatin 1200mg daily. •Quercetin 1000 with bromelain 750mg if food allergies. •Niacin therapy 250mg daily.

5—Rebuild food absorption ability: •Crystal Star DR. ENZYME™ with protease and bromelain caps; •Kal COLOSTRUM 1-3 tabs daily; •Apple pectin capsules 3 daily. •Planetary TRIPHALA caps as directed.

—For occasional and traveler's diarrhea: •Homeopathic: Nux Vomica, Hylands Diarrex, Chamomila. •Crystal Star TRAVELERS COMFORT™ drops with ginger; •Bee pollen, or •Beehive Botanical POLLEN PLUS; kelp tabs 6 daily.

—All-in-one diarrhea aid: •Crystal Star GREEN TEA CLEANSER™ with ¼ tsp. *ginger* powder, 15 drops *myrrh extract* and 1 tsp. Bragg's LIQUID AMINOS added.

—For antibiotic-induced diarrhea: •American Health ACIDOPHILUS liquid, or •UAS DDS-PLUS + FOS, or •Transformation Enzyme PLANTADOPHILUS.

—Superfood therapy: Choose one or two recommendations.
•Crystal Star RESTORE YOUR STRENGTH™ or Nature's Path TRACE-LYTE replace lost electrolytes. •Salute ALOE VERA JUICE with HERBS. • Lewis Labs FIBER YEAST daily.

Can't find a recommended product? Call the 800 number listed in Product Resources for the store nearest you.

Diverticulosis

Diverticulitis, Inflamed Bowel Disease

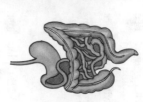

Diverticular disease is common today, affecting almost 50% of Americans over 60. It mimics many symptoms of Irritable Bowel Syndrome (page 378) - like the abdominal pain, cramping and distention due to inflammation of the colon mucous membranes from unpassed food residues and gas. **Diverticulosis** is characterized by small hernias that look like worn out tire bulges protruding through the weakened walls of the sigmoid colon. At its worst, a prolapsed colon structure can even result. **Diverticulitis** occurs when these small sacs become infected and inflamed. A constipated colon is most at risk for the pouch-y hernias (diverticula) which trap toxic waste to protect the body from infection. Studies link diverticular disease to the Western diet of heavily refined, low fiber foods (rare in countries where people eat a high fiber, whole foods diet) that lead to fermented, uneliminated food residues and chronic constipation or alternating constipation and diarrhea. If the condition continues, the pouches become painfully infected, and may even perforate leading to contamination in the abdominal area and sometimes severe bleeding from the rectum. 200,000 people are hospitalized each year because of complications from diverticulitis. *See also the CONSTIPATION CLEANSING DIET page 382.*

Diet and Lifestyle Support Therapy

Nutritional therapy plan:

1—Diet improvement is the best solution: Start with a short juice diet for 3 days (pg. 196). Use carrot, apple, grape or carrot/spinach juice.

2—Fiber is the diet key: to prevent constipation: Add oat or rice bran and take 2 tbsp. molasses with a banana and plain yogurt daily. Eat prunes for occasional constipation.

3—Add mild fruits and vegetables like carrots, bananas, potatoes, yams, papayas, broccoli, well-cooked black beans.

4—As inflammation subsides and healing begins, add brown rice, millet, cous cous, tofu, baked fish or seafood as lean protein sources.

5—Eat plenty of cultured foods for healthy G.I. flora: yogurt, kefir, miso, sea greens for EFAs.

6—Eliminate dairy products, fatty and sugary foods, red meats and fried foods during healing. Avoid wheat and dense grains, nuts and seeds during healing.

7—Drink 6 to 8 glasses of water and apple juice, cranberry juice or ginger ale (add New Chapter GINGER WONDER syrup to any drink).

—Bodywork:

•Avoid drugstore antacids. They eventually make the problems worse by causing the stomach to produce more acids.

•Take Chlorophyll liquid, 1 tsp. in water before meals

•Take peppermint, fenugreek, or catnip enemas once or twice a week for bowel cleansing and rebalancing. If desired, add 1 cup sesame oil to loosen and flush out impacted wastes.

•Massage therapy treatments often help.

•Active people are less prone to diverticular disease. Take a brisk walk every day possible. Walk outdoors to get a vitamin D boost.

•Apply wet hot ginger compresses to abdomen and lower back to stimulate systolic/diastolic action.

Herbal, Superfood and Supplement Therapy

Interceptive therapy: Choose 2 to 3 (Liquid or chewable supplements preferable.)

1—Heal bowel tissue: •Crystal Star BWL TONE IBS™ caps with wild yam 3x daily for 3 months (wild yam is a specific for diverticular disease). •*Evening Primrose Oil* for EFAs to normalize bowel function. •*Pau d'arco or uña da gato* tea 3 cups daily or Planetary TRIPHALA caps for a month.

2—Ease gas and flatulence: •B-complex vitamins, like Nature's Secret ULTIMATE B, •Source Naturals Co-ENZYMATE B complex, or •Real Life Research TOTAL B liquid sublingual (highly recommended), to curb stomach gas and rumbling as fiber combines with minerals.

3—Reduce inflammation and pain: •Crystal Star ANTI-FLAM™ caps (fast acting). •Crystal Star MUSCLE RELAXER™ caps for spasmodic cramping, or other cramp bark combo. •*Alfalfa-mint* tea, *Slippery elm* tea, *Comfrey-fenugreek* tea or Solaray ALFA-JUICE caps 6 daily; •Nature's Way CELL-MEND with *cat's claw* and IP6.

4—Control infection: •Crystal Star ANTI-BIO™ drops in water, or other •*Echinacea-goldenseal* combination; •*garlic* extract caps 6 daily.

5—Soothe stress leading to diverticular spasms: •Crystal Star STRESS OUT™ drops or *wild yam* extract drops in water. (usually results in 20 minutes or less.).

6—Enzyme therapy is important: •Nutricology PERM A VITE powder, a specific for diverticular disease, 1 hour before or after meals meals for bowel rebalance. •Crystal Star DR. ENZYME™ with protease and bromelain; UAS DDS-PLUS or Transformation Enzymes PLANTADOHILUS ½ tsp. with each meal; •Nature's Plus chewable BROMELAIN 40mg or chewable PAPAYA ENZYMES at each meal; •Enzymatic Therapy DGL chewables (especially if Candida is also present).

—Superfood therapy: Choose one or two recommendations.

•All One TOTALLY FIBER COMPLEX.

•Pure Planet CHLORELLA 20 tabs daily.

•Green Foods BARLEY ESSENCE.

•AloeLife ALOE GOLD drink to gently aid bowel action.

Can't find a recommended product? Call the 800 number listed in Product Resources for the store nearest you.

Down Syndrome

Genetic Mental Retardation, Mongolism

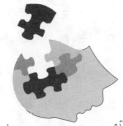

Down syndrome victims, born with an extra 21st chromosome (a defect that occurs in 1 out of every 700 births), are both physically and mentally retarded. For most children, this means poor muscle and connective tissue which causes weak, and slow motor functions. Gland and hormone deficiencies mean learning disability, and poor behavior with people. Down's thyroid disease can result in a "retarded," mongoloid appearance. Most sufferers have lung infections, and leukemia susceptibility. Studies show that some retarded behavior is learned, not inherited, and that Down's victims have immune dysfunctions like marked free radical damage from excess SOD production thought to be largely responsible for Down's accelerated aging process. Most Down victims don't live very long lives, and almost always fall prey to Alzheimer's disease. Untreatable by conventional medicine, vanguard work shows promising results from nutritional therapies which address the hypoglycemia, excess water fluoridation or heavy metal poisoning and allergies often involved. *Nutri-Chem's MSBPlus Version 6 has shown good results. Find out more: www.nutrichem.com or call 888-384-7855. Nutritional therapy has helped some Down's children improve height, facial appearance, memory and speech problems. See the HYPOGLYCEMIA DIET page 463 and ALZHEIMER'S page 317.*

Diet and Lifestyle Support Therapy

Nutritional therapy plan: *Better nutrition can improve IQ and physical health, both a glycogen storage and protein metabolism problem.*

1—Eat fresh foods for 3 days to clear out toxic waste, and provide a good working ground for nutrition therapy. Then, insist on a high nutrition diet of fresh, whole foods, rich in vegetable proteins, magnesium and EFA rich foods like leafy greens, seafoods and sea veggies (2 tbsp. sprinkled daily on soup, rice or salad are a therapeutic amount).

2—Eliminate all fast foods, refined sugary foods, dairy foods (esp. milk and cheese) and alcohol. Reduce high gluten foods.

3—Take Alacer MIRACLE WATER for brain potassium.

4—Mix nutritional yeast, lecithin and wheat germ; sprinkle 2 tbsp. daily on cereal.

5—*Chamomile* tea at night helps relax spasms. Crystal Star TINKLE TEA™ gently reduces fluid retention.

—Lifestyle measures:

• Music bypasses the brain to touch our emotional core. Play soothing classical or new age music in the home. I have seen it work wonders to calm behavioral stress problems.

• Avoid pesticides, heavy metals, (cadmium, lead and mercury), and aluminum.

• Ethical Nutrients ZINC STATUS, can check for deficiency.

—Bodywork:

• More oxygen and increased circulation help better brain function. New Chapter GINGER WONDER syrup helps circulation. Build more brain circuits by reading and playing games. Do deep breathing exercises to oxygenate the brain.

• Expose the body to early morning sunshine daily if possible for vitamin D.

• Massage therapy helps circulation and tissue strength.

• Stay interactive with other people and especially animals.

—Reflexology:

• Pinch the end of each toe. Hold 5 seconds. Squeeze all around the hand and fingers.

Herbal, Superfood and Supplement Therapy

Interceptive therapy plan: Choose 2 to 3 recommendations.

1—**Thyroid balance is key:** • Crystal Star OCEAN MINERALS™ iodine, potassium, silica; Green Foods ION-KELP tabs; • Eidon SELENIUM liquid help convert T4 to T3.

2—**Fortify nerves, boost brain acetylcholine:** • Solaray CENTELLA ASIASTICA caps for nerves. • Choline 600mg 4 daily, or phosphatidyl choline (PC 55), or phosphatidyl serine (PS) as directed. • Country Life MAXI-B with taurine, and extra B₆ 100mg for nerve strength; • PSP Marketing VITAL PSP PLUS (sometimes dramatic results).

3—**Lower homocysteine levels:** 1) B vitamins help, B-complex 50mg daily. Add 50mg extra B₆ and 400mcg extra folic acid to help break down homocysteine. • Or, royal jelly paste, 2 tsp. daily. 2) • Garlic caps, 4 daily to maintain aortic elasticity; • Ginkgo biloba extract daily; 3) Take daily ginger to inhibit an enzyme that makes blood prone to stickiness, or try New Chapter GINGER WONDER syrup.

4—**Antioxidants counteract free radical damage:** • Royal Bodycare MICROHYDRIN PLUS, one of the most potent free radical fighters available; • CoQ₁₀ 60mg daily, • Vitamin E 400IU with selenium 200mcg. • Ester C 550mg with bioflavonoids all help Down Syndrome. Premier GERMANIUM with DMG (half dose for children).

5—**Amino acid therapy is cutting edge Down's therapy:** Ask your naturopath how to best use: • Country Life RELAXER caps with Taurine 500mg; • Acetyl-carnitine (20mg for every 2C-lbs. of body weight). • GABA; • L-glycine and • L-glutamine.

6—**Nourish the brain with EFA's and produce better collagen:** • Evening Primrose Oil daily for 3 months. and • Flora VEGE-SIL caps help the body produce collagen.

—Superfood therapy: Down Syndrome may be a metabolic disease rather than in-herited. Enzyme therapy from superfoods is critical. Some good ones: Transformation DIGESTZYME with each meal, • Fit for You MIRACLE GREENS (enzymes and octacosanol). • Crystal Star RESTORE YOUR STRENGTH™, • Floradix CAL., MAG., VITAMIN D & ZINC liquid, • Green Kamut JUST BARLEY, • Unipro PERFECT PROTEIN and • Knudsen organic VERY VEGGIE juice.

Can't find a recommended product? Call the 800 number listed in Product Resources for the store nearest you.

Earaches

Excessive Earwax, Otitis Media, Otitis Externa (Swimmer's Ear)

Americans spend eight billion dollars a year treating ear infections! The most common ear infection in adults is swimmer's ear (inflammation of the outer ear canal), accompanied by thickness, even temporary loss of hearing. Middle ear infections are most common in children (accounting for a third of all childhood doctor visits) whose eustachian tubes have not fully formed and are easy breeding areas for infection. (A ruptured eardrum can result from a hard slap on the ear, a loud explosion or a serious middle ear infection.) Lavish use of antibiotics for ear infections is almost never justified, because common use often results in thrush in children, and candidiasis in adults. In fact, new research shows antibiotics are ineffective for most childhood ear infections! I'd also question having medical drainage tubes placed in your child's ears. They may damage hearing. Breast feed your baby; breast fed kids have far less ear infections during infancy, and as they grow up. Nursing mothers - avoid dairy foods if your baby is prone to ear infections, (problem signs: unusually fussy, with extremely tender earlobes). Enhance immune defenses to control chronic earaches in both adults and children. *See COLD INFECTIONS page 374 and FLU page 417 for more info.*

Diet and Lifestyle Support Therapy

Nutritional therapy plan for prevention:

1—Many ear infections are the result of food allergy reactions to foods like wheat. Eliminate MSG, and check for food additives and preservatives like sulfites, the biggest offenders. If earaches are chronic, keep the diet low in fats and reduce mucous-forming foods like dairy products.

2—During healing, eliminate all dairy foods, sugars and protein-concentrated foods, like peanut butter. Dilute sweet fruit juices. Their high natural sugars may feed bacteria.

3—Drink lots of water and diluted juices to keep mucous secretions thinned. Drink *Chamomile* tea to calm throbbing.

—**For pain:** Use ice packs (not heat) on ear to relieve pain.
•An onion poultice is a traditional remedy for earache pain. Press out and strain onion juice onto a small cotton plug. Place in the ear for fast relief and infection fighting.
•Mix warm vegetable glycerine and witch hazel. Soak a piece of cotton and insert in the ear to draw out infection.

—**An aromatherapy ear massage:** Add to 1-oz. vitamin E oil: 6 drops *chamomile* oil, 3 drops *tea tree* oil, 3 drops *lavender* or *calendula* oil. Rub around ear, massage neck.

—**Bodywork:**
•Massage ear, neck and temples. Pull ear lobe 10 times on each ear. Fold ear shell over and back repeatedly until blood suffuses area. Apply warm *lobelia* extract in the ear.
•Ear candles are effective used as directed but may remove protective ear wax coating.
•Most childhood earaches can be treated at home. Get medical help if you see these signs: —acute pain and loss of hearing within 48 hours. —fever that does not abate within 3 days. —dizziness, difficult breathing or vomiting, bloody discharge, or redness around the ear.

—**For excess earwax:** Have ear flushed at a clinic. Or put 3 drops of warm olive oil in ears to soften wax; flush with syringe and warm water. •Then press firmly but gently behind, then in front of the ear. Pull lobe up and down to work wax out. Fold ear shell in half. Open and fold repeatedly for circulation.

Herbal, Superfood and Supplement Therapy

Interceptive therapy plan: Choose 2 to 3 recommendations.

1—**Control the infection:** •Crystal Star ANTI-BIO™ capsules 4 to 6 daily, or extract 4x daily to clear infection. (ANTI-BIO extract may also be used as ear drops morning and evening.) •XLEAR nasal wash helps flush out bacteria and allergens that cause infections (highly recommended); •Nutribiotic GRAPEFRUIT SEED extract to clear infection.
•Echinacea extract internally. •Mix 1-oz. white vinegar and 1-oz. 70% isopropyl alcohol; drop in the ear for 30 seconds. Rinse out - three times daily.

2—**Reduce inflammation:** •Crystal Star ANTI-HST™ caps shrink swollen membranes. (Good results before flying to relieve ear congestion.) Chew •Xylitol gum to help open swollen ear canals. •Herbs, Etc. LYMPHATONIC to flush lymph glands.

3—**Relieve pain and throbbing:** •Crystal Star ANTI-FLAM™ 4 at a time for inflammation and EAR DEFENSE™ drops (highly recommended for both children and adults).

—**Effective ear drops:** •Mullein oil or •Herbs Etc. MULLEIN-GARLIC ear drops; Gaia's Children EAR DROPS; •Turtle Island warm EAR OIL drops; •*St. John's Wort Oil* drops; •*Calendula* oil drops; warm •*garlic* or olive oil. For swimmer's ear: boric acid-alcohol solution; food grade 3% H_2O_2 cleanses infection. •Take garlic tabs 4x daily, too.

4—**Enhance immune defenses:** •Crystal Star ZINC SOURCE™ spray or Zand ZINC HERBAL lozenges. •Gaia's ECHINACEA for children; •Liquid chlorophyll in water 3x daily.
•Vitamin C 500mg for each year of child's age daily; •Acidophilus pwdr. 1/4 tsp. in juice 4x daily, or •UAS DDS-PLUS with FOS (esp. if on antibiotic therapy).

5—**Homeopathic remedies:** Research shows homeopathy reduces ear infection pain and fever. Consider these: •NatraBio EARACHE; •*Pulsatilla* for mucous; •*Chamomilla* for irritability; •*Belladonna* for throbbing; •*Aconite* for sudden onset.

—**Superfood therapy:** (Choose one or two recommendations.)
•Jarrow GENTLE FIBERS drink.
•Alacer EMERGEN-C drink mix with electrolytes (very good preventive).
•Crystal Star RESTORE YOUR STRENGTH™ broth mix.

Can't find a recommended product? Call the 800 number listed in Product Resources for the store nearest you.

Eating Disorders

Anorexia Nervosa, Bulimia

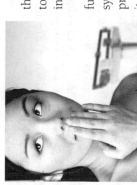

Almost 15% of Americans have some type of eating disorder. For 35% of women, and over 75% of American teenage girls, looking good means bone thin. Fashion models are seen as the aesthetic standard AND the health standard. Striving to meet this abnormal standard means thinness at any cost, leading to eating disorders that are extremely hard to overcome which can be fatal. (The mortality rate has improved, however. New statistics show that 30 years after initial diagnosis, anorexics now have a mortality rate of 7%, much better than the 20-40% death rate in the 1960s.)

Men are not completely exempt. Bodybuilders, male models and men in show business compete with ever-thinner rivals, and can suffer reduced testicular function from starving. *Bulimia* is a binge-purge cycle - consumption of huge amounts of food in a very short time and then vomiting to purge it from the system. It is usually first diagnosed by dentists because frequent vomiting erodes tooth enamel. *Anorexia* is self-starvation, distorted body image, extreme preoccupation with food, sometimes binge eating. *Orthorexia* is an eating disorder where the person becomes obsessed with dietary purity to the point where it becomes self-destructive.

Do you have an eating disorder? Is food running your life?

Eating disorders are usually caused by complex cultural or emotional problems that end up turning into a form of compulsive psychosis. Sometimes anxiety disorders, yeasts or celiac disease are involved. A genetic predisposition may play a role.

Ask yourself if you have any of these signs of an eating disorder:

• Do you always feel fat regardless of your actual weight?
• Do you try again and again but fail to lose weight?
• Do you still think you're fat even after losing a substantial amount of weight?
• Do your weight loss goals match what weight charts suggest for your height?
• Do you fast or put yourself on incredibly strict diets where you become totally preoccupied with food?
• Do you have a rigid eating routine?
• Do you eat when you are under stress or depressed?
• Are you a vegetarian solely to be thin, or for other reasons?
• Do you prepare food for others but refuse to eat it yourself? *(Anorexics often do this.)*
• Has your personality changed since you started your strict diet program? Are you more belligerent, aggressive, short-tempered or impolite to others. Do you feel extremely weak?
• Have your body processes changed since you started your strict diet program? Slower pulse rate? Hard stools? Bloating and fluid retention? Cold hands and feet? Cessation of menses? Lower metabolism?
• Have your looks changed since you started on your strict diet program? Dry skin? Dull, brittle hair? Yellow teeth? Tooth decay? Bone loss?
(Anorexics may develop a layer of thin, downy hair (lanugo) which helps them keep warm when body fat becomes dangerously low.)
(Bulimics have a swollen neck, broken blood vessels on the face and eroded tooth enamel from excessive vomiting.)
• Do you sometimes binge, or eat large amounts of food in a short period of time?
• Have you ever tried to "undo" the damage of eating by vomiting, taking laxatives or fasting?
(Bulimia victims are often extremely malnourished as well as extremely thin, because vomiting and excessive laxative use discharge most nutrients.)
• Do you feel guilty when you eat meat and dairy, or even high calorie or high-fat vegetarian foods?
• Do you try to hide your eating habits from others?
• Is there a relationship between eating and your self-esteem? • Do you feel you have lost control of your life?
• Do you exercise compulsively? Do you feel guilty or fat if you miss a regular exercise schedule?

For more information on recovering from eating disorders, contact the National Eating Disorder Association (800) 931-2237.

Can't find a recommended product? Call the 800 number listed in Product Resources for the store nearest you.

Eating Disorders

Diet and Lifestyle Support Therapy

Nutritional therapy plan:

1—Emphasize optimal nutrient foods to help your body rebuild itself. Eat a high vegetable protein diet, with high complex carbohydrates like brown rice and fresh veggies. Don't skip breakfast - try whole grain cereals (esp. oats), fruit and yogurt.

2—Carrot juice or Green Foods CARROT ESSENCE daily. •Alfalfa juice or nutritional yeast broth before meals can stimulate stronger appetite. Artichokes fill a need for anorexia.... they're delicious with a yogurt sauce.

3—NO junk foods, heavy starches or sugars. They disrupt the ability of your body to normalize its chemistry as you heal.

4—Eat slowly; chew well; have small meals often for best absorption.

5—Boost B vitamins to reduce stress: Make a mix of Red Star NUTRITIONAL YEAST, bee pollen granules, toasted wheat germ, molasses; take 2 tbsp. daily with any food or drink. **6**—Healthy meal replacement shakes are well-accepted by the bodies of people struggling with eating disorders.

—Bodywork:

Consider natural progesterone therapy to regain ovarian function if you have stopped menstruating.

•Since there is a high correlation between sexual abuse and eating disorders, psychological counseling is often helpful. It can also help in understanding the universal problem of low self-esteem that triggers this behavior. Therapy during healing reinforces the idea that destructive thinking and behavior can change, and the self-confidence of the sufferer reestablished. However, from experience I know it is almost impossible for an anorexic or bulimic person to seek help until they are almost beyond help.

•To improve self-esteem, cultivate relationships with positive people. Keep company with those in whose company you feel good about yourself.

•Get some mild exercise every day for lung, heart and muscle rebuilding... as well as for attitude improvement.

•Get regular massage therapy treatments.

•Consider meditation to reduce stress. Daily affirmations can boost self-esteem.

Herbal, Superfood and Supplement Therapy

Interceptive therapy plan: Choose 2 to 3 recommendations.

1—Normalize appetite and metabolism: •Zinc is a key. Severely zinc-deficient people can't manufacture a key protein that allows them to taste. Zinc lozenges help, or •Floradix CAL/MAG liquid with Zinc; •Crystal Star ZINC SOURCE™ extract with DR. VITALITY™ caps or tea; (Add extra tyrosine 500mg if desired.)

2—Herbal serotonin boosters help regulate mood-appetite brain chemicals: •Pacific BioLogic FOOD MOODS to help balance serotonin and GABA; •Natural Balance 5-HTP CALM, 100mg daily. •Crystal Star RELAX CAPS™ 4 daily (especially for bulimics) to rebuild nerve structure; •New Life TRYPTOZEN helps lower cortisol.

3—Control stress reactions: B-complex helps: like •Nature's Secret ULTIMATE B or •Country Life SUBLINGUAL B-12 3000mcg with folic acid 200mcg for healthy cell growth and energy; •take extra B-1 for extra stress control. •GABA compounds relieve stress. •Jarrow THEANINE relaxes and improves concentration. •Maitake Products REISHI caps restore the glands and balance emotions. •Artichoke caps are proving excellent for anorexia. •Centaury also has successful testing.

4—Stimulate appetite, digestion and nutrient assimilation: •Transformation DIGESTZYME speeds digestion, takes stress off enzyme reserves; •Ginseng-Gotu Kola caps, 4 daily; •Rainbow Light ADVANCED ENZYME SYSTEM; •Acidophilus complex powder ¼ tsp. 3x daily or •UAS DDS-PLUS with FOS.

5—Ginseng is a key for energy and balance without calories: •Root To Health POWER PIECES (panax ginseng in honey); •Prince of Peace Red Ginseng, Royal Jelly vials; •Crystal Star FEEL GREAT NOW!™ caps with ADRENAL ENERGY BOOST™ caps, 2 each daily; or •Pure Essence ENERGY PLUS for a feeling of well-being and strength.

—Mineral therapy is effective: The minerals people with eating disorders lose through vomiting are the ones that help control their weight - potassium and iodine stimulate the thyroid to keep metabolism and calorie-burning strong. (Minerals also help restore normal menstrual periods.) •Crystal Star OCEAN MINERALS™ caps (Iodine, Potassium, Silica from the sea) for new collagen growth; •New Chapter OCEAN HERBS (with sea greens); •Flora VEGE-SIL caps. •Futurebiotics VITAL K - liquid potassium.

—Superfoods are lifesavers (choose 2 or 3 recommendations.):
•Crystal Star RESTORE YOUR STRENGTH™ drink.
•Protein drinks: •Unipro PERFECT PROTEIN, •Pure Form WHEY PROTEIN with chunks of real fruit, or •Garden of Life GOATEIN if there is also dairy allergy.
•Green drinks help rebuild healthy blood: •Pure Planet 100% PURE SPIRULINA, or •Crystal Star ENERGY GREEN RENEWAL™.

Can't find a recommended product? Call the 800 number listed in Product Resources for the store nearest you.

Eczema and Psoriasis
Rosacea, Atopic Dermatitis

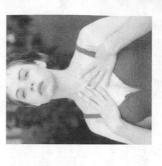

Eczema is an intense, itchy, inflammatory skin disease found on the elbows, knees, wrists and neck. It is most common in infants and children. People who are afflicted have trouble converting essential fatty acids. They also have low hydrochloric stomach acid which causes bad digestion, leaky gut syndrome, and most notably, poor absorption of calcium, the mineral that calms emotional distress, marked in eczema sufferers. Eczema is aggravated by food allergies to eggs, soy foods, wheat and milk. Depression and emotional stress can cause and aggravate psoriasis flare-ups.

Atopic dermatitis, a severe type of eczema, is usually caused by allergies to chemicals, plants, topical medicines, or jewelry metals. A diet with too many fatty foods and poor protein digestion, aggravates the allergies and so is also involved. Eczema and dermatitis, both systemic, spread, but neither condition is permanent and may be reversed by eliminating the offending allergen, improving digestion and boosting EFA intake.

Rosacea is a skin disorder related to adult acne occurring mainly in middle-aged people of Celtic descent. There is no known cure for acne rosacea. Doctors treat it in much the same way as other forms of acne, with oral and topical antibiotics. Eliminating food triggers, particularly spicy foods and alcohol, and avoiding excessive emotional stress, sun, dehydration and environmental pollutants is key to controlling rosacea breakouts.

Psoriasis, a troublesome, chronic skin disorder, affecting 7 million Americans, is on the rise. It's marked by silvery, yellowish skin scales on knees, elbows, buttocks, scalp or chest (normal skin cells mature within a month, a psoriatic skin cell takes only three to six days), psoriasis skin is always dry and thick even when not in the weeping, blistered stages. Arthritis and hypothyroidism frequently accompany psoriasis. Thin bowel walls allowing wastes elimination through the skin are usually involved. In extreme cases, large areas of skin are lost, leaving the body susceptible to severe secondary infections like staph infections and herpes outbreaks. Heredity plays a role in psoriasis, but a recent study links psoriasis more often to immune system malfunction. Psoriasis isn't contagious but its effects can be severe. Every year, about 400 people die from complications due to severe psoriasis. Drugs can offer dramatic short-term results, but the problem reappears if they are discontinued. Natural therapies, which usually take several months to produce consistent improvement, focus on stress reduction to get to the root of the problem, and anti-inflammatories for symptom relief. EFA supplementation with omega-3 fatty acids produces good results for psoriasis relief in clinical studies. See also SKIN INFECTIONS page 544 for more information.

What does your skin rash mean?

Your skin is the mirror of your lifestyle. Imbalances in your body often reveal themselves as skin disorders. Skin problems may start with internal toxicity, allergies, hormone problems or poor digestion. Overuse of drugs (especially antibiotics), stress and a poor diet clearly contribute to skin disorders. Check the signs below to determine what your skin rash may mean. •Use Coca's Pulse test, pg. 316 to determine food allergies that may be aggravating flare ups.

Signs that you may have eczema or dermatitis:
• Reddish, angry patches of skin, frequently on the cheeks, ankles or wrists?
• Crusting and tiny blisters on the skin? Itching, weeping skin?
• Tingling, unpleasant skin prickling? Bumps and scaling on the skin?

Signs that you may have psoriasis:
• Inflamed white, scaly skin lesions, on the scalp, knees, elbows, hands or feet?
• Intense skin sloughing (severe erythrodemic psoriasis)? Pitting or "oil drop" stippling of the nails
• Joint inflammation with arthritic pain (10% of people with psoriasis have psoriatic arthritis)

Signs that you may have rosacea: See also Rosacea under SKIN HEALING, page 546.
• Flushing and redness of the cheeks, chin, nose, and forehead with acne-like bumps and pimples?
• Dilated blood vessels on the face? Bloodshot eyes or gritty feeling in eyes?
• Small, hard bumps on both eyelids?

Can't find a recommended product? Call the 800 number listed in Product Resources for the store nearest you.

Eczema and Psoriasis

Diet and Lifestyle Support Therapy

Nutritional therapy plan:

1—A healthy, low fat diet is a key to psoriasis. Most severe psoriasis sufferers are overweight.

2—A high fiber, high mineral diet with lots of vegetable protein is the key to clearing and preventing eczema.

3—Go on a 3 day skin cleansing diet (pg. 208) to release acid wastes. Take 1 tbsp. psyllium husk, Sonné bentonite or AloeLife ALOE JUICE with herbs morning and evening.

4—Take three cranberry or apple juices daily. Chamomile tea reduces inflammation.

5—Eliminate fatty or fried foods, alcohol and red meats. Avoid nightshade plants like tomatoes, eggplant, potatoes, and peppers. Then follow a sugar-free, milk-free, low-fat diet with 60-70% fresh foods, whole grains (avoid wheat), seafood and sea vegetables like dulse for iodine therapy.

6—Make a skin health mix of lecithin granules, nutritional yeast, and unsulphured molasses and take 2 tbsp. daily.

—Bodywork:

• Exercise keeps circulation healthy; releases body wastes.

• Acupuncture treatments produce good results.

• Expose affected areas to early morning sunlight daily for healing vitamin D.

• Swim or wade in the ocean, or take kelp foot baths for iodine therapy (or a seaweed bath for even better effects).

• Take a catnip or chlorophyll enema once a week to release toxins that come out on the skin.

• For child eczema: bathe areas with strong chamomile tea, then apply an oatmeal paste, let dry. Repeat 4 days until clear.

Stress management is a key: Meditation seems to relieve psoriasis outbreaks.

• Overheating therapy (pg. 182) is effective for psoriasis.

—Effective skin applications:

• *Tea tree* or *Manuka* oil, or zinc pyrithione spray (Blue-Cap) for psoriasis. Capsaicin cream reduces psoriasis itching.

• Apply aloe vera gel or *nettles* extract, •Abkit CAMO-CARE cream, •Calendula-St.John's wort salve.

• Hot *ginger*, *goldenseal* or fresh *comfrey* leaf compresses.

• Jojoba oil with drops peppermint oil (very effective for scalp psoriasis).

• Emu oil, kukui nut or Crystal Star ANTI-BIO™ gel reduce lesions and *tamanu oil* to prevent scarring.

• Dreamous BIOPATHIC SERUM produces good results.

Herbal, Superfood and Supplement Therapy

Interceptive therapy plan: Choose 2 to 3 recommendations.

1—Control the infection: •Take Crystal Star ANTI-BIO™ caps, or •ANTI-BIO™ extract; •*Una da gato* caps 6 daily; • Nutricology Perm-A-Vite if there is leaky gut syndrome. •*Echinacea* extract or *Pau d' arco tea* or • Jarrow JARRO-DOPHILUS with FOS for 3 months as a lymphatic cleanser.

2—Reduce inflammation and scaliness: •MSM, up to 1000mg with MSM lotion; •*Turmeric* extract therapy - 4 to 6 caps daily for 6 weeks. (Often dramatic results in new skin without recurrence). Apply •*Mahonia bark* ointment to heal psoriasis plaques. For excellent results with eczema: •*Licorice root* caps with *red raspberry tea* or *burdock tea*; apply •*witch hazel* or *chickweed tea* relieves eczema itching. •Diamond HERPANACINE capsules (highly recommended) •New Chapter GREEN & WHITE TEA caps, or •Crystal Star DR. VITALITY™

• Take *Gotu kola* as a tea or in caps daily for anti-inflammatory green and white tea blend; properties and to normalize nerve tissue. •Homeopathic *Calc Sulph* for conditions where there are yellow discharges or scabs. •Homeopathic *Graphites* 6x for psoriasis. •Lifespan Nutrition SNEEZE-EZE organic nasal spray shows excellent results for eczema sufferers.

3—Minerals help heal the skin: Take •Crystal Star BEAUTIFUL SKIN™ tea 2 cups daily, and apply with soaked cotton balls. Or apply •Crystal Star HEALTHY SKIN™ gel to lesions •Zinc picolinate 50mg daily; with •vitamin E 400IU and selenium 200mcg (or mix zinc oxide with pricked vitamin E oil capsules and apply to sores). •Add copper caps 2mg 3x daily for 2 months; •Nutricology GERMANIUM 150mg daily. For psoriasis, •Take Alta Health SILICA with bioflavs. Apply •Body Essentials SILICA GEL.

4—Reduce scaling and itching with EFAs: For 3 - 6 months •*Evening primrose oil* 4000mg daily; •Barlean's lignan-rich *flax* oil 3x daily; •Health from the Sun TOTAL EFA's; •Spectrum NORWEGIAN FISH OIL for Omega 3 oils; •Lane Labs BENE-FIN shark cartilage caps 3 daily for 3 months. •Ayurvedic *Coleus forskholii.*

5—Reduce stress to help psoriasis: •Crystal Star ADRENAL ENERGY BOOST™ caps help form adrenal cortex; •Crystal Star RELAX CAPS™ ease stress.

6—Nourish the skin to prevent recurrence: Crystal Star BEAUTIFUL SKIN™ caps; •Ester C with bioflavonoids 3000mg daily for tissue regrowth and less histamine reactions. •Beta carotene 100,000IU daily, or •PHYCOTENE MICRO-CLUSTERS mixed carotenes and sea greens; •vitamin A & D 1000/400IU 4 daily. •B-complex 100mg with extra pantothenic acid 500mg, PABA 1000mg. Keep the liver healthy: •*Milk Thistle seed* extract 2x daily; •*yellow dock root tea* 2 cups daily.

—Superfood therapy: Take a green drink daily.
• **For EFAs:** Nutricology PROGREENS, •Green Foods GREEN MAGMA, Crystal Star ENERGY GREEN RENEWAL™. •Pure Planet AMLA C PLUS to help tissue integrity.

Can't find a recommended product? Call the 800 number listed in Product Resources for the store nearest you.

Emphysema - COPD

Smoker's Chronic Obstructive Pulmonary Disease

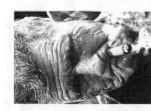

Emphysema, a wasting pulmonary disease, affects smokers almost exclusively, and kills 3 to 5 million people every year according to the World Health Organization. The severity of emphysema is often underestimated because both pneumonia and heart attack death is often triggered by underlying COPD. Smoking damages air sacs so that lungs lose their elasticity and dilation ability. In COPD, this situation is so severe that the sacs burst. The lung exchange of oxygen and carbon-dioxide is seriously affected to the point of extreme breathlessness. Breathing becomes ever more difficult, the sufferer feels asphyxiated and struggles for every breath as the lungs progressively scar and remaining lung tissue thickens. Severe pneumonia bouts almost always accompany emphysema, as do chronic bronchitis and continuing post-nasal drip, coated tongue and congestion. Most people today need portable oxygen generators to maintain some semblance of their lives. Natural therapies can help, but if a COPD sufferer continues to smoke, emphysema is usually fatal (for 50,000 men alone each year). See STOP SMOKING, page 548 in this book. All emphysema sufferers have a constant hacking cough, especially during exhalation and speaking. Energy and general vitality are low because of lack of oxygen. Emphysema is aggravated by allergies to chemicals and dairy foods, exposure to household and garden pesticides or heavy metal pollutants from industry.

Diet and Lifestyle Support Therapy

Nutritional therapy plan:

1—Eliminate mucous-forming foods that provide storage for the allergens, like pasteurized dairy, (mucous), red meats (saturated fat). Go on a short mucous cleansing juice diet for 3-5 days (pg.175). *Note:* Crystal Star IODINE, POTASSIUM, SILICA extract with 1 tsp. olive oil in juice dissolves mucous.

2—For 2 weeks, have a daily green drink: like •Wakunaga KYO-GREEN drink or •Pure Planet CHLORELLA drink, then have a glass of fresh carrot juice every day for a month, then every other day for a month.

3—Make sure your diet is low in sugars and fats to reduce breathlessness. Eat largely fresh foods. Increase your vegetable protein from whole grains, tofu, nuts, seeds and sprouts. Add vitamin B rich foods like brown rice, fresh greens and eggs frequently. Have a green salad with perilla oil dressing every day, (add Rainbow Light GARLIC & GREENS caps, too).

4—Add extra protein to your diet from seafoods like salmon, and sea veggies 2TBS daily, for more B$_{12}$.

—Bodywork:

•Avoid smoke, including smog and other air pollution. Use Enzymatic Therapy NICO-STOP to help stop smoking. Consider Nebulized, Inhaled Glutathione treatment by a holistic physician (recommended by Dr. Jonathan V. Wright).

•Do deep breathing exercises for 3 minutes every morning when rising to clean out the lungs. Take a brisk deep breathing daily walk to boost oxygen. (Carnitine 1000mg daily helps breathing during exercise.) •Get some early sunlight on the body every day possible.

•Steam head and nasal passages with eucalyptus and wintergreen herbs or Yogi BREATHE DEEP tea.

•Use 1 tsp. food grade 3% solution H$_2$O$_2$ in 8-oz. water in a vaporizer at night.

Herbal, Superfood and Supplement Therapy

Interceptive therapy plan: Choose 2 to 3 recommendations.

1—**Control the infection:** •Crystal Star ANTI-BIO™ caps 6 daily followed by •Propolis extract, or •Beehive Botanicals PROPOLIS TINCTURE 65%, 3x daily. •Crystal Star ANTI-FLAM™ caps reduce lung inflammation.

2—**Thin, loosen, expel phlegmy mucous:** •Crystal Star D-CONGEST™ fast relief drops; or, Planetary MULLEIN LUNG COMPLEX. Add •NAC (*N-acetyl-cysteine*) 1000mg, or Nutricology NAC 500mg daily (good results in clinical tests).

3—**Help lungs detoxify:** •Vitamin C crystals with bioflavs ¼ tsp. every hour to bowel tolerance during the day for a month (an ascorbic acid flush neutralizes lung poisons, encourages tissue elasticity); then reduce to 5000mg daily for 3 months. •Crystal Star TOXIN DETOX™ caps for 2 months. For tobacco smoke: •Nature's Secret ULTIMATE RESPIRATORY CLEANSE (highly recommended); •Glutathione 500mg daily, •Crystal Star OCEAN MINERALS™ iodine, potassium, silica caps 3 daily.

4—**Boost circulation and lung muscle action to eliminate poisons:** •Carnitine 1000mg daily; •Eidon MAGNESIUM liquid or magnesium citrate 500mg daily. Add •Pure Planet AMLA C PLUS and •Crystal Star CALCIUM MAGNESIUM SOURCE caps or •Flora MAGNESIUM liquid for critical lung nutrients.

5—**Nourish lungs and bronchial tubes:** •High B-complex 150mg daily with extra pantothenic acid 500mg, and folic acid 800mcg. •*Mullein-lobelia* caps daily; •*Pleurisy root* tea; •Lycopene caps, 4 daily, (a carotene specific for the lungs). •Transformation Enzymes PUREZYME protease enzymes (excellent results for scarring). •Enzymatic Therapy THY-MUPLEX COMPLEX. •PCOs from grapeseed or white pine, 100mg 3x daily strengthen collagen and elastin tissue.

6—**Antioxidants are critical for lung tissue oxygen:** •Beta carotene 150,000IU or mixed carotenes like •PHYCOTENE NANOCLUSTERS, available royalbodycare.com, with copper 2mg daily for lung tissue elasticity; •Vitamin E 1000IU with selenium 400mcg daily; •CoQ-10 300mg 2x daily. •Crystal Star RESTORE YOUR STRENGTH™ drink, or •AloeLife ALOE GOLD juice daily.

Can't find a recommended product? Call the 800 number listed in Product Resources for the store nearest you.

Endometriosis

Pelvic Inflammatory Disease (PID), Polycystic Ovary Syndrome

Endometriosis inflammation is caused by endometrial tissue that is not shed during menstruation. The tissue escapes the uterus and spreads, attaching to other areas of the body — ovaries, lymph nodes, fallopian tubes, bladder, rectum, even kidneys and lungs. There, it grows as normal tissue in abnormal places, bleeding severely during the menstrual cycle, from the vagina or the rectum, or bladder or back through the fallopian tubes, instead of normally through the vagina. Endometriosis increases risk for uterine and breast fibroids. It is credited with up 35-50% of infertility cases in American women. It is often followed by Chronic Fatigue Syndrome or Fibromyalgia. An immune-enhancing program that addresses liver therapy, improves emotional stress, body trauma, and relieves pain is effective, but takes several months.

Note: Polycystic Ovary Syndrome, with many of the same menstrual disturbance symptoms and infertility issues as endometriosis, has a quite different basis.... excess androgens, instead of excess estrogens. The first signs include increased adult acne, pronounced along the jaw line, and excessive hair on the face and abdomen.

Do you have signs of endometriosis?

Most women say the first sign is severe menstruation with prolonged bleeding cycles, and brutal abdominal and rectal area cramping. Swelling and bleeding occurs just before menses, during ovulation and during sex. Irregular bowel movements and diarrhea are common during the long menstruation. The abdomen becomes very bloated, from fluid retention, enlarged ovaries, irritable bowel inflammation and gas. Nerves become pinched and painful. Sleep becomes very difficult.

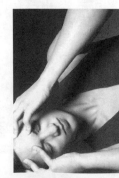

What puts you most at risk for endometriosis?

Causes are widely varied. Most experts cite high estrogen levels accompanied by low levels of progesterone as a primary hormone imbalance that causes abnormal behavior of the endometrium. Others link candida which create small perforations on the uterine wall, to endometriosis. The rise of sexually transmitted chlamydia, cervical dysplasia or vaginal warts in sexually active women has seen a commensurate rise in endometriosis. Chiropractors who treat endometriosis cases point to imbalances caused by hypoglycemia, oral contraceptives, X-Rays and immune dysfunction. New evidence shows exposure to dioxin is linked to endometriosis. A poor diet with too much fat, caffeine and alcohol, and low EFA and magnesium intake is regularly involved. Call the ENDOMETRIOSIS ASSOCIATION 1-800-992-ENDO for updated information.

An herbal "vag pack" can effectively detox the vaginal area

Boluses and vaginal packs are effective in drawing out internal infection from endometriosis, cysts, benign tumors, polyps and uterine growths, and cervical dysplasia. A cleansing herbal combination may be used as a vaginal pack by placing it against the cervix, or as a bolus inserted in the vagina. Both act as an internal poultice to draw out toxic wastes from the vagina, rectum or urethral areas. It takes 6 weeks to 6 months for complete healing, depending on the problem and severity. Use castor oil packs or the formula given below.

How to make a pack:

—**Formula #1:** Mix 1 part of each powdered herb with cocoa butter to form a finger-sized suppository: *squaw vine, marshmallow root, slippery elm, goldenseal root, pau d'arco, comfrey root, mullein, yellow dock root, chickweed, acidophilus powder.*

—**Formula #2:** Mix 1 part each powdered herb with cocoa butter to form a finger-sized suppository: *cranesbill powder, goldenseal root, red raspberry leaf, white oak bark, echinacea root, myrrh gum powder.*

Place suppositories on waxed paper in the refrigerator to chill and harden slightly. Smear on cotton tampon and insert, or insert as is, and use a sanitary napkin to catch drainage. Use suppositories at night; rinse out in the morning with *white oak bark* or *yellow dock root* tea to rebalance vaginal pH. Repeat for 6 days. Make sure there are long rest times between pack or bolus use – 1 week of use to 3 weeks rest. Repeat if necessary.

Can't find a recommended product? Call the 800 number listed in Product Resources for the store nearest you.

Endometriosis

Diet and Lifestyle Support Therapy

Nutritional therapy plan:

1—You can help your condition substantially with diet improvement. Go on a short 24 hour juice diet (pg. 173) to clear out acid wastes. (This helps you to work on the integrity of the liver and digestive system first. Repeat the cleanse for 24 hours before menses.) Add if desired

2—Decrease excess estrogen production with a low fat diet (20 grams daily). Especially avoid dairy foods.

3—Then follow a vegan diet for 3 months. (See *Robin Robertson's VEGAN PLANET* book for recipes.) Add cold water fish 3 times a week, especially wild (not farm raised) salmon. Eat cultured foods like yogurt, fresh fruits and green salads, whole grains and sea cereals until condition clears. Especially add soy foods, cruciferous vegetables and sea greens (2 tbsp. daily) for estrogen balancing power.

4—Follow with an immune power diet to prevent the condition from returning: Eliminate alcohol and caffeine foods during healing. Restrict refined sugars, red meats and dairy foods during healing. Keep all animal fats and high cholesterol foods low, to prevent excess estrogen production, a clear cause of endometriosis. Particularly avoid chocolate, tropical oils, fried and fast food of all kinds.

6—See the Hypoglycemia Diet, page 463 for better long term eating habits.

—Bodywork:

I know endometrial conditions are painful, but before you jump into surgery or any drastic treatment decision, endometriosis or fibroids may go away naturally when glands and hormones rebalance, such as after pregnancy and birth, or menopause. Question steroid drugs commonly given for endometriosis - especially prednisone.

• Use stress reduction techniques like massage therapy and acupuncture. Mild exercise works as a stress reducer. Get early morning sunlight on the body every day.

• Avoid all chloro-fluorocarbon products and any other known toxic chemical or environmental pollutants.

• Avoid IUD's. They are a major contributor to endometriosis.

—Cleansing douches:

• Garlic: infuse garlic cloves in 1 qt. water
• Mineral water - 1 qt.

—Reflexology point:

• Press both sides of the foot just below the ankle bone, 2x daily for 10 seconds each.

Herbal, Superfood and Supplement Therapy

Interceptive therapy plan: Choose 2 to 3 recommendations.

1—**Relieve pain and clear our wastes:** For 3 months: •Crystal Star WOMAN'S BEST FRIEND™ caps 6 daily, and *burdock* tea 2 cups daily, with •Transformation Enzyme PURE-ZYME tablets to dissolve adhesions of abnormally placed tissue (excellent results). Add if desired •Pure Essence FEM CREME rubbed on the abdomen. •*Black cohosh* extract; •Ascorbic acid flush: ascorbate vitamin C powder with bioflavonoids - ¼ tsp. in juice every hour until stool turns soupy; or •vitamin C 4000mg and *Evening Primrose Oil* 4000 daily. •Crystal Star PRO-EST BALANCE™ roll-on, controls pain, stimulates progesterone balance. •Pacific BioLogic GYNCEASE for abnormal bleeding; •Niacin 100mg every 3 hours to relieve uterine pain (ask your physician if you're on heart medication).

2—**Reduce inflammation and spasms:** •Crystal Star ANTI-FLAM™ caps, 4 at a time, or STRESS OUT™ muscle relaxer drops (fast acting relief), with DR. ENZYME™ with protease and bromelain, or •Enzymedica PURIFY protease, for pain during menses; •Enzymatic Therapy LYMPHO-CLEAR 3x daily.

3—**EFAs help metabolize, balance excess estrogen:** •*Evening Primrose Oil* caps 4000mg daily; •Omega-rich flax or fish oil; •Health from the Sun TOTAL EFA; •Barlean's ESSENTIAL WOMAN oils; •*Dandelion root* tea.

4—**Energy-building liver therapy:** •*Echinacea* and *Milk Thistle Seed* extracts; •Flo-radix GALLEXIER or •Crystal Star BITTERS & LEMON CLEANSE™. (*Note:* Bitters herbs can be excellent cleansers of pelvic congestion, but should be avoided during painful flare-ups.) •Nature's Secret ULTIMATE B, and extra folic acid 400mcg, and •Nature's Secret ULTIMATE GREEN with EFAs; •Floradix HERBAL IRON 3x daily.

5—**Balance hormones for long term relief:** •Crystal Star BREAST & UTERINE FIBRO DEFENSE™ caps for 3 months (highly recommended). •Choline 1000mg with inositol 500mg; •Crystal Star ADRENAL ENERGY BOOST™ caps for adrenal cortex balance; •Crystal Star IODINE, POTASSIUM, SILICA drops or •Bernard Jensen LIQUI-DULS for thyroid balance. •*Black cohosh, dong quai, cordyceps* combinations help dissolve scar tissue in the endometrium; •VITEX extract for pituitary support.

6—**For emotional stress and tension:** •Crystal Star RELAX CAPS™ for stress reduction - 2 at a time as needed (relief in about 25 minutes).

7—**Enhance immune response:** •CoQ-10, 300mg daily. •Solgar OCEANIC CARO-TENE 100,000IU daily; •Ester C with bioflavonoids 3000mg; •Future Biotics VITAL K liquid potassium 3 tsp. daily; •Vitamin E 400IU daily.

—Superfood therapy - greens are the key: (Choose one or more.)
• Fit for You, Intl. MIRACLE GREENS with sea greens.
• Crystal Star ENERGY GREEN RENEWAL™ drink.
• Crystal Star RESTORE YOUR STRENGTH™ drink or OCEAN MINERALS™ caps.

Can't find a recommended product? Call the 800 number listed in Product Resources for the store nearest you.

Energy

Increasing Stamina, Overcoming Fatigue, Nerve Exhaustion and Mental Burn Out

There's no doubt about it - stress and fatigue are becoming more a part of our lives - eight out of ten Americans say they feel tired on a regular basis. Some of us feel tired most of the time. Many of us don't have enough energy for our daily tasks. Almost all of us feel the need for a pick-me-up during a long day. Yet, turning to drugs or controlled substances for stimulation is asking for trouble. Overusing stimulants means dependency, irritability and lethargy, further reducing energy in a downward spiral. Even traditional food stimulants like caffeine, sodas or sugar usually end up making us feel more nervous and more restless. Natural energizers have great advantages over chemically processed stimulants. They don't exhaust the body, and are supporting rather than depleting. They can be strong or gentle as needed. Why do some people drag through their daily lives, while others run marathons or juggle demanding career and family responsibilities without blinking an eye? Sickness, body imbalances and dietary deficiencies; and prolonged stress, negativity, emotional depression and hopelessness all zap energy. *See my STRESS and ENERGY book for much more.*

What's sapping your energy? The 5 most common energy depleters.

—LACK OF SLEEP: Americans sleep 20% less today than our forefathers did at the turn of the century. Nearly 50 million Americans are chronically sleep-deprived. Almost 50% of the U.S. population has sleep-related problems like insomnia. A new study reports that an astounding 25% of adults feel that they cannot be successful and still get adequate sleep. Lack of sleep zaps our energy, reduces immune response, lowers our sex drive, and raises blood pressure. Cutting into your 8 needed hours of sleep time just by 90 minutes reduces daytime alertness up to 33%! **Signs that you may need more shut-eye:** 1) Cuts, scrapes, blemishes or other injuries heal slowly; 2) You have dark circles under your eyes; 3) You have difficulty getting up; 4) You are always tired; 5) Your memory is poor, your thinking fuzzy; 6) You find yourself relying on stimulants like coffee, tea, nicotine or other drugs to get through the day.

—STRESS: No one lives a completely stress free life. Stress depends on how you react to the changes and demands of your life. A little stress can even be good, motivating you towards meeting a goal. Too much stress can be disastrous to health. Chronic stress especially drains your energy, targeting organs like the adrenal glands and wiping out their energizing stores. It shows up in how you look and how you feel. The more "stressed out" you become, the more vulnerable you are to chronic health problems. **Signs you may be on stress overload:** 1) You get frequent headaches, chronic backaches or neck pain; 2) You have a tendency to "fly off the handle" easily; 3) You have fuzzy thinking and poor memory; 4) You have chronic indigestion; 5) You have chronic insomnia at night, and chronic fatigue during the day; 6) You have difficulty getting new ideas or performing creative projects; 7) You get frequent colds or flu.

—ADRENAL EXHAUSTION: Adrenal glands are the most affected by stress, emotional strain, anger or exhaustion. When you're under pressure, the adrenal medulla secretes adrenaline and norepinephrine to accelerate metabolism, heart rate, respiration and perspiration... responses vital to our survival, strengthening the body and increasing its resistance to stress. But when the adrenals release too few or too many hormones, exhaustion can result. **Body markers to watch out for:** 1) Constant fatigue or muscle weakness; 2) Mood swings, heart palpitations, panic attacks, anxiety spells; 3) Chronic heartburn and indigestion; 4) Unusual cravings for salt or sweets; 5) Extreme sensitivity to odors and/or noises; 6) Difficulty concentrating; 7) Chronic insomnia and headaches, particularly migraines; 8) Clenching or grinding your teeth, especially at night; 9) frequent yeast or fungal infections.

—THYROID MALFUNCTION: Your thyroid gland governs your metabolism, providing vital energy resources. Since World War II, an above average number of people have developed thyroid problems, largely it is thought, because of all the chemicals and pollutants in our environment. Today hypothyroidism (low thyroid) affects 15 million people, the vast majority of them women. **Signs to watch out for:** 1) Lethargy or fatigue in the morning; 2) Swollen ankles, hands and eyelids; 3) Bloating, gas and indigestion after eating; 4) Unusual depression; 5) Unusual hair loss, especially in women; 6) Unexplained obesity; 7) Breast fibroid growths; 8) Poor immune response.

—OVER-USE OF STIMULANTS LIKE CAFFEINE, SUGAR OR DRUGS: Americans want quick fixes and we often end up paying the price in terms of our health. Nine out of ten Americans use caffeine in some form, averaging 2 cups of coffee a day. The average American consumes 150 pounds of sugar a year, a whopping 1200% increase from a century ago. Caffeine and sugar overload raises blood sugar. In the effort to clean up the excess sugar in the blood, insulin, which regulates blood sugar, removes too much sugar, causing low blood sugar reactions, and more fatigue. Caffeine, a nervous system stimulant, is notorious for wiping out the adrenals, leading to low energy. Green tea has far less caffeine than coffee and offers 40mg l-*theanine* per cup, an amino acid that improves focus and reduces stress. **Clues you might be hooked:** 1) Frequent agitation, mood swings; 2) Headaches and exhaustion if stimulants are eliminated; 3) Increased tolerance to caffeine or sugar; constipation when caffeine is eliminated; 4) High blood sugar levels; 5) Exhausted adrenals; 6) Chronic insomnia.

Can't find a recommended product? Call the 800 number listed in Product Resources for the store nearest you.

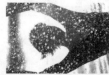

Energy

Diet and Lifestyle Support Therapy

Nutritional therapy plan:

1—Your high energy diet should consist of 65-70% complex carbohydrates, from fresh fruits, vegetables, whole grains and legumes; 20-25% protein, from nuts, seeds, whole grains, legumes, soy, yogurt and kefir, seafoods and poultry; 10-15% fats from sources like unrefined vegetable, nut and seed oils, eggs and low-fat dairy.

2—Foods that fight fatigue: potassium and magnesium-rich foods, complex carbohydrates, high vitamin B and C foods, and iron-rich foods.

3—Reduce sugar, caffeine (drains adrenals), and fatty dairy foods (produce clogging mucous).

4—Take a protein drink every morning, or PureForm WHEY PROTEIN. Add spirulina (or Pure Planet 100% PURE SPIRULINA) or bee pollen granules or Bragg's LIQUID AMINOS to any drink as a booster.

5—Drink plenty of healthy liquids. Dehydration's first sign is fatigue. I recommend PENTA bottled water, or Alacer EMERGEN-C granules in water for rapid rehydration, and Guayaki YERBA MATÉ tea for long range, non-jittery energy. Have a little wine at dinner for mental relaxation and good digestion. Don't overdo it though. Excess alcohol disrupts REM sleep and depletes B vitamins.

—Bodywork:

• If symptoms last more than 6 months, get a test for EBV, CFIDS, hypothyroidism or Candida albicans.

• Take a brisk walk every day; stimulates endorphins and replenishes oxygen in the entire body.

• Reflexology: with your knuckles, press center arch of your foot for 10 seconds. Stretch out for 5 minutes both morning and before bed to release energy blocks.

• Deep breathing helps oxygenate and energize the body.

• Get daily morning sunlight on the body when possible.

• Have a full spinal massage for increased nerve force.

• Take alternating hot and cold hydrotherapy showers to increase circulation.

• Good sleep and rest boost the amount of energy you have.

• Acupressure energizer: squeeze point between eyes where brows come together.

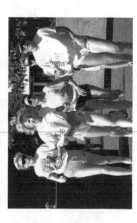

Herbal, Superfood and Supplement Therapy

Interceptive therapy plan: Choose 2 to 3 recommendations.

1—**Energizers for men:** •Crystal Star ATHLETIC PERFORMANCE ENERGY™ for men caps; •*Chinese red ginseng;* Jagulana JIAOGULAN PLUS energy formula; •Earth Power PHYTOCHI caps; •Always Young HGH WORKOUT FOR MEN spray with growth factors from velvet antler. •Zinc picolinate 50-75mg. •Prince of Peace GINKGO/RHODIOLA vials, or Natural Balance *Rhodiola* for stamina.

2—**Energizers for women:** •Crystal Star ADRENAL ENERGY BOOST™ caps; *Dong quai-damiana-ashwagandha* extract. •Pure Essence ENERGY PLUS w. 1000mg spirulina; •Jagulana JIAOGULAN Women's Relief formula (also for PMS); •Enzymatic Therapy THYROID–TYROSINE COMPLEX (excellent activity). •*Evening Primrose Oil* for fatigue; •Hawthorn extract for well-being. •Pacific BioLogic RECOVERY AMERICA MORNING FORMULA; •Nature's Secret ULTIMATE ENERGY.

3—**Ginseng is a natural energizer for both sexes:** •Crystal Star FEEL GREAT NOW™ caps with ginseng; •Rainbow Light TEN GINSENGS; *Siberian eleuthero* extract; •*Suma* caps, •Hsu's WILD AMERICAN GINSENG. •Prince of Peace GINSENG, ROYAL JELLY vials; •*Ashwagandha* 300-600mg nourish overworked adrenal glands.

4—**Mental energizers:** •Crystal Star MENTAL CLARITY™ caps; •*Ginkgo biloba* extract, or •Dr. Diamond DIAMOND MIND; • Planetary BACOPA-GINKGO BRAIN STRENGTH tabs; •NADH (a B-vit. derivative) 10mg boosts alertness, stamina, energy.

5—**Metabolic energizers improve body performance:** •Transformation PUREZYME capsules on an empty stomach and DIGESTZYME with meals if you have food sensitivities; •CoQ-10, 230mg daily or •Nutricology CoQ-10 with tocotrienols; •L-Carnitine 1000mg daily; •Alpha Lipoic acid 200mg daily; •B-complex 100mg with extra pantothenic acid 500mg daily.

6—**Nutrient boosters overcome fatigue:** •Cordyceps mushroom extract 30 drops daily overcomes adrenal fatigue or •Crystal Star OCEAN MINERALS™ caps for a thyroid nutrient boost. •Sublingual B-12, 2500mcg with folic acid 200mcg;(with tyrosine 500mg for best results). •Chromium picolinate 200mcg daily. •Source Naturals OPTI-ZINC or •Ethical Nutrients ZINC STATUS; •Trace Minerals Research CONCENTRACE minerals; •Eidon MAGNESIUM liquid for muscle fatigue.

7—**Antioxidant energizers:** •Vitamin C with bioflavs, 3000mg daily. • DMG sublingual tabs or •Unipro LIQUID DMG. •Diamond Formulas HEALTHY HORIZONS with alpha lipoic acid; •Nature's Secret BEYOND ENDURANCE. •*Gotu kola-peppermint-aralia* tea;

—Superfoods are a key to rapid energy:

•ALL 1 MULTIPLE VITAMINS & MINERALS drink.
•Crystal Star ENERGY GREEN RENEWAL™ drink, caps.

Can't find a recommended product? Call the 800 number listed in Product Resources for the store nearest you.

Epilepsy

Petit Mal, Partial Seizures

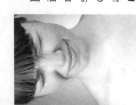

Epilepsy is a neurological disorder that acts like an electrical short circuit in the brain, causing seizures. 2 million Americans are affected by some form of epilepsy. 1) *Petit mal* - a short seizure with a blank stare and brief motor disability; most common in children; 2) *Grand mal* - a long seizure with falling, muscle twitching, incontinence, gasping, ashen skin, and sometimes loss of consciousness. Regardless of type, most victims have no memory of an attack. Many commonly prescribed anti-convulsant drugs are so strong and so habit forming that even non-epileptic people have bad reactions and seizures when cut off suddenly. Nutritional therapies can make drugs unnecessary. If you decide to use alternative methods, taper off drugs gradually and speak to your doctor. If seizures recur, return to the anti-convulsants briefly to let the body adjust. Causes of epilepsy are wide and varied, extending from poor waste elimination with a resultant overload on nerves, to heavy metal toxicity, allergies; EFA and mineral deficiencies; hypoglycemia and hormonal changes. Stress may trigger seizures. *Signs that a seizure is impending?* Victims report chest discomfort, nausea, dizziness, headaches, impaired speech, shortness of breath and numbness in the hands, lips and tongue. *See the HYPOGLYCEMIA DIET page 463 for more.*

Diet and Lifestyle Support Therapy

Nutritional therapy plan:

1—There must be a diet and lifestyle change for there to be permanent control and improvement. Consider a rotation diet to check for food allergy reactions. Over the long term, perhaps a Hypoglycemia Correction diet is best (page 463).

2—Start with a mild 3 day liquid diet (pg. 172) to release mucous and control system stress. Then follow a diet with at least 70% fresh foods. Have a green salad every day.

3—Add cultured foods like yogurt, kefir, tofu; brown rice or Amazake RICE DRINK.. Slowly add eggs, small amounts of low fat dairy foods, legumes, seafoods and sea veggies.

4—Take Red Star NUTRITIONAL YEAST drink or MISO soup before bed for B-vitamins and immune enhancement.

5—Eat organically grown foods if possible to avoid seizure triggers in pesticides. Eliminate foods with preservatives or colors; high fat foods, sugars, fried and canned foods, red meats, pork, alcohol, caffeine, MSG, aspartame and fatty dairy foods. Salmon is a good choice, but beware of farmed salmon, high in contaminates.

—**Bodywork:**

• Lemon juice or catnip enemas once a month keep the body pH balanced, toxin-free.
• Get daily outdoor exercise for healthy circulation.
• Biofeedback has been successful in limiting seizure attacks.
• New evidence shows that magnet therapy is effective in smoothing out the "electrical shorts" that accompany seizures.

What should you do in case of a seizure? Epileptic seizures are usually short, with quick consciousness recovery. Deep sleep usually follows a seizure.
—Do not attempt to restrain the person. Catch him if he falls. Loosen any constricting clothing. —Let the person lie down and get plenty of fresh air. Clear away sharp or hard objects. Cushion the head. —Squeeze the little finger very firmly during a seizure.
—Do not put anything in the person's mouth or throw water on the face. Turn head to let excess saliva drain out.

Herbal, Superfood and Supplement Therapy

Interceptive therapy plan: Choose 2 to 3 recommendations.

1—**Stabilize, nourish the nerves:** • Crystal Star RELAX CAPS™ and MUSCLE RELAXER™ caps as needed; • Glycine and Glutamine 500mg daily help control seizures (recommended). • Nature's Secret ULTIMATE B. • Anti-convulsants Taurine 1500mg daily and • B-6 250mg (good results for many). • Sublingual B-12 3000mcg with folic acid 200mcg; or • Eidon MANGANESE liquid with B-12 3000mcg.

2—**Natural sedatives help calm convulsions:** • *Lobelia* drops in water daily; • *Scull-cap* or *Catnip* tea, 2 cups daily. • Nutremedix CALM as directed. • Calcium 1000mg/magnesium 500mg or • Crystal Star CALCIUM-MAGNESIUM SOURCE™ caps to reduce nerve excitability, or • Country Life RELAXER caps with GABA and taurine 1000mg daily.

3—**Extra EFAs offer better brain balance:** • *Evening Primrose Oil* caps 4-6 daily for 2 months, then 3-4 daily for 1 month to balance body electrical activity.

4—**Protect your liver:** • Choline 600mg, or Choline-inositol or phosphatidyl choline for brain balance; • Reishi mushroom extract 2x daily; • Alpha Lipoic Acid 100mg. • Vitamin C, 500mg for each year of the child. • Crystal Star LIVER RENEW™ caps and • *Milk Thistle Seed* extract especially if you are taking Dilantin or other anti-seizure drugs.

5—**Minerals help rebalance body chemistry:** • Atrium LITHIUM 5mg as directed; • Trace Mineral Research CONCENTRACE tablets; or • Nature's Path TRACE-MIN LYTE; • American Biologics MANGANESE FORTE. Consider • Golden Pride FORMULA 1 oral chelation with EDTA.

—**For young child epilepsy:** • Floradix liquid vitamin-mineral complex. • Nature's Way ANTSP tincture, or • *lobelia* drops under the tongue as emergency measures. • Carnitine 250mg with folic acid 400mcg especially if taking Dilantin. • Nutricology SYMBIOTICS powder or • UAS DDS-JUNIOR for probiotic aid.

—**Superfood therapy:** • Crystal Star RESTORE YOUR STRENGTH™ drink. • Futurebiotics VITAL K drink. • AloeLife ALOE GOLD drink.

Can't find a recommended product? Call the 800 number listed in Product Resources for the store nearest you.

Eyesight

Weak Eyes, Blurred Vision, Bloodshot, Burning, Itchy, Watery Eyes

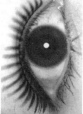

About 80% percent of what we learn during our lives we learn through sight. The eyes are not only the windows of the soul, but windows on our health as well, reflecting imbalances or poor health conditions elsewhere in the system. No other sense is so prone to poor health conditions. Your lifestyle profoundly affects your "eyestyle." U.S. eyestrain complaints have skyrocketed. Most of America's jobs are sedentary and involve computer use for much of the day, leading to blurring vision as the day goes on, frequent headaches and spots and floaters before the eyes. Environmental pollutants and the resultant rise in chemical allergies also affect eye health. Drugs of all kinds can react with your eyes. The worst offenders are cocaine, excessive use of chemical diuretics, sulfa drugs or tetracycline, aspirin, ibuprofen, acetaminophen, heartburn drugs, nicotine, phenylalanine and hydrocortisone. A diet high in sugar and refined carbohydrates can be a major eye offender, causing a more than 300% increase in the risk of vision problems! Your eyes age just before the rest of your body. The liver is the key to healthy eyes; keep it clean and well-functioning. The mind/body connection plays a big role in vision. Emotional harmony has an impact on the willingness to see. *Note: Techniques like Lasik eye surgery have led to dramatic vision improvements for thousands. But, the surgery is not for everyone. Major complications can occur. Investigate the Lasik technique carefully before undergoing surgery.*

Diet and Lifestyle Support Therapy

Nutritional therapy plan:

1—Increase protein from sea and soy foods (rich in omega-3 fatty acids): whole grains, low fat dairy foods, eggs (full of zeaxanthin), sprouts and seeds.

2—Increase vitamin A and high mineral foods: leafy greens (kale, arugula, chard), sea greens are loaded with carotenes and EFAs (2 tbsp. daily), orange and yellow veggies, broccoli, seafood, pumpkin seeds and parsley.

3—Add vision foods like broccoli, sunflower and sesame seeds, leeks, onions, cabbage and cauliflower, corn, barley, blueberries, watercress.

4—Take a vision drink 2x a week: 1 cup carrot juice, ½ cup *Eyebright* tea, 1 egg, 1 tbsp. wheat germ, 1 tsp. *rose hips* powder, 1 tbsp. honey, 1 tsp. sesame seeds, 1 tsp. nutritional yeast, 1 tsp. dulse powder.

5—Reduce sugar intake. Avoid chemicalized foods, especially fried and fatty foods, dairy foods and red meats. These foods cause the body to metabolize slowly, use sugars poorly, and form crystallized clogs.

—Eye relaxation techniques:

•Eye relaxation techniques are like eye yoga stretches to reduce eyestrain. (See the Bates Method book for more.)

•Look right; look up; look left; look down; look diagonally up down and to the sides. Rotate your gaze in a circle. (Don't do these exercise if you wear contacts).

•For eyestrain: Massage temples, pinch skin between the brows; then palm your eyes for 10 seconds at a time.

•Bathe eyes in a cool saline solution, witch hazel, apply black tea or chamomile tea bags; or bathe eyes in ice water. Then squeeze eyes shut for 3 seconds to increase blood flow to the area. Works almost immediately to reduce puffy eyes.

•For irritated eyes from smog or allergies: splash eyes with cool water. Then warm them with a hot washcloth over closed lids. Press eyes gently with fingertips and repeat.

•Chiropractic treatment helps for poor vision due to spinal misalignment.

Herbal, Superfood and Supplement Therapy

Interceptive therapy: Allow 2 to 3 months for effectiveness.

1—**Expand your eye power:** •Crystal Star EYES RIGHT™ extract or; •Esteem BRIGHT EYES caps (esp. for computer strained eyes); •Hyalogic EYEFACTOR HA (with hyaluronic acid, lutein, zeaxanthin, bilberry); Trimedica VISI CLEAR or NaturalCare Dr. Bob Martin's OPTIALL; •*Ginkgo biloba* extract stimulates circulation to the eye area. •Vitamin Research VINPOCETINE 30mg daily, has improved vision in 70% of test subjects.

2—**Bioflavonoids strengthen eye vessels:** •*Bilberry* extract or •Source Naturals VISUAL EYES with bilberry, lipoic acid, lutein; •Quercetin 1000mg w. bromelain daily; •PCOs (*grape seed or white pine*), 200mg daily; Nutricology OCUDYNE 2.

3—**Liver health for eye health:** •Crystal Star LIVER RENEW™ capsules 4-6 daily; •*Milk Thistle Seed* extract; •*Dandelion root* tea. •Chromium picolinate regulates sugar.

4—**Antioxidants boost eye health:** •*Parsley root* or *Eyebright* caps 4 daily; •Herbalist & Alchemist BLUEBERRY extract; •beta carotene 150,000IU daily, or •PHYCOTENE NANOCLUSTERS, sea greens carotenes available on royal-health.com; or •Source Naturals ASTAXANTHIN; •Alpha Lipoic Acid 150mg to boost glutathione; •Zinc 30-50mg daily; •Taurine 500mg daily; •Vitamin E 400IU w. selenium 200mcg; •Vitamin D 400IU.

5—**For itchy red eyes:** Swab inside of nose with •Aloe vera gel on a Q-tip. Take •Aloe vera juice daily; •B-complex 100mg; •Similasan EYE DROPS #2; •Boiron OPTIQUE.

6—**Clarifying eyestrain treatments:** (seeing sparks of light or color with eyes closed indicates stress): •BILBERRY extract 4x daily. •Bathe eyes in diluted *rosemary* tea (better than Visine). Place •*Raspberry* tea bags or *green tea* bags on bloodshot eyes; •*Borage seed* tea for sore eyes; •*Calendula* tea for scleroderma. •Similasan COMPUTOR EYES drops.

—Superfood therapy:

•Solgar EARTH SOURCE GREENS & MORE w. EFAs.
•Green Foods CARROT ESSENCE.
•Wakunaga HARVEST BLEND with kale.
•Crystal Star RESTORE YOUR STRENGTH™ drink.

Can't find a recommended product? Call the 800 number listed in Product Resources for the store nearest you.

Natural Therapy for Specific Vision Problems

—**CATARACTS:** See page 365. Consider Enzymatic Therapy CATA-COMP and Life Extension GLUTATHIONE, C, CYSTEINE caps for detoxification support.

—**GLAUCOMA:** caused by a build-up of pressure in the front compartment of the eye; may cause partial (or even full) blindness if not treated. See page 430.

—**CONJUNCTIVITIS INFECTION:** inflammation of the eyelid often caused by a viral infection.... extremely contagious. —**Alternative healing protocols:** • Take a pineapple-carrot juice daily; use •*Aloe vera* juice eyewashes, or *goldenseal root, mullein, yarrow or eyebright tea* eyewashes and •Zinc 50mg 2x daily; • *Bilberry* extract. •Palm eyes to release infection and stimulate circulation. •Apply yogurt, grated potato or apple to inflammation; or a calendula compress to draw out infection - just make a warm tea; soak a washcloth in the tea and press on the eye. Or, simply use an egg white and spread it on a cloth or bandage; then apply to affected area. Use •colloidal silver eyedrops, or • Boiron OPTIQUE remedy or homeopathic Belladonna 30C. Take •PCO's from grapeseed to help new tissue grow back, 200mg 2x daily. •Add ascorbate vitamin C 2000mg daily. •100,000 IU vitamin A for one month.

—**DRY EYES (Sjögren's syndrome):** a sudden onset problem, characterized by dry eyes and the inability to tear, dry mouth, dry skin and all mucous membranes. It often accompanies arthritis, scleroderma and systemic lupus. Caused by a vitamin A deficiency, low EFAs, and low immune response, it affects 9 times more women than men, usually after menopause. —**Alternative healing protocols:** Lower your intake of sugary foods and fatty foods, caffeine, red meat and dairy foods, corn, wheat, and nightshade plants (including tobacco and the drug Motrin, nightshade-based.) •Increase your green vegetable, whole grain and fiber intake. •Increase cold water fish, seafoods and calcium foods like broccoli. Increase water and healthy fluid intake like green and white tea. •Bathe eyes daily with *aloe vera* juice. Drinking aloe juice daily also moistens eyes. •Trimedica VISI CLEAR eye drops with lutein or •Similasan EYE DROPS #1 soothe and moisturize dry eyes; •Take high omega-3 flax or *Evening Primrose Oil* caps 4 daily or New Chapter SUPERCRITICAL DHA to improve tearing; • Take 3000mg ascorbate vitamin C daily; •emulsified vitamin A and E 25,000IU/400IU to clear tear pathways; •taurine 500mg 2x daily; •*Bilberry and Ginkgo Biloba* extracts act as natural antihistamines and increase circulation to the eyes; •*Ginseng* caps 2 to 3 daily for 3 months help your eyes produce moisture. • B complex 100mg with extra B₂, and zinc 30-50mg daily. Take •Crystal Star CALCIUM-MAGNESIUM SOURCE™ caps for extra absorbable calcium.

   For "computer" eyes: •Similasan COMPUTER EYES drops; Blink often to recoat your eyes with tears, to cleanse and lubricate. Press points under eyebrows; press points in inner corners of eyes; squeeze eyebrows; look up, down, right and left every half hour. •Tape page one of a newpaper to a wall about 8 feet from your computer. Every 30 minutes, look at the newspaper, bring the headlines into focus, then look back at your monitor. Yoga stretches help, too. •Clean your screen.

—**NIGHT BLINDNESS:** The inability of the eyes to adjust to changes in light intensity (usually a sign of a vitamin A deficiency). Blink rapidly for 5 seconds to help your eyes adjust. Use amber glasses for daytime driving. —**Alternative healing protocols:** •Add spinach and sea veggies several times a week to your diet. Take •BILBERRY or •GINKGO BILOBA extract capsules or liquid; •PCO's from grapeseed or white pine 100mg 3x daily; •CoQ-10 200mg daily; •Zinc 30mg daily; add •vitamin D 400IU daily. •Carotenoids, up to 200,000IU daily or •PHYCOTENE NANOCLUSTERS available from royal-health.com, or •vitamin A 25,000IU. Take for 1 month, then 10,000IU for 2 months. May improve night vision up to 65%! •For color blindness: Solgar oceanic carotene 25,000IU (from Dunaliella Salina). In some cases, night blindness is caused by blocked arteries. See my program for atherosclerosis on pg. 323.

—**MYOPIA (Nearsightedness):** only 2% of second grade children are nearsighted; by the end of high school, the figure is 40%; by the end of college, more than 60% of students are nearsighted! Alternative healing protocols: In addition to the recommendations for better eyesight on the previous page, use •vitamin C up to 5000mg daily; •Vitamin D 1000IU; •Crystal Star SUGAR CONTROL HIGH™ caps if you also have diabetic tendencies; •New Chapter SUPERCRITICAL DHA 100 to help improve distance vision. •Planetary TRIPHALA caps as directed; •BILBERRY extract or caps; •Enzymatic Therapy VISION ESSENTIALS capsules.

—**FLOATERS AND SPOTS BEFORE THE EYES:** extremely common in today's world, many are caused by drugs or a toxic overload from surgery or illness, candida yeast overgrowth or a polluted environment. A good liver detox can usually help floaters. Other floaters may be **Bitot's spots**, hard, elevated white spots on the whites of the eyes, bits of harmless debris that cast shadows over the retina, or **scotoma**, blind spots in the vision field because of retina trouble. To make debris floaters disappear, close your eyes and move your eyeballs up and down. —**Alternative healing protocols:** A diet to control hypoglycemia can help. See pg. 463. Take • bioflavonoids 1000mg daily and •Planetary TRIPHALA caps to cleanse the liver-3 months; •Vitamin K 100mcg 2 daily; •Vitamin A & D, 25,000IU/400IU, or •emulsified A & E 25,000IU/400IU to help remove lens particles; •pantothenic acid 500mg with B₆ 250mg; •Vitamin C or Ester C; rub Earth's Bounty O₂ SPRAY on the feet at night for several months; •*Dandelion* root tea and eyewash and a 2 month course of •MILK THISTLE SEED extract helps the liver.

Can't find a recommended product? Call the 800 number listed in Product Resources for the store nearest you.

—DARK CIRCLES UNDER THE EYES: usually caused by iron deficiency, but also an indication of liver or kidney malfunction, or chronic allergies. **—Alternative healing protocols:** •Take Floradix liquid iron; •Planetary TRIPHALA caps as directed for 3 months; •use chamomile or green tea teabags over the eyes for 15 minutes. Use Coca's Pulse test on pg. 316 to determine food allergies related to allergic "shiners."

—DYSLEXIA: a signal-scrambling learning disorder affecting over 40 million American children and adults! It may have more to do with the inner ear than the eyes. **—Alternative healing protocols:** Essential fatty acids are essential, especially •DHA and omega-3 rich fatty acids. Take •ginkgo biloba extract 3 to 4x daily; •ginger extract 3 to 4x daily; •lecithin caps 1400mg or choline 600mg; •Source Naturals DMAE 2 daily. Color therapy eyewear: Pick the color glasses that lets you read easiest. Wear for 30 minutes at a time.

—MACULAR DEGENERATION: AMD, age-related macular degeneration happens because oxidation to macular blood vessels causes the tissues to break down. People with light-colored eyes who are overweight are more at risk. Smoking increases risk of AMD up to 3 times over non smokers. AMD is often reversible with nutritional therapy. **—Alternative healing protocols:** Eat more green leafy veggies! Carotenoids, (specifically lutein and zeaxanthin) in dark greens can cut your risk up to 50%. See page 365.

—OVER-SENSITIVITY TO LIGHT (photophobia): Check your prescriptions. Many drugs cause increased sensitivity to sunlight. **—Alternative healing protocols:** •Ascorbate vitamin C 3000mg daily; •American Biologics A & E EMULSION as directed; or vitamin A & D 1000IU/400IU 4 daily; •Planetary TRIPHALA caps as directed •BILBERRY extract. Natural sunlight nourishes eyes. Face the sun with eyes CLOSED for 5 seconds. Then cover eyes with palms for 5 seconds. Repeat 10 times to relax eyes and reduce light sensitivity.

—PRESBYOPIA (middle age far-sightedness): If you have to wear glasses, try an under-corrected prescription to encourage your eyes to work with the glasses, not passively depend on them. **—Alternative healing protocols:** •Add B-complex vitamins like Nature's Secret ULTIMATE B daily; •taurine 600mg daily.

—RETINAL DETERIORATION: occurs when the retinal epithelium, the thin layer of cells located behind the receptor cells does not function properly in providing nutrients to or removing wastes from the crucial light receptor cells. The photo-receptors die and vision loss is irreversible. Alternative healing protocols: Take • carotenes like lutein and zeaxanthin, or PHYCOTENE NANOCLUSTERS from royalbodycare.com for absorbable carotenes from sea veggies. •GINKGO BILOBA and •BILBERRY extracts and •PCO's from grapeseed 100mg 3x daily have proven effective. •Gotu Kola or •Solaray CENTELLA ASIATICA caps help strengthen optic and retinal nerves.

—RETINITUS PIGMENTOSA: the progressive degeneration of the rods and cones of the retina. Common signs are night blindness and a narrow vision field. **—Alternative healing protocols:** Take •BILBERRY or •GINKGO BILOBA extract capsules or liquid. Take •CoQ-10, 100mg 2-3× daily (especially effective if the case is not severe); •PCO's from grapeseed or white pine 100mg 3x daily, taurine 500mg daily, •zinc picolinate 50mg daily. •Omega-3 fatty acids like flax or fish oils, or •Barleans' lignan-rich flax oil 3x daily; and •beta carotene 100,000IU or • vitamin A 15,000IU (Good clinical trial results. Use for one month.) Take •vitamin E 400IU 2x daily if retinitis is hemorrhagic.

—SHINGLES NEAR THE EYES (herpes zoster): **—Alternative healing protocols:** Merix RELEEV capsules and topical treatment works wonders around the eyes (do not use topical treatment in the eyes); high dose •vitamin C crystals ¼ tsp. in water every hour until the stool turns soupy - about 8000-10,000mg daily; •vitamin E 400IU with selenium 200mcg daily; •Country Life SUBLINGUAL B-12 3000mcg with folic acid 200mcg daily (See also HERPES page in this book).

—STYES & EYE INFLAMMATION: painful, pimple-like infections of the eyelids. Natural therapies work well when treatment is early. Origins stem from allergic, viral, or herpes-type infections. **—Alternative healing protocols:** use •buffered vitamin C eye drops (must be sterile solution) vitamin A, and zinc. If the cause is a bacterial infection, do not squeeze; use •Crystal Star ANTI-BIO™ extract drops in water (may also be used to bathe the affected area); or bathe eyes in •aloe vera juice eyewash, •chamomile tea, •raspberry leaf tea, •eyebright tea, •yellow dock tea or goldenseal root tea. •Mix one drop aged garlic extract in 4 drops distilled water and drop into infected eye. •Take vitamin A and D capsules 25,000IU/400IU and •omega-3 flax oil. Use •Boiron OPTIQUE homeopathic eye irritation remedy. •Alternating hot and cold compresses on affected area to stimulate drainage of infection. Or use a •calendula flowers compress to draw out a stye infection - just make a warm tea; soak a washcloth in the tea and press on the eye. •Eye inflammation compress: 1 tbsp. eyebright herb, ½ tbsp. powdered comfrey rt. or parsley root, ½ tbsp. powdered goldenseal root, 1 pint boiling water. Add herbs and steep for 30 minutes, covered. Apply to cotton balls and then to affected areas. Or simply use •the white of an egg and spread it on a cloth or bandage; then apply to affected area. (If an eyelash is in the infected follicle, gently pull it out after drawing the pus to a head with the hot compress; the pus will be released.)

Can't find a recommended product? Call the 800 number listed in Product Resources for the store nearest you.

Fevers

Nature's Cleansers and Healers

A slight fever is often your immune system's way of clearing up an infection or toxic overload quickly. Your body naturally raises its temperature on its own to "burn out" harmful poisons, to throw them off through heat and then through sweating. The heat from a fever can also de-activate virus replication, so unless a fever is exceptionally high (over 103° for kids and 102° for adults) or long lasting (more than two full days), it is sometimes a wise choice to let it run its natural course, even with children. Often they will get better faster. Don't over-medicate. *Fevers are usually a result of the problem and a part of the cure.* Bathe morning and night during a feverish illness. Infection and wastes from the illness are largely thrown off through the skin. If not regularly washed off, these substances lay on the skin and become partially reabsorbed into the body. There is usually substantial body odor during a cleansing fever as toxins are being eliminated, so frequent baths and showers help you feel better, too.

A cleansing, healing fever is characterized by hot, dry, flushed skin, followed by chill followed by fever, followed by lethargy and the desire to lie down. See your doctor if it looks more serious than that, because a lingering, or higher fever is sometimes a sign of more serious problems, such as mononucleosis, Epstein-Barr virus, or diabetes. *See Infections page 473-475 for more.*

Diet and Lifestyle Support Therapy

Nutritional therapy plan:

1—Administer plenty of liquids during a fever, and to the daily diet all during the illness - diluted juices, water, broths. Stay on a liquid diet during a fever to maximize the cleansing process: bottled water, fruit juices, broths and herb teas.
2—Carrot/beet/cucumber juice is a specific to clean the kidneys and help bring a fever down.
3—Sip on lemon juice with maple syrup and a pinch of cinnamon (very cleansing) all during the morning; grapefruit juice during the evening.
4—After a fever breaks, take enzyme therapy drinks, and Crystal Star DR. ENZYME™ caps with protease and bromelain.

Watchwords for fevers and kids: It's probably OK unless:
1) you have an infant with a temperature over 100°;
2) the fever has not abated after three days, and is accompanied by vomiting, a cough and trouble breathing;
3) your child displays extreme lethargy and looks severely ill;
4) your child is making strange, twitching movements.

—Bodywork:
•A cup of hot *bayberry* or *elderflower* tea, or *cayenne* and *ginger* capsules, speeds up the cleansing process by encouraging sweating and by stimulating circulation.
•*Catnip* enemas cleanse the elimination channels.
•Use cool water sponges, or alcohol rubdowns to reduce.
•Apply *peppermint* tea cooling compresses to the head.
•Add Dead Sea Salts to your bath to reduce aches and pains.
•Take ECHINACEA extract drops in water several times daily (good results) to encourage the lymph glands to throw off toxins.
•Take a sauna to sweat toxins out. Then sponge off with cool water, and follow with a brisk towel rub.

Herbal, Superfood and Supplement Therapy

Interceptive therapy plan: Choose 2 to 3 recommendations.
Don't forget - use child dosage for kids. See page 230.
1—**Control the infection:** •Crystal Star ANTI-BIO™ caps or drops; •*Lobelia* tincture drops in water every few hours and •Planetary ELDERBERRY SYRUP™ with *echinacea.*
•*Fenugreek* tea with lemon and maple syrup. •Vitamin A 10,000IU or beta carotene 25,000IU every 6 hours.
2—**Use a fever to fight a cold or flu.** Encourage sweating: Take •*Calendula* tea, •*Elderflower-sage* tea or •*Boneset-elder fl.-white willow-yarrow-ginger* tea or •*thyme* tea (especially for kids) until sweating occurs, usually within 24 hours.
3—**Help your body normalize from a fever and speed up healing:** •Vitamin C crystals ¼ tsp. every ½ hour in juice or water to bowel tolerance as an ascorbic acid flush.
•Add *garlic* capsules 3x daily.
4—**If you decide to reduce the fever:** Do not give aspirin to children to reduce a fever. Herb teas are much gentler and work very well, •like *peppermint, cilantro* or *catnip.*
•Herbs for Kids TEMP ASSURE extract for kids' fevers (highly recommended).
5—**Rebuild immune strength:** •American Biosciences IMMPOWER caps.

—Effective homeopathic remedies: •Bioforce Fiebresan drops; •Natra-Bio Fever tinc-
ture; •Hylands Hylavir flu or cold tablets. Homeopathic remedies for sudden fever onset:
•*Arsenicum album,* •*Belladonna,* •*Aconite.*

—Superfood therapy: (Choose one or two recommendations.)
•Crystal Star RESTORE YOUR STRENGTH™ drink.
•Solgar WHEY TO GO - lactose-free with probiotics.
•New Chapter GINGER WONDER syrup.
•AloeLife ALOE GOLD concentrate, 2 tbsp. in water as an anti-inflamma-tory (for adult fevers).

Can't find a recommended product? Call the 800 number listed in Product Resources for the store nearest you.

Fibroids

Breast (Cystic Mastitis), Uterine (Myomas or Fibromas)

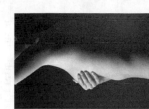

Up to 40 percent of American women 35 and older have fibroids. **Breast fibroids**, more common than blue eyes, are benign growths between the size of a walnut and an orange, that appear on uterine walls. They cause excessive menstrual bleeding, abdominal pain, bladder infections, painful intercourse and infertility. Excess estrogen that isn't metabolized smoothly by the liver, and an under-active thyroid are the normal cause for fibroids. Fibroids are not cancer, and have less than one-half of 1% chance of becoming cancerous before menopause. Benign growths usually cease after menopause; new growths after menopause may mean breast or uterine cancer. Natural therapies are consistently successful in helping women avoid fibroid surgery. Breast swelling and painful uterine bleeding have disappeared within weeks after a change to a low fat, vegetarian diet. Care for your liver which processes estrogens, to prevent fibroids. Avoid synthetic estrogens if possible. They can keep fibroids growing even after menopause. *Note: If considering uterine artery embolization (UAE) to remove fibroids, it may increase the risk of complications during pregnancy later.* Italian research says that eating red meat doubles the risk of uterine fibroids; eating plenty of vegetables cuts fibroid risk in half.

Diet and Lifestyle Support Therapy

Nutritional therapy plan:

1—Follow a low fat, vegetarian diet (50-60% fresh foods) to relieve symptoms. High fats mean unbalanced estrogen levels, a clear cause of fibroids. Obesity increases risk.

2—Coffee clearly aggravates fibroids. Avoid caffeine foods like chocolate and carbonated sodas. Avoid concentrated starches like pastries and fatty dairy foods. Avoid hormone-laden meats and refined sugars that can cause iodine deficiency. During menses, avoid fried, sugary and salty foods, especially smoked or preserved meats.

3—Get 60-70gm protein daily from largely vegetable sources to avoid unhealthy meat fats: grains, sprouts, soy foods, nuts, seeds, seafoods, hormone-free dairy and poultry.

4—Increase your intake of cruciferous veggies like broccoli, cauliflower, cabbage and brussels sprouts, and high fiber foods like apples which increase estrogen excretion.

5—Increase B vitamin-rich foods - brown rice, wheat germ and wheat germ oil (4 tsp. daily) and nutritional yeast.

6—Add miso, sea veggies, and dark leafy greens to neutralize toxins. Eat diuretic foods, like cucumber and watermelon to flush them out. Have fresh apple or carrot juice every day during healing. Drink plenty of water every day.

—**Bodywork:**

• The medical answer for rapidly growing fibroids is early detection, surgical biopsy, then removal. But tests are often inaccurate (15% false negatives and 30% false positives), and invasive medical procedures are painful and expensive. Even low dose radiation may mean increased risk of fibroids. Breast tissue is so sensitive that the time between a mammogram and fibroid growth is sometimes as little as three months. X-rays also contribute to iodine deficiency.

• Get outdoor exercise every day possible. No smoking.

• Apply poultices directly: green clay and castor oil packs.

• Try alternating hot and cold sitz baths to increase circulation to the uterus.

• Acupuncture has produced dramatic results for fibroids.

Herbal, Superfood and Supplement Therapy

Interceptive therapy plan: **Choose 2 to 3 recommendations.**

For breast fibroids: 1—Normalize hormone levels: •Crystal Star BREAST & UTERINE FIBRO DEFENSE™ caps for 3 months, then •Crystal Star FEMALE HARMONY™ caps or *Vitex* extract 2x daily with *Burdock* tea 2 cups daily. •*Evening Primrose Oil* 3000mg daily, or •vitamin E 800IU with folic acid 800mcg daily. •Nature's Way DIM-PLUS.

2—Dissolve adhesions: •Crystal Star CALCIUM SOURCE™ extract, •*Nettles* extract or •Calcium d-glucarate 1500mg daily. •Earth's Bounty O₂ SPRAY directly on fibroids, noticeable help in 3-6 weeks. Apply •Moon Maid Botanicals BREAST BALM to nodules. (highly recommended) •*Turmeric* extract. •Ester C powder w/ bioflav 5000mg daily.

—Drain excess lymph fluids: Herbs, Etc. LYMPHA-TONIC, •*Dandelion rt.* tea.

For uterine fibroids: 1—Normalize hormones: •Crystal Star WOMAN'S BEST FRIEND™ 6 daily, 3 months, then BREAST & UTERINE FIBRO DEFENSE™ for 3 months (highly recommended); or Crystal Star PRO-EST BALANCE™ roll-on for fibrous areas; or, •CORDYCEPS 750mg or •Pacific BioLogic GYNOEASE (not in pregnancy); •*Evening Primrose Oil* 3000mg daily. •Crystal Star BITTERS & LEMON CLEANSE™ to better metabolize estrogens.

2—Liver support balances hormone levels: •Crystal Star LIVER RENEW™ caps; •*Dandelion rt.* tea; •*Turmeric* extract. •B-complex 150mg daily; •CoQ-10 300mg daily.

3—Antispasmodics help pain: •Crystal Star STRESS OUT™ muscle relaxer extract. •*Centella asiatica.* •Magnesium 400mg daily.

4—Dissolve adhesions: •Transformation PUREZYME protease. High doses may be necessary. Ask your natural health practitioner if protease therapy is right for you. •Nature's Path TRACE-MIN-LYTE, •Crystal Star IODINE, POTASSIUM SILICA™ extract, or •Bernard Jensen's LIQUI-DULSE for iodine therapy. Take with •vitamin E 400IU.

—**Superfood supplements:** •Crystal Star ENERGY GREEN RENEWAL™ drink. •Pure Planet CHLORELLA drink. •Floradix LIQUID IRON if heavy menstrual bleeding.

Can't find a recommended product? Call the 800 number listed in Product Resources for the store nearest you.

Fibromyalgia

Immune Compromised Musculo-Skeletal Pain, Rheumatism Myalgia

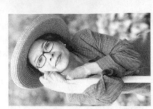

Fibromyalgia is an arthritic muscle disease that researchers say affects up to ten million Americans (mostly mid-life women). Our parents and grandparents called it rheumatism. The whole body feels pain with tender spots that hurt significantly when pressed. A stress-related immune disorder, the central cause seems to be a low level of serotonin in the brain and reduced growth hormone. Fibromyalgia symptoms are wide and diffuse, sharing many nerve and anxiety signs with Chronic Fatigue Syndrome (CFS), TMJ, and rheumatoid arthritis. The considerable depression that accompanies fibromyalgia often involves deep-seated resentment with nerve and hormone imbalances that impair sleep. Aluminum toxicity and cortisol deficiency may be linked; magnesium deficiency, a virus, hypoglycemia, and immune system breakdown may be involved. Most sufferers complain of dizziness, weakness, fatigue and confusion, migraine headaches, chronic diarrhea and irritable bowel. Most have digestive problems and shortness of breath. Other symptoms include cardiovascular problems like mitral valve prolapse and allergies. Being overweight and a smoker compounds fibromyalgia. *Labeled untreatable because NSAIDS drugs do not help, FM can be helped by natural therapies. Access the FIBROMYALGIA/ CHRONIC FATIGUE SYNDROME Network for more (800) 853-2929.*

Diet and Lifestyle Support Therapy

Nutritional therapy plan:

1—The HYPOGLYCEMIA diet page 463 is a good place to start diet improvement. Use Coca's Pulse test on pg. 316 to determine food allergies, common in FM sufferers.

2—Go on a short 3 day cleansing diet (page 173); then keep your diet at least 50% fresh foods during intensive healing. A largely vegetarian diet has a beneficial influence on blood toxins and fibrinogen that affects coagulation. Add cruciferous veggies like broccoli for 3-indole carbinole to reduce pain.

3—Avoid fatty foods, sugary foods, red meats and caffeine.

—**Lower your homocysteine levels:** Take 4 garlic capsules (1200mg a day) to maintain aortic elasticity. Take B₆, 50mg and folic acid 800mg to help break down homocysteine. Add red wine, 1 glass with dinner.

—**Bodywork:** More muscle strength is critical to healing. Build up your fitness with a low-impact aerobic exercise program, 20 minutes a day for body oxygen and muscle tone. Add light weight bearing exercise for 10 minutes a day to start. Water aerobics can be especially beneficial.

—**Relaxation techniques are crucial:**

•Choose from meditation, guided imagery, yoga, biofeedback, and progressive muscle relaxation - all of which have had success with fibromyalgia in developing a positive mind/body stance to work with the disease.

•Regular monthly massage therapy and acupuncture treatments have good success.

•Gentle heat applications are effective, especially with a massage, and Biochemics PAIN RELIEF lotion, B & T ARNIFLORA or Wakunaga FREEDOM ARTHRITIS RELIEF cream. Relieve pain with a massage oil made of 10 drops Angelica oil in 1-oz almond oil.

•Natural thyroid replacement shows good results in some cases. Contact Nutricology/ Allergy Research (800-545-9960) for more info about natural thyroid replacement.

Herbal, Superfood and Supplement Therapy

Interceptive therapy: Choose 3 or 4 recommendations.

1—**Reduce inflammatory pain:** •Dreamous FULL SPECTRUM GH spray (good reports for pain); •MSM caps 800mg daily; •Crystal Star DEPRESS-EX™ caps as a serotonin balancer; •Nutricology NATTO-ZYME to help break down and remove fibrin deposits; •Quercetin 1000mg and bromelain 1500mg with •*Turmeric* extract.•New Chapter ZYFLAMEND COX-2 inhibitor (AM and PM formulas and topical recommended). •Crystal Star ANTI-FLAM™ caps daily.

2—**Balance brain chemistry and nerve transmission:** •*Ginkgo Biloba* 3x daily; •Crystal Star RELAX CAPS™, 6 daily as needed. •*Gotu kola* caps or *Black cohosh* extract for nerves, 3x daily. •Crystal Star ADRENAL ENERGY BOOST™ caps 2 daily. •Rosemary tea, a memory booster.

3—**Improve musculo-skeletal system:** •Acetyl-Carnitine 1000mg daily. •Glucosamine-chondroitin, 1500/1200mg 6 daily. •Crystal Star MUSCLE RELAXER™ caps (fast relief). •For women: Planetary *Ashwagandha* drops with *una da gato* caps with *Burdock* tea for best results.

4—**Raise serotonin levels:** •SAMe (*S-adenosyl methionine*) 800mg daily boosts serotonin-dopamine levels. •*St. John's wort*, 300mg daily; •Natural Balance 5HTP.Calm for better mood. •Naturewell MIGRASPRAY for headaches; •Herbs, Etc. DEEP SLEEP.

5—**Add magnesium and B-vitamins:** •Magnesium 400mg 2x daily or •Ethical Nutrients MALIC/MAGNESIUM to alleviate tender points; •B-complex 150mg 3x daily, or •Nature's Secret ULTIMATE B tabs.

6—**Boost immune response:** •Tri-Medica Colostrum or •Nutricology LAKTOFERRIN; •glutathione 100mg daily; •Grapeseed PCO's 300mg daily; •Vitamin C up to 5000mg daily with extra bioflavonoids 500mg; •CoQ-10 200mg daily or Douglas Labs CoQMELT chewables (high activity).

—**Superfood therapy:** •Pure Planet CHLORELLA packets. •All One GREEN PHYTOBASE drink for pain. •Aloe Life ALOE GOLD drink. •Lane Labs TOKI collagen replacement drink (highly recommended).

Can't find a recommended product? Call the 800 number listed in Product Resources for the store nearest you.

Flu

Severe Viral Respiratory Infection

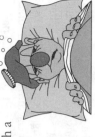

Each year, over 90 million Americans get a bout of flu. For many, the flu hits hard. We spend over 192 million days in bed because of it, and complications from flu kill 36,000 people each year. Like a cold, the flu is an upper respiratory infection caused by a rhino-virus. Unlike a cold, flu infections are more severe, longer-lasting, highly contagious, and today highly virulent. The elderly and those with weak immune systems are especially vulnerable. Recovery from flu is often slow with a pronounced period of weakness. Natural flu therapy offers body dynamics to help your body fight the flu.... warming against chills and aches, soothing a sore throat, releasing mucous congestion, and relieving feverishness by promoting perspiration....all without overwhelming the body's own natural immune response like antibiotics do. Flu treatment works best in stages. For the ACUTE, infective stage, (aches, chills, prostration, fever, sore throat, etc.), use a program for 2 to 4 days. The RECUPERATION, or healing stage, replenishes the body's natural resistance. Follow this phase for 1 to 2 weeks. Follow the IMMUNE SUPPORT stage for 3 weeks, especially in high risk seasons. *Note: antibiotics are ineffective against flu viruses and taking them inappropriately can lead to the development of drug-resistant disease strains. Flu shots and pain killers can affect immune response. Beware! See COLDS page 374 for extra help.*

Diet and Lifestyle Support Therapy

Nutritional therapy plan:

1—During the acute stage: take only liquid nutrients - plenty of hot, steamy chicken soup, hot tonics and broths to stimulate mucous release. Vegetable juices and green drinks rebuild the blood and immune system. Have ginger-garlic broth every day.

2—During the recuperation stage: follow a vegetarian, light, "green" diet. Have a salad every day, cultured foods like yogurt and kefir help you replace friendly flora; eat steamed vegetables with brown rice for strength.

3—For immune support: Avoid fast foods, sugary foods and dairy foods; they increase mucous clogging and allow a place for the virus to live. Avoid alcohol and tobacco; they are immune suppressors. Avoid caffeine foods; they inhibit iron and zinc absorption.

4—If you just can't seem to "get over it," try this effective remedy... make up 1 gallon of Crystal Star CLEANSING & PURIFYING™ tea, take 5 to 6 cups daily with 15 FIBER & HERBS COLON CLEANSE™ capsules daily until the virus is removed.

—Bodywork:

• During the acute stage: Sweating is effective at the first sign of infection. 1) Take 1 cayenne cap and 1 ginger cap. 2) Take a hot bath with *tea tree oil* drops. 3) Go to bed for a long sleep, so the body can focus on healing. 4) During the next several days, take a hot sauna or hot bath to help deactivate viruses: (see page 183), or a ginger foot bath to raise body temperature, and boost circulation.

• Gargle with a few drops *tea tree oil* in water, or *ginger root tea*; or use New Chapter GINGER WONDER SYRUP, 1 tsp. in water (great for kids).

• Nasal irrigations disinfect mucous membranes and clear breathing quickly: add ½ tsp. sea salt to 1 cup warm water. Fill a dropper with liquid, tilt your head and fill each nostril; then blow your nose. Or, use XLEAR nasal wash, a favorite of our whole staff.

• Take a *catnip* enema to cleanse flu virus from intestines.

• Massage therapy cleanses remaining pockets of toxins, and clears body meridians. Plus it makes you feel so good again!

Herbal, Superfood and Supplement Therapy

Interceptive therapy plan: Choose 2 to 3 recommendations.

1—For acute stage: • Ester C or ascorbic acid crystals: ¼ tsp. every half hour to bowel tolerance to flush and neutralize toxins. • Crystal Star VIREX™ caps to raise body temperature to reduce virus replication. (Take with • DR. ENZYME™ with protease and bromelain for best results. • Health from the Sun FLU GUARD (antiretroviral boxwood) or Merix Health Prdts C & F caps (fast acting), or • East Park FLU BAN olive leaf caps, or • Life Rising YIN CHIAO; • Andrographis drops, take at first signs for best results, • Homeopathic • Boiron homeopathic OSCILLOCOCCINUM (very effective).

2—During infection fighting stage: • Crystal Star ANTI-BIO™ extract or caps every 2 hours until improvement. • Nature's Path Silver-Lyte (ionized silver, a powerful infection fighter); • Garlic-ginger tea 2 cups daily, or Wakunaga AGED GARLIC extract. • Nature's Way SAMBUCOL, elderberry syrup, or • Zinc lozenges deactivate throat virus activity.

...**Congestion cleansers:** Cayenne-ginger; Echinacea-goldenseal (for stomach flu). Cayenne-garlic caps, peppermint tea.

...**Effective anti-virals:** • Andrographis tabs, take within first 24 hours. • Usnea extract, or • Propolis extract; • Echinacea extract; • St. John's Wort; • Osha root tea.

3—Speed recovery time: • Glutamine 2000mg daily; • Astragalus or Reishi mushroom extract 4x daily; • Cayenne-bayberry caps normalize glands; Lane Labs ADVACAL reduces achiness (a sign the body is drawing on bone calcium); • Chamomile tea (effectively relieves pain); • Wisdom of the Ancients SYMFRE tea. • Nutricology Germanium 150mg.

4—Establish immune response: • NAC, a powerful immune booster 1000mg daily; • Siberian eleuthero, panax ginseng, or astragalus extract boost lymphocytes and interferon; Ethical Nutrients ZINC STATUS. • Eidon SELENIUM liquid (to prevent virus mutations); • Nutricology LACTO-FERRIN with colostrum. • Planetary CORDYCEPS POWER CS-4.

—**Superfood therapy:** (Choose one) • Crystal Star RESTORE YOUR STRENGTH™ drink returns body vitality. • Wakunaga KYO-GREEN. • Green Foods GREEN MAGMA. • Pure Planet CHLORELLA.

Can't find a recommended product? Call the 800 number listed in Product Resources for the store nearest you.

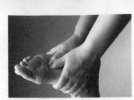

Foot Problems

Bone Spurs, Plantar Warts, Calluses, Corns, Bunions

Women have four times as many foot problems as men, largely pain and inflammation from of a lifetime of wearing high heels. **Bunions:** thickened skin on the side of the big toe. **Calluses:** thick, dead skin pads your body builds up on heels and balls of feet. **Corns:** painful hardened skin found on toe joints (hard corns) or between toes (soft corns). **Plantar warts:** painful, sometimes ingrowing, warts on the foot sole. **Bone spurs:** calcium deposit out-growths on the heel, reflecting acid/alkaline imbalance. They often accompany rheumatoid arthritis, alkalosis or tendonitis because people with these conditions have low stomach acid and enzyme production. *Note: If you try magnets for relief (successful for 90% of diabetic DPN foot problems), most tests show that when the magnets are removed, the problem reappears.* What causes foot growths? Poor calcium elimination (usually a result of constipation), a staph or strep type infection, body pH imbalance, a diet with too little vegetable protein, and too many sweets, caffeine and saturated fats (which leads to excess sebaceous gland output causing poor skin elimination of wastes), poor circulation, (especially from diabetes), a low acid diet that aggravates liver congestion (Note: Griseofulvin™ tabs for nail fungus can affect liver function). *See NAIL FUNGUS page 504 and GOUT page 431 for more.*

Diet and Lifestyle Support Therapy

Nutritional therapy plan:

1—Go on a 24 hour vegetable juice diet (pg. 173) to clear out acid wastes. Then eat plenty of fresh raw foods for a month. Have a green salad every day. Eat two apples a day.

2—Drink black cherry juice daily. Take a green drink every 3 days to flush the kidneys and re-balance your body pH.

3—Make sure your diet is rich in whole foods, vegetables and fiber, low in sugars, meat, dairy foods and saturated fats. Avoid acid-forming foods - red meats, caffeine, chocolate, carbonated sodas. Eliminate hard liquor and fried food.

4—Effective enzyme balancing foods: miso soup, lecithin 2 tsp. daily, fresh vegetables, nutritional yeast, cranberry juice.

—Healing foot soaks: Soak for 15 minutes.
• For blisters, add 2 tbsp. *Aloe Vera* gel to 1 gallon hot water. Apply *calendula* salve after blister heals.
• For stinky feet: 1 pot black tea; tannic acid eliminates odor.
• For ingrown nail, soak in Epsom salts bath.
• A paraffin wax treatment soothes and softens feet.

—Soak feet in warm water first, then apply: •Biochemics PAIN RELIEF; •Miracle of Aloe FOOT REPAIR or •Hemp seed foot lotion. **For corns,** •*tea tree* oil 2-3x daily, olive oil or lemon compresses, **For bunions,** •a weak goldenseal root-aloe vera juice solution; or •castor oil poultice. •Apply CAPSAICIN cream. **For plantar warts and bone spurs:** Soak feet in the hottest water you can stand for as long as you can; then apply: •Home Health CASTOR OIL PACKS; •Earth's Bounty O₂ SPRAY on wart 2x daily. Removal takes 2 months. Apply celandine tincture. •DMSO helps dissolve crystalline deposits. •Mix vitamin C crystals and water to a paste. Apply to spur; secure with tape. Leave on all day for several weeks. •Take homeopathic *thuja* 30c, apply *thuja* oil topically. Take with •*arnica* 30c 3x daily if there is also shooting pain. **Burning feet,** acupuncture works. *Replace shoes regularly. Degraded shoes contribute to foot and back problems.*

Herbal, Superfood and Supplement Therapy

Interceptive therapy plan: Choose 2 to 3 recommendations.

1—Dissolve crystalline deposits and flush them out: •Crystal Star DR. VITALITY™ caps with •BITTERS & LEMON™ extract each morning; add •*Echinacea* extract or apply BioForce ECHINACEA cream. •Country Life LIGA-TEND for at least 1 month; •Enzymatic Therapy ACID-A-CAL tabs. Apply •Nutribiotic GRAPEFRUIT SEED skin spray or ointment and take the capsules 2x daily. •Apply •Eidon SILICA MOISTURIZING LOTION or Hemphoria FOOT FRENZY.

2—Reduce pain, inflammation: •Quercetin 2000mg with Bromelain 1500mg daily;
•Crystal Star ANTI-FLAM™ caps 4 at a time; •Boiron ARNICA gel (excellent results!).

3—For calluses: apply •*Celandine* tincture or •*Calendula* ointment to dissolve hard skin.
•Vitamin A 25,000IU (not beta carotene) 3x daily for 3 months; •Barleans high lignan flax oil.

4—For bone spurs: •MSM 2500mg 2x daily shows good results; Mix • Vitamin C crystals with water to a paste. Apply and take vitamin C up to 5000mg daily with extra bioflavonoids 500mg. Take •Lane Labs ADVACAL ULTRA (excellent results) or •Cal/mag/ zinc 4 daily with •B-complex 100mg 4 daily.

5—For cracked, occasionally bleeding heels: Apply •SKIN-LASTIC MOISTURIZING MIST. For 3 months take •zinc picolinate 100mg daily; •vitamin E 600IU, 2 tbsp. each flax oil and snipped dried sea greens daily in your salad dressing for essential fatty acids (EFAs). Add •B-complex 100mg or •Nature's Secret ULTIMATE B for EFA metabolism.

6—Heel pain (often a low thyroid problem): •Evening Primrose oil 3000mg, add 2 tbsp. dry sea greens daily. Add •Crystal Star OCEAN MINERALS™ caps and magnesium 800mg.

7—Enzyme therapy to reduce inflammation, burning feet: •Prevail VITASE; •Crystal Star DR. ENZYME™ with protease; •Betaine HCl for calcium uptake; •Floradix GALLEXIER. •Vitamin C 5000mg for 1 month, Lipoic acid daily; EPO 3000mg daily.

—Superfood therapy: (Choose one or more) •Crystal Star ENERGY GREEN RENEWAL™ drink. •Sun Wellness CHLORELLA packets or tabs. •Kyolic KYO-GREEN with EFAs. •Aloe Life ALOE GOLD drink. •Solaray ALFA-JUICE tabs.

Can't find a recommended product? Call the 800 number listed in Product Resources for the store nearest you.

Frostbite

Chillblains, Possibility of Gangrene

Frostbite is the freezing of body extremities, due to prolonged exposure of the feet, hands, ears and face to severe cold and its effects of redness, swelling, blistering, numbness, etc. Circulation slows, causing skin to become hard, blue-white and numb. If untreated, severe frostbite of the extremities can turn into a gangrenous condition, in which blood flow stops, tissue becomes oxygen-deprived, numbs and dies.

In **dry gangrene**, the fluid between the cells freezes, causing them to rupture, and slough off into nearby blood vessels. There is dull, aching pain and coldness in the area. Rubbing accelerates the skin damage. Pain and skin pallor are early signs of dry gangrene. As the flesh dies, pain can be intense; once it is dead, the flesh becomes numb and turns dark. If treated right away however, dry, non-infected gangrene responds successfully to natural self-therapy.

Wet gangrene is the result of an infected wound, arteriosclerosis, or a diabetic condition, which prevents drainage and deprives the affected tissues of cleansing blood supply and oxygen. See an emergency clinic if you have wet gangrene. *See also Shock page 538.*

Diet and Lifestyle Support Therapy

Nutritional therapy plan:

1—For frostbite: paint on, but do not rub in, warm olive oil. Massage in for gangrene.
2—Paint on honey to arrest infective bacteria development and stabilize skin balance.
3—Give the person warm drinks or green drinks and plenty of water, but **no alcohol**. It constricts blood flow.
4—Eat a high protein diet for the two weeks after exposure, with plenty of whole grains to speed recovery.

—Immediate procedures:

• Get the exposed person to a heated room immediately. Cover warmly, so frostbitten areas will warm up gradually. Warm the entire body with hot drinks, dry clothing or human body heat.
• Gently stroke the kidneys toward the middle of the back.
• If the frostbite case is severe, wrap in gauze so blisters don't break. Elevate legs. Do not rub blisters.
• Use alternating warm and cool hydrotherapy to stimulate circulation. No hot water bottles, hair dryers, or heating pads. Don't rub a frostbite. It makes it worse. Slow warming is the key.
• If case is very severe, immerse areas in warm water and massage very gently under water for 5 to 10 minutes.

—Stimulating and healing oils:

• *Cajeput* oil
• *Mullein* oil
• *Tea tree* oil, which sloughs off old, infected tissue, and leaves healthy tissue intact.
• Biochemics PAIN RELIEF
• Aloe Life SKIN GEL (excellent to heal necrotic tissue)

Herbal, Superfood and Supplement Therapy

Interceptive therapy plan: Choose 2 to 3 recommendations.

1—Enhance circulation: •Nelson BACH RESCUE REMEDY every 5 minutes under the tongue as needed for shock. •*Ginkgo Biloba* extract every 2 hours, and •CoQ-10 60mg 3x daily; •Apply *Butcher's broom* extract mixed in water (also take internally, temporarily only). •*Sage* tea 2 cups daily.

2—Help raise body temperature: •Apply CAPSAICIN cream or a •*Ginger-Cayenne* powder compress mixed in olive oil.

3—Control infection: •Myrrh gum extract; •Witch Hazel; •Black Walnut Hulls extract; •Nutricology GERMANIUM for wound healing, 150mg for 2 months. Spray on •Earth's Bounty O₂ SPRAY, rub on affected area several times daily until healing begins. Herbal applications: •*Calendula-comfrey* salve, or •*Slippery elm* or •*Comfrey/plantain* compresses mixed with olive oil.

4—Repair damaged tissue: •Vitamin C powder with bioflavs. and rutin, ¼ tsp. every half hour for 6 days for collagen and tissue rebuilding. •Vitamin E 400IU. Take internally and prick a capsule - apply oil to affected areas. •Apply AloeLife ALOE SKIN GEL often to affected areas. •Body Essentials SILICA GEL

5—Enhance immune response: •PCO's from grapeseed or pine, 100mg 3x daily; •Enzymatic Therapy ORAL NUTRIENT CHELATES. Then follow with a full-spectrum multi-vitamin complex for 1 month to help redevelop tissue.

—Superfood therapy: (Choose one recommendation.)
•Crystal Star RESTORE YOUR STRENGTH™ drink and capsules.
•Pines MIGHTY GREENS drink.
•Prince of Peace GINSENG-ROYAL JELLY vials.
•Pure Planet CHLORELLA 1 pkt. tablets daily.
•Futurebiotics VITAL K 3 tsp. daily.

Can't find a recommended product? Call the 800 number listed in Product Resources for the store nearest you.

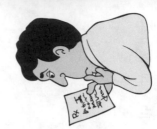

Fungal Skin Infections

Athlete's Foot, Ringworm, Impetigo

You can recognize a fungal skin infection by its characteristic moist, weepy, red skin patches. Although opportunities for risk of these types of infections seem to be everywhere, (new evidence even points to involvement with sinusitis), they don't take hold when there is good immune response. Enhancing immunity is the key to controlling fungal infections. Athlete's foot (ringworm of the feet) and other funguses of all kinds thrive in dampness and warmth. Make sure that any concurrently occurring fungal infections (like athlete's foot and "jock itch") are both treated, so that infection is not bounced from one area to another. Avoid drug overuse, particularly long courses of antibiotics and cortisones. Broad spectrum antibiotic and steroid drug use can kill friendly digestive flora and lower immune defenses allowing fungus micro-organisms to keep growing. **Is your itchy skin a fungal infection?** If it is, the area will be scaly, cracked, bleeding and tender, with a bacterial odor. Ringworm, foot and toenail fungus, mouth or nail infections and diaper rash in babies have moist thickened skin patches that do not dry out. Candida fungal infections have excessive belching from gas and allergy reactions, and persistent headaches. If your feet always burn, it can be a sign of low iron as well as a fungal infection. *See also Candida Albicans pg.358-363, and Nail Fungus pg. 504 for more.*

Diet and Lifestyle Support Therapy

Nutritional therapy plan:

1—Eat lots of cultured foods like yogurt, tofu and kefir to promote healthy intestinal flora and full nutrient absorption. Add lots of fresh fruits and vegetables to the diet.

2—Increase dietary protein for fastest healing: seafoods and sea veggies, sprouts, eggs, soy foods, poultry, whole grains.

3—Drink 6 glasses of water daily to keep elimination system free and flowing.

4—Avoid foods that promote a fungal growth environment: sugary foods are the biggest culprit, also red meats, dairy foods, cola drinks, caffeine and fried foods.

5—Reduce carbohydrates during healing: pasta, pastries, breads, nuts and all sugary foods, (vegetable carbs are OK).

—Bodywork:

•Fungal skin infections can be spread by shared towels and bathtubs. Disinfect shower area and wash towels regularly. Use different towels to dry off the infected skin area.

—For athlete's foot and toenail fungus:

•Keep feet and shoes aired and dry. Change socks daily. Go barefoot as much as possible where appropriate. •Dab with vinegar daily for athlete's foot/nail infection. •Apply *tea tree* or *manuka* oil; use *tea tree* oil soap. •Apply baking soda daily and soak your feet in warm epsom salts water for 10 minutes; dry then apply *witch hazel* or Crystal Star FUNGEX™ gel. •Expose affected areas to sunlight every day possible.

—For ringworm and impetigo:

•Apply Grapefruit Seed Extract skin ointment (excellent)
•Apply Earth's Bounty O₂ SPRAY.
•Pat on vinegar, or garlic vinegar or a strong goldenseal-myrrh tea.
•Apply a basil poultice to a ringworm patch.
•Take epsom salts baths for 20 minutes.

—For thrush: •Rinse mouth with *dilute tea tree* oil solution. Keep bathroom cup and toothbrush clean. Soak toothbrush in grapefruit seed extract solution.

Herbal, Superfood and Supplement Therapy

Interceptive therapy: Allow 2 to 3 months for effectiveness.

1—Control infection, destroy fungal organisms: Take •Crystal Star CANDIDA YEAST DETOX™ caps. •Apply Crystal Star FUNGEX™ gel, or ANTI-BIO™ gel with *una da gato*. Take •East Park OLIVE LEAF extract caps; or •Allergy Research OREGANO OIL caps. Apply •Nutribiotic GRAPEFRUIT SEED SKIN spray or gel (both highly recommended). •Colloidal silver- Nature's Path SILVER-LYTE as directed, or apply SILVER-LYTE topical spray. Apply •Well-in-Hand WART WONDER lotion.

2—EFA's stop skin peeling and heal skin: Apply •Barielle FOOT CARE cream or •hemp cream. Take •*Evening Primrose Oil* caps 4000mg daily for 2 weeks. Apply •Miracle of Aloe FOOT REPAIR; use •East Park OLIVE LEAF gel and •TOPICAL & CLEANSING BAR; or •*Mahonia* ointment.

3—Enzyme therapy and probiotics protect against funguses: •UAS DDS PLUS with FOS. 1) take acidophilus caps before meals, 2) dissolve acidophilus in water, apply to area. •Crystal Star DR. ENZYME™ with protease and bromelain or •Enzymedica PURIFY between meals.

4—Boost immune response to prevent recurring infection: •Crystal Star IRON SOURCE™ caps for burning feet. •Zinc 50mg 2x daily; •Lysine 1000mg daily.

—For ringworm: Apply •Nutribiotic GRAPEFRUIT SEED SKIN ointment (excellent results.) or •*Basil* tea skin wash; use •*Myrrh* or *Thuja* extract- internally and applied for both thrush and ringworm. •Earth's Bounty O₂ SPRAY.

—For athlete's foot: •Mix an antifungal paste: Crush or open in a bowl: B₂ 500mg, niacin 1000mg, pantothenic acid 500mg. Add 2 tsp. sesame oil and 2 tsp. nutritional yeast. Put on a sock to cover - leave on overnight. •Anti-fungal footbath: *tea tree* oil drops, *marsh-mallow root* and *black walnut hulls* extract. Soak feet for 20 minutes daily. •Take *Bloodroot* capsules, 4 daily.

—Superfood therapy: •Apply AloeLife SKIN GEL; drink aloe vera juice daily. •Balance your intestinal structure with Solgar WHEY TO GO protein drink.

Can't find a recommended product? Call the 800 number listed in Product Resources for the store nearest you.

Gallbladder Disease

Gallstones, Cholecystitis

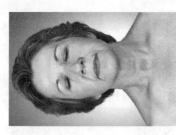

The gallbladder helps digest fats by producing bile (a compound of cholesterol, bile pigments and salts). But if you eat a lot of fatty and fried foods, gallbladder bile fluids may become saturated with cholesterol, the cholesterol precipitates into solid crystals, then accumulates into stones. The stones enlarge, the gallbladder becomes inflamed, and severe pain that feels like a heart attack ensues. It can be life threatening if left untreated. Stones may also block the bile passage, causing pain and digestive harm. About 20 million Americans have gallstones, and gallbladder cholecystitis (acute gallbladder inflammation); three fourths of them are women. High risk factors for gallbladder disease include a poor diet with high cholesterol and low bile acids, chronic indigestion and gas from too much dairy and refined sugars, obesity, certain drugs (notably HRT (hormone replacement therapy) drugs), age, and Crohn's disease. Yo-yo dieting increases risk of gallstones. (I personally knew a 64-year-old woman who died from her gallstones that became severe through twenty-five years of yo-yo dieting.) Gallstones are far easier to prevent than to reverse. New research shows eating just one large orange a day may reduce gallstone risk.

The sharp rise of three conditions in America affect our ability to digest cleanly.... 1) *food allergies* - because they affect our ability to digest (eliminate the offending food to stop attacks), 2) *parasite infections* - because they can lead to calcium composition stones 3) *lack of regular exercise* which stagnates digestive activity. Amazingly, research shows that even birth control pills or hormone replacement drugs, which charge estrogen balance, increase cholesterol production by the liver. See LIVER HEALING page 484 for more.

Do you have gallbladder problems? **You may not think it's serious, that it's just heartburn or indigestion, but if it's chronic, it's serious.**

• Do you have intense pain in the upper right abdomen during an attack, sometimes accompanied by fever and nausea (it may be gallstones)

• Do you have periods of nausea, vomiting, fever and intense abdominal pain that radiates to the upper back: (it may be cholecystitis, gallbladder inflammation)

• Do you have recurring abdominal pain, bloating and gas after you eat a heavy meal? along with headaches, sluggishness or nervousness? (it may be gallstones or Crohn's disease)

Do you have gallstones?

In the United States, high bile cholesterol levels are the main cause of gallstones, with most stones (80%) composed of cholesterol and varying amounts of bile salts, bile pigments and inorganic calcium salts. When bile in the gallbladder becomes supersaturated with cholesterol, it combines with other sediment matter present and begins to form a stone. Dietary factors like high blood sugar, high calorie and saturated fat intake that lead to obesity are also involved. A stone may grow for 6 to 8 years before symptoms occur. Continued formation of gallstones is dependent on either increased accumulation of cholesterol or reduced levels of bile acids or lecithin. It's easy to see that diet improvement will deter, even arrest, gallstones. **Gallstones can be serious.** Ninety-five percent of people suffering from cholecystitis have gallstones. If these symptoms sound like you, pay close attention and seek medical help immediately. An ultrasound test provides a definitive diagnosis.

Signs you may be prone to gallstones: **The biggest problem by far is obesity. If you are overweight, gallstone risk increases three to seven times.**

• Having high cholesterol levels contributes to increased gallstone risk.

• Your vitamin C intake is low — vitamin C plays a key role in the breakdown of cholesterol.

• Are you a yo-yo dieter? A recent study in Annals of Internal Medicine finds that women whose weight fluctuates by 10 to 19 lbs. at a time have more than a 30% higher risk of developing gallstones. When weight fluctuates more than 19 lbs. at a time, gallstone risk is 68% higher!

Do you need a gallstone cleanse?

In the United States, high bile cholesterol levels are the main cause of gallstones (bile cholesterol levels do not necessarily correlate with blood cholesterol levels). A stone may grow for 6 to 8 years before symptoms occur. Since continued formation of gallstones is dependent on either an increased accumulation of cholesterol or reduced levels of bile acids or lecithin, it's easy to see that anywhere along the way, diet improvement will deter, even arrest, stone development.

—**What else causes gallstones?** Other dietary factors like high blood sugar, and high calorie and saturated fat intake which leads to obesity are also involved. Gastrointestinal

Can't find a recommended product? Call the 800 number listed in Product Resources for the store nearest you.

problems like Crohn's disease and diverticulitis are warning signs. Drugs like oral contraceptives and some estrogen replacement drugs have been implicated. Blood cholesterol lowering drugs that contain fibric acid derivatives like *clofibrate* and *gemfibrozil* increase the level of bile cholesterol. Gallstones are present in 95% of people suffering from cholecystitis (gallbladder inflammation). There may be no identifiable symptoms, except for periods of nausea and intense abdominal pain that radiates to the upper back. Ultrasound provides a definitive diagnosis.

Important note:

Although I have personally seen several gallstone sufferers use the 9 day program on this page pass gallstones without surgery, I recommend it only under the supervision of a qualified health professional. The liver and gallbladder are interconnecting, interworking organs. Problems with either affect both. Before undertaking a Gallstone Flush to pass gallstones, have an ultrasound test to determine the size of the stones. If they are too large to pass through the urethral ducts, other methods must be used.

The Nine-Day Gallstone Flush Plan: Have a sonogram before embarking on a flush to determine the size of the stones.

Traditional naturopathic medicine has relied on natural gallbladder cleansing flushes as an effective method for passing and dissolving gallstones. Depending on the size of the stones and the length of time they have been forming, the flushing programs may last from 3 days to a month. If your sonogram shows that your gallstones are too large to pass through the bile and urethral ducts (less than 1% of cases), they must be dissolved first. Try using the Crystal Star STONE-X™ herbal program for 1 month (2 caps 3x daily with 3 to 5 cups of Chamomile tea). If pain and symptoms do not improve, you should consult a health professional. Surgical methods may be necessary. *Note:* If olive oil is hard for you to take straight, sip it through a straw. See my book COOKING FOR HEALTHY HEALING for a complete diet program to help prevent gallstones.

Three day Olive Oil and Lemon Juice Flush:

—*On rising:* take 2 tbsp. olive oil and juice of 1 lemon in water. Sip through a straw if desired.
—*Breakfast:* have a glass of organic apple juice.
—*Mid-morning:* have 2 cups of chamomile or cascara tea.
—*Lunch:* take another glass of lemon juice and olive oil in water; and a glass of fresh apple juice.
—*Mid-afternoon:* have 2 cups of chamomile or cascara tea.
—*Dinner:* have a glass of carrot/beet/cucumber juice; or a potassium juice or broth (pages 291).
—*Before bed:* take another cup of chamomile tea.

Follow with a 5 day Alkalizing Diet:

—*On rising:* take 2 tbsp. cider vinegar in water with 1 tsp. honey; or a glass of grapefruit juice.
—*Breakfast:* have a glass of carrot/beet/cucumber juice, or a potassium broth or juice.
—*Mid-morning:* have 2 cups of chamomile tea, and a glass of organic apple juice.
—*Lunch:* a vegetable drink with Pure Planet CHLORELLA, or Crystal Star ENERGY GREEN RENEWAL™ drink, a green salad with lemon-olive oil dressing and a cup of dandelion tea.
—*Mid-afternoon:* have 2 cups of chamomile tea, and another glass of apple juice.
—*Dinner:* have a small green salad with lemon-oil dressing, add daikon radish shreds as a gentle diuretic flusher; and another glass of apple juice.
—*Before bed:* 1 cup chamomile or dandelion tea.

End with a One Day Intensive Olive Oil Flush:

At 7 p.m. on the evening of the 5th day of the alkalizing diet, mix 1 pint olive oil and 10 juiced lemons; take ¼ cup every 15 minutes until used. Lie on right side for best assimilation.

...The key to preventing gallstones is diet improvement. Increase your fresh fruit and vegetable intake for more fiber. It keeps bad cholesterol deposits from forming and keeps food moving naturally through your system instead of developing deposits which may turn into stones. Vegetable proteins from foods like soy, oat bran and sea greens help prevent gallstone formation. Reduce your intake of animal protein, especially dairy foods (casein in dairy products increases formation of gallstones). Avoid fried foods, fast foods and sugary foods altogether if you are at risk for gallstones.

Can't find a recommended product? Call the 800 number listed in Product Resources for the store nearest you.

Gallbladder Disease

Diet and Lifestyle Support Therapy

Nutritional therapy plan:

1—The primary gallstone culprit is a diet high in saturated fats and trans fats, especially from red meats and dairy foods, the kind of fats that end up as fatty deposits around your middle and in your arteries. A low fat, high fiber vegetarian diet is the best choice.

2—Go on a short juice and gallbladder flush fast for 3 days. (*See previous page.*) In the acute pain stage, all food should be avoided. Only pure water should be taken until pain subsides.

3—After your gallbladder flush, take a glass of cider vinegar and maple syrup in water each morning.

4—Add 1 tbsp. lecithin grains before each meal, 1 tbsp. nutritional yeast and 1 tbsp. olive oil daily.

5—Avoid all dairy foods, (especially eggs and milk). Yogurt and kefir are OK. Add artichokes, pears and apples to your diet. Bitter veggies like dandelion greens, escarole, chard and endive are highly recommended to improve bile quality.

6—A new study shows coffee lowers the risk of gallstone disease - for some men 2 cups a day reduces risk by 30 to 40%. New research, especially for women, shows eating just one large orange a day may reduce gallstone risk. Having a large daily grapefruit also appears to help prevent gallstone formation.

7—Eat small meals frequently. No large meals. Drink 6 glasses water daily.

—Bodywork:

• Take coffee, garlic or catnip enemas every 3 days until relief.

• Take olive oil flushes for 2-3 weeks until stones pass.

• Apply castor packs or cold milk compresses to the abdomen area.

• A sedentary lifestyle is a major high risk factor. Mild regular exercise is more effective than strenuous exercise to reduce your body fat to keep gallstones away. Tests show that for women 2 to 3 hours of moderate exercise like light jogging per week can reduce gallstone surgery risk by 30%. Tests on men show 2 to 3 hours of moderate running a week reduces risk of gallstone formation by 40%.

• Acupuncture and acupressure have been successful for gallbladder disease.

• Try Coca's Pulse test on pg. 316 to determine possible food allergies that bring on attacks. Eggs, pork and onions are common offenders.

Herbal, Superfood and Supplement Therapy

Interceptive therapy plan: Choose 2 to 3 recommendations.

1—Increase bile solubility to reduce cholesterol levels: •Nature's Way enteric coated peppermint oil caps •PEPOGEST; •Crystal Star BITTERS & LEMON CLEANSE™ extract to help dissolve bile solids. •Herbal Answers ALOE VERA JUICE with herbs daily, with •MILK THISTLE SEED extract drops added to each glass.

—Enzyme therapy: •Alta Health CANGEST, •Rainbow Light ADVANCED ENZYME SYSTEM or •Transformation Enzyme LYPOZYME or •Crystal Star DR. ENZYME with Protease and Bromelain; •Acidophilus helps: •UAS DDS-PLUS with FOS before meals, or •UAS DDS-PLUS with FOS, and 1 HCL tablet with pepsin after meals; •Vitamin C up to 3000mg daily with bioflavonoids.

2—Bitters herbs increase bile flow and help the gallbladder expel small stones: •*Artemesia* extract drops; •*dandelion root* tea, 3 cups daily; •*Wild yam root* capsules 6 daily; •Crystal Star LIVER CLEANSE FLUSHING™ tea; •NatureWorks SWEDISH BITTERS, or •Gaia SWEETISH BITTERS extract; •Taurine 1000mg daily helps keep bile thinned.

3—Reduce inflammation and pain: •*Turmeric* extract (curcumin) 2x daily.

4—Help dissolve stones: •*Chamomile* tea, 5-7 cups daily for a month to dissolve stones (excellent results); or •Gaia HYDRANGEA ROOT extract; take •Crystal Star STONE-X™ capsules with lemon juice and water.

5—Prevent stone formation: •Ascorbate vitamin C or Ester C 550mg with bioflavonoids 6 daily; •Solaray ALFAJUICE caps. Fiber supplements reduce the risk of stones. •Futurebiotics COLON GREEN; •Planetary TRIPHALA INTERNAL CLEANSER; •All One WHOLE FIBER COMPLEX.

6—Balance excess blood sugar to keep stones from forming: •Spirulina caps in be-ween meals with •vitamin B complex 100mg helps stabilize blood sugar with •Biotin 600mcg; •Glycine caps and •Chromium picolinate 200mcg daily regulate blood sugar; •Gynemna sylvestre capsules, 2 before meals.

7—Lipotropics control and regulate cholesterol overload: •Choline-Inositol 2 daily; •Phosphatidyl choline 500mg daily, or •Solgar PHOSPHATIDYL-CHOLINE triple strength; with •Omega-3 flax seed oil 3x daily; •Vitamin A 25,000IU & D 1000IU.

•Methionine tablets before meals; •Solaray LIPOTROPIC 1000.

—Superfood therapy: (Choose one) *Note:* Since a predisposing factor for gallstones is excessive sugar consumption, avoid highly sweetened protein powder drinks.

•Jarrow GENTLE FIBERS drink morning and evening.

•AloeLife FIBER MATE drink.

The Gall Bladder

Can't find a recommended product? Call the 800 number listed in Product Resources for the store nearest you.

Gastric Diseases

Chronic Gastritis, Gastroenteritis, Gastric Ulcers

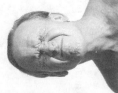

Gastric diseases refer to ulcerative disorders of the upper gastrointestinal tract. Stomach acids and some enzymes can damage the lining of the G.I. tract if your body's protective factors aren't functioning normally. Medical treatment focuses on reducing stomach acidity - a symptom - rather than addressing the cause of the problem. Many drug treatments are extensive, with definite side effects, and a tendency to alter the normal structure of digestive tract walls. The wholistic approach rebuilds integrity of the stomach lining, normalizes G.I. tract pH and function. Tagamet and Zantac, drugs prescribed regularly (one billion dollars in sales yearly) for gastric problems can be addictive, may inhibit bone formation and liver function. **Are you at risk for gastric diseases?** The biggest culprit is eating too much, too fast, too often.... especially fried, fatty foods, sugary foods and very spicy foods. Too much coffee and alcohol, overuse of NSAIDS and steroid drugs, Candida yeast overgrowth, *H. pylori* infection and food allergies are all implicated. If you have intestinal parasites (experts say 1 in 6 Americans do), your risk is higher. **Signs you may have a gastric disease:** Poor digestion, with sharp abdominal and chest pains, heartburn with breathing trouble similar to asthma. Acid bile reflux in the throat, usually with irritable bowel symptoms. Some have nausea, vomiting blood or a coffee ground-like material. See DIVERTICULITIS, COLITIS AND CROHN'S DISEASE pages for more.

Diet and Lifestyle Support Therapy

Nutritional therapy plan:

1—Emphasis should be on alkalizing foods. Include plenty of fiber foods, whole grains, brown rice, fresh fruits and vegetables. Eat cultured foods for friendly G.I. flora. Have a green salad daily. Alkalize with miso soup or •Red Star NUTRITIONAL YEAST in your diet. •Aloe vera juice, or •Herbal Answers ALOE FORCE JUICE (very soothing) each morning both cleanses and alkalizes.

2—Avoid alcohol, except a little wine at dinner. Eliminate caffeine, tobacco, aspirin and all fried foods. Chemicalized foods and most peppers are irritants.

3—Avoid dairy products, except cultured foods; they contribute to stomach acidity.

4—Have a glass of non-carbonated mineral water every evening. Add •ROYAL JELLY, 4 tsp. daily, or Prince of Peace ROYAL JELLY-GINSENG vials for 1 month for best results.

5—Eat small meals more frequently. No large meals. Chew everything well.

—Juices for stomach acid balance: •Carrot juice, or •Green Foods CARROT ESSENCE for healing vitamin A. •Carrot/cabbage, a stomach healer. •Pineapple-papaya for extra enzymes. •Liquid chlorophyll 1 tsp. in water before meals is also effective.

—Teas to soothe intestinal distress: •*Pau d'arco-Peppermint* tea combo; •*Calendula* tea; •*Plantain* tea; •*Slippery elm* tea; •*Chamomile* tea; •*Ginger* tea, or •New Chapter GINGER WONDER syrup tones intestinal walls.

—Bodywork:
•Avoid cortico-steroid drugs. They often result in ulcers. Antacids offer minor symptomatic, or no relief. Excess use of aspirin increases gastric problem risk.
•Techniques like biofeedback are successful for many gastric problems.
•Take a "constitutional" walk after meals. Don't eat when upset, angry or anxious.

—Acupressure points:
Pull middle toe on each foot for 1 minute.

Herbal, Superfood and Supplement Therapy

Interceptive therapy plan: Choose 2 to 3 recommendations.

1—**Reduce pain and inflammation:** •MSM caps 800mg 2x daily or •Futurebiotics MSM caps 2 daily; •Enzymedica GASTRO as directed; •*Una da Gato* capsules 6 daily, or Nature's Way CELL MEND with *una de gato* and IP-6; •*Goldenseal/myrrh* extract 3x daily curbs infection (gently effective). •*Ginkgo Biloba* extract 3x daily; •Planetary TRIPHALA caps (highly recommended); •Holistic PROPOLIS LOZENGES.

2—**Calm nerve - intestinal distress:** •Crystal Star RELAX CAPS™ as needed; *Ho-Shou-Wu* (Fo-Ti) extract drops in water; •*Pau d'arco* or *Ginseng* extract drops in water.

3—**Soothe the stomach lining and lessen bleeding:** •Lane Labs NATURE'S LINING chewables (highly recommended). •*Turmeric* extract (curcumin) capsules; •Nature's Herbs DGL-POWER; •Magnesium, or •Country Life magnesium-potassium-bromelain caps soothe membranes. •Jarrow BIOSIL drops in warm water, or •Flora VEGE-SIL caps.

4—**Balancing stomach pH helps the body cleanse:** •Crystal Star BITTERS & LEMON™ extract balances gastrointestinal region; •gamma-oryzanol (from rice) 300mg reduces abdominal distention; Flora FRUTIN protects esophagus from stomach acid damage.

5—**Protease enzymes help curb leaky gut syndromes:** •Enzymedica PURIFY as directed (good results even in serious cases). •Glutamine 500mg 4x daily (or 1 tsp. glutamine powder in juice 3x a day); •Crystal Star DR. ENZYME™ with protease and bromelain; •Nutricology PERMAVITE decreases permeability of small intestine to increase absorption.

6—**Digestive enzymes and probiotics rebalance the gastric area:** •Prevail ACID-EASE tablets; •UAS DDS-PLUS with FOS before meals or •Nutricology SYMBIOTICS. •Betaine HCl for stomach acid; •Activated charcoal releases gas; •Pancreatin helps digest fats; Schiff ENZYMALL with ox bile (good results); •Enzymatic Therapy DGL chewable tablets after meals, and especially after taking ant-acid drugs.

—Superfood therapy: (Choose one or two)
•Crystal Star RESTORE YOUR STRENGTH™ drink or •Crystal Star ENERGY GREEN RENEWAL™ drink. •Solgar WHEY TO GO protein drink.

Can't find a recommended product? Call the 800 number listed in Product Resources for the store nearest you.

Gastric Diseases

GERD (Gastro-esophageal Reflux Disease), Hiatal Hernia

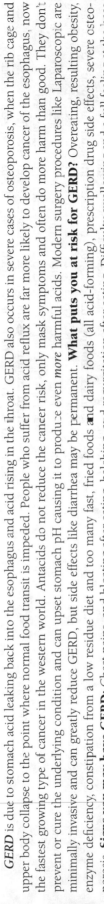

GERD is due to stomach acid leaking back into the esophagus and acid rising in the throat. GERD also occurs in severe cases of osteoporosis, when the rib cage and upper body collapse to the point where normal food transit is impeded. People who suffer from acid reflux are far more likely to develop cancer of the esophagus, now the fastest growing type of cancer in the western world. Antacids do not reduce the cancer risk, only mask symptoms and often do more harm than good. They don't prevent or cure the underlying condition and can upset stomach pH causing it to produce even *more* harmful acids. Modern surgery procedures like Laparoscopic are minimally invasive and can greatly reduce GERD, but side effects like diarrhea may be permanent. **What puts you at risk for GERD?** Overeating, resulting obesity, enzyme deficiency, constipation from a low residue diet and too many fast, fried foods and dairy foods (all acid-forming), prescription drug side effects, severe osteoporosis. **Signs you may have GERD:** Chest pains, and bloating after eating, belching, and regurgitation after eating. Difficulty swallowing and a full feeling at the base of the throat, leading to chronic hoarseness; raised blood pressure accompanied by gastro-intestinal bleeding, and sometimes by a stomach ulcer. *Hiatal hernia* occurs when part of the stomach protrudes through the diaphragm wall, causing difficult swallowing, burning reflux in the throat, and great anxiety. Hiatal hernia is common in the U.S. today.

Diet and Lifestyle Support Therapy

Nutritional therapy plan: See previous page, INDIGESTION and HEARTBURN pages for more.

1—Eat only raw or lightly steamed vegetable-source fiber foods during healing. Take 2 glasses of mineral water or aloe vera juice daily. •To prevent night time reflux, elevate head off bed 6 to 8 inches. Don't eat within two hours of your bedtime.

2—Drink 2 glasses of fresh carrot or apple juice every day, or •Aloe vera juice daily; Try •AloeLife or Saluté ALOE VERA juice. Try Apple Cider Vinegar (organic) 1 tbsp. per day in the morning if you have low HCl (contraindicated if you have ulcers).

3—When digestion has normalized, follow a low fat, low salt, high fiber diet. Use •All One TOTALLY FIBER complex drink for gentle cleansing fiber.

4—Eat smaller meals more frequently. No large meals. No liquids with meals. Eat slowly so that you are less likely to swallow air and belch. •Don't lie down after eating.

5—Foods that aggravate a hiatal hernia: coffee, chocolate, red meats, hard alcohol drinks, sodas. Wear yellow color therapy eyewear during meals until hernia is gone.

6—Eliminate fried and spicy foods because they slow the rate at which your stomach empties, allowing food to travel backwards to the esophagus. Refined carbohydrates and sugary foods should be eliminated as they boost gastric acidity. Avoid nuts, seeds, acidic juices and gas-producing foods during healing.

—Juices for stomach acid balance: •Carrot juice, or •Green Foods CARROT ESSENCE for healing vitamin A. •Carrot/cabbage, a stomach healer. •Pineapple-papaya for extra enzymes. •Liquid chlorophyll or Sun Wellness CHLORELLA, 1 tsp. in water before meals is also effective.

—Bodywork: Avoid all tobacco. Nicotine affects gastric functions •Have a chiropractic adjustment to the area or a massage therapy treatment at least once a month. (I have personally seen massage therapy work for many people.) •Apply a green clay pack to the upper abdominal area. •NAET (Nambudripad Allergy Elimination Technique) helps eliminate food allergy reflux.

Herbal, Superfood and Supplement Therapy

Interceptive therapy plan: Choose 1 or 2 recommendations.

1—Lessen spasm and pain: •Glutamine 500mg 4x daily (or 1 tsp. glutamine powder in juice 3x a day) decreases permeability of small intestine to increase absorption. (Relief often within 30 minutes.) •Transformation GASTROZYME; •UAS DDS-PLUS with FOS, along with •Crystal Star ANTI-FLAM™ caps 4 daily, or •MUSCLE RELAXER™ caps 2 with each meal, or •PMS RELIEF™ extract ½ dropperful at a time as needed for pain and spasms. •Propolis extract ½ dropperful every 4 hours during an attack.

2—Soothe inflamed tissue of the stomach lining and esophagus: •Lane Labs NATURE'S LINING chewables (highly recommended to heal erosions caused by aspirin therapy). •Chamomile tea; •Pau d'arco tea; •Licorice root extract; •Slippery elm or marshmallow tea as needed. •Bromelain 1500mg as needed; or •Source Naturals ACTIVATED QUERCETIN or Quercetin 5 daily to reduce inflammation, with bromelain and vitamin C. •Enzymatic Therapy GASTRO-SOOTHE as directed (recommended). •Zinc gluconate lozenges under the tongue as needed. •Schiff EMULSIFIED A 25,000IU 2x daily to rebalance digestive tract.

3—After initial stages, bitters herbs stimulate the secretion of stomach acid, cleanse the stomach and balance its functions: •Crystal Star BITTERS & LEMON™ extract to balance gastrointestinal region (fasting acting); or •MILK THISTLE SEED extract for 1 to 3 months; •Planetary TRIPHALA caps as directed; •Crystal Star DR ENZYME™ with protease and bromelain for enzyme therapy.

4—Protease enzymes help curb leaky gut syndromes: •Enzymedica PURIFY as directed (results even in serious cases). •Glutamine 500mg 4x daily (or 1 tsp. glutamine powder in juice 3x a day) decreases permeability of small intestine to increase absorption. Try •Transitions EASY GREENS drink.

5—Digestive enzymes and probiotics rebalance the gastric area: •Herbal Products and Development POWER PLUS FOOD ENZYMES; •Nature's Herbs DGL-POWER as needed; •Pancreatin 1400mg with meals; •American Health ACIDOPHILUS liquid; •Alta Health CANGEST caps or powder 3x daily.

Can't find a recommended product? Call the 800 number listed in Product Resources for the store nearest you.

425

Gastric Diseases - Ulcers

Stomach, Peptic, Duodenal

One in ten Americans now have, or have had, an ulcer. Every year, ten thousand people die of ulcer complications. A **stomach** or **gastric ulcer** is in the upper stomach lining with pain right after eating. A **duodenal ulcer,** is in the duodenum, the first part of the small intestine, so pain comes two or three hours later. A **peptic ulcer,** the most common, is an erosion of the lower stomach lining, small intestine or esophagus. Most ulcers are caused by *H. pylori,* a stomach bacterium which liberates copious amounts of damaging ammonia and carbon dioxide if the body's protective intestinal devices fail. Natural therapy helps re-establish intestinal balance. **Do you have an ulcer?** An ulcer is an open sore in the stomach or duodenum wall. Burning and the urge to vomit are common. If the vomit is bright red, and the feces very dark, it is a bleeding ulcer. **What gives you an ulcer?** Our lifestyle habits make us prime ulcer candidates. For most people it's stress creating an acid system, or irritants like coffee, alcohol and nicotine, and NSAIDS drugs (the latest figures show Americans take 85 million aspirin a day!) Food sensitivities, very sugary foods, anemia, Candida albicans, hypoglycemia, and excessive use of antacids are common. Calcium carbonate antacids, like Tums and Alka-2 actually produce more gastric acid secretions when medication is stopped, and may cause kidney stones. Sodium bi-carbonate antacids, like Alka-Seltzer and Rolaids elevate blood pH levels, interfering with metabolism, and may increase blood pressure. Aluminum-magnesium antacids, like Maalox and Mylanta can cause calcium depletion and contribute to aluminum toxicity.

Diet and Lifestyle Support Therapy

Nutritional therapy plan:

1—Go on a short liquid diet (pg. 173) to cleanse the G.I. tract. Take 3 juices of your choice daily: 1) Potassium broth (pg. 291); 2) Aloe vera juice each morning or •Herbal Answers ALOE FORCE juice w. herbs. 3) Cabbage/celery/parsley juice; 4) Apple-alfalfa sprout juice with 1 tsp. spirulina powder. Add 2-3 glasses mineral water daily.

2—Add easily digestible, fresh alkalizing foods, like leafy greens, steamed vegetables, whole grains and non-acidic fruits. Cooked unripe plaintain is especially healing. Have a small raw cabbage salad daily during healing. Using rosemary in cooking is helpful.

3—Include cultured foods, such as yogurt, kefir and buttermilk for friendly G.I. flora.

4—Avoid sugary, fatty foods (interfere with buffer activity of protein and calcium), pasteurized dairy foods, red meat, heavy, spicy foods. Reduce alcohol (a little wine is ok). Avoid cola drinks (provoke acid production).

5—Chew all food well. Eat small meals. No large, heavy meals. Avoid late night snacks.

Note: Tagamet and Zantac drugs (over 1 billion dollars in sales yearly) suppress stomach HCL formation, may cause later liver damage. Both drugs interfere with the liver's ability to process and excrete toxic chemicals, exposing vulnerability to poisons from pesticides, herbicides, etc. Take DGL (deglycyrrhizinated licorice) to normalize after these drugs.

—Bodywork:
•A mild olive oil flush: sip 2 tbsp. oil through a straw before retiring, for a week.
•Avoid smoking, caffeine, NSAIDS drugs and aspirin - key culprits in aggravating ulcers. Smoking inhibits a natural bicarbonate secretion that neutralizes harmful acids.
•Take a catnip or garlic enema once a week during healing to detoxify the G.I. tract.

Herbal, Superfood and Supplement Therapy

Interceptive therapy plan: Choose 2 to 4 recommendations.

1—**Reduce pain and inflammation:** •Transformation GASTROZYME caps as needed in place of antacids; •*Ginger* capsules before meals or •New Chapter GINGER WONDER syrup–1 tbsp. in 8-oz. water 2x daily; •Jarrow Formulas CURCUMIN-97 capsules; •*Goldenseal-cayenne* caps; •NAC (N-acetyl-cysteine) 600mg or Source Naturals N-ACETYL-CYSTEINE as directed (for alcohol-induced ulcers); Eidon ZINC liquid for pain relief.

—**For duodenal ulcers:** •Crystal Star MUSCLE RELAXER™ caps to calm; and •Gamma Oryzanol (GO), a rice bran extract, as directed; •Planetary TRIPHALA caps as directed. •*Bilberry* extract 15 drops in *calendula* tea 3x daily.

2—**Overcome H. pylori infection:** •Crystal Star ANTI-BIO™ caps 6 daily or Nutricology MASTICA (mastic gum); Wakunaga AGED GARLIC EXTRACT has potent activity against H. pylori; •Olive Leaf extract as directed; •Kal COLOSTRUM 1-3 tabs daily; •*Una da gato* tea, 3 cups daily; •Quercetin 1000mg with bromelain 1500mg daily. •Propolis tincture as needed. •Evening Primrose Oil 2000mg daily or •Omega-3 flax oil, 2 tsp. daily retard H. pylori growth.

—**Herbal flavonoids inhibit H. pylori bacteria:** •*Ginkgo Biloba* extract; •*Goldenseal-myrrh* extract; •*Garlic* or *garlic-parsley* capsules 8 daily.

3—**Soothe ulcerated areas:** •Nature's Herbs DGL-POWER before meals; •*Slippery elm* tea heals inflamed tissue; •*Chamomile* tea 3 cups daily; •*Marshmallow root* tea. •Stress B-complex 100mg with extra pantothenic acid 500mg and B-6, 50mg.

5—**Restablish, improve integrity of the gastrointestinal mucosa:** •Glutamine 500mg 3x daily. •CHLORELLA-GINSENG extract rebuilds mucosa. •Ester C, 3000mg daily for 3 months. •Vitamin E 400IU 2x daily; •Schiff emulsified A 100,000IU for 6 days; •Lane Labs NATURE'S LINING chewables (highly recommended).

6—**Rebuild immune response:** •Wakunaga KYO-GREEN with EFAs; •Sun Wellness CHLORELLA tabs 15 daily, or liquid chlorophyll 3 tsp. daily; •Chromium picolinate 200mcg; •UAS DDS-PLUS with FOS or •Jarrow JARRO-DOPHILUS.

Can't find a recommended product? Call the 800 number listed in Product Resources for the store nearest you.

Gland Health

An overview of the major endocrine glands with specific recommendations for maintaining their health.

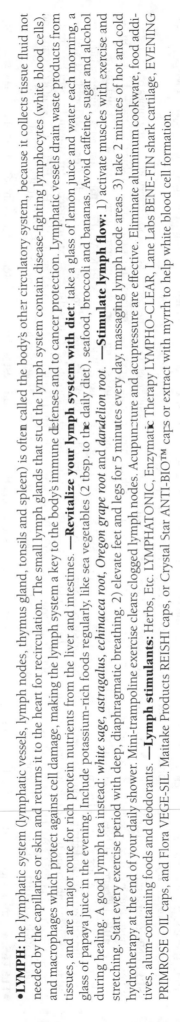

There are two types of glands in the body — exocrine (glands regulated by the hypothalamus, that secrete their fluids through ducts, like the salivary and mammary glands); and endocrine (glands that emit their secretions directly as hormones into the bloodstream). Endocrine glands are involved with almost every body function. They are integral to hormone balance, proper metabolism, high energy and immune response. Deep body balance is dependent on the vitality of your glands. Invariably, your glands suffer the most from a lifestyle high in stress and low in rest and nutrition. Glandular malfunction leads to a wide array of health problems today: from thyroid malfunction, to hair loss, to exhaustion, to diabetes.

•**ADRENALS:** composed of two distinct parts — the adrenal medulla and the adrenal cortex, the medulla secretes the hormones epinephrine (adrenaline) and norepinephrine in the "fight or flight" response. The adrenal cortex secretes corticosteroid hormones, formed from cholesterol. Normally, adrenal glands are about the size of a lima bean, but when overstressed they can grow 4 times that size. Many menopausal woman who complain of chronic low back pain actually have swollen adrenals! Adrenal stimulating herbs: *licorice root, schizandra, wild yam root, panax ginseng, bupleurum, Siberian eleuthero* and *turmeric.* See page 300 for a complete program for adrenal health.

•**HYPOTHALAMUS:** located just behind the pituitary gland. Hormones secreted by this small group of nerve cells are involved in breast milk production, body temperature, sleep and wakefulness, mood, water balance and smooth muscle contraction. Adaptogen herbs like *gotu kola, panax ginseng, astragalus* and *Siberian eleuthero* help keep the hypothalamus balanced. Pacific BioLogics EMOTIONAL RESCUE Day and Night formulas offer premier support for the entire limbic system, including the hypothalamus.

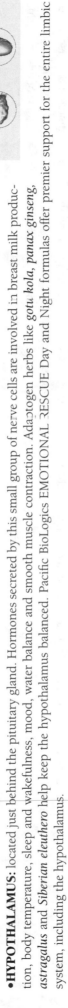

•**LYMPH:** the lymphatic system (lymphatic vessels, lymph nodes, thymus gland, tonsils and spleen) is often called the body's other circulatory system, because it collects tissue fluid not needed by the capillaries or skin and returns it to the heart for recirculation. The small lymph glands that stud the lymph system contain disease-fighting lymphocytes (white blood cells), and macrophages which protect against cell damage, making the lymph system a key to the body's immune defenses and to cancer protection. Lymphatic vessels drain waste products from tissues, and are a major route for rich protein nutrients from the liver and intestines. —**Revitalize your lymph system with diet:** take a glass of lemon juice and water each morning, a glass of papaya juice in the evening. Include potassium-rich foods regularly, like sea vegetables (2 tbsp. to the daily diet), seafood, broccoli and bananas. Avoid caffeine, sugar and alcohol during healing. A good lymph tea instead: *white sage, astragalus, echinacea root, Oregon grape root* and *dandelion root.* —**Stimulate lymph flow:** 1) activate muscles with exercise and stretching. Start every exercise period with deep, diaphragmatic breathing. 2) elevate feet and legs for 5 minutes every day, massaging lymph node areas. 3) take 2 minutes of hot and cold hydrotherapy at the end of your daily shower. Mini-trampoline exercise clears clogged lymph nodes. Acupuncture and acupressure are effective. Eliminate aluminum cookware, food additives, alum-containing foods and deodorants. —**Lymph stimulants:** Herbs, Etc. LYMPHATONIC, Enzymatic Therapy LYMPHO-CLEAR, Lane Labs BENE-FIN shark cartilage, EVENING PRIMROSE OIL caps, and Flora VEGE-SIL. Maitake Products REISHI caps, or Crystal Star ANTI-BIO™ caps or extract with myrrh to help white blood cell formation.

•**OVARIES:** the ovaries produce the female eggs for reproduction, and two hormones, estrogen and progesterone, responsible for maintaining secondary sexual characteristics, and preparing the uterus and breasts for the reproductive cycle. See Hormone Health and Balance pages 455-461 for specific balancing recommendations.

•**PITUITARY:** called the body's master gland, the pituitary regulates all gland activity. Stress is a direct contributor to pituitary deficiency symptoms, especially mental burn-out, poor healing, erratic blood sugar levels and body fluid imbalance. Stimulate the pineal with acupressure: press for 10 seconds, 3x each, over the left eyebrow for pituitary stimulation; on the forehead where the eyebrows meet for pineal stimulation. —**Diet help:** eat plenty of green leafy vegetables. Have a veggie drink like Knudsens VERY VEGGIE or Futurebiotics VITAL K drink, or Crystal Star ENERGY GREEN RENEWAL™ drink twice a week. Eat complex carbohydrates like broccoli, potatoes, sprouts, peas, dried fruits, whole grains and brown rice. Drink fresh fruit juices each morning, 6 glasses of bottled water daily. Avoid beer, sweet wines, refined carbs, sugar, heavy pastries, and canned foods. Avoid all MSG-containing foods and preserved foods. —**Supplement help:** include a multi-mineral, like MEZOTRACE sea mineral complex or Trace Mineral Research CONCENTRACE, Ester C with bioflavonoids and rutin, Country Life sublingual B-12, 2500mcg, Glutamine 500mg 4x daily for growth hormone, B-complex 100mg daily, Flora VEGESIL caps and Enzymatic Therapy RAW PITUITARY (good activity). —**Herbal help:** Crystal Star OCEAN MINERALS™ caps (iodine, potassium and silica from sea veggies). Sea greens of all kinds work synergistically with the pituitary in glandular formulas. Solaray ALFA-JUICE caps; Prince of Peace AMERICAN GINSENG, BEE POLLEN, ROYAL JELLY vials daily, and *gotu kola-damiana* caps.

Can't find a recommended product? Call the 800 number listed in Product Resources for the store nearest you.

•**PANCREAS:** the pancreas is both an exocrine and an endocrine gland, secreting hormones into the bloodstream and digestive enzymes into the small intestine. Its hormone, glucagon, controls blood sugar levels and digestive enzymes. Today, pancreas glandular therapy is used for digestive disorders, low blood sugar and heart problems, and as an antimicrobial and anti-inflammatory. The Islets of Langerhans are tiny but important glandular clusters in the pancreas that produce insulin. Their destruction or impairment results in diabetes or hypoglycemia. Alcoholism, excessive use of prescription drugs, and poor nutrition can lead to painful inflamed pancreatitis. Avoid sugary foods if you have a weak pancreas. Maintain pancreatic health with chromium picolinate 200mcg daily, phosphatidyl choline to aid in fat digestion, Nutricology PANCREAS Organic Glandular, and pancreatin, a digestive enzyme.

•**PINEAL GLAND:** Lying just under the pituitary gland, behind the eyes, the pineal gland is the body's light meter. Many health problems result from our modern day indoor lifestyle, in which we receive distorted light waves from sunglasses, eyeglasses, window glass, fluorescent lights and contact lenses. Both pineal and pituitary glands benefit from 20 minutes a day of early morning sunlight. The pineal helps balance the endocrine system, regulating our body rhythms, sleep patterns, fertility and the development of consciousness. Small doses of melatonin (.3 to .5mg) can help rebalance pineal gland function for persons who are travelling between time zones and for people who are blind. Ask your natural health practitioner.

•**PROSTATE:** the prostate is a large male gland that lies just below the neck of the bladder, and around the top of the urinary tract. The primary function of the prostate is to help the semen move through the urethra during ejaculation. It also produces an alkaline fluid which carries the sperm from the testes into the vagina. This fluid greatly enhances the chances of fertilization because it balances the acid environment of the uterus for the sperm. The prostate enlarges during sexual arousal. If there is prolonged arousal without ejaculation, the pressure from the prostate on the testicles becomes very uncomfortable. See Benign Prostatic Hyperplasia page 526 for more information.

•**SPLEEN:** the largest mass of lymphatic tissue in the body, the spleen produces lymphocytes, destroys worn-out blood cells, and serves as a blood reservoir. During times of great stress or hemorrhage, the spleen can release its stored blood to prevent shock. Depletion symptoms include anemia, pallor, extreme slimness, poor memory and sluggishness. —**Diet help for spleen health:** Take a carrot-beet-cucumber juice every day for 1 week, then every other day for another week to "spring clean" the spleen of stored toxins. Then, build up red blood cells with a potassium broth (pg. 291), a mixed veggie drink, Green Foods GREEN ESSENCE drink, or Crystal Star ENERGY GREEN RENEWAL™ drink, and a leafy green salad every day. Include brown rice and alfalfa sprouts frequently. —**Herbs for spleen health:** Crystal Star FEEL GREAT NOW!™ caps, *red root tea, hawthorn, yellow dock root* for blood building and tone. Spleen enhancing tea: *4-oz. hawthorn, 1-oz. cardamom, 1-oz. safflowers, 1-oz. lemon balm, 1-oz. red sage;* take 2 cups daily. —**Supplements for spleen health:** Enzymatic Therapy LYMPH-SPLEEN COMPLEX, or GOLDEN SPLEEN 500, Nutricology IMMOPLEX Glandular, Vitamin E 400IU daily, Nature's Way ALIVE WHOLE FOOD ENERGIZER, marine carotene 50-100,000IU daily, liquid chlorophyll 3 tsp. daily with meals, and Nutricology SYMBIOTICS, ½ tsp. in water 2x daily or American Health ACIDOPHILUS liquid.

•**TESTES:** a man's testicles are the workhorses of his reproductive system, producing sperm and the male hormone testosterone. Testosterone causes the development of male secondary characteristics - face and body hair (and the male pattern receding hairline), body odor, voice change, enhanced muscles, male sexual organs and the increased oiliness and coarseness of a man's skin (a factor that means men's skin ages about ten years *behind* the skin of women). Testosterone also establishes the male sex drive, but has nothing to do with male erection. Some men do experience a decrease in testosterone production as they age, especially if his diet and lifestyle are not conducive to healthy gland function. The symptoms of this endocrine imbalance are similar to a woman's menopause and are called andropause. See pg. 251 for a complete lifestyle program for Male Andropause.

•**THYMUS:** the "master gland" of the immune system, vital to the production of T-lymphocyte cells and thymic hormones, critical to cell-mediated immunity, the thymus gland shrinks with age and is easily damaged by oxidation and free radicals. Thymus gland extracts help against infections, food allergies, hair loss and cancer growth. —**Antioxidants for thymus health:** vitamin E with selenium, beta-carotene, zinc, vitamin B₆ and vitamin C, Nutricology THYMUS Organic Glandular help produce thymic hormones. —**Herbs for thymus health:** *Echinacea root* and *echinacea-goldenseal-myrrh* compounds boost activity of white blood cells and interferon production. *Panax ginseng* and *licorice* help regulating thymus activity.

•**THYROID:** the thyroid secretes the high iodine hormone thyroxin involved in growth, digestion, metabolism (vital energy resources for every body activity), body temperature, reflexes, and heartbeat. The two most common thyroid disorders are hypothyroidism, (as in Hashimoto's disease) where the thyroid doesn't produce enough thyroxin (a rising problem in our polluted environment), and hyperthyroidism, secretion of too much thyroxin (as in Grave's Disease). **Signs of an underactive thyroid:** depression, fatigue, hair loss (especially in women), obesity, intolerance to cold, breast fibroids and poor immune response. **Signs of overactive thyroid:** feeling "wired" for no reason, rapid heartbeat, diarrhea, insomnia, bulging eyes or double vision, light menstrual period, feeling warm, and unexplained weight loss. Iodine and potassium, rich in sea greens and herbs are some of the best nutrients to take for thyroid health. The glands produce parathyroid hormone which raises calcium levels in the blood. The parathyroid glands embedded in the thyroid gland help maintain the proper level of nutrients in the body. Raised calcium levels caused by excess parathyroid production can contribute to kidney stones and kidney failure. See pages 480-482 for more.

Can't find a recommended product? Call the 800 number listed in Product Resources for the store nearest you.

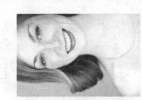

Gland Health

Deep Body Balance

Your glands and hormones work at your body's deepest levels - involved with almost every body function and biochemical reaction. They're a key to good health, especially as you age. *Exocrine glands*, like salivary and mammary glands, regulated by the hypothalamus, secrete their fluids through ducts; 2) *Endocrine glands*, like the pituitary, pineal or ovaries, emit hormone secretions directly into the bloodstream and lymph system. Hormones are chemical messengers exerting wide-ranging effects throughout our bodies. Secretions like adrenaline, insulin, and thyroid hormone are dramatically affected by nutritional deficiencies, environmental pollutants, chemicalized foods and synthetic hormones. In fact, glands and hormones are affected first by harmful toxins and poor nutrition. A mineral deficiency, something that plagues most Americans, undermines the health of almost every gland and organ. The chronic stress loads most Americans live under directly affects hormone balance (like low levels of steroidal hormones produced by our "stressed-out" adrenals). **Signs your body needs a gland cleanse:** unexplained weight gain and sluggish metabolism (low thyroid activity); blood sugar problems (imbalanced insulin levels); poor assimilation of nutrients (low enzymes from a congested pancreas); fatigue, mental fuzziness, dizziness when you get up quickly, heart palpitations (adrenal exhaustion); cold hands and feet; hair, skin and nails problems; or menstrual problems (thyroid malfunction).

Diet and Lifestyle Support Therapy

Nutritional therapy plan:

1—Begin with a 3 day juice-liquid diet and follow with 1 to 3 days of all fresh foods.

2—*The night before* your gland cleanse.... take a gentle herbal laxative, like Zand CLEANSING LAXATIVE tabs; or Yogi DETOX tea. *The next day...* if in season, go on a watermelon juice only cleanse. Drink throughout the day to rapidly flush and alkalize. If watermelon is not available, start with the following:

On rising: take lemon juice in water with 1 tsp. honey. Add 2 tsp. nutritional yeast.

Breakfast: have a carrot juice with 1 tbsp. any green superfood (next column).

Mid-morning: take a carrot or mixed veggie drink. Add 1 tsp. dulse flakes.

Lunch: have miso soup with dulse flakes and nutritional yeast flakes sprinkles.

Mid-afternoon: have a mixed vegetable-tomato base juice (like Knudsen's Very Veggie).

Dinner: have a high mineral broth: Simmer 30 minutes: 3 carrots, 1 cup parsley, 1 onion, 2 potatoes, 2 stalks celery. Strain.

Before Bed: have an apple or pineapple/papaya juice. If desired, blend in 1 fresh fig. Or try Jarrow GENTLE FIBERS drink (an excellent gland balancer).

—Bodywork:

• Enema: Take an enema during your gland cleanse to help release toxins.

• Exercise: Take a regular 20 minute "gland health" walk every day.

• Environmental: Avoid air and environmental pollutants as much as possible. Your glands are the first to feel the damaging effects.

• Acupressure points: Stroke the top of the foot on both feet for 5 minutes each to stimulate endocrine and hormone secretions.

• Massage therapy: Have a massage therapy treatment to stimulate circulation and re-establish clear meridian pathways in the body.

• Thump the thymus point briskly each morning 6 times for immune response.

Herbal, Superfood and Supplement Therapy

Interceptive therapy plan: Choose 2 to 3 recommendations.

1—**Deep clean your glands:** •Gaia Herbs SUPREME CLEANSE: Planetary Herbs PAU D'ARCO DEEP CLEANSER.

2—**Enhance your gland functions:** Use herbal compounds that contain phytohormone-rich herbs, like *ginseng, licorice root, sarsaparilla, dong quai,* and *black cohosh*. For gland homeostasis, •Crystal Star FEEL GREAT NOW!™ with ginseng and ADRENAL ENERGY BOOST™ formulas. •Planetary Formulas SCHIZANDRA ADRENAL SUPPORT; use •Crystal Star TOXIN DETOX™ caps or N-acetylcysteine 1000mg daily if you are regularly exposed to toxic pollutants.

—**Raw gland extracts offer biochemical support for gland stress and fatigue:** •Premier Labs RAW MULTIPLE GLANDULAR; •Nutricology ORGANIC THYMUS and ADRENAL CORTEX glandulars.

3—**Essential fatty acids are essential:** •Barlean's Organic OMEGA TWIN FLAX/BORAGE COMBO, •Futurebiotics VITAL K LIQUID, •Lane Labs OMEGA MULTI caps.

4—**Enzymes and probiotics assist detoxification and protect from toxins:** •Source Naturals LIFE FLORA; •Arise & Shine FLORA GROW; •Transformation Enzyme PUREZYME, or •Enzymedica DIGEST for adrenal exhaustion; •Crystal Star DR. ENZYME™ with protease and bromelain and UAS DDS-PLUS FOS.

5—**Electrolytes expedite a gland cleanse:** •Nature's Path TRACE-LYTE LIQUID MINERALS; •Arise & Shine ALKALIZER.

—**Your glands need greens! Chlorophyll rich superfoods:** •Body Ecology VITALITY SUPERGREEN; •Solgar EARTH SOURCE GREENS & MORE; •Crystal Star ENERGY GREEN RENEWAL™ or RESTORE YOUR STRENGTH™ drink; •Nutricology PRO GREENS with EFAs; •AloeLife ALOE GOLD JUICE; •Prince of Peace ROYAL JELLY-GINSENG vials daily.

Can't find a recommended product? Call the 800 number listed in Product Resources for the store nearest you.

Glaucoma

Eyeball Fluid Pressure and Hardening

Glaucoma, build up of pressure in the eyeball, affects up to 3 million people over 65 in America. Now the 2nd leading cause of blindness in Hispanics and African Americans. Usually asymptomatic in early stages, it often goes undetected for years, but if the pressure is not relieved, the eyeball may harden, harm the retina and progressively damage eyes and optic nerve. Side vision becomes limited; if untreated, blindness can result. Collagen, the most abundant and necessary protein in the eye, is responsible for eye tissue strength and integrity. Improved collagen metabolism can be a key to the relief of eye pressure. **Signs you may have glacoma:** Colored halos around lights, blurred, hazy vision, eye inflammation (red eyes), loss of peripheral or nightime vision, the inability to tear; fixed, dilated pupils, chronic pain and tunnel vision around the eyes (acute closed-angle glaucoma is a serious eye emergency with severe, throbbing pain and loss of vision if pressure is not relieved within 36 hours). **Causes of glaucoma?** Overusing steroids and other drugs like certain antihypertensives and antidepressants, diabetes and arteriosclerosis, food allergies, poor collagen metabolism, too much caffeine and sugar, long emotional stress, adrenal exhaustion, liver malfunction, thyroid imbalance. *See Liver Cleansing page 199 and Eyesight page 411 for more.*

Diet and Lifestyle Support Therapy

Nutritional therapy plan:

1—Go on a fresh foods diet for 2 weeks to clear the system of inorganic crystalline deposits. Take one of the following every day during these 2 weeks: •Crystal Star BITTERS & LEMON CLEANSE™ extract drops in water; •Carrot/beet/cucumber/parsley juice; •Fresh carrot juice. •Potassium broth (pg. 291)

2—Avoid sugary foods, caffeine and foods with caffeine. Avoid known food allergens.

•**Vitamin A-rich foods for eyes:** Endive and leafy greens, carrots, sea foods and sea vegetables, broccoli.

•**Vitamin C foods for eyes:** Citrus and carrot juice, bell peppers, cucumbers, beets.

•**Eye nourishing drinks:** •AloeLife ALOE GOLD JUICE 2x daily, also dilute and use as an eyewash. •Pure Planet CHLORELLA- 2 tsp. daily in water; •Solgar EARTH SOURCE GREENS & MORE drink.

—**Glaucoma healing eye washes:** Bathe eyes daily with a dilute water ascorbate C/bioflavonoid solution to reduce pressure. •Crystal Star EYEBRIGHT COMPLEX™ tea; •Weak *goldenseal* solution; •*Chamomile* tea; •*Fennel* seed compresses.

—**Lifestyle measures:**

•Relax more. Strive for a less stressful lifestyle.

•Practice deep breathing exercises to reduce eyeball pressure. Hyperbaric oxygen chambers are beneficial.

•Stop smoking. It constricts eye blood vessels and increases pressure.

•Certain drugs tend to inhibit or destroy collagen structures in the eye. Drugs to avoid if you have glaucoma: steroid drugs, tranquilizers, epinephrine-like or atropine drugs, aspirin and over-the-counter antihistamines.

•Get a good spinal chiropractic adjustment or regular massage therapy treatments.

•Life Extension BRITE EYES eye drops with L-carnosine.

Herbal, Superfood and Supplement Therapy

Interceptive therapy plan: Choose 2 to 3 recommendations.

1—**Vitamin C therapy reduces intra-ocular pressure:** •Ascorbate Vitamin C with bioflavonoids and rutin, 10,000mg daily, or to bowel tolerance, for 1 month. Or, as an intensive ascorbic acid flush, take ¼ tsp. at a time in water every hour. Add •Quercetin 1000mg with bromelain 750mg 6 daily. Add •Lane Labs BENE-FIN shark cartilage.

2—**Lower intra-ocular pressure:** •Crystal Star EYEBRIGHT COMPLEX™ 4 daily with natural carotenes and vitamin C; •Enzymatic Therapy Ayurvedic *coleus forskohlii* extract; •Nature's Secret ULTIMATE B, •Prince of Peace GINSENG-ROYAL JELLY vials. •Golden Pride FORMULA ONE with EDTA.

3—**Improve liver function:** •Spirulina 6 daily or •Solaray ALFAJUICE caps - a liver cleanser. •Planetary TRIPHALA INTERNAL CLEANSER.

4—**Enhance eye circulation:** •GINKGO BILOBA extract or *cayenne* capsules, 2 daily to normalize circulation to the optical system. •Magnesium 400mg (Nature's calcium channel blocker) or Flora MAGNESIUM liquid daily (improves blood flow).

5—**Improve collagen metabolism:** •Lane Labs TOKI - a collagen replacement drink (highly recommended). •BILBERRY extract several times daily; or •Solaray VIZION caps with bilberry; •Source Naturals VISUAL EYES; •Herbal Magic GOTU KOLA-GINSENG caps 4 daily. •Vitamin E 400IU daily to help remove lens particles.

6—**Antioxidants are critical to healing:** •Alpha lipoic acid 300mg daily; •Nutricology OCUDYNE II w. lutein; •OPCs from grapeseed or white pine, 300mg daily; •Glutathione 50mg 2x daily or NAC (N-acetylcysteine) 600mg 2x daily; •Beta carotene 150,000IU daily or •PHYCOTENE MICROCLUSTERS available at Healthy House.

7—**Protect against glaucoma:** •Carnitine 1000mg daily; •Crystal Star OCEAN MINERALS™ for iodine imbalance; •Transformation PUREZYME to optimize protease activity; •Nature's Life I-SIGHT 2x daily.

—**Superfoods are important** (the eyes require a great deal of nourishment.) •Pure Planet CHLORELLA- 2 tsp. daily in water. •Crystal Star ENERGY GREEN RENEWAL™.

Can't find a recommended product? Call the 800 number listed in Product Resources for the store nearest you.

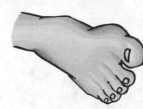

Gout

Arthritis of the Toe and Peripheral Joints

Gout is a common type of arthritis suffered 90% by overweight, middle-aged males (affects 1 out of a hundred). It's a metabolic disorder where tiny, needle-like crystals of uric acid in blood and body fluids cause pain in the joints. Although known as a toe problem, tendons, fingers and kidneys are also gout sites. Gout gets increasingly worse with gradual joint destruction, and longer and longer attacks. The natural healing approach is simple and successful. Gout therapy involves diet change to eliminate high purine foods and heavy alcohol that causes sediment. It reduces dietary fat for weight loss and cholesterol reduction. It advocates kidney cleansing to normalize uric acid levels in the blood. **What causes gout?** Overeating is the hallmark of gout... especially too much red meat, fried food, alcohol, sugars (especially fructose), and caffeine. Overloaded kidneys don't excrete properly, causing uric acid build-up. Overuse of some drugs, like thiazide diuretics cause potassium deficiency. Obesity, hypoglycemia and hypothyroidism all appear to be factors. **Do you have gout?** Onset of gout is often rapid with chills and fever, and excruciating pain. If you have extremely painful red, swollen joints in the foot and big toe, it's an almost certain sign. Resveratrol (a constituent found in grape skins and the herb *Polygonum cuspidatum*) show good results against gout in vitro tests. Corns and calluses contribute; take care of them when they appear. *See ARTHRITIS THERAPY page 324.*

Diet and Lifestyle Support Therapy

Nutritional therapy plan:

1—Gout is clearly caused by dietary factors. Reduce caffeine, white flour foods, fried foods, and fatty foods, especially red meats. Avoid high levels of fructose in any food or drink. Eliminate alcohol during healing; it inhibits uric acid secretion from the kidneys. Highly recommended: •Crystal Star DR. VITALITY™ green and white tea, or •Aloe vera juice each morning.

2—Go on a bladder/kidney liquid cleansing diet (pg. 197) to rid the body of sediment wastes. Barley grass juice, like •Green Kamut JUST BARLEY drink is a specific for gout.

3—Follow with a diet of 75% fresh foods for a month to balance uric acid formation.

4—Drink 4 glasses of black cherry juice (or try •Jarrow GENTLE FIBERS drink daily) and 6 glasses of water daily. Eat cherries and other dark fruits.

5—Eat high potassium foods: fresh cherries of all kinds and cherry juice, bananas, strawberries, celery, broccoli, potatoes, green and sea veggies to put acid crystals in solution so they can be eliminated. Or try •Potassium broth (page 291).

6—Avoid high purine foods: red meats, rich gravies, broths, sweetbreads, organ meats, mushrooms, asparagus, legumes (esp. peanuts), spinach, rhubarb, sardines, anchovies, nutritional yeast, lobster, oysters, clams.

—Lifestyle measures:

•Lose weight to ease pressure on feet and legs. But lose it slowly. Rapid weight loss shocks your metabolism and may trigger a gout attack.
•Check your high blood pressure medicine. Several of them cause formation of inorganic crystal sediments. •Avoid aspirin. It can raise uric acid levels.
•A visit to a natural hot springs can provide effective pain relief.

—Bodywork: wiggle and rotate toes to boost circulation.

•Apply plantain (good results), ginger, or fresh comfrey compresses to inflamed area.
•Apply topical DMSO with aloe vera to painful area to help dissolve crystalline deposits (usually 2 to 4 days before results.) or •Apply Boiron ARNICA GEL for pain relief.

Herbal, Superfood and Supplement Therapy

Interceptive therapy plan: Choose 2 or more recommendations.

1—Take down inflammation and pain: •Crystal Star DR. ENZYME™ caps with protease and bromelain, or ANTI-FLAM™ capsules (with white willow), with ADRENAL ENERGY BOOST caps daily. •Enzymatic Therapy CHERRY JUICE extract (good results). •Quercetin 1000mg with bromelain 1500mg 3x daily until relief. •Ho-Shou-Wu (*Fo-Ti*). •Nutricology GERMANIUM 150mg reduces pain and swelling. •B-complex 100mg with extra B₆ 250mg and folic acid 800mcg 3x daily inhibits xanthine oxidase.

Herbal diuretics reduce swelling without potassium loss: •Crystal Star BLAD-DER-KIDNEY COMFORT™ caps or TINKLE™ tea; or *Buchu* tea.

2—Reduce uric acid accumulation: •Vitamin C therapy for almost immediate relief - take ascorbate Vitamin C with bioflavonoids and rutin, ¼ tsp. at a time in water every 4 hours for 1 week, then 5000mg daily for 3 weeks. Take with •lithium orotate, 5 to 10mg for best results. •Take Enzymatic Therapy ACID-A-CAL caps; •Enzymedica PURIFY, protease enzymes balance pH levels; •DEVILS CLAW extract reduces uric acid and cholesterol build-up. •*Dandelion* and *Sarsaparilla* tea 2 cups daily flush acids.

3—Essential fatty acids inhibit leukotriene production: •Omega-3 rich flax oil 2 tbsp. daily; •Evening Primrose oil 3000mg daily.

4—Enrich your body flavonoids: •*Hawthorn* or *Bilberry* extract 4x daily; •PCO's from grapeseed and white pine bark, 100mg 3x daily.

5—Rebalance thyroid (hypothyroidism is involved in gout): •Take sea greens 2 tbsp. daily, or •Crystal Star OCEAN MINERALS™ caps, or Solaray ALFAJUICE tabs, or •FutureBiotics VITAL K 3 tsp. daily to normalize thyroid activity.

6—Regulate blood sugar, increase circulation: •Glycine 500mg daily. with chromium picolinate 200mcg; •Biotech CELL-GUARD with SOD, 6 daily; •Niacin 50mg.

—Superfood therapy: (Choose one or two recommendations.)
•Crystal Star RESTORE YOUR STRENGTH™ for iodine and potassium. •Alacer EMERGEN-C drink mix. •Pure Planet TART CHERRY CONCENTRATE.

Can't find a recommended product? Call the 800 number listed in Product Resources for the store nearest you.

Graves' Disease

Hyperthyroidism, Hyper-parathyroidism

Graves' disease is a result of too much thyroid (thyroxine) secretion. It means an overactive metabolism, and every body process speeds up - digestion, nervous energy, impatience, perspiration, the inability to rest even though tired, hair loss, unhealthy weight loss, rapid heartbeat, climate sensitivity, even aging. Graves' disease affects women far more than men (65,000 women a year), and younger people far more than the elderly. **Hyperparathyroidism**, too much PTH secretion, affects blood calcium levels and can lead to kidney stones and osteoporosis. **Signs you may have an overactive thyroid:** Bulging eyes and blurred vision (thyroid-related ophthalmopathy), nervous tension and irritability are common. Restlessness with insomnia, sweating and tremors; itching, burning eyes and skin; along with arthritis-like joint swelling are frequent. Most sufferers experience unhealthy weight loss with diarrhea, extreme sensitivity to light, mood swings, and sometimes mental psychosis during a "thyroid storm." Younger victims often have a goiter; older victims have heart palpitations. **What causes overactive thyroid?** Autoimmune traits may be inherited, but for most women, it's stress, overuse of diet pills, mental burnout and fatigue that are the triggers. A few have a bacterial infection in the thyroid gland (Mycoplasma). *See GLAND HEALTH page 427 for more. Or call the American Thyroid Association 800-849-7643.*

Diet and Lifestyle Support Therapy

Nutritional therapy plan: *An overactive thyroid responds well to natural therapies.*

1—For the first month of healing, follow a diet of about 75% fresh foods. Include plenty of vegetable proteins from sprouts, sea greens, soy foods and whole grains. Have a daily potassium drink (pg. 291) or green drink, like •Crystal Star ENERGY GREEN RENEWAL™ drink, with sea veggies and green superfoods like spirulina.

2—Add B vitamins and complex carbohydrates from brown rice and vegetables.

3—Eat plenty of cultured foods for friendly G.I. flora - yogurt, kefir, raw sauerkraut (cultured veggies).

4—Make a mix of nutritional yeast, toasted wheat germ, lecithin; take 2 tbsp. daily in a fresh fruit smoothie.

5—Drink 8 glasses of water daily, and carrot juice 3x a week; take papaya juice for adrenal support. Avoid stimulants like caffeine and sodas.

—**Thyroid-balancing foods:** raw cruciferous vegetables, like cabbage, cauliflower, broccoli and kale, beets, spinach. (Cooking inactivates most thyroid lowering ability.)

—**Bodywork:**
•Exercise daily to the point of breathlessness and mild sweating.
•Get some early morning sun on the body every day possible. Wade and swim in the ocean frequently to access naturally-occurring thyroid minerals.
•Acupressure points: press points on both sides of the spinal column at the base of the neck, 3 times for 10 seconds each.

Note: Conventional medicine relies on radioactive iodine to kill the cells that produce thyroid hormone. After treatment, patients use synthetic thyroid durgs (Synthroid) linked to bone loss, headaches, insomnia and tachycardia (rapid contractions of the heart) for the rest of their life. Ask your doctor plainly about drug interactions if you take synthroid for overactive thyroid. Some drugs, like over-the-counter diet pills, can both bring on and aggravate a thyroid problem.

Herbal, Superfood and Supplement Therapy

Interceptive therapy plan: Choose 2 or more recommendations.

1—**Help balance thyroid and metabolism:** •Crystal Star TOXIN DETOX™ caps with bugleweed and sea veggies helps reduce T-4 by inhibiting thyroid stimulating antibodies (sometimes dramatic results); may be used with •Crystal Star OCEAN MINERALS™ capsules 2-4 daily or •Futurebiotics VITAL K daily. •Gaia Herbs BUGLEWEED-MOTH-ERWORT extract; •*Ginkgo Biloba* extract; •*Mullein-Lobelia* extract; •Enzymatic Therapy THYROID/TYROSINE COMPLEX 4 daily (highly recommended). •*Astragalus* extract capsules 4 daily; •Holy Basil extract helps reduce T4.

2—**Calm thyroid storms:** •Calcium citrate 4 daily; •EVENING PRIMROSE OIL or *borage* oil caps 500mg 4 to 6 daily; •Transformation Enzyme CALMZYME. •Lecithin 1900gr daily; or •Vitamin E 800IU daily; •Crystal Star RELAX™ caps; •*Hawthorn* leaf, berry and flower extract; Niacinamide 100mg daily for thyroid-related ophthalmopathy.

3—**Support the liver:** •Crystal Star LIVER CLEANSE FLUSHING™ tea for 1 month, then •*Milk Thistle Seed* extract for 2 months. Then LIVER RENEW™ caps or •Enzymatic Therapy LIQUID LIVER caps, or •Siberian eleuthero extract capsules 2000mg.

4—**Ease stress and sleeplessness:** •Stress B-complex with extra B$_2$ 100mg, and B$_6$ 100mg. •Nature's Secret ULTIMATE B; •Rainbow Light ADAPTOGEM caps; •Country Life STRESS "M."

5—**Establish immune health:** •CoQ-10, 200mg daily; •Marine carotenes, Solgar OCEANIC CAROTENE 100,000IU, or •Royal Bodycare PHYCOTENE MICROCLUSTERS with 17 carotenoids from *spirulina* and *dunaliella* algae; •Ester C with bioflavs. 6 daily; •Zinc picolinate 50-75mg daily. •Diamond Herpanacine HEALTHY HORIZONS with natural vitamin E and alpha lipoic acid effectively fights Grave's free radical damage.

—**Superfood therapy:** (Choose one or two recommmedations.)
•Crystal Star RESTORE YOUR STRENGTH™ drink for absorbable iodine and potassium.
•Nutri-Tech ALL ONE vitamin-mineral drink.
•CC Pollen POLLEN ENERGY.
•Futurebiotics VITAL K, 2 tsp. daily.

Can't find a recommended product? Call the 800 number listed in Product Resources for the store nearest you.

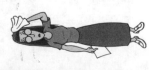

Hair Growth
Healthy Hair, Graying Hair

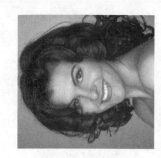

We all want it... thick, gorgeous hair. Your scalp has at least 100,000 hairs (normally shed about 25 to 50 hairs a day) so you have a lot to work with. Your hair is one of the mirrors of your health and your diet. Hair consists of protein layers called keratin. In healthy hair, the cell walls of the hair cuticle lie flat like shingles, leaving hair soft and shiny. In damaged or dry hair, the cuticle shingles are broken and create gaps that make hair porous and dull. **Hair problems?** They're never isolated conditions, but the result of more basic body imbalances. In fact, changes in hair are often the first indication of nutritional deficiencies. Too dry or too oily hair; lots of falling hair; dull hair; flaky deposits on the scalp; brittle hair with split ends; lack of bounce and elasticity can all signal body imbalance. **Bad hair causes?** Multiple mineral deficiencies, lack of usable protein, poor circulation, recent illness and drug residues, liver malfunction resulting in loss of hair. Be careful of the hair dyes you use. A new study shows that permanent hair dyes more than once a month double the risk for bladder cancer. Using the dyes for 15 years or longer tripled the risk! •Concerned about lead-based hair dyes? Natural henna is non-carcinogenic and used for centuries to color. Works best on thin, light, porous hair, often offering dramatic body. *See next page and* DANDRUFF *page 386 for more.*

Diet and Lifestyle Support Therapy

Nutritional therapy plan for prevention:

1—A good diet is the real secret to great hair. Feed hair a vegetable protein diet. Mix these hair foods and take 3 tbsp. daily in juice: wheat germ (oil or flakes), blackstrap molasses, Red Star nutritional yeast (B-vitamins and for color) and sesame seeds.

2—Hair foods: Carrots, bell peppers, lettuces, bananas, strawberries, apples, peas, onions, cucumber, sprouts, Aloe vera juice, green or white tea. •A protein drink each morning can have dramatic effects on dry hair: Unipro PERFECT PROTEIN, or Solgar WHEY TO GO.

3—Avoid saturated fats, sugars and highly processed foods. They show up in hair health. A diet high in essential fatty acids (healthy fats) like seafood, sea greens, cantaloupe, spinach, perilla or flax oil, adds shine and increases volume.

4—Poor liver function equals unhealthy hair. Too much alcohol, caffeine and drugs put a heavy load on the liver and rob the body of B vitamins.

—**Kitchen cosmetics for hair:** 1) Wet hair, blot, apply 4 tbsp. mayonnaise or mashed avocado. Wrap in a towel for 30 minutes. Rinse/shampoo. 2) Mix yogurt and an egg; apply to hair. Wrap in a towel for 30 minutes. Rinse /shampoo. 3) Mix 1 egg yolk with your second shampoo for bounce. 4) Condition dry, limp hair: mix olive oil (try Home Health olive oil) with drops of essential lavender and rosemary oil and rub in hair. Leave on 5 minutes and rinse. 5) Super hair texture: Make 8-oz green tea and 8-oz. rosemary tea (with fresh sprigs if possible). Strain each. Add 1 tbsp. lemon juice and 1 tbsp. white vinegar. Work through hair and leave on 1 minute. Rinse.

—**Bodywork:**
•Massage scalp each morning for 3 minutes to stimulate hair growth.
•Sunlight helps hair grow, but too much sun dries and damages.
•Wash hair in warm, not hot water. Rinse in cool water for scalp circulation.
•Chlorine residue? Add 2-3 tbsp. cider vinegar to your shampoo to clarify hair.
•Shampoos rich in EFAs: Henna, Aloe Vera, Neem oil or Babassu palm shampoos.
•Rinse hair in sea water or kelp water for body.

Herbal, Superfood and Supplement Therapy

Interceptive therapy plan: Choose 2 to 3 recommendations.

1—**Minerals from herbs and sea greens are dramatic for hair growth:** •Crystal Star BEAUTIFUL HAIR & NAILS™ high sea greens caps (also a good rinse for shine). Natural silica boosts hair strength: Horsetail extract; or Flora VEGE-SIL capsules. Clinically proven: •MSM 4000mg daily for 6 weeks. •Thyme, Cedarwood essential oils; or •Rosemary or Lavender sprigs steeped in wine. Amazing for hair growth: •2 tbsp. daily dried snipped sea greens (use dulse if there is also iron deficiency- affects blood flow to the scalp), or •Crystal Star OCEAN MINERALS™ caps 4 daily, (highly recommended); •Lane Labs TOKI collagen replacement drink; •Eidon ZINC liquid for enhanced collagen production; •New Chapter OCEAN HERBS; •Nature's Path TRACE-MIN-LYTE.

2—**Prevent early gray:** Lane Labs TOKI COLOR hair color support caps, with •Crystal Star ADRENAL ENERGY BOOST™ (results noticeable in about 3 months); •Green Nutrition INDIUMEASE (excellent results); •Ho-Shou-Wu or Gotu kola extracts; •Bio-Tech SHEN-MIN caps or; •Cat's Claw extract for 3 months to return hair to original color.

3—**EFAs are imperative for damaged hair:** plant-based products with sage and calendula for body, wheat germ oil or jojoba for condition. •Crystal Star RESTORE YOUR STRENGTH™ drink (EFAs from sea greens). •Evening Primrose oil 2000mg daily. Rub in Jojoba oil daily until sebum deposits disappear. •Use Hemp or Henna shampoo.

4—**Restore hair color and growth after illness or radiation treatments:** 1 each daily: PABA 1000mg, molasses 2 tbsp., pantothenic acid 1000mg, folic acid 800mcg, B-complex 100mg with extra B₆ 100mg and folic acid 800mcg, Country Life sublingual B-12, 2500mcg a day. New hair visible noticeably in about 3 weeks. •Biotin 600mcg daily.
•Tyrosine 1000mg daily; •Vitamin C with bioflavs 6 daily; •Cysteine 1000mg;

—**For oily hair:** plant-based astringent products with witch hazel or lemon balm. Rinse hair with white vinegar after your shampoo. Or, try Lamas WHEATGRASS DEEP CLEANSING shampoo.

—**Enhancers for dry hair:** plant-based products with burdock, nettles and rosemary. Ayurvedic BRAHMI oil (infuse gotu kola in sesame oil, then strain and apply from scalp to ends, rinse after 10 minutes); Camocare concentrate, for dazzle.

Can't find a recommended product? Call the 800 number listed in Product Resources for the store nearest you.

Hair Loss

Alopecia, Male Pattern Baldness

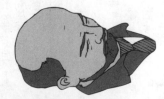

Over 40 million men and 20 million women have thinning hair. *Alopecia areata* affects 2.5 million people, and may be triggered by a glitch in the immune system. Heavy hair loss may signal of an early heart attack. Female pattern baldness, related to heredity, thyroid disease and hormonal changes, represents 50% of women who have permanent hair loss. Although hereditary pattern baldness is not easily reversible, other factors are involved in most hair loss that can be improved for thickness and regrowth. Hair health depends on blood circulation and nutrition. Your therapy choice must be vigorously followed. Occasional therapy has no effect. Two months is usually the minimum for really noticeable growth. **Are you at risk for permanent hair loss?** Poor circulation is one of the most common causes. Poor diet with too much salt and sugar, and too little protein is always involved. For women, a primary cause is thyroid gland imbalance and overproduction of male sex hormones, from postpartum changes or discontinuing birth control pills. Hair loss above the temples in women can mean a possible ovarian or adrenal tumor. Contributors: dandruff or seborrhea sebum plugs, high cholesterol, chemotherapy and high blood pressure drugs which sap B vitamins, prolonged emotional stress, anemia from severe illness, and mineral deficiencies. *See previous page and Menopausal Hair Loss page 494 for more.*

Diet and Lifestyle Support Therapy

Nutritional therapy plan:
1—Most important diet tip: eat sea greens every day for EFAs. 2 tbsp. dried, snipped sea greens over rice, soup or salad daily (produces real results).
2—Eat foods rich in silica and sulphur: beets, parsley, sea greens, garlic and onions, sprouts, horseradish, green leafy veggies, carrots, bell peppers, eggs, apricots, cucumbers, rice, and seeds. •ALL 1 MULTIPLE drink with green plant base.
3—Eat foods rich in iodine and potassium: sea greens and seafoods for thickness. Try •Crystal Star RESTORE YOUR STRENGTH™ drink for absorbable minerals and sea greens.
4—Add soy foods for phyto-hormones, plant protein, EFAs and vitamin E.
5—Add biotin-rich foods: brown rice, lentils, oats, soy foods and walnuts.
6—Drink 6 glasses of water daily. PENTA bottled water is ideal for absorption.
7—Reduce salt, sugar and caffeine; avoid animal fats, fast foods and preserved foods.
—**Take a hair protein mix to stop the shedding:** wheat germ flakes, nutritional yeast, pumpkin seeds, chopped dulse; take 2 tbsp. daily in food.
—**Active scalp conditioners:** 1) Jojoba oil and shampoo relieves sebum build-up - Hobe ENERGIZER TREATMENT shampoo; 2) Aloe vera oil; 3) CURETAGE shampoo- conditioner with cayenne for alopecia.

—**Bodywork:**
•Be careful of tight hairstyles and curlers, hot rollers, and chemicals for perming or straightening. Discontinue commercial hair coloring, flat irons, hot hair dryers.
•Stress is clearly a contributor: Get a massage therapy treatment once a week (with scalp massage). Get outdoor exercise every day possible for body oxygen.
•Rinse hair with sea water, a rosemary-dulse tea or kelp "tea" for thickness.
•Aromatherapy oils for alopecia: *lavender, cedarwood, rosemary,* and *thyme* blended with jojoba and grapeseed oil. (Good clinical results.)
—**Head circulation is a key:** •Finger massage scalp vigorously for 3 minutes each morning. •Brush hair for 5 minutes daily. •Rinse for several minutes with alternating hot and cold shower water. •Use a slant board once a week.

Herbal, Superfood and Supplement Therapy

Interceptive therapy plan: Choose 2 to 3 recommendations.
1—**Natural silica boosts hair strength:** Crystal Star BEAUTIFUL HAIR & NAILS caps; •horsetail tea, or •Flora VEGE-SIL capsules. •Futurebiotics HAIR, SKIN AND NAILS for men and women; •Green Nutrition INDIUMEASE (for new hair growth).
2—**Sea greens feed your hair:** •2 tbsp. daily dry snipped sea greens like kelp, or •Crystal Star OCEAN MINERALS™ caps 4 daily, or •Green Foods ION KELP tablets daily; or •Arise & Shine liquid ORGANIC SEA MINERALS; •New Chapter OCEAN HERBS; •Nature's Path TRACE-MIN-LYTE with sea greens.
3—**EFAs are imperative to hair growth:** •Evening Primrose Oil 3000mg or *borage* oil caps, •Omega Nutrition OMEGA PLUS caps; •Spectrum high lignan FLAX OIL, 3 caps daily (results within 6 weeks). •Omega Nutrition Coconut Butter; •GINSENG/REISHI extract.
4—**Stimulate your scalp:** •Ginkgo Biloba - regrowth; •White sage tea - thinning hair; •*Sage* oil - hair restorative properties; •CoQ-10, 200mg daily, plus •*Cayenne-Ginger* tea rub on, leave in 10 minutes for scalp circulation. Or, 4 tbsp. aloe vera gel, 1 tbsp. jojoba oil, 1 tsp. rosemary essential oil, ¼ tsp. ginger powder.
5—**Feed your hair amino acids:** •Cysteine 2000mg daily with •zinc 75mg daily with •zinc 75mg daily with zinc deficiency. •Anabol Naturals AMINO BALANCE caps for regrowth (highly recommended).
6—**Treat your prostate to treat your hair loss:** Male pattern baldness emanates from testosterone levels. •Prostate remedies - *saw palmetto, pygeum, potency wood,* and *panax ginseng* or •Crystal Star PROSTATE PROTECTOR™ caps or •New Chapter PROSTATE 5lx softgels; •Copper 2mg help inhibit 5 alpha-reductase enzymes.
7—**Hormone balancing herbs help women's hair loss:** •A *black cohosh, dong quai, burdock* combination, or •Crystal Star EST-AID™ caps; •Pure Essence Labs FEM CREME for hair loss after pregnancy (due to low progesterone).
8—**B-vitamins help hair growth** (noticeable within 3 months): •2 tbsp. or more black-strap molasses daily; •B-complex 150mg daily with extra niacin 50mg daily, B6 50mg daily; •AMAZAKE rice drinks for B vitamins.

Can't find a recommended product? Call the 800 number listed in Product Resources for the store nearest you.

Hashimoto's Disease

Chronic Lymphocytic Thyroiditis

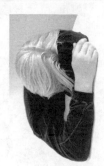

An autoimmune disorder where the immune system suddenly attacks healthy tissue, Hashimoto's is the most frequent cause of hypothyroidism (low thyroid), and the most common cause of enlarged thyroid (goiter) in America. Most prevalent in menopausal women who live high stress lives, almost one in ten women over the age of 65 have early-stage hypothyroidism clearly linked to Hashimoto's! At its worst, Hashimoto's can completely destroy the thyroid gland. **Are you at risk for Hashimoto's?** Symptoms are wide ranging and seemingly unrelated… painless thyroid enlargement, great fatigue and loss of enthusiasm for life, unusual weight gain, high cholesterol and triglycerides, sensitivity to cold, dry skin, brittle nails and thin, falling hair. **Do we know what causes Hashimoto's?** Iodine depletion from X-rays or low dose radiation like mammograms may be a prime factor in its development. Hashimoto's hypothyroidism can be easily determined by a simple blood test. Conventional medical treatment is a lifelong prescription of synthetic thyroid hormone. But for many women, synthroid is linked to severe headaches, insomnia, bone loss and rapid heart contractions. An unbalanced thyroid invariably causes over-production of estrogen for women, leading to other problems. Shifting emphasis toward natural therapies can greatly raise your own healing capacities.

Diet and Lifestyle Support Therapy

Nutritional therapy plan:

1—A largely fresh foods, immune-boosting diet full of fruits and vegetables is the mainstay of treatment for this disease. Take a mixed veggie drink or a potassium broth (pg. 291) several times weekly. Or try •Fit for You, Intl. MIRACLE GREENS with dulse, or •Body Ecology VITALITY SUPER GREENS; •Sun Wellness CHLORELLA drink or •Crystal Star RESTORE YOUR STRENGTH™ drink or caps daily for 2 to 3 months.

2—Avoid "goitrogen" foods that prevent your body's use of iodine, like cabbage, turnips, peanuts, mustard, pine nuts, millet, tempeh and tofu. (Cooking these foods inactivates the goitrogens.) Note: Cancer of the thyroid has been linked to highly fluoridated water. Watch for bottled brands; some contain fluoride.

3—Avoid table salt, (use an herb salt instead), but eat plenty of iodine-rich foods: sea greens (2 tbsp. daily over rice, soup or a salad), seafoods, fish, mushrooms, garlic, onions and watercress.

4—Especially eat vitamin A-rich foods: yellow vegetables, eggs, carrots, dark greens, raw dairy. Avoid fluorescent lights and fluoride toothpaste. They deplete vitamin A in the body. If you work under fluorescents, take Emulsified A 25,000IU 3x daily, or beta carotene 100,000IU daily, with vitamin E 400IU daily.

5—Avoid fatty foods, fast foods, sugars, white flour and red meats.

—Bodywork:

• Take a brisk half hour walk daily; exercise increases metabolism and stimulates circulation.
• Apply alternating hot and cold packs on the thyroid gland 3x a week to stimulate circulation.
• Sun bathe in the morning. Sea bathe and wade whenever possible.
• The drug levothyroxine, frequently given for hypothyroidism can cause significant bone loss. Ask your doctor. Avoid antihistamines and sulfa drugs.
• For dry skin from thyroid malfunction, apply Herbal Answers ALOE FORCE GEL.

—Acupressure point:

• Press hollow at base of the throat to stimulate thyroid, 3x for 10 seconds each.

Herbal, Superfood and Supplement Therapy

Interceptive therapy plan: Choose 2 or more recommendations.

1—**Raw glandular therapy helps dramatically:** •Nutricology TG-100 capsules (highly recommended); •Gaia Herbs THYROID SUPPORT caps; •Enzymatic Therapy THYROID-TYROSINE COMPLEX (recommended); or •Tyrosine 1000mg with Lysine 1000mg daily; •Raw Adrenal glandular or •Country Life ADRENAL SUPPORT w. tyrosine. *Note:* If you take thyroid hormone medication for Hashimoto's, don't take iron supplements along with the medicine. Iron binds up thyroxine, rendering it insoluble.

2—**Balance thyroid function:** Your thyroid needs iodine to produce its hormones. Low thyroid invariably means too much estrogen with numerous problems for women. Herbal iodine, especially sea herbs, is effective without side effects. •Crystal Star IODINE, POTASSIUM, SILICA extract or •OCEAN MINERALS™ caps 2x daily, kelp tablets or •Green Foods ION KELP (recommended); •New Chapter OCEAN HERBS; •Solaray ALFA JUICE caps; •Burdock or dandelion rt. tea 3x a week supports the liver (involved with T3 production); •Nutricology GUGGUL LIPIDS help fight thyroid-related weight gain.

3—**Enhance adrenals:** •Crystal Star ADRENAL ENERGY BOOST™ caps (almost immediate energy) or •THYROID META MAX 6 daily; •Planetary SCHIZANDRA ADRENAL complex.; •Sarsaparilla extract; •Evening Primrose oil caps 3000mg daily; •Eidon ZINC liquid.

4—**Treat constipation:** low thyroid can lead to body toxicity and immune system impairment. Gentle bowel cleansers like aloe vera, triphala or slippery elm are good choices. •Crystal Star BWL-TONE IBS™ caps, 2 caps 3x daily; •Nutricology PERMAVITE drink mix with slippery elm; Ascorbate vitamin C with bioflavonoids 3000mg daily.

5—**Protect cardiovascular health:** Hypothyroidism accelerates atherosclerosis! Tone with •Hawthorn and •Ginkgo Biloba extracts; add •CoQ₁₀ 100mg or Esteem CARDIOLIFE with CoQ10 daily and •Country Life sublingual B-12 2500mcg; and Omega 3 fish oil.

6—**Boost circulation and repair nerves:** •Gotu kola extract caps, up to 6 daily; •Siberian eleuthero extract 2x daily; •Cayenne-Ginger caps 3 daily.

—**For goiter:** paint •BLACK WALNUT extract on throat, and take ½ dropperful 2x daily; drink 2 cups burdock tea daily, apply •calendula compresses daily for a month.

Can't find a recommended product? Call the 800 number listed in Product Resources for the store nearest you.

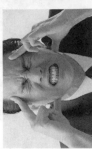

Headaches - Vascular

Migraines, Vascular Headaches, Cluster Headaches

Migraines are more than just bad headaches. They're a total body assault. Almost 30 million Americans suffer from migraines. Migraines in young women who have estrogen dominance are up 56% since 1979. **Classic migraines** mean constriction/dilation of brain, scalp and face blood vessels and throbbing pain, lasting anywhere from 4 hours to two days, several times a month. They are preceded by an aura, sudden sensitivity to smell and light, nausea, vomiting, chills and fever... and can last up to 3 or 4 days. **Common migraines** have no aura, but the same pain and visual disturbances, distorted taste and smell, weakness and confusion. **Cluster headaches** mean two or more sudden, extremely painful headaches *a day*, accompanied by nausea and great sensitivity to light and movement. They cluster over the forehead or eyes causing distorted vision. They usually affect men and appear to be connected to testosterone imbalance, repressed anger and histamine reactions. Raised blood fats during attacks reduce serotonin levels, causing dilation of blood vessels in the brain and thus migraine pain. Prescription drugs can reduce migraine frequency and severity, but may also cause rebound headaches when the drugs are discontinued. If you have a history of heart problems, ask your doctor before taking migraine medicines that constrict blood vessels. Common causes include estrogen or testosterone imbalance, and reaction to drugs like Viagra.

Diet and Lifestyle Support Therapy

Nutritional therapy: *Nutritional awareness is a must for prevention.*

1—Food allergies are the biggest migraine triggers. The most common are allergies to wheat, dairy and sensitivity to caffeine (withdrawal can be a precipitator). Avoid known triggers: Nitrate foods like pickled fish or shellfish, smoked meats, aged cheeses, red wine, avocados, chocolate, pizza, sourdough bread, refined sugars or aspartame. Avoid red meats, sodas (phosphorus binds up magnesium), MSG, soy sauce, citrus, peanuts, tomatoes and hard liquor. See the Hypoglycemia Diet page 463 to help blood sugar regulation.

2—At the first signs of a migraine: take 1-2 cups of strong coffee to prevent blood vessel dilation (not if caffeine sensitive), or a glass of carrot-celery juice.

3—Eat pain preventers: High magnesium foods reduce throbbing: leafy greens, fresh seafoods and sea greens, nuts, whole grains, molasses. •Vitamin C rich foods: pineapple for bromelain. •Turkey for serotonin. Drink green tea daily or Crystal Star GREEN TEA CLEANSER™ as a preventive.

—Bodywork:

•ICE IT. Chill a head wrap and slip it on, or put an ice pack on the back of the neck to reduce swelling; or put your feet in cold water to draw blood from the head. Staying in a cool room provides relief.

•Almost immediate results: a coffee enema to stimulate liver and normalize bile activity; a bowel movement may relieve vomiting.

•Physical therapies: 1) Chiropractic manipulation 2) Acupuncture and acupressure 3) Massage therapy 4) Biofeedback 5) Deep breathing exercises, 6) Magnet therapy is effective for migraines.

—Reflexology therapy: Apply lavender essential oil to temples. Then 1) Apply pressure to inside base of the big toe 3 times for 10 seconds each time. 2) Massage temples for 5 minutes. Breathe deeply. 3) Do 10 neck rolls. Pull ear lobes for 5 seconds. Rub all around ear shell. 4) Hold hand open, palm down; massage flesh between thumb and forefinger with other hand. Pain begins to recede immediately.

Herbal, Superfood and Supplement Therapy

Interceptive therapy: *A colon cleanse is very effective in stopping vascular headaches.*

1—**Help control the pain:** *For Migraines:* •Crystal Star ANTI-FLAM™ caps; •NatureWell MIGRA SPRAY (usually works in 7 minutes or less); •Feverfew extract caps. Try LifeSpan SNEEZE-EZE 3 days a week to prevent migraines. •Gaia MIGRA-PROFEN. •Weber & Weber PETADOLEX with *butterbur* extract shows good results. •DLPA 1000mg for pain control. •Wakunaga AGED GARLIC extract fights accompanying *H. pylori. For Cluster Headaches:* •One ginger cap at first sign of visual disturbance. Then take •Crystal Star STRESS OUT™ extract, (usually results in 25 minutes). Rub •CAPSAICIN cream on temples or take •*Capsicum-Ginger* capsules 4 daily. •Ethical Nutrients ZINC STATUS and •New Chapter GINGER WONDER SYRUP to reduce nausea.

2—**Magnesium checks release of pain-producing chemicals:** •magnesium citrate 800mg daily; •Floradix MAGNESIUM liquid; or •Nature's Plus QUERCETIN PLUS 1000mg daily with magnesium 1000mg daily for nerves. •Glutamine 1000mg 2x daily.

3—**Calm stress reactions:** •5-HTP, 50mg (proven results) or •Natural Balance HTP Calm; •Crystal Star RELAX CAPS™ for painful spasms. •Esteem Products MELLOW OUT before bed; •Twin Lab GABA PLUS, or •Country Life RELAXER caps for brain stress.

4—**B-vitamin therapy:** •Stress B-complex 100mg or •Nature's Secret ULTIMATE B; •Country Life sublingual B-12 2500mcg. •Royal jelly, up to 50,000mg daily. •Niacin for migraines: up to 500mg daily (not recommended for cluster headaches).

5—**Add EFAs:** •Evening primrose oil, 4000mg daily; Omega-3 flax caps 3 daily. •Nutricology PRO-GREENS with EFAs.

6—**For hormone-related migraines:** •*Dong quai-damiana-ashwagandha* caps. •Rub on temples Pure Essence FEM CREME.

7—**Antioxidants are a key:** •Detox to help migraines related to chemical overload: Vitamin C 5000mg, 800mg glutathione and 400mg alpha lipoic acid; •Nutricology GER-MANIUM 150mg; •Melatonin an antioxidant hormone .3mg at night for cluster headaches, 1 week on, 1 week off. •MICROHYDRIN PLUS, especially for migraines.

Can't find a recommended product? Call the 800 number listed in Product Resources for the store nearest you.

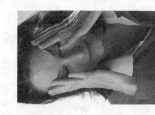

Headaches - Stress and Tension

Sinus Headaches, Nervous Headaches

Headaches don't fit into neat little diagnostic boxes. There seem to be as many kinds of headaches as people who have them. *Tension headaches* are muscle contraction headaches in the temples or back of the head, usually caused by stress or fatigue, may last for hours or days. ... your head feels like it's in a vise; it's hard to sleep. Tension headaches respond well to treatments like massage, acupressure, and cold compresses. **Do you get lots of headaches?** Headache causes span the range of our modern lifestyles: emotional stress, food allergies, computer eyestrain, pinched nerves, constipation; too much caffeine, salt, sugar or MSG; hypoglycemia, PMS, artificial sweeteners like Aspartame (Nutrasweet, Equal); a sluggish liver, arthritis, Candida albicans or herpes simplex infection, and heavy metal poisoning are some of the more common headache generators. Flickering fluorescent light bulbs can bring on a blinding headache. **Beware.** Overusing drugstore headache drugs can cause rebound headaches and health problems over the long term. Acetaminophen can damage the liver, especially when taken with alcohol. NSAIDS drugs like buprofen and aspirin, commonly used to relieve headaches, can cause serious gastrointestinal problems. In fact, NSAIDs send 76,000 people to the hospital and kill 7,600 people every year!

Diet and Lifestyle Support Therapy

Nutritional therapy plan: See also SINUSITIS page 539 AND STRESS page 553.

1—Go on a short 24 hour juice fast (pg. 173) to remove congestion. Drink lots of water and lemon, veggie drinks (like Knudsen's VERY VEGGIE) or potassium broth. (pg. 291). Or try •Nutricology PRO-GREENS w. EFAs or•Solgar EARTH SOURCE GREENS & MORE with EFAs, or •Crystal Star RESTORE YOUR STRENGTH™ drink with sea veggie EFAs.

2—Follow with an alkalizing diet: apples and apple juice, cranberry or cherry juice, sprouts, salads and some brown rice. Make a mix of nutritional yeast, lecithin granules, cider vinegar and honey; take 2 tbsp. daily in juice to restore body balance:

3—*Avoid headache trigger foods:* •Additive, sulfites, MSG laced foods. •Salty, sugary, wheat-based foods. •Overuse of high caffeine foods. •Cheese. •Nitrate preserved meats. •Overusing alcohol, beer, wine. Hot peppers help open up sinuses.

4—Apply cold black tea bags to eyes for 15 minutes, or just have some black coffee.

5—Use salicin from almonds...just 12 to 15 almonds can relieve a headache.

6—When you feel a headache come on, immediately take ginger capsules, drink ginger tea, or eat some crystallized ginger. Or try New Chapter GINGER WONDER syrup.

—Lifestyle measures:

•ICE IT. Apply an ice pack on the back of the neck and upper back. Add a hot foot bath and pain reduction is dramatic. Or try alternating hot and cold showers.

•Take a brisk walk. Breathe deeply. The more brain oxygen, the fewer headaches. Stay well hydrated to decrease muscle spasms that lead to headaches.

•Onion or horseradish poultices applied to the nape of the neck or soles of the feet relieve headache inflammation.

•Use a HEPA (high efficiency particulate air) filter to clean indoor allergens.

•Apply lavender or peppermint aromatherapy oils on the temples.

•At home technique: Apply pressure to the sorest points on your neck, shoulder and upper back for 10 seconds. Follow by massaging the area and •Dip a cold, wet washcloth into cold witch hazel, or catnip-sage tea and use on your forehead.

Herbal, Superfood and Supplement Therapy

Interceptive therapy plan: Choose 2 or 3 recommendations.

1—**Relax, relieve tension**: •Crystal Star STRESS OUT™ drops (fast acting, usually works in 25 minutes); •Bromelain 1500mg, acts like aspirin without stomach upset. •Pacific BioLogic CHILL OUT or •Bach Flowers RESCUE REMEDY combat stress headache; •*Valerian-Wild Lettuce* or *Scullcap* extracts; •Homeopathic Hylands *Calms Forte.*

2—**Enhance nerve health:** Mineral-rich herbs provide key bio-chemical ingredients for neurotransmission. •Crystal Star RELAX™ caps, help rebuild nerves (relief in about 25 minutes). •Nature's Plus QUERCETIN PLUS 1000mg daily with magnesium 1000mg daily, prevent nerve twitches.; Medicine Wheel STRESS EASE; •Jarrow THEANINE caps.

3—**Magnesium and B-vitamin therapy:** Crystal Star CALCIUM-MAGNESIUM SOURCE™ caps; •Floradix CALCIUM, MAGNESIUM liquid; •Magnesium citrate 800mg daily with •Country Life MAXI-E with taurine. •Niacin therapy: 100mg as needed daily.

4—**Balance your body with tonics and EFAs:** •Guayaki YERBA MATÉ green tea, an almost immediate tonic for stress headaches. •Chinese Hepataplex formula; •Ginkgo Biloba extract capsules 6 daily. •Crystal Star DR. VITALITY™ green and white tea caps or tea; New Chapter GREEN & WHITE TEA softgels. Apply •Evening Primrose Oil 2000mg; rub •Chinese WHITE FLOWER oil or •TIGER BALM on forehead and temples.

5—**For hormone-related headaches:** •Crystal Star FEM-SUPPORT CFS STAMINA™ with ashwaganda. Apply •Pure Essence Labs FEM CREME to temples or back of the neck; •*Chamomile* tea as needed.; Herbal Magic RELAXA-HERBAL caps.

—**For sinus headaches:** Crystal Star •ANTI-HST™ 2 caps 3x daily; •Pure Essence Labs ALLER FREE caps; •Xlear, Inc. XLEAR nasal wash; or •Baywood ORIGINAL ALLERGY FORMULA Drink •*rosemary* tea. or mix rosemary essential oil in hot water and inhale as a steam; or take the extract under the tongue. Rub •CAPSAICIN cream on temples or take •*Capsicum-Ginger* capsules 4 daily.

—**For stress or caffeine headaches:** •Crystal Star STRESS-ARREST™ tea or ANTI-FLAM™ caps. •DLPA 1000mg, or •Country Life RELAXER caps with GABA for brain relief. •Gaia Herbs INFLA- PROFEN; Homeopathic •Nux vomica for caffeine withdrawal.

Can't find a recommended product? Call the 800 number listed in Product Resources for the store nearest you.

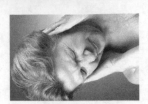

Hearing Loss

Tinnitus, Excess Wax, Ear Malfunction

Experts say one in ten Americans suffer some hearing problem. Hearing loss is the third most common health problem for people over 65. For men, it starts much earlier. A 23 year study by the National Institute on Aging says men start losing their hearing in their twenties; women don't have noticeable hearing loss until their sixties. (A lot of women are right... their husbands really *don't* hear them.) Even worse, hearing loss is becoming more common in kids. A recent JAMA study shows nearly 15% of school-aged kids have hearing problems. 85% of hearing loss involves tinnitus (ringing in the ears), a common high-dose aspirin side effect. Much of the rest is noise-induced. Natural therapies can help externally or nutritionally-based causes (as opposed to internal bone fusions that need surgery). Most hearing loss is marked by a feeling of fullness and ear clogging, no pain, but an extremely annoying ringing sound in the head. **What causes hearing loss?** arteriosclerosis and high blood pressure, gluten sensitivity, poor circulation and poor digestion (low HCL), thickening of ear passages or congestion in the middle ear, nerve damage, bronchial mastoid and sinus infections, some antibiotics or heart medication reactions, hypoglycemia, raised copper levels but low calcium levels, Crohn's disease, excess ear wax, and smoking (limits blood flow to the inner ear). Check your toothpaste. It should be sodium-lauryl-sulfate free. See EARACHES page 400 and TINNITUS page 557 for more.

Diet and Lifestyle Support Therapy

Nutritional therapy plan: See Hypoglycemia Diet page 463 for more diet suggestions.

1—Eat light to hear better - plenty of vegetable protein, sprouts, whole grains, fruit, cultured foods. A glass of wine at night is a good idea.

2—Lose excess weight. Fat clogs the head, too. Reduce dietary fats, cholesterol and mucous-forming foods. Avoid refined sugars, heavy starches and concentrated foods.

3—Take fresh grated horseradish in a spoon with lemon juice. Hang over a sink to release excess mucous and clear head passages.... almost immediately.

—For ringing in the ears:

• Go on a short 3 day mucous cleansing diet (pg. 202). Eat fresh foods for the rest of the week....plenty of salads and citrus fruits. Have lemon juice and water each morning.

• Then, for a month eat a mildly cleansing diet. Avoid fatty foods. Reduce dairy foods. Add plenty of vegetable fiber foods. A glass of wine at night is a good idea.... can help tinnitus right away sometimes. Add •New Chapter GINGER WONDER 2 tbsp. daily.

• Keep diet very low in sugars, salt, and dairy foods, high in calcium leafy greens. Drink bottled water. Add betaine HCl with pepsin to aid nutrient absorption (not if you have a peptic ulcer). Add •*Cayenne-Ginger* for circulation.

—Bodywork:

• For ringing in the ears: Massage neck, ear and temples. Pull earlobes - top front and back to clear passages of excess wax or mucous. •Get a cranial sacral massage to relieve eustachian tube drainage.

• Chiropractic adjustment; misaligned vertebra can compromise blood flow to the ears and worsen hearing.

• Avoid continuous loud noise. (Listening to loud rock music through headphones on a regular basis results in major ear problems.)

• Acupressure point: Squeeze joints of the ring finger and 4th toe, covering all sides for 3 minutes each day. For ear ringing: stroke gently downward from top of the temple to bottom of the cheek with nails for 30 seconds on each side.

Herbal, Superfood and Supplement Therapy

Interceptive therapy plan: Choose 2 to 3 recommendations.

1—**Improve blood flow to the hearing apparatus:** •*Ginkgo Biloba* extract 200mg daily for 3 months or more. •Metabolic Response Modifiers CARDIO-CHELATE with EDTA to open clogged arteries (highly recommended). •Niacin therapy: 500mg daily.

2—**Dissolve excess wax:** •Put 6 drops *garlic* oil and 3 drops *goldenseal* extract in the ear, leave 2 minutes. Repeat daily for a week. Flush with vinegar and water. •Or put 4 drops white vinegar and 3 drops 70% isopropyl alcohol in ear; leave 30 seconds; flush with water. Repeat daily for a week. —**Ear drops:** Dilute in water; use as drops: •*Lobelia* extract; •*Mullein* oil drops relieve pain; •Herbs, Etc. MULLEIN-GARLIC ear drops.

3—**Relieve pressure, open ear canals:** •Nature's Answer BIOEAR (highly recommended); •Crystal Star ANTI-HST™ caps; •Dr. Bob Martin's HEARALL caps; Clear Products CLEAR TINNITUS caps; •*Echinacea* extract drops and •Mega C therapy: Use Ester C crystals ¼ tsp. every hour to bowel tolerance for 1 week.

4—**Calcium and silica are key nutrients:** Lane Labs ADVACAL, 6 daily; •Floradix CALCIUM, MAGNESIUM liquid; •Crystal Star CALCIUM MAGNESIUM SOURCE™ caps. •Flora VEGE-SIL; •Body Essentials SILICA GEL 1 tbsp. in 3-oz. liquid 3x daily.

5—**Antioxidants may prevent hearing loss:** •Nutricology GERMANIUM 150mg daily; •Beta carotene 150,000IU and •Vitamin C with bioflavonoids, 5000mg daily for 3 months; •Grapeseed or white pine PCOs 300mg daily. •Sun CHLORELLA drink daily.

6—**For age-related deafness, one each daily:** Emulsified A 25,000IU; Ester C 1000mg with bioflavs; Magnesium 800mg; Glutamine 1000mg; Calcium 1500mg with vitamin D; Nature's Secret ULTIMATE B for regrowth of damaged ear canal hairs; •Green Foods BARLEY ESSENCE enhances SOD production.

—**Ringing in the ears:** •*Ginkgo Biloba* extract 200mg daily, 3 months; take with 1 dropperful •Crystal Star ANTI-BIO™ if a low grade ear infection (fast results). •Sublingual B-12 2500mcg; calcium 1500mg daily for earbone softness; •Clear Products CLEAR TINNITUS caps; •VINPOCETINE 30mg 2x daily. •N-acetyl-cysteine (NAC) drains congesting fluid; •Histidine caps, 1000mg daily.

Can't find a recommended product? Call the 800 number listed in Product Resources for the store nearest you.

Heart Arrhythmias

Palpitations, Tachycardia, Atrial Fibrillation

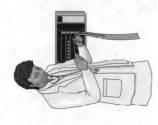

Arrhythmias: Electrical disruptions that affect the natural rhythm of the heart. *Palpitations:* the heart beating out of sequence. *Atrial fibrillation:* episodic heart flutter, shortness of breath, uncomfortable awareness of a racing heart often accompanied by dizziness or fainting, which may predispose a person to having a stroke. *Atrial tachycardia:* too rapid contractions of the heart coming on in sudden attacks; usually associated with coronary artery disease. May increase the risk of congestive heart failure. *Digoxin,* often given for arrhythmias has side effects, like gastric irritation, hearing and visual disturbances, headaches and dizziness. Lifestyle and diet change are better ways to avoid arrhythmias. If your pulse is over 80 and remains that way, you should make some diet improvements and get a further heart diagnosis. *Do you have heart arrhythmias?* Irregular and/or rapid heartbeat, uncomfortable awareness of your heartbeat, skipped heartbeats and shortness of breath; a feeling that you cannot breathe; light-headedness; often chest discomfort. Common Causes: Poor diet with too much refined sugar and saturated fat; lack of exercise/aerobic strength; obesity; smoking; stressful lifestyle; alcohol or drug abuse; high blood pressure; diabetes. *See also* ANXIETY--PANIC ATTACK *page 320 for more information.*

Diet and Lifestyle Support Therapy

Nutritional therapy plan:

1—A green drink once a week esp. during initial healing. •Pure Planet CHLORELLA packets, •Eidon POTASSIUM liquid, or •Nutricology PRO-GREENS with EFA's are effective. Keep your diet low in fats, salt and calories. Have a daily green salad, seafood and sea veggies every day. Add often, sunflower and sesame seeds, miso soup, rice, oat bran, and leafy vegetables. Reduce dairy. •Pure Form WHEY PROTEIN drink instead.

2—Make a stable heart mix of lecithin granules, toasted wheat germ, nutritional yeast, chopped sea vegetables; sprinkle 2 tbsp. daily on a salad, soup or protein drink.

3—Arrhythmias can be aggravated by coffee, alcohol, or nicotine. •Avoid soft drinks. The phosphorus binds up magnesium, making it unavailable for heart regularity. Drink a bottle of mineral water with 1 tsp. •New Chapter GINGER WONDER syrup every day.

Take your own pulse: Your pulse refers to the number of beats your heart has per minute. Taking your own pulse can help tell you whether you're at risk for tachycardia, atrial fibrillation or other types of irregular heartbeat. A normal resting pulse reading for adults and teens ranges between 60 to 100 beats per minute. Pulse readings for children and infants are slightly higher. Children ages 7-10 range between 70 to 110 beats per minute; A normal infant pulse rate may reach up to 150 beats per minute. Most physicians advise NOT allowing your heart rate to reach more than 200 beats per minute.

—Take your pulse in the morning.

1: Place your index and middle finger around the back of your wrist. 2: Use your index and middle finger to locate the radial artery in your wrist. Use light pressure to feel for your pulse. It should be easy to find. 3: Count the number of beats your pulse has in 30 seconds. Multiply those results by 2 to calculate your pulse rate per minute. Follow the procedure a second time. Note irregularities like pauses (or no pauses) between beats, or skipped beats. Report them to your physician. These may be warning signs of undiagnosed heart abnormalities.

Bodywork: •Plunge face into cold water when arrhythmia occurs to stop palpitations.

Herbal, Superfood and Supplement Therapy

Interceptive therapy plan: Choose 2 to 3 recommendations.

1—Regulate heart action: Heart regulating herbs usually work within 1 minute for simple palpitations. •Hawthorn extract as needed (about 800mg daily); or *Hawthorn-arjuna-passionflowers* extract; •Cayenne extract drops; •*Siberian eleuthero* extract drops; •Prince of Peace GINSENG-ROYAL JELLY vials. •*Valerian* extract. •Herbal Magic HAWTHORN HEART with motherwort, a preventive; •Gaia Herbs LINDEN/HAWTHORN extract; •Magnesium 800mg daily, esp. if you have had heart surgery. •*Astragalus* extract if heart problem is related to a virus; •*Ginkgo Biloba* and *Cat's Claw* extracts help prevent ischemia-caused fibrillation.

2—Help remove fatty deposits may cause arrhythmias: •Berberine-containing herbs, *goldenseal root, coptis, Oregon grape root, barberry.* Add •taurine 500mg 2x daily with •Ester C 550mg 2x daily; •Wakuanaga AGED GARLIC EXTRACT.

3—Normalize circulation: •*Butcher's broom* tea (for 2 to 3 weeks); •*Rosemary* tea (or *rosemary* wine sips); •*Ginkgo biloba* extract; •*Ginger* capsules 2 daily; •*Peppermint-Sage* tea. •Solaray CHROMIACIN 3x daily (don't take high doses of isolated niacin).

4—Calm and stabilize heartbeat: •Stress B Complex 150mg with extra B-6, 100mg; •Pacific BioLogic CHILL OUT capsules and •Country Life CALCIUM-MAGNESIUM-POTASSIUM capsules. •*Cayenne-Ginger* caps or Solaray COOL CAYENNE 2 daily, or •Crystal Star RESTORE YOUR STRENGTH™ drink for daily potassium to increase heart strength gradually. •Deter atrial fibrillation: •Floradix MAGNESIUM liquid; •Crystal Star CALCIUM-MAGNESIUM SOURCE™ caps, •Country Life CAL-MAG-BROMELAIN.

5—Essential fatty acids (EFAs) help protect against arrhythmias: •*Evening primrose oil* 2000mg daily, or Omega-3 flax oils 3 daily, or Spectrum NORWEGAIN FISH OIL 3-6 daily; •Crystal Star OCEAN MINERALS™ caps, iodine, potassium from sea greens.

6—Antioxidants - key preventives: •OPC's from white pine or grapeseed 100mg daily; •Futurebiotics VITAL K; •CoQ-10, 200mg daily (noticeably strengthens heart muscle); •Carnitine 1000mg 2 daily; •Vitamin E 400IU with selerium 200mcg. daily; •MICROHYDRIN PLUS helps remove fatty build-up on arteries (royal-health.com).

Can't find a recommended product? Call the 800 number listed in Product Resources for the store nearest you.

Heart Disease

Cardiovascular Diseases, Angina, Coronary, Heart Attack, Stroke

Of all the world's people, Americans are at the highest risk for heart disease. It's still our biggest killer. A million of us die each year because of heart problems. Yet, experts tell us most heart disease is 100% preventable with changes in diet and lifestyle. Heart disease was almost unknown before the turn of the twentieth century. Today, two-thirds of America suffers from some kind of cardiovascular disease. Natural therapies are proving to reduce mortality better than aggressive medical intervention or even the most advanced drug treatment. Many cholesterol-lowering drugs can cause liver toxicity, stomach distress and vision impairment. They may deplete CoQ-10, an essential co-enzyme that strengthens the heart, by up to 50%. Beware of calcium channel blockers (top selling blood pressure drugs), increase heart attack risk up to 60%! They block many body functions and are implicated in aggravated cardiovascular problems. Research also shows that they raise suicide risk. Actively explore magnesium, Nature's calcium channel blocker, with your physician.

Is heart disease contagious?

New research points to the infectious bacteria *Chlamydia pneumoniae*, as a possible factor in heart disease development. *C. pneumoniae* is a different species of the same bacteria that causes the STD, Chlamydia. It's a common cause of pneumonia, sinusitis and bronchitis — most people are infected by it 2 or 3 times during their lives. The heart connection? Blocked blood vessels are 20 times more likely to carry *C. pneumoniae* than unblocked vessels. Scientists speculate that *C. pneumoniae* creates inflammation that plays a role in the progression of atherosclerosis, too. Important note: a recent month-long clinical trial found that antibiotic therapy reduced the number of heart attacks and deaths in hospitalized heart patients. Herbal antibiotics are a safe and effective natural alternative. If you are recovering from a heart attack or have coronary heart disease, a month long course of *Echinacea/Goldenseal* extract or Crystal Star's ANTI-BIO™ caps may flush out infectious bacteria trapped in blocked lymph glands and blood vessels.

Are your homocysteine levels too high?

Homocysteine is big news today. But the connection between heart disease and homocysteine isn't new. Homocysteine is a body substance that helps manufacture proteins and assist with cellular metabolism. It's a harmless amino acid, but in excess, can cause blood platelets to clump and vein walls to break down, leading to atherosclerosis and coronary disease. Research linking heart disease to high homocysteine plasma levels began in 1969, when a Harvard pathologist, found severe atherosclerosis in children with very high homocysteine levels.

What we know about high homocysteine today: A recent New England Journal of Medicine study shows that people with high homocysteine levels are 4½ times more likely to die of heart disease than other people. New estimates are that 1 in 5 cardiac cases can be attributed to high homocysteine levels. High homocysteine levels may be especially dangerous for women. Women with high homocysteine levels and low folic acid in the blood are twice as likely to have a heart attack as women with normal levels.

Factors that contribute to high homocysteine levels:

—Too much protein: Protein-rich foods have the amino acid methionine which converts to homocysteine; consider if you are on a high protein "Zone" diets.

—Vitamin B deficiency: (especially B_6, B_{12} and folic acid the body needs to break down homocysteine). Prescription drugs deplete B vitamins: Methotrexate, diuretics used to treat high blood pressure, the cholesterol-lowering medicine Questran, nitrous oxide, azaribine, most oral contraceptives, and even aspirin suppress folic acid.

—Genetic defect: A defect in a reductase enzyme triggers a need for more folic acid than is normally required to prevent elevated homocysteine levels.

—Aging along with thyroid hormone deficiency: Homocysteine levels increase by about one micromole per liter for every 10 years of age.

—Coffee and Nicotine: Smokers have higher levels of homocysteine. Norwegian research suggests heavy coffee drinking elevates homocysteine levels.

Balance your homocysteine levels naturally. A simple 3 point program shows protection in one to three months.

1: B vitamins come to your rescue. A high intake of folic acid and B_6 lowers risk for cardiovascular disease 45% in women (February 1998 Journal of the AMA). Try B Complex, 100mg daily. Add 50mg extra of B_6 and 400mcg extra of folic acid to help break down homocysteine.

2: Four garlic capsules (1200mg a day) maintain aortic elasticity.

3: Take daily ginger. If you take aspirin to prevent a stroke or heart attack because aspirin inhibits an enzyme that makes the blood prone to dangerous stickiness, know that ginger not only inhibits this same enzyme but it does so without aspirin's side effects like gastric bleeding.

Can't find a recommended product? Call the 800 number listed in Product Resources for the store nearest you.

Considering heart surgery? Can heart surgery and drugs protect you? Here are the risks:

Many experts think drugs and surgical techniques to protect your heart are based on big bucks instead of health. Heart surgery procedures alone cost Americans over $50 billion each year. Clearly, lives have been saved and extended, but drugs and surgery carry serious risks. They are highly invasive, expensive, traumatic procedures. Many are questioning some of the techniques, saying that often the cure may be worse than the disease. It's true that sometimes heart surgery can be the beginning of the end of a normal, natural, lifestyle. The latest study from New England Journal of Medicine reveals heart surgery patients fare worse than heart patients who only undergo medical therapy. In fact, heart disease patients actually have 98.4% chance of survival WITHOUT surgery. By-pass surgery, the most popular surgical heart disease "solution," benefits less than 10% of heart patients. Many don't live 6 or 7 years after their first operation. Most of us know someone for whom bypass surgery or a pacemaker was the beginning of the end. My late father-in-law was one. If you're considering heart surgery, talk to your doctor at length and get all the information about your prospective procedure — the advantages, the healing risks and requirements, and the long term problems.

Information you should know about commonly performed heart surgeries:

...**Pacemaker Implant Surgery:** For people who suffer from a slow heart rate — $25,000. Pacemakers battery-powered devices implanted just under the skin send out electrical impulses to stimulate heartbeat. Research from the Mayo clinic and The Heart Institute in St. Petersburg shows electrical devices like cell phones, medical equipment, even security devices at shopping malls interfere with pacemakers, creating fluctuations in heartbeat that can lead to drowsiness, shortness of breath or blackouts. The battery in a pacemaker eventually wears out, so it must be continually monitored for effectiveness.

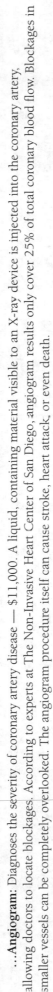

...**Angiogram:** Diagnoses the severity of coronary artery disease — $11,000. A liquid, containing material visible to an X-ray device is injected into the coronary artery, allowing doctors to locate blockages. According to experts at The Non-Invasive Heart Center of San Diego, angiogram results only cover 25% of total coronary blood flow. Blockages in smaller vessels can be completely overlooked. The angiogram procedure itself can cause stroke, heart attack, or even death.

...**Bypass Surgery:** For people with blocked coronary arteries — $45,000. Blocked portions of the coronary arteries are bypassed with grafts taken from veins in the legs. But, the veins of the leg aren't designed to withstand the high pressure blood flow from the heart. There's just too much wear and tear, so many patients don't live beyond 6 or 7 years after their first operation. Only a small percentage of heart disease patients (less than 10%) actually benefit from bypass surgery. According to Julian Whitaker M.D. in his newsletter, nearly 1 in 25 people die during the bypass surgery itself. Bypass surgery is still the most popular heart disease surgery with over 573, 000 operations performed on men and women each year.

...**Balloon Angioplasty:** A balloon-tipped catheter is used to "inflate" or open up blocked arteries — $15,000. An angioplasty causes a heart attack in 4% of people having the procedure. In 5%, the blockage is actually made worse. Statistics show that 35% of treated blockages actually return to their pre-op severity in less than a year. I personally know two people who had to have another angioplasty within a year. Doctors from the University of Texas hope to improve angioplasty success rates by using clot busting drugs directly on clot-prone areas during the procedure which may help prevent future blockages. Incidentally, new studies show fish oil capsules after a balloon angioplasty can help prevent re-clogging...a big problem.

Diagnosing your cardiovascular problem:

Signs that you are suffering a heart attack or a stroke: 1) severe chest pain or sudden weakness or numbness of the face, arm and leg, usually on one side of the body; 2) trouble talking or understanding speech; 3) fluctuating state of consciousness, with tingling sensations; 4) dimness or loss of vision, particularly in one eye; 5) sudden severe headache and dizziness, leading to unsteadiness or a sudden fall. A heart attack or stroke does most of its damage in the first six hours. Call an emergency room immediately if you feel you are having a heart attack of any kind.

Can herbs help in a heart attack emergency?

Sometimes they can. Until the nineteenth century, tincture of cayenne was a traditional healer's emergency method to bring a person out of a heart attack. About 5 droppersful (approx. 30 drops each) have been able to stop an attack. If the victim is unconscious, begin with two droppersful and add more as response begins. Up to 10 or 12 droppersful may be needed, but reports from healers even today are miraculous for this technique. When taken at the onset of symptoms, studies show the amino acid l-carnitine, about 1000mg daily, lessens the severity of a heart attack and reduces complications. Stronger, liquid carnitine can sometimes be used in an emergency. Ask your health practitioner. Remember herbs (and most natural healing remedies) are best used for degenerative, chronic ailments. If you live near a clinic of any kind, get there immediately. Modern medicine is at its best in just this kind of emergency.

ANGINA: A warning sign of a heart attack. —**Signs and symptoms:** recurring, sudden, intense chest pains, lasting 30 seconds to 1 minute, with a vise-like grip of pressure across the chest. People usually feel initial angina attacks during physical exertion because one or more arteries are partially clogged, with the blood supply to the heart reduced, functioning

Can't find a recommended product? Call the 800 number listed in Product Resources for the store nearest you.

441

inefficiently and painfully. Do not ignore this sign as "just indigestion." May also be brought on by emotional stress, exposure to cold, or overexertion. —**Alternative healing protocols:** Follow a vegetarian diet. •*Salvia miltiorrhiza* (Chinese red sage)- better than nitrates for angina. Take 1000mg Carnitine, 2000mg Arginine, 2000mg Lysine and 800IU vitamin E daily to scour arteries; •CoQ-10, 300mg daily; •*cayenne/ginger* caps, 2 daily; or •*Ginkgo Biloba* extract capsules, up to 240mg daily to increase blood flow to the brain; •Omega-3 flax oil 3x daily; •Vitamin C 3-5000mg daily with bioflavonoids; •Bromelain 1500mg daily; •Flora MAGNESIUM liquid; •Esteem Products CARDIOLIFE; •Metabolic Response Modifiers CARDIO-CHELATE, oral chelation w. EDTA. Explore Enhanced External Counterpulsation (EECP) therapy, a non-surgical, non-drug approach to increase circulation with your physician.

ACUTE MYOCARDIAL INFARCTION, (CORONARY): This is a heart attack, with permanent damage to the heart muscle, and death. The heart stops beating; the blood supply to the brain is cut off. Plaque build up in the coronary arteries, eventually narrows one to total obstruction. Instantly the part of the heart served from that artery is without blood supply. In just five minutes, it will suffer damage, even death from the cut off of oxygen. —**Signs and symptoms:** excruciating pain, starting in the lower chest and spreading throughout the upper half of the body - weak, rapid pulse with perspiring, pale skin. Blood pressure drops dangerously, there is dizziness, then unconsciousness. High fever usually follows an attack. If you feel you're having a heart attack, call 911 immediately and unless you're allergic, chew aspirin. It may save your life. —**Alternative healing protocols:** Antioxidants are a key. •Liquid carnitine for myocardial infarction during an attack (see previous page). Use •NAC, (N-acetyl-cysteine). •vitamin C 1000mg daily and •Enzymatic VITALINE, CoQ-10 chewables and •Lipoic Acid 600mg daily to inhibit heart damage from free radicals after an infarction. Use •Magnesium 400mg 2x daily to help prevent coronary; •folic acid 400 mcg to keep homocysteine levels down, with •B-6 100mg and •Country Life sublingual B-12, 2500mcg •Fo-Ti root to increase heart vigor. •For men, L-Arginine 1000mg daily helps blood vessels widen. •For women, a DHEA supplement is a preventive after menopause. Take •HAWTHORN extract or ARJUNA drops as needed, to normalize heart rate. Protectors: •ginger and garlic 6, caps each, •Spectrum NORWEGIAN FISH OIL and •a cup of green or white tea or Crystal Star DR. VITALITY™ tea and •ginkgo biloba extract daily. Proteolytic enzymes prevent inflammation, like Crystal Star DR ENZYME™ with protease and bromelain. •MICROHYDRIN PLUS 3 caps daily, available at royal-health.com.

STROKE and TIAs: Stroke, blocked blood supply to the brain, is the third leading cause of death in the U.S. and a major cause of disability. Experts say that stroke deaths may double by 2032. Similar to a coronary, the difference being oxygen-deprived brain tissue which dies within minutes. —**Signs and symptoms:** temporary loss of speech or vision, disordered behavior, thought patterns and memory, to paralysis, coma and death. See previous page for signs you may be having a stroke. Ask for a stethoscope neck check (for a bruit sound) if you think you are at risk. *Note:* Modern medicine suggests a daily aspirin to prevent life-threatening strokes. Aspirin inhibits a specific enzyme that makes the blood less prone to dangerous clots. Ginger not only inhibits the same enzyme, but it does so without side effects. —**Alternative healing protocols:** Up to 80% of strokes are preventable. Take •a cup of green tea, or •Crystal Star GREEN TEA CLEANSER™ each morning. Eat anti-stroke seafoods and fish twice a week- salmon is highly recommended. Eat more fruits and vegetables for fiber. Have a green salad every day. Reduce caffeine and alcohol, salty and sugary foods. Snip dry sea greens over any food or eat sushi often (loaded with vitamin K). Take •2000mg carnitine daily and *Hawthorn* extract as needed. •Nutricology BEST BLOOD OXYGENATION FORMULA; Use •Metabolic Response Modifiers CARDIO-CHELATE, oral chelation w. EDTA. •Vitamin C 3000mg daily with rutin and bioflavs, 500mg; •CoQ10 240mg effective against TIA's. Take •Lane Labs PALMVITEE for protection against second stroke- good clinical trial results. Other second stroke protectors: •B-complex 100mg daily with extra •folic acid 400 mcg; •magnesium 400-800mg daily and •alpha lipoic acid 100mg daily; •VINPOCETINE for faster rehabilitation. Meditation and acupuncture show success against stroke. Ginseng shows promise for memory enhancement after stroke. Consider •Crystal Star FEEL GREAT NOW! caps with ginseng. Consider Constraint-Induced (CI) Movement Therapy to improve partial paralysis after a stroke. Call Taub's Training Clinic to request an information packet, 205-975-9799.

MITRAL VALVE PROLAPSE (MVP): The mitral valve is one of the gates within the heart that regulates oxygen-rich blood flow. A prolapse (elasticity loss) of the gate valve is the most common heart abnormality.... thought to be genetic, affecting about 3% of Americans. However, MVP may be as high as 30% in women ages 14-35. Mitral valve prolapse is benign in the majority of cases, but is linked to stroke and other complications in a few people. —**Signs and symptoms:** palpitations or rapid heart rate, anxiety attacks or night panic attacks, shortness of breath, along with physical weakness. Though common, the uneven flow of blood increases likelihood of clot formation in people under 45, who also have a higher rate of stroke during their younger years. 85% of people with MVP have a magnesium deficiency that affects the collagen structures throughout the body. Small, thin women are more likely to have a mitral valve prolapse. —**Alternative healing protocols:** Add •magnesium 800mg daily for protection; •1000mg L-carnitine 3x a day relieve symptoms; •*Hawthorn* extract as needed, and Lane Labs PALM VITEE (both highly recommended). •Crystal Star HEART PROTECTOR™ capsules for women, or •*Ginkgo Biloba* to normalize circulation; •Crystal Star FEMALE HARMONY™ with phyto-estrogen herbs. Relaxation techniques like meditation, shiatzu and biofeedback are a good idea, and daily mild exercise, like leisurely swimming or a brisk walk.

CONGESTIVE HEART FAILURE: CHF occurs when a weak, dilated heart, damaged by arteriosclerosis or disease like hypothyroidism, ceases to pump effectively. Circulation becomes poor, organs and tissues become clogged with blood. Most common in women after menopause, possibly because of high iron stores. —**Signs and symptoms:** great energy depletion,

Can't find a recommended product? Call the 800 number listed in Product Resources for the store nearest you.

dizziness and shortness of breath after exertion; swollen ankles and feet, with nausea and gas. Later symptoms are greater heart exhaustion and fluid in the lungs. —**Alternative healing protocols:** •Crystal Star HEART PROTECTOR™ caps for women, and •DR. ENZYME™ w. protease and bromelain to reduce inflammation; • Nutricology COMPLETE HEART; •Magnesium, 800mg daily for better muscle performance. •Flora MAGNESIUM liquid or •Country Life CALCIUM-MAGNESIUM™; •Douglas Labs CoQMelt daily (highly recommended); an herbal combination with •Arjuna herb, •Astragalus, or Ayurvedic •*Coleus Forskohlii* (highly recommended); •vitamin E 800IU daily and •Maitake Products REISHI capsules for boosting antioxidants; •HAWTHORN extract (impressive results in clinical tests); •Creatine 100mg 4x daily to improve heart muscle metabolism; •Vitamin C 3000mg daily w. bioflavonoids; •BILBERRY extract daily. •Stress B-complex 100mg with extra thiamine (B-1), 200 mg and pantothenic acid 250mg daily. • A daily dry sauna improves arterial blood flow. Exercise helps rid the body of excess iron.

CARDIOMYOPATHY: An insidious type of heart failure where an enlarged, severely weakened heart muscle pumps only a fraction of the blood the body needs. —**Signs:** great fatigue, and great trouble breathing. —**Alternative healing protocols:** Reduce risk by reducing caffeine and nicotine. Use •CoQ-10, 300mg daily. •Douglas Labs CoQMelt (highly recommended for absorbability). •*Hawthorn* extract, or Fo-Ti (*Ho-Shou Wu*) extract; •*Ginkgo Biloba* or *ginger* capsules daily to normalize circulation; •Wakunaga KYOLIC FORMULA 106 for better blood flow; •Nutricology BEST BLOOD OXYGENATION formula; •magnesium 800mg daily or•Country Life CAL-MAG-BROMELAIN 1500 mg; •L-carnitine 1000mg daily; •taurine 500mg daily.

ISCHEMIA: Reduced blood flow to the heart and cell oxygen starvation, caused by atherosclerotic plaques along the artery walls. Ischemia leads to angina, coronary or congestive heart failure. —**Signs and symptoms:** high blood pressure; poor circulation; aching feet, legs and muscles, or numbness on one side, speech difficulty, double vision and vertigo. —Alternative healing protocols: Nutricology BEST BLOOD OXYGENATION formula; •HAWTHORN extract as needed; •BILBERRY extract protects integrity of microvessel walls; •CoQ-10, up to 300mg daily; •garlic cap 6 daily; •ginger capsules 4 daily to inhibit platelet aggregation or •New Chapter GINGER WONDER syrup– 1 tbsp. in 8-oz. water 2x daily; •PHYCOTENE MICROCLUSTERS, potent mixed carotenes, available at royalbodycare.com; •Vitamin E 800IU with selenium 200mcg daily; •Nattokinase enzyme therapy shows good results.

ARRYTHMIAS: *Tachycardia:* heartbeat so rapid that the heart cannot deliver blood efficiently. It can be fatal. *Palpitations:* the heart beating irregularly. *Fibrillation:* more serious than tachycardia, it includes a further weak, irregular quiver to the heartbeat. See page 439.

ATHEROSCLEROSIS: Atherosclerosis results in-high blood pressure, page 452. (See Atherosclerosis page 323 and Cholesterol page 368.)

Quick Heart Rehabilitation Check Program   **This program has proven successful against heart disease recurrence.**

This program is designed especially for those of you who have survived a heart attack, or major heart surgery. Coming back is tough. Beginning and sticking to a new lifestyle that changes almost everything about the way you eat, exercise, handle stress, and even the smallest details of your life, is a challenge. The following mini-rehabilitation program is a blueprint that you can use with confidence. It addresses the main preventive needs - keeping your arteries clear and your blood slippery - goals that clearly can be achieved through a good diet and exercise.

—*Reduce saturated fats to 10% of your diet;* less if possible. Limit polyunsaturated oils to 10%. Avoid trans fats and refined carbohydrates to keep triglycerides in check. Add monounsaturates (olive oil, avocados, nuts and seeds). Add EFAs (fish, flax oil, etc.).

—*Eat potassium-rich foods for cardiotonic activity:* spinach and chard, broccoli, bananas, sea greens, molasses, cantaloupe, apricots, papayas, mushrooms, tomatoes, yams, etc. or take a potassium drink (pg 291), Crystal Star RESTORE YOUR STRENGTH™ drink, or Futurebiotics VITAL K (a serving of high potassium fruits or vegetables offers about 400mg of potassium, a serving of the above drinks offers approx. 100-125 mg of potassium).

—Eat plenty of complex carbohydrates: broccoli, peas, whole grain breads, vegetable pastas, potatoes, sprouts, tofu and brown rice. Have a green salad every day.
—Have 3 to 4 servings of seafood each week: fish, seafood, sea veggies, soy foods like miso for EFAs and high omega-3 oils, like fish oil caps, perilla oil or flax oil in dressings.
—Have a glass of wine at dinner for relaxation: and better digestion so heartburn doesn't occur. Add herbs like ginger, peppermint or rosemary to keep your body pH balanced.
—Eat magnesium-rich foods for heart regulation: tofu, wheat germ, oat or rice bran, broccoli, potatoes, lima beans, spinach and chard.
—Eat high fiber foods for a clean system and alkalinity: whole grains, fruits and vegetables, legumes and greens.

Choose several of the following supplements as your individual daily micro-nutrients:
• *For clear arteries:* Solaray CHROMIACIN; selenium, omega-3 flax or fish oils 3x daily; Golden Pride FORMULA ONE, oral chelation w. EDTA 2 packs a.m./p.m.
• *For heart regulation-stability:* Pure Planet CHLORELLA tabs; magnesium 400 mg; carnitine 500 mg; Crystal Star HEART HEALTH™ drops; *hawthorn* or *gotu kola* extracts.
• *For antioxidants:* Wheat germ oil raises oxygen level 30%; Pure Planet CHLORELLA tabs; vitamin E 400IU with selenium 200 mcg; CoQ-10, 200 mg, *Gingko Biloba* extract.
• *Cardiotonics:* Hawthorn extract; *cayenne* or *cayenne-ginger* capsules; garlic; *Siberian eleuthero* extract; *gotu kola* extract; PHYCOTENE NANOCLUSTERS available at royal-health.com.
Can't find a recommended product? Call the 800 number listed in Product Resources for the store nearest you.

- *Anti-cholesterol-blood thinning*: Ginger or *cayenne-ginger* caps 4 daily; taurine 500 mg; Golden Pride FORMULA ONE, oral chelation w. EDTA; MRM CARDIO-CHELATE.
- *For healthy blood chemistry*: Chromium picolinate; Ester C 500 mg with bioflavonoids daily especially if you have had bypass heart surgery.
- *For preventing TIA's (small strokes)*: CoQ-10, 60 mg 2 daily; ascorbate or Ester C with bioflavonoids, up to 500 mg daily for arterial integrity; vitamin E 400IU and selenium 200 mcg.
- *Natural calcium channel blockers*: magnesium 1200 mg daily; parsley caps 2 daily; carnitine 1000 mg daily.

Is our 21st century lifestyle so bad that we are literally killing ourselves?

Perhaps. There's our still sad American diet. Less than 25% of us get the recommended 5 servings of fruits and vegetables a day that protect against heart disease. Even worse, 25% of the "vegetables" we do eat in America are french fries- the most damaging for cardiovascular health! Low fiber is a big problem, (despite all the media attention). The typical American eats less than one-third of the daily fiber recommended for cardiovascular health! There's our sedentary lifestyle. Lack of exercise makes us a wide open target for heart disease. Regular moderate exercise cuts risk for heart attack and stroke almost in half. Our computers have changed our lives at every level. New statistics from the National Institute of Health show an astounding 58% of adult Americans get no exercise at all! Third: Americans are "stressed out." Chronic stress is a part of the American lifestyle. Most Americans feel overwhelmed. Financial or work-related stress in common. A recent survey finds over 25% of the baby boomers (at the peak of their careers and earning power) still feel out of control in their lives! Chronic stress causes coronary arteries to constrict, blood pressure to soar and cholesterol to build on artery walls. It's no wonder our hearts are about to explode!

Getting to the heart of the matter. You can carve out heart health with your own knife and fork.

The single most influential key to heart health is your diet. Almost all cardiovascular disease can be prevented and treated by improvements in nutrition. In general, high fat, high calorie foods create cardiovascular problems, and natural foods relieve them. Most Americans get over half their calories from processed foods that are high in calories and low in nutrients. Fried foods, salty and sugary foods, low fiber foods, dairy foods, red meats, preserved meats, tobacco and caffeine all contribute to clogged arteries, LDL cholesterol, high blood pressure and heart attacks. The following diet is easy to live with, has all the elements to keep arteries clear, and heart action strong. It emphasizes fresh, whole fiber foods, high minerals with lots of potassium and magnesium, anti-inflammatory fruits like cherries and berries, and oxygen-rich green vegetables, sprouts and wheat germ (wheat germ oil can raise the oxygen level of the heart as much as 30%), and vegetable proteins. (Vegetarians have less heart disease than meat eaters… perhaps because produce contains the anti-inflammatory compound, salicylic acid.) It all adds up to today's definition of living well, a longer, healthier life, and control over your life. Pleasure comes from better health and vitality instead of rich food and drink.

On rising: A high protein vitamin/mineral drink, like All One MULTIPLE with green plant base or Fit for You, Intl. MIRACLE GREENS in orange or grapefruit juice, or a cup of green tea.

Breakfast: Make an EFA mix of 2 tbsp. each: lecithin granules, wheat germ, nutritional yeast, sesame seeds and a little honey. Sprinkle 2 tsp. every morning on fresh fruits or mix with yogurt; and/or have a poached egg with bran muffins or whole grain toast and kefir cheese; or some whole grain cereal or pancakes with a little maple syrup.

Mid-morning: have a potassium drink (see page 291), or Pines MIGHTY GREENS drink, or Crystal Star RESTORE YOUR STRENGTH™ drink, or all natural V-8 juice or a cup of antioxidant tea like rosemary or peppermint tea; and/or some crunchy raw veggies with kefir cheese or yogurt dip; or a cup of miso soup with sea greens snipped on top.

Lunch: have a cup of fenugreek tea, add 1 tsp. maple syrup and a healthy pinch of ginger; then have a tofu and spinach salad with some sprouts and bran muffins; or a high protein salad or sandwich with nuts and seeds and black bean or lentil soup; or an avocado, low fat cheese or soy cheese sandwich on whole grain bread; or a seafood pasta salad.

Mid-afternoon: have peppermint tea; or a cup of miso soup and a hard boiled egg, or whole grain crackers, or carrot juice or KNUDSEN'S VERY VEGGIE juice.

Dinner: have a broccoli quiche with whole grain crust; or baked seafood with brown rice and peas; or a veggie casserole; or a stir fry with soup and rice; or grilled fish or seafood and a green salad and baked potato. A glass of wine before dinner is good for things that help your heart….relaxation, digestion and tension relief. Wine has an enzyme that breaks up blood clots.

Before bed: have another cup of miso soup, or a cup of Red Star nutritional yeast paste broth in hot in water (delicious), apple or pear juice, or chamomile tea.

Notes: 1) Avoid commercial antacids that neutralize natural stomach acid and invite the body to produce even more acid, thus aggravating stress and tension.
2) Preventive heart care works. People who exercise are strikingly free of circulatory diseases. For heart and artery health, heart rate and respiration must rise to a point of mild breathlessness for 5 minutes a day. A daily walk or exercise like dancing or swimming enhances the whole cardiovascular system, and reduces stress, an underlying cause of all disease.

Can't find a recommended product? Call the 800 number listed in Product Resources for the store nearest you.

Can you care for your heart by caring better for your teeth and gums?

A new 5-year study by the NIH links periodontal disease and heart attacks.

People with periodontal disease are 2.7 times more likely to have a heart attack than people with healthy gums! Researchers suspect that gum disease allows toxic bacteria from excess plaque to enter the bloodstream, causing blood platelets to clump up, accelerating atherosclerosis! If you already have gum disease or periodontitis, add • CoQ-10, 120mg to your diet. It's a specific for teeth, gums, and your heart; brush with •MICROBRITE powder daily, available at royal-health.com and rinse with •Nature's Answer PERIOWASH anti-infective mouthwash.

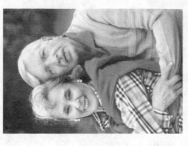

Heart problems for men and women are different

Until very recently, men and women's heart disease was considered largely the same. New research shows that men and women face very different challenges of heart disease. I've worked extensively to create natural healing programs that address the unique heart needs of men and women. Men's heart disease has been the focus of conventional medicine study. Until the mid-1990's women were largely left out of heart census taking. Yet, while about 500,000 men died each year from heart disease, over 550,000 American women fell victim and died. Even more frightening, studies reveal women receive less medical treatment despite having more cardiac symptoms. Today, though the death rate for men is still high, male children now have a lower heart attack fatality rate than their fathers did. Heart disease is still the leading cause of women's death in America, accounting for half of all women's deaths and killing 5 times more often than breast cancer. Heart disease for women, as for men, is linked to obesity, too little exercise and high cholesterol (even though tests show women have 60-70% *less* artery clogging plaque than men).

Many studies point to emotional health, as well as the traditional causes of stress, anger, and overwork, as major triggers of heart attacks for men. A Harvard School of Medicine study shows that men with the highest anger scores on personality tests are three times more likely to develop heart disease. Male pattern baldness and a protruding stomach also indicate a higher risk of heart disease. High blood pressure and atherosclerosis are the top cardiovascular problems that men face. High triglycerides (blood fats), largely related to a high fat diet and an overworked liver, can double a man's heart attack risk! High blood pressure, often called "the silent killer," affects 1 in 3 of all American adults. Coronary heart disease is 3 to 5 times more likely in people with high blood pressure! Men are more at risk for HBP than women until about age 55. High blood pressure is most dangerous for African American men. When blood pressure is high, the heart and arteries work overtime, and atherosclerosis speeds up. Atherosclerotic plaques on your arteries restrict blood flow to organs and tissues leading to heart attacks, strokes, even gangrene.

Can donating blood regularly prevent a heart attack for a man? Yes, it can! Men have twice as much iron in their bodies as women. Iron acts as a catalyst in oxidizing cholesterol, which is linked to artery hardening and scarring. Recent studies show that men cut their risk for heart attack or stroke *by up to a third* when they reduce their excess iron stores by regularly donating blood. Amazing.

Does oral chelation reverse men's heart disease? Intravenous chelation therapy with EDTA has largely been ignored by mainstream medicine, but it has been successful for blood vessel diseases like arteriosclerosis for over 40 years. Chelation with EDTA (*ethylenediamine tetra acetic acid*, a synthetic amino acid) binds to and flushes out arterial plaque and calcium deposits that cause artery hardening. Intravenous chelation is powerful but expensive therapy. Oral chelation is cheaper and more convenient than IV chelation, a good option for men that improves blood flow and may even reverse some cardiovascular problems. Consider Golden Pride oral chelation FORMULA #1 or Metabolic Response Modifiers CARDIO-CHELATE.

The newest research shows heart attack symptoms are different for men and women!

Even with all the health information we have today, men and women still ignore heart attack symptoms..... and, sadly, lose the first hours when treatment is so critical. *Heart attack symptoms are <u>always</u> worth repeating. Here are the warning signs men should watch for:*

• Pressure, or pain in the center of the chest lasting more than a few minutes
• Pain and numbness spreading to the face, neck or arms, usually on one side.
• Severe headache with light-headedness, sweating, nausea, skin paleness or shortness of breath.

Can't find a recommended product? Call the 800 number listed in Product Resources for the store nearest you.

A Man's Healthy Heart Program

1) Men tend to overeat- especially fatty foods. Hardening of the arteries is strongly tied to a diet high in animal fat, especially from butter, red meat, ice cream and eggs, the very foods many men overeat! Over-consumption of salt, a high stress lifestyle with little "downtime," and smoking are key factors. A low fat, high fiber diet is important for heart protection. It is essential for overcoming high blood pressure. Reduce fatty dairy foods like ice cream and rich cheeses. Cut back on red meat, especially pork. A better choice? Eat seafood at least twice a week. An 11 year study covering over 22,000 male physicians found that eating seafood just once a week cuts men's risk of sudden cardiac death by 52%!

2) Use olive oil instead. You can't fry in olive oil, but fried foods are so bad for your heart that this is a plus. Olive oil boosts healthy HDL cholesterol levels and removes fats from the blood. Try Spectrum Naturals organic olive oil. Eat more SUPERGREEN foods - spinach, chard and sea greens, for magnesium therapy and EFAs, keys to heart regulation and health.

3) Men at risk for heart disease need more fiber! Fiber has proven in many studies to reduce arterial plaque. Herbs are a good source of cleansing fiber for the male system. An herbal fiber drink mix daily like Jarrow GENTLE FIBERS along with *artichoke* extract helps reduce cholesterol, lower blood fats (triglycerides) and cleanse fatty build-up.

4) Add healing spices like garlic, onions, turmeric and cayenne peppers to your diet. Garlic thins the blood, normalizes blood pressure, helps reduce serum cholesterol and arterial plaque build-up. Both onions and garlic stimulate healthy circulation. Cayenne peppers strengthen all cardiovascular activity, dilate arteries and reduce blood pressure. Tumeric, an anti-inflammatory spice, helps decrease cholesterol levels and prevents progression of atherosclerosis. Don't like spicy recipes? Consider a garlic product like Wakunaga's KYOLIC FORMULA 106, with garlic, vitamin E, hawthorn and cayenne pepper. Boost circulation to thin "sticky blood" with Futurebiotics CIRCU-A.V.

5) Eat vitamin C rich foods like citrus fruits, broccoli or peppers. Low blood levels of vitamin C are linked to progressing atherosclerosis and to increased heart attack risk. A new study shows that men with no pre-existing heart disease who are deficient in vitamin C have 3.5 times MORE heart attacks than men who are not deficient in vitamin C.

6) Herbal stress busters are a good choice for men. They reduce anxiety linked to high blood pressure. Herbal formulas like Crystal Star HEART PROTECTOR FOR MEN™ with *gotu kola, passionflower* and *scullcap* calm stress reactions. I recommend *Siberian eleuthero*, a ginseng-like adaptogen that builds resistance to stress and restores nervous system health.

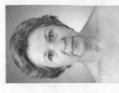

A Woman's Healthy Heart Program

Heart problems in women are different than those of men; they are hormone-dependent. A woman's highest risk for heart disease is during menopause. The risk rises noticeably every year for a woman in peri-menopause and goes on rising as she ages. Hundreds of thousands of hormone replacement therapy prescriptions are written every year by doctors trying to protect menopausal women from heart disease. Yet, the use of HRT to protect against heart disease is highly debatable. There is no conclusive evidence that estrogen protects against heart disease. The International Meeting on Atherosclerosis concludes that the heart protective benefits attributed to estrogen may result from population selection or changes towards healthier lifestyles during studies. Research shows that HRT does NOT prevent heart attacks for women who already have heart disease. In fact, the latest studies show women who take HRT for over 5 years suffer 24% MORE heart attacks than women who don't, and the risk is highest (a whopping 81% increase) during the first year on HRT. I believe there are better solutions for preventing heart disease naturally that don't carry these risks of HRT, with its links to uterine and breast cancer, blood clots and gallbladder disease.

Facts you need to know if you're thinking about beginning hormone replacement therapy to prevent heart disease:

1) The most commonly prescribed hormone replacement drug, Premarin, actually suppresses folic acid, contributing to high homocysteine levels, a known risk factor for heart disease. New research shows synthetic progestins in combination with HRT drugs may cause dangerous coronary vasospasms linked to heart attack.

2) Tests with some estrogen contraceptive pills actually increase a woman's risk of heart disease, heart attack, stroke and serious blood clotting problems.

3) Some reports suggest that SERMs (*selective estrogen receptor modulators*) like Evista may protect against heart disease. But Evista should not be taken by women with congestive heart failure. Evista also increases risk of serious blood clots in the legs, lungs or eyes, particularly if you're sedentary for long periods of time.

What are the *biggest heart problems for women?*

—**Heart attacks** are especially serious for women. Statistics show that a woman is 50% MORE LIKELY to die from a heart attack than a man! Women have heart attacks at older ages when they are in poorer health, with arteries less able to compensate for the partial death of heart muscle caused by a heart attack. Heart attack symptoms may be different. Women don't always have intense chest pains during a heart attack. Heart attack symptoms women should watch for: shortness of breath, palpitations, fatigue; tooth, jaw and ear pain, even back pain.

—**Congestive Heart Failure**, where the heart is unable to efficiently pump blood is a big problem. Over two million menopausal women today have CHF, and their risk for sudden

Can't find a recommended product? Call the 800 number listed in Product Resources for the store nearest you.

cardiac arrest and death is up to 9 times higher than the general population! High iron stores after menopause may increase risk. Further, new research shows NSAIDs (Non-steroidal anti-inflammatory drugs) may cause up to ⅕ of all heart failure cases. Alpha blocking blood pressure drugs may also be to blame. Symptoms to watch for: extreme fatigue and water retention (particularly bloated ankles). Consider •Crystal Star HEART PROTECTOR FOR WOMEN™ caps, and •creatine 3000mg daily or •Natural Balance CREATINE 3000 to 5000mg daily.

—*Atrial Fibrillation*, a dangerous irregular heartbeat is a huge threat…. 90% of women who have it are more likely to die than those who don't. If you're affected by atrial fibrillation, a cardiotonic, herbal heart protector with *arjuna* and *hawthorn* like Crystal Star HEART HEALTH™ drops can help regulate heartbeat and strengthen the cardiovascular system.

Are you having a Panic Attack or a Heart Attack? *If symptoms persist, seek a qualified health practitioner.*

Women may confuse panic attacks with heart attacks during menopause because the symptoms seem so severe. Menopausal heart palpitations and nighttime anxiety attacks are extremely common. When I first began menopause, I remember waking up terrified that I was having a heart attack, but found out later that it was a panic attack.

Panic attack signs to look for: *If you have these symptoms, you're probably suffering from a panic attack. It will more than likely pass quickly.*

• hyperventilating, feeling short of breath, or bolting upright out of bed, especially in the early morning hours.
• racing heartbeat, dizziness or feeling faint.
• feeling like you're "going crazy" or losing control, or being full of fear that has no basis in reality and the fear interfering in the normal functioning of your life.
Herbs offer relief from nighttime panic attacks. I keep heart stabilizing herbs like hawthorn, arjuna, ashwagandha and passionflowers by my bed at night for immediate relief.

Heart attack signs to look for: *If you're having these symptoms, seek medical attention immediately! Ignoring symptoms could mean risking your life.*

In a recent report, <u>less than 30%</u> of women experienced the intense chest pains that are classic in men's heart attack (the reason researchers believe women are more reluctant to seek treatment). In addition to the symptom list for men (see page 445), women should watch for the following symptoms which can appear up to a month before the attack!

• Unexplained, unusual fatigue
• Poor sleep, usually accompanied by anxiety
• Unexplained shortness of breath, often without pain
• Unusual attacks of indigestion, often followed by or accompanied by, back pain, or teeth, jaw or ear pain

The same report showed the following symptom list indicate a heart attack may be imminent for a woman:

• Shortness of breath, often with palpitations and breaking into a cold sweat
• Extreme fatigue and weakness, usually accompanied by dizziness

A Woman's Healthy Heart Program

1: Sea veggies act as total body tonics to restore female vitality during menopause. Sea veggies are loaded with fat-soluble vitamins like D and K that help our bodies make steroidal hormones like estrogen and DHEA which protect against heart disease during menopause. Sea veggies also dissolve fatty deposits in the cardiovascular system that precipitate heart disease.

2: Phytoestrogen foods like soy help maintain normal vascular function. Soy foods not only lower cholesterol, but along with herbs, soy is a rich source of phytoestrogens for female vitality and heart protection during menopause. My favorite phytoestrogen heart protector for post-menopausal women is a *dong quai/damiana/ashwagandha* extract combination

3: Have cold water fish 3 times a week for heart-healthy omega-3 oils and EFAs. Salmon is one of God's gifts, a rich source of omega-3 fatty acids and vitamin E. Wild salmon is a better source of EFAs than farmed salmon, and is much lower in hormone-disrupting PCB's (polychlorinated bi-phenols).

4: Use natural vitamin E (400IU) daily. Even though it's old news, vitamin E, like Lane Labs PALM VITEE with tocotrionols daily, cuts heart attack risk 77%!

5: Take a daily herbal heart tonic to protect against congestive heart failure, especially if you have reached menopause. Use a heart toning combination like Crystal Star HEART PROTECTOR FOR WOMEN™ with herbs like *hawthorn, bilberry, motherwort, ashwagandha, dong quai, gingko biloba, astragalus, red sage,* and *ginger root* for 6 months as circulatory support; or try HEART FOOD CAPS by Heart Foods or COMPLETE HEART by Nutricology.

6: CoQ-10, up to 300mg daily, or Douglas Labs CoQmelt strengthens the heart muscle and helps it work more effectively. (CoQ-10 is also a protector against breast cancer.)

7: EFAs (essential fatty acids) are important to women's heart health, because they are critical for hormone balance, thought to be a big part of women's heart problems. EFAs help decrease the "stickiness" of blood platelets. Evening primrose oil provides top quality EFAs for women. Spectrum Naturals high lignan Organic Flax Oil is a good diet/salad dressing choice.

8: Eat brown rice regularly for heart smart B vitamins. Brown rice as a valuable source of fiber, vitamins and minerals is superior to refined grains for heart health.

Can't find a recommended product? Call the 800 number listed in Product Resources for the store nearest you.

Heart Disease

Diet and Lifestyle Support Therapy

Nutritional therapy plan:

1—Your diet is your greatest asset in preventing heart disease. A healthy heart diet has plenty of magnesium and potassium rich foods: fresh greens, broccoli, cantaloupe; sea-foods and sea greens; flavonoids from pitted fruits, green tea and wine, soy, brown rice, whole grains, garlic and onions. Try •Crystal Star RESTORE YOUR STRENGTH™ drink with highly absorbable potassium from sea greens, or •Eidon POTASSIUM liquid.

2—Reduce saturated fats to no more than 10% of your daily calorie intake. Especially limit fats from animal sources and hydrogenated oils. —Pay conscious attention to avoid-ing red meats, caffeine foods, refined sugars, fatty, salty and fried foods, prepared meats and soft drinks. The rewards are worth the effort. Keep fats cleansed with •ALOE VERA juice with herbs each morning.

3—Eat 70% of daily calories from complex carbohydrates like vegetables and grains; 20% of calories from low fat protein sources. Add salmon to your diet at least once a week. It contains CoQ-10 to strengthen weak heart muscles (noticeable activity).

4—Eat less than 100mg per day of diet cholesterol. Keep cholesterol below 160.

5—Add 6 glasses of good water daily to your diet.... the best diuretic for a healthy heart. (Chlorinated/fluoridated water destroys vitamin E in the body.)

6—A glass or two of wine with dinner can relieve stress and raise HDLs. Try Crystal Star DR. VITALITY™ tea with green and white tea, ginger and hawthorn can quickly help regulate heartbeat and normalize circulation (highly recommended).

7—Make a hearty morning mix of lecithin granules, red yeast rice, toasted wheat germ, nutritional yeast, snipped dry sea greens, molasses, take 2 tbsp. daily with food. Or try •New Chapter GINGER WONDER syrup– 1 tbsp. in 8-oz. water 2x daily.

—Watchwords:

•Bite down on the tip of the little finger to help stop a heart attack.

•Apply hot compresses and massage chest of the victim to ease a heart attack.

•Chewing an aspirin with water immediately following symptoms of a heart attack, may be able to reduce mortality through its ability to rapidly reduce arterial blockage.

•Take alternate hot and cold showers frequently to increase circulation.

•Smoking constricts arteries and can cause blood pressure to skyrocket, too. Research-ers estimate that 150,000 heart disease deaths could be prevented each year if Americans just quit smoking! Need more? One in 4 smokers has a gene abnormality that triples the risk of a coronary heart attack.

•Take some mild regular daily exercise. Do deep breathing exercises every morning for body oxygen, and to stimulate brain activity.

•Consciously add relaxation and a good daily laugh to your life. A positive mental outlook does wonders to reduce stress.... and boost immune response.

Herbal, Superfood and Supplement Therapy

Interceptive therapy plan: Choose several recommendations.

1—**In a heart emergency:** •1 tsp. *cayenne* powder in water, or *cayenne* tincture drops in water may help bring a person out of a heart attack; or take liquid carnitine as directed.

•One-half dropperful *Hawthorn* extract every 15 minutes; or •Crystal Star HEART PRO-TECTOR™ formulas for men and women (highly recommended)

2—**Superhero nutrients tone your heart muscle:** •NutriCology CoQ-10 with TOCO-TRIENOLS and COMPLETE HEART caps. •Lane Labs PALMVITEE tocotrienols; •Esteem CARDIOLIFE caps with CoQ10; •Ester C with bioflavonoids, up to 5000mg daily for interstitial arterial integrity-elasticity, and to prevent TIAs (little strokes). —**EFA therapy:** •EVENING PRIMROSE oil 3000mg daily; •Flora UDO'S PERFECTED OIL BLEND caps;

•Health from the Sun TOTAL EFA also balance prostaglandins that regulate arterial muscle tone; •Magnesium rich herbs: motherwort, maca, parsley; or •Flora MAGNESIUM liquid, or Magnesium 800mg, or •Country Life CALCIUM-MAGNESIUM-BROMELAIN.

3—**Improve blood flow:** •Metabolic Response Modifiers CARDIOCHELATE w. EDTA; •Wakunaga KYOLIC FORMULA 106; •red sage tea or Gingko Biloba extracts are vasodilators, 2-3x daily; •Natural Balance CREATINE 3000mg daily; MICROHYDRIN, available at Royal Bodycare.

4—**Antioxidants strengthen the cardiovascular system and keep it clear:** •Crystal Star HEART PROTECTOR FOR MEN™ and HEART PROTECTOR FOR WOMEN™ caps caps; •Grapeseed PCO's 100mg 3x daily; •Alpha lipoic acid 200mg daily; N-acetylcysteine 100mg daily; •Biogenetics BIO-GUARD with wheat sprout complex and selenium.

5—**Boost your thyroid to reduce heart disease risk:** •Spirulina, liquid chlorophyll, or Pines MIGHTY GREENS drink; or •2 tbsp. dry sea greens daily.

6—**Cardiotonics help the heart beat stronger and steadier:** •Douglas Labs CoQMelt daily, or Enzymatic Therapy COQ-10 chewable tabs (work quickly and effectively);

•Carnitine 1000mg daily; •*Cayenne-Ginger* caps or *Garlic* capsules 6 daily; or •Heart Foods HEART FOOD Cayenne caps; •*Siberian eleuthero* caps 2000mg or tea 2 cups daily;

•Prince of Peace GINSENG-ROYAL JELLY vials. •Wheat germ oil caps boost tissue oxygen (highly effective).

7—**Phyto-estrogen heart protective herbs for menopausal women:** •Crystal Star FEMALE HARMONY™ caps, or •*Ginkgo Biloba* extract help prevent ischemia-caused fibrillation. •Crystal Star HEART PROTECTOR for WOMEN™ with *dong quai*; •*Vitex* extract; •*Licorice root* tea; •*Ginseng-licorice* drops.

8—**Heart disease preventives:** •Folic acid to keep homocysteine levels down, with •B-6 100mg and •Country Life sublingual B-12, 2500mcg. •Flora MAGNESIUM liquid to help prevent stroke.

9—**Reduce blood stickiness to prevent a heart attack:** •Bromelain 1500mg regularly increases fibrinolysis; •Chromium picolinate or Solaray CHROMIACIN for arterial plaque and insulin resistance. •Omega-3 oils, or Lane Labs OMEGA MULTI 3x daily.

Can't find a recommended product? Call the 800 number listed in Product Resources for the store nearest you.

Hemorrhage

Internal Bleeding, Excessive Bleeding, Blood Clotting Problems, Nosebleeds

The suggestions on this page refer to first aid for minor or non-life threatening bleeding problems. Obviously, you should get to an emergency room or call an ambulance if there is an emergency situation. Nosebleeds, bleeding gums and urinary tract bleeding are types of bleeding that can be addressed with these remedies. Most remedies are astringents (tighteners) or styptics (stoppers) that may also be used for swollen veins or hemorrhoids. Once the bleeding has been arrested, the idea with natural remedies is, as always, to address the underlying causes (like weak membranes or fragile capillary structure) that allow bleeding to be excessive. **Do you have excessive bleeding?** Do you: clot even small wounds with difficulty? experience internal pain from a rupture or ulcer? bruise easily? have numerous broken blood vessels? have black stools with a stomach ulcer? If you have nausea, dizziness, enlarged pupils, drowsiness, confusion, or convulsions after an accident to an artery or your head, hemorrhage is usually involved. **Bleeding causes:** Broken blood vessels from weak vein and vessel walls, internal wounds from an accident; lack of vitamin K in the body, (especially from eating irradiated foods which deplete your body vitamin K), over-use of aspirin or other blood thinning drugs; arterial plaque accumulation. An English study shows that hemorrhage may be prevented by taking daily PCOs. See SHOCK TREATMENT page 538 for more.

Diet and Lifestyle Support Therapy

Nutritional therapy plan: *Don't use aspirin or other blood-thinner drugs like Heparin if you are at risk for internal bleeding.*

1—Make a variety of sprouts a regular part of your diet for natural vitamin K to help clotting and optimize healthy intestinal flora. Other high vitamin K foods: kale, spinach and all dark green veggies, broccoli, cauliflower, and eggs.

2—Take a cup of green tea every morning, or try Crystal Star DR. VITALITY™ with green and white tea. (I am prone to excessive bleeding, but since I started a green tea regimen, the condition has normalized.) Green tea catechins control hemorrhage by activating coagulants.

3—Have a glass of carrot-spinach juice, or a mixed vegetable drink once a week. Try Crystal Star ENERGY GREEN RENEWAL™ drink, or •Green Foods MAGMA PLUS, or liquid chlorophyll 3 tsp. daily once a week to build healthier blood balance.

4—Eat plenty of papayas. Use citrus peel directly on the bleeding area.

—Bodywork:

• **Styptics to apply directly:** •Make a clotting paste with crushed plantain leaves and water and apply.

• **Body pressure points:**

—Press insides of the thighs with fingers just above knees, for 10 seconds at a time.

—Hold arm in the air on the side of the bleeding to decrease pressure.

—Pull knuckle of middle finger on either hand until it pops, to lower blood pressure.

—To help arrest bleeding of a vein or artery: apply direct pressure with cold compresses or ice packs. Get to a doctor and treat for shock.

—For a nosebleed: blow once vigorously to clear the nose, then pinch the sides of the nose together. Place a cold compress on nose. Apply pressure and hold firmly for 10 minutes.

• **Astringents to apply directly:** Cold cloths or ice packs. •Witch hazel or Yarrow compresses. •Calendula salve or poultice. •Propolis tincture.

Herbal, Superfood and Supplement Therapy

Interceptive therapy plan: Choose 2 to 3 recommendations.

1—When bleeding just won't stop: •Take capsicum, take 1 tsp. in a cup of hot water to stop bleeding. (Take with an eyedropper on the back of the tongue if it is too hot to swallow; or •take 2 dropperfuls *bilberry* extract and 2 *cayenne* capsules (also apply directly; it will burn but it works) and get to a clinic. •Take 2 *turmeric* extract capsules.

•Apply *Panax notoginseng* (Tienchi) extract directly to cut bleeding time in half.

2—For better clotting: •Crystal Star DR. VITALITY™ caps with green and white tea; •Solaray CALCIUM CITRATE caps. Make a •clotting tea combo: *Licorice root, comfrey root, shepherd's purse, goldenseal root, cranesbill;* —**Homeopathic remedies,** especially for clotting difficulty from dental or cosmetic surgery: •*Ferrum Phos.*: bright red bleeding; •*Arnica:* bleeding with bruising, or nosebleeds; •*Phosphorus*: persistent bleeding.

3—Astringents tighten veins and capillaries. (Use externally and internally to check bleeding). • *White oak bark* or *yarrow* tea; •*Myrrh* extract; •*Bilberry* extract; •Solaray CRANESBILL blend capsules; •*Goldenseal* extract; •*Nettles* tea and capsules.

4—For bloody urine: •take 4 *turmeric* extract caps; or make an •astringent tea: *plantain leaf, calendula flowers, horsetail* and *bugleweed.* (Also use as an effective compress.)

5—For intestinal and stomach bleeding: 2 cups daily •*Pau d' arco,* or *white oak bark* tea; •*Turmeric* extract capsules; •*Comfrey root* or *ginger root* tea; or *Shepherd's purse* capsules. •Vitamin K 100mcg 3x daily to maintain micro-flora integrity. •Crystal Star DR. PROBIOTICS™ with FOS to help with vitamin K production.

6—For nosebleeds: •*Arnica* ointment (specific for nosebleed); *white willow* tea compresses; •Vitamin C 3000mg daily for nosebleeds (especially if you also bruise easily).

7—High flavonoids strengthen veins and capillaries: •OPCs from grapeseed or white pine 300mg daily; •Quercetin 1000 with bromelain 1000mg, 2 daily; •Vitamin C bioflavonoids and rutin boosts collagen and interstitial tissue formation, try Ester C or ascorbic acid crystals up to 5000mg daily, or Twin Lab CITRUS BIOFLAVONOID caps, or •Jarow GENTLE FIBERS drink with extra bioflavs to increase tissue integrity. •Prince of Peace GIN SENG-ROYAL JELLY vials for stronger blood.

Can't find a recommended product? Call the 800 number listed in Product Resources for the store nearest you.

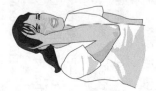

Hemorrhoids

Piles, Anal Fissure

Hemorrhoids, also called piles, are swollen, inflamed veins and capillaries around the anus that often painfully protrude out of the rectum. In the year 2000 alone, 75 million Americans visited their doctor for hemorrhoids. There is usually constipation and because of straining, rectal bleeding. New research also shows a link with diarrhea and hemorrhoids. The pain and discomfort of hemorrhoidal itch and swelling are well known. *Anal fissures* are often misdiagnosed as hemorrhoids, but they are not swollen veins, instead they are tiny tears in the lower part of the intestine. They are very painful and often require surgery (over 40,000 surgeries a year) to fix. A change in diet composition and natural therapies can help you avoid drugs and surgery for either hemorrhoids or anal fissures. **Do you have hemorrhoids?** You probably do if you have chronic pain, itching and rectal bleeding with your bowel movements, protruding anal swellings, or an extremely inflamed anal fissure. **What causes hemorrhoids?** A fast food diet with too many over-refined, fried, fatty, low residue foods and not enough healthy hydrating liquids is the prime culprit; most sufferers are chronically constipated with habitual straining, or suffer with chronic diarrhea from too many antacids and laxative abuse. Other causes involve body chemistry imbalances from overeating and consequent liver exhaustion, lack of exercise (really too much sitting), and vitamin B₆ deficiency, especially from drugs like anti-depressants and pain killers. Pregnancy usually brings short term hemorrhoids. *See also COLON HEALTH & CONSTIPATION page 381 for more.*

Diet and Lifestyle Support Therapy

Nutritional therapy plan:

1—Diet improvement is the key to permanently reducing hemorrhoids. Avoid refined, low fiber foods, and acid forming foods, like caffeine and sugar.

2—Take 1 tbsp. olive oil or flax seed oil before each meal. Include plenty of fiber foods in your diet, particularly lots of vegetable cellulose (dried fruits, brans and vegetables).

3—Include daily sprouts and dark greens for vitamin K to inhibit bleeding.

4—Include lots of berries and cherries for PCO's, or try •Jarrow GENTLE FIBERS to strengthen veins and capillaries.

5—Take 2 tbsp. cider vinegar mixed with 2 tbsp. maple syrup, or •New Chapter GINGER WONDER syrup every morning for a month.

6—Drink plenty of healthy liquids throughout the day - juices and mineral water, •AloeLife ALOE GOLD drink, or Guayaki YERBA MATÉ green tea.

7—Keep meals small, so the bowel and sphincter area won't have to work so hard.

8—Apply papaya skins or lemon juice directly to inflamed area to relieve itching.

—**Bodywork:** •Take a good half hour walk every day. •Put feet on a stool when sitting on the toilet to ease strain. •Soak in a hot tub to reduce inflammation and stop itching.

—**Effective enemas remove congestion:** •Nettles; •Chlorella or spirulina; •Nutribiotic GRAPEFRUIT SEED extract - 20 drops per gallon of water (very effective).

—**Effective rectal applications:** •Ice packs; •Witch hazel as needed; •MotherLove RHOID BALM or SITZ BATH; •Open and apply a vitamin E capsule; •Epsom Salts sitz baths; •Earth Mama Angel Baby BOTTOM BALM; •ALOE LIFE ALOE SKIN GEL.

—**Effective compresses:** •Alternating hot and cool water, or cold water compresses every morning; •Horsetail tea - frequently; •Elderberry tea.

Herbal, Superfood and Supplement Therapy

Interceptive therapy plan: Choose 2 to 3 recommendations.

1—**Relieve inflammation and encourage healing:** •Crystal Star HEMR-EZE™ capsules for 2 weeks (may also open, mix with aloe gel and use as an effective suppository). Apply. •Crystal Star HEMR-EZE™ gel; •St. John's wort oil, or •calendula ointment, and make a hemorrhoid tea: mix equal parts *comfrey root, wild yam* and *cranesbill.* Take internally and apply directly. •Take *stone root tea,* 3 cups daily for a month.

—Use homeopathic remedies: •Hylands HEMMOREX, •Hippocastanum, •Boiron homeopathic HEMORRHOID SUPPOSITORIES, or •homeopathic *Collinsonia canadensis* to relieve itching and burning.

2—**Encourage vascular tone:** •*Ginkgo Biloba* or *bilberry* extract for PCO's; •Solaray CENTELLA ASIATICA caps for vascular tone. Add •Crystal Star LIVER CLEANSE FLUSHING™ tea for sluggishness, and •BWL-TONE IBS™ caps or •*butcher's broom* tea for gentle healing. •Evening primrose oil caps 4 daily; • *Ho-Shou-Wu* (Fo-Ti) capsules.

3—**Strengthen vein and capillary walls with flavonoids:** •Vitamin C therapy for collagen and interstitial tissue formation: use Ester C or ascorbic acid crystals with bioflavs. and rutin - take up to 5000mg daily; (also make a solution in water to apply directly). •Source Naturals activated QUERCETIN with bromelain 4 daily.

4—**Herbal suppositories are easy and work almost right away.** (mix herbs with cocoa butter as the delivery medium): •*Goldenseal-Myrrh; Bee Pollen* granules; •*Slippery elm; Garlic-Comfrey; Cranesbill; Yarrow; White oak bark.* •Use NatureAde SOFT-EX tablets to soften stool short term.

5—**Nutrients help rebuild colon and rectum health from the inside:** •PCO's from grapeseed or white pine, 2 daily; •Bromelain 1500mg caps; lecithin caps 1900gr daily; •Vitamin K 100mcg 2x daily with vitamin B-6 250mg daily.

—**For anal fissure:** take internally and apply •Crystal Star ANTI-BIO™ caps; or apply •Crystal Star ANTI-BIO™ gel (with una da gato). Take •Liquid chlorophyll 3 tsp. daily in 8-oz. water daily and •Enzymatic Therapy HEMTONE capsules.

Can't find a recommended product? Call the 800 number listed in Product Resources for the store nearest you.

Hepatitis

Severe Viral Liver Infection

Hepatitis has reached epidemic status in the U.S. Millions are unaware they're infected! *Type A:* a viral infection passed through blood and feces or by contaminated food. (The CDC says fully 1/3 of Americans have evidence of present or past infections). *Type B:* sexually transmitted via blood, semen, saliva, dirty needles (infects 325,000 Americans a year). *Type C:* a post-transfusion virus, affects 4.5 million Americans - 230,000 new cases each year. *Type D:* caused by Epstein-Barr virus and cytomegalovirus. *Non-A, Non-B:* higher mortality viruses passed by transfusions. Hepatitis ranges from chronic fatigue to serious liver damage, even to death from liver failure or liver cancer. Liver cancer rates have jumped 70% in the last 20 years largely due to the surge in hepatitis. The medical approach, only beneficial in 40% of cases, relies on intravenous interferon therapy which can cause infertility, depression, psychosis and severe fatigue. Natural therapies, in contrast, have had great success in hepatitis cases, both in arresting viral replication and in regenerating the liver. **Signs of hepatitis?** Great fatigue, flu-like exhaustion and diarrhea, an enlarged, tender, congested liver, loss of appetite to the point of anorexia, nausea, dark urine, gray stools; skin pallor and histamine itching, depression, irritated bowel and digestive problems; skin jaundice; cirrhosis of the liver. **How do you get hepatitis?** Almost 90% of intravenous drug users infected. Medical workers are at risk. Yet, hundreds of thousands of people with hepatitis C are not in any high risk group, leaving experts to believe that the disease may have triggers we haven't discovered yet.

Diet and Lifestyle Support Therapy

Nutritional therapy: Get plenty of bed rest, especially during the acute infectious stages.

1—Hepatitis Healing Diet: For 2 weeks: Eat only fresh foods - salads, fruits, juices, bottled water. Have a glass of roasted dandelion tea each morning. Take a glass of carrot/beet/cucumber juice every other day. Take a glass of lemon juice and water every morning. Take Sun Wellness CHLORELLA drink or granules daily. •Use detoxifying chlorophyll twice weekly the first two critical weeks of healing. Take 1 tsp. powder in water 2-3x daily for 7 days; then 1 tsp. 4x daily at meals and bedtime for 7 days.

Then for 1 to 2 months: Take roasted dandelion tea every day, carrot-beet-cucumber juice every 3 days, and papaya juice or AloeLife ALOE GOLD drink with 2 tsp. spirulina each morning. Eat lots of vegetable proteins, with steamed vegetables (esp. dark greens), brown rice, tofu, eggs, healing mushrooms like shiitake or maitake, whole grains and yogurt. Avoid red meats. EFAs from seafood are beneficial. Eat light at night to reduce the workload on the liver. •Crystal Star BITTERS & LEMON CLEANSE™ each morning. Then for 1 more month: Take 2 glasses of tomato juice/lemon juice or roasted dandelion tea every day. Take a daily glass of apple-alfalfa sprout juice or a green drink like Nutricology PRO-GREENS with EFAs, or Crystal Star RESTORE YOUR STRENGTH™ drink. Continue with vegetable proteins, cultured foods, fresh salads and complex carbs for strength. Important! Avoid refined, fried, fatty foods, sugars, heavy spices, alcohol and caffeine during healing. Add Crystal Star DR. VITALITY™ green and white liver cleansing tea to any meal.

—Get tested for Hepatitis C if: 1) you had a blood transfusion before 1992. 2) you inject illegal drugs. 3) you are on dialysis. 4) you've had multiple sex partners. 5) you have body piercing/ tattoos. 6) you contact blood. 7) your live-in partner has Hepatitis C.

—Lifestyle measures: •Count on 2 weeks for emergency detox measures; 1-3 months for healing the liver, rebuilding blood and body strength. •Overheating therapy can be effective for Hepatitis. See page 182. A steam bath or sauna removes much toxicity through the skin. •Acupuncture treatments help restore a sense of well being.
•Avoid all alcohol, amphetamines, cocaine, barbiturates, or tobacco of any kind.

Herbal, Superfood and Supplement Therapy

Interceptive therapy: Choose 2 to 3 recommendations.

1—Cleanse the liver of toxins: •Alpha Lipoic acid 600mg daily (excellent liver detoxifier); •Jarrow SAMe 200, 3 daily; •Crystal Star LIVER RENEW™ capsules 4 to 6 daily, with LIVER CLEANSE FLUSHING™ tea 2 cups for 1 month. Reduce dose to half the 2nd month. •Planetary Formulas BUPLEURUM LIVER CLEANSE (use with roasted dandelion tea for best results) •*Oregon grape-red clover* detox tea; •Colloidal Silver (good results against hepatitis C). •Dreamous IMMUNOVATION; •Herbasway LIVER ENHANCER tea (good results against hepatitis B); •Nutricology LIVERCEL; •Take Vitamin C crystals, up to 10,000mg daily in water, to bowel tolerance for 1 month and •CoQ10, 300mg daily.

2—Inhibit viral replication, stimulate interferon: •Vitamin E 800IU with Selenium 400mcg or E don SELENIUM liquid; Interferon therapy: *Astragalus-Reishi-Shiitake-Echinacea* compound; •Royal Bodycare MICROHYDRIN PLUS (can significantly reduce elevated liver enzymes); •*Echinacea-St. John's wort:* take 4 days *echinacea* extract then 4 days *St. John's wort* extract. •PSP Marketing VIRAMAX, 2 caps 4x daily (highly recommended).

3—Heal liver tissue: Cholesterol drugs deplete glutathione, vital for liver detox. •Acetyl-L-carnitine 2000mg daily; •Solaray LIPOTROPIC PLUS caps; •Crystal Star Dr. ENZYME™ with protease and bromelain helps soften hardened liver tissue; •Ayurvedic *Phyllanthus amarus* for hepatitis B; •Transformation PUREZYME caps. •Nutricology GERMANIUM 150mg daily.

4—Take normalizing liver tonics for 1 month: •Nutricology NAC (N-acetyl-cysteine) 1500mg daily; •Maitake mushroom extract caps; or •Dandelion root extract or roasted *dandelion* tea, or •*astragalus* extract or •*lobelia* extract drops in tea; *turmeric* extract caps or *bayberry–cayenne* capsules, 6 daily to control inflammation. •Crystal Star ANTI-HST™ caps to control histamine reactions, for 1 month. Reduce dose to half 2nd month.

5—Long term liver support: Use •Futurebiotics MSM 1000mg, •Beta carotene 150,000IU daily; •MILK THISTLE SEED extract. —**Probiotics re-establish immunity:** •Nutricology SYMBIOTICS with FOS if detection is early. •Natren BIFIDO FACTORS daily for 1 month or •UAS DDS-PLUS with FOS.

451

Can't find a recommended product? Call the 800 number listed in Product Resources for the store nearest you.

High Blood Pressure

Hypertension

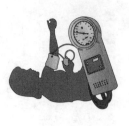

High blood pressure is a major health problem in America's fast-paced, high-stress world. High blood pressure affects 1 out of every 3 U.S. adults today. It's the leading health problem for American women. The newest research shows that middle aged Americans actually have a 90% chance of developing high blood pressure! Less than half have their blood pressure under control, largely because only half of them know they have a problem! HBP causes 60,000 deaths a year and directly relates to more than 250,000 deaths from stroke. It is a silent condition that steals health and can steal life. It increases risk for heart attack, for congestive heart failure (especially in women) and kidney malfunction. It accelerates atherosclerosis (hardening of the arteries), damages the heart and blood vessels and, according to a recent study published in the journal Stroke, speeds up the aging process of the brain!

What causes high blood pressure? Most cases of high blood pressure are caused by arteriosclerosis and atherosclerosis (clogging arterial fats and increased fat storage), 90% of which in turn may be the result of a calcium, magnesium or fiber deficiency - factors that can be controlled by diet and lifestyle improvement. Most sufferers are greatly overweight due to a high fat, high sugar diet; most have a high consumption of salt and red meat which overly raises critical copper levels. A high stress lifestyle, usually linked to smoking, excess alcohol and too much caffeine is also involved. This type of life contributes to key markers for high blood pressure: thickened blood with excess mucous and waste, insulin resistance from poor sugar metabolism, thyroid metabolic imbalances, exhausted kidneys and varying degrees of auto-toxemia from chronic constipation.

Clinical studies show that people with hypertension who make good life changes fare much better than those on anti-hypertensive prescription drugs. Vegetarians have less hypertension and fewer blood pressure problems. Exercise is a key.

Do you have high blood pressure?

Ideal blood pressure stays below 120 (systolic-the pressure exerted when the heart pumps) over 80 (diastolic-the pressure when the heart rests between beats) or slightly less. If the reading goes over 140/90, hypertension is usually indicated. **If the diastolic (or bottom) number goes over 104, severe hypertension is diagnosed.** Your physician will gladly check your blood pressure for you. In addition, most pharmacies have convenient on site testing or home blood pressure test kits you can buy. Even small changes in blood pressure may be serious. Persons with blood pressure levels of 120 over 80, once thought to be safe, are now considered at risk for hypertension. Ask your physician.

Warning signs of high blood pressure:

—frequent headaches and irritability? chronic constipation? (from calcium and fiber deficiency)
—dizziness and ringing in the ears? frequent heart arrhythmias? flushed complexion? red streaks in your eyes? (from auto-toxemia)
—great fatigue along with sleeplessness? depression? kidney malfunction? (from insulin resistance and poor sugar metabolism)
—chronic respiratory problems? (from excess mucous and wastes)
—uncontrolled weight gain and fluid retention? (thyroid imbalance from increased fat storage, too much salt, red meat, and lack of exercise)
—swollen ankles (poor mineral/water balance- also a sign of congestive heart failure)

Do you have to take high blood pressure drugs for life?

Calcium channel blockers inhibit the entry of calcium into heart cells and smooth muscle cells of blood vessels. Without calcium, the cells cannot contract and the result is lowered blood pressure. But calcium is an important mineral for heart health! Calcium regulates the contraction and relaxation of the heart, and inhibits heart spasms. Calcium is most beneficial when it is brought into the body with a balanced ratio of magnesium through foods. I always say magnesium is "Nature's calcium channel blocker." Magnesium naturally blocks the entry of calcium into heart muscle cells and vascular smooth muscle cells, reducing vascular resistance in order to keep blood pressure normal. Good food sources include: dark green veggies (or sea greens), whole grains, nuts and seeds, beans and poultry.

Beta blockers work to impede the action of the body's beta receptors, adrenaline response modifiers between the heart and brain. The theory is that the brain can't notify the heart to constrict the arteries, so it slows down, regardless of its need.

Americans are told that if they have high blood pressure, lifetime drug therapy is the best solution. But over the long-term, side effect hazards may outweigh the benefits of these drugs. New studies in the journal *Circulation* find that calcium channel blockers increase heart attack risk by up to 60%. British studies show they raise the risk of suicide! For men, impotence commonly results. The drugs are also linked to breast cancer and memory loss. Some side effects of beta blockers are dizziness, nausea, asthma, impotence in men and joint pain.

Can't find a recommended product? Call the 800 number listed in Product Resources for the store nearest you.

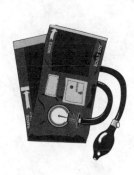

Try one of the new home blood pressure monitors. It could give you a more accurate picture.

Chronic high blood pressure, or hypertension, is a major risk factor for heart disease and stroke, which together account for almost half of U.S. deaths. If you are more than 30 pounds overweight, have a history of hypertension, heart disease, or stroke, or have a family history of cardiovascular disease, you might give serious thought to investing in a home blood pressure monitor for peace of mind.

For some people, home blood pressure testing is more accurate than professional testing, because the anxiousness of being in a doctor's office raises their blood pressure. Home testing eliminates this "white coat hypertension," and the medications that might be unnecessarily prescribed to treat it.

Simply slip your arm into the provided cuff and fill it with air using the bulb-shaped hand pump. When you release the air, the monitor determines your pressure electronically and displays it digitally. (Although available and more convenient, finger cuffs are not as accurate as the arm cuffs.)

Can natural therapies lower blood pressure? The newest information shows that most people don't require medication to control their disease. Millions can reverse high blood pressure with simple diet and lifestyle therapy. 1997 Harvard Medical School research finds a low-fat diet may lower blood pressure as much as drugs. New research from the West Oakland Health Center finds that meditation for 20 minutes, twice daily is as effective as drug therapy to lower blood pressure.

High Blood Pressure Prevention Diet

Eighty-five percent of high blood pressure is preventable without drugs. In fact, a good diet is your best bet to control high blood pressure. Reduce and control salt use. (See Low Salt Diet, pg. 154.) Drink plenty of water to balance your body salts. When your body perceives that it is becoming dehydrated, it responds by retaining sodium to reduce further water loss, starting a vicious cycle of craving for salty foods and liquids that ends in high blood pressure. (Constantly taking diuretics for high blood pressure aggravates this cycle.) Start by eliminating foods that provoke high blood pressure – canned and frozen foods, cured, smoked and canned meats and fish, commercial peanut butter, soy sauce, bouillon cubes and condiments, fried chips and snacks, dry soups. Rewards are high – a longer, healthier life – and control of your life. Avoid antacids that neutralize natural stomach acid and invite your body to produce even more acid.

On rising: Have lemon water with maple syrup or a high vitamin/mineral drink. like All One MULTIPLE with green plants, or Crystal Star RESTORE YOUR STRENGTH™ drink.

Breakfast: Make a mix of 2 tbsp. each: lecithin granules, toasted wheat germ, nutritional yeast, sesame seeds and a little honey. Sprinkle some on fresh fruit or mix with yogurt; or have a poached or baked egg with bran muffins or whole grain toast, and kefir cheese or unsalted butter; or some whole grain cereal or pancakes with a little maple syrup.

Mid-morning: Have a veggie drink, like Knudsen's VERY VEGGIE or Crystal Star ENERGY GREEN RENEWAL™ drink, or Green Foods GREEN MAGMA, or natural V-8 juice or peppermint tea: or a cup of miso soup with sea greens snipped on top: or low-sodium ramen noodle soup; and/or some crunchy raw veggies with a kefir cheese or yogurt dip.

Lunch: Have one cup daily of fenugreek tea with 1 tsp. honey; then have a tofu and spinach salad with some sprouts and bran muffins; or a large fresh green salad with a lemon oil dressing. Add plenty of sprouts, tofu, raisins, cottage cheese, nuts, and seeds as desired; or have a baked potato with yogurt or kefir cheese topping, and a light veggie omelet; or a seafood and vegetable pasta salad, or some grilled or braised vegetables with an olive oil dressing and brown rice.

Mid-afternoon: Have a mineral water, a cup of peppermint tea, or a cup of miso soup with a hard boiled egg, or whole grain crackers; or dried fruit snack (especially figs which prevent arterial damage), and an apple or cranberry juice.

Dinner: Have a baked vegetable casserole with tofu and brown rice, and a small dinner salad; or a baked fish or seafood dish with rice and peas, or a baked potato; or a vegetable quiche (such as broccoli, artichoke, or asparagus), and a light oriental soup; or some roast turkey and cornbread dressing, with a small salad or mashed potatoes with a little butter; or an oriental vegetable stir fry, with a light, clear soup and brown rice. A little wine is fine with dinner for relaxation, digestion and tension relief.

Before bed: Have a cup of miso soup, or Red Star NUTRITIONAL YEAST broth, apple juice, or some *chamomile* tea.

Can't find a recommended product? Call the 800 number listed in Product Resources for the store nearest you.

High Blood Pressure

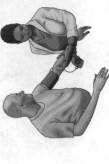

Diet and Lifestyle Support Therapy

Nutritional therapy plan:

1—Keep body weight down. One of the biggest risk factors is excess fat storage. Go on a juice diet for 1 day every week for 2 months to improve body chemistry and reduce extra blood fats. Have a veggie green drink, like Sun Wellness CHLORELLA drink daily, or Knudsen's VERY VEGGIE juice, or carrot juice at mid-day. Have citrus juices or a potassium drink (pg. 291) in the morning. Have apple, pear or papaya juice before dinner. Chamomile tea or Sovex yeast broth at bedtime.

2— Then follow the *High Blood Pressure Diet* on the previous page: eat lots of vitamin C, magnesium, potassium foods: broccoli, bananas, oranges, dried fruits (esp. figs), potatoes, seafood, bell peppers, avocados, celery, brown rice and leafy greens to help rebalance sodium levels. Add •New Chapter GINGER WONDER syrup to any juice or recipe.

3—Eat smaller meals more frequently; consciously undereat. Avoid caffeine, salty, sugary, fried, fatty foods, smoked meats, heavy pastries and soft drinks. All cause potassium depletion and allow arterial plaque build-up. Drink plenty of pure water to improve sodium balance.

4—Cut the fat. Harvard Medical School research reveals a low-fat diet can lower blood pressure as much as drugs. Cutting back on hard, saturated fats (from meats and dairy) and trans fats (highly processed fats in snack foods and fried, fast foods) is highly recommended. But don't cut out the good fats. Include EFA rich foods like olive oil, seafood (esp. salmon), sea greens (like nori, kelp or wakame), herbs like evening primrose and flax seed oil regularly. Make a mix of wheat germ, flax oil, nutritional yeast; take 2 tbsp. daily.

—Bodywork:

•You have high blood pressure if you have a repeated reading over 150/90mmHg. Monitor your progress often with a home or free drugstore electronic machine reading.
•Avoid all tobacco to dramatically lower blood pressure. Smoking constricts blood vessels making your heart work harder. Smoking aggravates high blood sugar levels.
•Phenylalanine, especially as found in Nutra-Sweet, and over-the-counter antihistamines can aggravate high blood pressure.
•Eliminate caffeine and hard liquor. They cause adrenaline rushes that make blood pressure soar. (A little wine with dinner can actually lower stress and hypertension.)
•Exercise is important. Take a brisk 30 minute walk every day. Breathe deep.
•Relaxation techniques are important. Meditation and massage are two of the best.
•Use a dry skin brush all over the body frequently to stimulate better blood flow.

—Reflexology: •Pull middle finger on each hand 3x for 20 seconds each time, daily.

Herbal, Superfood and Supplement Therapy

Interceptive therapy plan: Choose 2 to 3 recommendations.

1—Help regulate your blood pressure: •Crystal Star HEARTSEASE H.B.P.™ caps daily, or •Esteem CARDIOLIFE (noticeable activity). •Vitamin E therapy: Take 1 100IU capsule daily for 1 week, then 4 capsules daily for 1 week, then 2 400IU capsules daily for 2 weeks. Add 1 selenium 200mcg, and 1 Ester C with bioflavs each time, for hypertension caused by toxic heavy metals. Add mixed carotenes for uptake. •Nutricology PROLIVE caps (olive leaf extract). •Optimal Health PRESSURE FX (88% effective in a Brazilian study). *Salvia miltiorrhiza* (Chinese red sage) helps reduce HBP in women.

2—Tone your arterial system with flavonoids: Take •HAWTHORN extract as needed, especially if you have palpitations. •Ginkgo Biloba extract for extra circulation; •Cayenne-ginger caps 4 daily, or Wakunaga AGED GARLIC extract; •Grifron MAITAKE or REISHI caps •Bilberry extract, or •organic Grapeseed PCOs 100mg as needed; •Garlic, or onion-garlic caps 6 daily. •Siberian eleuthero extract caps, 2000mg daily. •Hibiscus tea lowers blood pressure (clinical results 1999 Journal of Ethnopharmacology).

3—Naturally reduce edema swelling: •Crystal Star TINKLE™ caps and TINKLE™ tea; •*Dandelion* extract drops in tea (fast acting). Most high blood pressure medicines cause potassium-magnesium loss. If you are taking diuretics, take •vitamin C 1000mg daily, potassium 99mg daily or •Crystal Star OCEAN MINERALS™ caps (Iodine, Potassium and Silica from the sea) and •B-complex 100mg.

4—Reduce your risk of a stroke: •Crystal Star GREEN TEA CLEANSER™ each a.m. •Rainbow Light CALCIUM PLUS caps w. high magnesium, 6 daily. •Nutricology NATTOZYME (*nattokinase*) is a specific.

5—Reduce stress to control hypertension: •Nature's Secret ULTIMATE B daily with extra B₆ 100mg, niacin 100mg 3x daily. Crystal Star •RELAX CAPS™. •Hyland's homeopathic CALMS FORTE tabs. •CoQ₁₀ 60mg 3x daily; •Suma caps 6 daily; •Crystal Star ADRENAL ENERGY BOOST™ caps 4 daily and •CALCIUM-MAGNESIUM SOURCE™ caps or drops.

6—Boost your essential fatty acids: •Omega-3 fish or flax oils 3 daily; Spectrum NORWEGIAN FISH OIL. •Evening Primrose Oil 3000mg daily.

7—Digest fats and dairy foods better to help high blood pressure: •Bromelain 1000mg. daily; •Chromium picolinate 200mcg. daily to combat insulin resistance. •Transformation LYPOZYME; •Crystal Star DR. PROBIOTICS™ with FOS; •Planetary TRIPHALA caps as directed (very good results). •Metabolic Response Modifiers CARDIO-CHELATE with EDTA.

—Superfood therapy: (choose 1 recommendation.)
•Futurebiotics VITAL K drink daily.
•All One TOTALLY FIBER COMPLEX drink.

Can't find a recommended product? Call the 800 number listed in Product Resources for the store nearest you.

Hormone Imbalances – Women

Estrogen Disruption, Hysterectomy Aftermath, Environmental Hormone Effects

A healthy female system works in an incredibly beautiful, complex balance. It is an individual model of the creative universe. A woman is usually a marvelous thing to be, but the intricacies of her body are delicately tuned and can become unbalanced or obstructed easily, causing pain and poor function. From child-bearing age, to premenopause, to menopause, to post-menopause, many women are affected by fluctuations in their hormones that rattle their lives. Female hormone imbalances are involved in myriad health problems including: fibroids, endometriosis, headaches, PMS, depression, low libido and infertility. Hormones help regulate everything from energy flow, to inflammation, to a woman's monthly cycle. Tiny amounts can cause big reactions, both good and bad. Maintaining hormonal balance in today's world isn't easy. Every day, we are bombarded with man-made hormones — widespread hormone-mimicking pollutants, hormone drugs and hormones injected in our foods. A high stress lifestyle which depletes the adrenal glands is a major factor in hormonal problems for women. A hormone balancing lifestyle program is something most of us can benefit from. Using lifestyle therapy to rebalance hormone ratios gently harmonizes your body, rather than regulating hormones by injection, which sometimes stops natural hormone production by the endocrine glands entirely. Natural hormone balancing therapies after trauma, stress or serious illness, or after a hysterectomy, childbirth, or an abortion allow your body to achieve its own hormone levels and bring itself to its own balance at its deepest levels.

Your hormones may be out of balance if: You have painful, difficult menstruation, or absence of menstruation. You have spotting between periods. You're often depressed, irritable and moody for no reason. You have frequent water retention.

What causes hormone problems? Birth control pills and hormone replacement therapy are primary culprits. Stress, which leads to adrenal exhaustion (the adrenal glands produce most hormones). Severe dieting or serious body building, surgery or long illness and nutrient deficiencies, especially protein, calcium and iodine deficiency, low B Complex or EFAs.

What about environmental hormones?

Environmental hormones are so commonplace in modern society that there is no way to completely avoid them. They come from pollutants, drugs, hormone-injected meats and dairy foods, plastics, pesticides, pesticides, and hormone replacement drugs for both sexes. Only in the last ten years has anyone realized how common environmental estrogens are in today's world. Nearly 40% of pesticides used in commercial agriculture are suspected hormone disrupters. The problem is so huge that in 1996 the Environmental Protection Agency began implementing a congressionally mandated plan through EDSTAC (Endocrine Disrupter Screening and Testing Advisory Committee) to test 87,000 compounds to determine their effect on the reproductive systems of humans and animals. However, due to the enormous scope of the project, a lack of funding and strong opposition from the chemical industry, very little real progress has been made.

The threat these chemicals have on human health and the environment is very real, and growing. Estrogen-mimicking pollutants may, in fact, be changing the face of evolution. New reports show the devastating effect of hormone disrupting pollutants on our wildlife and human health. Pallid sturgeons, found only in the Mississippi river, are now condemned to extinction as decades of exposure to pollutant PCB's (*polychlorinated biphenyls*) and DDT (*dichloro-diphenyl-trichloroethane*) have resulted in no new species birth for more than 10 years. Studies done on turtles at the University of Texas find that even when environmental factors (like heat) are controlled to determine a male outcome, females or intersex turtles are hatched from just a small amount of PCB's are painted on the eggs. The newest research shows Atrazine, a weed killer, causes wildlife to develop the wrong sex organs. More shocking: Atrazine use is so commonplace that it now contaminates the water in states where it isn't even used.

The effects of estrogen disruption mean maintaining female hormone balance is clearly a challenge.

One of the biggest health threats facing the health of women today is the excess estrogen assault from our environment. Hormone disrupters affect your entire endocrine system, all the communication system of your glands, hormones and cellular receptors in your body. They alter the production and breakdown of your own hormones, and the function of your hormone receptors — disrupting hormone balance at its developmental core. They can compete for hormone receptor sites in the body and bind to them in place of natural hormones, causing major fluctuations in hormonal levels in the body. They are a serious concern for women in early pregnancy because a developing embryo is highly sensitive to estrogen disrupter toxicity. Compounding the problem, these chemicals may increase in potency when they're combined inside your body from several different sources, like from hormone-injected meats and pesticide-sprayed produce. Women aren't the only ones endangered by the estrogen-mimics. Substantial evidence shows that man-made estrogens threaten male reproductive health, too. Most alarming statistics relate to sperm count and hormone driven cancers.

Can't find a recommended product? Call the 800 number listed in Product Resources for the store nearest you.

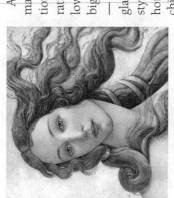

456

Science is just beginning to accept, even though naturopaths have known for some time, that man-made estrogens can stack the deck against women by increasing their estrogen levels hundreds of times over normal levels. (The hormone replacement drug for women, Premarin, is one of the top-selling drugs in America!) Although many scientists still believe that there is no significant difference between man-made and natural hormones, it seems apparent from the evidence of thousands of women, that even if a lab test can't tell the difference, their bodies can. There is grim news about estrogenic chemicals and developing human fetuses, too. Male and female hormones must remain in balance in an embryo for sexual organs to develop normally. In early stages, a fetus is capable of developing either set. Hormone balance determines whether the child will be male or female. Exogenous estrogens can upset this balance, resulting in children with stunted male sex organs or with both sets of sex organs.

There is a link between pesticides and breast cancer. Pesticides, like other pollutants, are stored in body fat areas like breast tissue. Some pesticides including PCB's and DDT compromise immune function, overwork the liver and affect glands and hormones the way too much estrogen does. One study shows 50 to 60% more *dichloro-diphenyl-ethylene* (DDE) and *polychlorinated bi-phenols*, (PCB's) in women who have breast cancer than in those who don't. The quantity of DDT in body tissues is also higher. Some researchers suggest that the reason older women are experiencing a higher rate of breast cancer may be that these women had greater exposure to DDT before it was banned. The dramatic rise in breast cancer is consistent with the accumulation of organo-chlorine residues in the environment. Israel's recent history offers a case study. Until about 20 years ago, both breast cancer rates and contamination levels of organo-chlorine pesticides in Israel were among the highest in the world. An aggressive phase-out of these pesticides has led to a sharp reduction in contamination levels, followed by a dramatic drop in breast cancer death rates.

Other women's diseases associated with long exposure to estrogen mimics in the environment: —reproductive organ cancer, —breast and uterine fibroids, —polycystic ovarian syndrome, —endometriosis, —pelvic inflammatory disease.

Are *hormone disrupters impacting you?* Signs that you may have estrogen disruption:
• Breast inflammation and pain that worsens before menstrual periods, usually followed by heavy, painful periods.
• Weight gain: especially in the hips.
• Head hair loss — facial hair growth.
• Hot flashes: a sign of estrogen disruption in the brain.
• Endometriosis: now linked to dioxin, an airborn hormone disrupter.
• Breast and uterine fibroid development, ovarian cysts, and pelvic inflammatory disease.
• Breast, uterine and reproductive organ cancer: up to 60% more DDE, DDT and PCB's, known estrogen disrupters, in women with breast cancer.
• Early puberty: nearly half of African-American girls and 15% of Caucasian girls now begin to develop sexually by age 8, a clear indicator of estrogen disruption.

Are you at risk of exposure to estrogen disrupters? You may be especially exposed if: 1) you live in a high agricultural area; you eat a high fat diet (fatty areas of your body store pesticides and other agricultural chemicals); 2) you eat hormone-injected dairy foods or meats regularly; 3) you're on prescription HRT drugs or birth control pills.
For saliva hormone testing: visit http://www.salivatest.com, or call ZRT Laboratory, 503-466-2445. Address: ZRT Laboratory, 1815 NW 169th Pl. Suite 5050, Beaverton, OR 97006.

Is there any way to reduce your exposure?
First, cut back on fat! Hormone disrupters accumulate in body fat.... the reason a high fat diet is a major risk factor for long term exposure to them, and why it may lead to increased risk for hormone-driven cancers.

Second, eat sea veggies like wakame, nori and dulse regularly. Algin, a gel like substance in sea greens, protects against chemical overload (often involved in breast cancer) by binding to chemical wastes so they can be eliminated safely from the body. Eat cruciferous veggies regularly to improve estrogen metabolism.

Third, avoid hormone-injected commercial meats, especially beef and pork. Choose hormone-free dairy products, too.

Fourth, use hormone-disrupting drugs like HRT drugs for menopause, and birth control pills only when all other options have been ruled out. Avoid hormone-mimicks in personal care products, like placenta-containing hair rinses and conditioning treatments.

Are the new designer estrogens, the SERMs (*selective estrogen receptor modulators*), estrogen disrupters?
SERMs are a part of the new revolution in estrogen replacement drugs. Under the name raloxifene, (brand name Evista) SERMS were developed to fight what are perceived as menopausal diseases like osteoporosis, heart disease, even Alzheimer's disease, without increasing breast and uterine cancer risk, like traditional HRT drugs.
Can't find a recommended product? Call the 800 number listed in Product Resources for the store nearest you.

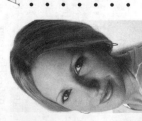

Designer estrogen SERMs seem promising at first glance. Early reports suggested that Evista (the most widely prescribed SERM) may prevent breast cancer without increasing risk for other cancers, and may protect against heart disease. Further, studies showed that Evista does increase bone density in women with osteoporosis. But Evista comes with its own set of drawbacks. Evista may not prevent fractures, the very problem women fear most, and it does not prevent bone loss in the spine. Twenty-five percent of patients in one study reported more hot flashes, a sign of estrogen disruption, while using Evista. Evista also increases risk for serious blood clots in the legs, lungs and eyes - especially for sedentary women. Its effects on circulation are so powerful many women discontinue therapy because leg cramps caused by the drug are so severe. Scientists are even concerned that Evista may increase risk for Alzheimer's disease because it seems to act as an anti-estrogen in the brain, (hot flashes may be a sign of falling hormone levels in the brain). In Alzheimer's, where natural estrogen appears to provide protection, anti-estrogen activity in the brain is obviously not desirable. Evista should not be taken by women with a history of congestive heart failure (faced by many women after menopause), pregnant women or individuals with active cancers. Drug-resistance to Tamoxifen (an anti-breast cancer drug) may develop if you take Evista because the two drugs are so closely related. New evidence suggests that SERMs can affect the glue-like molecule that holds cells together, potentially making cancers that develop later in life more aggressive!

The bottom line at this point on SERMS? We may have more knowledge about our bodies than we did 50 years ago, but we still don't understand hormones well. Hormones have widespread effects that are poorly understood. Although doctors are ecstatic about SERMs, these drugs still work at the hormone level and early reports suggest these drugs, like other HRT drugs, still disrupt delicate hormone balance. Phytohormone-containing herbs like *wild yam, red clover* and *dong quai* are really natural SERMs, which safely control menopause symptoms and may even help protect women from diseases like osteoporosis or heart disease after menopause.

Many women are finding that herbs are a better choice for hormone balance.

Many of the phytoestrogen containing herbs, like *black cohosh* for instance, are not just natural (instead of chemical) estrogen balancers. As living medicines, they can work intelligently with your body. In many cases, these herbs don't compete for receptor sites or have a direct estrogenic activity in the body. In fact, they work mainly as adaptogens which balance glandular activity and normalize body temperature fluctuations. They do what herbs always do best no matter what the problem is ..... they are body normalizers.

—**For hot flashes and night sweats:** •Crystal Star EST-AID™ capsules, 4 to 6 daily; •Moon Maid Botanicals PRO-MENO wild yam cream; •Pure Essence Labs FEM CREME; •VITEX extract; vitamin E 800IU; •Evening Primrose Oil caps 3000mg daily; •Nature's Secret ULTIMATE B daily and •Ester C 3000mg daily.

—**For side effects from synthetic hormones or birth control pills:** •Vitamin E 800IU; •New Chapter EVERY WOMAN'S ONE DAILY; •B-complex 100mg daily, with extra B₆ 250mg, •Country Life sub-lingual B-12, 2500mg and folic acid 800mcg daily; •Emulsified A & D 25,000IU/1,000IU; •Ester C 550mg with bioflavonoids, 6 daily; •Lane Labs ADVACAL tablets, 3-6 daily; •Esteem WOMEN'S COMFORT caps..

—**To rebalance prostaglandin formation:** (Prostaglandin imbalance can lead to breast and uterine fibroids, arthritis, eczema, menstrual difficulties, high blood pressure and cholesterol, and a tendency to gain weight.) Avoid saturated fats, especially from red meats and pasteurized, fatty dairy foods. Take •high omega-3 oils from cold water fish or flax seed oil 3x daily. Or use •Evening Primrose 3000mg daily or •Nature's Secret ULTIMATE OIL capsules 4-6 daily for 3 months.

Is hormone replacement therapy always necessary after a hysterectomy?

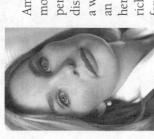

More than a half million American women have hysterectomies every year. The surgery is major, requiring a month or more of recovery time. Still, 50% of American women will have a hysterectomy in their lifetime. One in 1,000 women actually die as a result. Endometriosis, uterine fibroids or heavy periods are common reasons for a hysterectomy, but new research shows that just 10 percent of hysterectomies are really medically necessary. According to one UCLA-Rand study, 14 percent of women who have a hysterectomy have no symptoms that warrant surgery. The surgical removal of a woman's uterus or ovaries (or both) can mean major disruptions in hormonal health, premature menopause and usually a lifelong prescription of hormone replacement drugs. In many cases, natural therapies can help a woman avert surgery and help her body normalize naturally. Vitex extract and natural progesterone creams help manage heavy, abnormal bleeding. Herbs are also an excellent choice to boost hormone production by the adrenal glands (and energy) if surgery has already been done. By supporting endocrine health, the rainforest herb Maca (highly recommended) can control hysterectomy-induced symptoms like depression, low libido, constipation and hot flashes. Maca Magic HRT is an energizing formula with herbs like wild yam and vitex known for balancing hormones and increasing libido.

Can't find a recommended product? Call the 800 number listed in Product Resources for the store nearest you.

457

Hormone Imbalances - Men

Andropause, Impotence, Environmental Hormone Effects

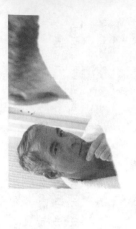

Low testosterone affects an astounding 1,000,000 American men! Yet in a recent survey, 68% of men cannot name a single symptom caused by low testosterone. Only 15% named low sex drive as a symptom of low testosterone; 6% named fatigue; 3% named a decrease in muscle mass; and less than 1% linked low testosterone to men's osteoporosis. Clearly, many men are in the dark about how hormone imbalances affect their health. Men's hormone changes have been much less publicized and researched than women's, but hormone disruption is as much a part of a man's life as it is a woman's. Some men are more attuned to their hormonal fluctuations than others. Some report clear monthly changes in their energy levels, mood, work and sports performance that they attribute to their equivalent of a "period." Blood levels of testosterone fluctuate dramatically at different times in life- from 250 to 1,200 nanograms, and these changes affect a man's performance, mood and sexuality. While a man's hormone fluctuations are less dramatic than a woman's, testosterone levels start to decline around age 40, falling up to 10% each decade. This phenomenon called "andropause" is now recognized by almost eight in ten family physicians as a real condition that affects quality of life for men. More physicians are becoming increasingly interested in TRI, or testosterone replacement therapy for andropausal men, but I find most men benefit the most from a detailed lifestyle program emphasizing natural foods, bodywork therapies and supportive herbs and supplements designed to meet their changing needs. See pg. 251 of this book for more information.

Your hormones may be out of balance if: You have prostate pain and inflammation with poor urinary control. You have a pouchy tummy with poor abdominal tone. You have reduced sex drive.

What causes male hormone problems? Synthetic steroid use. Stress, which leads to adrenal exhaustion (the adrenal glands produce most hormones). A vasectomy. Severe dieting or serious body building, surgery or long illness and nutrient deficiencies, especially protein, calcium and iodine deficiency, low B Complex or EFAs.

For saliva hormone testing: Dr. David Zava, Ph.D., ZRT Laboratory, 503-469-0741, fax 503-469-1305, Address: ZRT Laboratory, 12505 NW Cornell Rd., Portland, OR 97229.

Andropause

The needs of the male body increase as a man approaches andropause. Men need a high energy diet to keep active as they grow older, plenty of nutrients to retain sexual potency, and proteins to maintain muscle mass. If you're in andropause, consider natural therapies as an effective way to renew vitality. Men I've talked to who are using them report better energy, increased stamina and more sexual satisfaction.

Are you in andropause? Signs to watch for:
—Is your energy unusually low lately? Is your work output or sports performance less than you're used to?
—Have you lost height? Are your shoulders slightly hunching? (a sign of early osteoporosis) Get a side view in your mirror.
—Has your beard or head hair growth slowed? Is your chest hair getting sparse but ear hair increasing?
—Have you lost muscle mass? Has your strength or endurance decreased? (a sign of lower testosterone.)
—Is your urination frequent and/or difficult, especially at night? (a sign of an enlarged prostate)
—Are your erections less strong or less frequent? Is your sex drive lower than normal for you?
—Are you anxious about your well-being and your future?

Nutritional therapy can renew male vitality. **Diet improvements (even if your diet is okay) are essential.**
1: Eat smaller, more frequent meals. Overeating can suppress hormone production.
2: Drink in moderation. Heavy drinking can lead to prostate problems and impaired erections.
3: Limit consumption of fatty dairy foods and meats (especially beef), notoriously high in hormone-disrupting chemicals. Chicken is also loaded with antibiotics. Buy organic poultry (Try Petaluma Poultry ROSIE THE ORGANIC CHICKEN, DIESTEL and COLEMAN NATURAL PRODUCTS). Reduce fried foods, caffeine and sugar – they deplete the adrenals and drain male energy. Don't go too far though. An extremely low fat diet is disastrous for andropausal health. Recent studies find it may reduce testosterone levels almost to preadolescent levels — not good news for an older man! Include healthy fats from seafood instead, and hormone-free turkey and chicken regularly. Flax seed oil is a healthy oil to use in salad dressings. (Use about 1 tbsp.)
4: Add soy foods (tofu, tempeh, soy milk, etc.) for hormone normalizing isoflavones. Add high energy foods like complex carbohydrates from whole grains, legumes, fresh fruits and vegetables. Add a superfood drink each afternoon like •Crystal Star ENERGY GREEN RENEWAL™ drink or Fit for You, Intl. MIRACLE GREENS to reduce craving for fatty junk foods.

Can't find a recommended product? Call the 800 number listed in Product Resources for the store nearest you.

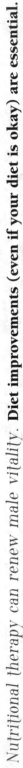

5: Drink green tea to flush out fats that harbor hormone disrupting chemicals. Add hormone balancing-energizing superfoods for stamina, like Nature's Secret BEYOND ENDURANCE

6: Increase your intake of zinc to renew sexual potency. Zinc, highly concentrated in semen, is the most important nutrient for male sexuality. Eat high zinc foods like liver, oysters, nutritional yeast, nuts and seeds regularly. Add zinc-rich spirulina to your superfood supplement list, and try •Ethical Nutrients ZINC STATUS (checks for deficiency and is a supplement).

7: Limit your use of microwaves. Microwaving foods kills enzymes. Enzymes are an important tool for glandular and hormone metabolism.

8: Wash produce thoroughly to reduce hormone disrupting pollutant residues. Use Healthy Harvest FRUIT & VEGETABLE RINSE.

Bodywork techniques are critical for male vitality and balance. **Exercise is vital to male hormone health at any age.**

•Exercise is a vital component of male hormone balance and sexuality. It makes your body stronger, function better and endure longer. In one study, 78 healthy, but sedentary men were studied during nine months of regular exercise. The men exercised 60 minutes a day, 3 days a week. Every single man reported significantly enhanced sexuality.... increased frequency, performance and satisfaction. Rising sexuality was even correlated with degree of fitness improvement. The more fitness the men were able to attain, the better their sex life! •Do deep abdominal breathing - page 250 with yoga stretches every morning. Get morning sunlight on the body, on the genitalia if possible. •Massage therapy restores unblocked energy meridians and increases circulation. •Don't smoke if you want your libido in top condition. Smoking disrupts hormone activity. •Muscle Testing (Applied Kinesiology) can determine which hormonal herbs or supplements are specific to your problem. Once you learn the simple technique (see page 378), a nutritional consultant, a chiropractor, a massage therapist), you can do it yourself to decide which products are right for you.

What about environmental hormones and male hormone problems?

Women aren't the only ones endangered by the estrogen-imitating effects of chemicals and pesticides. There is substantial evidence that man-made estrogens threaten male health and fertility, too. An unusually large number of male babies (both animals and human) are showing up with male feminization (small testicles, low sperm count, and miniature penises), a trend many scientists believe is directly related to chemicals in our environment. Shocking research from Taiwan shows a group of women who unknowingly consumed hormone-disrupting PCB contaminated rice oil over a period of ten months, then gave birth to boys who later developed reduced penises.... direct evidence that PCBs cause serious birth defects in humans.

The dramatic rise in prostate cancer deaths over the last 40 years is another wake-up call to change our environment for health. While the rate of prostate cancer has doubled since World War II, male sperm counts have declined by half - a trend that has led to speculation that environmental, dietary, and lifestyle changes in recent decades are interfering with a man's ability to make sperm. Semen analysis tests over the last few decades show undeniably that total sperm count as well as sperm quality of the general male population has been deteriorating. In 1940, the average sperm count was 113 million per ml. In 1993, that value had dropped to 65 million. In the US, we now have a normal count of 20 million! Today men have only about 82% of the sperm counts they had in 1940. For the first time in America's history, one in six married couples of childbearing age has trouble conceiving and completing a successful pregnancy. Are estrogen disrupting hormones to blame? New evidence suggests the answer is yes. In tests, pregnant rats who were exposed to "minute quantities" of DES (diethylstilbestrol) and other synthetic estrogens showed a 5% to 15% decline in sperm count in their male offspring when they matured.

Pollutants used to be considered strictly estrogenic, like poly-chlorinated bi-phenols (PCBs), or dioxin and pesticides used for agriculture. New reports reveal environmental androgens in pollutants (substances that mimic male sex hormone) are much more widespread than previously thought. Vanderbilt University School of Medicine found that of ten pollutants, 5 bound to the androgen receptor while only 2 bound to the estrogen receptor. Men can really benefit from adding more dietary fiber from whole grains, fresh fruits and vegetables that can bind to and eliminate hormone-disrupting pollutants lodged in their bodies. Always wash commercial produce thoroughly to reduce harmful pollutant residues and buy organic whenever possible. The produce sections in health food stores are like gold, not just in terms of taste and local freshness but in the concept that good food really is good medicine!

What about male impotence? Impotence affects 52% of U.S. men between 40 and 70 years of age!

Blood vessel disease and diabetes account for nearly 60% of impotence cases. Viagra, one of the first designer drugs to be marketed directly to the public, is promoted as a sex aid for impotent men. Today, over 16 million men worldwide have taken Viagra. Its phenomenal success says a lot about the state of male reproductive health today. Viagra enhances the physical mechanism for erection, producing smooth muscle relaxation and increasing circulation to the penis. Viagra's manufacturer is developing faster acting versions of the drug. Other drug companies are developing a Viagra rival to tempt both the male and female libido. *Does Viagra really mean better sex?* More than 5 years into the Viagra craze we see that enhancing sexuality through drug chemistry is not all we thought. The fact that it is a powerful, potentially dangerous drug has been vastly understated in its advertising. Side effects and risks surfaced almost immediately. At this writing there have been over 564 Viagra-related deaths- from massive cardiac arrest, stroke, cardiovascular complications or drug interactions. Although manufacturers Viagra maintains it's safe if used properly, I urge caution, especially for men with a history of heart problems or who take other prescription drugs.

Can't find a recommended product? Call the 800 number listed in Product Resources for the store nearest you.

Can natural therapies help impotency?

Unless you have a clear medical condition, better libido results not from a pill, but from a good lifestyle.

Many sexual difficulties begin in the dining room, from stress and a poor diet, not the bedroom. Atherosclerosis, clearly related to diet, can block blood supply to the penile artery, and is the primary cause of impotence in 50% of men over 50! Diabetes, smoking, overuse of alcohol or sedatives, and anti-depressant drugs or high blood pressure medicines, regularly cause impotence. Sexual function depends on healthy glands and organs to produce sex hormones. Herbs work through the glands to rebalance and nourish. Herbs enhance and enrich sexual feelings and activity, yet they do not overwhelm, like some drugs. Ginkgo biloba improves circulation, increases vascular strength and reverses atherosclerosis impotence. In one study, ginkgo was 30% more effective than drug injections with over 50% of patients showing regained potency. Take the whole herb extract, 15 drops under the tongue, 2 or 3 times a day. Peruvian maca has been used by traditional healers for centuries to treat impotence and is highly recommended. Animal studies confirm maca can boost fertility and sexual activity. The men I talk to who use it are delighted with their results (so are the women!) Dosage? Around 3,000mg daily, in extract or tablets.

Natural therapy plan for male potency

—Take care of your prostate. Many men don't realize how much they can relieve prostate problems without drugs. The pharmaceutical industry isn't going to tell them! In Europe, botanical medicines are the first-choice treatments for men instead of drugs. Some prostate drugs, like Proscar, can cause impotence and decreased libido! For the majority of prostate problem, drugs are unnecessary. Herbs like *saw palmetto* and *pygeum* show excellent results in wide clinical trials. Here's why: As men grow older they tend to accumulate more of the rogue testosterone, dihydrotestosterone (DHT), which causes cells to multiply and the prostate to enlarge. The Quarterly Review of Natural Medicine finds *saw palmetto* reduces the symptoms of BPH by blocking DHT, inhibiting the enzyme 5-alpha reductase related to prostate enlargement. Consider •Crystal Star PROSTATE PROTECTOR™ or •New Chapter PROSTATE 5LX to help reduce prostate enlargement and dribbling urine symptoms. (Usually improvement in 48 hours.) Check your alcohol intake. Heavy drinking can lead to prostate problems and impaired erections. Dr. Howard Peiper's book Natural Solutions For Sexual Enhancement, says "alcohol, especially beer, elevates levels of DHT in the body and can be a contributing factor in sexual dysfunction." DHT elevation is linked to testosterone decline and elevation of female hormones.... definitely undesirable for men.

—Build muscle mass. Take a protein drink each morning to build muscle mass and stamina. •Pure Form WHEY PROTEIN, chunks of real fruit and branch-chain amino acids, leucine, isoleucine and valine - ideal for building muscle protein. Before you turn to a drug-based growth hormone supplement, consider •Glutamine 3000mg daily. It helps your pituitary stimulate your own growth hormone - for some men dramatically. Add a glutamine fortified body builder like •Metabolic Response Modifiers L-GLUTAMINE to improve muscle tone.

—Renew sexual potency. Try the Aurvedic herb •*tribulus terrestris*, to boost libido. Athletes like its benefits of increased strength and stamina. Try •Natural Balance TRIBULUS TERRESTIS, or •Natural Balance COBRA, or •Crystal Star MALE PERFORMANCE™ caps (long history of success for enhancing libido and overcoming impotence). **—For low sperm count:** •Lane Labs FERTIL MALE caps (clinically shown to improve sperm count and mobility); Carnitine 2000mg daily helps sperm cells reach their destination; •B$_{12}$ 6,000 mcg. daily.

—Feed your adrenals. Men need healthy adrenals to keep energized as testosterone levels begin to decline. I've talked to many men over 40, working stressful jobs with major family responsibilities who just can't keep it up anymore because their adrenals are shot from years of abuse. If you tend to eat fast foods on the run, drink a lot of coffee and get little sleep you're setting your body up for an adrenal crash. Adrenal exhaustion for men sometimes precipitates depression and severe stress reactions. Crystal Star •ADRENAL ENERGY BOOST™ caps have a long history of success in restoring a man's vitality. **—Normalize production of steroid hormones with EFAs:** •Evening primrose oil 3000mg daily. •Superior Trading GINSENG BEE SECRETION. •Health from the Sun TOTAL EFA caps. •Nature's Secret ULTIMATE OIL. •Omega Nutrition ESSENTIAL BALANCE OIL caps and liquid.

—Boost hormone production, improve physical performance. •Glutamine 2000mg daily naturally stimulates rejuvenating growth hormone; •Crystal Star MALE PERFORMANCE™ for 3 months. •Maca Magic EXPRESS ENERGY caps or liquid. •*Siberian eleuthero* extract. •American panax ginseng and potency wood. •Panax ginseng-Damiana. •Ginseng-Licorice-Dandelion. •Golden Pride REJUVENATE FOR MEN and •CoQ-10, 200mg daily. •Nutricology ANDROBALANCE. **—Raw glandular therapy:** raw pancreas, raw orchic, raw pituitary.
—Hormone tonics for more energy: •Crystal Star ADRENAL ENERGY BOOST™ •Prince of Peace RED GINSENG, ROYAL JELLY vials.

What about vasectomies? **Over half a million vasectomies are perfomed every year.**

Science has long debated whether a vasectomy, the contraceptive procedure which severs or seals off the vessel that carries sperm from the testes, increases the risk of prostate cancer in men. In one study of 73,000 men, 300 of the men developed prostate cancer between 1986 and 1990. Men with vasectomies had a 66% greater risk of prostate cancer than did the men without vasectomies. In a separate study, vasectomies increased the risk of prostate cancer by 56%. Other research does not confirm a vasectomy-prostate cancer link. Still, the procedure has clear drawbacks for men. As sperm builds up in the sealed-off vas deferens after a vasectomy, the body re-absorbs the cells. This confuses the immune system, making it less alert to tumor cells. Sometimes the body's immune defenses try to mount an allergic response against its own tissue. Post vasectomy pain syndrome is a primary result for some men. A vasectomy also affects testicle secretions and lowers prostatic fluid. When the natural movement of sperm and hormones is artificially prevented, a host of male health problems can result.

Can't find a recommended product? Call the 800 number listed in Product Resources for the store nearest you.

Uncovering the truth about the new "superhormones."

There is a "superhormone revolution" sweeping the U.S. today. Drug companies are selling hormones like they were vitamins or beauty aids! Every day they tempt us to try new and different hormones. They're selling big promises: beauty, a long life span or recharged sexuality. Some "hormone authorities" even recommend taking a concoction of several hormones, called a hormone cocktail. Americans are loading up on hormones to deal with today's lifestyle disorders. Thousands of us are swallowing down a mouthful of hormones.... DHEA, melatonin, pregnenolone, human hGH growth hormone, testosterone, estrogen, progesterone, and thyroid hormone – all in the hope of finding the silver bullet to protect our health and our looks. Drug companies tell us that superhormones will enable us to be healthy and live to the ripe-old age of 120. Some once-conservative medical doctors even say that the money spent on diet, exercise, herbal remedies and drugs is wasted...and that superhormone supplements are the sole pillar for vital health....a sensationalized spin that's truly created a hormone circus!

What's driving the superhormone revolution? America's baby boomers are the force behind the billion dollar hormone dance. As they cross the 50-yard line of life, the realities of aging are staring boomers in the face. They're demanding new answers- and lots of change. So it shouldn't come as a surprise that hormones are a megabucks business. The #2 prescribed drug in the U.S. today is Premarin, an estrogen replacement drug. DHEA, pregnenolone and ANDRO are rising stars in the supplement hormone world, already generating over $325 million in sales annually. Don't be fooled. They may be sold over-the-counter, but these hormones are drugs with hidden dangers and big reactions! Regard them with respect and caution.

There is no doubt that hormones play a dramatic role in human health or that hormone production slows down with age. But I don't believe a cabinet full of superhormone supplements and drugs is the best choice for most people. Hormones are incredibly minute glandular secretions, produced from body chemical substances called steroids which affect the part of the brain that influences sexual behavior. Hormones regulate everything from energy flow and mood, to inflammation, to a woman's monthly cycle, to a man's hair growth. Tiny amounts can cause big reactions, both good and bad. While there are times when taking supplemental hormones is okay.... for an acute situation or a short term need, hormone drugs often disrupt hormone balance further and can lead to many hormone-driven problems including breast and uterine cancer.

Why are our hormones so imbalanced? Hormone imbalance disorders are raging through this country. We see hormone imbalance in women's disorders like PMS, endometriosis and fibroids, and men's disorders like impotence, prostate enlargement and male andropause. Women with hysterectomies are only beginning to see the harm that removing delicate glands, or treating fragile hormones with drugs can do. Bone loss in both sexes is related to hormone imbalance. Hormone imbalance disorders come from hormone disrupting chemicals in foods, drugs and pollutants (nearly 40% of pesticides used in commercial agriculture are suspected hormone disrupters!). A poorly functioning liver (the liver metabolizes excess estrogen), and a high fat diet (excess fat harbors hormones) are almost always implicated, as is a diet high in refined "non food" chemicalized foods that the body rejects or ignores.

Facts you may not know about superhormones...

—*fiction*: Over-the-counter superhormones like DHEA, melatonin and ANDRO are natural substances.

fact: ALL over-the-counter hormone supplements are produced in a lab, even when they start out with a plant extraction or animal glandular material.

—*fiction*: They are safe for regular use.

fact: Side effects are common with superhormones. Long range effects on human health are unknown. Deep hormone balance can be affected. Taking hormones as if they were vitamins is playing Russian Roulette with your health, especially for athletes who usually combine more than one highly concentrated, stimulant or hormone (both legal or illegal).

—*fiction*: Superhormones will make a man a superman or a woman a love slave.

fact: Superhormones can boost libido, but the benefits are short term and may come with side effects like mood swings or agitation. I believe that advertising hormones as cosmetics is both irresponsible and misguided. Carelessly taking high doses of superhormones may be counterproductive, even dangerous, as we have seen with Viagra. When you begin mixing hormone-like steroidal substances in your body, you are changing your natural body chemistry. I have seen some of the unpleasant side effects like female chest hair growth and bloody urine for myself. I believe a better choice is subtle, safe foods or herbs that contain plant hormones, especially for healthy people with normal hormone levels. Many are remarkably similar to human hormones, gentle, and can even be taken up by human hormone receptor sites!

What about Plant or Phyto-Hormones? Plant or phyto-hormones are remarkably similar to human hormones. They can be accepted by hormone receptor sites in our bodies, and, at only 1/400 to 1/1000 the strength of human hormones, they are extremely gentle and safe, exerting a tonic effect rather than drug-like activity. Although used for centuries by both men and women, we are just beginning to understand their power. Studies on soy foods and herbs like ginseng, black cohosh and wild yam clearly show hormone-normalizing effects.

Can't find a recommended product? Call the 800 number listed in Product Resources for the store nearest you.

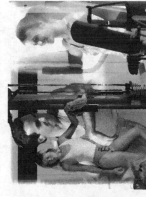

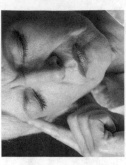

Hypoglycemia
Low Blood Sugar

Hypoglycemia and diabetes stem from the same causes. Hypoglycemia is often a way station on the road to diabetes. Often called a "sugar epidemic" today, hypoglycemia is caused when we repeatedly eat too much sugar and refined carbs like pastries and desserts; this causes the pancreas to overreact by producing too much insulin - the excess insulin then lowers blood sugar too much in an effort to normalize body sugar balance. Hypoglycemia is particularly harmful to the brain, which requires glucose as an energy source to think clearly. Small fluctuations in brain function disturb our feeling of well-being. Large fluctuations cause anxious feelings of depression, mood swings, fatigue, even aggressive behavior. Sugar balance is also needed for muscle contractions, digestive system and nerve health.

Hypoglycemia in children is widely acknowledged as a cause of both hyperactivity and learning disorders. Chronic negativity, mood swings, aggressive behavior, and obstinate resentment to all discipline are reasons for at least taking the self-test below, as well as a Glucose Tolerance Test from a physician. For children, hypoglycemia can only be managed by a diet from which all forms of concentrated sugars have been removed, including fruit juices.

You can check for low blood sugar: Correct diagnosis and treatment of sugar instabilities is essential.

Our bodies have a complex set of checks and balances to maintain proper blood glucose levels. Low blood sugar is the biological equivalent of a race car running on empty. Some of the symptoms can be helped right away by eating something, but this does not address the cause. The following questionnaire, can help you decide, in cooperation with a health care professional, whether you need low blood sugar support, and whether other professional help is necessary. Mark the symptoms as they pertain to you: (1) for mild symptoms, occurring once or twice a year; (2) for moderate symptoms, occurring several times a year; (3) severe symptoms, occurring almost constantly. A score of 6 or more signifies a need for sugar balance nutritional support. A score of 12 -18 indicates a need for therapeutic measures several times daily. *Questionnaire reprinted with permission from the Enzymatic Therapy Notebook.*

( ) Irritability, constant phobias, fears, extreme fatigue, exhaustion
( ) Unexplained depression and restlessness, anti-social behavior, often violence
( ) Craving for sweets, general ravenous hunger, digestive problems
( ) Frequent headaches, usually with blurred vision, crying and weak spells
( ) Manic/depressive psychological states, swinging between lethargy or hyperactivity

( ) Poor concentration, mental confusion, spaciness, forgetfulness, indecisiveness
( ) Constant worry and anxiety, nervousness (even nervous breakdown)
( ) Nightmares, insomnia; inability to return to sleep after waking; night time urination
( ) Cold sweats, shakiness and trembling, twitching, involuntary muscle jerks
( ) Heart and pulse racing; faintness, dizziness, trembling

Hypoglycemia sufferers beware! Sugar and sweeteners are in almost everything you eat today.

Hidden sugars like "high fructose corn syrup," (in most sodas and juices today), are a health hazard for hypoglycemics. Studies show that sodas sweetened with high fructose corn syrup cause mineral loss, especially phosphorous and calcium, which may contribute to osteoporosis. Studies from Israel reveal that rats fed a high fructose diet age faster with premature skin wrinkling and sagging. Worse, studies show artificial sweeteners like aspartame have received more complaints about adverse reactions than any other food ingredient in FDA history. Over 5,000 food products contain NutraSweet and Equal, and since the patent has recently expired, you'll more than likely be seeing even more aspartames in foods soon. Read labels carefully! Some people have serious reactions — extreme dizziness, headaches, throat swelling, allergic reactions and retina deterioration are just a few documented side effects. The American College of Physicians says aspartame is causing a plague of neurological diseases in the U.S.

Aspartame, 200 times sweeter than sugar, keeps blood sugar levels out of control by disrupting the way your body uses insulin. Diabetes and hypoglycemia may progress and worsen. Some diabetic patients suffer severe reactions after switching to aspartame sweeteners. Pregnant and lactating women, toddlers or allergy-prone children, and those with PKU, should avoid aspartame products. Using aspartame for weight control can actually increase appetite, especially for sweets!

In 1999, the World Environmental Conference showed that if aspartame's temperature exceeds 86° F, its wood alcohol converts to formaldehyde. Formaldehyde causes methanol toxicity in the body, accumulating in the retina causing blurred vision, bright flashes or black spots and even retinal bleeding. Pilots report seizures and visual disturbances while flying after drinking sodas sweetened with aspartame. Over time, body methanol toxicity can mimic the symptoms of multiple sclerosis (MS), lupus and fibromyalgia. Scientists say that many cases of M.S. and lupus may actually be misdiagnosed "aspartame disease." Aspartame also alters delicate brain chemistry (brain tumors rates have increased by 10% since aspartame was added to our food supply), leading to memory loss and aggravating Parkinson's disease and increasing Alzheimer's risk. This is especially critical for the elderly who consume chemically sweetened beverages at record levels. Eliminating aspartame offers complete remission of symptoms for some people.

Amazingly, Gulf War Syndrome may be directly related aspartame poisoning! Sodas sweetened with aspartame were left sitting in the blistering desert heat for weeks at a time for our troops in Desert Storm. By the time our soldiers drank them, aspartame's chemical structure was so altered by the heat, the soldiers got sick almost immediately.

Can't find a recommended product? Call the 800 number listed in Product Resources for the store nearest you.

Hypoglycemia

Diet and Lifestyle Support Therapy

Nutritional therapy: Diet for Hypoglycemia Control: A healthy diet is critical.

Nutrient deficiencies always accompany hypoglycemia. Overeating sugar and refined carbohydrates, in foods like pastries and desserts, quickly raises glucose levels, causing the pancreas to over-compensate and produce too much insulin, which then lowers body glucose levels too far, too fast. The diet below supplies your body with slow even-burning fuel that prevents sudden sugar elevations and drops. Eat 6 to 8 mini meals, with plenty of fresh foods to keep sugar levels in balance. Avoid all sugary foods, alcohol and caffeine. Try a diet like this for 2 to 3 months until blood sugar levels are regularly stable. Don't go on long, severely restrictive weight loss diets during healing.

Diet changes for hypoglycemia pay off for total health, too. Eat: 1) potassium-rich foods: oranges, broccoli, bananas, tomatoes. 2) chromium-rich foods: nutritional yeast, mushrooms, whole wheat, sea foods, beans and peas. 3) high quality vegetable protein at every meal. Get some exercise every day to work off unmetabolized acid wastes.

On rising: take a "hypoglycemia cocktail." 1 tsp. each in apple or orange juice to control morning sugar drop: glycine powder, powdered milk, protein powder, nutritional yeast. Or try a protein/amino drink, like Pure Planet CHLORELLA, Wakunaga HARVEST BLEND, or Crystal Star RESTORE YOUR STRENGTH™.

Breakfast: very important for hypoglycemia, with 1/3 of daily nutrients. Have oatmeal with yogurt and fresh fruit; or poached or baked eggs on whole grain toast with butter or kefir cheese; or whole grain cereal or pancakes with apple juice, soy milk, fruit sauce, yogurt, nuts; or tofu scrambled "eggs" with bran muffins, whole grain toast and butter.

Mid-morning: have a mixed veggie drink, Green Foods GREEN MAGMA with 1 tsp. Bragg's LIQUID AMINOS, or Crystal Star ENERGY GREEN RENEWAL™ drink as a liver nutrient; or a sugar balancing herb tea, such as *licorice, dandelion*, or Crystal Star DR. VITALITY™ tea; and some crisp, crunchy vegetables with kefir or yogurt cheese;

Lunch: a fresh salad with cottage cheese or soy cheese, nuts, noodle or seed toppings, and lemon oil dressing; or a seafood and chicken sandwich on whole grain bread, with avocados, low fat cheese; or a bean or lentil soup with tofu or shrimp salad or sandwich, or a vegetarian pizza on a chapati crust with low fat cheese.

Mid-afternoon: have a hard boiled egg with sesame salt, and whole grain crackers with yogurt dip; or licorice or dandelion root tea, or another green drink, or yogurt with nuts and seeds.

Dinner: have steamed veggies with tofu, or baked or broiled fish and brown rice; or Asian stir fry with seafood, rice and veggies; or a vegetable pasta with verde sauce and hearty soup (add green beans for pancreatic support); or Spanish beans and rice, or a veggie quiche and a small mushroom and spinach salad.

Before bed: have a cup of miso broth; or papaya juice with a little yogurt.

Herbal, Superfood and Supplement Therapy

Interceptive therapy plan: Choose several recommendations.

1—Help your body rebalance sugar levels: •Crystal Star SUGAR CONTROL LOW™ caps. •Crystal Star FEEL GREAT NOW!™ caps with ginseng helps remove sugar from the blood. •Jarrow GENTLE FIBERS™ or other fiber cleanse morning and evening absorbs excess carbohydrates and balances sugar curve. •Vitamin C 3000mg with bioflavonoids. (Take vitamin C immediately during an attack, either in foods like cranberry juice or oranges or in tablets-highly recommended). Note: Some oral contraceptives can cause glucose intolerance and poor sugar metabolism. Ask your doctor.

2—Adrenal tonics help the body handle stress: •Crystal Star ADRENAL ENERGY BOOST™ caps nourish exhausted adrenals; •Prince of Peace RED GINSENG-ROYAL JELLY vials; •*Gotu kola* caps, 2 daily. •Source Naturals GLUCO SCIENCE; •Transformation BALANCEZYME PLUS with MASTERZYME to support adrenals; •Nubricology ADRENAL CORTEX extract; •*Evening Primrose Oil* caps 2000mg daily; •B Complex 200mg daily with extra PABA 100mg, and pantothenic acid 500mg.

3—Help stabilize blood sugar swings: •Glutamine 500mg daily. •1 tsp. each: spirulina granules and bee pollen granules in a fruit juice, or •Pure Planet SPIRULINA, between meals. •Take AloeLife ALOE GOLD concentrate 1 tsp. 3x daily before meals (add pinches of cinnamon, ginger and nutmeg to help control cravings-good results).

4—Enzyme therapy increases protein synthesis and glucose homeostasis: both depend on a wide range of micro-nutrients in short supply in the American diet. •CoQ-10 200mg daily for 3-6 weeks; •Pancreatin 1200mg with meals; •Crystal Star DR. EN-ZYME™ with protease and bromelain; •Prevail GLUCOSE FORMULA; •UAS DDS-PLUS with FOS, especially if candida yeast is also a problem, which it frequently is); •Ayurvedic TRIPHALA or Amla fruit tonic.

5—Chromium may be critical: Chromium therapy choices include •GTF Chromium 200mcg; •Solaray CHROMIACIN; •Chromium picolinate 200mcg daily; •Premier Labs VANADIUM, 25mcg; •Country Life DMG B₁₅, 125mg sublingual.

6—Add minerals to overcome body basic deficiencies: •Mezotrace SEA MINERAL COMPLEX daily or •Nature's Path TRACE-LYTE liquid minerals in juice. •Trace Mineral Research CONCENTRACE liquid or tabs.

—Effective superfoods: protein drinks help build a "floor" under a sugar drop.
•Metabolic Response Modifers WHEY PUMPED.
•Crystal Star DR. VITALITY™ tea.
•Crystal Star ENERGY GREEN RENEWAL™ drink.
•Red Star NUTRITIONAL YEAST (B-complex).
•Nature's Answer BIOSTRATH immune enhancing drink.
•Fit for You, Intl. MIRACLE GREENS with spirulina

Can't find a recommended product? Call the 800 number listed in Product Resources for the store nearest you.

Hypothyroidism

Sluggish Thyroid, Wilson's Syndrome, Goiter

Hypothyroidism (low thyroid) is a common problem, aggravated by the strain pollutants in our environment put on glandular health. Today, thyroid disease affects nearly 15 million people, most of which are women. Among women over 65, one of ten has early-stage hypothyroidism. In hypothyroidism, the thyroid gland does not produce adequate thyroid hormone to meet body demands. Metabolism slows, affecting virtually every cell in the body. In infants, poor thyroid function is called cretinism, marked by mental retardation and dwarfism. At its worst, hypothyroidism can completely destroy the thyroid gland. Conventional treatment is a lifelong prescription of thyroid hormone, levothyroxine (Synthroid), linked to severe headaches, insomnia, bone loss and tachycardia (rapid contractions of the heart). In 1999, Synthroid, a synthetic thyroid drug, overtook the HRT drug Premarin as the top-selling prescription drug in the U.S. Note: New research shows that calcium carbonate may reduce absorption of Synthroid.

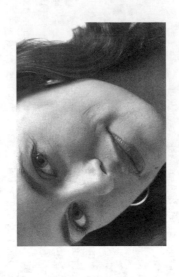

What causes hypothyroidism? 1) Hashimoto's thyroiditis, becoming more common (see page 435). 2) Iodine deficiency from X-rays or low dose radiation (like mammograms); 3) Excessive dieting, especially in the U.S. 4) Exposure to environmental pollutants like fluoride (thyroid cancer has been linked to highly fluoridated water). Long use of HRT drugs.

What is Wilson's Syndrome? Many women suffer from sub-clinical hypothyroidism called Wilson's syndrome. This syndrome has all the symptoms of hypothyroidism listed below but cannot be detected by standard laboratory tests. Unlike true hypothyroidism, Wilson's syndrome is not caused by a deficiency of thyroid hormone. Instead, it's caused by irregular processing of thyroid hormones. A stressful event like childbirth, loss of a loved one, or divorce usually precedes this syndrome. A chronically low body temperature (below 98.6) is a major warning sign. A physician knowledgeable in natural therapies can diagnose Wilson's syndrome.

Is your thyroid low and metabolism poor? Since World War II, an above average number of people have thyroid problems.

Metabolism is something of a mystery; we may never know exactly how it functions. We do know thyroid metabolism provides vital energy resources to every part of the body. Researchers speculate that the enormous amount of chemicals that came into our culture during and after WW II (some not well-tested for safety) affected thyroid health.

Signs you may have hypothyroidism and low metabolism:

• great, unrelenting fatigue, especially in the middle of the day, weak muscles
• hormonal imbalances (like PMS, delayed or absent menstruation, or unusually heavy menstruation)
• bloating, gas and indigestion immediately after eating
• unusual depression, usually with markedly reduced libido and poor immune response
• unexplained hair loss in women, often accompanied by breast fibroids
• unexplained weight gain or obesity, with frequent constipation and bloating
• unusual sensitivity to cold, especially hands, feet and ears; yellowish color on hands and feet
• slow heart rate; unusually high LDL "bad" cholesterol levels
• appearance of goiter (swelling of the thyroid gland) with low selenium levels
• puffy face and eyelids; dull, dry hair; dry, itchy skin; easily broken nails
• poor memory and concentration, unexplained mood swings and changes in personality.

Note: If you think you might have hypothyroidism, a simple blood test from your physician can confirm diagnosis.

Take your basal body temperature to help judge your metabolic rate:

Your body temperature is a reflection of your metabolic rate, governed by the thyroid gland. Imbalances in thyroid hormone production reveal themselves in changes in basal body temperature. Normal basal body temperature is 98.6°. If your basal body temperature is chronically low, it can be a sign of low thyroid function or Wilson's syndrome. If it is high, it may indicate an overactive thyroid gland or hyperthyroidism. See Graves' Disease pg. 432 for more. You need a thermometer to perform this test.

1. Before bed, shake down a thermometer to below 95°F and put it in a safe place overnight. 2. On rising, place the thermometer in your armpit for 10 minutes. For best results, lie down and stay still while performing the test. 3. After 10 minutes, read your temperature and note it with the day's date. 4. Repeat your temperature test for 3-5 consecutive mornings. Women who are menstruating should take this test on the 2nd, 3rd, and 4th days of their monthly period. Post-menopausal women, and men can take the test any time.

Can't find a recommended product? Call the 800 number listed in Product Resources for the store nearest you.

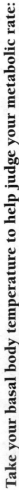

Hypothyroidism

Diet and Lifestyle Support Therapy

Nutritional therapy plan:

1—Follow a 75% fresh foods diet for a month to rebalance metabolism. Have a green salad daily.

2—Eat plenty of iodine-rich foods: sea greens, seafoods, fish, mushrooms, garlic, onions and watercress. Use iodine-rich herb salt or sea greens instead of table salt. Try •Crystal Star RESTORE YOUR STRENGTH™ drink for 3 months, rich in thyroid-enhancing iodine and potassium from sea veggies, or •Fit for You MIRACLE GREENS with sea greens.

3—Eat vitamin A-rich foods: yellow vegetables, eggs, carrots, dark green vegetables, raw dairy.

4—A mixed veggie drink like Knudsen's VERY VEGGIE or a potassium broth (pg. 291) twice a week. (See superfoods below.)

5—Avoid refined foods, saturated fats, sugars, white flour and red meats.

6—Avoid "goitrogens," foods that prevent the use of iodine: cabbage, turnips, peanuts, mustard, pine nuts, millet and soy products. (Cooking these foods inactivates the goitrogens.)

7—Take 2 tbsp. lecithin granules daily over whole grain cereal for memory boosting nutrients.

8—Stop drinking fluoridated water. It is a thyroid antagonist that depresses thyroid activity.

•The drug levothyroxine, frequently given for hypothyroidism can cause significant bone loss. Ask your doctor. Avoid antihistamines and sulfa drugs.
•Low thyroid levels affect your child's IQ. Studies show children born to mothers with underactive thyroids have IQ's 7 points lower than children born to healthy mothers!

—Bodywork:
•Take a brisk half hour walk daily to increase metabolism and stimulate circulation.
•Sun bathe in the morning. Sea bathe and wade whenever possible. Take a Crystal Star HOT SEAWEED BATH™ twice a week for thyroid boost. Bonus: Smooths skin and reduces cellulite, too.
•Color therapy: for hypothyroid, wear orange glasses 30 minutes; switch to blue for 5 minutes.
•Avoid fluorescent lights and fluoride toothpaste. They deplete vitamin A in the body.

—Acupressure point:
Press hollow at base of the throat to stimulate thyroid, 3x for 10 seconds each.

Herbal, Superfood and Supplement Therapy

Interceptive therapy: (Choose 2 to 4 recommendations) *Don't take iron with thyroid medication. It binds up the thyroxine, rendering it insoluble. Hormone replacement drugs can depress thyroid health and worsen hypothyroidism.*

1—Increase thyroid activity: The thyroid needs iodine to produce its hormones. An imbalanced thyroid causes excess estrogen production with many problems for women. Herbal iodine sources are effective without side effects: •Crystal Star IODINE, POTASSIUM, SILICA™ extract or •OCEAN MINERALS™ caps 2x daily, or •THYROID META-MAX™ 2 daily. Use with *ashwagandha* extract and HCl 600mg for best results (this previous program is highly recommended); •Gaia Herbs THYROID SUPPORT phytocaps; •Ethical Nutrients THYRO-VITAL; •Solaray ALFA JUICE caps; or •Enzymatic THYROID/TYRO-SINE COMPLEX (highly recommended); or •Tyrosine 500mg with L-lysine 500mg 2x daily, or •Taurine 500mg with L-lysine 500mg 2x daily. •Kelp tabs 8 daily, with cayenne 3 daily, or •Green Foods ION KELP tabs. •Nutricology GUGGUL LIPIDS to aid in T_3 (Tri-iodothyronine) production and reduce thyroid-related weight gain.

—Natural glandular therapy: Natural thyroid hormone replacement more closely resembles human thyroid hormones. •Nutri-PAK thyroxin-free double strength thyroid.
•Nutricology TG100 (under the supervision of a health professional); •Raw Thyroid complex; or •Raw Thymus glandular.

2—Support your adrenals to help your thyroid: •Crystal Star ADRENAL ENERGY BOOST™ caps 2x daily; or •Country Life ADRENAL COMPLEX with tyrosine. •Evening Primrose oil, 2000mg daily. •*Siberian eleuthero* extract 2000mg daily, or •Rainbow Light ADAPTOGEM, or •Planetary Formulas SCHIZANDRA ADRENAL COMPLEX; •CC Pollen ROYAL JELLY caps; •Vitamin C 5000 mg daily to help convert cholesterol to adrenal hormones.

3—Stop thyroid destruction with antioxidants: •CoQ$_{10}$ 100mg daily; Royal Bodycare MICROHYDRIN PLUS; •Country Life sublingual B-12, 2500mcg daily; •Emulsified A 25,000IU 3x daily; •Vitamin E 400IU daily.

4—For goiter: apply •BLACK WALNUT extract as a throat paint, and take ½ drop-perful 2x daily; apply •calendula compresses twice a day for a month.

5—Improve memory and mental function with EFAs: For women, •EVENING PRIMROSE OIL 3000 mg daily; For men, •flax seed oil 2 tbsp. daily. •Ginkgo Biloba extract 2x daily. Try •Wakunaga KYO-GREEN with EFAs. •Herbal Magic GINSENG-GINKGO REJUVENATOR twice daily. •Country Life Magnesium-potassium-bromelain, 2 daily, •Zinc 75mg daily.

—Superfood therapy:
•Body Ecology VITALITY SUPER GREEN.
•Sun Wellness CHLORELLA drink or tabs daily.

Can't find a recommended product? Call the 800 number listed in Product Resources for the store nearest you.

Immune Response

Building Stronger Immunity

Your immune system is your bodyguard. It works both pro-actively and protectively to shield you from anything in your world that threatens your life and limb. The main elements of the immune system are the thymus gland, bone marrow, the spleen, the complement system of enzymatic proteins, and the lymphatic system with white blood cells and lymphocytes, the backbone of immune defenses. Your immune system is ever-vigilant, constantly searching for proteins, called antigens, that don't belong in your body. It can deal with a wide range of pathogens - viruses, funguses, bacteria and parasites. It can even recognize potential antigens, such as drugs, insect venoms and chemicals in foods; and malignant cells and foreign tissue, like transplanted organs or transfused blood. **Is your immune response?** Probably, if you get chronic, continuing infections, colds, and respiratory allergies. **Why do you have low immune response?** In today's world, it's usually because of poor diet and nutrition. Other big factors: prolonged use of antibiotics, steroid drugs or recreational drugs, (long-term use can depress immunity to the point where even minor illness can become life-threatening); staph infections; Candida yeast infections; environmental and heavy metal pollutants all figure in. Have a good stress-relieving laugh every day!

Diet and Lifestyle Support Therapy

Nutritional therapy plan for prevention:

1—The American diet of processed foods, 20% sugars and 37% fat, suppresses immunity. Saturated fats in pastries, fried foods, and red meats are the worst culprits. Refined sugar is a major immune system depressant, destroying the ability of white blood cells to kill germs for up to 5 hours after consumption. Reduce dairy foods to keep the body free flowing.

2—Consider a green superfood drink each day. Green superfoods like Pure Planet CHLORELLA or SPIRULINA, Green Foods GREEN MAGMA, or Crystal Star ENERGY GREEN RENEWAL™ to supply a "mini-transfusion" to detoxify your bloodstream.

3—Eat plenty of fresh foods, fiber foods, whole grains, seafoods, eggs and cultured dairy foods, like yogurt and kefir for friendly G.I. flora. Eat organically grown foods whenever possible. Drink bottled water. City tap water may contain as many as 500 different disease-causing bacteria, viruses and parasites.

4—Food enzymes are basic to immune response. Include a cup of green tea or •Crystal Star DR. VITALITY™ green and white tea, fresh fruits and vegetables every day. Especially include enzyme-rich sprouts, garlic, fresh vegetable juices, papaya and sea greens.

—Bodywork:

•Relaxation techniques are immune-enhancers. A positive mental attitude makes a big difference in how your body fights disease. Creative visualization establishes belief and optimism. Biofeedback or massage therapy reduce stress.

•Regular aerobic exercise keeps system oxygen high. Disease does not readily overrun a body where oxygen and organic minerals are high in the vital fluids.

•Immune power builds the most during sleep. Use aromatherapy immune oils like lavender or rosemary oil before bed.

•Tobacco in any form suppresses immunity. The cadmium content causes zinc deficiency. It takes 3 months to rebuild immune response even after you quit.

•Stimulate immunity with early morning sunlight every day. Avoid excessive sun. A sunburn depresses immunity.

Herbal, Superfood and Supplement Therapy

Interceptive therapy plan: Choose 2 to 3 recommendations.

1—**Stimulate white blood cell activity:** •Crystal Star ANTI-BIO™, or •Allergy Research LACTOFERRIN caps with colostrum; •Lane Labs NOXYLANE 4 (clinically shown to triple natural killer cell activity); Beta glucan formulas: •Grifron MAITAKE D-Fraction; •Immudyne MACROFORCE; •Olive Leaf extract; •Ester C with bioflavs 3000mg; •Herbs Etc. ECHINACEA-ASTRAGALUS softgels; •Nature's Way CELL MEND with IP-6; •NAC (*N-acetyl-cysteine*) 600mg daily. —**Medicinal mushrooms enhance interferon production:** Reishi, shiitake and maitake mushrooms; •Planetary Formulas REISHI SUPREME; •Herbs Etc. DEEP HEALTH with Reishi/Shiitake Complex.

2—**Immune modulators are response tonics:** •Natural Balance MODUCARE caps. •Source Naturals WELLNESS CELL RESPONSE caps (transfer factors); •Siberian eleuthero, •Panax ginseng, or •Jagulana JIAOGULAN caps or tea; •Propolis caps 4 daily (good during high risk seasons); •BioStrath YEAST ELIXIR w. HERBS; •Herbal Magic IMMUNE SYSTEM KIT™; •Zand HERBAL INSURE extract; •Futurebiotics VITAL K.

3—**Restore immune strength:** •Royal Bodycare MICROHYDRIN PLUS; Diamond Herpanacine HEALTHY HORIZONS with alpha lipoic acid; •Jarrow JARRO-DOPHILUS with FOS; Transformation Enzyme PLANTADOPHILUS; •UAS DDS-PLUS. •vitamin E 400IU with selenium 200mcg; •CoQ$_{10}$ 200mg daily; •Nutricology GERMANIUM 150mg.

—Enhance thymus gland activity: •Raw thymus glandular; •Nature's Path THY-LYTE; •Enzymatic Therapy THYMULUS; •Nutricology ORGANIC THYMUS. (Tap thymus with knuckles each morning to stimulate thymus.)

4—**Enzymes are basic to immune response:** •Biotec CELL GUARD w. SOD, or Solgar SOD 2000 units for 6 weeks; •Crystal Star DR. ENZYME™ with protease; •Transformation PUREZYME caps (excellent results); *Milk Thistle Seed* extract; or •Goldenseal - Oregon grape root; •Licorice root tea for a month.

5—**Sea plants help your body detox:** Sea greens, 2 tbsp. daily, with algin to purify your body; or take •Crystal Star •OCEAN MINERALS™; •Nature's Path TRACE-MIN-LYTE.

Can't find a recommended product? Call the 800 number listed in Product Resources for the store nearest you.

Understanding Immune Response: *The immune system is the body's most complex, delicately balanced infrastructure.*

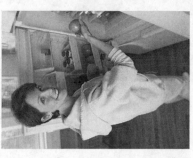

We hear about immune system breakdown. Yet, most of us don't know very much about the immune system or how it works. It's really an amazing part of our bodies. While the workings of other body systems have been well known for some time, the complex nature and dynamics of the immune system have been largely a mystery. One of the problems in comprehending immune response is its highly individual nature. Each and every one of us has our own personal body blueprint. Health for each of us is entirely individual…. and it's most evident in our immune response. We have a personal defense system that comes charging to our rescue at the first sign of an alien force, like a harmful virus, fungus, parasite or pathogenic bacteria. This personal response shows us that health and healing response are so much more than the latest wonder drug. It shows us that we are truly the ultimate healer of ourselves.

Most Americans today don't have good immune response to fight off illness. Pollution, drug overload and nutrient-poor diets compromise our immune health even in good weather. So we're already pre-disposed to a life of frequent colds and flu when bad weather rolls in. Stress is a big culprit that lowers immune response because it affects the production of interferon, your body's natural antiviral agent. People who are under continuous stress from work or their personal lives are 2 and a half times more likely to get a cold or flu infection than other people. You may think you're protected if you've had a flu shot, but think again. Flu shots are only effective for *specific* flu viruses…… you may be exposed to a different one, or even a brand new one (flu viruses mutate rapidly). That means your shot won't be effective. In any case, follow-up studies show flu shots are only effective for 24% of the population.

Drugs aren't the answer for immune enhancement. The immune system is not responsive to drugs for healing. Even doctors admit that most drugs really just stabilize the body, or arrest a harmful organism, to allow the immune system to gather its forces and take over. The unique nature of each person's unique immune response system makes it impossible to form a drug for each person. Antibiotics used to fight infections actually depress the immune system when used long-term. Long courses of tetracycline and erythromycin are some of the most common and some of the worst for immune health. But natural nutritive forces, like healing foods and herbal medicines can and do support the immune system. They enhance its activity, strengthen it, and provide an environment through cleansing and detoxification for it to work at its best. I believe the only way to stay healthy during high risk times is to prepare your body for the defenses it's going to need. Even if you've improved your diet, take another look at it because a super nutritious diet is imperative when you're under attack.

What does the immune system really do?

Immune defense is autonomic, using its own subconscious memory to establish antigens against harmful pathogens. It's a system that works on its own to fend off or neutralize disease toxins, and to set up a healing environment for the body. It is this quality of being a part of us, yet not under our conscious control, that is the great power of immune response. It is also the dilemma of medical scientists as they struggle to get control of a system that is all pervasive and yet, in the end, impossible to completely understand. It is as if God shows us his face in this incredibly complex part of us, where we are allowed to glimpse the ultimate mind-body connection.

Maintaining strong immune defenses in today's world is not easy. Much in our modern life challenges our immune systems. Devastating, immune compromised diseases are rising all over the world. Reduced immunity is the main factor in opportunistic diseases, like candida albicans, chronic fatigue syndrome, lupus, HIV, hepatitis, mononucleosis, herpes II, sexually transmitted diseases and cancer. These diseases have become the epidemic of our time, and most of us don't have very much to fight with. An overload of antibiotics, antacids, immunizations, cortico-steroid drugs, and environmental pollutants eventually affect immune system balance to the point where it cannot distinguish harmful cells from healthy cells.

I see traditional medicine as "heroic" medicine. Largely developed in wartime, its greatest strengths are emergency measures - the ability to arrest a crisis, destroy or incapacitate pathogenic organisms, reset and re-attach broken body parts, and stabilize the body so it can gather its healing forces. Because drugs work in an attempt to directly kill harmful organisms, it is easy to see that their greatest value would be for emergency measures, and for short term use.

But, with prolonged drug use: three *unwanted* things often happen: 1) Our bodies can build up a tolerance to the drug so that it requires more of it to get the same effect. 2) The drug slowly overwhelms immune response so the body becomes dependent upon it, using it as a crutch instead of doing its own work. 3) The drug misleads our defense system to the point that it doesn't know what to assault, and attacks everything in confusion. This type of over-reaction often happens during an allergy attack, where the immune system may respond to substances that are not really harmful. Most of the time, if we use drugs wisely to stimulate rather than over kill, if we "get out of the way" by keeping our bodies clean and well nourished, the immune system will spend its energies rebuilding instead of fighting, and strengthen us instead of constantly gathering resources to conduct a "rear guard" defense.

The very nature of immune strength means that it must be built from the inside out. The immune system is the body system most sensitive to nutritional deficiencies. Giving your body generous, high quality, natural remedies at the first sign of infection improves your chances of overcoming disease before it takes serious hold. Powerful, immune-enhancing superfoods and herbs can be directed at "early warning" problems to build strength for immune response. Building good immune defenses takes time and commitment, but it is worth it. The inherited immunity and health of you, your children and your grandchildren is laid down by you.

Can't find a recommended product? Call the 800 number listed in Product Resources for the store nearest you.

What depresses immune response?

...**Long term courses of drugs:** *antacids* reduce nutrient assimilation, *antibiotics* destroy friendly bacteria vital to GI immunity, *anti-inflammatory drugs* (like acetaminophen, aspirin and ibuprofen) inhibit white cells that fight infection.

...**Long term exposure** to smoke, chemicals and pollutants put a strain on the body's natural detoxification system and lead to genetic mutations that cause cancer.

...**A diet high in fast, chemicalized "non-food" foods:** I call these foods "foods in a box," that your body generally rejects or ignores. Fake fats like olestra that rob cancer-fighting carotenoids are especially disrupting.

...**Repeated exposure to allergens** (from foods, chemicals or environmental allergens) causes the immune system to take a dive because immune defenses are all channeled to deal with the allergen rather than to fight infection. (In turn, allergies are usually the result of impaired immunity.)

...**A diet high in saturated fats, refined sugars or trans fats:** they're in deep fried foods, fast foods and almost all snack foods. Trans fats increase LDL (bad) cholesterol and decrease HDL (good) cholesterol, and are regularly found at high levels in women with breast cancer. Saturated fats interfere with prostaglandin E1 which regulates efficient T-cell activity. Excessively sugary foods suppress white blood cell activity for up to 5 hours! Eating these foods regularly may mean your immune system is taking a nose dive all day long!

...**Low intake of protective, antioxidant and enzyme-rich fruits and vegetables.**

...**Excessive dieting or low nutrient intake** which depresses interferon activity. Overeating also depresses immune response.

...**A lifestyle low on rest.** Natural killer cell activity is reduced by as much as 28% when sleep is cut by 4 hours (clinical tests at U. CA. San Diego School of Medicine).

...**Having parents who smoke, drink to excess or abuse drugs.** Children born to addicted parents have more genetic predisposition to illness and infections.

...**Not being breast-fed as a child.** Breast milk is rich in antibodies, essential fatty acids and interferon that strengthen a child's developing immune system.

...**A poor outlook on life or severe, long lasting depression.** In addition, people who overextend themselves may be unusually susceptible to immune system malfunction.

Does your immune system need a boost? **It isn't easy to measure immune health.**

Each one of us is different and the character of immune response varies widely. I've worked for years to develop ways people can communicate with their bodies. Here's a personal quiz to monitor your immune status: If you answer yes to more than 3 of these questions, your immune system is probably sluggish.

1: Do you get long lasting, chronic infections, colds, respiratory problems or allergies?
2: Do you have or have you had in the past any immune-deficient diseases, like chronic fatigue syndrome, Hashimoto's or fibromyalgia?
3: Do you have a history of malabsorption problems, like irritable bowel syndrome (I.B.S.), or chronic diarrhea or constipation?
4: Do you have diabetes or liver disease?
5: Do you have bouts of systemic candida or yeast infections that don't seem to go away even after conventional treatments?
6: Do you have a skin disorder like adult acne or Rosacea?
7: Have you recently undergone surgery, chemotherapy or radiation treatment?
8: Have you ever been the recipient of an organ transplant?
9: Have you undergone long-term treatment with antibiotics or steroid drugs?
10: Do you have periodontal disease?
11: Do you drink 2 or more drinks of hard alcohol 4 to 5 times a week or take recreational drugs on a regular basis?
12: Are you a smoker or are you exposed to second-hand smoke on a regular basis?
13: Do you live in an area where there is smog or heavy pesticide use?
14: Are you regularly exposed to industrial heavy metals, like cadmium, asbestos or mercury?
15: Do you drink untreated tap water or eat produce sprayed with pesticides?
16: Do you regularly eat meats, like pork or beef that are injected with antibiotics and hormones?
17: Do you have circulation problems or a history of claudication?
18: Do you suffer from chronic stress, anxiety, panic attacks or depression?
19: Do you suffer from chronic insomnia? Are you always tired?

Can't find a recommended product? Call the 800 number listed in Product Resources for the store nearest you.

Look on the bright side.
Laughter lifts more than your spirits.
It also boosts your immune response.
Laughter lowers cortisol, an immune suppressor, allowing better immune activity.

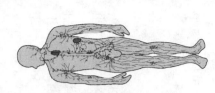

Lymphatic system health is the foundation of good immune response.

The lymphatic system, including lymphatic vessels and nodes, the thymus gland, tonsils and spleen, acts as your body's secondary circulatory system. It's a network of tubing, millions of tiny vessels, ducts and valves that flush and filter waste products from cells and tissues, and carry them to the elimination organs. The lymph nodes are also the factory for crucial white blood cells (lymphocytes) that produce the powerful antibodies which form the overall defense of your body against infections. A major player in your health, the lymph system is a key to your body's immune defenses because it can render harmful bacteria harmless.

As lymph flows around your body, large, eater cells called macrophages in the lymph nodes engulf foreign particles like harmful bacteria and cellular debris. Swollen lymph nodes (often really infected lymph nodes) are caused by an overload of pathogens the lymphatic system cannot keep under control. The lymphatic system doesn't have a pump, like the heart. The valves of the lymph system can keep lymph fluid moving along, but they depend on your breathing and muscle movement to drive them. It's one of the reasons I recommend exercise and deep breathing as an important part of any immune enhancing program. Exercise improves lymphatic circulation so it can remove waste materials that block immune response. The health of your lymphatic system depends to a large extent on the health of your liver. The liver produces most of the body's lymph fluid, which is rich in lymphocytes, special white blood cells which form overall body defenses. A sluggish liver invariably means a congested lymph system. Lymph is also a major route for nutrients from the liver and intestines, so it's rich in fat soluble nutrients, like protein, produced in the liver.

Is your lymphatic system congested? Signs and symptoms that your lymph system is congested:

• Your body looks uncharacteristically soft and pudgy or has newly noticeable cellulite. Inadequate lymph flow is a key factor in cellulite development.
• You get frequent colds and flu. A congested lymph system means reduced defense against pathogens that cause infections.
• You feel extremely sluggish, with low energy or poor memory. You are under chronic stress. Your skin is extremely pale or you are extremely thin.
• You use aluminum cookware or alum-containing deodorants, or eat alum-containing foods (some condiments). Chronic exposure to aluminum puts a strain on lymphatic health.
• You eat a diet high in saturated fat and refined carbohydrates. These foods compromise glandular health and congest your lymphatic system.
• You live a very sedentary lifestyle with little or no exercise. Optimum lymphatic flow depends on regular physical activity.

Lymph healing protocols for immune health:

—**Boost nutrients.** Protein and B$_{12}$ deficiency especially effect lymphatic efficiency. Take a lymph builder drink: 1 handful parsley, 1 garlic clove, 5 carrots, and 3 celery stalks. Add 2 tsp. green superfood like •Crystal Star ENERGY GREEN RENEWAL™ drink or •Wakunaga of America KYO-GREEN. Eat lymph boosting vegetables: cabbage, kale, carrot, bell pepper, collards; or lymph-enhancing fruits: apple, pineapple, blueberries and grapes. Include potassium-rich foods regularly — sea veggies, broccoli, bananas and seafood. Spicy foods like natural salsas, cayenne pepper, horseradish and ginger boost a sluggish lymph system. Take a glass of lemon and water regularly in the morning and Crystal Star DR. VITALITY™ tea in the afternoon for lymph revitalization. Avoid coffee, sugar, dairy products and alcoholic drinks. They contribute to lymphatic stagnation.

—**Optimize liver health:** Herbal bitters like turmeric, cardamom and lemon peel regenerate both liver and lymphatic system. Try •Crystal Star LIVER CLEANSE FLUSHING™ tea; or •Gaia Herbs SWEETISH BITTERS ELIXIR, or •Crystal Star's BITTERS & LEMON™ extract, or a •white sage, astragalus, echinacea root, Oregon grape root, dandelion root tea.

—**Cleanse your lymphatic system for optimum defense:** •Echinacea, one of the best herbal lymph cleansers I know, flushes the lymphatic system beautifully. •Red root and Astragalus, powerful lymph cleansers, are synergistic with echinacea. For serious immune deficient disease, •Gaia Herbs SUPREME CLEANSE. Electrolytes detoxify lymph glands: •Nature's Path TRACE-LYTE liquid minerals. Improve lymphatic filtration with •Zinc picolinate; •Vitamin E; •B-complex, 100mg daily, B-12 sublingual, 2500mcg; •vitamin C, 3,000mg daily.

—**Boost lymphocyte formation:** •Crystal Star ANTI-BIO™ caps; •Herbs Etc. LYMPHATONIC reduces lymphatic swelling and congestion; •Nature's Apothecary LYMPH CLEANSE; •Gaia Herbs ECHINACEA-RED ROOT SUPREME. Enzymes reduce inflammation and maximize healing results: Crystal Star DR. ENZYME™ with protease and bromelain is a specific. Silica plays an integral role in lymphatic health. Silica therapy can lead to dramatic increases in phagocytes (the cells that kill pathogens). Silica is especially beneficial for people with lymphatic diatheses (malfunction of the lymphatic system). •Crystal Star IODINE, POTASSIUM, SILICA drops; •Eidon SILICA MINERAL SUPPLEMENT; or •Jarrow BIO-SIL.

—**Stimulate lymphatic circulation:** •A seaweed bath is a quick way to stimulate lymphatic drainage and rid your body of disease-causing toxins. In a bath, the electromagnetic action of seaweed releases excess body fluids and wastes from congested cells through the skin, replacing them with vital, immune boosting minerals. Unpolluted, shoreline waters are hard to find. •Crystal Star offers a blend of packaged seaweeds in a HOT SEAWEED BATH™. (See page 184 for more info.) •A mineral bath is also effective. Add 1 cup Dead Sea salts. 1 cup Epsom salts, ½ cup regular sea salt and ¼ cup baking soda to a tub; swish in 3 drops lavender oil, 2 drops juniper oil, 2 drops marjoram oil and 1 drop ylang ylang oil. Stir water briskly to disperse evenly. •Take an alternating hot and cold hydrotherapy treatment at the end of your daily shower. •**Lymph supporting therapies:** massage therapy (elevate feet and legs for 5 minutes every day, massaging lymph node areas). Mini trampoline exercises and dry skin brushing with a natural bristle brush are both specifics for optimum lymph health.

Can't find a recommended product? Call the 800 number listed in Product Resources for the store nearest you.

469

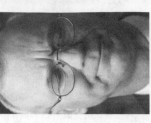

Indigestion and Heartburn

Gas, Bloating, Flatulence

Indigestion plagues up to 40% of Americans. 50 million Americans suffer nighttime heartburn at least once a week that is severe enough to disrupt their sleep. Digestion problems go beyond the symptoms of heartburn, gas and bloating. Energy is reduced, constipation results from metabolic byproducts that aren't eliminated, allergic reactions, diarrhea and fatigue can all ensue. If you have chronic indigestion, you're probably aging faster than normal, your immune defenses are low, and you may be at risk for infections like candida yeasts to take hold. As we age, digestion weakens. Our bodies make less stomach acid (a 65 year old has 85% less HCl than they did at 35). Without enough HCl to activate natural pepsin, proteins don't digest well, so you may become deficient in critical amino acids.

Heartburn means gnawing, burning pain, tenderness and difficulty swallowing directly after you eat. Indigestion means abdominal distention and excess intestinal gas. Both indigestion and heartburn are caused by poor food assimilation, usually from low enzymes. Gas forms when bacteria acts on undigested carbohydrates. Poor food combining, eating too much food, or too many fatty, spicy foods, and allergies to sugar, wheat or dairy all contribute. Too much caffeine, sodas and alcohol are heartburn triggers, amazingly so are fluoridated water or toothpaste. Chronic constipation or diverticulitis (from lack of fiber), candida yeast overgrowth and HCl deficiency are regularly involved.

Have you become a victim of antacids?

Acid blocking drugs may mean that important B vitamins (especially B-12), minerals and trace minerals aren't assimilated well. A new survey finds that 15 million Americans have heartburn every day! We spend $1.7 billion on indigestion remedies each year! Yet antacids are designed to provide temporary relief. Evidence is piling up that excessive use of over-the-counter antacids may wreak havoc on digestive health. They may even themselves become a health problem because they radically change your digestive chemistry.

Do any of these antacid problems pertain to you?

1) *The tolerance effect:* The more you use antacids, the more you need them. Antacids either neutralize stomach HCl (hydrochloric acid), that you need for digestion, or they block it, confuse the body and disrupt its normal processes. If you take a lot of antacids, your body overcompensates, producing excess stomach acid.

2) *Antacids disrupt pH balance:* Optimum pH is between 7.35 and 7.45. If you take lots of antacids, your GI tract fluctuates between over alkaline and over acid, leading to problems like diarrhea or constipation, gallbladder problems, hiatal hernia, even malnutrition. A friend thought his heartburn symptoms would improve if he doubled up on his acid blocker dosage. He ended up in the bathroom all night, passing completely undigested food. Disrupting body pH alters bowel ecology, too, potentially causing dramatic overgrowth of candida yeasts.

3) *Pernicious ingredients:* Many antacids contain aluminum which causes constipation and bone pain. Others overdose you on magnesium, causing diarrhea. Some contain both aluminum and magnesium, confusing your body with alternating constipation and diarrhea. Antacids full of sodium may cause water retention. Most have chemical coloring agents that can cause allergic reactions in some people, or lead to mood changes if taken regularly...... the way many people take them.

4) *Some drugs interact with antacids:* People on drug therapy for HIV know antacids decrease their HIV drug absorption by up to 23%. Oral contraceptives may lose their effectiveness if taken with antacids. People using NSAIDS drugs for arthritis along with antacids suffer 2½ times more serious gastrointestinal complications than those taking a placebo! Antacids not only block drug absorption, they also block your food absorption of nutrients, especially B₁₂, necessary for virtually all immune responses.

5) *Some antacids build up in the body, impeding body processes:* I know a woman who was hospitalized three times for kidney stones until her physician finally advised her to stop taking her over-the-counter antacids because the unabsorbed calcium in them was causing the kidney stone formation.

The Secrets to Better Digestion: 5 Easy Steps To Less Indigestion, Heartburn and Gas

1. Take **ENZYMES.** We are born with a limited supply of enzymes which become depleted with age. But enzymes can be easily brought into your body through fresh foods. If all your food is cooked, microwaved, or processed above 118° Fahrenheit, all of its enzymes are destroyed. Enzymes are especially critical for digestion. If the foods you eat do not contain enough enzymes for digestion, the body has to pull from its reserves in your liver or pancreas, weakening enzyme dependent processes in these areas like detoxification or hormone secretion.

When you lack enzymes for digestion, bacteria feed off the undigested food in the GI tract. This can produce symptoms like gas, bloating, heartburn and constipation. I have worked with thousands of people over the years with digestive problems. In literally every case, when an otherwise healthy person added more plant enzymes to their diet (either through fresh foods or enzyme supplements), digestive problems were drastically reduced. People carrying extra weight from body congestion often drop 10 lbs. Enzymes even overcome food allergies. Supplementating with amylase, the plant enzyme which digests starches, renders gluten-rich grains like wheat and rye harmless to people with gluten enteropathy, a severe intestinal

Can't find a recommended product? Call the 800 number listed in Product Resources for the store nearest you.

malabsorption syndrome caused by an allergy to gluten-rich grains. Fresh, enzyme-rich foods smooth out both digestion and elimination. Have a green salad every day! Consider supplemental enzymes, too. Transformation DIGESTZYME is an excellent choice for digestive problems. For therapeutic enzyme therapy to improve immune response and target inflammatory disorders like arthritis or injuries, Crystal Star's DR. ENZYME™ with protease and bromelain is highly recommended. See page 92 for a complete discussion of enzyme therapy.

2. **Take PROBIOTICS.** Literally meaning "life", probiotics are "friendly bacteria," like Lactobacillus acidophilus and Bifidobacteria bifidum, that inhabit your digestive tract and maintain the inner ecology critical to digestion and health. They keep out pathogens like viruses, yeast and harmful microorganisms by competing with them for space in the gastrointestinal tract. Research from the University of Delaware finds that bifidobacteria actually have the ability to remove cancer cells or the enzymes which lead to their formation! Probiotics are a powerful preventive against digestive problems like diarrhea, constipation and even more serious problems like inflammatory bowel disease, even colon cancer.

Chemicals in your food or environment (like chlorine in drinking water), fast food, a stressful lifestyle, excessive alcohol consumption, cigarette smoking and certain prescription drugs all deplete your body's supply of probiotics. Antibiotics, by far, are the biggest offender in probiotic depletion. (In France, Japan and India, doctors routinely recommend acidophilus when they prescribe antibiotics.)

Probiotics are constantly at work to keep you healthy and energized and your digestion smooth. I recommend eating more cultured foods rich in these organisms, like yogurt, kefir or raw sauerkraut. High quality probiotic supplements are widely available. Consider American Health ACIDOPHILUS liquid or UAS DDS-PLUS for probiotic therapy for optimum digestion.

3. **Practice good FOOD COMBINING.** Sometimes, it's not what you eat that's making you sick, it's how you combine the foods you eat. Proper food combining can still make all the difference for your digestion. Different foods need different enzymes to digest well. Your intelligent body activates the proper enzyme when the food reaches your mouth. Eating foods that are not compatible can cause fermentation in the stomach, leading to gas, constipation or diarrhea- clear signs that food is not being assimilated well.

Most experts think human enzyme assimilation was developed very early, when our species ate almost all fresh or dried foods. Foods we might have eaten together were naturally compatible because of harvest times and seasons. We traditionally ate certain foods at the same time, and we developed the capacity to digest them at the same time. Today we can eat any type of food we want when our taste-buds want it..... and that gets us into trouble. Enzymes which digest one type of food but are incompatible with another type in the same meal are either blocked or get confused, and we get the non-compatible food signs of gas and bloating.

Our digestive systems have adapted somewhat over the millenia. Unless your digestion is seriously compromised, you may not need to follow all the food combining rules all the time. Sometimes we let these things control our lives and lose the pleasure of eating.

For myself, I try to follow just two principles: I eat fruits alone and on an empty stomach in the morning. I don't eat fruits and vegetables together. To learn more, please refer to a good "Correct Food Combining Chart" available in most health food stores.

4. **Eat more FIBER.** By now, most of you know that fiber is good for you. Boosting fiber intake from grains like oats can lower harmful LDL cholesterol levels linked to heart disease. It speeds weight loss by suppressing the appetite and reducing colon congestion. It also improves glucose tolerance for people with diabetes and provides protection against breast and colon cancer development. And, of course, fiber is vital for your digestion. Fiber keeps the entire digestive system running smoothly by decreasing the transit time of food in the intestines. (Food is more likely to ferment and putrefy causing indigestion the longer it remains in your gut!) **Fiber is a system regulator, not a laxative.** It relieves both constipation and diarrhea by increasing the weight and frequency of stools. Increasing fiber intake is a primary treatment for even serious digestive problems like diverticulitis and Irritable Bowel Syndrome.

But, most people don't get enough fiber from their diets. In fact, today's statistics tell us that most Americans need to double their fiber intake to get the 30 to 35 grams a day recommended by health professionals. Six half-cup servings of whole grains, cereal or legumes and 4 servings of fresh fruits and vegetables each day can give you the fiber you need to stay regular and healthy. Fiber supplements are also a good choice as an addition to a balanced diet. I like Nature's Secret ULTIMATE FIBER and Jarrow GENTLE FIBERS.

5. **Eat more ALKALINE FOODS.** The typical American diet relies on too many acid-forming foods. The body, by design, is slightly alkaline, with a pH of 7.4. When the body becomes too acidic, it pulls alkaline minerals like sodium, calcium, potassium and magnesium from its reserves to restore an alkaline state. Over the long-term, this becomes dangerous. Mineral are the building blocks of life. Even small deficiencies are linked to depression, osteoporosis and premature aging. An acidic body condition is the primary cause of GERD (Gastro-Esophageal Reflux Disorder) the most common cause of heartburn for 40 million Americans. GERD is also implicated in chronic fatigue syndrome, arthritis, cancer, allergies and fungal infections. Bringing more alkaline foods into your diet not only eases your indigestion and heartburn, it may prevent the onset of serious disease later!

•ACID-FORMING FOODS to limit: refined sugar, white flour, alcohol, soft drinks, coffee and caffeine containing foods, red meat, and fried, fatty foods.
•ALKALINE FORMING FOODS to increase: mineral water, land/sea vegetables, sea salt, herbal teas, miso, brown rice, honey, fruits and fruit juices.

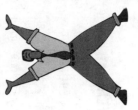

471

Can't find a recommended product? Call the 800 number listed in Product Resources for the store nearest you.

Indigestion and Heartburn

Diet and Lifestyle Support Therapy

Nutritional therapy plan:

1—Eat an alkalizing diet, with plenty of cultured foods like yogurt, kefir and miso soup, high fiber foods like whole grains, fresh vegetables, fruits, and enzyme-rich foods like papaya and pineapple.

2—Avoid fatty, spicy, sugary and acid-forming foods. Omit fried foods, red meats, fatty dairy products, dried fruits, sodas and caffeine. Switch to herbal teas, like Crystal Star DR. VITALITY™ green and white tea blend with ginger for better digestion, instead of acid-forming coffee.

3—Eat smaller meals. Chew food very well.

4—If you get frequent bouts of hiccups because of poor digestion - very common today - try Wild Cherry tea (sometimes dramatic help).

—Cleanse the digestive system and establish good enzymes:

• Start with a cleansing, pectin mono diet of apples and apple juice for 2 days. (For people that really suffer, this makes them feel better almost right away.) Then for 4 days use a diet of 70% fresh foods and steamed brown rice for B vitamins. Add fresh veggies and high fiber foods gradually if digestion is delicate.

—Watchwords:

• If 1 tsp. cider vinegar in water relieves your heartburn you need more stomach acid.
• If you are bloated, take ½ tsp. baking soda in water to ease distension.
• If you have flatulence, take a catnip or slippery elm enema for immediate relief.
• If your stomach is sour, settle it with lime juice and a pinch of ginger.
• If you absorb poorly, a glass of wine can offer better absorption.
• At first sign of heartburn, take 2-oz. ALOE VERA juice.
• Indigestion triggers: late night snacks, chocolates, fatty fried foods, rich desserts or sauces, alcohol, smoking, coffee, lots of sugar-free sorbitol candies (cramping and diarrhea).

—Bodywork:

• Commercial antacids neutralize stomach acid, inviting the stomach to produce even more acid, often making the condition worse in the long run. New tests even show that chronic use of aluminum-containing antacids causes bone loss. Avoid over-using antibiotics. They destroy friendly flora in the digestive tract, too, which you'll need to replace with probiotics.
• Apply hot ginger compresses to abdomen and over liver area (upper right abdomen).
• Lie on your back and draw knees up to chest to relieve abdomen pressure.
• Try to eat when relaxed. Meals eaten in a hurry or under stress contribute to poor digestion. Life isn't going to slow down on its own. Make a conscious effort to lessen digestive stress. Try a short walk before eating.

Herbal, Superfood and Supplement Therapy

Interceptive therapy plan: Choose 2 or more recommendations.

1—**Bitters herbs help the cause of heartburn:** • Crystal Star GERD GUARD™ caps before and after meals; • BITTERS & LEMON™ extract each morning as a preventive. • Gaia Herbs SWEETISH BITTERS.

2—**Get to the heart of heartburn:** • L-glutamine 1500mg daily for long-term relief; • Lane Labs NATURE'S LINING to strengthen the stomach wall (highly recommended); • Prevail ACID EASE or • Betaine HCl capsules after meals; • Turmeric extract (curcumin).

3—**Soothe the burn:** • Slippery elm tea or tablets; • Marshmallow tea; • Hylands homeopathic Indigestion after meals; • Umeboshi plum paste. For acute indigestion: • Nature's Herbs DGL POWER; • Rainforest Remedies BELLY BE GOOD; • 2 tbsp. Aloe vera juice.

4—**For gas and bloating:** • Ginger capsules 2 to 4 as needed; Homeopathic remedies work very well: BioForce Indigestion Relief, or Nux vomica, • Ignatia 6c, or • Dioscorea 6c work for bloating. Take 2 to 4 peppermint oil drops in water or Heather's Tummy Tamers PEPPERMINT OIL capsules. (Also helpful for irritable bowel syndrome). • Activated charcoal - short term.

—Relieve gas quick: • pinches cinnamon, nutmeg, ginger, cloves in water- drink down.

5—**For belching and burping:** • AkPharma BEANO drops; • Prevail BEAN-VEGI formula; • Country Life DIGESTIVE formula; • Transformation GASTROZYME, a natural antacid.

6—**For cramping and diarrhea:** • Activated charcoal tabs (short term help); • Apple pectin tabs (long term help); • Body Essentials SILICA GEL; • Nutricology PERM A VITE to reduce gut permeability; • Crystal Star STRESS OUT™ muscle relaxer drops (fast activity); • Crystal Star STRESS ARREST™ tea (gentle activity).

7—**Complete digestion with digestive teas:** • Peppermint, spearmint or alfalfa-mint tea; sage, thyme, dill, caraway ease digestion. • Catnip-fennel-lemon peel tea; • Chamomile tea; • Wild Yam tea, especially if you have eaten too much refined sugar.

8—**Effective enzyme therapy:** • Bromelain 1500mg daily, or • Nature's Plus chewable bromelain 40mg; • Biotec Goods BIO-GESTIN; • American Health PAPAYA CHEWABLES; • Transformation DIGESTZYME with meals; • Pancreatin capsules 1400mg; • Garlic/parsley or ginger caps.

9—**Probiotics for friendly flora:** • Nutricology SYMBIOTICS + FOS, dairy free; • UAS DDS-PLUS + FOS; • Jarrow Formulas JARRO-DOPHILUS.

—Superfood therapy: Choose 1 or 2 recommendations.

• Crystal Star ENERGY GREEN RENEWAL™ drink.
• C'est Si Bon CHLORENERGY (chlorella).
• Nature's Answer SEACENTIALS GOLD (highly recommended).
• Aloe Life STOMACH PLUS FORMULA (fast heartburn relief).
• Sun Wellness CHLORELLA

Can't find a recommended product? Call the 800 number listed in Product Resources for the store nearest you.

Infections

Staph Infections, Viral Infections, Bacterial Infections

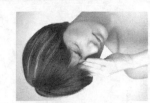

A *staph infection* involves a staphylococcus micro-organism, is usually virulent, and often food-borne. Antibiotic measures are effective. In minor cases, the infection can be resolved through natural means. A *bacterial infection* involves pathogenic microbial bacteria (Don't take iron supplements during an infection. They may make the bacteria grow faster.) Antibiotic agents are normally effective. A *viral infection* involves virus organisms that infiltrate the deepest regions of the body and live off the body's cell enzymes. Virus infections are virulent, deep-reaching, tenacious. Antibiotics are not effective. Antiviral treatment must be vigorous, since viruses can both mutate and move to escape being overcome. All types of infections regularly cause painful inflammation as the body reacts to overcome them. Chronic recurring infections may indicate low thyroid or liver function. **Is it an infection?** If there's inflammation, (like boils, sores, and abscesses), often with a high temperature and a cough or sore throat (a sign your body is actively working to throw off the infection), along with breakdown of tissue into waste matter, like mucous or pus, it may be. Most sufferers have extremely reduced energy and fatigue. **What commonly causes an infection?** Low resistance from a low nutrition diet with too many refined foods, too few green vegetables, over-using antibiotics, or an allergy reaction. *See Also Fungal and Parasite Infections pages 420 and 519.*

Diet and Lifestyle Support Therapy

Nutritional therapy plan:

1—For any infection: an enzyme therapy detox is effective: use 3 parts water to 1 part fresh pineapple juice; drink 8 glasses in 24 hours; or •Crystal Star DR. VITALITY™ tea.

2—Take 6 glasses of mixed vegetable juices like Knudsen's VERY VEGGIE, or potassium broth (pg. 291) or •Aloe vera juice, morning and evening, over the next 24 hours. Then eat only veggies and brown rice for 3 days to keep the body acid free and free flowing.

3—Take a glass of lemon juice and water each morning to stimulate kidney filtering.

4—Include vegetable source proteins for faster healing: sea greens and seafoods, whole grains, sprouts, and soy foods. Avoid foods that feed infections: all sugars, refined foods, caffeine, colas, tobacco and alcohol (except for a little wine) during healing.

—**Help remove infections through the skin:**
•Earth's Bounty O₂-SPRAY: staph infections. •Crystal Star ANTI-BIO™ gel: skin infections. •Apply *ginger-cayenne* compresses to take down swelling. •Eucalyptus and tea tree oil: staph and fungal infections. •Nutribiotic GRAPEFRUIT SKIN SPRAY. •Green clay packs for inflammation. •Honey keeps skin infections from spreading. •Herbal Answers HERBAL ALOE FORCE gel.

—**Bodywork:** Sleep. Healing is at its peak during sleep.
•Overheating therapy is effective in deterring virus replication (use a sauna to raise blood temperature). Even slight temperature increases can lead to considerable reduction of infection. See page 183 for the technique.
•Activate kidney cleansing with a chamomile or chlorophyll enema.

—**For children:** •Osha root tea or Hylands *HYLAVIR* tablets. •Anti-infection aromatherapy for children 1 year and up: 1 drop tea tree oil, 1 drop essential oil of lavender, 1 drop calendula oil in juice. •Make an anti-infective salve: equal parts garlic powder, goldenseal powder, zinc powder - mix into calendula ointment.

Herbal, Superfood and Supplement Therapy

Interceptive therapy: Herbs can help infections that are resistant to medical treatment.
—**For a staph infection:** •Nutribiotic GRAPEFRUIT SEED extract. •Olive leaf extract, •East Park OLIVE LEAF extract; and •Echinacea extract, or •Herbs. Etc. ECHINACEA TRIPLE SOURCE (acute)or PHYTOCILLIN (chronic); reduce inflammation with •Bromelain 1500mg daily, or •Crystal Star ANTI-BIO™ extract and caps (excellent activity against a broad range), and •Vitamin C crystals with bioflavs., ½ tsp. in water every hour in acute stages, reducing to 5000mg daily. —Thymus defense: •raw thymus 3x daily;
—**For a bacterial infection:** Destroy the active microbe with •Oregano oil, as directed; Use •Grifron MAITAKE D-Fraction, Beta Glucan for resistant bacteria; •CoQ-10, 300mg daily; •Olive leaf extract as directed. •Nutribiotic GRAPEFRUIT SEED extract. Flush lymphatic toxins with •Crystal Star ANTI-BIO™ caps or drops every 4 hours, and •Vitamin C crystals with bioflavs 5000mg daily. Reduce inflammation with •Crystal Star DR. ENZYME™ w. protease and bromelain, or bromelain 3000mg and Lysine 2000mg daily, or •Lane Labs BENE-FIN shark caps. Boost immunity with •*Propolis, Garlic, Echinacea.*
—**For a viral infection:** •Olive leaf extract caps, 4 daily and and •Vitamin C crystals with bioflavs. ½ tsp. in water every hour in acute stages. •Health from the Sun FLU GUARD with boxwood leaf powder; or •Garlic (both gram negative and gram positive viruses), or •Germanium 150mg; •Propolis or •St. John's wort extracts or •Oregano oil as directed; •Beta Glucan 75mg before meals.•Merix RELEEV (excellent for herpes);
•Vitamin A (not beta-carotene) 100,000IU daily for 3 days only. Prevent serious irfection wiuth Transfer Factors like •Source Naturals WELLNESS CELL RESPONSE. Raise immunity with •reishi or maitake mushrooms; Lane Labs MGN-3 (highly recommended) or •Planetary ASTRAGALUS JADE SCREEN. •Restore homeostasis with •Planetary TRIPHALA caps (help for chronic infections); and•MICROHYDRIN available at royalbodycare.com.

—**Superfood therapy choices:** •Crystal Star RESTORE YOUR STRENGTH™, daily during healing; then ENERGY GREEN RENEWAL™ for body chem balance. •Nutricology PRO-GREENS w. EFAs. •C'est Si Bon CHLORENERGY (chlorella). •Futurebiotics VITAL K drink.

Can't find a recommended product? Call the 800 number listed in Product Resources for the store nearest you.

Infections have taken on an uglier face. *Are you prepared for the supergerm assault?*

Our antiseptic, prescription drug lifestyle hasn't saved us from infectious disease. Germ warfare is out of control all over the world. Supergerms like *e. Coli, salmonella*, SARS (Severe Acute Respiratory Syndrome, see pg. 487 for more), antibiotic-resistant pneumonia, and staph infections are a real and present danger in the U.S. At least 30 new diseases from supergerms have emerged in the last 20 years. Experts believe hundreds more are on the way. In the last fifteen years, infections from supergerms jumped from the fifth leading cause of death to the third leading cause in the U.S. Over-use of antibiotics in the medical community and the agriculture industry is a common thread at the base of these infections. Last year the Institute of Medicine called for a global effort to fight the problem of antibiotic overloading. Deadly flus are killing people in Hong Kong. Mystery respiratory illnesses are claiming Native American lives in the Southwest U.S. Mad Cow disease from contaminated beef has killed more than 20 people in Britain and has spread to Canada. Mad cow has now been found in U.S. beef, too. Devastating *Ebola* virus has attacked thousands in Africa. Many experts believe it is just a matter of time before *Ebola* makes it to the U.S. via an infected airline passenger!

Strains of drug-resistant tuberculosis and pneumonia are targeting people with compromised immune systems, like those with HIV - itself a supervirus unheard of until the 1940s! Staph infections (increasingly acquired during hospital visits), once easily treated by penicillin, are now 95% resistant to conventional treatment! Virulent staph organisms are resistant to the most powerful new antibiotics. Food borne supergerms are leaping on the U.S. radar with a death toll of 5,000 Americans each year. *E. coli* contaminated beef and other foods have sent thousands to the hospital! The problem is so severe that FDA food safety inspectors say they can't keep up with demand. Blame is placed on substandard conditions in the agriculture industry, exposure to infected animals and contaminated foods, and low immune response rising from pollution, chemical toxins and poor diet.

Has antibiotic therapy backfired? **Germs are getting smarter, mutating into more deadly strains that conventional antibiotics can't touch.**

Penicillin and antibiotics during World War II were a boon for fighting infectious disease. Clearly antibiotic therapy has saved many lives - from wartime injuries, strep infections, meningitis and pneumonia. But antibiotics should not be taken casually or indiscriminately. Some experts estimate that as much as HALF of all antibiotic use is inappropriate or unnecessary. Children may be especially affected. A 1996 survey shows that 70% of kids have taken at least one course of antibiotics by the time they're six months old. When they are overused or misused antibiotics can be a recipe for disaster! Thousands of antibiotics are prescribed every year to treat the viruses that cause colds and flu. If you're taking an antibiotic to get rid of a virus or an allergy-related condition like chronic bronchitis, not only is it largely ineffective, but often reduces the ability of that antibiotic to treat your future bacterial infections.

A strange phenomenon: The more antibiotics you take, the more an infection will find a *new way* to attack. Some bacteria can create 72 new generations with the same antibiotic resistant gene in just one day! Even the latest, most robust antibiotics hardly survive a year before the microbe they were designed to arrest, develops, mutates and grows stronger against them.…. For instance, the newest report reveals the antibiotic Cipro, widely prescribed in the anthrax attacks of 2001, is becoming less and less effective because of overuse! Ampicillin and tetracyclin, used extensively in the 30s, are practically useless today. Another problem with grave consequences: Some people, quite understandably, in an effort to limit their antibiotic intake, stop taking their antibiotics before the prescription is completed. If you don't take the full recommended course of antibiotics, you are unknowingly giving germs that haven't been destroyed the opportunity to mutate and form a defense against the drug…. one of the big reasons why doctors need ever more powerful antibiotics to quell supergerm infections.

Another phenomenon: even Third World countries, without a long history of antibiotic use, are suffering. With the best will in the world, America has sent carloads of antibiotics to these countries in an effort to control some of their virulent infections. The antibiotics were distributed liberally without prescriptions and their overuse has now spurred the development of hundreds of new drug-resistant strains — and the strains are migrating around the world as infected people travel or move.

Even if you don't take antibiotics regularly, you're not immune. People are getting low dose antibiotics daily from commercial meats, dairy foods and produce without knowing it. About 40% of the antibiotics produced in the U.S. each year are fed to cattle, pigs and chickens to fight diseases that break out in overcrowded feed lots. A 1998 Harvard Medical School study shows that an astounding 300,000 pounds of antibiotics was sprayed on fruits like apples and pears to prevent a blight! The FDA has pulled two antibiotics widely used by poultry farmers because of the risk that antibiotic resistance to deadly *campylobacter* could be transferred to humans through eating the meat! Even more worrisome, new household cleaning supplies contain antibiotics to keep your home "germ-free," but a study published in the journal Nature finds that *triclosan*, a widely used antibacterial household chemical, can cause certain bacteria to mutate into new strains resistant to treatment and also disrupts essential fatty acid synthesis, vital for healing.

Can you fight supergerms? *Check out my herbal program on the next page to help solve the antibiotic resistant drug problem.*

1) Use antibiotics only when needed and as directed. Ask your physician if an antibiotic is really right for your infection. (Antibiotics are ineffective for common colds and most ear infections.) 2) For basic household cleaning, use grapefruit seed extract to disinfect cutting boards and countertops, and as a soak to disinfect vegetables, fish and poultry. 3) Reduce antibiotic exposure and overload with organic meats and dairy. I primarily eat foods from the sea because they aren't affected by rampant hormone and antibiotic injection. Free range turkeys have a more natural diet than commercial animals and their meat is antibiotic free.

Can't find a recommended product? Call the 800 number listed in Product Resources for the store nearest you.

Herbs to the rescue! *We think of herbs as so gentle and subtle. How can they work when drugs can't?*

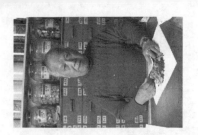

Herbal antibiotics may become some of our best weapons against drug-resistant diseases. Herbal antibiotics work differently than antibiotic drugs. In essence, herbs work with each person's individual immune system. Drugs work against the harmful organism. As heroic medicine, drugs often work best for short time use, to arrest a virulent pathogen and give your body a chance to stabilize so your own immune response can take over. But antibiotic drugs target all bacteria in your body, not just the harmful ones. So they wipe out friendly bacteria in the intestines, important for immune strength and protection against *Candida* yeast overgrowth, *E. Coli* and *Salmonella* infections. Antibiotics taken over a long time also weaken immune response. Research from Baylor School of Medicine reveals that antibiotics actually prevent your immune system's white blood cells from attacking and killing pathogenic bacteria.

—Herbs with antibiotic properties work with your body's own immune defenses. They help flush the lymphatic system of disease toxins, and stimulate immune response so your body can neutralize or eliminate the pathogens without harming healthy tissue. Herbs are living medicines that interact with our bodies in a very complex way. We may never understand all their healing power, but one way is to remind ourselves that whole herbs are foods. Herbs work with our enzyme and digestive functions just as foods do. As with foods, you don't get the interactions with drugs like you might when you combine different drugs. Think about it, would you stop eating spinach, for instance, just because you're taking an antibiotic? Herb healing pathways are different than drugs - even for drugs that originally started as plants.

There are the three categories of herbal antibiotics you can use for your natural supergerm arsenal:

1: **Immune Boosters:** They are not direct germ killers, but they illustrate how herbs like echinacea and astragalus with antibiotic activity work as opposed to drug antibiotics.

—*Echinacea*, a potent immune system stimulant, increases phagocytosis, the process where your immune system engulfs pathogens. Echinacea increases levels of antiviral interferon in the body. Echinacea prompts the thymus, bone marrow and spleen to produce more immune cells for more protection. Echinacea helps cleanse the blood and boost lymphatic filtration and drainage making it a powerful detoxifier for removing infective organisms, especially when combined with goldenseal and myrrh as in Crystal Star's ANTI-BIO™ formulas.

—*Astragalus* boosts natural killer activity and enhances interferon production against pathogens. It is highly beneficial for respiratory illnesses, promoting the regeneration of bronchi cells. Astragalus is ideal for travelers exposed to drug-resistant disease strains. Consider Herbs Etc. ECHINACEA/ASTRAGALUS Complex or Planetary ASTRAGALUS JADE SCREEN.

2: **Lymph Flushers:** They work with the lymphatic system, your immune system's circulatory process, to flush, filter and engulf pathogens, rendering them innocuous.

—*Echinacea* flushes the lymphatic system to rid the body of toxins. Echinacea extract is, by far, one of the best lymph cleansers I know to build body defenses against disease.

—*Seaweed baths* stimulate lymphatic drainage to rid you of toxins via the skin, replacing them with immune boosting minerals. Try Crystal Star HOT SEAWEED BATH™.

—*Bitters herbs* like *turmeric, cardamom* and *lemon peel* regenerate the liver and lymphatic system to enhance immune response. Consider Crystal Star BITTERS & LEMON™.

3. **Organism Killers:** super powerful herbs that may be the best or only tool to wipe out supergerms.

—*Olive leaf extract* is effective against 56 different pathogens. East Park Research finds that olive extract may remedy as many as <u>120 illnesses.</u> Even serious infections like herpes, tuberculosis and pneumonia respond to olive leaf. Olive leaf extract is ideal for people traveling to third world countries. Planetary OLIVE LEAF extract or Nutricology PROLIVE caps.

—*Tea tree oil* has new studies showing that it can kill antibiotic-resistant staph infections even at low concentrations. Adding 1-3 drops of tea tree oil to an infuser and breathing deeply can fight off many respiratory infections. *Note: Do not take 100% pure tea tree oil internally unless under the guidance of a health professional experienced in the use of essential oils.*

—*Garlic* has a powerful antibiotic punch against infections like dysentery and *H. pylori*, responsible for the majority of ulcers, including antibiotic-resistant strains. In one study, immune cell activity rose 140% in people who ate 2 bulbs in a two-day span and 156% in people who took 1800 mg of aged garlic. Consider Wakunaga Kyolic AGED GARLIC EXTRACT.

—*Oregano oil* contains over 50 compounds with organism killing actions. It can inhibit candida yeast, bacteria, viruses and parasites, and may help prevent food borne illness. Allergy Research OREGANO OIL. *Note: Direct contact to pure oregano essential oil can cause mild burns.*

—**Propolis**, the natural protective casing of beehives, inhibits the growth of life-threatening staph and strep species. Lab tests find it actually works better than some antibiotics in killing these bacteria. In addition, propolis can enhance the effectiveness some antibiotics like streptomycin. It has antiviral properties against today's super flu strains, fights cavities and shows promise as an anti-cancer agent. I like Beehive Botanicals PROPOLIS THROAT SPRAY. *Honey* itself is even effective against deadly staph, *E. coli, shigella* and *salmonella*, and can stop *H. pylori*, responsible for most ulcers, after just three days of treatment. Other research shows unprocessed honey fights fungi and bacteria linked to wound and surgical infections. Royal Jelly, a powerful natural antibiotic, is highly effective for herpes, flu, and skin and intestinal infections.

—**Probiotics** like acidophilus suppress virulent strains of *E. Coli, staph, candida* and *salmonella* in the intestines- as effective as the drug Neomycin Sulfate against *E. Coli.* Results are even effective against breast cancer; which studies show slows up to 85% by *Lactobacillus.* Consider UAS DDS-PLUS with FOS.

—**Selenium** therapy enhances immune cell defense against super viruses. In a Chinese study hemorrhagic fever patients (like Ebola virus), death rates decreased from 100% to 36% with selenium! In another study, selenium significantly reduced infections in 74% of AIDS patients. Try 200mcg selenium or Eidon SELENIUM liquid.

Can't find a recommended product? Call the 800 number listed in Product Resources for the store nearest you.

Infertility

Difficulty Conceiving Children - Men and Women

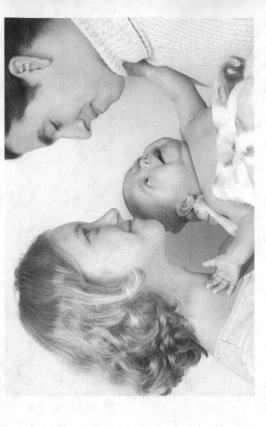

For the first time in history, incredible numbers of people are having trouble conceiving and bearing a child. An amazing 20% of married couples in the U.S. today are affected by some kind of infertility problem. Difficulties seem to be somewhat evenly divided between men (about 35-40%) and women (over 35-40%). In 20-30% of cases, both the man and woman have fertility problems. Over 6 million women of childbearing age in the U.S have problems conceiving. Twenty million U.S. men are characterized as semen infertile. Millions more are described as semen sub-fertile. The fertility industry grosses $2 billion a year!

Unfortunately, current conventional fertility treatments have many drawbacks. In vitro fertilization often results in multiple pregnancies and tough decisions for expectant parents. (To correct this problem, a new technique called "blastocyte transfer" is in the works to reduce risk of multiple births.) Evidence also shows Intracytoplasmic Sperm Injection (ICSI), introduced in 1993 to boost sperm count in infertile men, may cause abnormalities in embryos and even slow development in children. Bladder defects are common in babies born through in vitro fertilization.

More worrisome, a 1999 study in the journal Lancet shows women treated with fertility drugs have TWICE the risk of developing breast cancer — and over 5 TIMES the risk for uterine cancer as other women! Another study reports women who have never been pregnant before increase their risk for ovarian cancer 27 times when they use fertility drugs. Over use of NSAIDs (Non-steroidal anti-inflammatory drugs) like ibuprofen can induce "luteinized unruptured follicle syndrome," a syndrome in which eggs are never released for conception. Some "infertile" women have been able to complete successful pregnancies just by stopping their NSAIDs use!

What causes infertility?

Poor nutrition (especially a fast food diet) and stress are at the base of most fertility problems. Increasingly, environmental hormone mimics from pollutants and chemicals are linked to infertility in both sexes. **For men:** low sperm count or poor sperm quality are the most prevalent common denominators, followed by zinc deficiency, and heavy metal toxicity. Bacterial infections (unless they're long term or virulent) cause temporary infertility which is usually resolved once the infection stops. Too much alcohol or marijuana beget long term problems that last for years. However, the type of underwear men wear may not influence fertility as previously thought. 1999 research shows sperm count and testicular temperature is no different in men who wear briefs than in men who wear boxers. **For women:** anxiety or depression can change body balance enough to impede pregnancy, especially if the emotional stress is about the fertility problem itself. Physical problems like severe anemia, polycystic ovary syndrome and endometriosis must be dealt with for pregnancy to occur.

Home Ovulation Predictors: **An ovulation test can help women get pregnant.**

Conception only occurs during part of the monthly menstrual cycle, for a week or so after ovulation. Ovulation occurs about the midpoint between periods, but many women have irregular cycles, making it difficult for them to know when they are fertile. Ovulation predictors enable women to pinpoint their fertile days by measuring the concentration of luteinizing hormone (LH) in urine. The level of LH increases significantly 12 to 24 hours before ovulation. Ovulation tests instruct women to test their urine daily for several days early in the menstrual cycle with activating strips. The strips turn a color, to establish an LH baseline. When LH rises, shortly before ovulation, the test strip turns a different color. A woman can then better plan sexual intercourse for conception.

Home fertility test: **There are natural ways to stay informed about your ovulation cycle.**

The Ovu Tech Fertility Detector is a completely natural personal fertility health system. It allows you to find out when you're most fertile by licking a tiny slide and viewing crystallization patterns which determine your fertile periods with a microscope. Watching your reproductive cycle in your own home can be informative, interesting and it's easy. For more information on the OvuTech Fertility Detector, visit http://www.johnleemd.com/store/more_ovu-tech.html.

See HORMONE IMBALANCE *page 455*, HEALTHY PREGNANCY section *page 212 for more.*

Can't find a recommended product? Call the 800 number listed in Product Resources for the store nearest you.

Infertility

Diet and Lifestyle Support Therapy

Nutritional therapy plan: Diet is all-important. The body does not readily allow conception without adequate nutrition. Consciously follow a healthy diet and lifestyle for at least six months before trying to conceive. See my book, *Do You Want To Have A Baby? Natural Fertility Solutions & Pregnancy Care* for a complete diet and supplement program.

—For women:
• Reduce dairy products, (especially full fat milk), fried and fatty foods, sugary and junk foods.
• Avoid tobacco, alcohol, except moderate wine, caffeine, red meats (they may have synthetic hormones), and chemical-laced foods.

—For men:
Make a mix of nutritional yeast, bee pollen granules, wheat germ, pumpkin seed - blend 2 tsp. into any superfood drink below.
• Eat zinc foods: oysters, wheat germ, onions, sunflower and pumpkin seeds.
• Emphasize organic foods (especially tomatoes for a lycopene boost). Lancet research shows men who eat organic foods produce 43% more sperm than those who do not.

—For both sexes:
• Eat plenty of whole grains, cultured foods like yogurt, seafoods and sea vegetables, fresh fruits and vegetables. Limit fat intake.
• Have a cup of green tea (men) or white tea (women) every morning. Or try Crystal Star DR. VITALITY™ green and white tea blend.

Lifestyle measures:

—For both parents:
Do not smoke; avoid secondary smoke. Avoid areas with smog and pollutants as much as possible.
• Get daily mild exercise. Too much intense exercise can actually hamper fertility.

—For women:
anxiety and infertility are linked. Relax more. Acupuncture, guided imagery, deep breathing (page 250) are successful for women as relaxation techniques.
• Consider massage therapy. Research from Florida's Clear Passage Therapies shows 4 out of 8 infertile women were able to deliver healthy, full-term babies after deep massage therapy treatments.
• Vaginal pH balance douche right before intercourse: use baking soda/honey for over-acid condition, vinegar/water for over-alkaline.
• Alternate hot and cold sitz baths to stimulate circulation.
• Consider OvuTech home fertility kit to determine your most fertile times by viewing patterns in saliva.

—For men:
avoid hot electric blankets, and hot water beds.
• Sun bathe in the early morning, nude if possible for 15 minutes.
• Stress and abnormal sperm production are linked. Relax more.

Herbal, Superfood and Supplement Therapy

Interceptive therapy plan: Choose 2 or 3 recommendations.

1—For women:
Preconception (normalize menstrual cycle)- •VITEX extract promotes ovulation; •Crystal Star FEMALE HARMONY™ caps 4 daily with EVENING PRIMROSE OIL for EFAs, 4 daily; or •Crystal Star PRO-EST BALANCE™ roll-on or Moon Maid PRO-MENO wild yam cream for 1 month with extra B₆ to reduce chance of miscarriage. •Pure Essence Labs FEM CREME natural progesterone cream to help avoid miscarriage caused by luteal phase failure; •High potency royal jelly 2 tsp. daily, try •Prince of Peace RED GINSENG, ROYAL JELLY vials; •aromatherapy rose oil; or •Histidine 1000mg daily for more sexual enjoyment. •*Red raspberry* tea to tone uterus, *(excellent results)*. •*Licorice* extract or Maitake SX-FRACTION for hormone balance if you have Polycystic Ovary Syndrome.

—**Women's fertility nutrient boosters:** •Crystal Star CONCEPTIONS™ tea, (add *Ashwaganda* extract drops for extra activity); •Herbs America MACA MAGIC caps for a fertility and libido lift (highly recommended); •Crystal Star OCEAN MINERALS™ caps (iodine, potassium, silica from sea veggies) to guard against birth defects. •Vitamin E 400IU 2x daily; •B-complex, like Nature's Secret ULTIMATE B with extra B₆ 100mg, PABA 1000mg and folic acid 800mcg daily. •Country Life sublingual B-12, 2500mcg daily. •Lane Labs ADVA-CAL ULTRA with magnesium (highly recommended). •*Cayenne-ginger* caps, *Motherwort* tea, *Hawthorn* extract 4x daily for a feeling of well-being.

2—For men:
Effective ginseng boosters: •Crystal Star MALE PERFORMANCE™ caps or •*ginseng/damiana* 4 caps daily. To boost sperm quality and amount •*Siberian eleuthero* extract (increases almost 30%); •Lane Labs FERTIL MALE (clinically shown to promote sperm count and mobility); •Tribulus terrestris 750mg 3x a day; •L-carnitine 3000mg daily if subfertile; •Arginine 1500mg daily (unless you have herpes); •Vitamin C 3000mg daily and niacin 500mg *(good results for low sperm count or sperm clumping)*; •chromium picolinate 200mcg daily; and •Zinc 50 -75mg daily. To remove heavy metals, especially lead from pesticides •Crystal Star TOXIN DETOX™ caps 6 daily, with •sublingual B-12, 3500 mcg and folic acid 800mcg. •Pycnogenol 200mg for three months (a specific to improve sperm quality).

—**Men's fertility nutrient boosters:** •Vitamin E 400IU with selenium 200mcg daily (tests show pregnancies rise 21%). •Ethical Nutrients ZINC STATUS; Folic acid 800mcg daily (a key fertility nutrient for men, too); •Solaray MALE CAPS w. orchic extract, or •Country Life MAX with raw orchic. •the carotene Lycopene (excellent results).

—**Superfood therapy:**
•Pure Planet AMLA C PLUS or •Green Foods MAGMA PLUS drink.

Can't find a recommended product? Call the 800 number listed in Product Resources for the store nearest you.

Insect Bites and Stings

Bees, Wasps, Mosquitoes, Non-Poisonous Spiders

Insects are the most successful life form on Earth today. They eat up to a fifth of our food supply, but supply food themselves to most of the world's other animals. They're hard for us to live with, because they defend themselves by biting and stinging, but they pollinate the world's plants. Insect bites can be annoying, painful, even dangerous, because of the diseases they transmit. Killing insects wholesale isn't the answer. We need them for the health of the planet. Chemical repellents rack up many reports of toxic side effects. Try natural ways instead, that provide time-proven defense against insect bites and stings. The following are recommendations for people mildly affected by insect poisons. If you are violently allergic, with chest tightness, wheezing, hives or intense pain and severe swelling, get emergency medical treatment immediately. **Watch for these signs of insect bites and stings:** Pain, swelling, itching and redness around a bite area. More severe reactions can be nausea, dizziness, headache, chills, fever, allergic and histamine side-effects (itchy rashes). Unless really allergic, most children can handle about 1 bee sting per pound if there are multiple stings, before it becomes an emergency. A spider bite can be more serious. Try to get a look at the biting spider so you can describe it to a clinic nurse and get the best treatment. *See also Bruises, Cuts and Abrasions page 342 for more information.*

Diet and Lifestyle Support Therapy

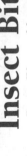

—**Household helpers to ease insect bites:** •Apply AloeLife ALOE SKIN GEL (good activity); •wheat germ oil and chlorophyll liquid; •ice pack; •raw onion slices or vinegar (wasp stings and mosquito stings); •raw potato slices; •lemon juice; •tobacco and water paste; •toothpaste; •rubbing alcohol neutralizes protein in bee venom to ease pain and itching; •honey mixed with 1 drop peppermint oil; •baking soda mixed with water; •charcoal tabs or burnt toast

—**Avoid:** ...consuming meats and sweets and alcohol for 24 hours before going into mosquito territory. They attract insects and you'll get faster healing, too. Alcohol causes the skin to swell and flush, aggravating bites and stings.... bananas and nuts and other serotonin-rich foods that attract insects.

—**Environmental preventives:** •Sprinkle garlic or eucalyptus powder around the house. •Sprinkle sassafras tea or dried tomato leaves around the house. •Sprinkle vanilla water around the house. •Burt's Bees HERBAL INSECT REPELLANT. •Wear light colors. Avoid flowery perfumes to escape bees. They think you are a source of pollen!

—**Once bitten.....** •Apply cold or ice pack compresses, and see shock page in this book if reaction is severe. •To lessen the effect of a bite, keep quiet, and keep the affected area below the level of the heart. •Pull a bee stinger out sideways with tweezers or by dragging you fingernail across the stinger. Apply a wet mud paste to take down inflammation.

—**Natural repellent oils:** Re-apply often - repellency is based on aroma. Don't use on fine fabrics. •Citronella for mosquitoes, ticks and flies. •Cedarwood for fleas and ticks. •Tea tree oil for mosquitoes. •Eucalyptus for most flying insects. •Lemon-Eucalyptus for mosquitoes. •Lemon grass for a broad range of insects. •Pennyroyal for fleas (do not use if pregnant). •Peppermint, rosemary, thyme, geranium and lavender for flies, mosquitoes and fleas.

Herbal, Superfood and Supplement Therapy

—**Interceptive therapy plan: Choose 2 to 3 recommendations.**

1—Natural antihistamines take down inflammation: •Crystal Star ANTI-HST™ 2 to 6 daily, and •ANTI-FLAM™ caps with DR. ENZYME™ with protease and bromelain take down rash or swelling (very effective). Or every 4 hours, •Quercetin Plus with bromelain or •Source Naturals ACTIVATED QUERCITIN. •Vitamin C therapy: Use calcium ascorbate powder. Take ¼ tsp. every 15 minutes right after the bite, then ¼ tsp. every few hours until pain and swelling are gone. Also mix some powder to a paste with water and apply directly. •Or take vitamin C capsules 1000mg with Pantothenic acid 1000mg, several times daily as an antihistamine. —**Add** •Bach Flower RESCUE REMEDY drops and cream to reduce stress from a bite or sting.

2—Stop the sting with herbal applications: •B&T STING STOP gel or apis ointment for stinging and swelling; •Comfrey leaf poultice; •Turmeric powder paste; •Witch hazel; •Tea tree oil. Dissolve •PABA or papaya tablets in water and apply. •Apply neem or tamanu oil.

3—Draw out the poisons with herbal compresses: •Hot parsley leaf; •Black cohosh; •Chamomile; •crushed fresh ivy leaves applied to sting; •green clay packs.

4—Flush poisons from your system: •Take a few drops of cayenne extract in warm water every ½ hour to boost circulatory defenses. Use •Echinacea extract every few hours to flush lymph glands. •C'est Si Bon CHLORENERGY helps reestablish body balance.

—**For prevention:** Take vitamin B-1, 100mg for kids, 500mg for adults, or •Source Naturals CO-ENZYMATE B for a month during high risk seasons. •Rub fresh elder leaves or *elder-chamomile* tea on area. •Mix 1 tsp. each *citronella, pennyroyal, eucalyptus* oils in a base of safflower oil and apply to exposed skin (especially against fleas). •Avon SKIN SO SOFT deters biting flies. Use •Organix NEEM lotion, Neem Oil spray, or Heart Foods TICKWEED PLUS with neem oil, or •Quantum BUZZ AWAY (Deet free).

—**Homeopathic remedies:** •Ledum tincture to relieve swelling and stinging; •Apis ointment for puffiness; •Urtica for itchiness; •Cantharis for inflammation.

Can't find a recommended product? Call the 800 number listed in Product Resources for the store nearest you.

Insomnia

Sleep Disorders, Sleep Apnea, Snoring

Fifty-eight percent of Americans regularly experience insomnia symptoms. We take a million and a half pounds of tranquilizers annually - yet we sleep 20% less than our ancestors did. Sleep deprivation is a health problem because we only during rest do bone marrow and lymph nodes produce substances that empower immune response. Most people need 7-9 hours of sleep every night. Sleep involves blood glucose levels. A blood sugar drop will awaken you. Commercial sleeping pills interfere with the ability to dream, and interrupt natural sleep patterns. They interact adversely with alcohol because the nervous system never really relaxes. They lose their effectiveness in as little as 3-5 days of use. 45% of adults snore regularly (usually related to poor food digestion), often at a tone of 38 decibels of sound…as loud as highway traffic! Don't worry about "making up" lost sleep. One good night's sleep repairs fatigue. **Have trouble falling asleep? Staying asleep all night? Do you snore or have sleep apnea, a serious disorder, linked to high blood pressure, irregular heartbeat, headaches and fatigue?** Insomniacs have less work productivity, impaired thinking and memory, are irritable during the day, and get sick more often. Insomnia itself is due largely to psychological factors, like stress, tension and anxiety, the inability to turn your mind off (women) too much caffeine, alcohol, salt and sugar (men). Many insomniacs have a B vitamin deficiency, reaction to drugs (check your prescriptions), asthma or allergies, or too high copper levels.

Diet and Lifestyle Support Therapy

Nutritional therapy plan:

1—A carbohydrate rich meal, like pasta with vegetables induces sleep. A meal with both proteins and carbohydrates (adding meat to the pasta) keeps you awake. Avoid salty and sugary foods before bed. Don't eat too late. •Go to bed earlier.

2—Eat only a light meal at night. Good late-night "sleepytime" snacks about an hour before bedtime: bananas, celery and celery juice, wheat germ, walnuts (serotonin source), brown rice, lemon water and honey, nutritional yeast, Red Star NUTRITIONAL YEAST broth, or miso soup with 1 tbsp. Bragg's LIQUID AMINOS added. Have a small glass of bottled mineral water or cherry juice (a good source of melatonin) at bedtime.

3—Have a glass of wine at dinner for minerals, digestion and relaxation.

4—Don't take caffeine drinks except in the morning. Crystal Star's DR. VITALITY™ tea offers a clean energy boost and is a great alternative to a morning cup of coffee.

—**Pay attention to a snoring problem.** You may be at higher risk for high blood pressure and heart disease. Snoring is caused by 1) an obstruction or narrowing of the airways, alcohol, sleeping pills or smoking. 2) sleep apnea - breathing ceases because the tongue blocks the throat.… a common problem in overweight men. •Get off your back. •Elevate your head. •Lose weight. •Cut back on alcohol at night. •Drip a dilute MSM solution into nostrils before bed, for up to 80% less snoring. •Drink chamomile tea before bed.

—**Stress reduction techniques:**

•Biofeedback, acupressure, yoga, hypnotherapy, massage therapy treatments help.

•Exercise in the morning, outdoors if possible; a "sunlight break" promotes sleep 12 hours later, and keeps circadian rhythm regular. Take a "constitutional walk" before bed.

•Before bed breathing stretch: take 10 deep breaths; wait 5 minutes; take 10 more.

•Use a "white noise," sleep sound machine.

•Take an epsom salts bath before bed. Enough of the natural magnesium will enter your skin to relax your muscles and help you sleep.

Herbal, Superfood and Supplement Therapy

Interceptive therapy plan: Choose 2 to 3 recommendations.

1—**Nervine relaxers ease tension that deters sleep:** •Crystal Star RELAX CAPS™ 2 as needed; or •NIGHT CAPS™ 2 as needed. •*Passionflower* extract, helps relax your mind especially if weaning off sleeping pills. •*Valerian-lemon balm* tea to improve sleep and daytime mood; •*Gotu kola* caps, or •Herbs, Etc. DEEP SLEEP for nerve tension (highly recommended) or Pacific Biologic RECOVERY evening formula, to calm racing thoughts.

—**Homeopathic sleep remedies:** •B&T ALFALCO, before bed. •Hyland's CALMS FORTE; •*Chamomilla*; •*Nux vomica* if you've over-indulged; •Boiron QUIETUDE.

2—**Adaptogens help normalize glands and hormones:** •Planetary REISHI MUSHROOM SUPREME. •Melatonin .3mg for sleep disorders, if your melatonin is low, on a temporary basis, to reset your biological clock. —**Herbal melatonin sources:** •St. John's wort, •feverfew, and •scullcap (especially if you have a headache at bedtime).

3—**Muscle relaxers ease tightness, let you relax:** •Crystal Star MUSCLE RELAXER caps with Jamaican dogwood (fast acting) ; •Jarrow Formulas KAVA caps if under stress.

4—**Natural sedatives:** •Chamomile tea; •Valerian caps 2 before bed, or •Flora FLORA-SED. —**For restless legs:** •Vitamin E 400IU before bed; •Folic acid 800mcg daily.

5—**Improve sleep quality, dream recall:** •5-HTP 50 to 200mg before bed to rebalance serotonin, enhance dream recall. •If you're in pain, take one each: DLPA 500mg, Calcium-magnesium capsule. •If hypoglycemic, take GABA 500mg and Glycine 500mg capsules before bed. Aromatherapy •Chamomile or lavender oils on temples, pillow, bottoms of feet. •Or make a *hops-rosemary* sleep pillow to reduce insomnia (recommended) .

6—**For better calcium - magnesium blood balance:** (so you won't wake up at night and not be able to return to sleep.) •Crystal Star CALCIUM MAGNESIUM SOURCE™; •Floradix CALCIUM and HERBAL REST liquids; •Lane Labs ADVACAL ULTRA with high cal/mag; •Rosemary Gladstar's *Valerian-Hops* formula. •B Stress complex 100mg.

8—**For nightmares:** •Nelson Bach Flower Remedies; •Nature's Secret ULTIMATE B to help prevent nightmares. •B-ccmplex with extra B₁ 500mg at night for 1 to 2 months; •Niacinimide 500mg. •*Catnip/lemon* balm tea.

Can't find a recommended product? Call the 800 number listed in Product Resources for the store nearest you.

Kidney Disease

Nepritis, Kidney Stones, Bright's Disease

Kidney infections are usually severe, serious, and should be addressed immediately. *Nephritis* involves chronic inflammation of kidney tissues. In *Bright's disease*, the blood becomes toxic from an overload of unfiltered wastes. Inflammation develops with blood in the urine, high blood pressure and water retention. Diabetes is a forerunner of Bright's Disease. *Kidney stones* are extremely painful (most people say worse than a heart attack), but preventable. (See the following cleanse.) In fact, prevention through improved diet and exercise is the best medicine. Kidney caution - elderly people who chronically use NSAIDs drugs (like Advil, Motrin, and Aleve) often have high blood levels of creatinine, a sign that kidney function is impaired. Chronic kidney and bladder disease can have disastrous consequences. Today over 300,000 Americans are on kidney dialysis to filter the impurities from their blood that their kidneys and bladder can no longer handle. Sadly, only ¼ of patients are still alive after 5 years on dialysis as the procedure severely weakens and imbalances body chemistry.

What causes kidney disease? Mostly a result of diet overload... overeating sugary foods, red meat, carbonated drinks and caffeine.... and/or drug overload... overuse of prescription or pleasure drugs, aspirin, salt and chemical diuretics. Diabetes, or latent diabetes is regularly involved. Drug and diet excesses lead to deficiencies, especially essential fatty acids (the good fats that keep bad fats in check), B-vitamins and magnesium that keep your body systems normal. Heavy metal poisoning from lead or cadmium (cigarettes) and excess aluminum often show up on kidney disease tests. Hypothyroidism and multiple allergies may also play a role.

Do you have signs of kidney disease? Kidney disease means painful, frequent urination, chronic lower back pain and fatigue, chills and fever; fluid retention. Most people have deep purple circles or lines under their eyes. You may have kidney stones but show no apparent symptoms except a dull ache in the lower back... that is until the stone blocks the urinary tract, which results in excruciating, radiating pain. This is then followed by very painful urination or blood in the urine, along with nausea, fever and vomiting.

Do you have kidney stones?

Kidney stones have long afflicted mankind. Evidence of kidney stones has recently been found in a 7,000 year-old Egyptian mummy! Still, in every decade since World War II, the U.S. has seen a steady rise in kidney stone cases. Today 10% of American men and 5% of American women have a kidney stone by the time they're seventy. Kidney stones are a diet-related illness. They are directly linked to low dietary fiber, high fats from large amounts of animal protein, sugary foods, and too much alcohol and salt. Notable amounts of unabsorbed calcium (usually from dairy sources or antacids), also play a part.

What causes kidney disease? The above symptoms parallel the rise of the Standard American Diet, full of fat, fried foods, rich dairy products and sugar. Excessive use of antacids and adrenal exhaustion also contribute to kidney stones. Kidney stones form when minerals that normally float free in kidney fluids combine into crystals. When inorganic mineral waste overloads and the body has too little fluid, kidney stones form. There are three types of kidney stones: those composed of calcium salts, the most common type (75-85%), struvite, or non-calcium-containing crystals (10-15%), and uric acid crystals, at about 5-8% occurrence. It takes from 5 to 15 hours of vigorous, urgent treatment to dissolve and pass even small stones.

Can you prevent kidney stones? A vegetarian diet, low in proteins and starches, that emphasizes fresh fruits, vegetables and cultured foods to alkalize the system, is the key to avoiding kidney stone formation. This type of diet is high in fiber to reduce urinary calcium waste. Eliminate caffeine foods, salty, sugary and fried foods and soft drinks that inhibit kidney filtering. Avoid clogging, mucous-forming foods like dairy foods, heavy grains, starches and fats, to relieve irritation and inhibit sediment formation. Note: Do not use TUMS for indigestion symptoms. They may increase risk for stone formation.

Is your body showing signs that it needs a kidney stone cleanse?
There may be no apparent symptoms at first except a dull ache in the lower back. When the stone(s) become large enough to block the urinary tract, there is excruciating, radiating pain with extremely painful urination and constant urgency to urinate. The abdomen becomes distended. Women who have heavy menstrual bleeding or anemia, signs of a vitamin K deficiency, should be especially careful since it can lead to stones. As infection sets in, there are chills, nausea, vomiting and fever.

Can't find a recommended product? Call the 800 number listed in Product Resources for the store nearest you.

The Kidney Stone Cleanse

Note: Drink plenty of water, 8-10 glasses of bottled water each day of your cleanse so that waste and excess minerals are continuously flushed and urine flow does not stagnate. Dehydration is a key factor in kidney stone formation.... causing a reduction in urine volume and increasing excretion of stone constituents.

The night before your kidney stone cleanse....Take a cup of chamomile tea. The next day... Take 2 tbsp. olive oil through a straw every 4 hours to help dissolve stones.

—*On rising:* take cranberry juice (from concentrate) in water with 1 tsp. maple syrup; or 2 tbsp. apple cider vinegar in water with 1 tsp. honey; and a cup of chamomile tea.

—*Breakfast:* have a glass of cranberry juice, fresh unsweetened lemonade or fresh watermelon juice, or watermelon chunks, or Crystal Star GREEN TEA CLEANSER™.

—*Mid-morning:* 1 cup watermelon seed tea (grind seeds, steep in hot water 30 min., add honey); or *dandelion* tea, or Crystal Star BLADDER-KIDNEY COMFORT™ tea.

—*Lunch:* have a carrot/beet/cucumber juice, and a green leafy salad with cucumbers and sprouts.

—*Mid-afternoon:* have a cup of chamomile tea; and asparagus stalks and carrot sticks with kefir cheese; or fresh apples with kefir or yogurt dip.

—*Dinner:* have brown rice with steamed veggies or steamed asparagus with miso soup and snipped, dry sea greens; or a baked potato with kefir cheese and a green leafy salad.

—*Before Bed:* take a glass of aloe vera juice and another cup of chamomile tea; or miso/ginger soup with sea greens snipped on top.

After your cleanse: As you return to solid foods, make sure you eat plenty of fresh fruits and vegetables. Even meat eaters have a lower incidence of stones when they add extra fresh fruits and vegetables. Keep salt and protein low for at least 3 weeks. Establish a diet with plenty of fiber. Vitamin K plays a key role in your body's natural inhibition of kidney stone formation. Make sure you add plenty of green leafy vegetables, sprouts and sea greens, high in vitamin K.

Supplements to consider:

Kidney stone cleansers: Ascorbate or Ester C powder in water; ¼ tsp. every hour to bowel tolerance until stones pass – about 5000mg daily; Alpha Lipoic acid 100 to 150mg daily. Herb Pharm KHELLA extract to reduce pain from acute attacks.

Mineral balancers to prevent stones: Flora VEGE-SIL caps 2 daily; Eidon MAGNESIUM liquid, Magnesium 500mg and B6 daily 10mg help prevent calcium oxalate stone formation.

To avoid stones: Vitamin C 3000mg with bioflavs helps acidify urine; Futurebiotics VITAL K or vitamin K 100mcg daily; quercetin 1000mg with bromelain 1500mg. Consider Himalaya's URICARE Ayurvedic formula to help pass existing stones and prevent new formation (highly recommended).

Enzyme support: Protease helps break apart protein-based viscid matter that cements salts into stones. Transformation PUREZYME and Crystal Star DR. ENZYME™ with Protease.

Dissolve sediment wastes: Enzymatic Therapy ACID-A-CAL; green tea, chamomile, rosemary, or dandelion/nettles tea - 5 cups a day for one to 2 weeks.

Green superfoods inhibit stone growth: Crystal Star ENERGY GREEN RENEWAL. Wakunaga HARVEST BLEND, Aloe Falls ALOE-GINGER, C'est Si Bon CHLORENERGY.

Fiber supplements reduce risk of stones: All One WHOLE FIBER COMPLEX; Nature's Secret ULTIMATE FIBER; Jarrow GENTLE FIBERS.

Heat therapy: Apply wet, hot compresses and lower back massage when there is inflammation flare up. especially lobelia, turmeric or ginger fomentations.

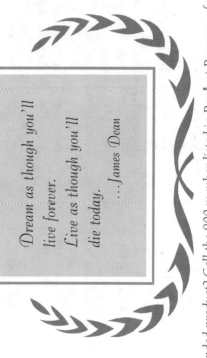

Dream as though you'll live forever.
Live as though you'll die today.
...James Dean

Can't find a recommended product? Call the 800 number listed in Product Resources for the store nearest you.

Kidney Disease

Diet and Lifestyle Support Therapy

Nutritional therapy plan:

1—Try a short 3 day kidney cleanse to remove toxic infection and help dissolve stones: Each morning take 2 tbsp. cider vinegar or lemon juice in water. Take one each of the following juices daily: carrot-beet-cucumber, cranberry, potassium broth (pg. 291), and a mixed greens (your choice) veggie drink. Add •Spirulina 1 tsp. powder daily, especially if kidneys have drug damage. Try •Rainbow Light HAWAIIAN SPIRULINA powder.

Take 2 cups watermelon seed tea daily if there are kidney stones.
Take aloe vera juice before bed, or •Aloe Falls ALOE JUICE with ginger.
Take 8-12 glasses of water each day.

2—Then, follow a simple low salt, very low protein, vegetarian diet with 75% fresh foods for a week.

3—Avoid all fried, fatty foods, colas and sodas during healing. Avoid salts, sugars, and caffeine-containing foods. Eliminate dairy products. Reduce animal protein to less than 15% of your diet. Choose moderate amounts of seafood for your protein instead of red meat.

4—Add sea veggies (any kind) and bee pollen, 2 tbsp. each for healing amino acids daily that provide kidney friendly protein to heal.

—Bodywork:

• Take a daily brisk walk to keep kidney function flowing.
• Avoid commercial antacids during healing.
• Avoid NSAIDS drugs. They have been implicated in kidney failure cases.
• Avoid smoking and secondary smoke.
• Apply moist heat packs, comfrey compresses, and/or alternating hot and cold compresses on the kidney area.
• Apply Chinese white flower oil or tiger balm to kidney area 2-3x daily.
• Apply compresses to kidney area, like hot ginger/oatstraw, cayenne/ginger, mullein/lobelia.
• Use capsicum, spirulina or catnip enemas 2-3x weekly to stimulate better kidney function.

Herbal, Superfood and Supplement Therapy

Important note: Eliminate iron supplements during healing. Avoid L-cysteine, it aggravates crystallization in the kidneys. If you're taking strong diuretics (such as hydrochlorothiazide) for kidney problems, be sure you add a balanced mineral supplement to discourage calcium crystal build-up.

Interceptive therapy plan: Choose 2 to 3 recommendations.

1—Control the infection: •Crystal Star ANTI-BIO™ capsules 6 daily until infection clears; then •STONE-X™ capsules for a month to help dissolve stones; or •Planetary STONE FREE. Then, •Herbs Etc. KIDNEY TONIC every morning for another month. Use Crystal Star DR. ENZYME™ with protease and bromelain for extra dissolving action.

2—Healthy kidney flushing support: Take •Dandelion tea, 2 cups daily; or •Crystal Star BLADDER KIDNEY COMFORT™ caps or tea; try •Uva Ursi, Couchgrass or Watercress tea. Take with Crystal Star OCEAN MINERALS™ caps (with iodine-potassium-silica from the sea) if taking diuretic drugs.

3—Normalize kidney activity: •Cleavers tea; •Parsley-cornsilk tea (very good results); •St. John's wort extract caps (especially if incontinent); •Solaray ALFAJUICE caps daily; •vitamin K 100mcg daily; •Lane Labs ADVACAL ULTRA 4 daily; •Gotu Kola caps 4 to 6 daily.

4—Reduce kidney inflammation: •Quercetin 1000mg daily with bromelain 1500mg daily; •B-complex 100mg; extra B-6, 100mg daily and •magnesium 800mg daily. •Enzymatic Therapy LIQUID LIVER with GINSENG and RENATONE 2x daily. •High omega-3 flax oil daily, •Solaray LIPOTROPIC PLUS daily, or •Choline/Inositol caps 4x daily. •Tranformation Enzyme EXCELLZYME.

5—Reverse kidney damage: •GINKGO BILOBA extract as needed; •Licorice tea 2 cups daily; •Evening primrose oil caps 4 daily. •MICROHYDRIN PLUS, available at royalhealth.com; •Crystal Star DR. ENZYME™ with protease and bromelain or •Transformation PUREZYME protease caps (highly recommended) . •Enzymatic Therapy VITALINE COQ10 chewables to improve kidney functioning and reduce free radicals in cases of kidney failure. •Jarrow LIQUID CARNITINE for dialysis patients (ask your physician).

6—Kidney cleansers and detoxifiers: •Burdock root tea, 2 cups daily; •Echinacea extract 4x daily; •garlic-cayenne caps 8 daily; •Alpha Lipoic acid up to 600mg daily (excellent detoxifier); •Dandelion extract especially for nephritis. •Gaia Herbs PLAINTAIN-BUCHU SUPREME caps; •Golden Pride FORMULA ONE oral chelation with EDTA; •Planetary TRIPHALA tabs to reduce bowel toxicity.

—Superfood Therapy: Choose 1 or 2 recommendations.
•Crystal Star ENERGY GREEN RENEWAL™.
•Futurebiotics VITAL K drink daily.
•C'est Si Bon CHLORENERGY 2 pkts. daily.

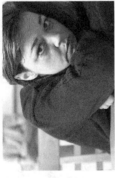

Can't find a recommended product? Call the 800 number listed in Product Resources for the store nearest you.

Leukemia
Blood and Bone Marrow Cancer

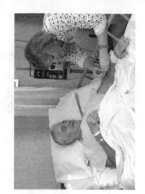

Leukemias, cancers characterized by excessive production of white blood cells, originate in damaged bone marrow, spleen and lymph node tissues. 30,000 Americans are diagnosed each year with leukemias; 30% are children. Once deadly, the survival rate for leukemia has improved - over two-thirds of its victims survive. Natural treatments in conjunction with new cytotoxic drugs shows great promise. **Do you have symptoms of leukemia?** The rapid increase in white blood cells, with no red blood cell production means extreme tiredness, weakness and pallor, easy bruising, nosebleeds, bone pain, thinness, fever, chills and chronic infections - especially in children. Spleen, liver, lymph nodes and gums become swollen; there are red spots under the skin. **What causes leukemia?** Pesticide exposure, water overfluoridation, or high levels of arsenic in water, and indiscriminate use of X-rays and some drugs, especially in children and pregnant women. Severe malnutrition, exposure to second hand smoke and thyroid malfunction play a role. *See the CANCER DIET in this book, or DIETS FOR HEALTHY HEALING by Linda Page.*

Diet and Lifestyle Support Therapy

Nutritional therapy plan:

1—Food healing value is lost quickly. Make sure your diet is very nutritious.

2—Start with a gentle cleansing/detoxification brown rice diet (pg. 178) for 7 days, taking AloeLife ALOE VERA GOLD daily, or Sun Wakasa GOLD, liquid CHLORELLA daily. Follow with a modified macrobiotic diet program, using organically grown foods (pg. 348) for 3 to 4 months with no animal protein and lots of alkalizing foods.

3—Vegetable proteins are the key after initial detoxification. Eat lots of green leafy vegetables for red blood cell formation. Include potassium and beta carotene-rich foods.

4—To clean vital organs, take a glass of carrot/beet/cucumber juice, or Green Foods CARROT ESSENCE and GREEN MAGMA drinks, every day for the first month of healing; every other day for the second month; once a week the third month. Include wheatgrass juice or Rainbow Light HAWAIIAN SPIRULINA at least three times a week for enzyme therapy. Add a potassium broth every other day (pg. 291).

5—Take 2 glasses of cranberry juice (or pomegranate juice) daily.

6—Avoid alcohol, fast foods and chemicalized foods, refined sugars and red meats.

—Bodywork:

•Overheating therapy is effective for leukemia. See page 182 in this book.
•Add a wheat grass enema or implant therapy for best results (pg. 189).

•Avoid smoking, pesticides, X-rays, microwaves, electromagnetic fields from power lines and radiation of all kinds if possible. There seems to be a clear link between these and leukemia, especially in children.

•Chemotherapy treatment for other cancers has sometimes been implicated in the development of leukemia.
•Relaxation techniques are effective: meditation, imagery, acupuncture, reflexology.

—Lymph-Flow Bath to restart immune response: Put ½ pound each baking soda and sea salt in the tub. Soak for 20 minutes. Dunk head 5 times. Drip dry; stay warm: then shower.

Herbal, Superfood and Supplement Therapy

Interceptive therapy plan: Choose 2 to 3 recommendations.

1—**Help detoxify the blood:** •Crystal Star DETOX BLOOD PURIFIER™ caps 2 daily with GREEN TEA CLEANSER™ 2x daily, or •*burdock* tea or *nettles/yarrow* tea 2 cups daily for 1 month •Natural Energy CAISSE'S TEA, •Flora FLOR-ESSENCE Essiac liquid, or •*Pau d'arco* tea for 2 months. •Vita Carte BOVINE CARTILAGE or •Nutricology MODIFIED CITRUS PECTIN to stimulate glutathione (recommended)

2—**Help reduce organ swelling:** •Turmeric capsules (*curcumin*) 8 daily; •Crystal Star LIVER RENEW™ capsules with •MILK THISTLE SEED extract for 2 months to revitalize liver function. •Enzymatic Therapy LIQUID LIVER with SIBERIAN GINSENG 4 daily.

3—**Help kill the cancer:** •Nutricology GERMANIUM 150mg daily with •Glutathione 50mg 4x daily; •Eidon COLLOIDAL SILVER liquid; •Earth's Bounty O₂ caps as directed. •American Biologics DIOXYCHLOR for detoxification. •St. John's wort is a specific for leukemia caused by radiation treatments. Consider •New Chapter ST. JOHN'S WORT SC27. (Recommended. Ask your physician if you're on chemo drugs.)

4—**Help rebuild marrow and red blood:** •PHYCOTENE NANOCLUSTERS available at royal-health.com. •Folic acid 800mcg daily, especially if taking chemotherapy. •Floradix LIQUID IRON; •*Siberian eleuthero* extract; •*Garlic/cayenne* caps 8 daily; or *Yellow Dock* tea; •Crystal Star IRON SOURCE BLOOD BUILDER™ caps and extract. •Country Life sublingual B-12, 2500mcg for body balance/strength. •Transformation PUREZYME.

5—**Normalize blood cells and lymphatic system:** •Nutricology CAR-T-CELL liquid; •Enzymatic Therapy THYMUPLEX tablets; •Maitake Products REISHI caps, or •C'est si Bon CHLORENERGY for 2 months. •*Pau d'Arco* or *Echinacea* extract.

6—**Strengthen blood and immune system:** •ASTRAGALUS extract (fast working); •HAWTHORN extract; •Niacin therapy: 250mg 4x daily during healing with •B Complex 100mg, 4x daily, with extra folic acid, and B₆ 250mg. •Crystal Star OCEAN MINERALS™ 4 daily (recommended). •Ascorbate vit. C or Ester C powder, up to 10,000mg daily with bioflavonoids and rutin for several months. •Beta carotene 150,000IU daily for at least 6 weeks. •Vitamin E 800IU daily with selenium 200mcg; •zinc 50mg.

Can't find a recommended product? Call the 800 number listed in Product Resources for the store nearest you.

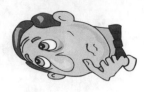

Liver Disease, Liver Health

Cirrhosis, Jaundice, Renewal and Revitalization

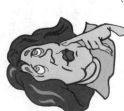

Be good to your liver. The health of every body system depends to a large extent on the health of the liver. It is the body's most complex and amazing organ - a powerful chemical plant that converts everything we eat, breathe and absorb into life-sustaining substances. The liver filters out toxins at a rate of over a quart of blood per minute. It manufactures bile to digest fats and prevent constipation. It is a vast storehouse for vitamins, minerals and enzymes that it releases to build and maintain healthy cells. The liver produces interferon, the body's natural germ killer, and is responsible for more than 1500 functions that directly maintain your immune system. It also metabolizes hormone excesses.

Cirrhosis, or scarring, of the liver tissue is a serious, degenerative condition, preventing the liver from its proper function. It is the second biggest killer of people between 45 and 65 in America today. Usually a consequence of alcohol abuse, it is also almost always a part of other severe liver infections, such as hepatitis, EBV, and AIDS related syndromes. *Jaundice*, the yellow discoloration of the skin and eyelids due to excess concentrations of bilirubin, is a symptom of liver congestion, not a disease. If your diet is nutrient poor, the liver becomes exhausted, and even more serious debilitation results. Unfortunately, the U.S. diet is loaded with calories, fats, sugars, alcohol, and unknown amounts of toxic substances, so almost everyone has some degree of liver malfunction. Smoking is terrible for liver health. Try even harder to quit all forms of tobacco. It almost goes without saying that alcohol must be eliminated.

Do you have sluggish liver signs? The first signals are great tiredness, bouts of general depression, anger or irritation, unexplained weight gain, poor digestion, and food and chemical sensitivities. PMS, constipation and congestion are regular signs; some people get skin itching, nausea and shakes; most have faint jaundiced skin and some liver spots. *See also* HEPATITIS *page 451 and* LIVER DETOX DIET *page 199.*

Check yourself for these signs of underlying liver congestion:

•Indigestion and mild nausea after meals. Especially indigestion after fatty foods. Distention in the stomach (liver area).
•Unexplained head and body aches.
•Sluggishness, reduced energy, usually along with constipation alternating to diarrhea.
•Slightly yellow look to the skin and eyelids; skin itching or irritation.
•Body fluid retention and swelling, usually accompanied by bags under the eyes.

What contributes to liver problems? Overeating... especially rich foods like heavy meats, cheeses and sugars, and excessive alcohol intake all contribute to long term poor nutrition...and long term liver problems. Excessive use of prescription drugs —especially non steroidal anti-inflammatory drugs and acetaminophen for pain, and antibiotics and tranquilizers are big factors today. Exposure to toxic environmental chemicals and pollutants can cause liver toxicity, especially a problem if the diet is also low in fiber and vegetables that provide protection. *See Liver Detox page 199 for more.*

Is your liver exhausted?

In today's world, protecting your liver from toxic overload and exhaustion is not easy. In the United States, liver disorders, largely a result of a lifestyle that includes lots of toxins, are responsible for more than 50,000 deaths annually. Fortunately, the liver has amazing regenerative powers. A complete liver renewal program takes from three months to a year.

Signs that your liver may be exhausted:

• Liver cirrhosis or chronic hepatitis. If you have liver cirrhosis, you'll see increasing weakness, jaundice and abdominal distention. As cirrhosis progresses, you may have anemia and large bruise patches.
• Frequent, unexplained fatigue and headaches. Frequent cold and flu infections, and a high incidence of allergic reactions (like sinus infections).
• Thick, coated tongue (yellowish or white), usually accompanied by chronic constipation, and often a candida yeast infection.
• Jaundice or yellowish tint to the skin, eczema, psoriasis, acne rosacea or several age spots.
• Gas or discomfort that worsens after a fatty meal. (The liver is responsible for fat metabolism.) Or unusually high cholesterol levels.
• A man who is thin everywhere else but who has a protruding stomach (liver area).

Can't find a recommended product? Call the 800 number listed in Product Resources for the store nearest you.

Liver Health and Wellness

Diet and Lifestyle Support Therapy

Nutritional therapy: Optimum nutrition is the best liver protection, and the key to liver healing. Keeping fat low in your diet is crucial for liver vitality and regeneration.

1—If condition is acute, go on a 3 day liquid detoxification diet (see Liver Detox, page 199) to clean out toxic waste. Take aloe vera juice or AloeLife ALOE GOLD drink each morning. Drink 6-8 glasses of water and 2 cups of roasted dandelion tea daily. Take a carrot/beet/cucumber juice daily for 1 week, then every other day for a week, then every 2 days, then every 3 days, etc. for a month. Include two glasses of carrot juice daily for a month, or Green Foods CARROT ESSENCE, or C'est Si Bon CHLORENERGY drink daily. Make a mix of lecithin, nutritional yeast and wheat germ oil; add 2 tsp. to any drink.

2—Then follow an alkalizing, rebuilding diet for a month with high quality vegetable protein. Take daily during healing: 1 tbsp. each lecithin granules and nutritional yeast, 2-3 glasses cranberry, pomegranate, or apple juice and 8 glasses of bottled water. Take a daily liver rebuilding tonic for a month: Mix 4-oz. *hawthorn* berries, 2-oz. *red sage*, 1-oz. *cardamom*. Steep 24 hours in 2 qts. of water. Add honey. Or take superfood liver drinks like Wakunaga KYO-GREEN with EFAs, Fit for You, Intl. MIRACLE GREENS or Crystal Star RESTORE YOUR STRENGTH™ drink. A good bile stimulating tea might include: *ginger, orange peel, dandelion root, fennel, mint* and *coriander seed* (recommended).

4—Avoid all alcohol, fried, salty or fatty foods, caffeine (except green tea), sugar and tobacco. Avoid red meats, refined starchy foods and dairy foods during all healing phases. Reduce sugars, saturated fats and fried foods permanently. Eat smaller meals, minimize late night eating.

Liver health and support foods:
- Vegetable fiber foods that absorb excess bile and increase regularity.
- Potassium-rich foods: seafoods, dried fruits.
- Bitter foods: artichoke, beet, endive, radish, arugula, dandelion greens, turmeric.
- Chlorophyll-rich foods: leafy greens, sea greens.
- Enzyme-rich foods: yogurt and kefir.
- Sulphur-rich foods: eggs, cruciferous vegetables, garlic and onions.
- Vegetable protein foods: sprouts, whole grains, tofu, wheat germ, nutritional yeast.

—Bodywork:
- Take one coffee enema during your detoxification cleanse; (1 cup coffee to 1 qt. distilled water.) Wheat grass, chlorella implants are also effective.
- The liver is dependent on enough oxygen coming into the lungs. Exercise, air filters, time spent in the forest and at the ocean, and drinking pure water are important. Take a daily walk on each day of your cleanse. Breathe deep to help the liver eliminate toxins.
- Take several saunas if possible during a liver cleanse for faster, easier detoxification.
- Apply castor oil packs to the liver area three times a week to aid liver detoxification.

Herbal, Superfood and Supplement Therapy

Interceptive therapy plan: Choose 2 to 3 recommendations.

1—**Gently cleanse the liver:** •Crystal Star GREEN TEA CLEANSER™ daily; •Pau d'Arco tea, or *roasted dandelion root* tea for 3 to 6 months. Add •Planetary BUPLEURUM LIVER CLEANSE or •Crystal Star LIVER RENEW™ caps 6 daily and •Jarrow JARRO-DOPHILUS with FOS or •UAS DDS-PLUS daily to cleanse and restore liver tissue. If there's jaundice: take •*Barberry* tea or LIVER CLEANSE FLUSHING™ tea, 3 cups daily, with •Alpha Lipoic Acid 300-600mg daily until clear. Take •SAM-e 400-800mg, or •Nature's Apothecary LIVER CLEANSE a day to counteract damage from alcohol or drugs. •Acid B-complex 100mg (if not included in your supplement).

—Lipotropics prevent liver fat accumulation, help balance hormone levels: •Choline 600mg or •Country Life PHOSPHATIDYL CHOLINE 600mg 4x daily; or •Solaray LIPOTROPIC PLUS caps esp. if taking contraceptives; or •Choline/inositol 100mg; •Methionine 2x daily. Or take •Pure Form WHEY PROTEIN or AloeLife FIBERMATE powder and mix in 1 tsp. high omega-3 flax seed oil daily.

2—**Prickly herbs heal and enhance liver activity:** Take one or a combination of the following drops in water 3x daily: •*Milk thistle seed* extract in aloe vera juice, or •*Artichoke* extract, or •*Dandelion Root* tea or extract, or •*Burdock Root* tea 2 cups daily.

3—**Bitters herbs boost liver and bile production:** •Crystal Star •BITTERS & LEMON™ extract each morning; •Solaray TURMERIC extract caps (curcumin) 4 daily, or •*barberry-turmeric* capsules 6 daily; •Gaia SWEETISH BITTERS; •*dandelion* extract. •Enzymatic Therapy SUPER MILK THISTLE complex with artichoke.

4—**Enhance liver vitality:** •Reishi or Maitake mushroom extracts (highly recommended); •Bupleurum or cat's claw extract (especially if immune compromised); •Royal jelly 2 tsp. daily, or •Prince of Peace royal jelly-ginseng vials. •SAMe 800mg daily. •Lipoic Acid 600mg daily; or MRI ALPHA-LIPOIC ACID; •Enzymatic Therapy LIQUID LIVER w. Siberian Ginseng. •Vitamin C 500mg every hour in cleansing stage, then 3000mg daily. •N-acetylcysteine 600mg boosts immune enhancing glutathione; take with ascorbate vitamin C 500mg every hour during cleansing stage, then 3000mg daily.

—Help heal internal scarring: •Gotu Kola or •Schizandra extract daily (powerful liver protection); •Crystal Star DR. VITALITY™ tea or •Crystal Star DR. ENZYME™ with protease and bromelain (highly recommended).

5—**Boost liver antioxidants to overcome free radicals:** •Carnitine 1000mg; •Beta-carotene 100,000IU, or •PHYCOTENE NANOCLUSTERS from royal-health.com; •CoQ$_{10}$ 100mg daily; •PCO's from grapeseed or white pine 100mg daily (for 2 to 3 months). •Ascorbate vitamin C crystals 5000mg daily or to bowel tolerance. •Nutricology GER-MANIUM 150mg. •Solaray ALFAJUICE caps. •Vitamin E 800IU with selenium 200mcg 2x daily; •Country Life sublingual B-12, 2500mcg daily for energy. •MICROHYDRIN PLUS from royal-health.com (highly recommended). •Glutamine 2000mg daily.

Can't find a recommended product? Call the 800 number listed in Product Resources for the store nearest you.

Low Blood Pressure

Hypotension, Hypoadrenalism

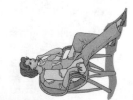

Even though we hear less about low blood pressure, it's also a threat to good health. Low blood pressure is generally recognized as 100/60 or below, an abnormal reading that registers malfunction of the circulatory system's systole/diastol action. **What brings about low blood pressure?** Causes are wide ranging, from a reaction to drug medication (a common problem for the elderly who over-use drugs that lower immunity), to an electrolyte-loss response to a disease, or an endocrine or nerve disorder. LBP is also a sign of weak arterial system walls, where blood and fluid can leak and abnormally distend tissues, preventing good circulation. A poor diet that lacks vitamin C and bioflavonoids can cause this type of "run-down" condition, along with weak adrenal action from emotional stress, and weak kidney action which may cause system toxemia. Natural treatment works well for symptoms like dizziness or light-headedness upon standing up, indicating a reduction of cerebral flow. **Do you have signs of low blood pressure?** Great fatigue after even mild exercise, and low energy are primary signals, sometimes dizziness and lightheadedness, especially on standing quickly. Intolerance to heat and cold, nervousness, low immunity and high susceptibility to allergies and infections, particularly opportunistic disease like candida yeast overgrowth.

Diet and Lifestyle Support Therapy

Nutritional therapy plan: *See ADRENAL HEALTH page 300 and CHRONIC FATIGUE SYNDROME page 370 for more diet information.*

1—Eat a fresh foods diet for a week - mixed veggie drinks, potassium broth (pg. 291), nutritional yeast (especially important), green salads. Take a lemon and water drink each morning with 1 tsp. maple syrup.

2—Then, follow a modified macrobiotic diet for 2 months, focus on vegetable proteins, green salads with celery (natural sodium), miso, onions, garlic (natural sulphur), and other alkalizing foods, and dried or fresh fruits. —Include strengthening complex carbohydrates, such as peas, broccoli, potatoes and whole grains.

3—Bioflavonoids help strong blood vessels: Citrus juices like pineapple or grape juice; green tea or •Crystal Star GREEN TEA CLEANSER™ or DR. VITALITY™ green/white tea (highly recommended).

4—Reduce all high cholesterol, starchy foods. Avoid caffeine, canned and refined foods, animal fats, red meats. Try protein drinks instead like Unipro PERFECT PROTEIN or Metabolic Response Modifiers WHEY PUMPED (highly recommended).

5—Add minerals for strength: Crystal Star RESTORE YOUR STRENGTH™ drink or caps for absorbable minerals. Try Natural salts to help hypoadrenalism: try Knudsen RECHARGE electrolyte drink, or Alacer MIRACLE WATER.

—Bodywork:

•Acupressure, chiropractic spinal manipulation and shiatsu therapy are all effective in normalizing circulatory function.
•Alternating hot and cold hydrotherapy (pg. 185) revs up circulation.
•Aromatherapy circulation blend: Aromaland THERATONE.
•Avoid tobacco and secondary smoke.
•Consciously try to relax your body once a day with meditation, yoga exercises and rest.
•Do deep breathing exercises (pg. 250) to stimulate circulation and oxygenate tissues.
•Stand up slowly to allow blood pressure to normalize.

Herbal, Superfood and Supplement Therapy

Interceptive therapy plans: Choose 2 or 3 recommendations. *Note: Avoid the amino acids phenylalanine and tyrosine if your blood pressure is low.*

1—**Normalize blood pressure:** •Crystal Star HEART PROTECTOR FOR WOMEN™ or HEART PROTECTOR FOR MEN™ caps 2-4 daily for a month, with •8 garlic caps daily; or Heart Foods CAYENNE HEART FOOD caps. •Vitamin E therapy for 8 weeks: work up from 100IU daily the first week, to 800IU daily, adding 100mg daily each week (short term, ask your physician); •COQ-10 200mg daily. •Dandelion root caps 4 daily.

2—**Support better metabolism:** •Crystal Star BITTERS & LEMON CLEANSE™ extract for metabolism support; •Green Foods ION KELP tablets or •Biotec SEA PLASMA tablets 10 daily; •Siberian eleuthero extract caps, 4-6 daily; or •Imperial Elixir SIBERIAN GINSENG or Prince of Peace ELEUTHERO vials.

3—**Boost and regulate circulation:** •Nutricology BEST BLOOD OXYGENATION FORMULA; •Cayenne/ginger caps 4 to 8 daily. •Magnesium 400mg 4x daily, or •Solaray CAL/MAG CITRATE, 1000mg calcium and 1000mg magnesium, or •Rainbow Light CALCIUM PLUS with high magnesium.

4—**Tone blood vessels with flavonoid-rich herbs:** •HAWTHORN or BILBERRY extracts 2-3x daily; •Gotu kola extract or Rosemary for nerve balance; •Lemon peel, Hibiscus, Rose hips tea. •Vitamin K 100mcg 2 daily for capillary strength, or •Futurebiotics VITAL K, 6 tsp. daily.

5—**Normalize adrenal function:** •Crystal Star ADRENAL ENERGY BOOST™ capsules 2x daily for a month with extra •Ginkgo Biloba or Hawthorn or Licorice extract 4x daily; or •Nutricology ORGANIC ADRENAL CORTEX; •DHEA 25mg daily for 3 months.

6—**Enhance liver function to normalize blood pressure:** •Enzymatic Therapy LIQUID LIVER with Siberian Eleuthero. •B Complex 100mg daily with extra B₁ 100mg and pantothenic acid 500mg. •Floradix LIQUID IRON.

7—**Antioxidants are important:** •PCO's from grapeseed and white pine, 100mg daily, or •BD Herbs GRAPE SEED organic extract for extra high flavonoids. •Germanium 150mg 2x daily. •Vitamin C with bioflavonoids and rutin 3000mg daily. •Extra zinc 30mg 2x daily.

Can't find a recommended product? Call the 800 number listed in Product Resources for the store nearest you.

Lung Disease

Tuberculosis, Sarcoidosis, Cystic Fibrosis, SARS

Chronic pulmonary diseases have increased dramatically in the last decade. Three that are especially worrying..... **Sarcoidosis** is a systemic viral infection with widespread, grainy lesions on tissue or organs. The liver, as well the lungs are affected, with a deep chronic cough and difficult breathing. **Tuberculosis**, a contagious, bacterial infection recently declared a global emergency by the World Health Organization, is on the rise in America, too. It is characterized by bloody sputum, a chronic cough, shortness of breath and fatigue, night sweats, serious weight loss and chest pain. **Cystic fibrosis** is an inherited childhood abnormality that can destroy the lungs and cause serious impairment to the liver and pancreas. It's characterized by recurring lung infections and severe malnutrition from low nutrient absorption. Cystic fibrosis symptoms include very salty sweat from dysfunctional sweat glands.

All have similar symptoms of constant coughing, inflammation and pain, and difficulty breathing; difficulty performing even simple activities without shortness of breath. Most have common causes, too, environmental and heavy metal pollutants, such as chlorofluorocarbons and smoke, and general malnutrition along with vitamin A deficiency. Suppressive over-the-counter cold and congestion remedies become a factor in aggravating problems when they don't allow the lungs to eliminate harmful wastes properly. Some medications damage the lungs. Check your prescriptions and consult *http://www.pneumotox.com/* for more information on drug-induced lung diseases.

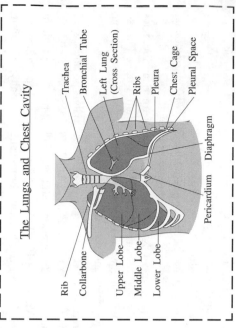

The Lungs and Chest Cavity

Trachea
Bronchial Tube
Left Lung (Cross Section)
Ribs
Pleura
Chest Cage
Pleural Space
Diaphragm
Pericardium
Lower Lobe
Middle Lobe
Upper Lobe
Collarbone
Rib

Are you at risk for SARS (Severe Acute Respiratory Syndrome)?

Severe Acute Respiratory Syndrome, or SARS, is a highly contagious respiratory supergerm which first emerged in Asia around November of 2002. Three hundred cases and 5 deaths were reported from China's Guangdong Province in February. The numbers grew to 1,323 cases with 49 deaths by March. Panic ensued, a world travel warning was issued and world commerce markedly slowed. By the time the outbreak ended in late July, there were 8,098 reported, many more unreported, and 774 deaths. Southeast Asia and Canada were the hardest hit. One hundred and ninety-two probable cases were reported in the U.S with no fatalities. No new cases were reported until January 2004, with no deaths, but infectious disease experts fear SARS could strike hard again unless protective drugs are tested soon.

SARS is a member of the coronavirus family, the same virus that causes the common cold, but SARS is a strain never before seen in humans. While experts aren't sure how SARS originated, many suspect it jumped from civet cats (who carry the virus in their stool and respiratory secretions) to humans through the practice of eating cats in Southern China. Major SARS risk factors include: having close contact with someone (living with them or caring for them) who has probable or confirmed SARS, having a history of travel to a SARS affected area, or living in a SARS affected area.

What are SARS symptoms? Initial signs: fever, cough, chills, chest pain, difficulty breathing and pneumonia. The newest research suggests that people with the STD chlamydia are at a high risk for SARS complications.

Although recovery is difficult and long, statistics show 90% of people who contract SARS eventually do recover. The other 10% become seriously ill. Overall mortality rate is 3-4%, similar to the mortality rate of West Nile virus.

The most successful medical treatment known today for SARS relies on a combination of intravenous antiviral drugs (Ribavirin), corticosteroid drugs (hydrocortisone) and broad spectrum antibiotics. Anti-HIV medications are also being considered in the SARS medical arsenal. Natural therapies for SARS focus on prevention through reducing risk factors and building immune strength (see the Immunity diet, pg. 469 of this book). In addition, although they have not been FDA approved to treat SARS, herbal antibiotics and antiviral supplements like usnea, echinacea, goldenseal, humic acid, oregano oil, lomatium and olive leaf extract may be useful. However, because of the virulence of this disease, it is not recommended for anyone with a suspected SARS infection to self-medicate. If you suspect SARS, seek immediate medical attention.

Can Avian Flu affect you (H5N1 Virus)?

A highly contagious, virulent Asian respiratory supergerm, avian flu is a feared pandemic threat, but as of this update (May 2006), is still only widespread among birds. Cases in humans are still rare. Its symptoms are similar to SARS - flu symptoms; extreme chest congestion where the person eventually is suffocated by the contents of their own lungs.

See the ASTHMA DIET page 328 or my book "Diets For Healthy Healing" for a complete lung healing diet.

Can't find a recommended product? Call the 800 number listed in Product Resources for the store nearest you.

Lung Disease

Diet and Lifestyle Support Therapy

Nutritional therapy plan:

1—Go on a short mucous cleansing liquid diet (pg. 175). Then, use the following lung cleansing diet for two weeks:

Lemon or grapefruit juice and water each morning with 1 tsp. maple syrup; or water-diluted pineapple juice to act as a natural expectorant.

Fresh carrot juice, like Green Foods CARROT ESSENCE, or a potassium drink (pg. 291) daily.

Eat two apples and two fresh green salads daily.

Have steamed vegetables with brown rice and tofu or seafood for dinner.

Take cranberry, pomegranate or celery juice before bed.

Add your choice of the following healing drinks daily: •Salute ALOE VERA JUICE with herbs, •Rainbow Light HAWAIIAN SPIRULINA, or •Crystal Star RESTORE YOUR STRENGTH™ drink (highly recommended...sometimes results in 24 to 36 hours).

2—High quality protein is needed to heal lung diseases. The diet should be high in vegetable proteins and whole grains, low in sugars and starches.

Include cultured foods such as yogurt and kefir for friendly G.I. flora.

Add lung specific fruits, like apricots, apples, peaches, plums.

Include nutritional yeast 2 tsp. daily.

Take a protein drink each morning, like Unipro PERFECT PROTEIN.

—Bodywork:

•Avoid all CFCs (chloro-fluoro-carbons). They are as harmful to your lungs as they are to the atmosphere.

•For Tuberculosis: Calendula ointment chest rub.

•Get plenty of fresh air and sunshine, away from air pollution.

•Scratch the arm lightly, for 5 minutes daily, along the meridian line from the shoulder to the outside of the thumb to clear and heal lungs.

•For cystic fibrosis, use gentle percussion on the chest to keep mucous from clogged airways. Add •UAS DDS-JUNIOR with FOS daily to normalize GI environment (good results for children).

•Take a catnip or chlorophyll enema once a week to clear body toxins out faster.

•Apply a mustard plaster to the chest area every evening to open up airways and release congested wastes. See pg. 76 for preparation technique.

•Believe it or not, playing a harmonica exercises and strengthens weakened lungs.

Herbal, Superfood and Supplement Therapy

Interceptive therapy plan: Choose 2 or 3 recommendations.

1—Help control lung infection: •Crystal Star ANTI-BIO™ caps 6 daily for 1 week; then 2 daily with *Usnea* extract or Crystal Star •D-CONGEST™ fast relief drops daily for 1 month. •OLIVE LEAF extract caps 3x daily. •Herbs, Etc LUNG TONIC; •Eidon SELENIUM for virus protection; •Immudyne MACROFORCE beta glucan (noticeable difference).

2—Help remove pollutants from lungs: •Crystal Star TOXIN DETOX™ caps 4 daily for 2 months; PSP Marketing DESTROXIN (zeolite); •Nature's Secret ULTIMATE RESPIRATORY CLEANSE; •Nutricology GERMANIUM 150mg (highly recommended) .

3—Help heal the lungs: •Pau d'arco tea 3 cups daily; •Evening Primrose Oil 6 daily. •B-complex 150mg, extra B-12, 2500mcg for anemia; •Now OREGANO OIL soft gels.

4—Antioxidants for the lungs: (May give to children in lower dose as protection.) •Beta-carotene 150,000IU daily; •Royal Bodycare MICROHYDRIN PLUS; •Lycopene 5-10mg; •CoQ-10 100mg 3x daily; •Grape seed or white pine PCOs 100mg 3x daily; •Carnitine 1000mg 2x daily; •Vitamin C 5000mg (or more) with bioflavonoids daily.

—H₂O₂ therapy: •Earth's Bounty OXY-CLEANSE caps, or •American Biologics DIOXYCHLOR for 1 month. Rest for a month; resume if needed. There will be intense and prolonged coughing, as accumulated waste is released. H₂O₂ works to destroy chronic infection in the lungs and provide nascent oxygen to the tissues.

—Natural help for tuberculosis: •Olive Leaf extract caps; •High potency royal jelly 2 tsp. daily; •Silica is a specific: Try •Crystal Star IODINE, POTASSIUM, SILICA™ drops or •Eidon SILICA liquid; and Body Essentials SILICA gel chest rub. Use •Mullein tea or •Chlorella 20 tabs daily. •Vitamin A 100,000 daily (one month under practitioner). •CoQ-10, 100mg 3x daily; •Quercetin 1000mg with Bromelain 1500 daily; •Vitamin C 5000mg daily with Ho Shou Wu extract 30 drops daily.

—Natural help for sarcoidosis: •Planetary TRIPHALA INTERNAL CLEANSER caps; •Crystal Star DR ENZYME™ with protease and bromelain to reduce scar tissue; •Melatonin .3mg or as directed to reduce inflamed nodules; •Futurebiotics VITAL GREEN tabs; •Garlic caps 8 daily; •Immudyne MACROFORCE beta glucan (good results).

—Natural help for cystic fibrosis: •Crystal Star DR. ENZYME™ with protease and bromelain; •Transformation PUREZYME protease; •CoQ-10 200mg daily; •Echinacea/goldenseal caps 6 daily or •*Usnea* extract; •Spectrum NORWEGIAN FISH OIL daily; •Solaray ALFA-JUICE caps 6 daily; •Nutricology GERMANIUM 150mg; •Healing tea blend: *licorice, osha root, astragalus, thyme, coltsfoot;* •Ginseng is a specific- •Consider Crystal Star FEEL GREAT NOW!™ caps with ginseng fortifiers, or •Herbs Etc. GINSENG SEVEN SOURCE.

Can't find a recommended product? Call the 800 number listed in Product Resources for the store nearest you.

Lupus

Systemic Lupus Erythematosis

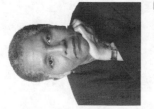

Lupus is a multi-system, auto-immune, inflammatory, viral disease affecting close to 2 million Americans, more than 80% of them black and Hispanic women. The immune system becomes disoriented and develops antibodies that attack its own connective tissue. Joints and connective are affected producing arthritis-like symptoms. Kidneys and lymph nodes become inflamed; in severe cases heart, brain and central nervous system degenerate. Orthodox treatment has not been very successful for lupus. In fact, a study published in the New England Journal of Medicine reveals up to 10% of cases may be caused by drug reactions! Natural therapies help rebuild a stable immune system and relieve some associated stress. Our experience shows that you feel worse for 1 or 2 months until toxins are neutralized. Then, suddenly, as a rule, you feel much better. A natural program works, but requires many months. **Signs of Lupus?** Great fatigue and depression, rough, red skin patches, chronic nail fungus (red at cuticle base), inflammation around the mouth, cheeks and nose, light sensitivity, dry eyes, low grade chronic fever; rheumatoid arthritis symptoms, migraines, anemia, amnesia, even psychosis. **Common causes?** Viral infection, the result of taking too many antibiotics or prescription drugs from Hydrazine derivatives, food allergies, emotional stress, latent diabetes, Candida albicans infection or chronic fatigue syndrome.

Diet and Lifestyle Support Therapy

Nutritional therapy plan:

1—Diet therapy, especially eliminating food allergens reduces the symptoms of lupus. Follow the Arthritis Diet, page 326 for 3 months: Eat 60-75% fresh foods during this time. Avoid nightshade plants that aggravate lupus, like eggplant, tomatoes, tobacco. *Note:* Alfalfa-containing or wheat products may aggravate some lupus cases.

2—A potassium drink, pg. 291 daily for 1 month, then every other day for 1 month, then once a week the 3rd month (sometimes dramatic results).

3—Then follow a modified macrobiotic diet (pg. 348) until blood tests clear, (sometimes 2-3 years, but I've seen good healing success). Take aloe vera juice 1 to 2 glasses daily, or AloeLife ALOE GOLD JUICE 2x daily. Drink green tea every morning or Crystal Star GREEN TEA CLEANSER™ to re-establish homeostasis.

4—A low fat, vegetarian diet is strongly recommended to increase essential fatty acids and decrease fats. Avoid red meats, sugars, starchy foods. Include organic sea greens like Maine Coast SEA VEGETABLES and seafoods (esp. salmon) for "good" fats.

4—Add green drinks at least once a week for a year. We've seen results with Wakunaga KYO-GREEN drink, Crystal Star RESTORE YOUR STRENGTH™ drink, Nutricology PRO-GREENS with EFAs. Or try C'est Si Bon Company CHLORENERGY tabs.

—**Bodywork:** The risk of lupus is 40% more likely in users of oral contraceptives than in women who have not used them. Smokers are also at a higher risk. Penicillin, allergenic cosmetics, and phototoxins from UV rays may also result in a flare-up of lupus.

•Get plenty of rest. Removing amalgam fillings may help alleviate symptoms.

•Apply Crystal Star ANTI-BIO™ gel with una da gato to heal roughened skin patches. Use with 250,000IU beta carotene for fast results.

•Effective stress reduction techniques for lupus: biofeedback, meditation, yoga, tai chi and acupuncture. Take a walk every day for exercise and stress reduction.

•Over-medication for lupus, especially by cortico-steroid drugs is dangerous; they weaken the bones, cause excess weight gain and eventually suppress immune response.

Herbal, Superfood and Supplement Therapy

Interceptive therapy plan: Choose 2 to 4 recommendations.

1—**Reduce inflammation and manage pain:** •Homeopathic Hormonegetics HGH 2c-30c; •MSM caps 800mg daily or •Futurebiotics MSM caps or MICROHYDRIN PLUS with MSM from royal-health.com; •Gotu kola extract or Solaray Centella Asiatica caps 6 daily. •Quercetin 1000mg and bromelain 1500mg daily, or •Solaray TURMERIC (curcumin) caps •Vitamin E 800IU daily •Maitake Products MAITAKE D-FRACTION.

2—**Relieve arthritis-like symptoms:** •Acetyl-L-Carnitine 1000mg daily. •Chondroitin 1200 and Glucosamine 1500mg daily. •Evening Primrose oil 3000-4000mg daily or Barleans HIGH LIGNAN FLAX OIL for inflammation: •Crystal Star DR. ENZYME™ with protease and bromelain is a specific; •Burdock tea 2 cups daily, blood cleanser for muscles; •Nutricology GERMANIUM 150mg (noticeable results).

3—**Add magnesium, B-vitamins ease muscle pain:** •Magnesium 800mg daily, or •Ethical Nutrients MALIC/MAGNESIUM; •B-complex 150mg 3x daily, or •Nature's Secret ULTIMATE B tabs for EFAs. •Folic acid 400mcg daily if taking methotrexate.

4—**Relieve lupus stress:** •SAMe (S-adenosyl methionine) 800mg daily; •Maitake Prdcts REISHI MUSHROOM caps; •Kava extract or Crystal Star RELAX™ caps with kava relieves muscle spasms. •Siberian eleuthero extract or Crystal Star ADRENAL ENERGY BOOST™ caps relieve adrenal stress; •St. John's wort 300mg daily for lupus depression.

—**Hormone balancers:** DHEA is a specific for lupus (helps patients decrease prednisone): •Nutricology DHEA 50mg daily; •Crystal Star PRO-EST BALANCE™ roll-on.

5—**Heal the liver:** •Crystal Star LIVER RENEW™ caps and LIVER CLEANSE FLUSHING™ tea daily for 1 month; •bupleurum extract 2x daily or Planetary BUPLEURUM LIVER CLEANSE; •Country Life sublingual B-12, 2500mcg daily.

6—**Boost immune response:** •Astragalus extract 4x daily; •Nutricology LAKTO-FERRIN w. colostrum; •Glutathione 100mg daily; •PCOs from grapeseed 300mg daily; •Vitamin C 5000mg daily; •CoQ-10 300mg daily; •Nutricology PERM A VITE formula for leaky gut syndrome; •Beta-carotene 150,000IU daily; •High potency royal jelly, 40,000mg or more. •Rainforest Remedies STRONG RESISTANCE drops.

Can't find a recommended product? Call the 800 number listed in Product Resources for the store nearest you.

489

Lyme Disease

Lyme Arthritis

Lyme disease is a serious illness caused by a micro-organism transmitted by the deer tick.... no bigger than a freckle. Over 100,000 Americans have been infected, mostly in the upper East Coast, upper Midwest, Northern California, and the Oregon coast. A steadily debilitating disease, with symptoms much like those of arthritis, Lyme disease is difficult to guard against. Antibiotics are the current medical treatment, and seem to work in the initial phases; but symptoms usually recur after the drugs are withdrawn, and they do not work in the later stages at all. Natural therapies that address the disease as if it were a virus, used after a course of drug antibiotics, have had good success. Note: The Lyme disease vaccine *Lymerix* is 78% effective in preventing Lyme disease after receiving three doses, but may cause reactions like arthritic joint pain and facial paralysis in up to 30% of the population. *Do you have Lyme disease?* Watch for a large red "bulls-eye" rash with a light center, that grows as large as 10 to 20 inches. Check for initial flu-like symptoms of stiff neck, chills and aches, and unusual fatigue or lethargy, head aches and joint pain, especially in children. Later symptoms of heart arrhythmias, muscle spasms with racking pain, meningitis (brain inflammation), bladder problems, arthritis, facial paralysis and other numbing nerve dysfunctions, extreme fatigue and memory loss. Lyme disease mimics other disease conditions. Get a simple test at a health care clinic if you feel you are at risk. *Contact www.lyme.org. or American Lyme Disease Foundation (800-886-LYME).*

Diet and Lifestyle Support Therapy

Nutritional therapy plan:

1—A modified macrobiotic diet (pg. 348) is recommended for 2-3 months to strengthen the body while cleaning out and overcoming the disease.

2—Take a potassium drink (pg. 291) twice a week. Green drinks like Green Foods GREEN MAGMA drink, Sun Wellness CHLORELLA, 2 pkts. daily, or Crystal Star ENERGY GREEN RENEWAL™ are good defense.

3—Have a veggie drink like Knudsen's VERY VEGGIE or a green salad every day.

4—Take 1 tsp. each daily: wheat germ oil for body oxygen, EGG YOLK LECITHIN, royal jelly 40,000mg or more.

5—Avoid alcohol, tobacco, all refined and caffeine-containing foods, and sugar foods. Omit red meat, high gluten and starchy foods.

—**Bodywork:** Treat Lyme Disease early. Time is critical. The longer the tick is attached, the greater the risk of serious disease. Symptoms show up 3 weeks after tick bite.
• Use natural tick repellents on exposed body areas. A few drops of eucalyptus oil on a tick will cause it to fall out (immediately effective).
• Remove the tick with tweezers as close to the head as possible. Pull straight up. Do not squeeze or twist it. (Gut contents will empty into you.) Never touch the tick with your hands. Apply alcohol to bite area to disinfect.

—**Prevention is the key:** Strong immune response is the best defense. DEET chemical repellent, while effective, can be fatal if ingested and cause adverse reactions in children.
• Keep shrubbery to a minimum where children play. Check outdoor pets for ticks regularly.
• When walking through tall grass or brush, wear long-sleeve shirts and pants, and tape pant legs into socks. Wear shoes and boots that cover entire foot.
• Put suspicious clothing in dryer to kill ticks by dehydration. Washing clothes is not effective.
• Do a meticulous, daily body inspection if you have been in the woods or live in an infested area. Have a partner inspect for louse-size arachnids or dark freckle-sized nymphs behind knees, in scalp and pubic hair, in armpits and under watchbands.

Herbal, Superfood and Supplement Therapy

Deer ticks also transmit the even more serious pathogen, *Ehrlichia*, that causes HGE, which can be fatal. Rigorously check for tiny deer ticks if you live in an infested area. Use natural therapy *after* a course of medical antibiotics.

Interceptive therapy plan: Choose 2 to 4 recommendations.

1—Herbal anti-virals show the best results: Clean the tick bite with: •*tea tree* oil, •*calendula* extract, •*echinacea/goldenseal* extract, or •*St. John's wort* extract 2-3x daily. Then take •OREGANO OIL or OLIVE LEAF extract caps, 3x daily, or •*Usnea* extract 2x daily, one week on, one week off to overcome the infecting microbe, or •Nutribiotic GRAPEFRUIT SEED extract, 10 drops 3x daily in water. Take •Nutricology GERMANIUM 150mg daily; •Eidon COLLOIDAL SILVER as directed.

2—Reduce inflammation, repair nerve damage: •Crystal Star DR. ENZYME™ with protease and bromelain; •Crystal Star ANTI-FLAM™ caps, or turmeric (*curcumin*) caps 6 daily. •Crystal Star RELAX CAPS™ to rebuild nerve structure. •Solgar oceanic carotene 100-150,000IU daily with quercetin and bromelain as an anti-inflammatory.

3—Enhance lymph and liver activity: •Crystal Star ANTI-BIO™ caps or extract 6x daily or *echinacea* extract to cleanse lymph glands; •Crystal Star LIVER RENEW™ caps daily boosts liver activity for a month. •*Garlic* capsules 6 daily; •Vitamin C or Ester C powder, ¼ tsp. every hour to daily bowel tolerance as toxin neutralizer, especially during acute attacks or recurrence; •*Chaparral* tea as directed only by a clinical herbalist.

4—Boost immune response: •N-acetyl-cysteine (NAC) 2000mg daily; •Maitake Products REISHI caps or •*suma* extract or *astragalus* extract to re-establish homeostasis. •Lane Labs BENE-FIN shark cartilage enhances leukocytes with •Nutricology THYMUS ORGANIC GLANDULAR caps. • Crystal Star ZINC SOURCE™ throat rescue drops.

5—Probiotics reestablish homeostasis: •Pure Essence FLORALIVE or •Jarrow JARRO-DOPHILUS for damage from long courses of antibiotics and to restore intestinal health. •Solaray pancreatin 1300mg 4x daily on an empty stomach.

—**To repel Lyme ticks:** Use •*myrrh* or *pennyroyal* oil topically.

Can't find a recommended product? Call the 800 number listed in Product Resources for the store nearest you.

Measles
Rubella

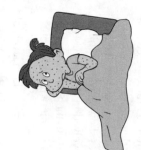

Measles is a highly contagious, but rare viral infection that attacks a vulnerable immune system. Most communicable in the early stages, initial symptoms appear as a feverish, upper respiratory cold or flu, followed by a red rash. Usually a childhood disease, measles also affects adults whose immunity to the virus has not been established. (After-effects of measles are rare in children but may be permanent in adults. Women are often left with chronic joint pain.) *Rubella* (German measles), characterized by swollen lymph glands and then a rash, is a more severe, more contagious measles virus that can cause birth defects. Measles vaccinations have a number of side effects for children - be wary. *See Childhood Diseases page 236 for more information. Do you have measles?* You may if you have a fever and cough, with sneezing, runny nose, red eyes, headache, and swollen lymph nodes. You can be sure if the fever is followed by a red rash on your face and upper body which sloughs off when the fever drops. With rubella, there is heavy coughing, a rash covers the body, light hurts the eyes, white spots appear in the mouth and throat, and you'll probably get an ear infection (sometimes hearing is affected permanently). *Why do you get measles?* Measles comes with low immunity from a poor diet, or too many immune-depressing antibiotics or cortico-steroid drugs.

Diet and Lifestyle Support Therapy

Nutritional therapy plan for prevention: Keeping your immunity high is the best defense against measles.

1—Start with a liquid foods diet for at least 24 hours to increase fluid intake as much as possible. Use fresh fruit and vegetable juices, miso soup, bottled water and herb teas such as catnip, chamomile or rosemary, that will mildly induce sweating and clean out toxins faster.

2—Then follow with a simple, basic diet featuring vitamin A and C-rich fresh fruits and veggies.

3—Give 1 tsp. acidophilus liquid in citrus juice each morning. Offer fresh fruits with yogurt all through the morning. Or try Jarrow GENTLE FIBERS drink 2x daily.

4—Have a fresh green salad each day.

5—Have a cup of miso or clear soup with 1 tsp. nutritional yeast and 1 tbsp. snipped sea greens daily. Or have a cup of miso (or Ramen) soup each day, and a cup of Red Star NUTRITIONAL YEAST extract broth or BioStrath original LIQUID YEAST before bed.

—Bodywork:

• Use hydrotherapy baths with *comfrey* or *calendula* flowers to induce sweating, and reutralize body acids.

• Herbal body washes soothe and heal the skin: make into tea, soak a washcloth and wipe down a rashy body. *Elder* flower; *Peppermint;* or *Ginger* root.

• Apply *ginger-cayenne* compresses to the rash. Apply *calendula* gel to sores.

• Frequent hot baths will often release poisons through the rash.

• Take tepid oatmeal baths to relieve skin itch and rash.

• Eyestrain and photosensitivity are common. Keep children especially in a darkened room.

• Pat *aloe vera* gel on sores, also put aloe vera juice in bathwater for skin healing.

• Take a garlic or *catnip* enema during acute stage to lower fever and clean out infection fast (person should be 8 years or older.)

Herbal, Superfood and Supplement Therapy

Interceptive therapy plan: Choose 2 to 3 recommendations.

1—Curb the viral infection: • Planetary YIN CHIAO-ECHINACEA COMPLEX to break out fever and rash, and start the healing process (excellent results) . • Herbalist & Alchemist VX COMPOUND with *lomatium* and *St. John's wort* daily, or • *St. John's wort* extract or capsules, or • *mullein-lobelia* tincture in acute stage (for kids); • Crystal Star ANTI-FLAM™ caps with Crystal Star DR. ENZYME™ with protease and bromelain to reduce inflammation; or • Herbs, Etc. PHYTOCILLIN, or • Enzymedica PURIFY.

2—Deal with the skin rash: Use • *marjoram, catnip, yarrow* or *chamomile* teas, 3-4 cups daily to break out rash; • *raspberry, gotu kola* or *lobelia* tea to heal sores (apply and drink); • apply *marjoram* tea to sores to soothe itching; or • PHYCOTENE CREAM from royal-health.com.

3—For eyestrain and discomfort: Make a dilute tea from • Crystal Star EYEBRIGHT TEA™; Use as an eyewash to soothe. Or, • Similasan EYE DROPS #3 for eye strain and fatigue.

4—To control an accompanying middle ear infection: • Crystal Star ANTI-BIO™ caps 4 to 6 daily, or extract drops 4x daily to clear infection. (May also be used as ear drops morning and evening.) • Nutribiotic GRAPEFRUIT SEED extract to clear infection. Warm • *lobelia* extract in the ear (for kids); • *garlic* oil caps, 2 daily.

5—For a cough and sore throat: • Crystal Star ZINC SOURCE™ throat rescue herbal drops (almost immediate sore throat relief). Use • *licorice* tea or • *coltsfoot* tea, or • *ginseng-licorice* extract as an expectorant. • Zinc gluconate lozenges, esp. • Zand HERBAL ZINC lozenges for kids. Try • New Chapter GINGER WONDER syrup - 1 tbsp. in 8-oz. water 2x daily, (soothes sore throat, provides healing benefits).

6—To speed recovery: Short-term vitamin A therapy is a key: • Emulsified vitamin A & D 10,000IU/400IU for children as soon as rash appears. Use a stronger dose for rubella, up to 100,000IU in divided doses. • Vitamin C therapy is important: • Alacer effervescent EMERGEN-C, 2 to 4x daily in juice, or ascorbate vitamin C, 1/4 tsp. 3 to 4x daily in juice or water. • Enzymatic Therapy VIRAPLEX complex.

Can't find a recommended product? Call the 800 number listed in Product Resources for the store nearest you.

Menopause

Taking Control of your Life Change

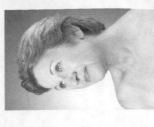

By 2015, almost half of all American women will be in menopause. Will the temperature of the planet rise from all the hot flashes?!

Menopause is intended by Nature to be a gradual reduction of estrogen by the ovaries with few side effects. In a well-nourished, vibrant woman, the adrenals and other glands pick up the job of estrogen secretion to keep her active and attractive after menopause. While almost 90% of women experience some normal menopausal body changes and hormonal fluctuations, most only last a year or two and are not severe enough to interrupt their lives. Still, our modern stressful lifestyles and poor eating habits mean that many women reach their menopausal years with prematurely worn out adrenals and poor liver function where estrogen is not being processed correctly, so hormone fluctuations are magnified. Keeping your adrenals healthy, changing old habits to support your adrenal energy can eliminate many unpleasant menopausal symptoms. (See page 300 for specifics.) For some women however, erratic estrogen and other hormone secretions cause chronic hot flashes, insomnia and fatigue. Libido is reduced, irritability increases, mood swings come to the fore as a woman's hormone balance changes, frightening heart palpitations may occur, calcium metabolism disturbances may increase risk for osteoporosis; skin and vaginal tissue may become dry, occasional male characteristics may appear. It's disconcerting to say the least. Some women say they'll do anything to stop menopause symptoms. So should you try hormone replacement therapy?

Hormone Replacement Therapy.... There's a firestorm of controversy about synthetic hormone replacement.

Premarin, an estrogen replacement drug for menopausal women made from pregnant mare's urine, is one of the top selling drugs in the U.S. The threat of breast and uterine cancer is dramatically increased with HRT, and the risk increases as a woman ages. In an action that received wide media attention, U.S. government scientists halted a July 2002 study on hormone replacement because it was such a threat to the participants' health. Increased risk of invasive breast cancer, heart disease, stroke and pulmonary embolism (blood clots in the lungs) were all cited as reasons for halting the study. The drugs being tested included Premarin, Prempro and Provera. Scientists have known since the late 1980s that HRT could increase the risk of breast cancer. Studies released in the last few years detail the connection between HRT and breast cancer even further. A 2000 study showed women taking HRT for just five years have a 40% greater risk of developing breast cancer. A newer study found that long-term HRT raises the odds of one of the most dangerous types of breast cancer as much as 85%. In hopeful news, some research finds that the higher risk for breast cancer diminishes, even largely disappears when a woman is off HRT treatment for five years. Drug companies and much of the medical community, for whom synthetic hormones are an incredibly profitable business, continue to justify the risks because of the perceived advantages to osteoporosis and estrogen management. Yet, the newest research reveals that benefits for these problems are not validated over the longterm.

—**Does HRT really protect against menopausal heart disease?** Using hormone replacement therapy or ERT to protect against heart disease is highly debatable. There is no conclusive evidence that estrogen protects against heart disease. A 1997 review concluded that the heart protective benefits attributed to estrogen may result from population selection bias or even changes towards healthier lifestyles during the studies. A more recent report shows that HRT does not help treat or prevent heart disease in menopausal women. In addition, HRT drugs can deplete folic acid, raising homocysteine levels, a known risk factor for heart disease, and destroy vitamin E, a heart protective antioxidant. With its links to uterine and breast cancer, I don't believe HRT should be considered as a long-term preventive for heart disease. There are better solutions for preventing heart disease that don't carry these risks.

—**What's the HRT connection to osteoporosis?** Long considered a woman's problem because of its female hormone involvement, osteoporosis affects from 35 to 50 percent of women in the first five years after menopause. HRT is still strongly promoted for osteoporosis prevention. Many menopausal women are so afraid of osteoporosis that with a little coaxing from their physicians they begin taking hormone drugs right away. Of those, about 60% discontinue the therapy because of side effects or fear of cancer! There is no question that hormones are involved in bone-building and bone loss, but declining estrogen levels after menopause do not by themselves cause osteoporosis. Although some studies show estrogen inhibits bone cell death, the newest tests reveal that as many as 15% of women on estrogen therapy continue to lose bone! Moreover, estrogen isn't the only hormone involved in bone building. The hormone progesterone actually increases bone density in clinical tests. Low androgen levels of DHEA and testosterone also play a role in bone loss, particularly in men's osteoporosis. Osteoporosis prevention is a program not a pill. There are clear lifestyle factors that increase your risk of this devastating disease. See also OSTEOPOROSIS page 509 for more information.

—**Are there environmental consequences with so many women on HRT drugs?** The latest studies show there may be. Studies on the Las Vegas sewage wash reveal high levels of synthetic hormones from human urine in waters where male fish show signs of hormone disruption. In these waters, male carp produce the egg laying protein associated with females.

Can't find a recommended product? Call the 800 number listed in Product Resources for the store nearest you.

If, as suspected, HRT or birth control drugs are to blame, we have a huge problem on our hands. Billions of pounds of "treated" sewage are released in discharge waters where wildlife make their home! Hormones, caffeine, antidepressants and painkillers have been found in streams all across the nation! More research is currently being done to determine the long term effects of hormones from human urine on our environment. Check out environmental estrogen disrupters (xenoestrogens) on page 459 for more information on this disturbing trend.

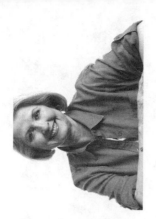

Menopause the natural way:

80 percent of postmenopausal women in the U.S. do not use any form of HRT at all! Beyond increased cancer risk, HRT has many unpleasant side effects. Women taking hormone drugs report weight gain (especially fatty deposits on the hips and thighs), heavy bleeding (worse than former menstrual periods), PMS-like pain, severe leg cramps, migraine headaches, uterine and breast fibroids, and low libido. Unless you have specific, extenuating circumstances (only about 6% of American women do), a natural menopause may be the best. Even women who don't have a symptom-free menopause say they feel younger and more energetic when they address menopausal changes, naturally. If you are about to be confronted with the great HRT choice, consider carefully before you agree. Aggravating symptoms which often accompany menopause are due to the body's difficulty in adapting to its new hormone functions. Many are positively influenced with natural therapies. If you're experiencing a raging hormone roller coaster, with hot flashes, mood swings, vaginal dryness and low libido, check out these pages for the natural way to "keep the change!"

Natural Therapies for Specific Problems Associated with Menopause

Research shows that plant estrogens and isoflavones from herbs help increase bone density to reduce osteoporosis risk, and reduce high cholesterol to enhance heart and artery health.

—**HOT FLASHES and NIGHT SWEATS:** The body's temperature-regulating mechanism becomes unstable during the shifting hormone balance of menopause. As estrogen levels drop, the pituitary responds by increasing other types of hormones to re-establish hormone homeostasis. Hot flashes generally last 2 to 4 years after menstruation ends, and subside as the body adjusts to its new hormone levels. Stress, too much caffeine and alcohol trigger hot flashes. —**Alternative therapy protocols:** •Crystal Star EST-AID™ caps 4 to 6 daily as needed (excellent results, usually within 1 week); Note: many women add 2 RELAX CAPS™ for stress and symptoms (results in about 25 minutes). •Moon Maid Botanicals PRO-MENO cream or •Pure Essence Labs TRANSITIONS; or •Source Naturals HOT FLASH tabs; •Gamma oryzanol (GO), 100 mg 3x daily; •*sage* or *motherwort* tea, 3 cups daily; •VITEX extract 2x daily; •*dandelion* tea to strengthen the liver (noticeable difference); • EVENING PRIMROSE OIL, 3000mg daily. •Prince of Peace AMERICAN GINSENG, BEE POLLEN, ROYAL JELLY vials 1 daily (noticeable energy rise).

—**SAGGING INTERNAL TISSUE and ORGANS:** Herbal compounds are well-suited to elasticizing tissue and toning prolapsed organs. —**Alternative therapy protocols:** •Crystal Star WOMEN'S BEST FRIEND™ caps, 6 daily or •Vitex extract, or Rainbow Light VITEX SUPERCOMPLEX; •Jarrow GLUCOSAMINE SULFATE; •Crystal Star OCEAN MINERALS™ caps (iodine, potassium and silica from the sea); •Crystal Star CELLULITE BODY-SHAPER™ roll-on or •Weleda BIRCH CELLULITE OIL to help tone sagging tissue on arms, knees and neck (great for cellulite, too).

—**LOW LIBIDO, PAINFUL INTERCOURSE, DRY VAGINA:** Reduced estrogen levels can cause vaginal mucous membranes to become dry, resulting in painful intercourse - just at a time of life when you want to be more spontaneous, without fear of pregnancy. —**Alternative therapy protocols:** •Prince of Peace RED GINSENG, ROYAL JELLY vials; or •panax ginseng tea 1 cup daily or panax ginseng caps 2 daily with tsp. high potency royal jelly; •apply Moon Maid VITAL VULVA salve before intercourse; or •apply vitamin E oil or use Vitamin E suppositories; •Evening Primrose Oil, 3-4000mg daily for EFAs, with B-6, 250mg. •Rub Transitions PRO-GEST cream on abdomen as directed (good results); •Crystal Star WOMEN'S DRYNESS™ extract (fast acting when taken before intercourse); or •Maca herb caps 2 daily for 1 to 2 weeks (for noticeable difference); and •Crystal Star LOVE FEMALE™ caps or Esteem WOMAN ALIVE for more responsive libido. •Nutricology ADRENAL CORTEX ORGANIC GLANDULAR; or •Enzymatic Therapy THYROID - TYROSINE caps, 4 daily.

—**POOR CIRCULATION, TINGLING in the LIMBS:** A common menopausal condition, especially evident when one takes a deep breath. —**Alternative therapy protocols:** Make a daily circulation drink for almost immediate improvement: Mix ½ cup tomato juice, ½ cup lemon juice, 6 tsp. wheat germ oil, 1 tsp. nutritional yeast; Hawthorn extract or Ginkgo Biloba extract as needed; •PCOs from grapeseed or white pine 200mg daily; gotu kola or cayenne/ginger 4 caps daily; •Zand HAWTHORN HEART tabs; or •Natural Balance GREAT LEGS formula, or •Futurebiotics CIRCU A.V. caps.

Can't find a recommended product? Call the 800 number listed in Product Resources for the store nearest you.

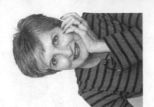

—DEPRESSION, IRRITABILITY, INSOMNIA, FATIGUE: Psychological symptoms distress many normally practical, well-balanced women. Many women feel that their lack of energy during menopause is the number one disruption in their lives. **—Alternative therapy protocols:** magnesium-rich foods, like leafy greens, almonds, apricots, avocado, carrots, citrus fruits, lentils, and salmon counteract depression and anxiety; reduce caffeine intake (it affects mood more during menopause). •Planetary GINSENG REVITALIZER; •*Dong quai-dami-ana-ashwagandha* drops offers balance. •Crystal Star DEPRESS-EX™ with *St. John's Wort*, or RELAX™ caps, or •Gaia Herbs PHYTO-PROZ SUPREME; •Nature's Secret ULTIMATE B COMPLEX helps emotional anxiety. •Aromatherapy essential oils help menopausal depression: try Bergamot, Geranium, Neroli, Clary Sage, and Jasmine by Wyndemere; •Homeopathics are a good choice: •Boiron IGNATIA for grief and black moods; •GOOD MOODS, RESTFUL SLEEP, or STRESS RELIEF, by Nature's Apothecary.

—BODY SHAPE CHANGES and MENOPAUSAL WEIGHT GAIN: Women have a gynoid pattern of fat distribution that accumulates fat around hips and buttocks, making it hard for them to lose fat in these areas. Estrogen in the female body directs the storage of "sex-specific fat" on the buttocks, hips and thighs for child-bearing and hormone functions. As women get older, the problem escalates. Estrogen reduction during menopause generates another change in fat distribution. Menopausal women develop more fat storage in the deep abdominal cavity than menstruating women. This is because the fat cells in the stomach help to produce estrogen when production slows down in the ovaries - another reason why very thin women often have a difficult menopause. Small, focused changes in diet and lifestyle can help solve the weight problems for menopausal women. See *Weight Loss After 40*, pg.567 for more information. **—Alternative therapy protocols:** Now is the time to start exercising - at least 3x weekly to retain muscle and gain body tone; for weight control without overstimulation. Weight training along with moderate aerobic exercise and pre-workout stretches 3 times a week realizes excellent results, along with •Prince of Peace AMERICAN GINSENG, BEE POLLEN, ROYAL JELLY vials; •Crystal Star THERMO THINNER (alternate with THYROID META MAX™ or TUMMY BULGE™ caps); or •Gaia Herbs DIET SLIM. Use any formula with •Transformation LIPOZYME to optimize fat metabolism. Note: Take calcium along with any weight loss supplement to insure success.

—FACIAL HAIR GROWTH-HEAD HAIR LOSS: An extremely common menopausal condition, female pattern baldness is a disconcerting problem involving genetics, vitamin-mineral uptake, and stress. The slow-down and change in estrogen production affects the activity of hair follicles, and results in the head hair loss and facial hair growth women hate. Excess (DHT) in women can cause hair follicles to become dormant as in men. Balanced thyroid hormone production is critical to normal hair growth. Hypothyroidism leads to coarse, lifeless hair which easily falls out. Hyperthyroidism causes soft, thinning hair and hair loss. **—Alternative therapy protocols:** •sea greens make a big difference -most women notice better hair growth and texture in 3 to 4 weeks. Take at least 2 tbsp. daily of dried chopped sea greens, and eat lots of sushi. Reduce animal fats to unclog hair follicles; add soy foods for plant protein (hair is 97% protein!); •Crystal Star BEAUTIFUL HAIR & NAILS™ caps for noticeable hair regrowth; •Evening Primrose Oil 4000 mg daily; •Crystal Star CALCIUM MAGNESIUM SOURCE™ or •Flora CALCIUM, MAGNESIUM liquid with zinc and vitamin D for hair growth. •B Complex 100mg with extra B₆ daily; •Country Life sublingual B-12, 2500mcg every other day. Mix fresh blender-ground ginger with aloe vera gel and apply to hair; leave on 15 minutes. • VITEX extract, or •Nature's Path TRACE-MIN-LYTE also stimulate hair growth. *Saw Palmetto* herb reduces facial hair growth. Note: Use any formula with Betaine HCl if hydrochloric acid is low.

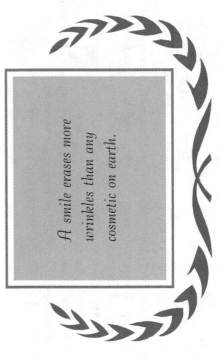

A smile erases more wrinkles than any cosmetic on earth.

Can't find a recommended product? Call the 800 number listed in Product Resources for the store nearest you.

Menopause

Diet and Lifestyle Support Therapy

Nutritional therapy plan:

1—A good diet is crucial to sailing through the second half of life disease-free and full of vitality. Limit fatty dairy products and meats, especially beef, high in hormone disrupting chemicals (buy organic chicken and turkey, now widely available). Reduce sugars and alcohol. (A little wine with dinner is fine.) Avoid caffeine. It taxes adrenal glands, upsets hormone levels. Steam and bake foods - never fry. Add B-vitamins through superfoods like CC Pollen ROYAL JELLY 2 tsp. daily or take Prince of Peace AMERICAN GINSENG-BEE POLLEN-ROYAL JELLY vials.

2—Especially eat cold water fish like salmon, and tuna for EFAs and to cut heart disease risk. Or try C'est Si Bon CHLORENERGY or Nutricology PROGREENS with EFAs, Crystal Star ENERGY GREEN RENEWAL™ with EFAs from sea greens.

3—Add soy foods like miso and tofu, and avoid spicy foods to reduce hot flashes. Balance estrogen levels by boosting boron-containing foods, like green leafy veggies, fruits, nuts, legumes. (Boron also helps harden bones.)

4—Add bioflavonoids, structurally similar to the body's estrogen. Whole grain fiber (or •Jarrow GENTLE FIBERS or All One TOTALLY FIBER COMPLEX) can reduce hot flashes. Fresh fruits and veggies also regulate estrogen levels and reduce mood swings.

5—Eat calcium foods: root vegetables, dark greens, non-fat dairy foods. Eliminate carbonated drinks loaded with phosphates that deplete calcium. Drink mineral water instead.

—Lifestyle changes for better body balance during menopause:

• Exercise regularly outdoors to get the advantages of natural vitamin D for bone health. A daily brisk walk keeps the system flowing.

• Do deep stretches on rising and each evening before bed. Yoga for body toning.

• Weight training 3 times a week along with aerobic exercise is a perfect way to keep skin from sagging. Weight training helps you keep the muscle while you lose the fat. In a natural menopause, when estrogen levels drop naturally, so does some body fat and excess fuids.

• Get a massage therapy treatment once a month for energy restoration, a body tune-up and a feeling of well-being.

• Smoking contributes to breast cancer, emphysema, osteoporosis, wrinkling and early menopause. Now is the time to quit!

• Twenty minutes in a sauna daily significantly cuts night sweats for menopausal women (helps normalize both sugar levels and excess, or disruptive estrogen levels.)

Herbal, Superfood and Supplement Therapy

Interceptive therapy plan: Choose several recommendations.

1—**Crystal Star's highly successful menopause program:** •EST-AID™ caps 4-6 daily the first month, 2 daily for 2 months, to control hormone imbalances; •CALCIUM-MAGNESIUM SOURCE™ caps for bone weakness accompanying estrogen changes; •EASY CHANGE™ caps or roll-on for the years of the change; •ADRENAL ENERGY BOOST, or •FEMALE HARMONY™ for a feeling of well-being. •MILK THISTLE SEED extract to help normalize estrogen levels through long term liver balance.

2—**For hot flashes:** •Ester C with bioflavs 4x daily - helps hot flashes, excess menses bleeding. •Vitamin E 800 daily; •Gamma oryzanol 300mg daily; •CoQ10 200mg daily. •Pure Essence Labs FEM CREME or •Moon Maid PRO-MENO wild yam cream as directed; •Pure Essence Labs TRANSITIONS or •Vitex extract (most commonly prescribed menopause remedy in Europe). Scullcap extract helps hot flashes and anxiety reactions.

3—**Boosting adrenal activity is a key to balance:** 1: Add Vitamin C 5000mg daily to maintain adrenal integrity and convert cholesterol to adrenal hormones. 2: Add sea greens to your diet, at least 2 tbsp. dry, chopped sea greens (any kind) daily. Or add 6 to 12 pieces of sushi to your weekly diet. Sea vegetables are a rich source of fat-soluble vitamins like D and K which assist with production of steroidal hormones like estrogen, and DHEA in the adrenal glands. 3: *Licorice*, *Sarsaparilla* and *Siberian eleuthero* work specifically to stimulate the adrenal glands to regulate body energy after menopause. Consider Crystal Star ADRENAL ENERGY BOOST™ caps 2 daily. 4: Royal jelly daily is a rich source of adrenal boosting pantothenic acid.

4—**Bone builders:** •Trace Minerals Research TRANSCEND for WOMEN; Lane Labs ADVACAL PLUS (clinically proven); •Metabolic Response Modifiers OSTEO-MAX.

5—**For sleep disturbances, anxiety:** •1 gram niacinamide at bedtime to stimulate serotonin; •Planetary RHODIOLA ROSEA full spectrum tabs; •5-HTP, 50-100mg with •Crystal Star NIGHT CAPS™ 1 at bedtime (excellent results); or •Herbs, Etc. DEEP SLEEP gels (also good results). •Homeopathic *Nux Vomica*, •*Kava kava* or •Herb Pharm PHARMA KaVA drops (not with alcohol); •Liddell LETTING GO homeopathic spray.

6—**Elevate mood and increase energy:** •Ginkgo biloba extract; •Herbal Magic GINSENG-GINKGO REJUVENATOR; •Siberian eleuthero extract; •Planetary GINSENG REVITALIZER tabs; •Nature's Secret ULTIMATE B; •Stress B-complex 100mg; •Barlean's high lignan flax oil 3 daily.

7—**Iodine therapy for thyroid-metabolism balance:** •Sea greens, 2 tbsp. daily or sushi daily to your diet; take •Crystal Star OCEAN MINERALS™ caps or •New Chapter OCEAN HERBS; or •Bernard Jensen LIQUI-DULS; or •Kelp tabs 8 daily.

Can't find a recommended product? Call the 800 number listed in Product Resources for the store nearest you.

Menstrual Problems

Excessive Flow (Menorrhagia), Inter-period Bleeding (Metrorrhagia)

Progesterone hormone assures uniform shedding of the uterine lining - low levels of progesterone means tissue will build up. A high estrogen level also stimulates growth of the uterine lining, causing uneven and more endometrial tissue formation. The combination of these two factors leads to abnormally heavy flow during menstruation, and/or spotting between periods as excess tissue is shed. A low progesterone-to-estrogen ratio also causes PMS bloating, irritability and depression. Mild to moderate hypothyroidism is usually involved in menorrhagia; good response is often dramatic with herbal iodine therapy. **Do you have excessive menstrual bleeding?** Heavy bleeding for 2 or more days of your period, with large dark clots and spotting between periods. An abnormal (but non-cancerous) PAP smear may occur. **What causes menorrhagia?** Hypothyroidism (sluggish thyroid) is almost always implicated. Uterine fibroids are commonly involved, often from a low nutrition diet with too much caffeine, salt and red meat, which aggravates hormone - gland imbalances. Endometriosis, or pelvic inflammatory disease or hyperplasia from too much estrogen are other major factors. Excess aspirin or blood-thinning medications may add to the problem along with a calcium or chronic iron or Vitamin K deficiency. Note: some contraceptive pills cause breakthrough bleeding. *See Menopause pages 492-495 for more information.*

Diet and Lifestyle Support Therapy

Nutritional therapy plan:
1—Consciously work on nutrition improvement, with emphasis on vegetable proteins, mineral-rich foods, like carrot juice or Green Foods CARROT ESSENCE, and high fiber foods like Jarrow GENTLE FIBERS drink daily for tissue strength. Add iodine foods like sea vegetables (2 tbsp. daily) for excessive menstrual flow.
2—Eat plenty of dark leafy greens like spinach, kale, dandelion greens or collard greens to build blood. Green drinks like C'est Si Bon CHLORENERGY or Crystal Star ENERGY GREEN RENEWAL™ drinks help breakthrough bleeding. Include cayenne as a natural hemostatic.
3—Increase Omega-3 rich foods: salmon, cold water fish, sea greens, flax seed oil for EFAs that help regulate metabolism.
4—Add sulphur foods like garlic, onions and turmeric spice.
5—Restrict intake of animal foods, especially cheese and red meats (many are loaded with hormone drugs).
6—Reduce fried, saturated fatty foods, sugars, and high cholesterol foods.
7—Avoid caffeine and caffeine-containing foods, hard liquor (a little wine is fine).
8—Make a mix of nutritional yeast flakes, wheat germ flakes, amaranth grain (astringent) lecithin granules; add 2 tbsp. to the diet daily.

—Bodywork:
•Acupressure: Press on the insides of the legs about 5" above the knees; 5 minutes on each leg to decrease bleeding.
•Apply ice packs to the pelvic area.
•Get extra sleep during this time.
•Get daily regular exercise to keep system and metabolism flowing.
•Avoid drugs of all kinds, even aspirin and prescription drugs if possible. Many inhibit Vitamin K formation.

Herbal, Superfood and Supplement Therapy

Interceptive therapy plan: Choose 2 or more recommendations.
1—Address underlying hypothyroidism to arrest excess bleeding: •Crystal Star OCEAN MINERALS™ (Iodine, Potassium, Silica from the sea) caps, or •IODINE, PO-TASSIUM, SILICA extract; •Bernard Jensen LIQUI-DULS iodine drops or •Premier raw thyroid. •Bee pollen caps 1000mg 2 daily and •Prince of Peace GINSENG-ROYAL JELLY vials add absorbable B vitamins. •Enzymatic Therapy THYROID/TYROSINE, or •Nature's Path TRACE-MIN-LYTE. Add •Black Haw extract to any choice (very good results).
2—Help shorten periods: •Enzymatic Therapy FEM-TROL capsules if periods are too frequent; •*Nettles* extract, ¼ tsp. 2x daily; •Vitamin K 100mcg 2 daily; •Vitamin A normalizes heavy bleeding: up to 100,000IU for 2 to 3 weeks only, then reduce to 10,000IU. Add •Crystal Star DR. ENZYME™ with protease and bromelain for pain relief.
3—Lengthen luteal phase to curtail long bleeding periods: •EFAs from Evening Primrose Oil 6 daily, or •Flax seed oil for spotting or •Lane Labs OMEGA MULTI for cramps. •Crystal Star FEMALE HARMONY™ caps 2 daily with 2 bayberry capsules, daily for 2 months to normalize cycle, especially if pre-menopausal. (good results for this protocol).
4—Balance progesterone: •Pure Essence FEM CREME, •Moon Maid PRO-MENO, or •Crystal Star PRO-EST BALANCE™ roll-on applied as directed.
5—Astringents help moderate blood loss: •Make an astringent tea - take a cup 3x daily, during and before your period: *shepherd's purse, cranesbill, red raspberry, periwinkle, agrimony* work well, or try •Crystal Star GREEN TEA CLEANSER™ each morning.
6—Tone the reproductive system: •Crystal Star WOMAN'S BEST FRIEND™ caps 6 daily (good results), with •VITEX extract as a tissue toner; •MILK THISTLE SEED extract helps stop spotting. •*Red raspberry* tea helps relax uterine cramps.
7—Balance body iron: •Crystal Star IRON SOURCE BLOOD BUILDER™; •Floradix LIQUID IRON. •Country Life B-12, 2500mcg, •folic acid 400mcg for iron uptake.
8—Strengthen connective tissue with bioflavs and silica: •Eidon SILICA liquid or Flora VEGE-SIL, or •Kal BIOFLAVONOID COMPLEX. •Rainbow Light CALCIUM PLUS capsules 4 at a time daily. •Nature's Plus Vitamin E 800IU.

Can't find a recommended product? Call the 800 number listed in Product Resources for the store nearest you.

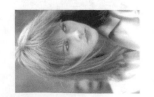

Menstrual Problems

Suppressed, Delayed, Irregular Flow, Peri-Menopause

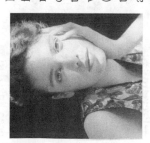

Irregular menstrual periods are among the most common disorders women suffer. Most are related to gland health and lifestyle. Intense body building and training for marathon or competition sports affects menstruation (sometimes to the point of cessation) because a woman's body fat is extremely reduced. The body will not slough off tissue when it feels at risk in forming more. In young girls, menses may be delayed because of abnormally low estrogen levels due to low blood calcium levels, or to eating disorders and crash dieting. Irregular menses due to prolonged emotional stress should be addressed with relaxation and exercise techniques. **Do you have menstrual problems?** If you don't menstruate, or haven't yet, even though you've reached puberty, or your menses are irregular, with a feeling of continual heaviness and bloating. **What causes are involved?** Poor health or poor diet with very low protein and low blood calcium levels (often from weight loss diet foods), gland and hormone imbalance (especially young girls), too much caffeine or too many carbonated drinks, lack of exercise or too much exercise (marathoner's syndrome), hypoglycemia. IUD-caused cervical lesions or cysts, venereal disease, stress, emotional shock, adrenal exhaustion and the birth control pill also cause irregularities. *See PMS page 515 for more info and natural cramps therapy.*

Diet and Lifestyle Support Therapy

Nutritional therapy plan:

1—Make sure your diet is very nutritious, with plenty of vegetable proteins and complex carbohydrates. (Your body may not menstruate regularly if it is malnourished).

2—Eat brown rice and other B-complex-rich foods like sea greens (loaded with EFA's, too), or add Prince of Peace GINSENG-ROYAL JELLY vials for metabolic balance.

3—Avoid red meats. Switch to Omega-3 rich protein foods: salmon, cold water fish, sea greens, flax seed, sesame seeds.

4—Avoid caffeine and caffeine-containing foods, such as chocolate and sodas.

5—Have a green veggie drink like Crystal Star ENERGY GREEN RENEWAL™, or Nutricology PROGREENS with EFA's, or Rainbow Light HAWAIIAN SPIRULINA, several times a week for healthy blood building. Try Green Foods VIBRANT WOMAN with B-complex 100mg for very good results.

6—Make a mix of toasted wheat germ, lecithin granules, and nutritional yeast; take 2 tbsp. each daily for adrenal support.

7—Drink plenty of pure water daily.

—Help remove infections through the skin:

• Pelvic compresses: especially seaweed compresses. Crystal Star HOT SEAWEED BATH™ is also indicated and successful in many cases.

• Horehound compresses on the pelvis.
• Ginger compresses on the pelvis.
• Alternating hot and cold sitz baths to stimulate pelvic circulation.
• Regular mild exercise to keep system free and flowing.
• Do knee-chest position exercises for retroverted uterus.
• Consciously get adequate rest and a reasonable schedule until periods normalize.
• Acupuncture, meditation and massage therapy treatments have all been effective for irregular menses.

Herbal, Superfood and Supplement Therapy

Interceptive therapy plan: Choose 2 to 4 recommendations.

1—**Help normalize menstrual flow:** •*Cramp bark-spearmint-squaw vine-sarsaparilla* tea 2 cups daily to normalize. •Black cohosh caps, Black Haw tea or Plum Flowers STASIS IN THE MANSION OF BLOOD teapills for suppressed menstrual discharge. •Pure Essence Labs FEM CREME, or •Moon Maid PRO-MENO wild yam cream (take as directed or periods may be very irregular). •Herbal Magic FEMSTRUATION; Enzymatic •THYROID/TYROSINE for accompanying hypothyroidism.

2—**Balance hormones to normalize cycle:** •Crystal Star FEMALE HARMONY™ caps and tea with •*burdock* tea 2 cups. •Rainbow Light VITEX-BLACK COHOSH SUPERCOMPLEX for abnormal cycles. •*Una de Gato* caps for irregular menses. •Esteem WOMEN'S COMFORT formula (great for PMS, too, see page 515).

   —**Balancing EFA sources (correlated with irregular, painful periods):** •EVENING PRIMROSE oil 4000mg daily, or Spectrum EVENING PRIMROSE oil 1300mg caps; •Flax seed oil 3 daily; •Nature's Secret ULTIMATE OIL.

3—**For healthy blood composition:** •Crystal Star IRON SOURCE BLOOD BUILDER™, •Turmeric (curcumin) extract caps 6 daily help move stagnant blood. •Nature's Plus Vitamin E 800IU. •B-complex 100mg daily, with extra folic acid 400mcg and •Country Life sublingual B-12, 2500mcg every other day.

   —**Tone uterine tissue:** •Blue cohosh caps for 1 month (good results).

4—**Support exhausted adrenals:** •Crystal Star ADRENAL ENERGY BOOST™ 2 capsules daily; •CC Pollen HIGH DESERT ROYAL JELLY; •Medicine Wheel FOUNTAIN of YOUTH, or •Planetary SCHIZANDRA ADRENAL COMPLEX.

   —**For teenage delayed menses:** •*Dong quai/damiana* caps or extract 2x daily (excellent results), with an herbal calcium formula such as •Crystal Star CALCIUM MAGNESIUM SOURCE™, or a good •calcium/magnesium supplement with •zinc 50mg daily and •kelp tabs or Greer Foods ION KELP 8 daily for 2 months.

Can't find a recommended product? Call the 800 number listed in Product Resources for the store nearest you.

Miscarriage

Miscarriage Prevention, False Labor

Between 1 in 6 and 1 in 3 pregnancies end in miscarriage. Spontaneous miscarriage, most likely to occur in the first trimester, frequently happens before a woman even recognizes she's pregnant. **What causes miscarriage?** Miscarriage is often Nature's way of dealing with an abnormal embryo (such as development of extra fetal chromosomes, or improper fixing of the fetus to the womb walls) that could not have lived a normal life if the pregnancy had been brought to full term. Rarely is miscarriage the fault of the mother's actions (such as stress, a fall or exercise), except when her nutrition (especially protein) is very poor, or if she is addicted to drugs or nicotine. Even then, Nature tries hard to avoid conception under dangerous conditions. Aside from the early discomforts of pregnancy, miscarriage is the greatest threat during this time, especially if the mother is over 35 and has had difficulty becoming pregnant. Rarely chronic infections, diabetes, poor uterine muscle tone or weak blood vessels and capillaries may play a part. **Are you at risk for miscarriage?** Spotty to profuse bleeding during pregnancy, usually with cramps, lower back pain and severe abdominal pain is the first sign. Take a prenatal formula all through pregnancy for a healthier baby and to help prevent miscarriage. *See my book, Do You Want To Have A Baby? Natural Fertility Solutions and Pregnancy Care for more information.*

Diet and Lifestyle Support Therapy

Nutritional therapy plan:

1—A good prevention/building diet should include plenty of magnesium and potassium-rich foods; leafy greens, brown rice, cooked green and yellow veggies, tofu, sprouts, molasses, etc. Add sea greens for natural vitamin B_{12}. Be sure you get enough vegetable protein for the baby's growth: whole grains, sprouts and seeds, low fat dairy foods and seafoods.

2—Limit intake of goitrogen foods that impair thyroid function like raw cruciferous vegetables (cooked is OK), peanuts, mustard, pine nuts, millet and soy products.

3—Avoid alcohol, caffeine, drugs. Reduce sugars and refined foods of all kinds. NO soft drinks; they bind magnesium and make it unavailable.

4—Avoid a restricted raw foods diet. Include warming foods like nutritional broths and soups, herbal pregnancy teas, whole grains, and steamed vegetables often.

5—Mix of 1 tsp. lecithin, 4 tsp. toasted wheat germ, 1 tsp. nutritional yeast and 2 tsp. molasses; take 2 tbsp. daily over cereal or in a green drink. Note: I consider green drinks to be one of the keys to a healthy pregnancy. Try •Crystal Star ENERGY GREEN™, •Green Kamut JUST BARLEY or •All ONE MULTIPLE green plant base daily.

—Preventives:

•A medical sonogram and fetal heart monitoring are recommended in every case. If miscarriage is inevitable, seek medical or midwife guidance to ensure it is complete. Retained tissue can cause serious infection. Abnormal vaginal discharge or a fever are infection warning signs to watch for.

•Smokers are twice as likely to miscarry and have low birth weight babies.

•Avoid X-rays; they can damage the fetus. Stay at least four feet away from home appliances like TV's, microwaves, vacuums, and toasters.. Try to stay at least 2 feet away from computer monitors and hard drives. Electromagnetic radiation from these appliances has been linked to an 80% increase in the risk of miscarriage.

• Avoid physical strain at time of conception to aid implantation of the fertilized egg.

Herbal, Superfood and Supplement Therapy

Interceptive therapy plan: Choose 2 to 3 recommendations.

1—**Traditional help for threatened miscarriage:** In every case, ask your healthcare provider or midwife first. •Have the woman lie very still and give a cup of *false unicorn* tea every ½ hour. As hemorrhaging decreases, give the tea every hour, then every 2 hours. Add 6 *lobelia* extract drops as a relaxer to the last cup. •Or give *wild yam/red raspberry* tea hourly until bleeding is controlled; or give •*hawthorn* extract ½ dropperful and bee pollen 2 tsp. hourly until bleeding is controlled. —**For false labor:** •Magnesium therapy helps reduce false labor. To help stop bleeding, take •2 caps each *cayenne;* or add •*lobelia* (small amounts) and *cayenne* extracts to *nettles* tea. Get to a hospital or call your midwife immediately. •Take Crystal Star MUSCLE RELAXER™ caps 4 at a time, or PMS QUICK RELIEF drops, for pain. •Take *cramp bark* or *scullcap* for afterpain.

2—**To prevent miscarriage:** John Lee M.D. recommends transdermal progesterone 40mg a day to help prevent miscarriage caused by luteal phase failure. After your first month, increase dose gradually to 60mg per day. Ask your healthcare professional. Whole *wild yam* creams and *sarsaparilla* (progesterone activity) may also help prevent miscarriage due to hormonal insufficiency. Consider •Pure Essence FEM CREME, and take emulsified A & D daily. •Selenium deficiency may increase miscarriage risk. Consider •Eidon SELENIUM liquid. Take •Red Raspberry-Catnip tea blend all through pregnancy; and kelp tabs 6 daily. •Vitamin E 400IU and vitamin K 100mcg 2 daily during pregnancy help protect against miscarriage. (Discontinue Vitamin E two weeks before due date.) •*Black haw* tea in small doses throughout pregnancy helps prevent spontaneous abortion.

3—**Tone the uterus:** Use • *squaw vine* and *false unicorn root* as uterine tonics. Use •*Mother-wort* tea to reduce anxiety. Take •vitamin E 100IU with selenium 200mcg. Add •Jarrow GENTLE FIBERS drink daily for tissue strength.

4—**Vitamin C and bioflavonoids can lessen risk of pre-eclampsia:** •Vitamin C or Ester C with bioflavs. and rutin strengthen, 2-3000mg daily. •American Health ACEROLA PLUS with rose hips or •Solaray QBC with bromelain and C.

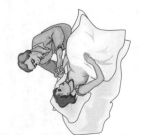

Can't find a recommended product? Call the 800 number listed in Product Resources for the store nearest you.

Mononucleosis

Epstein-Barr Virus Infection

Mononucleosis, a chronic fatigue syndrome, was one of the first acute, infectious diseases to be recognized as an immune-compromised group of symptoms in young adults. Today, mono is associated with the Epstein-Barr virus or the cytomegalovirus (both herpes-type viruses). New Danish studies link mononucleosis infection to increased Hodgkin's disease risk. The virus is virulent and highly infectious. Immune response is very weak. Medical antibiotics are not effective. It's an opportunistic disease allowed by a weak immune system and contagion (often sexual) from an infected carrier; overuse and abuse of pleasure drugs and/or alcohol and consequent liver malfunction. Fatigue is long term, even after acute symptoms have been overcome. **Do you have mono?** Symptoms occur in 4 to 7 weeks of exposure. The first symptoms are extreme tiredness, followed by severe flu-like, swollen lymph nodes in the neck, high fever and sore throat, skin rashes or bruises and loss of appetite. Mono is in fact a totally run-down condition - glands, lymph nodes, bronchial tubes, liver and spleen are all greatly debilitated. The spleen enlarges with pain on on the upper left side of the abdomen. The skin is pale, then jaundiced as the liver throws off body poisons. Concentrate your efforts on revitalizing liver, lymph and spleen systems for healing. You'll need at least three months of rebuilding to restore strength. *See LIVER CLEANSING DIET and CHRONIC FATIGUE SYNDROME for more information.*

Diet and Lifestyle Support Therapy

Nutritional therapy plan: Do not fast. Strength and nutrition are too low.

1—High quality vegetable proteins are a key to healing. Begin healing with plenty of cleansing/flushing fruit juices and bottled water for 1 week to relieve fever and sore throat. Key: •Vitamin C powder with bioflavs, ¼ tsp. every 2 hours in water or to bowel tolerance daily for 1 month. Reduce dosage 2nd and 3rd month but continue C program.

2—Particularly use apple/alfalfa sprout, papaya/pineapple, and pineapple/coconut juices for strength and enzyme enhancement. Or consider •Futurebiotics VITAL K drink daily.

3—Follow with a week of green drinks, like Crystal Star ENERGY GREEN RENEWAL™, a potassium broth (pg. 291), and vegetable juices to cleanse, strengthen and rebuild liver function.

4—Eat a diet high in vegetable proteins; (brown rice, tofu, nuts, seeds, sprouts, etc.), and cultured foods: (yogurt, kefir, etc.) for friendly flora.

5—Add vitamin A and vitamin C rich foods, like fruits and vegetables.

6—Take your choice of superfood drinks to be used during entire 3 month healing time. We have used superfoods with success for exceptionally weak conditions like this: •AloeLife ALOE GOLD drink, •Sun Wellness CHLORELLA WAKASA GOLD (excellent results) , •Crystal Star RESTORE YOUR STRENGTH™ drink, •Nutricology PRO-GREENS with EFAs and •Solaray ALFA-JUICE.

—Bodywork:

• Bed rest during the acute stages, and regular mild exercise during the rebuilding stages are critical to successfully overcoming mono.

• Get early morning sunlight on the body every day possible.
• Overheating therapy has been effective for mono in curbing the advance of the virus. See page 183 for correct home technique.
• Biofeedback has also been successful.
• Avoid all pleasure drugs, caffeine and chemical stimulants. These are often the substances that reduce immunity to its infective point.

Herbal, Superfood and Supplement Therapy

Interceptive therapy plan: This program has had notable success.

1—**Address the viral infection:** •Crystal Star ANTI-BIO™ caps or extract, 6x daily for 2 weeks, or VIREX™ (stronger for viruses); •OLIVE LEAF extract and •OREGANO OIL are effective •*Echinacea/goldenseal rt.* and *garlic* clear lymph gland infection. •Crystal Star CLEANSING & PURIFYING™ tea helps normalize blood composition; •Herbalist & Alchemist VX COMPOUND with *lomatium* and *St. John's wort* daily; •Pure Planet RED MARINE ALGAE 4 tabs daily for 1 month (excellent results for EBV). •MICROHYDRIN from royalbodycare.com.

2—**Cleanse and enhance liver and spleen functions:** •Alpha lipoic acid 300-600mg daily, •Crystal Star LIVER RENEW™ caps 6 daily; •MILK THISTLE SEED extract 3-4x daily for 3 months. •Enzymatic Therapy LYMPH-SPLEEN complex.

3—**Rebuild adrenal response:** •Crystal Star ADRENAL ENERGY BOOST™ caps or Planetary SCHIZANDRA ADRENAL COMPLEX; Then add Superior ELEUTHERO Extract for body homeostasis. •Prince of Peace GINSENG-ROYAL JELLY vials.

4—**Re-establish body strength:** •Nutricology GERMANIUM 150mg (noticeable results); •Country Life sublingual B-12, 2500mcg daily for 1 month, then every other day for a month; •Crystal Star FEEL GREAT NOW™ caps 2 daily for 2 months.

5—**Enhance immune response:** •Herbs, Etc. LYMPHATONIC softgels flush lymph glands; •*Siberian eleuthero* extract. •*Astragalus* extract; •*Cordyceps* extract (highly recommended) •Reishi mushroom capsules; •Planetary REISHI MUSHROOM SUPREME. •Biotec CELL GUARD 6 daily. •Nutricology THYMUS ORGANIC GLANDULAR caps; •Enzymatic Therapy THYROID-TYROSINE capsules.

6—**Amino acids, proteolytic enzymes, probiotics help rebuild body essentials:** •Anabol Naturals AMINO BALANCE for critical essential protein. •Bee pollen capsules, 8 daily; •Biotec Pacific SEA PLASMA tabs 10 daily. •Crystal Star DR. ENZYME™ with protease and bromelain; •CoQ10 300mg daily. Add •American Health ACIDOPHILUS LIQUID, or •Nutricology SYMBIOTIC powder, ¼ tsp. in water

Can't find a recommended product? Call the 800 number listed in Product Resources for the store nearest you.

Motion Sickness

Jet Lag, Inner Ear Imbalance

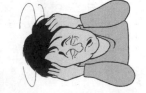

Motion sickness happens when the brain can't respond properly to a motion it doesn't understand. Inner ear imbalance is usually at the root of motion sickness symptoms. (Deaf people do not get motion sickness). Lack of oxygen at heights can play a role. *Jet lag* is the inability of internal body rhythm (circadian rhythm), to resynchronize after sudden shifts in sun time over more than 2 time zones. Our internal clocks are set by hypothalamus-controlled hormonal rhythm and by the pineal gland's sensitivity to light. Our bodies instinctively try to maintain stability by resisting time change, causing psycho-physiological impairment of well-being and performance. Natural remedies are very successful, without the side-effects of standard Dramamine-type drugs. Get enough sleep, don't drink alcohol before traveling. Stay in the center of a boat to minimize the rocking motion. **Do you get motion sickness?** You do if you get an upset stomach, queasiness, a cold sweat and/or vomiting during a vehicle trip; or if you're in a bad mood with increased heart rate, unusual sleepiness, dizziness, and poor appetite while traveling. You're in jet lag if you can't sleep well, are lethargic, dehydrated, and have poor performance after a trip. Within 48 hours of landing, some people experience chronic low-grade fever, cough and headaches. *See also* VERTIGO *and* DIZZINESS *page 557 for more information.*

Diet and Lifestyle Support Therapy

Nutritional therapy plan:

1—Before departure: Take a cup of miso soup with 2 pinches of ginger added, or try 1 tsp. •New Chapter GINGER WONDER syrup; or a bowl of brown rice mixed with 3 tbsp. nutritional yeast; Or take a cup of strong green tea or •Crystal Star DR. VITALITY™ tea.

2—During the trip: Suck on a lemon or lime during the trip whenever queasiness strikes. Munch on soda crackers to soak up excess acids. Take sugar-free, carbonated sodas. Avoid fried, salty, sugary or dairy foods. They can cause digestive imbalance.

3—For jet lag: Drink water, juices and herb teas to combat dehydration on a flight - but avoid alcohol when flying. It can upset nervous system biochemistry. During readjustment, eat high vegetable protein meals when you are trying to stay awake; high carbohydrate meals when you are trying to sleep. Eat complex carbohydrates if you are traveling to high altitudes. For irregularity, have a leafy green salad and an apple every day, or try •Nature's Secret ULTIMATE GREEN tabs, 6 to 10 daily.

4—Boost body stability with fiber. Try •Jarrow GENTLE FIBERS drink before departure.

—Bodywork: During an attack: Massage knee caps for 3 minutes. Massage little finger for 10 minutes. Massage back of head at base of skull, and behind ears on mastoids. Massage legs and extremities frequently on a long plane flights. Breathe deeply for 1 minute. Get fresh air and oxygen as soon as possible.

—For jet lag:
•Take a few drops of •GINGER extract in water for almost immediate relief during or after a flight.
•Shift your sleep/wake cycle in advance to the new time. Schedule a stop-over if you can. On arriving, get in the sunlight to help reset your biological clock.
•Stay away from smoke in the airport. It can keep you toxic for hours.
•Walk about in the plane to promote circulation, prevent blood stagnation.
•Wear a •SpringLife POLARIZER. (Excellent results for chronic sufferers.)

Herbal, Superfood and Supplement Therapy

Interceptive therapy plan: Choose 2 to 3 recommendations.

1—Prepare your body equilibrium before a trip: •Crystal Star GREEN TEA CLEANSER™ each morning for a week before a trip, and during a trip for stomach enzyme balance. •*Ginger* caps, 4 caps before a trip, 2 to 4 during a trip; or *ginger/cayenne* caps (better than Dramamine). •GINKGO BILOBA extract before and during traveling for inner ear balance. •Imperial Elixir SIBERIAN GINSENG 5000 as a preventative. Use for several days before your trip and while you travel; Take •Biotec Foods JET STRESS.

2—Soothe nerve stress, boost your minerals: •Crystal Star OCEAN MINERALS™ caps about a month before a trip for body balance. Take •*Peppermint* or *chamomile* tea; •Crystal Star RELAX™ caps, or •Enzymatic Therapy KAVA-TONE. •Homeopathic Hyland's *Calms Forte.*

3—Ginseng is effective for body balance: •*Siberian eleuthero* extract before and as needed during a trip; •Crystal Star FEEL GREAT NOW! caps as needed. •Chinese *Sheng mai san* to help prevent altitude sickness.

4—B's for better balance: •Vitamin B-1, thiamine 500mg acts like Dramamine before a trip. •Vitamin B-complex 100mg for several weeks prior to travelling, extra folic acid 400mcg; •Country Life sublingual B-12, 2500mcg; or •Nature's Secret ULTIMATE B.

5—Soothe your digestion: •Nutribiotic GRAPEFRUIT SEED extract helps overcome the effects of bad food and water or a trip. •Crystal Star DR. ENZYME™ with protease and bromelain for body balance and inflammation relief.

—For jet lag: Before a long flight: Take •Glutamine 500mg and 1 *echinacea/goldenseal* cap, 2 vitamin C with bioflavonoid tabs, 1 beta-carotene caps, 1 GINKGO BILOBA extract capsule for inner ear balance. •Tyrosine 500mg 2 to 3 daily a few days before a trip and during the trip as needed. •Melatonin therapy: take 3mg before retiring on your trip and for two to three days after for best results. •Medicine Wheel MOTION STOP drops as needed. •Homeopathic Nux vomica for nausea and indigestion. —**During your trip take:** •GINKGO BILOBA extract drops as needed, and •6 vitamin C 500mg chewables with •B-complex 100mg daily.

Can't find a recommended product? Call the 800 number listed in Product Resources for the store nearest you.

Multiple Sclerosis

M.S. and A.L.S. (Amyotrophic Lateral Sclerosis)

For 500,000 Americans, **Multiple Sclerosis** is a progressive, central nervous system disease in which the myelin sheath wrapping the nerves is damaged. Triggered in a strange way by an auto-immune reaction (where the immune system attacks itself) to viruses like herpes or Epstein Barr, the immune system creates antibodies to the brain's myelin which bears an uncanny resemblance to the viruses. Other research links low essential fatty acids to myelin sheath degeneration and MS. (Myelin is naturally high in essential fatty acids.) M.S. must be treated vigorously. A little therapy does not work, but long lasting remission is possible. Natural therapies take 6 months to a year (time well spent as MS drug treatments often fail and have severe side effects). Strong immune defense is essential. **A.L.S. (Lou Gehrig's disease)** is a disease of the skeletal muscle nerves that results in progressive muscle wasting as the muscles lose their nerve supply. Treat both M.S. and A.L.S. for nerve damage first, then work on restoring muscle function and immune health. Transdermal histamine therapy (*Prokarin*) shows good results. *(Contact EDMS at 360-654-0448 or check out www.prokarin.com)* **Are you at risk for M.S?** Initial onset of numbness, tingling and fatigue usually occurs between age 30 and 45, more often in women. Visual loss, preceded by blurring, double-vision and eyeball pain, follows. Breathing difficulty, slurred speech, a staggering gait, tremors, dizziness, and bladder and bowel problems result from paralysis or partial paralysis onset. Men become sexually impotent as nerves degenerate. Symptoms mimic Lyme disease. Malnutrition and stress often precede M.S.

Diet and Lifestyle Support Therapy

Nutritional therapy plan: A healthy diet deters the onset of M.S. attacks.

1—Follow a cleansing diet for 2 months, similar to one for Candida albicans (see pg. 358). Then, follow a modified macrobiotic diet (pg. 348) for 6 months. Take potassium broth (pg. 291) twice a week. Kombucha mushroom drink, along with a mild liver detox has led to marked improvement in several cases because it cleans out trigger toxins. Take •Alpha lipoic acid 300-600mg. •Crystal Star LIVER RENEW™ caps 6 daily and LIVER CLEANSE FLUSHING™ tea and •Vitamin C, ¼ tsp. every hour to bowel tolerance, daily for a month. (Reduce to 5000mg daily after the cleanse). Take a catnip enema or spirulina implant once a week for several months.

2—Reduce saturated fats from red meats and dairy products, and increase healthy essential fatty acids from food like seafoods and sea greens. The diet should be 70-80% fresh foods, with plenty of salads and green drinks,15-20% fresh fruits, and 5-10% vegetable proteins from sprouts, legumes and seeds. Eat fish and sea veggies with a bowl of brown rice every day for B vitamins and EFAs. Also try •Nutricology PROGREENS, or •Crystal Star RESTORE YOUR STRENGTH™ drink with EFAs from sea greens. •Pure Planet CHLORELLA stimulates immune B and T cells.

3—Keep sugar levels low. Avoid all refined and fried foods, full-fat dairy foods, and caffeine foods. Eliminate meats except fish. Reduce high gluten foods. Especially avoid artificial sweeteners (aspartame), and MSG foods. Eliminate pectin-containing candies like gummy bears or fruit jellies.

—**Bodywork:** Sunlight and vitamin D influences the remission of M.S. There are far less incidences of the disease in sun-belt regions. Mild daily exercise, guided imagery, massage therapy and mineral baths are useful.

•Bee venom therapy can produce dramatic results, even in advanced cases. Contact the American Apitherapy Society at 800-832-3460.

•Remove mercury amalgam fillings. •C'est Si Bon CHLORENERGY helps if you have amalgam fillings removed.

Herbal, Superfood and Supplement Therapy

Interceptive therapy plan: Choose 2 to 3 recommendations.

1—**Rebuild strong nerve structure:** •Crystal Star RELAX caps (highly successful). •All One GREEN PHYTOBASE, or Source Naturals MYELIN SHEATH formula with oatseed tea for nerve pain; •*Ashwagandha* drops counter fatigue; •Solaray CENTELLA ASIATICA for nerve repair; •*Ginkgo biloba* extract for tremor and brain boost. •Chondroitin sulfate-A 1200mg for spine help, with magnesium 400mg 3x daily; •Pacific Biologic ADAPTRIN; •Jarrow GENTLE FIBERS drink helps nerve tissue.

2—**Preserve brain cells with amino acid therapy:** •NADH, 10mg in the morning; •Phosphatidyl serine 300mg daily/ 3 months; •Lysine 500mg daily; •Acetyl-Carnitine 1000mg; •Country Life AMINO MAX •Threonine for spasticity. •CoQ$_{10}$, 260mg daily. —**For** •MICROHYDRIN available from royalbodycare.com. •Glutathione 100mg daily. **A.L.S:** Amino acid therapy may slow deterioration rate up to 75% (better than drugs). I recommend a full spectrum formula like •Anabol Naturals AMINO BALANCE 3x daily.

3—**Essential fatty acids a key:** •EVENING PRIMROSE OIL caps 4-6; •Nature's Secret ULTIMATE OIL or Omega-3 rich flax oil 3x daily. •Green Foods WHEAT GERM extract with EFAs; •Crystal Star PRO-EST BALANCE™ a wild yam source for hormone balance; •DHA 200mg daily, or Source Naturals FOCUS DHA, with •Beta carotene 150,000IU. •EGG YOLE LECITHIN and cold water fish oils 3x daily, for M.S.-related eye damage. Use enzyme therapy for inflammation: •Transformation PUREZYME or Crystal Star DR. ENZYME™ with protease and bromelain.

4—**Boost B-vitamins and minerals:** •Sublingual B-12, 2500mcg 2 daily for 1 month w. GERMANIUM 150mg, then every other day for 2 months; •Nature's Secret Ultimate B or B-complex 150mg daily; •extra folic acid 400mcg 2x daily. •Niacin therapy: 500mg 3x daily, with B$_6$ 500mg. •Crystal Star CALCIUM MAGNESIUM SOURCE™ caps with sea greens or •Lane Labs ADVACAL ULTRA with vitamin D. •CC Pollen ROYAL JELLY 2 tsp.

5—**Enhance the adrenals:** •Vitamin K 100mcg daily; •American Biologics SUB-ADRENE; •Crystal Star ADRENAL ENERGY BOOST with sea greens.

Can't find a recommended product? Call the 800 number listed in Product Resources for the store nearest you.

Muscle Cramps, Spasms, Twitches

Leg Cramps and Restless legs

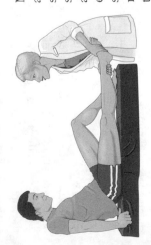

Muscle spasms, cramps, twitches and tics are usually a result of vitamin and mineral deficiencies or imbalances. Most cramping occurs at night as minerals move between the blood, muscles and bones. A good diet and natural supplements have been very successful in fortifying and strengthening the body against nutrient shortages. Improvement is noticeable within two weeks. Acupressure is highly successful. See Acupressure page 33 in this book. **What causes muscle cramps?** Metabolic insufficiency of calcium, magnesium, potassium, iodine, trace minerals, and vitamins E, D and B$_6$; lack of sufficient HCL in the stomach. Vitamin C and silicon deficiency causes poor collagen formation, vital to muscle elasticity. Food allergies to preservatives and colorants may be involved. Note: If you take high blood pressure medicine and have continuing muscle spasms, ask your doctor to change your prescription. Some have sodium imbalance that upsets mineral salts in the body. Leg cramps are usually the result of poor circulation. **Do you get frequent muscle cramps, pulls and spasms?** Leg cramps are uncontrollable, very painful spasms and twitches, especially acute at night. Facial tics are embarrassing muscle twitches, etc. *See also SPORTS INJURIES page 551 for more information.*

Diet and Lifestyle Support Therapy

Nutritional therapy plan:

1—Eat vitamin C-rich foods: leafy greens, citrus fruits, especially kiwi, brown rice, sprouts, broccoli, tomatoes, bell peppers, etc.

2—Eat potassium-rich foods; bananas, broccoli, sunflower seeds, beans and legumes, whole grains and dried fruits. Or try •Futurebiotics VITAL K 3 tsp. daily.

3—Add 2 tbsp. sea greens daily for iodine and potassium - a difference in about a week. Or try •Sun Wellness CHLORELLA with 1 tsp. kelp or •Crystal Star RESTORE YOUR STRENGTH™ drink with sea greens, or •Rainbow Light HAWAIIAN SPIRULINA.

4—Eat magnesium-rich foods; lettuce, bell pepper, green leafy vegetables, molasses, nuts and seafoods. Take a veggie drink like Knudsens VERY VEGGIE 2x a week. Or try •Green Foods GREEN MAGMA/ barley grass, or •Green Kamut JUST BARLEY. •Crystal Star ENERGY GREEN RENEWAL™ drink (works well for men).

5—Muscles need healthy fluids to contract and relax. (Penta water is a favorite.) Take an electrolyte drink, like Knudsen's RECHARGE for good mineral salts transport.

6—Avoid refined sugars, processed and preserved foods. Food sensitivities to these substances are often the cause of twitches and spasms.

—Bodywork:

•Aromatherapy: apply rosemary or juniper essential oils.

•Vinegar or Epsom salts baths (2 cups to bath water), or apply a hot salt pack. Heat sea salt in pan, funnel into an old sock; apply to affected area.

•Topical applications: —*Arnica* gel; —*Lobelia* extract.

•For leg cramps: Massage legs; elevate the feet; slap soles and legs with palm to stimulate circulation. Take brisk walk every day to relieve leg cramps at night.

•Use alternating hot and cold hydrotherapy, or hot and cold compresses applied to the area to ease pain, promote circulation and healing.

•Shiatsu and massage therapy are effective in re-aligning the body's "electrical" impulses, and relieving muscle cramps.

Herbal, Superfood and Supplement Therapy

Interceptive therapy plan: Choose 2 to 3 recommendations.

1—**Reduce cramping:** •Crystal Star MUSCLE RELAXER™ caps 4 at a time, or STRESS OUT™ muscle relaxer extract (usually results in 25 minutes). •Alacer EMERGEN-C drink (very fast and effective); •*Lobelia* extract drops for cramping; •*Valerian*-wild lettuce or Medicine Wheel SERENE drops calm muscle spasms; •Floradix HERBAL IRON for leg cramps. —**Homeopathic remedies for muscles:** •Hyland's Mag Phos to reduce pain. •Arnica Montana tincture and ointment for recovery.

2—**Reduce inflammation:** •Crystal Star DR. ENZYME™ with protease and bromelain; •Quercetin 1000mg with bromelain 1500mg; •Acetyl-L-Carnitine 1000mg daily. •Glucosamine-chondroitin, 6 daily; •Nuricology ENZOCAINE, Source Naturals INFLAMAREST (excellent results) •Crystal Star ANTI-FLAM™ caps, 4 at a time as needed.

3—**Reduce pain and aches:** •MSM caps 800mg daily or •Trimedica MSM caps; Crystal Star •*Ginseng-licorice* extract, (cortisone-like properties without side effects).

—For men: •Country Life LIGATEND as needed (very effective), •MAXI-B COMPLEX w. taurine; Nature's Path CAL-LYTE with electrolytes; •Magnesium-potassium-bromelain 3 daily, with •zinc 75mg, and chromium 100mcg to rebuild muscle strength.

—For women: •Solaray CAL/MAG CITRATE 4-6 daily, with vitamin D 1000IU; •Magnesium 400mg 2x daily or •Ethical Nutrients MALIC/MAGNESIUM to alleviate tender points; •CoQ-10, 60mg 3x daily.

4—**Restore nerve health:** •Crystal Star RELAX CAPS™ daily 4 to 6. •EVENING PRIMROSE OIL 4 daily for EFAs; •*Passionflower* or *Scullcap* tea as needed.

5—**Help rebuild strong muscle tissue:** •Crystal Star IODINE, POTASSIUM, SILICA drops or •Flora VEGE-SIL silica caps 3-4 daily for collagen and tissue regeneration; •*Horsetail/oatstraw* tea; •Solaray ALFA-JUICE caps. •Vitamin C or Ester C, up to 5000mg daily with bioflavonoids for collagen formation.

—For leg cramps at night: •B-complex 100mg daily, with extra B$_6$ 250mg and pantothenic acid 250mg for nerve repair. Take extra B$_6$ before bed at night as needed; •Calcium/Magnesium 1000/500mg; or •Flora MAGNESIUM liquid; •Vitamin E 400IU; •PCO's 100mg daily; Futurebiotics VITAL K with magnesium.

Can't find a recommended product? Call the 800 number listed in Product Resources for the store nearest you.

Muscular Dystrophy and Myasthenia Gravis

Muscle Wasting Diseases, Facial Tics (Bell's Palsy), Spina Bifida

Muscular dystrophy is severe weakening of muscle and nerve growth due to abnormal childhood development. MD affects mostly very young children, where muscle and nerve degeneration prohibits their ability to support body weight. **Myasthenia gravis**, largely a woman's problem, is a debilitating muscle and immune disorder, where immune antibodies turn against normal tissue. Myasthenia gravis is characterized by progressive fatigue, exhaustion and paralysis, beginning with muscles and nerves of the lips, tongue and face. Emergency symptoms include great difficulty breathing and swallowing. **Bell's palsy** is a facial nerve disorder beginning with muscle weakness (sometimes from an infection) on one side of the face and the inability to close one eye. **Spina bifida** involves a genetic defect in nerve development of the spinal column. Children born with spina bifida have poor motor ability, and essentially paralyzed from the waist down. **Muscle wasting symptoms?** All show noticeable muscle and nerve weakness and atrophy, tremor, palsy, especially a degenerating ability to walk, with falling and stumbling. Poor reflexes, chronic constipation (which keeps toxins in the body) and some loss of bladder control are usual. There may be mild mental retardation. **What causes muscle wasting?** Muscular dystrophies and spina bifida may result from a defective gene, or a folic acid or other micronutrient deficiency in the mother during pregnancy. Myasthenia gravis relates to a body chemistry deficiency like choline or prostaglandins between nerves and muscles causing poor neurotransmission and chronic blood sugar imbalances.

Diet and Lifestyle Support Therapy

Nutritional therapy plan: Natural therapies have been successful in increasing nutrient assimilation, in overcoming EFA deficiency, in rebuilding nerve and muscle tissue, and sometimes in arresting progressive muscle wasting. Remission shows marked success from an improved diet.

1—Avoid nightshade plants: tomatoes, eggplant, white potatoes, green peppers, etc.

2—Eat vitamin C-rich foods; leafy greens, citrus fruits, brown rice, sprouts, broccoli, or add •Aloe Life ALOE GOLD drink.

3—Eat potassium-rich foods; bananas, broccoli, sunflower seeds, beans and legumes, whole grains and dried fruits.

4—Add sea greens daily for iodine and potassium. See a difference in about a week

5—Eat magnesium-rich foods; lettuce, bell pepper, green leafy vegetables, molasses, nuts and seafoods. Take a mixed veggie drink 2x a week. Or try some green superfood-veggie drinks like •Crystal Star ENERGY GREEN RENEWAL™ with barley grass, •Fit for You, Intl. MIRACLE GREENS, Green Kamut JUST BARLEY, Sun Wellness CHLORELLA packets or tabs. We've seen All One GREEN PHYTOBASE drink help against pain.

6—Take 2 tsp. wheat germ oil daily in juice or water.

—Bodywork:

•Avoid smoking, secondary smoke, and oxygen-depleting pollutants as much as possible to lessen breathing problems.

•Get some mild outdoor exercise every day for fresh air, and aerobic lung and muscle tone.

•Relaxation techniques like yoga and foot massage are especially helpful because stress aggravates myasthenia gravis symptoms.

•Overall body massage therapy and shiatsu are both effective in increasing oxygen use and strengthening nerves and muscles (excellent results for several symptoms in these diseases).

Herbal, Superfood and Supplement Therapy

Interceptive therapy plan: Choose 2 to 3 recommendations.

1—**Help rebuild stronger muscles:** •MSM caps 800mg daily or •Futurebiotics MSM caps with chromium picolinate 200mcg; or •MSM with MICROHYDRIN from royal-health. com. •Crystal Star RELAX CAPS™ 6 daily as needed (good response activity).

2—**Balance thyroid action for rapid improvement:** •Pure Essence FEM CREME as directed, with a thyroid booster like •Enzymatic Therapy THYROID/TYROSINE. Add •Crystal Star OCEAN MINERALS™ caps for more thyroid help. •Country Life DMG sublingual.

3—**EFAs help repair neurotransmitters and nerves:** •EVENING PRIMROSE OIL caps 4000mg daily; •NADH - 10mg in the morning; •EGG YOLK LECITHIN (excellent results). •Choline 600mg, •Phosphatidyl choline (PC 55), or •Phosphatidyl serine (PS) 100mg 3 daily/3 months, or •DHA 200mg daily with magnesium 400mg 3x daily; •High potency royal jelly 40-50,000mg daily. •Biotec PACIFIC SEA PLASMA tabs 8 daily; •Glycine 500mg daily.

4—**Increase circulation:** •GINKGO BILOBA extract 3x daily for muscle tremor. Apply •cayenne and ginger compresses to affected areas to help prevent atrophy or *cayenne/ginger* capsules 2 at a time as needed. •SIBERIAN ELEUTHERO extract 3-4x daily.

5—**Relieve pain:** •Baywood TOPICAL SUPER COOL RELIEF™ (helps muscle tics, too); •Acetyl-L-Carnitine 1000mg daily. •Glucosamine-chondroitin, 1500/1200mg 6 daily; •Vitamin E 800mg. •Biochemics PAIN RELIEF lotion.

6—**Proper elimination is important to release toxins:** •Crystal Star FIBER & HERBS COLON CLEANSE™ caps 4-6 daily for 3 weeks.

7—**Add magnesium and B-vitamins:** •Magnesium 400mg 2x daily or •Ethical Nutrients MALIC/MAGNESIUM to alleviate tender points; •B-complex 150mg 3x daily, or •Nature's Secret ULTIMATE B; •Solaray 2000mcg B_{12} or •Source Naturals Dibencozide 10,000mcg. Or try •Prince of Peace AMERICAN GINSENG-BEE POLLEN-ROYAL JELLY vials (noticeable difference).

8—**For eye tics:** CoQ$_{10}$, 100mg daily, or Douglas Labs CoQMELT chewables.

Can't find a recommended product? Call the 800 number listed in Product Resources for the store nearest you.

Nails

Nail Health and Nail Fungus

Nails are wonderfully useful as an "early warning system" to diagnose illness and evaluate health. If the eyes are the "windows of the soul," the nails are the "windows of the body." One of the last body areas to receive nutrients carried by the blood, nails show signs of trouble before other, better-nourished tissues do. Healthy nails are pink, smooth and shiny.

Nail Signs: *White spots:* zinc or thyroid deficiency; *White bands or ridged nails:* zinc, iron or protein deficiency, injury; *Discolored nails:* vitamin B_{12} deficiency, kidney or liver problems; *Yellow nails:* vitamin E deficiency; poor circulation, lymph congestion, too much polish, possible diabetes or lung disease; *Green Nails:* fungal infection; *Blue nails:* lung, heart problems, drug reaction, silver or copper toxicity; *No half moons:* vitamin A deficiency, kidney disorder; *Split, peeling nails:* Vitamin A & D, iron, calcium, biotin or HCl deficiency; poor circulation, thyroid problems, drug reaction; *Hang nails:* folic acid deficiency; *Poor shape:* iron-zinc deficiency; *Spoon-shaped nails:* anemia, B_{12} deficiency; *Pitted nails:* alopecia, vitamin C or protein deficiency; *Raised nails:* fungal infection, drug reaction, thyroid problems; *Hammered looking nails:* hair loss; *Down-curving nails:* heart and liver disorders; *White nails with pink tips:* liver cirrhosis; *Pale pink/half white:* possible anemia, kidney failure; *Brown Nails:* psoriasis; *Red Nails:* vascular disease; *Slow growing:* diabetes, respiratory problems.

Diet and Lifestyle Support Therapy

Nutritional therapy: *Most nail problems are diet-related. Blood, gland, and organ disorders as well as nutritional deficiencies show up in nail conditions.*

1—Good nutrition is the key for nail health. Give your program a month to show improvement. Nothing seems to happen for 3 weeks; noticeable changes appear in the 4th week. Give yourself 3 to 6 months to achieve nail health.

2—Eat vegetable protein and calcium foods to strengthen nails - whole grains, sprouts, leafy greens, molasses, and seafood. For basic "green," use •Pure Planet CHLORELLA.

3—Eat sulphur-and-silicon-rich foods, like onions, sea vegetables, broccoli and fish.

4—For splitting nails; take 2 tbsp. •Red Star NUTRITIONAL YEAST for B vitamins, or 2 tsp. wheat germ oil daily for a month. For weak, peeling nails; soak daily for 5 minutes in warm olive oil or cider vinegar. For brittle nails: massage castor oil into nails.

5—For discolored nails, rub lemon juice on nail base. Take papaya enzymes daily. White vinegar removes dark polish stains. Use just once a week to avoid drying nails out.

6—For color and texture; mix honey, avocado oil, egg yolk, and a pinch of salt. Rub on nails. Leave on ½ hour. Rinse off. Mix and apply a •mud face mask in water

—Bodywork:

• Nail enamels are among the most toxic environmental polluters. Fake nails or tips add weight to the nails and prevent them from thickening naturally. Don't keep nails constantly polished. Allow them to breathe at least 1 day a week. Nail color dyes penetrate the nail to the skin, often causing allergic reactions. A simple manicure without polish - with beeswax spread on the nails, then buffed to a shine leaves nails naturally beautiful.

• To tint nails naturally: make a thin paste of red henna powder and water. Paint on and let dry in the sun. Rinse off for long lasting, pretty pink nails with no chipping.

•Sunny Brae Bodyworks NAIL CUTICLE OIL with neem (good, fast results).

• A paraffin hand dip restores nail and skin elasticity. When wax hardens, put on old mittens or socks for ten minutes. (Wax does not adhere.) Peel off for satiny hands and feet.

•Acupressure treatment: Press 3x for 10 seconds on the moon of each nail to stimulate circulation and bring up color.

Herbal, Superfood and Supplement Therapy

Interceptive therapy plan: *If both toenails and fingernails look bad, it's probably an internal condition. Changes in shape, color, texture reflect skin or nail diseases.*

1—**Plant minerals - the best choice for nails:** Silica is key: For 2 months, take •*Horsetail* or *dandelion* tea or extract 3x daily; or •Flora VEGESIL caps or Eidon SILICA liquid; •Body Essentials SILICA GEL. •Trace Mineral Research CONCENTRACE.
•Futurebiotics HAIR, SKIN and NAILS tabs. •Nature's Path TRACE-MIN-LYTE. •Rainbow Light Hawaiian SPIRULINA for zinc.

—**Mineral nail soaks for strength** *(may also be taken internally):* •*Dulse-oatstraw* tea; •*Pau d'arco* tea; •*Kelp* tea, take 6-8 tabs daily.

2—**Strengthen, grow nails:** •Lane Labs TOKI collagen drink (outstanding). Barielle NAIL STRENGTHENER CREAM (made to strengthen horse hooves, great for nails).
•Crystal Star OCEAN MINERALS™ caps or •MSM 4000mg daily for 6 weeks; •Nature's Plus ULTRA NAILS with biotin 600mcg daily for split nails.

3—**EFAs nourish nails:** •Evening primrose or borage oil caps 4 daily. •Crystal Star BEAUTIFUL HAIR & NAILS™ caps.

4—**For nail fungus:** Apply •castor oil or •tea tree oil daily for 6 weeks; soak nails in •Nutribiotic GRAPEFRUIT SEED extract solution, 4 drops in 8-oz. water until fungus clears (4 weeks). Mix •BORIC ACID with water to a paste, paint on nails only (not skin) with Q-Tip, leave on overnight. Massage in •oregano oil; or use •1 part diluted DMSO solution mixed with ½ part each oregano oil and olive oil. Take •Pure Essence FLORALIVE with CANDEX or Crystal Star CANDIDA YEAST DETOX™ caps or *Bloodroot* caps. *Note:* prescription Griseofulvin™ tabs for nail fungus can affect liver function.

—**For nail problems:** •Zinc 50mg daily for spots/poor growth. Apply •Vitamin E oil or jojoba oil for broken or hang nails; •Vitamin A & D for poor growth, ridges and crusty skin around nails; •Biotin 600mcg 4 daily and vitamin A oil for brittleness, splitting or white spots; •Raw thyroid extract for spots or chipping; •A green clay poultice draws out a nail infection; •use wild alum (*cranesbill* herb) paste with water to relieve inflammation from ingrown or hangnails.

Can't find a recommended product? Call the 800 number listed in Product Resources for the store nearest you.

Narcolepsy

Chronic Sleeping Disorder, Sleeping Sickness

Narcolepsy is a neurological sleep disorder involving sleep-wake mechanisms in the brain. Victims are unable to control their sleep spells, and suddenly fall asleep, sometimes in dangerous situations like driving. Sleeping attacks are erratic, recurrent, overwhelming, and can happen at any time - day or night, no matter what the person is doing. Sufferers are easily awakened, although they fall asleep again within an hour or two. Narcoleptics may also experience complete loss of muscle control. There may be up to 200,000 people in the U.S. with narcolepsy (men and women equally). Symptom onset generally occurs between the ages of 10-20 years. **Do you have narcolepsy?** Symptoms usually begin during the teens with uncontrolled, excessive drowsiness, inappropriate, erratic periods of sleep and longer than normal sleep during regular sleep hours. There is loss of muscle control (cataplexy) when awake sometimes triggered by strong emotions. Some have nightmare-like sleep paralysis, unable to move while awake. Some have memory loss or dream-like hallucinations. **What causes narcolepsy?** Symptom onset generally occurs between the ages of 10-20 years, and a type involving a B_6 deficiency of the dopaminergic system and poor use of body oxygen. There are two types of the disorder - DDD (dopamine dependent depression), irregular work/sleep schedules that throw off the body clock, coupled with hypoglycemia or food allergies, vitamin B_6 or tyrosine deficiency, and poor thyroid function. Chronic stress, accompanying poor brain and adrenal function, are factors that often lead to depression. See FOOD ALLERGY page 311, HYPOGLYCEMIA page 463 and THYROID HEALTH page 464 for more.

Diet and Lifestyle Support Therapy

Nutritional therapy plan:

1—Food allergies are thought to be involved with narcolepsy. See FOOD ALLERGY page 311. A rotation/elimination diet may be helpful. See a nutritional health professional, and start by eliminating common allergens like wheat, corn, potatoes, and dairy foods.

2—The diet should be low in fats and clogging foods, such as dairy products and animal proteins; high in light cleansing foods, such as leafy greens and sea vegetables, or add •Biotec PACIFIC SEA PLASMA tabs 8 daily (good results).

3—Eat nutritional yeast and foods high in B vitamins, like brown rice regularly.

4—Eat tyrosine-rich foods: wheat germ, poultry, oats, eggs for better brain connection.

—Superfood therapy: Choose one or two recommendations.
•Sun Wellness CHLORELLA 2pkts daily for natural germanium.
•Nature's Life SUPER GREEN PRO-96, or Nutricology PRO-GREENS, with EFAs.
•Pure Planet SPIRULINA.

—Bodywork:
•Establish circadian rhythms (day/night) for your body. Regular sleep habits are important for a person with narcolepsy. Soothing chamomile aromatherapy or lavender baths can help at first. Apply •Rosemary aromatherapy applied on the temples.

•Take regular daily exercise for circulation and tissue oxygen.
•Biofeedback and chiropractic adjustment are effective in correcting the "electrical -shorts" involved in brain-to-motor transmission.
•Hallucinations and dreams are so real in narcolepsy that the person often cannot tell fantasy from reality. Avoid hallucinogenic drugs - they aggravate frightening nightmares and the experience of sleep paralysis where a narcoleptic person is unable to move even though awake. Sometimes a dangerous panic reaction sets in.

Herbal, Superfood and Supplement Therapy

Interceptive therapy plan: Choose 2 to 3 recommendations.

1—Boost circulation to the brain: •Ginkgo biloba extract or •Wakunaga GINKGO BILOBA PLUS as needed; Rainbow Light GINKGO SUPERCOMPLEX.

2—Ginseng helps regulate sleep patterns and are key brain nutrients: •Crystal Star FEEL GREAT NOW™ caps with ginseng are effective. •Ginseng/licorice extract helps balance critical sugar use; (•chromium picolinate 200mcg daily, and •Magnesium 800mg daily also regulate sugar); or use •SIBERIAN ELEUTHERO extract drops or •Imperial Elixir SIBERIAN GINSENG and •Prince of Peace GINSENG-ROYAL JELLY vials.

3—Normalize serotonin levels: •St. John's wort extract as needed; •Enzymatic Therapy TYROID/TYROSINE caps, 4 daily as an anti-depressant (good results). •For bad moods, add 5-HTP 50mg at night for serotonin connection. •Stress B-complex 150mg daily, with extra B_6 200mg daily; or •Anabol Naturals AMINO BALANCE; •Country Life AMINO MAX caps with B_6 daily for at least 2 months for additional brain protein.

4—EFAs help body "electrical" alignment and neurotransmission: •EVENING PRIMROSE OIL caps 4-6 daily; •Omega 3 flax oils 3-4x daily; •EGG YOLK LECITHIN 2-3x daily (excellent results). •Choline 600mg, or Phosphatidyl serine (PS) 100mg 3 daily/ 3 months; •High potency royal jelly 40-50,000mg 2 tsp. daily; •Glycine 500mg daily.

5—Normalize body chemistry: •Maitake Products, Inc. REISHI caps; ginseng-gotu kola caps 4 daily; •MICROHYDRIN from Royal Bodycare as directed.

6—Antioxidants are critical for brain balance, energy: •Alpha Lipoic Acid neutralizes toxins, recycles glutathione for better use, (or take •Glutathione 100mg daily). •NADH 5 to 15mg daily; •Nutricology GERMANIUM 150mg; •CoQ_{10} 200mg daily; (Take with vitamin E 400IU for best results.) •PCOs 100mg 4x daily; •Country Life DMG B_{15} daily, or •Unipro DMG liquid, under the tongue.

7—Support thyroid and adrenals: •Crystal Star THYROID META-MAX™ or •OCEAN MINERALS™ caps with ADRENAL ENERGY BOOST™ 2 each daily •Enzymatic Therapy ADRENAL COMPLEX.

Can't find a recommended product? Call the 800 number listed in Product Resources for the store nearest you.

Nausea

Vomiting, Upset Stomach, Morning Sickness, Infant Colic

Nausea can be caused by many factors - motion sickness, vertigo, exposure to toxic chemicals, even psychological shocks. Over 50% of pregnant women experience frequent morning sickness nausea during the first trimester. While pregnancy's sudden hormone and metabolic changes are a big contributor to morning sickness, soothing natural treatments can lessen its severity. Infant colic and nausea causes from allergic reactions, infection or nervous reactions can also be helped with natural, soothing therapies. **Are you nauseated?** Morning Sickness: nausea and vomiting morning or night during the first trimester of pregnancy; gland and hormone upset causing digestive imbalance; sensitivity to food substances. Colic: Excess gas and abdominal discomfort; incessant crying; burping; hiccups. **Why are you nauseated?** Morning Sickness: gland and hormone imbalance as the body adjusts to a new biorhythm. For infants: mother's acidity during breast feeding; mineral deficiency in the milk formula; introduction of protein foods too soon (may form lifelong allergies); colic if poor food absorption. Unidentified nausea: congested liver if yellow bile is vomited; enzyme deficiency; candida albicans yeast; low blood sugar; chronic constipation, or poor food combining. *See MOTION SICKNESS page 500 for more.*

Diet and Lifestyle Support Therapy

Nutritional therapy plan:

—**For nausea:** A 24 hour diet of plenty of mild liquids and herb teas. Mix ¼ tsp. baker's yeast in warm water to quell non-pregnancy nausea. Take lemon and maple syrup in water. Cultured foods like yogurt or Rejuvenative Foods VEGI-DELITE.

—**For morning sickness:** Keep soda crackers or dry toast by the bed; take before rising to soak up excess acids; eat ice chips to calm spasms; drink a little fresh juice for alkalinity. Cucumbers soaked in water and eaten relieve stomach congestion fast.

For breakfast: slowly sip orange juice or ginger ale sweetened with honey; then a little bran cereal. Or take vanilla yogurt in the morning; friendly flora settles digestive imbalance.

Daily: take 2 tbsp. nutritional yeast flakes in juice or on a salad for absorbable, non-toxic B vitamins. Get fiber from vegetables and whole grains to keep bowels clean and flowing.

—**For colic:** A nursing baby's digestion is dependent on yours. Avoid cabbage, brussels sprouts, onions, garlic, yeast breads, chocolate, fried or fast foods. Refrain from red meat, alcohol, refined sugar and caffeine until a colick-y child's digestion improves. Give a catnip enema once a week, or as needed - instant gas release. For chronic colic: usually indicates a dairy allergy. Reconsider cow's milk - goat's milk or soy milk are better alternatives. Give papaya or apple juice.

—**For simple nausea:** •Massage the abdomen with aromatherapy oils like peppermint, chamomile or lavender. •Mix pinches from your spice cupboard in a cup of water - nutmeg, ginger, cinnamon, turmeric, basil, mace, etc. Drink straight down.

—**Bodywork for morning sickness:**

•Deep breathing exercises every morning, and a brisk deep breathing walk every day for body oxygen.

•Acupressure points: Press the hollow of each elbow 3x for 10 seconds each.

•Biofeedback and hypnotherapy have been effective. See a qualified chiropractor or massage therapist, esp. if nerve reactions are part of the cause.

•Soft classical or new age music in the morning help calm you and the baby.

Herbal, Superfood and Supplement Therapy

Interceptive therapy plan: Choose 1 or 2 recommendations.

—**For morning sickness:** Take •*ginger* caps or extract on rising, or make *ginger* tea or •*ginger/peppermint* tea (or homemade ginger ale), sip slowly with crackers. •Acidophilus powder, ¼ tsp. 3x daily, or •chewable papaya enzymes to settle gastrointestinal imbalance. •Stress B complex 50mg daily, with •magnesium 400mg. •Vitamin B₆ shots are sometimes effective for severe morning sickness.

—Rebalance your hormones: •Earth Mama Angel Baby HEARTBURN tea daily; or •red raspberry tea daily. (Helpful all during pregnancy). •Y.S. ROYAL JELLY, one tsp. each morning on rising.

—Decongest your liver: •MILK THISTLE SEED extract; •*Dandelion/yellow dock* root tea. •*Rose hips* tea daily. •*Catnip* tea with 1 goldenseal cap on rising.

—**For nausea:** •New Chapter GINGER WONDER syrup does wonders for any kind of stomach upset; or make a •*ginger* tea or •*ginger/peppermint* tea and drink slowly with crackers. Other anti-nausea teas: •*Peppermint* or *spearmint* tea with a pinch of ginger, or •*catnip/peppermint* tea; •*sweet basil* tea, or •*alfalfa/mint* tea. Take ¼ tsp. umeboshi plum paste, especially from over-indulgence in sweet, rich foods. •Activated charcoal tabs 500-1000mg as needed. •Vitamin B₆ 50-100mg daily; •Acidophilus powder - ¼ tsp. 3x daily, or chewable papaya enzymes to settle gastrointestinal imbalance. •Homeopathic Nat. Sulph.; Nux Vomica.

—**For infant colic:** •Apply warm ginger compresses to the stomach and abdomen; •give very dilute *fennel* tea or *catnip* tea, 1 tsp. in water with a little maple syrup. •Natren LIFE START ¼ tsp. in water or juice 2-3x daily, or •Solaray BIFIDO-BACTERIA powder for infants; •Solaray BABY LIFE for mineral and B Complex deficiency; •Hylands Homeopathic Colic or Mag. Phos. tabs; •small doses of papaya enzymes dissolved in juice. •B-complex liquid for children, dilute doses in water about once a week.

Can't find a recommended product? Call the 800 number listed in Product Resources for the store nearest you.

Nerve Problems

Nervous Tension, Anxiety, Numbness

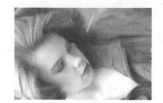

Along with the brain, your nervous system is the chief (and first) means of receiving input messages from your body and the outside world. Beyond our world of frayed nerves, poor nerve health can spawn a host of physical disorders — Alzheimer's and Parkinson's disease, inflammatory meningitis, loss of, or impaired muscular movement and control. The nervous system also affects mental balance - weak nerves result in neurosis, tension or anxiety. **Do you have nerve health problems?** Extreme nervousness and irritability, the inability to relax (usually with back pain), yet with lack of energy; chronic headaches and stiff neck, dizziness, heart palpitations often with high blood pressure may mean you do. Some people experience periodic numbness in various parts of the body; hands, and fingers may itch, toes may "go to sleep" or tingle. Temporo-mandibular joint misalignment (TMJ) is common. Some people have double vision or a blind spot in the visual field. **What causes nerve problems?** Beyond damage from stroke, M.S., a blow or an accident like a whiplash injury or a pinched nerve; poor circulation, thyroid dysfunction and psychic inhibitions can all figure in. Too many chemicalized foods, especially sugars, unrelieved mental or emotional stress, metabolic imbalance from an infection may be involved. Bottle fed babies have a 46% higher risk of developing neurologic abnormalities than breast-fed babies. See Parkinson's Disease page 320 and Diabetic Neuropathy page 393 for more.

Diet and Lifestyle Support Therapy

Nutritional therapy plan:

1—Diet improvement is a key to nerve health: If your nerves are damaged, try a short 24 hour liquid diet. Include high chlorophyll green drinks like carrot/celery juice for nerve restoration, Crystal Star ENERGY GREEN RENEWAL™, or Green Foods GREEN MAGMA for nerve restoration. Make a mix of nutritional yeast, kelp granules and unsulphured molasses and add 2 tsp. to any drink for absorbable B vitamins. Then, eat only fresh foods for 3 days to alkalize and clean the blood. Drink 2 cups green tea daily or Crystal Star DR. VITALITY™ green and white tea blend (excellent for anxiety reactions). Then add lightly cooked foods to your 75% fresh foods diet for the rest of the week.

2—For 3 months: add regularly, high fiber foods, B vitamin foods like nutritional yeast (or Biostrath LIQUID YEAST), miso soup, bee pollen, 2 tsp. daily, brown rice, leafy greens, whole grains, (or wheat germ oil 1 tsp. daily, or •Green Foods WHEAT GERM ESSENCE). and sulfur foods like onions, garlic, oat bran, lettuce, cucumbers and celery. Have a daily green salad every day for magnesium. Keep your diet low in salt and saturated fats. Avoid red meats, caffeine, sodas (the phosphorus binds up magnesium, making it unavailable). Try •Sunflower seeds and molasses for thiamine and iron.

—Lifestyle measures: •Alcoholic drinks seem to worsen symptoms. •Tobacco and obesity aggravate nerve disorders. Lose weight and stop smoking. •Hot and cold hydrotherapy (pg.185) boosts circulation. Baths with baking soda or sea salt calm jangled nerves. •Aromatherapy nerve relaxers: *lavender, rosemary, cinnamon, peppermint* oils.

—Topical nerve applications: Capsaicin creme; •*Cayenne/ginger* or turmeric compresses; •St. John's wort oil. •Baywood SUPER COOL RELIEF; •B&T TRIFLORA analgesic gel.

—Stress reduction techniques offer excellent results: Biofeedback for neuro-muscular feedback, yoga, acupuncture, massage therapy, shiatsu, and chiropractic adjustment. •A brisk walk with deep breathing every day for body oxygen. •Acupressure sandals help clear reflexology meridians. •Gardening, crossword puzzles, hobbies, artwork, etc. all relieve tension and anxiety. •Laughter is the best relief of all.

Herbal, Superfood and Supplement Therapy

Interceptive therapy plan: Choose 2 to 4 recommendations.

1—Repair and restore nerves: •Crystal Star RELAX CAPS™ 2-4 at a time to rebuild nerves. STRESS OUT™ MUSCLE RELAXER extract (works to calm nerves in 25 minutes); •Deva Flowers ANXIETY drops, or •Pacific BioLogic CHILL OUT caps; •Crystal Star HEARTSEASE-H.B.P.™ caps 4 daily. •Excellent extracts: *Siberian eleuthero, Black Cohosh* and *St. John's wort* help regenerate nerve tissue. •Alpha Lipoic Acid 500mg daily with •*Gotu kola* caps 4 daily for nerve damage repair (excellent results). •Vitamin C 5000mg daily with bioflavs and rutin helps rebuild nerve connective tissue; •Crystal Star DR. ENZYME™ with protease and bromelain eases nerve inflammation pain.

2—Neurotransmitter nutrients calm nerve spasms and tics: •Crystal Star RELAX™ caps with *St. John's wort* (highly successful); •CoQ₁₀ 200mg daily; •*Ginkgo biloba* extract for tremor; •L-Glutamine 1000mg daily. •Chondroitin sulfate-A 1200mg for spine improvement; •Country Life RELAXER with GABA 100mg and taurine, or •Twin Lab GABA PLUS with 500mg GABA; •B-complex 150mg with extra B₆ 500mg daily, if extremities are periodically numb; •Wakunaga NEURO-LOGIC. •Niacin therapy: 500mg daily. •TYROSINE 500mg 2x daily. •Devil's claw extract drops 2x daily (good results).

3—Nerve tonics regenerate nerves: •Crystal Star MENTAL CLARITY™ caps with ginseng and kava. Helpful extracts: •*Siberian eleuthero,* •*Reishi mushroom,* •*Rosemary* or •*Ginkgo Biloba* extract 2x daily for motor nerves; •Country Life MAXI B complex with taurine; •Ester C 3-5000mg daily with bioflavonoids and rutin 500mg each for collagen development. •Helpful teas: *Passionflowers, Catnip, Chamomile* and *Scullcap* tea. •Liddell LETTING GO homeopathic for feelings of overwhelm. •Royal jelly 50,000mg 2tsp. daily.

4—Minerals and EFA's nourish nerves: •Lane Labs ADVACAL ULTRA; •Rainbow Light CALCIUM PLUS with high magnesium, 4 daily; •Crystal Star OCEAN MINERALS with sea greens; •Trace Mineral Research CONCENTRACE; •Nature's Path TRACE-MIN-LYTE daily. EFAs: •Evening Primrose oil 4000mg daily; •Phosphatidyl Choline (PC55); •EGG YOLK LECITHIN 3x daily (excellent results). •DHA 200mg daily with magnesium 1200mg day or; •Biotec PACIFIC SEA PLASMA tabs 8 daily; •Glycine 500mg daily.

Can't find a recommended product? Call the 800 number listed in Product Resources for the store nearest you.

Neuritis

Trigeminal Neuralgia

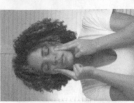

Generally regarded as a syndrome of motor, reflex and sensory nerve symptoms; neuritis (peripheral neuropathy) is an inflammation of a nerve or nerves. It's usually a deterioration process, often part of a chronic, degenerating illness, such as diabetes or leukemia. *Trigeminal neuralgia* is characterized by sudden, sharp, severe pain that shoots along the course of a nerve often as a result of pressure on the nerve trunks, or poor nerve nutrition and an over-acid condition. **Do you have neuritis?** If you have a combination of muscle weakness along with poor muscle reflexes; if you have nerves and muscles that tingle or burn; if you have periodic numbness in the muscles or nerve area; if you have facial tics; nerve inflammation; temporary blindness from optic neuritis.

What contributes to neuritis? Causes are wide ranging... from a pinch or lesions in the spine, to effects of excess alcohol or prescription drugs, to a B-vitamin deficiency (common), to a diabetic neuropathy reaction, to a herpes or shingles infection, to poor circulation, to a multiple sclerosis-type weakness and numbness; to kidney and gallbladder malfunction, to arthritis, lupus, chronic migraines, even heavy metal poisoning. *See Nerve Health on the previous page for more information.*

Diet and Lifestyle Support Therapy

Nutritional therapy plan:

1—Go on a short 24 hour liquid diet (pg. 173) to rebalance body acid/alkaline pH.

2—Then, for the rest of the week eat mostly fresh foods, with plenty of leafy greens, sprouts, celery, sea vegetables, and enzyme foods such as apples and pineapple. Take a glass of lemon juice and water every morning. Have a potassium broth (pg. 291) every other day or •Aloe Life ALOE GOLD drink. •Futurebiotics VITAL K 3 tsp. daily.

3—Make a mix of lecithin granules, sesame seeds, nutritional yeast (or •Biostrath LIQUID YEAST with herbs), and wheat germ; sprinkle 2 tbsp. over food or in a drink daily.

4—Add essential fatty acids from the sea for nerve restoration: seafoods and sea greens daily for 2 months, or •Crystal Star ENERGY GREEN RENEWAL™ drink with sea greens.

5—Keep B-vitamin foods high: like brown rice, bee pollen granules, leafy greens, whole grains or •Prince of Peace GINSENG-ROYAL JELLY vials.

6—Drink 6 glasses of water daily with a slice of lemon, lime or cucumber, or •Crystal Star GREEN TEA CLEANSER™ 2 cups daily. Or try •C'est Si Bon CHLORENERGY daily.

7—Keep salts, saturated fats and sugars low. Avoid caffeine especially (a trigger), hard liquor and soft drinks (bind up magnesium).

—**Topical nerve help applications:** Rub on capsaicin creme, or •Nature's Way CAYENNE PAIN RELIEVING OINTMENT; •*Cayenne/ginger compresses*; •*St. John's wort oil.*
•Apply B&T TRIFLORA analgesic gel.

—**Bodywork:**

•Get some regular mild exercise every day for body oxygen and circulation.
•Use hot and cold hydrotherapy to stimulate circulation (pg. 185).
•Do 10 neck rolls as needed at a time to relieve nerve trauma.
•Stress management techniques should be a part of any healing program.
•Acupuncture, chiropractic adjustment, shiatsu, and massage therapy are all effective in controlling nerve disorders.

Herbal, Superfood and Supplement Therapy

Interceptive therapy plan: Choose 2 or more recommendations.

1—**Help repair and restore nerves:** •Crystal Star RELAX CAPS™ as needed to help rebuild nerve sheath, 4 daily (rapid noticeable results); •Crystal Star OCEAN MINERALS™ caps 2 daily to help restore nerve health. •BILBERRY extract - tissue-toning, flavonoids or •Ascorbate or Ester C with bioflavonoids and rutin, 5000mg daily, to rebuild connective tissue. •Country Life LIGATEND as needed. •Taurine 500mg daily.

2—**Relieve nerve spasms:** •GINKGO BILOBA extract for facial neuralgia; •Crystal Star MUSCLE RELAXER™ caps for spasms pain; •Scullcap tea daily controls facial tics. •DLPA 750mg relieves pain (good results). •Homeopathic: Hylands, Calms Forte or Nerve Tonic.

3—**Reduce nerve inflammation:** •Solaray Curcumin (*turmeric* extract) or •Crystal Star ANTI-FLAM™ caps 4 daily to take down inflammation with Crystal Star DR. EN-ZYME™ with protease and bromelain, or Bromelain 1500mg daily. •Devil's claw extract drops in water daily; •Lane Labs ADVACAL ULTRA with high magnesium, 4-6 daily (good results usually within 2 months); •Quercetin 1000mg; •Homeopathic: *Aranea Diadema* - radiating pain, •Mag. Phos. - spasmodic pain, •Hypericum - heal nerve injury.

4—**Effective herbal nerve tonics:** •Lobelia extract drops (short term); •*Passionflowers* or *scullcap* tea; •*valerian/wild lettuce* extract (powerful nerve relaxant); or make a nerve soothing tea: *St. John's wort, peppermint, lavender, valerian, lemon balm, blessed thistle.* •Niacin therapy: 500-1500mg daily to stimulate circulation.

5—**Essential fatty acids nourish the nervous system:** •Evening Primrose oil 4000mg daily; •Barleans high lignan flax oil, or •Omega Nutrients OMEGA-PLUS caps 3 daily; •Phosphatidyl Choline (PC55); •Nature's Plus EGG YOLK LECITHIN 3x daily.

6—**Strengthen circulation:** •Butcher's broom tea daily for 1 month to clean out circulatory wastes; •GINKGO BILOBA or •HAWTHORN extract, 2 to 4x daily, or •Heart Foods HEART FOOD PLUS; •Cayenne/ginger caps 4 daily, •Metabolic Response Modifiers CARDIOCHELATE with EDTA, a.m. and p.m.

7—**Neural nutrients for long term restoration:** •Country Life sublingual B-12, 2500mcg daily; and •Stress B-complex 100mg with extra B_6 250mg and folic acid 400mcg.

Can't find a recommended product? Call the 800 number listed in Product Resources for the store nearest you.

Osteoporosis

Osteomalacia, Ankylosing Spondylitis

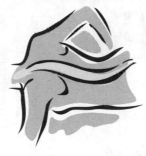

Osteoporosis is a disease that robs bones of their density and strength, making them thinner and more prone to break. Eventually, bone mass decreases below the level required to support the body. Long considered a woman's problem, because of its female hormone involvement, osteoporosis affects from 35 to 50% of women in the first 5 years after menopause. Osteoporosis also affects men, just at a later age and with less ferocity. Over 28 million Americans suffer from osteoporosis today, and experts from the National Osteoporosis Foundation predict over 40 million Americans will suffer from osteoporosis by the year 2015. For women, osteoporosis is greater than the combined risks of breast, uterine and ovarian cancers. Half of all women over 50 will suffer an osteoporosis-related fracture in their lives. (One in eight men will suffer an osteoporosis-related fracture.) *Osteomalacia* involves lowered calcium in the bone. *Ankylosing spondylitis* is a type of osteoporosis where spine vertebrae fuse together in bone spurs. Nutritional therapy offers a broad base of both treatment and protection.

Are you at risk for osteoporosis? Check the following risk factors. They affect a lot of women.
1) Are you post-menopausal with a family history of osteoporosis? (especially high risk for menopausal women who have not had children)?
2) Are you over 75 years, with a history of calcium and vitamin D deficiency?
3) Do you smoke? drink coffee regularly? eat red meat regularly?
4) Do you over use cortico-steroid drugs? Research indicates that over a long period of time steroid drugs tend to leach potassium from the system, weakening the bones.
5) Have you used synthetic thyroid drugs for long periods of time? The drug Synthroid can increase risk for both osteoporosis and high cholesterol, may also aggravate weight gain.
6) Did you have your ovaries removed before menopause? Did you have an early menopause, before 45 years old? Do you have a history of irregular or no menstrual periods?
Note: You can test yourself for probable osteoporosis. Use pH paper (sold in most college book stores), and test your urine. A habitual reading below pH 7 (acid) usually means calcium and bone loss. Above pH 7 (alkaline) indicates a low risk. *See* Bone Health *page 337 for more information, and call Eidon (800-700-1169) for their new mineral test and balancing program.*

You can arrest or avoid post-menopausal bone loss
Osteoporosis is far more complex than was thought even just 5 years ago. Bone and cartilage are an ever-changing infrastructure. Bone is living tissue, and like other body systems requires a wide variety of nutrients. Osteoporosis is partially a result of reduced nutrient (particularly mineral) absorption, which is highly bound to enzyme activity. High levels of phosphorous in meat, soft drinks and other common processed foods deprive the body of calcium. Lack of vitamin D from sunlight, and too little exercise also contribute to bone porosity. You don't have to let osteoporosis steal your health! You can start today to build up your bones, even if you've already been diagnosed with the disease. I've seen natural therapies literally transform people crippled by osteoporosis who are living active, full lives after rigorously following natural therapies. After more than 15 years of working with osteoporosis, I find the most successful treatment involves not only normalizing hormone levels, but also improving lifestyle and dietary habits that we know accelerate bone loss. It's not just a case of adding estrogen. Successful osteoporosis treatment is a complete lifestyle program, not just a pill!

What about calcium? *Over 50% of American women suffer from calcium deficiency alone.*
Calcium is a cornerstone of medical world treatment for osteoporosis. Calcium is the most abundant mineral in the body, and 98 percent of all calcium is stored in the bones. But osteoporosis is the result of much more than a calcium deficiency, so calcium isn't the whole answer, or even the only mineral involved in bone health. Two-thirds of the body's magnesium is also contained in the bones. Osteoporosis involves both mineral and non-mineral components of bone, so your bones need a full range of supportive nutrients. Getting your minerals from mineral-rich veggies like broccoli, kale and collard greens, and herbs like lamb's quarters, oatstraw, kelp, dulse, burdock, dandelion, borage seed and lobelia may be a better choice. Unlike dairy foods, mineral-rich herbs and veggies come without heavy protein, and they offer many more nutrients for bone building, especially high levels of vitamin K, which helps calcium attach to bone tissue, and magnesium and potassium. For bones of steel, I recommend ditching high fat dairy products and considering more veggies.

Still there are always two sides to every story. We know modern farming techniques leech minerals from the soil, so hardly anyone gets enough minerals from foods. Massive water fluoridation across the U.S. means many Americans are losing some calcium with every sip of their tap water. Today, I'm a firm believer in high quality plant mineral supplements for maximum bone building. Calcium supplements can't stand on their own as a viable treatment. In fact, bone strength is best enhanced when calcium is used with other nutrients, like B vitamins (esp. B6), magnesium, silica, manganese and boron, especially for older women who don't retain calcium very well by itself.

Can't find a recommended product? Call the 800 number listed in Product Resources *for the store nearest you.*

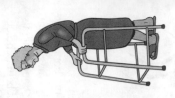

How do you know if you have a calcium deficiency? Calcium deficiencies show up pre-menstrually as back pain, cramping, or tooth pain. (Take a calcium supplement before your period to see if this is your problem.... supplementation helps these symptoms disappear.) But, avoid calcium-containing antacids that block stomach acids, causing reduced bone growth.

There is a clear link between high protein consumption and osteoporosis, too. Amino acids from excess protein cause excretion of large amounts of minerals by the kidneys especially calcium, released from bone material to neutralize the acidity of the protein amino acids. Animal protein is an even bigger danger. Long term studies of vegetarians and meat eaters from age 60 through 90, reveal that the minerals in meat eater's bones decreased 35% over time - minerals in a vegetarian's bones decreased only 18%. High levels of phosphorous in meat and soft drinks also deprive the body of calcium. Soda consumption has doubled since the 1970s, a major reason many believe for the alarming growth of osteoporosis incidence in our society.

The Fosamax Deception

Over 800,000 women in the U.S. today take Fosamax (*Alendronate sodium*), the first non-hormonal drug approved to treat osteoporosis. Fosamax belongs to a class of drugs called "bisphosphonates" which inhibit the action of osteoclasts, the cells in the skeleton that break down bone. When Fosamax was FDA approved in April of 1997, the public was ecstatic. Preliminary reports found Fosamax could reduce height loss and risk of fractures without any serious side effects. However, as Fosamax made its way into the American public, its problems became glaringly clear. Esophageal injury caused by this drug is a real threat. There are at least 250 reports linking Fosamax to esophageal injury. Of these, 51 cases were considered serious. I have heard from at least 2 of these women myself. Ulcers in the esophagus, severe chest pain, blurry vision, difficulty swallowing, headaches, and gastrointestinal distress are other side effects. The latest research shows that if left untreated, eye inflammation resulting from Fosamax can lead to blindness! Taking Fosamax with NSAIDs (non steroidal anti-inflammatory drugs) or aspirin is a really bad idea. Risk for gastrointestinal problems can skyrocket from both drugs! Leading health experts now believe Fosamax actually blocks bone resorption, the process which removes weakening bones to allow space for new healthy bone growth, a definite concern for people trying to build strong bones. Over time, women using this drug may actually see an increase in fractures due to bone weakening. Fosamax stays in the body 10 to 15 years after taking it, so residual effects may continue to surface for years!

How do hormones fit into the bone building picture?

A man's testosterone supply protects against osteoporosis. For a woman, osteoporosis involves thyroid malfunction and poor collagen protein, as well as progesterone/estrogen balance. Progesterone is a key factor in laying down and strengthening bone. Many doctors prescribe a combination of Premarin, (from pregnant mare's urine), conjugated man-made estrogens, and Provera, a synthetic progesterone to address menopausal bone loss. (See also page 456 on the new SERM drugs for osteoporosis.) However, new research shows that neither Premarin nor Provera prevent osteoporosis; they can sometimes slow it, but after 5 or 6 years on the therapy, bone loss continues at the same rate and cancer risk is greatly increased. Taken orally, these drugs pass through the liver where much of the substance is lost or altered. For this reason, and because hormones are readily absorbed through the skin, the estrogen patch has also become popular. My experience has been that neither work as well as natural, plant-derived progesterone therapy, delivered in herbal combinations. Early tests on women over 60 show that plant progesterone, such as that found in wild yam, along with a good diet and supplements and regular exercise, may even reverse osteoporosis, something that no synthetic hormone in any combination has been able to demonstrate.

What about progesterone creams derived from wild yam roots?

Can they really stave off osteoporosis? Progesterone actually enhances bone formation, something estrogen cannot do. In one study on women with osteoporosis, a bone scan showed up to 5% new bone density in an eighteen month period after the women used a natural wild yam progesterone cream, along with a good nutritional program. Other research shows that plant progesterone creams increase bone density up to 29% for women after 3 years or less of therapy. Adding a germanium supplement orally accelerates the bone building benefits.

Is crash dieting bad to the bone?

A recent study shows that for each 10% decrease in weight, there is a two-fold increase in the risk of hip fractures in older women. When blood calcium levels become too low from crash dieting, your bones release their calcium to keep the rest of the body running smoothly. In addition, women who diet to excess regularly show up with estrogen deficiency, also involved in bone loss. Even taking calcium supplements is not enough to maintain bone mass during dieting. The test was very discouraging because almost all the women gained the weight back. I find better results are obtained for dieters when minerals are added via green drinks and vegetable juices. Women who take in minerals from these sources don't gain the lost weight back, either as quickly or as much. Since a majority of American women admit to being on a weight control diet most of the time, it seems maintaining a broad spectrum of low fat foods, and adding high mineral drinks from food or herb sources to avoid bone loss while dieting is a better choice. Note: Hormone and calcium deficiencies appear regularly in women with irregular menstrual cycles, notably when they result from excessive exercise or eating disorders.

Can't find a recommended product? Call the 800 number listed in Product Resources for the store nearest you.

Is your lifestyle putting you at risk for osteoporosis? A low nutrition, processed foods diet sets the stage for bone loss.

—Low mineral intake means a lack of structural support and impaired digestion. Minerals are critical for a strong skeletal system, and they are the bonding agents between you and your food. A lack of minerals means low thyroid function and poor collagen protein development, also part of osteoporosis.

—Osteoporosis is highly bound to food-enzyme activity. It is at least in part, a result of poor digestion and enzyme deficiency. If you don't eat enough fresh plant foods, you probably have low enzymes and poor digestion. I find this is especially true for older men who try to correct digestive problems with handfuls of antacids.

—Too much protein.... There is a clear relationship between high protein consumption and osteoporosis. According to The Journal of the American Dietetic Association when protein consumption is doubled, calcium loss increases 50%!

—Over-acid blood from overeating red meats, sodas, caffeine foods and alcohol puts you at risk for bone loss. As much as 60mg of alkaline minerals like calcium can be leached from the skeleton every day to help neutralize overly acidic blood pH. Over time, this mineral loss can translate in to major bone loss from demineralization! Soda warning: USDA research finds that men who consume five cans of cola a day for three months absorb less calcium, increasing risk for bone deterioration and injuries or breaks!

Beyond diet, your lifestyle influences osteoporosis.

—Too little exercise stunts healthy bone development. Too little sunlight means less vitamin D is available for bone building.

—Smoking interferes with your body's calcium and estrogen production. Women smokers have 10% lower bone density and are more vulnerable to fractures than non smokers.

—Depression may cause bone loss. Research shows that people with a history of severe depression have 15% less bone density in their lower spines than non-depressed people.

—Women who suffer from chronic stress may be at a higher risk. High cortisol levels from chronic stress inhibit bone building, suppress the production of androgens that help build bones and decrease mineral absorption, key to healthy bone structure.

—Overusing steroids, antibiotics or tobacco, and too much alcohol severely reduces mineral absorption.

—Drinking fluoridated water is a risk factor! New studies link hip fractures to fluoridated water. Here's why: Fluoridated water literally leaches calcium from the bones.

—Ovary removal puts you at greater risk for osteoporosis.

It is difficult to detect osteoporosis without a bone mineral density (BMD) measurement, but there are early warning signs to watch for.

1: Bone loss is greatest in the spine, hips and ribs, so osteoporosis begins to show up as chronic back and leg pain. Bone pain may also occur in the spine, affecting the cranial nerves.

2: Look for loss of bone in the jaw and tooth sockets. Bone may draw away from the teeth, causing them to loosen, or fall out. Look for unusually frequent dental problems, too.

3: Vision defects or facial tics may also occur due to bone marrow obliteration.

Note: Consider an **osteoporosis urine test**. Use pH paper (sold in most laboratory supply stores or college book stores). A habitual reading below pH 7 usually means calcium and bone loss. Above pH 7 indicates a low risk.

You can also get a **bone mineral density (BMD) measurement** test through your doctor or local pharmacy. The new DEXA (Duel Energy X-ray Absorptiometry) bone density tests enable doctors to measure bone strength without being confused by muscle, fat or skin. By doing this, the DEXA method is able to more accurately measure bone strength in the spine and hips, where the majority of disabling fractures occur.

Can pumping iron stop bone loss?

Studies find people who do regular weight bearing exercises have denser bones than those who don't. It seems your bones can rebuild themselves, but only when they're used. A sedentary lifestyle increases osteoporosis risk. Power walking is good for bones, so are aerobic workouts, like Tae Bo, or weight bearing exercise 3-4 times a week (especially for men and women under 35 whose bone mass is still growing). You can use your own body weight in bone building exercises, especially outside in the sun to increase production of bone building vitamin D.

Here are two of my favorites: 1: For your upper arms - do mini push up against the wall. Just stand at arm's length away from a wall, with your hand flat against the wall. Then just lean in and push back about 10 or 20 times for each arm. 2 For your lower back and legs. Stretch as high as you can. Then lean over as far as you can toward your toes and hold for 5 seconds.

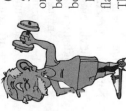

Can't find a recommended product? Call the 800 number listed in Product Resources for the store nearest you.

Osteoporosis

Diet and Lifestyle Support Therapy

Vegetarians have lower risk of osteoporosis with stronger bones after menopause and in later life.

Nutritional therapy plan:

1—Eat vitamin C foods: kiwis, oranges, grapefruit, potatoes for collagen production.

2—Skip the iodized salt and add sea greens like nori, wakame, dulse, kombu or kelp (2 tbsp. daily, snipped on salads, soups, rice, pizzas), for bone minerals and vitamins D and K that boost hormones like estrogen, progesterone and DHEA, prime bone supports.

3—Eat calcium, magnesium and potassium-rich foods - broccoli, fish and seafood, eggs, yogurt, kefir, carrots, dried fruits, sprouts, miso, beans, leafy greens and sea greens, tofu, bananas, apricots, prunes, molasses, etc. Or try •Futurebiotics VITAL K drink. •**Try these Bone Strength Snack Balls:** Mix 1 c. sesame tahini, ½ c. honey or maple syrup, 2 tbsp. powdered ginseng, 3 tbsp. powdered dong quai, 3 tbsp. bee pollen granules, 1 tbsp. spirulina or barley grass powder, ½ c. ginseng-royal jelly-honey blend, ½ c. chopped walnuts, ½ c. raisins. Roll into a paste. Form balls. Chill. Then roll in a blend of toasted amaranth, grapenuts, and 3 tbsp. dry dulse flakes.

4—Reduce protein intake from red meat and dairy foods. They disrupt pH balance and lead to mineral loss. Get protein from soy, fresh fish, legumes, vegetables and sea greens instead. (Note: pasteurized milk is not a good source of absorbable calcium, and can actually interfere with mineral assimilation.) Drink juices like carrot and orange instead. One 8-oz. glass of fresh carrot juice has 400mg bioavailable calcium. An 8-oz. glass of fortified milk has 250mg with low assimilation.

5—Avoid sugar, high salt foods (snackfoods and processed foods), hard alcohol, caffeine foods (except green and white tea or Crystal Star DR. VITALITY™ which has bone building properties), tobacco, and nightshade plants that interfere with calcium absorption.

—**Bodywork:**

•Smoking cigarettes causes bone loss in women. Smoking a pack a day during adulthood results in a 10% loss in bone density, leaving bones more subject to fracture than than those of non-smokers. Smoking also appears to interfere with estrogen production.

•Get early morning sunlight on the body every day possible for vitamin D.

•Avoid fluorescent lighting, electric blankets, aluminum cookware, non-filtered computer screens, etc. All tend to leach calcium from the body.

•Exercise is a nutrient in itself. Weight-bearing exercise is a good way to build bone and prevent bone loss. Duration of exercise is more important than intensity. Note: if you already have low bone density, I suggest starting on a weight bearing exercise program after improvements from diet changes are seen in your bone scans in order to avoid injury. The water limits overdoing it. I've found the best ones are often water workout exercise. Consult with a qualified health professional to find out what exercises are right for you.

Herbal, Superfood and Supplement Therapy

Interceptive therapy plan: Choose 2 or 3 recommendations.

1—**Balance your hormones (don't just add estrogen):** •Ipriflavone 600mg daily, or •Metabolic Response Modifiers OSTEO-MAX 200mg ipriflavone with 200mg MCHC (*microcrystalline hydroxyapatite concentrate*). *Plant hormones are effective:* •Crystal Star EASY CHANGE™ daily. (Use with •evening primrose oil 3000mg daily, for maximum mineral absorption and hormone balancing EFAs); •Pure Essence FEM CREME. Take with •Nutricology GERMANIUM 150mg daily for best results (good activity).

2—**Boost your minerals (not just calcium):** •Lane Labs ADVACAL ULTRA FAST RELEASE (clinically proven to increase bone density in the spine).•Calcium citrate 1500mg /magnesium 1000mg and boron 3mg for absorption (too much boron alone actually causes bone loss.) •Flora VEGE-SIL for 6 months; or •Ethical Nutrients BONE BUILDER with silica. •Crystal Star CALCIUM MAGNESIUM SOURCE™ and •IODINE, POTASSIUM, SILICA extract (silica helps collagen-calcium production). •Enzymatic Therapy OSTEOPRIME; •Trace Mineral Research CONCENTRACE; •Nature's Path TRACE-MIN-LYTE (contains 500mg sea plants and electrolytes); horsetail or nettles tea.

—**Boost important mineral absorption vitamins:** •Vitamin D 1000IU; •marine carotenes 100,000IU, and •zinc 30mg daily; •boron 3mg, and •vitamin K 100mcg.

3—**Boost bone health with EFA's:** •Crystal Star Evening Primrose oil pearls, 6 daily; •Spectrum Naturals Evening Primrose oil 1300mg; •high omega-3 flax oil 3x daily, or •Barlean's OMEGA TWIN flax-borage combo; or •Nature's Secret ULTIMATE OIL. •Crystal Star ENERGY GREEN RENEWAL™ with EFA's. •Nutricology PRO GREENS with EFA's.

4—**Enzymes boost nutrient absorption:** Men especially benefit from enzyme therapy; •Herbal Products Dvlpt. POWER PLUS ENZYMES; •Transformation DIGESTZYME; •Floradix CALCIUM, MAGNESIUM, VITAMIN D & ZINC herbal syrup. Note: Low stomach acid diminishes calcium absorption. Herbal "bitters" like Crystal Star BITTERS and LEMON CLEANSE™ extract encourage the body to produce more stomach acid.

5—**Bioflavonoids: important for hormone-like activity:** •Ester C with bioflavs. up to 5000mg daily for collagen development and connective tissue; or •Hawthorn, •Bilberry, or •Ginkgo Biloba extracts. •Ipriflavone 200mg 3x daily.

6—**B vitamins are important:** •B-complex 100mg daily with extra B₆ 250mg; •Country Life sublingual B-12, 2500mcg daily, •Nature's Secret ULTIMATE B.

7—**For bone pain:** •Glucosamine /chondroitin; •DLPA 750mg for bone pain.

—**Collagen and your bones:** A daily cup of fresh pineapple juice can deter osteoporosis by providing manganese, which the body uses to make collagen, the protein that forms the building blocks for bone and cartilage. Sea veggies are also good sources for manganese. Or try •Lane Labs TOKI collagen replacement drink (noticeable results for bones).

Can't find a recommended product? Call the 800 number listed in Product Resources for the store nearest you.

Ovarian Cysts

Polycystic Ovary Syndrome, Type II PAP Smear, Small Tumors

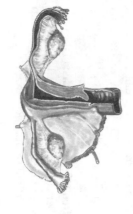

Ovarian cysts are showing up in record numbers, especially in women with menstrual difficulties, in women who have irregular or no periods, and for women who have excessive bleeding during their periods. The cysts are small, non-malignant, chambered sacs filled with fluid. As with so many women's problems, they are thought to be hormone-driven, usually from too much estrogen, and hypothyroidism. But they are not cancerous, nor are they cancer precursors. They normally cease to grow after menopause, but they are often painful, especially during intercourse, and can cause excessive menstrual bleeding and inter-period spotting. Medical treatment involves hormone therapy or removal, with accompanying hazards. Further, recent research published in the *Lancet* shows that surgical removal of ovarian cysts does not reduce cancer risk. Alternative treatment focuses on dietary measures to change habits that put you at risk, and herbal medicines. **Polycystic ovary syndrome (PCOS)** is far more serious and affects 1 in 15 women of childbearing age. Multiple cysts develop on both ovaries and menstruation becomes irregular. PCOS is almost always accompanied by obesity, insulin resistance, adult acne, excess facial hair growth and infertility. Chronic stress and eating disorders play a role in PCOS development. Natural hormone balancing, diet changes, stress reduction and regular exercise are keys to recovery. A *Type II Pap Smear* can be a sign of ovarian cysts as well as cervical dysplasia, cervical cancer and endometriosis. Herbal medicines can help stop these problems before they become full blown.

Do you *think* you *might* have *ovarian cysts?* They are difficult to diagnose without a medical exam. Signs to look for:

—acute or chronic pain or swelling in the fallopian tubes or ovaries, and usually the inability to conceive.
—an erratic menstrual cycle with unfamiliar pain, unusual swelling and discomfort in the lower abdomen and breasts.
—often profuse uterine bleeding because of endometrial hyperplasia that results from unbalanced estrogen stimulation.
—painful intercourse, heel pain, and constantly swollen breasts.
—unusual abdominal gas, fever and coated tongue.
—Some women also experience excess hair growth due to an imbalance between estrogen, progesterone and testosterone levels.
—Most sufferers also experience unusual weight gain because of low thyroid activity.

What *causes ovarian cysts?*

Too much estrogen is the most common cause of cysts. Some research points to long use of birth control pills or synthetic hormone replacement which may play a part because it upsets hormone balance. (Most sufferers are overweight, which also aggravates cysts.) Using, or having formerly used, an IUD, may be a factor. Frequent radiation treatments and X-rays that you may undergo for other problems may change cell structure and set up an environment for ovarian cyst growth. Diabetes, especially alcohol-induced diabetes, is a high-risk factor. A stressful lifestyle that encourages an over-acid system and poor waste elimination, sets up unhealthy body chemistry for cysts.

You *may not need surgery for ovarian cysts*

Endometriosis can also cause endometrial cysts on the ovaries. These are called "chocolate" cysts because they contain oxidized blood with the appearance of chocolate syrup. Endometrial cysts cause almost incapacitating pain in the uterus, lower back, and organs in the pelvic cavity prior to and during the menses. Painful intercourse, excessive bleeding, including the passing of large clots and shreds of tissue during the menses, and infertility are some of the other symptoms. Ovarian cysts are not cancerous and the need for surgery removal only arises not because of malignancy, but because the pedicle of the cyst can become twisted and gangrenous, or because of painful pressure on surrounding organs. Natural therapy focuses on normalizing hormone levels and correcting the unhealthy body chemistry. It has been quite successful, and offers you a choice before jumping into surgery. Give yourself from 4 to 6 months of healing on an herbal, hormone-balancing regimen for ovarian cysts. *See ENDOMETRIOSIS page 406 for more information.*

Can you *prevent ovarian cysts from returning?*

Preventive measures call for balancing estrogen levels as naturally as possible. Look to phyto-hormone-containing herbal compounds first. Phytoestrogen-rich herbs can prevent a woman's own or other estrogens from attaching to cell receptors. Phytoestrogens have 1/400 or less the estrogenic activity of human hormones. They can be used to "jam" the cellular receptor sites for estrogen, to prevent it from stimulating the cells. Soy foods, such as tofu and soy milk, buckwheat, citrus, and flax are also good sources of estrogen-blocking flavonoids.

Can't find a recommended product? Call the 800 number listed in Product Resources for the store nearest you.

Ovarian Cysts

Diet and Lifestyle Support Therapy

Nutritional therapy plan:

1—Reducing dietary fat intake is the first, best step to reducing cyst growth. High fats mean high circulating estrogen. Too much estrogen is the most common cause of cysts. Fats from red meats and dairy foods are the worst offenders. Get protein for healing from vegetable sources, whole grains, sprouts, soy foods and seafoods.

2—Over-acidity sets up an environment for ovarian cyst development. B vitamin rich foods, like leafy greens and other fresh vegetables, miso, brown rice, wheat germ, nutritional yeast, sea greens and green drinks, like Crystal Star ENERGY GREEN RENEWAL™ (with sea veggies for thyroid balance), help alkalize the system.

3—Especially avoid fried, salty foods, during menses. Eliminate heavy starches, full fat dairy foods, and hard liquor.

4—Eat iodine rich sea foods to overcome hypothyroidism. Avoid caffeine and refined sugars which deplete your body of iodine, a critical nutrient for healthy thyroid activity.

5—Drink bottled water. Chlorinated water tends to leach vitamin E from the body.

—Type 2 PAP smears? *An herbal program for a Type 2 PAP smear has had good results.* **1:** Take one herbal chlorophyll source drink like •Green Foods VIBRANT WOMAN daily. Chlorophyll is a prime agent for immune enhancement, especially as it naturally occurs in plants like green grasses and blue-green algae. **2:** Take 4 Lane Labs AngioPGM caps daily. **3:** Take about 400mg grape seed oil PCO tablets daily or MICROHYDRIN PLUS available at royal-health.com. **4:** Take EVENING PRIMROSE OIL 4000mg daily. **5:** Take antibiotic, anti-inflammatory herbs like Crystal Star WOMAN'S BEST FRIEND™ caps 6 daily, or *goldenseal/echinacea/myrrh* caps. **6:** Take *diindolylmethane* (DIM) 400mg daily. DIM helps fight abnormal cell growth by promoting proper estrogen metabolism. "Good" estrogen metabolites promote cell apoptosis, helping eliminate precancerous cells.

As cysts and pain reduce, switch to a 3-month preventive program. **1:** Take Crystal Star FEMALE HARMONY™ 2 capsules daily (a body balancing compound). Add VITEX extract for Polycystic Ovary Syndrome. Add *saw palmetto* 160mg 2x daily if you also have excess facial hair. **2:** Keep fat intake to 15% of your diet. Make fresh fruits and vegetables 50%. Have a green salad daily for chlorophyll and fiber. Avoid hard alcohol, tobacco and caffeine. **3:** Take vitamin E 400IU daily, as an estrogen antagonist. Take B-complex 100mg daily to help the liver metabolize estrogen. Take *evening primrose oil* 1000mg daily. **4:** Take vitamin C 2000mg daily with bioflavonoids. Bioflavs have estrogen-like effects to help balance the body's estrogen-progesterone ratio. **5:** Take an herbal iodine source twice daily, like Crystal Star OCEAN MINERALS™ caps (iodine-potassium and silica from the sea). Eat iodine-rich foods, like sea greens, seafoods, fish, mushrooms, garlic and onions. A hot seaweed bath using sea plants may be used for iodine therapy. The skin is the body's largest organ of ingestion. Iodine from sea vegetables is easily absorbed through the pores during a seaweed bath.

Herbal, Superfood and Supplement Therapy

Interceptive therapy plan: Choose 2 to 3 recommendations.

1—Help reduce and dissolve cysts: •Crystal Star WOMAN'S BEST FRIEND™ caps, 4 daily for 3 months, with •ANTI-FLAM™ caps and DR. ENZYME™ with protease and bromelain for inflammation pain. •Lane Labs AngioPGM as an anti-infective; •Black cohosh extract or •Enzymedica PURIFY help dissolve adhesions. •Pure Essence Labs FEM CREME rub on abdomen. (Good results in about 3 months.) •White peony rt. tea daily helps boost chances of ovulation in women with PCOS. •Maitake products MAITAKE SX-FRACTION™ reduces insulin resistance for PCOS (highly recommended).

—Draw out infection: •Make an effective vaginal pack: mix powders of *echinacea, goldenseal root, white oak, cranesbill, chaparral* and *red raspberry* in water and glycerine to make a solution. Soak a tampon in a strong water solution of these herbs. Insert in the vagina at night (wear a sanitary napkin to prevent leakage). Rinse vagina in the morning with a *goldenseal-myrrh* tea with 1 tbsp. vinegar. Use 1 week on/1 week off for 6 weeks. Use with a blood cleansing combination like •Crystal Star DETOX BLOOD PURIFIER™ caps, or a daily blood cleansing tea like •*dandelion-parsley root-raspberry-ginger* tea. (Often works in 6 weeks to dissolve small cysts.) Apply castor oil packs over the lower abdomen to help shrink cysts and reduce pain.

2—Add EFA's to take down inflammation: •*Evening Primrose oil,* 6 daily; •Spectrum Naturals 1300mg Evening Primrose oil; •Health from the Sun TOTAL EFA, or •Barlean's OMEGA TWIN flax-borage combo; or •Nature's Secret ULTIMATE OIL. •QUERCETIN 1000mg with BROMELAIN 1500mg daily.

3—Iodine therapy helps hypothyroidism, often effective in 3 months: (Take with vit. E, an estrogen antagonist, for best results.) •Bernard Jensen LIQUI-DULS; •Crystal Star OCEAN MINERALS™ caps. •Two tbsp. dry sea greens snipped over rice, salad, soup or a pizza are a therapeutic dose. •Gaia Herbs THYROID SUPPORT. •Nature's Answer SEACENTIALS GOLD.

4—Love your liver to better handle estrogen, flush excess estrogen secretions: •Milk Thistle Seed extract; •Dandelion or burdock tea; •B-complex 100mg daily; •C'est Si Bon CHLORENERGY 1 pkt. daily; Pancreatin 1300mg for fat metabolism.

5—Antioxidants that help: •PCOs from grapeseed, 400mg daily; •Nutricology germanium 150mg; •Vitamin E 400IU as an estrogen antagonist; or VITAMIN E CLUSTERS available from Royal Bodycare with selenium 200mcg or Eidon SELENIUM liquid; •Vitamin C 5000mg daily with bioflavonoids (for estrogen-like effects to balance estrogen-progesterone ratio).

—Superfood therapy can really help: •Crystal Star RESTORE YOUR STRENGTH™ drink or caps. •Fit for You, intl. MIRACLE GREENS with sea greens. •Nutricology PRO GREENS with EFAs. •Pines MIGHTY GREENS.

Can't find a recommended product? Call the 800 number listed in Product Resources for the store nearest you.

PMS

Pre-Menstrual Syndrome, Cramps, Dysmenorrhea

PMS is by far the most common women's health complaint. For some women, it disrupts their whole lives.

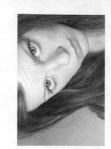

What's really going on with PMS?

The intricacies of a woman's body are delicately tuned, and can become unbalanced or obstructed easily, causing pain, poor function, and a disconcerting feeling of not being "together" that often results in physiological and emotional problems, especially during the menstrual cycle. PMS seems to be partly a consequence of modern women's emancipation. In times past, women were a silent, long-suffering lot, who felt that female disorders were just part of being a woman. Women were not out in the high profile workplace with men; they could go to bed and suffer alone. In times past, our diets consisted of more whole and fresh foods than they do today. Our environment wasn't full of chemicals, nor our foods full of junk. The modern women's lifestyle seems almost made to order for stress and imbalance. Today's foods and our environment are full of chemicals that clearly affect delicate hormone balance.

A whopping 90% of premenopausal American women experience some degree of PMS. Over 150 symptoms have been documented - new ones are being added all the time. Symptoms like headaches, adult acne, food cravings, bloating, irregular bowel movements, and mood swings can last anywhere from 2 days to as long as 2 weeks! Some women say their cycles make them feel out of control all month! While most women try to grin and bear PMS aggravation, up to 10% have symptoms serious enough to seek professional help.

What causes PMS?

The hormone shift in estrogen/progesterone ratios during the menstrual cycle is the major factor in PMS symptoms. (Women report the most symptoms in the two week period before menstruation, when the ratios are the most elevated.) Low brain serotonin, low thyroid, excess estrogen along with prostaglandin imbalance because of poor liver malfunction, and a diet loaded with too much salt, red meat, sugar and caffeine are all implicated in PMS. Most women who get PMS don't get enough regular exercise. Many have low B vitamins, don't get enough quality protein and have several mineral deficiencies. Stress or long term emotional distress can be a big factor.

But drugs and chemical medicines to take care of the symptoms, standing as they do outside a woman's natural cycle, usually do not bring positive results for women. The medical establishment, with highly focused "one-treatment-for-one-symptom" protocols, has not been successful in addressing PMS. For example, contraceptive drugs, regularly given to reduce symptoms, make PMS worse for some women. Antidepressant drugs like Prozac, the new rage for PMS treatment, mean insomnia and shakiness for many patients instead of relaxation.

PMS symptoms tends to get worse for women in their late thirties. Hormone imbalances after taking birth control pills, after pregnancy, and just before menopause magnify symptoms. For some women, a PMS problem becomes an endometriosis diagnosis as they move into their thirties. Switch from tampons to pads if you are very congested. Some research also shows that tampons may raise the risk of endometriosis. Up to 60% of women with severe PMS also struggle with allergies, especially to yeast. When the immune system attacks an allergen it produces inflammatory prostaglandins that trigger menstrual pain. Clearly there is no one cause and no one treatment for PMS. A holistic approach is more beneficial and allows a woman to tailor treatment to her own needs. *See next page, LIVER CLEANSING page 199 and HYPOGLYCEMIA DIET page 463 for more information.*

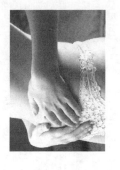

Do you get PMS? **Check out the following most common signs of PMS to see if they apply to you.**

...Do your friends and loved ones say you're unusually irritable, argumentative or tense at certain times each month?
...Do you notice moody swings, aggressive behavior, even depression at certain times during each month?
...Do you experience cyclical water retention, bloating, and constipation each month?
...Do you feel a noticeable energy drop before your period.... to the point where you don't want to get out of bed or do anything?
...Do you get regular monthly headaches or lower back pain before your period?
...Do you get sore, swollen breasts before your period?
...Do you get nausea attacks and heavy cramping just before and during your period?
...Do you get food cravings for salt and sweets before and during your period? Do you tend to binge during certain times of the month?
...Do you get acne and skin eruptions before and during your period?
...Do you get pre-period mouth sores? (Mouth sores with mood swings mean probable low progesterone or thyroid levels.)

Can't find a recommended product? Call the 800 number listed in Product Resources for the store nearest you.

The Natural Keys to Controlling P.M.S.

Menstruation is a natural part of our lives. PMS is not. Women can take control of PMS naturally and effectively.

Natural treatment is much more gratifying because it allows you to take more control of your life, and address the symptoms that are unique to you. It's an approach that emphasizes a highly nutritious diet, and herbal tonifiers to encourage the body to provide its own balance for relief. Natural therapies work well for most women because they address the full spectrum of factors involved, but they need time to work. A woman can expect a natural therapy program for PMS to take at least two months, as the body works through both ovary cycles. The first month shows noticeable decrease in PMS symptoms; the second month finds them dramatically reduced. Don't be discouraged if you need six months or more to gently coax your system into balance. Even after most of the symptoms are gone, continue with the diet recommendations, and smaller doses of the herb and vitamin choices to prevent PMS return.

—**Phytohormone-rich herbal compounds help balance body estrogen levels:** Phyto-estrogens are remarkably similar to human hormones. They can help raise body estrogen levels that are too low by stimulating the body's own hormone production, or by attaching to estrogen receptor sites. Plant estrogens can also lower estrogen levels that are too high. Even though they are only ¹⁄₄₀₀ or less of the strength of the body's own circulating estrogens, they are able to compete with human estrogens for receptor sites. When the weaker estrogens attach to receptors, the net effect is a lowering of too high estrogen levels. Phytohormone-rich plants like soybeans and wild yams, and hormone-rich herbs like black cohosh, ginseng, licorice root and dong quai, have a safety record of centuries. An herbal combination like •Crystal Star FEMALE HARMONY™ tea or capsules or •Esteem WOMEN'S COMFORT may be taken over a long period of time as a stabilizing resource for keeping the female system female, naturally. Progesterone creams, using natural, whole (not synthesized), wild yam, can control almost 90% of symptoms by some reports to keep you relaxed, prevent bloating and minimize unhealthy food cravings. Crystal Star PRO-EST BALANCE™ roll-on shows success against PMS pain by normalizing for estrogen-progesterone ratio balance.

—**Essential fatty acids balance prostaglandins.** Non- inflammatory, hormone-type prostaglandins act as transient hormones, regulating body functions almost like an electrical current. Foods like ocean fish (especially ahi tuna and salmon), olive and perilla oils, and herbs like Evening Primrose reduce pain by boosting your body's essential fatty acid supply. Add cherries, cranberries and blueberries to your diet to reduce PMS pain. Their anthocyanins have pain-relieving compounds up to 10 times stronger than aspirin or ibuprofen. Arachidonic acid in animal fats tends to deplete progesterone levels and strain estrogen/progesterone ratios. •Evening Primrose oil 3000-4000mg daily, along with a broad spectrum herbal balancing compound like Crystal Star FEMALE HARMONY™, shows excellent results against PMS.

—**Love your liver to balance estrogen and progesterone levels:** Lower your fat intake and reduce dairy foods to help your liver do its job. A high-fat diet hampers liver function. Many dairy foods are a source of synthetic estrogen from hormones injected into cows. At the very least, switch to non-fat dairy products. Estrogen is stored in fat; non-fat foods don't contribute to estrogen stores. Focus on high quality vegetarian protein to improve estrogen metabolism. On PMS days, avoid dairy foods altogether and include cruciferous vegetables like broccoli for estrogen balance at least twice a week. A cup of green or white tea, or a green tea blend like •Crystal Star GREEN TEA CLEANSER™ each morning relieves organ congestion and detoxifies the liver. Non-fat yogurt is a good food choice because it contains digestive lactobacillus. Reduce caffeine to one cup of coffee a day. Caffeine tends to deplete the liver and lowers B vitamin levels, contributing to anxiety, mood swings, and irritability. Fifteen to 30% of women with breast tenderness find quick relief by stopping caffeine use! A little wine is fine, but you'll suffer less from PMS if you avoid hard liquor. When your liver has to process strong alcohol, B vitamin levels are lowered and normal estrogen clearance is impaired, leading to bloating, cramps and pain. Consider •Planetary BUPLEURUM LIVER CLEANSE; or •MILK THISTLE SEED extract or •*dandelion root* tea daily.

—**Boost thyroid activity to reduce PMS:** Estrogen levels are controlled by thyroid hormones. If the thyroid does not have enough iodine, insufficient thyroxine is produced and too much estrogen builds up. Herbs from the sea are an excellent choice for thyroid balance because they are rich in potassium and iodine. Two tablespoons daily in a soup or salad, or over rice, or six pieces of sushi a day, are a therapeutic dose. Or try •Crystal Star OCEAN MINERALS™ caps; •Bernard Jensen LIQUI-DULS, or •Gaia THYROID SUPPORT phytocaps.

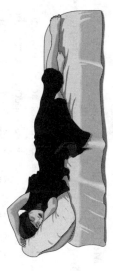

Can't find a recommended product? Call the 800 number listed in Product Resources for the store nearest you.

PMS

Diet and Lifestyle Support Therapy

Nutritional therapy plan: *Improve your diet first to control PMS. Women with severe PMS symptoms eat 60% more refined carbohydrates, 280% more sugars, 85% more dairy products, and 80% more sodium than women who don't get PMS.*

1—A low fat, vegetarian diet with regular seafood clearly diminishes symptoms. Add soy foods like miso, tempeh and tofu, and plenty of cruciferous veggies to reduce estrogen build-up linked to PMS. Try •Crystal Star RESTORE YOUR STRENGTH™ drink for iodine-balancing sea greens.

2—Try an anti-mood swing, anti-constipation drink: 2 cups fresh peaches, chunked; 2 frozen bananas, chunked; 1 cup apple juice.

3—Keep the diet low in salt and sugar. Eat plenty of cultured foods, like yogurt and kefir for friendly flora. Eat brown rice often or add Red Star NUTRITIONAL YEAST to any recipe for B vitamins. Eat smaller meals often for blood glucose balance. Have body balancing miso soup at night for relaxation and better sleep.

4—Avoid caffeine, red meat, sugars and saturated fat animal products. Eliminate dairy foods during PMS days. I like •Solgar WHEY TO GO for quality protein.

5—Drink 6 glasses of bottled water daily. Have fresh apple or carrot juice every day during PMS.

—Bodywork:

•Treat yourself to a good massage or shiatsu session before your period to release clogging mucous and fatty formations. Massage breasts and ovary areas to relax reproductive organs.

•Exercise is a must for female hormone balance. Exercise improves the way your body assimilates and metabolizes nutrients, especially hormones. It changes food habits, and decreases craving for alcohol or tobacco. It boosts beta endorphin levels in the brain. It improves circulation to relieve congestion. It encourages regularity for faster elimination of toxins.

•Stretching/relaxation exercises such as yoga with deep breathing and tai chi help. Acupuncture and reflexology are also effective.

•End your shower with a cool rinse to stimulate circulation and relieve lymph congestion.

•Meditate to banish PMS. Harvard studies show 57% improvement for women with PMS who meditate twice daily for 15-20 minutes.

•Be sparing with your schedule during premenstrual days. Give yourself some slack, take some time to read, listen to music and relax.

•Light is linked to PMS. Get out in the sunshine at least 20 minutes a day.

•Stop smoking and avoid second-hand smoke. Nicotine inhibits hormone function.

Herbal, Superfood and Supplement Therapy

Interceptive therapy plan: Choose 2 or 3 recommendations.

1—**Normalize hormone fluctuations:** Crystal Star's 2-month program is highly successful: •FEMALE HARMONY™ capsules 2 daily each month, with EVENING PRIMROSE oil 6 daily the 1st month, 4 daily the 2nd month. Before your period, drink green tea or •Crystal Star GREEN TEA CLEANSER™ each morning as a mini detox. Take •TINKLE TEA™ or caps for 5 days prior to your period to relieve pre-period edema. Use *Ashwagandha* extract for stress and to tonify; try •PRO-EST BALANCE™ roll-on to prevent cramping and pain (fast acting). During your period use MUSCLE RELAXER™ caps, 4 at a time; or PMS RELIEF CRAMP BARK COMPLEX™ extract as needed. (Apply •HERPEX™ LYSINE/LICORICE gel for PMS mouth sores.)

2—**Relieve estrogen build-up:** •Crystal Star OCEAN MINERALS™ caps and/or •*Burdock* tea 2 cups daily; •Herbal Magic FEMSTRUATION; •Mood Maid PRO-MENO wild yam cream or •Pure Essence FEM CREME natural progesterone w. •vitamin E 400IU.

3—**Boost minerals to relieve cramps and ease salt cravings:** Calcium can cut symptom severity in half! •*Chamomile* tea (absorbable calcium source) or •Crystal Star CALCIUM MAGNESIUM SOURCE™ caps, or •Lane Labs ADVACAL ULTRA tabs; chew 3 to 9 zinc lozenges daily; •Black Cohosh extract drops every 2 hours; Flora MAGNESIUM liquid or •Calcium 1200mg with magnesium 400mg relaxes the uterus.

—Pelvic applications for cramps: Ice packs to pelvic area; •Ginger compresses on pelvic area. •New Chapter ARNICA GINGER gel. •Aromatherapy compress: one drop each: oils of *chamomile, marjoram, juniper* and *helichrysum* in a quart of cool water; or mix 3 drops each *basil* and *lavender* oil in 2-oz. sweet almond oil and rub on abdomen.

4—**Ease mood swings and irritation:** •Esteem WOMEN'S COMFORT caps; •5-HTP, 50mg at night; •Crystal Star RELAX CAPS™ for stress, or DEPRESS-EX™ caps for anxiety reactions; •New Chapter ST. JOHN'S SC27; •Now SAMe caps. •Nature's Secret ULTIMATE B; •GABA 2000mg daily; •Vitamin C up to 5000mg daily to neutralize heavy metal toxins. **—Relieve period headaches:** Crystal Star RELAX CAPS™ and NatureWell MIGRA-SPRAY help even severe headaches. (Many good reports.)

5—**Relieve excessive flow:** •Bayberry capsules 4 daily; •Cranesbill/red raspberry tea; •Vit. C 3000mg w. bioflavonoids or •Bilberry for bioflavonoids, •vitamin K 100mcg.

6—**Relieve breast soreness and fluid retention:** •Crystal Star TINKLE™ tea as needed; •Roasted dandelion root tea (good liver decongestant and for calcium); •Ginkgo Biloba for better circulation; •Crystal Star VITEX extract; •Evening Primrose Oil 3000mg daily. •Gymnema sylvestre extract for sugar cravings. Try •Nature's Answer SEACENTIALS GOLD for detoxifying congestion help.

7—**Relieve back pain:** •Crystal Star STRESS OUT™ muscle relaxer drops (usually help within 25 minutes) . •Barleans Omega-3 rich flax oil 3 daily; •quercetin 1000mg and bromelain 1500mg. •Ginger tea or •New Chapter DAILY GINGER drops in water.

Can't find a recommended product? Call the 800 number listed in Product Resources for the store nearest you.

Pain Control

Using Pain's Information for Better Healing

Pain is a mechanism our bodies use to draw attention to a problem. Pain signals us to attend to its underlying cause. Every person feels and reacts differently to pain. It can stem from centers that control certain areas of the body, and from local areas that demand pinpoint action. There are different kinds of pain: physical, emotional, chronic, local, intermittent, throbbing, dull, spasmodic, sharp, shooting, etc. Pain can be your body's best friend. It alerts you when something is wrong and needs your attention. It identifies the location, severity, and type of problem, so that you can treat the right area. Pain can be your body's worst enemy. Constant pain saps strength and spirit, causes irrational acts and decisions, and alters personality. Pain killers allow you to think clearly, work and live, while addressing the problem. But strong pain killing drugs afford relief by masking pain or deadening certain body mechanisms. For many people, natural therapies are superior to drugs and their side effects. Herbal pain managers have broader actions than analgesic drugs. They work at a deeper level, to relax and soothe, letting you use pain's information about your body, yet not be overwhelmed by the trauma. **There are four basic pain centers:** 1: cerebro-spinal area, (nerve, lower back, cramping); 2: frontal lobe area, (ear, tooth and headaches over the eyes); 3: base of the brain (migraines, tension headaches); 4: abdomen, (menstrual cramping, digestive, elimination). **Common paths to pain:** Poor posture, poor nutrition, an acidic diet that eats away protective tissue, adrenal exhaustion, recovery from disease, injury or surgery, tumors or growths, repressed anger.

Diet and Lifestyle Support Therapy

Nutritional therapy plan:

1—A vegetarian diet, low in fats, high in minerals is the best support for all kinds of pain - back and menstrual pain, migraines, arthritis, muscle aches.

2—Eat plenty of complex carbohydrates and vegetable proteins for strength: whole grains, broccoli, peas, brown rice, legumes, seafoods, etc. Fermented soy foods like tempeh, miso, natto and tofu are a specific for inflammation relief.

3—Add anthocyanin foods like cherries and berries as anti-inflammatories (often up to 10 times better than aspirin).

4—Add high mineral foods to the diet. Emphasize magnesium and calcium foods for muscle strength. Include bioflavonoid-rich foods, like fresh fruits and vegetables.

5—Have a vegetable drink like Knudsen's VERY VEGGIE or •Crystal Star RESTORE YOUR STRENGTH™ broth mix, and a green leafy salad every day. Note: Dehydration worsens chronic pain. Be sure to drink 8 glasses of water daily. Try •PENTA bottled water (highly recommended).

6—Avoid caffeine, salty and sugary foods to eliminate an overacid condition.

—Bodywork:

•Acupressure: pinch and massage webs between the thumb and index finger.

•Chiropractic adjustment, biofeedback, acupuncture, magnet therapy, and massage therapy control pain. •Prolotherapy injections can be helpful in reducing pain and improving range of motion from injury. Contact American Association of Orthopedic Medicine at 800-992-2063 for a referral.

•**Pain-relieving compresses:** *Plantain-marshmallow; Wintergreen-cajeput* oil; *Comfrey* leaf; *Lobelia.*

•**Topical pain relievers:** Tea tree oil; TIGER BALM; DMSO with aloe roll-on; Chinese WHITE FLOWER oil; Biochemics PAIN RELIEF lotion; Capsaicin creme, or Nature's Way CAYENNE PAIN RELIEVING ointment; B&T ARNI-FLORA homeopathic gel; Baywood TOPICAL SUPER COOL RELIEF with menthol, emu oil, MSM cream, and boswellia (highly recommended).

Herbal, Superfood and Supplement Therapy

Interceptive therapy plan: Choose 2 to 3 recommendations.

1—**Herbal pain management:** •*Kava* extract, stress relief; •*Lobelia* drops, cramps; •*Valerian/Wild Lettuce* extract, sedative, anti-spasmodic; •*White willow*, anti-inflammatory/ analgesic; •*Cramp bark* or *Jamaican dogwood,* cramping, spasms; •*Passionflowers* or *scullcap,* gentle sedatives; •*St. John's wort*, nerve damage; •*Wild yam* and *cat's claw,* inflammation; •Capsaicin cream, nerve pain; •*Myrrh*, analgesic; •Calendula, injury pain; •*Black cohosh* and *cayenne*, neck pain.

—Crystal Star herbal pain relievers work better than single herbs for pain: •Crystal Star ANTI-FLAM™ and •MUSCLE RELAXER™ caps or STRESS OUT™ muscle relaxer extract, spasms-muscle pain; •STRESS ARREST™ tea, •RELAX™ caps, nerve pain.

2—**EFA's and enzymes reduce inflammation:** Use proteolytic enzymes: •Crystal Star DR. ENZYME™ with protease and bromelain; or •bromelain 1500mg. For better results, combine enzymes with •Quercetin 1000mg and •vitamin C with bioflavs 5000mg daily. •MSM 1000mg, or •Futurebiotics MSM or •MICROHYDRIN with MSM from royalbodycare. com; •Evening Primrose oil caps 3000mg daily; •Earth's Bounty NONI caps.

3—**Natural pain killers:** •Natural Balance SUPER FLEX BACK FORMULA caps for lower back/cerebro-spinal pain; •New Chapter ZYFLAMEND AM and PM COX 2 inhibitors; •Glucosamine 1500mg-chondroitin 1200mg complex; •*Boswellia serrata* 150mg. 3x daily; •DLPA 1000mg daily; •PCO's from grapeseed or white pine 300mg daily. •Country Life LIGATEND capsules as needed (good results); •Twin Lab GABA PLUS caps daily; •DLPA 1000mg as needed; •CoQ$_{10}$ 200mg daily; •Magnesium, muscle cramping pain, 800mg daily. •Vitamin K 100mcg daily, chronic pain.

4—**Magnet therapy for pain is effective:** Try •Magnalyfe products. •Spring Life POLARIZERS also show effective pain relief over a long period of time.

—Superfood therapy: Choose 1 or 2 recommendations.

•Jarrow GENTLE FIBERS drink for bioflavonoids.

•New Chapter GINGER WONDER SYRUP, a proven anti-inflammatory

•Wakunaga KYO-GREEN, or •Sun Wellness CHLORELLA, 1 pkt. daily.

Can't find a recommended product? Call the 800 number listed in Product Resources for the store nearest you.

Parasite Infection

Intestinal Worms, Amoebic Dysentery, Giardia

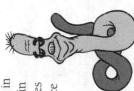

The human body is a host to over 130 different types of parasites! Worm and parasite infestations can range from mild and hardly noticeable to serious, even life-threatening in a child. Some experts estimate 50 million American children are infected with parasitic worms. Amoebas, a protozoan usually contracted from parasite infested water or food in third world countries, cause dysentery. Up to 50% of the U.S. water supply is contaminated with *giardia lamblia*, a protozoan that is not killed by chlorination. 2 million cases of Giardia are reported by the CDC every year. Other parasites move all over the body, including the brain, weakening the entire system. Nutritional therapy is a good choice for thread and pin worms, but not for heavy infestations. Short term conventional medical treatment is more beneficial for masses of hook and tape worms and blood flukes. (*Research shows that liver flukes may be a cause of cancer.*) **Do you have parasite signs?** *Round worms:* fever intestinal cramping. *Hookworms:* anemia, abdominal pain, diarrhea, lethargy. *Blood flukes:* lesions on the lungs, hemorrhages under the skin - typical in AIDS cases. *Protozoa (amoebae):* arthritis-like pain, leukemia-like symptoms, dysentery, pain, and dehydration. *Tapeworms:* intestinal obstruction (even from a single worm). Tapeworm eggs in the liver have been mistaken for and treated as if they were cancer. *Giardia:* diarrhea, weakness, weight loss, cramping, bloating and fever. *See DIVERTICULITIS, COLITIS AND CROHN'S DISEASE pages for more.*

Diet and Lifestyle Support Therapy

Nutritional therapy plan: *A strong immune system is the best defense for parasites, many of which have become drug-resistant - low nutrition = low immunity.*

1—Go on an apple and apple juice mono diet for 4 days. (1 day for a child). Take 8 garlic caps daily during the fast and chew fresh mango or papaya seeds mixed with honey. On the 3rd day, add papaya juice with 1 tbsp. wormwood tea, and 1 tbsp. molasses. On the 4th day, add 2 cups *senna/peppermint* tea with 1 tbsp. castor oil, and eat raw pumpkin seeds every 4 hours. Follow with a high resistance diet to prevent recurrence. Eat lots of onions and garlic. Avoid all sweets, dairy foods and junk foods. 3TBS amaranth or rice each morning helps remove parasites. Eat a daily green salad. Drink only bottled water. Take Pure Planet CHLORELLA, 2 tsp. daily. Garlic enemas or a high colonic irrigation helps clean the colon fast and address fungal infections, or yeast overgrowth conditions.

2—Herbal fast to expel tapeworms: Mix 4-oz. cucumber juice with honey and water. Take only this mixture for 24 hours. Follow with 3 cups senna/pumpkin seed tea. Drink down at once. •Drink at least 8 glasses water a day to flush out dead parasites.

3—For amoebic dysentery: Take a carrot/beet/cucumber juice daily for a week to clean the kidneys. Take a lemon juice/egg white drink each morning. Take 2 tbsp. epsom salts in a glass of water to purge the bowels. Then eat a high vegetable protein diet with cultured foods like yogurt, and bile stimulating foods like dandelion greens, artichokes, radishes.

Are you at risk for parasites? *Nationwide research conducted by the Centers for Disease Control over the last 25 years reveals that one in every six people selected at random had one or more parasites.* Most kissed and slept with their pets. Many frequently ate raw or smoked fish, or prosciutto or homemade sausages. (Note: Use toilet seat covers in public restrooms.)

—**Bodywork:** A purged stool test is helpful for diagnosing parasitic infections.

•Apply zinc oxide to anal opening. Then take a warm sitz bath using 1½ cups epsom salts per gallon of water. Repeat for 3 days. Worms often expel into the sitz bath.
•For crabs and lice - apply one of the following around anus: Thyme or sassafras oil, tea tree oil, (or myrrh extract and tea tree oil mixed).

Herbal, Superfood and Supplement Therapy

Interceptive therapy plan: Choose 2 to 3 recommendations.

1—Release and cleanse the parasites: •Crystal Star PARASITE PURGE™, or Nature's Secret PARASTROY; •Herbal Magic PARASITE KIT; •Arise & Shine WORM SQUIRM liquid or •Farmacopia IMMUN-NEEM capsules, 4 daily with 2 garlic caps, or 8 •*Cayenne/Garlic* capsules, after every meal for 2 weeks, and 4 cups fennel tea daily. (Or take garlic oil capsules in the morning. Refrain from eating or drinking until bowels have moved. Repeat for 3 days.) Then take •Creation's Garden PARASINE and keep intestines cleansed and flushed with •Crystal Star BITTERS & LEMON™ extract or Enzymedica PURIFY caps each morning. •Ayurvedic TRIKHATU tablets; •Uni-Key VERMA PLUS.

—**Anti-infectives:** •Crystal Star ANTI-BIO™ caps 4 daily as a lymph flush; •*Black walnut hull* or •*Myrrh* extract; •*Una da gato* caps 6 daily for a month; •*Basil* tea; •*Oregano* Oil caps 600mg for 6 weeks (good test results, but not during pregnancy); •*Witch hazel* leaf tea or •*dandelion* tea, 4 cups daily. •Uni-Key PARA SYSTEM or •East Park OLIVE LEAF EXTRACT, (a potent parasiticide).

2—Remove putrefactive fecal matter and mucous build-up: •Solaray GARLIC/ BLACK WALNUT caps; •Nature's Way HERBAL PUMPKIN; •Ayurvedic Concepts BITTER MELON; •AloeLife ALOE GOLD juice daily. •Homeopathic Ipecac. Relax bowels: •Valerian caps 4 daily; •Slippery elm tea 2 cups daily; •Magnesium 400-800mg daily.

3—For giardia: Nutribiotic GRAPEFRUIT SEED extract internally (read directions carefully); ELACK WALNUT or MYRRH extract, 10 drops under the tongue every 4 hours, or *tea tree* oil, 4 drops in water 4x daily, or *goldenseal* extract for 10 days.

4—Immune enhancers against parasites: •Earth's Bounty OXY CAPS. •Floradix HERBAL IRON liquid for strength during healing; •Beta carotene 50,000IU daily as an anti-infective; •B-complex 50mg daily.

5—Prob-otics are important to re-establish intestinal health: •American Health fermented soy-based ACIDOPHILUS liquid; •UAS DDS-PLUS with FOS; •Nutricology SYMBIOTICS powder, ½ tsp. 3x daily. •Garden of Life PRIMAL DEFENSE contains Homeostatic Soil Organisms- "prebiotics."

Can't find a recommended product? Call the 800 number listed in Product Resources for the store nearest you.

Parkinson's Disease

Central Nervous System Dysfunction

Parkinson's disease is a debilitating nerve disorder thought to be caused by neuro-toxic free radical damage to the brain ganglia that control muscle movement. The result is dopamine depletion in the brain, characterized by a slowly spreading muscle weakness and body rigidity. Posture is stooped, walking is shambling, motion is trembling and lifespan is shortened. Tragically, even though thinking processes often remain normal, the victim feels frozen, unable to move voluntarily. With over a million and a half cases in the U.S., Parkinson's affects men and women equally, usually between 50 and 75. L-dopa, the drug of choice for Parkinson's, has hallucinatory side effects and causes leg cramps. **Parkinson's signs?** Signs begin with a slight tremor in the hands or slight dragging of the foot, pronounced with fatigue; voluntary movement becomes increasingly difficult; walking becomes stiff and slow - the person may experience falls. Speech is difficult; vision problems ensue; the face may become expressionless and drooling develops because of muscle rigidity; there is numbness and tingling in the hands and feet. Depression (which can show dramatic improvement with supplementation) often sets in. **Parkinson's contributors?** Free radical damage from pesticide and aspartame residues, aluminum, mercury fillings and psycho tropic drugs are especially problematic. *Call (800) 457-6676 for Parkinson's information and practitioner referral.*

Diet and Lifestyle Support Therapy

Nutritional therapy helps re-establish normal biochemistry.

1—Go on a fresh organically grown foods diet for 3 days to cleanse and alkalize. Flora FLOR-ESSENCE tea aids detoxification. Then, follow a modified macrobiotic diet (pg. 348) for 3 to 6 months until condition improves. Eat 4-5 smaller meals a day. Keep meat protein low. Eliminate alcohol, caffeine and refined sugars of all kinds. Drink unfluoridated bottled water. Add one cup of •Crystal Star DR. VITALITY™ tea daily.

2—Go on a 24 hour juice fast (pg. 173) every two weeks during healing, with aloe vera juice or •AloeLife ALOE GOLD each morning to accelerate toxin release.

3—Live cell therapy from green drinks, like Crystal Star RESTORE YOUR STRENGTH™ drink, and chlorella for 2 months has been notably successful in reducing symptoms. Take vegetable drinks at least twice a week, or Sun CHLORELLA once a day.

4—Make a nerve mix of lecithin granules, toasted wheat germ, almonds, sunflower seeds, sesame seeds and nutritional yeast and take 2 tbsp. daily. Or, try •Red Star NU-TRITIONAL YEAST or •Green Foods WHEAT GERM extract.

5—New research shows that adding foods like eggs, chicken soup and shrimp helps normalize deficient brain-neurotransmitter biochemistry.

—Bodywork:

•Relaxation techniques like chiropractic treatment, massage therapy, acupuncture and acupressure have had notable success in reversing early Parkinson's.

•Catnip enemas once a month during healing to help liver/kidney function.

•Regular aerobic exercise is critical for outlook and muscle health. A brisk walk every day is highly recommended.

•Avoid aluminum (cookware, deodorants with aluminum chloride, condiments with alum, etc.)

•Fermented papaya preparation is being used with good results in Japan. Check out www.osatousa.com for information on how to purchase in the U.S.

• More information on natural Parkinson's disease protocols, visit: *http://www.cochran-foundation.org/*

Herbal, Superfood and Supplement Therapy

Interceptive therapy plan: Choose 1 or 2 recommendations.

1—**Rebuild nerve strength to ease tremor:** •Crystal Star RELAX CAPS™ 2 as needed, and •STRESS OUT™ muscle relaxer extract to ease shakiness (help within an hour); •Twin Lab GABA plus, or •Country Life RELAXER caps. •Threonine fights spasticity.

2—**Nourish brain and nerves:** Effective ginseng therapy: •Crystal Star MENTAL CLAR-ITY™ caps; Planetary BACOPA-GINSENG BRAIN STRENGTH; •Crystal Star MENTAL CLAR-ITY™ caps; Planetary BACOPA-GINSENG BRAIN STRENGTH; •Prince of Peace ROYAL JELLY/GINSENG vials. •Rainbow Light ADAPTO-GEM ginseng caps. •COQ10, specific for brain cell protection; •Enzymatic VITALINE COQ10 1200mg daily. •Lysine 500mg daily, •Anabol Naturals AMINO BALANCE, glutathione 100mg daily. (PD victims usually low.) •Scullcap tea daily (controls PD facial tics) or •Wakunaga NEURO-LOGIC daily.

3—**Increase body's dopamine biosynthesis:** •Sabinsa MUCUNA PRURIENS, a natural source of L-Dopa (goods results against PD); •NADH, 5-10mg in the morning; •Tyrosine 1000mg daily or •Enzymatic Therapy THYROID-TYROSINE daily;

4—**Enhance neurotransmitter activity:** •Phosphatidyl serine (PS) 100mg 3x daily; •Metabolic Response Modifiers NEURO-MAX; •Niacin therapy: 500mg 2x daily, with B-complex 100mg, extra B$_6$ 500mg daily if not taking L-dopa (if taking L-Dopa, do not take vitamin B$_6$; it can block L-Dopa to the brain), and •B-12, sublingual 2500mcg every other day. •Magnesium 800mg daily. •Creatine 3000mg daily for neuroprotection.

5—**Increase circulation:** •HAWTHORN extract as needed; •GINKGO BILOBA extract for leg cramps and tremor. •Solaray CAYENNE/GINSENG formula; •Golden Pride FOR-MULA ONE oral chelation with EDTA. •Add Crystal Star DR. ENZYME™ with protease and bromelain to take down inflammation.

6—**Critical EFA's for nerves and brain:** •EVENING PRIMROSE OIL 4-6 daily; •DHA 200mg daily or Neuromins DHA. DLPA 750mg helps depression.

7—**Antioxidants are critical in overcoming free radical brain damage:** •PCO's from grapeseed or white pine 300mg daily (also helps side effects from Sinemet); •Vitamin E 1000IU 2x daily with Selenium 200mcg; and•Vitamin C 5000mg daily with bioflavs; (as an ascorbic acid flush, pg. 193 for initial 2 weeks).

Can't find a recommended product? Call the 800 number listed in Product Resources for the store nearest you.

Phlebitis

Thrombo-Phlebitis, Embolism, Arterial Blood Clot

Phlebitis is vein inflammation, usually in the legs. It is a relatively common condition. An embolism is the obstruction of a blood vessel by a foreign substance or blood clot. Thrombophlebitis is the existence of a blood clot within the vascular system. Deep vein thrombosis is life-threatening because the clot can break free and occlude a vessel or lodge in the lung. Get medical help immediately!

Common Symptoms: Swelling, inflammation, redness and aching in the legs; fever with blood clots in the legs; pain and tenderness along course of a vein; swelling below obstruction. Elevate legs whenever possible. No prolonged sitting. Consciously stretch and walk frequently during the day.

Common Causes: Clogged and toxic bloodstream from excess saturated fats, especially from too much red meat and fried food; inactivity, lack of daily exercise, and sedentary lifestyle; poor circulation from constipation, obesity or weak heart; oral contraceptive side effect; prolonged emotional stress. Believe it or not, even too tight underwear or jeans can constrict circulation in the abdomen and groin where deep-vein phlebitis originates. Keep your weight down to relieve pressure on circulatory system instead of squeezing into tight clothes. *See the HEALTHY HEART DIET page 448 for more information.*

Diet and Lifestyle Support Therapy

Nutritional therapy plan:

1—Take one glass of each every other day: Black cherry juice, fresh carrot juice, a veggie drink like Knudsen's VERY VEGGIE, or Aloe Life ALOE FIBER MATE drink, or Jarrow GENTLE FIBERS, or Green Foods WHEAT GERM extract drink for venous integrity.

2—Have a daily cup of green tea or Crystal Star DR. VITALITY™ green and white tea.

3—Have a leafy green salad every day. Drink 6 glasses of bottled water daily.

4—Eat plenty of onions, garlic and other high sulphur foods. Have an onion/garlic broth at least 2-3x week.

5—Green drinks help circulation: Try •C'est Si Bon CHLORENERGY 1 packet daily, •Wakunaga KYO-GREEN, •Crystal Star ENERGY GREEN RENEWAL™ drink. Or make a circulation mix of lecithin granules and nutritional yeast and take 2 tbsp. daily. Or try Solgar WHEY TO GO protein drink to lower cholesterol.

6—Avoid starchy, fried and fatty foods. Avoid refined sugars, caffeine and hard liquor.

—Bodywork:

• Take a brisk half hour walk daily.
• Avoid smoking and secondary smoke. It constricts blood vessels and restricts oxygen use.
• Avoid anti-coagulants and oral contraceptives unless necessary.
• Take alternating hot and cold sitz baths, or apply alternating hot and cold ginger/cayenne compresses to stimulate leg blood circulation.
• Apply Earth's Bounty O₂ spray, or alcohol compresses.

Apply effective herbal compresses right to the legs:

•Plantain; •St. John's wort and St. John's wort oil; •Yarrow flowers and •Calendula flowers or •CALIFLORA gel, •B&T ARNICA, •Witch hazel, •Fresh comfrey leaf.

Herbal, Superfood and Supplement Therapy

Interceptive therapy plan: Choose 2 or more recommendations.

1—Help normalize blood composition and circulation: •Crystal Star HEARTSEASE HBP™ caps, or •Butcher's broom caps, or Natural Balance GREAT LEGS caps for 1 month.
•HAWTHORN extract 4x daily for 3 months to normalize circulation, or •Nutricology BEST BLOOD OXYGENATION formula; •Wakunaga KYOLIC 108 to reduce high homocysteine.
•Glucosamine/chondroitin caps for anti-thrombogenic, anti-coagulant activity. •Reishi mushroom extract capsules or •Planetary REISHI MUSHROOM SUPREME to rebuild immunity.

—**Niacin therapy:** 500mg 3x daily, with •Chromium picolinate 200mcg or Solaray CHROMIACIN.

2—Take down inflammation: •Crystal Star DR. ENZYME™ with protease and bromelain (helps reduce harmful blood clots), or •Enzymedica PURIFY protease (powerful blood purifier). •Nutricology NATTOZYME (specific for unhealthy blood coagulation).

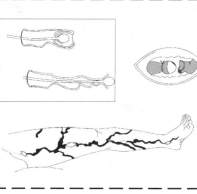

•Bromelain 1500mg daily with Quercetin 1000mg (anti-inflammatory and clot inhibitor for fragile veins). •Crystal Star GREEN TEA CLEANSER™ each morning on rising with ANTI-FLAM™ caps 4 as needed; •Evening Primrose Oil 4000mg daily; •Barleans lignan-rich flax oil 3x daily.

3—Strengthen veins and capillaries with flavonoids: •Crystal Star VARI-VEIN™ caps with grapeseed PCO's and horse chestnut, or •PCO's from grapeseed or white pine 300mg daily to strengthen arterial system.
•Esteem Products BEYOND RELIEF; GINKGO BILOBA or BILBERRY extract caps 6 daily. •Solaray CENTELLA-VEIN 3x daily.

4—Cleanse infection always present in phlebitis: •Nutricology GERMANIUM 150mg daily (highly effective); •ECHINACEA extract; •Ascorbate vitamin C crystals with bioflavs, ¼ tsp. daily to bowel tolerance for 2 weeks. •Biotec CELL GUARD 8 daily scavenge free radicals.

5—Help intermittent claudication *(atherosclerosis affecting the legs)*: •Pacific BioLogic ADAPTRIN - Ayurvedic Padma 28 (recommended); •Lane Labs PALMVITEE tocotrienols (Rapid improvement often noted).

Can't find a recommended product? Call the 800 number listed in Product Resources for the store nearest you.

521

Pneumonia

Bacterial Pneumonia, Viral Pneumonia, Pleurisy

Pneumonias and pleurisy are inflamed lung diseases caused by an array of viruses and other pathogenic organisms. *Bacterial pneumonia*, contracted mostly by children, is caused by staph, strep or pneumo-bacilli; it responds to antibiotics, both medical and herbal. *Viral pneumonia* is an acute systemic disease caused by virulent viruses which do not respond to antibiotics. Herbal antivirals show some success. *Pleurisy* is the inflamed pleura membrane surrounding the lungs, and often accompanies pneumonia. Pneumonias drastically weaken immune response. Typically, it can take 2 to 3 months to recover strength and up to 2 years to be able to resist a cold or flu without falling victim to another pneumonia bout. **Do you have pneumonia?** Sore, inflamed lungs and chest, with difficult breathing, heavy coughing and expectoration, worsening after 5 days. Fluid in lymph and lungs, back, muscle and body aches, chills, high fever and the inability to "get over it" all figure in. Great fatigue remains for 6 to 8 weeks even after recovery. *What causes it?* Low immunity from poor nutrition or a preceding respiratory infection, clogged lymph nodes, gum disease, chemical sensitivity to pesticides and herbicides. Body stress and fatigue from a long day outdoors in winter can be a trigger. *See LUNG DISEASE page 487.*

Diet and Lifestyle Support Therapy

Nutritional therapy plan:

1—Go on a mucous-cleansing liquid diet for 1 to 3 days during the acute stages. (pg. 202). Drink plenty of fruit juices, herb teas and pure water to thin mucous. Avoid alcohol.

2—Take a hot lemon and honey drink with water each morning, or a cup of green tea, or an aloe vera juice drink like Sun Wellness Chlorella WAKASA GOLD, or •AloeLife ALOE GOLD drink. Or have a fresh carrot juice, a potassium broth (pg. 291).

3—Then follow a largely fresh foods, cleansing diet for 1-2 weeks. Add a superfood drink once a day, like Barleans GREENS or Crystal Star RESTORE YOUR STRENGTH™.

4—Then eat a diet high in vegetable protein, low in meat and dairy foods, to allow easier healing. Add cultured foods: Rejuvenative Foods VEGGIE DELITE, yogurt, kefir.

5—As an emergency measure, take fresh grated horseradish root in a spoon with lemon juice. Hang over a sink immediately to expel large quantities of mucous.

—Lifestyle measures:

•Do not risk your health if you experience major difficulty in breathing. Short term heroic medicine may be necessary. Newer broad spectrum drugs can sometimes give your body a "breather" from the infection trauma and are less harmful to normal body functions than most primary antibiotics. Ask your physician.

•Get plenty of rest. Do diaphragmatic breathing, especially during recovery. Breathe in, pushing abdomen out, then from chest to completely fill upper and lower lungs.

•Apply a hot *cayenne/ginger* poultice: Mix powders - ½ tsp. *cayenne*, 1 tbsp. *lobelia*, 3 tbsp. *slippery elm*, 2 tbsp. *ginger* and enough water to make a paste. Leave on chest 1 hour.

•Apply a mustard plaster to chest to stimulate lungs, draw out poisons: Mix 1 tbsp. mustard powder, 1 egg, 3 tbsp. flour + water to make a paste; leave on til skin turns pink.

•Take an oxygen bath. Use 1 to 2 cups 3% H₂O₂ to a tub of water. Soak 20 minutes. •Overheating therapy helps for viral pneumonia to quell virus replication. See page 182. •Take hot and cold showers to stimulate lung circulation (pg. 185). Then use chest or back percussion with a cupped hand front and back to loosen matter.

Herbal, Superfood and Supplement Therapy

Interceptive therapy plan: Choose 2 to 3 recommendations.

1—Control the infection: •Olive leaf extract caps 2 to 6 daily; •Oregano oil 3 caps, 3x daily; •MICROHYDRIN PLUS, available at royalbodycare.com; •Crystal Star ANTI-BIO™ caps or extract (anti-viral support for viral pneumonia) 6x daily to flush toxins. Take your choice of herbal antibiotics with probiotics to rebuild immunity: •Pure Essence FLORALIVE or •Jarrow JARRO-DOPHILUS.

—**After crisis has passed**, take •Crystal Star •ANTI-HST™ caps, to encourage oxygen uptake. Add •Crystal Star MUSCLE RELAXER™ caps 6 daily, or •Herbs, Etc. LUNG TONIC softgels or *cayenne/ginger/goldenseal* caps 6 daily, or *mullein/lobelia* extract drops as broncho-dilating anti-spasmodics. •Quercetin 1000mg with bromelain, 1500mg daily takes down inflammation. Better oxygen uptake: •Hawthorn or Ginkgo Biloba extract. Diuretics reduce lung fluid: •*Uva Ursi/Cornsilk* or *Senna/Dandelion* tea.

2—Expectorants help remove excess mucous from the lungs: •Zand DECONGEST tabs; •*pleurisy root* tea or •*slippery elm* tea; •Crystal Star D-CONGEST™ fast relief spray with extra ginger pinches or •Yogi BREATHE DEEP tea.

3—Take powerful antioxidants: •Carnitine 1000mg 3x daily for 1 month; NAC (*N-acetyl-cysteine*) 500mg 3x daily; •CoQ-10, 300mg daily; •Nutricology germanium 150mg 2 daily (very effective). •PCOs from grapeseed or white pine 300mg daily.

4—Protect your lungs against further infection: •Vitamin C/antioxidant therapy: •Ascorbate vitamin C crystals with bioflavonoids and rutin, ¼ tsp. every hour to bowel tolerance, daily for 2 weeks; then every 2 hours for 2 weeks; then 3000mg daily for a month; or use •American Health MEGA ACEROLA PLUS with Vitamin C. •Zinc pico-linate 4x daily, or •Source Naturals OPTI-ZINC 30mg daily; •Vitamin E 400IU 2x daily; •GINSENG/LICORICE extract as a demulcent and adaptogen.

5—For pneumonia with pleurisy (*burning lungs, difficulty taking a deep breath, great fatigue even on a short walk*): •Source Naturals INFLAMA-REST (highly recommended); with Crystal Star ANTI-BIO™ extract; •Earth's Bounty O₂ CAPS and rub O₂ SPRAY rubbed on the chest twice daily; •Thyme extract drops in water as a decongestant.

Can't find a recommended product? Call the 800 number listed in Product Resources for the store nearest you.

Poisoning, Environmental Illness

Heavy Metals, Radiation, Chemical Contaminants, Gulf War Syndrome

Heavy metal poisoning is a major problem for modern societies. There seems to be no way to avoid toxic exposure. Chemical pollutants and toxic byproducts affect every facet of our lives, from our water and food supply to the workplace and our homes. Immune response is the first casualty of an unhealthy environment, especially in the way that the liver and kidneys are impacted. Periodic detoxification needs to be a part of our lives today to help the body use its own cleansing mechanisms to maintain healthy immunity. *Note: Hair analysis is helpful in determining nutrient deficiencies caused by environmental toxins.* **Signs you may be chemically toxic?** Do you wake up feeling lousy for no reason. Do you smell things like perfumes and strong cleansers more intensely than most? Does alcohol or certain medications, even some vitamins make you feel worse? Is your reaction time when driving noticeably poorer in city traffic? Do you experience schizophrenic-like behavior, unusual memory loss, infertility, impotence or insomnia? Do you have small black spots along your gum line? Do you have bad breath and body odor, premature graying or hair loss (from cigarette toxins)? **Chemical toxin causes?** Pollutant and toxic chemical build up from chemical-laced foods, insecticides, amalgam dental fillings, fluoridated water, hair dyes; aluminum cookware and deodorants, smoke, smog, cigarette and marijuana smoking (causes cadmium overload with zinc depletion) See page 53 on neutralizing effects of radiation.

Diet and Lifestyle Support Therapy

Nutritional therapy plan:

1—Don't go on an all-liquid diet when trying to release heavy metals or chemicals from the body. They enter the bloodstream too fast and heavily for the body to handle, and can poison you even more. Instead, go on a seven day brown rice and vegetable juice diet (pg. 178) to start releasing poisons. Have a glass of fresh carrot juice, fresh lemon in water, or •Aloe Answers ALOE FORCE juice with herbs, a potassium broth (pg. 291), or Futurebiotics VITAL K drink for potassium, and miso soup daily. Drink bottled or distilled water.

2—Green drinks are key detoxifiers and blood builders: •C'est Si Bon CHLORENERGY, (Zeolite), highly recommended for a heavy metal, petrochemical detox. For radiation a specific for heavy metal poisoning (mercury, cadmium, lead, arsenic) and radiation toxicity, or •Crystal Star ENERGY GREEN RENEWAL™.

3—Add lots of leafy greens and mineral-rich foods like sea greens. Eat organically grown foods when possible. Avoid canned foods. Avoid fried foods, red meats, pasteurized dairy foods, fatty and sugary foods. Avoid caffeine - it inhibits liver filtering.

4—Make a mix of ¼ cup *each*: wheat germ, molasses, lecithin granules and nutritional yeast - take 2 tbsp. daily in any dish or drink. Add spices: chili powder, turmeric and black pepper to protect against radiation. *Cilantro* excretes mercury; aluminum, lead toxicity.

—**Lifestyle measures:** •Protect against radiation syndromes: avoid foods labeled irradiated or electronically pasteurized. •Use an indoor air filter to remove toxins in the air. Use vinegar, baking soda and salt as household cleansers if you are very sensitive. •Protect against EMF fields: avoid non-filtered computer screens, electric blankets, microwave ovens. (Don't use plastic wrap in a microwave; its heat can drive the molecules into the food.) •Avoid smoke, pesticides (sprinkle pepper on anthills instead) and herbicides, phosphorus fertilizers, fluorescent lights, aluminum cookware and deodorants. •Take a walk every day, breathing deeply. Do deep breathing exercises on rising, and in the evening on retiring to clear the lungs and respiratory system. •Earth's Bounty O₂ SPRAY on soles of feet every 2 days to keep tissue oxygen high. •Take a hot seaweed bath for mineral therapy. •Spring Life POLARIZERS have notable success against environmental pollutants.

Herbal, Superfood and Supplement Therapy

Avoid commercial antacids - they interfere with enzyme production, and the ability of the body to carry off heavy metals. Use plant enzymes instead.

Interceptive therapy plan: Choose 2 or more recommendations.

1—**Release contaminants from the body:** •Crystal Star TOXIN DETOX™ or •DETOX BLOOD PURIFIER™ caps for 2-3 months; •For lead poisoning in children: take vitamin C with •CLEANSING & PURIFYING™ tea daily to release toxins through sweat; add •white pine PCOs. as a preventive for 3 months (good results). • PSP Marketing DESTROXIN poisoning: vitamin C powder with bioflavonoids ½ tsp. every hour to bowel tolerance. •Anabol AMINO BALANCE is a natural chelator of metals (recommended).

2—**Enhance liver activity:** •Alpha Lipoic Acid 600mg daily for 2 months. •Crystal Star LIVER RENEW™ caps with •*Milk thistle seed* extract or •*Dandelion* extract; •Crystal Star LIVER CLEANSE FLUSHING™ tea or Enzymatic Therapy LIVA-TOX caps; •EVENING PRIMROSE oil caps 4 daily; •Biostrath LIQUID YEAST.

3—**Boost thyroid activity** (esp. if you're in a fluoridated area): •Crystal Star IODINE, POTASSIUM, SILICA drops or OCEAN MINERALS™ caps, or Kelp 8-10 tabs daily, (for radiation poisoning). •Solaray ALFA-JUICE caps; •Bernard Jensen's LIQUI-DULSE.

4—**Build strong immune defenses:** •*Astragalus* extract; •*Propolis* extract or lozenges; •*Cat's Claw* extract for 2 months; •*Garlic* 6-8 caps daily; •*Siberian eleuthero* extract caps; •Spirulina = tsp. daily, or •Spirulina NANOCLUSTERS from Royal Bodycare (especially for radiation toxins); •CHLORELLA 2 tsp. daily for chemical toxins.

5—**Protect yourself with powerful antioxidants:** •Carnitine 1000mg 3x daily for 1 month; •NAC (N-acetyl-cysteine) 500mg 3x daily; •CoQ-10, 60mg 4x daily; •Nutricology GERMANIUM 150mg daily. •Beta carotene 150,000IU with extra lycopene 5-10mg; •PCO's from grapeseed or white pine 100mg 3 daily; •Vitamin E 400IU with selenium 200mcg; •Glutathione 100mg daily; •MICROHYDRIN PLUS available at royalbodycare. com; •Source Naturals OPTI-ZINC 30mg daily, and CHEM-DEFENSE; Enzymatic Therapy TI-YMUPLEX. •Biotec CELL GUARD 8 daily.

Can't find a recommended product? Call the 800 number listed in Product Resources for the store nearest you.

Poisoning, Food

E. Coli, Salmonella, Botulism, Arsenic, Campylobacter

The CDC estimates that every year in the United States 76 million people contract foodborne illness, 325,000 people are hospitalized and 5,000 die as a result. Even with government inspections, better packaging, refrigeration and preservatives, food poisoning is on the rise (mostly in children and the elderly). It's one of the places scientists point to illustrate the fast development of antibiotic-resistant disease strains. **Botulism** is poisoning by a micro-organism similar to that causing tetanus. (Do not give honey to infants for fear of botulism.) **Salmonella** is widespread (a new strain DT104 is responsible for nearly 10% of food poisoning cases) from bacteria found in hormone-injected beef and poultry. *E. coli*, a bacteria that attacks the kidneys sickens up to 20,000 American annually and kills several hundred. *Campylobacter bacteria* may infect up to ⅔ of chickens on the market today and causes 2.4 million food poisoning cases every year. **Do you have signs of food poisoning?** Many people get cold sweats after eating, severe abdominal pain and flatulence, headaches, chills, fever and rashy skin. *Salmonella* infects the intestines with diarrhea, nausea, cramps and vomiting. Botulism signs are weak, limp muscles 12 to 36 hours after eating, double vision, dry mouth, speech difficulty, vomiting, cramps, even respiratory failure. **Food poisoning risks?** Reaction to pesticides and fungicide residues, food additives, preservatives, sulfites and MSG; breathing noxious fumes; lack of proper food preparation and storage. Discard all bulging food cans. *Call the POISON CONTROL CENTER Hotline, 800-764-7661, for emergency information.*

Diet and Lifestyle Support Therapy

Nutritional therapy plan:

1—Take ½ cup olive oil very slowly through a straw to remove poison from the stomach or a glass of warm water with 1 tsp. baking soda. Take a green drink every 4 hours to normalize body chemistry: try Crystal Star ENERGY GREEN RENEWAL™ or Pure Planet CHLORELLA, 1 tsp. in water.

2—Take no milk, juice, alcohol or vinegar until poisons have moved from the stomach. Take ALOE VERA JUICE morning and evening for a week after poisoning.

3—Eat high fiber foods, citrus fruits, wheat germ, whole grains, green and yellow vegetables. These foods act as protectors against pesticides and poisons in food.

4—Balance your intestinal structure with Garden of Life GOATEIN Protein drink (from goat's milk- highly digestible), or Futurebiotics VITAL K, 2 tsp. daily.

— **Toxin neutralizing foods:**
1-2 heads of iceberg lettuce
Bamboo shoots
Strong black or green tea or lemon water
Burnt toast
2 raw eggs
Apple pectin caps (good results)

— **Bodywork and lifestyle measures:**
•Use emetic of Ipecac or strong *lobelia* tea with ¼ - ½ tsp. cayenne to vomit up poisons and empty the stomach. Follow with *white oak* tincture to normalize stomach.
•Use a coffee or catnip enema to flush bowels and stimulate liver detox function.
•Sweat out pesticides and chemical poisons from food in a long, low heat sauna. Or, home overheating therapy is effective. See page 182 in this book for correct technique.
•Spring Life POLARIZERS have notable success against food-borne pollutants.
•Use American Biologics DIOXYCHLOR or NutriBiotic GRAPEFRUIT SEED extract in water as directed to decontaminate produce or Healthy Harvest VEGETABLE RINSE.

Herbal, Superfood and Supplement Therapy

Interceptive therapy plan: Choose 2 or more recommendations.

1—If you think you have food poisoning: Take •Activated charcoal tabs to absorb poison, 3 to 5 every 15 minutes, or •Solaray CLAY & HERBS caps or bentonite clay powder to absorb poisons. Take •vitamin C powder, ½ tsp. every ½ hour (or vitamin C caps 500mg every hour) to bowel tolerance to flush and alkalize the tissues. •Niacin therapy helps sweat out poisons; 250-500mg every hour until improvement is felt (about 3-4 capsules).

2—Normalize your stomach and intestines: Take •Crystal Star CLEANSING & PURI-FYING™ tea 3 times daily, with •Pure Planet CHLORELLA tabs. 10 every 4 hours to neutralize toxins and normalize body chemistry. Use •Nelson Bach RESCUE REMEDY for rebalance. Take •Garlic caps 2 with each meal. For *salmonella:* take •Guarana water extract. For *E. coli* and *salmonella:* take •bee pollen granules. For *arsenic poisoning:* take •*Yellow dock-nettles* tea.

3—Detoxify your liver: •MILK THISTLE SEED extract is primary, (even used in Europe to fight liver disease caused by *Amanita*, death cap mushrooms). •Alpha Lipoic Acid 300-600mg daily (highly recommended); •Enzymatic Therapy LIVA-TOX caps or •SAMe 800mg daily with •Crystal Star LIVER RENEW™ caps 6 daily and LIVER CLEANSE FLUSHING tea, 2 cups daily; •Crystal Star BITTERS & LEMON™ extract each morning (very effective).

4—Sea greens are primary poison protectors: •Crystal Star OCEAN MINERALS™ caps 2 daily; Green Foods IONKELP tabs 12 daily. Nature's Path TRACE-MIN-LYTE with sea greens, 4 daily. Toxin neutralizing teas: *Plantain, Scullcap, Wormwood* tea.

5—Probiotics produce fatty acids and acidify the bowel to inhibit pathogenic organisms: including *salmonella* - Jarrow Products JARRO-DOPHILUS or •UAS DDS-PLUS. Take with •Crystal Star ANTI-BIO™ extract 4-6 daily for extra stomach cleansing anti-infective bitters.

6—Protective supplements against food poisons: •Vitamin E 400IU with selenium 200mcg; •Vitamin C, 3000mg daily; •Glutathione 100mg daily; •mixed carotenes PHY-COTENE NANOCLUSTERS from royalbodycare.com; •Biotec CELL GUARD 6 daily.

Can't find a recommended product? Call the 800 number listed in Product Resources for the store nearest you.

524

Poison Oak and Poison Ivy

Sumac

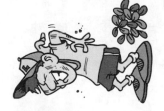

Urushiol, the toxic oleoresin responsible for the poison oak and ivy reactions, is one of the most potent external toxins on earth! One quarter ounce of urushiol has the potential to affect everyone in the world. Its toxicity can survive for 100 years after the plant is dead. Irritating resins are carried in smoke when the plant is burned, so don't burn it or try to uproot it. Even sap that has been diluted 50 million times can induce toxicity. Poison oak, poison ivy and sumac all react with the body's immune system T-lymphocytes to produce the itchy rash. Over 2 million people a year get a poison oak or ivy reaction, mostly in children. Over 60% of Americans are sensitive to it, but once you lose your sensitivity, an immunity sets in that remains for life.

Is your rash poison oak or ivy? Allergic reaction takes place within 72 hours after contact. The resin responsible for the allergic skin reaction must touch the skin or clothing of the person to cause the reaction. Reaction signs range from an annoying itch to a life-threatening condition. Itching blisters on the skin ooze, erupt and spread the systemic plant poisons. (Thankfully, the blisters don't contain the oleoresin, so you can't "pass it on.") There may be throat swelling, cramps and diarrhea. People with sun-sensitive skin are most susceptible. *See Skin, ITCHING, page 514 for more information.*

Diet and Lifestyle Support Therapy

Nutritional therapy plan:

1—Apply cider vinegar, denatured alcohol, and oatmeal paste or a cornstarch paste to blisters to control itching and neutralize acid poisons.

2—Follow a fresh foods diet during acute blistering to cleanse systemic poisons out of the bloodstream. No junk or fried foods.

3—Take several veggie green drinks during acute phase, like Green Foods GREEN ESSENCE or C'est Si Bon CHLORENERGY.

4—Then alkalize your body with ALOE VERA juice and apply aloe vera gel.

—**Bodywork:**

• *Artemesia* (mugwort) grows in the same vicinity as poison oak, and appears to be a naturally-occurring protective plant against it. Rub fresh mugwort leaves on any exposed skin before you go out in the woods or brush.

• Cover all exposed skin before going out. If you do become exposed, remove clothing for washing. Take a shower and lather up with regular blue dishwashing soap (DAWN). Excellent for poison oak prevention! Or, wash within 30 minutes of contact in cold water with a non-oil soap. (*Oil soaps spread the urushiol.*) If there's an ocean nearby, a swim is excellent effective, neutralizing therapy.

• If you see it on your property, kill poison oak and ivy with a systemic herbicide for best results.

—**Effective bath additions:** • 1 cup Epsom salts with 4 tbsp. green clay added and a few drops of peppermint oil. • Apple cider vinegar. • Baking soda or cornstarch. • Oatmeal (very effective, esp. for children).

—**Effective skin rash applications:** wash affected area in *cold* water first. • Aloe vera gel. • Witch hazel. • Rubbing alcohol. • Wet black tea bags. • Dr. Bronner's Natural peppermint liquid soap.

Herbal, Superfood and Supplement Therapy

Intercept ve therapy plan: Choose 2 or more recommendations.

1—Stop the itch: Apply a jewelweed poultice to calm the itch (excellent results) or • Crystal S ar ANTI-BIO™ gel as needed. Take • *Echinacea-Goldenseal-Mugwort-Yellow Dock* capsules as directed to help neutralize the systemic poison. • Homeopathic *Rhus Tox.* Spray with Earth's Bounty O₂ spray (a good medicine cabinet item).

2—Reduce swelling, promote healing: • Nutribiotic GRAPEFRUIT SEED extract caps as directed, or grapefruit SKIN SPRAY as needed (sometimes works overnight); • Enzymedica PURIFY, protease breaks down poison oak proteinaceous matter (very effective). • Emulsified vitamin A & E oil; • Apply • a paste of honey and goldenseal powder; cover with a bandage. • Vitamin E oil decreases healing time.

3—Calm the histamine reaction and soothe the nerve endings: • Crystal Star ANTI-HST™ capsules 6 daily until clear, to help curb histamine allergy reaction. • Vitamin C therapy is a natural antihistamine: take vitamin C crystals, ¼ tsp. every hour to bowel tolerance, until itching lessens, then reduce to ¼ tsp. 4x daily until clear. Take • magnesium 400mg 2x daily. Take • zinc 30mg daily.

4—Strengthen the adrenal glands against sensitivity: • Crystal Star ADRENAL ENERGY BOOST™ caps 2x daily or • Planetary SCHIZANDRA ADRENAL COMPLEX. • Hylands homeopathic *Poison Oak* tabs to build resistance protection (very effective).

—**Effective topical healers:** • Jewelweed tea, a specific - apply locally, take internally. • Tea tree oil, which sloughs off old, affected tissue, and leaves healthy tissue intact; • Comfrey/aloe salve; • B &T CALIFLORA gel; • Calendula ointment or calendula-goldenseal ointment, or Goldenseal solution in water; • Witch hazel; • Bioforce ECHINACEA cream; • Fresh plantain leaves, crush and rub on affected areas; • Sassafras tea; • Black walnut tincture, apply locally, take internally; • Oregon grape root, yerba santa or yellow dock root washes; • Floradix CALCIUM, MAGNESIUM liquid; • Chinese WHITE FLOWER OIL.

Can't find a recommended product? Call the 800 number listed in Product Resources for the store nearest you.

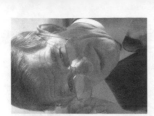

Prostate Enlargement

Benign Prostatic Hypertrophy, Chronic Prostatitis

Prostate disorders usually begin after age 35. Between the ages of 51 and 60, 50% of all men have an enlarged prostate - over 90% percent by age 80. Commonly prescribed drugs like PROSCAR and PROS-GUARD can cause side effects of decreased potency and libido (in some cases sexuality is stifled entirely). But men can help themselves naturally manage prostate problems without the highly adverse side effects (often as bad as the prostate problem itself), or limited success of the drug approach. Men who exercise regularly are less likely to develop prostate problems. Avoid chemical antihistamines. Overuse impairs liver and prostate function. **Is your prostate enlarged?** With BPH, the disease is basically the symptoms.... an inflamed, swollen, infected prostate gland; frequent, painful desire to urinate with reduced flow of urine or dribbling, especially at night, incontinence in severe cases; lower back and leg pain; impotence, loss of libido, and usually painful ejaculation. Most men also suffer insomnia and fatigue. **What's at the root of the problem?** A high fat diet puts a man at greatest risk, as does a poor diet with too little fiber, and too much alcohol and caffeine. Essential fatty acid and prostaglandin depletion lead to hormonal changes like increased estrogen levels and altered testosterone levels. Exhausted lymph system from too many antihistamines and lack of exercise figures in. *See PROSTATE CANCER page 351.*

Diet and Lifestyle Support Therapy

Nutritional therapy plan:

1—Take lemon juice and water every morning for two weeks to cleanse sediment; then add cider vinegar and honey in water daily for a month to prevent sediment recurrence. Add green tea daily. Follow a fresh foods, low fat, high fiber diet for 3 week, with plenty of green salads, fresh fruits, juices and steamed vegetables.

2—Watchwords should be: less saturated and trans fat, more fiber. Add whole grains, soy foods, seafoods and sea greens (2 tbsp. snipped dry daily) for more EFAs.

3—Make a mix: lecithin granules, toasted wheat germ, pumpkin seeds, oat bran, nutritional yeast, sesame seeds, crumbled dry sea greens; take 4 tbsp. daily over rice or miso soup.

4—Drink 6 glasses of water or cleansing fluids daily. Especially add 2 glasses of cranberry juice. Have a vegetable drink like Nutricology PRO GREENS with EFAs, or Crystal Star RESTORE YOUR STRENGTH™ drink for iodine and potassium nutrients, during healing.

5—Avoid red meats, caffeine, hard liquor, sodas, especially beer, during healing. Limit spicy foods that irritate your bladder. Avoid tobacco, fried, fatty and refined foods forever.

—**Bodywork:** Some studies show that a man should think twice before having a vasectomy, because of possible increased risk of prostate cancer among vasectomized men. As sperm builds up in the sealed-off vas deferens, the body reabsorbs it and sometimes tries to mount an autoimmune response to its own tissue. Also the testes are a powerful focal point of man's life force. When something interferes with the movement of sperm, energy flow is blocked, eventually resulting in stagnation and degeneration. A vasectomy can also result in liver blockage that leads to prostate inflammation, leg cramps, abdominal pain and irritability.

•Sexual intercourse during prostatitis irritates the prostate and delays recovery. After recovery, sex life should be normal in frequency with a natural climax.
•Overheating therapy shows some success for some men. See page 182.
•Use *chamomile* tea enemas once a week during healing as an acid cleanser. Or take warm chamomile sitz baths for 20 minutes at a time morning and evening.
•Ice packs reduce pain. A brisk daily walk helps. Warm baths soothe and relax.

Herbal, Superfood and Supplement Therapy

Interceptive therapy plan: Choose 2 or more recommendations.

1—**A highly successful anti-inflammatory herbal program:** •Crystal Star PROX™ PROSTATE PROTECTOR™ caps 6 daily, then 4 daily for 1 month; •Cerniline American can CERNILTONE flower pollen extract; •Crystal Star RELAX™ caps to ease urination; •EVENING PRIMROSE oil 4000mg daily for 1 month, then 2-4 daily for 1 month with •bee pollen caps 2 daily, and •ANTI-BIO™ caps 4 daily for 1 month. •Crystal Star DR. ENZYME™ with protease and bromelain or Bromelain 1500mg (faster healing).

—**A two-month prevention program:** •Zinc 100mg daily for 1 month, then 50mg daily for 1 month or Ethical Nutrients ZINC STATUS; •B-6, 200mg daily; •Glutamine 1000mg daily or •Anabol Naturals AMINO BALANCE (highly recommended).

Follow-up: •Crystal Star MALE PERFORMANCE™ for regeneration, •OCEAN MINERALS™ caps, or *kelp* tabs 10 daily for prevention, •New Chapter ZYFLAMEND or PROSTATE 5LX formulas to guard against prostate cancer (good results). Take •vitamin E 400IU; or *white oak bark* tea, or •Melatonin 3mg at night to decrease size of prostate.

2—**Rid the body of pathogens and congestive residues:** •Vitamin C crystals, ½ tsp. every hour to bowel tolerance for 2 weeks, then ½ tsp. 4x daily for 2 weeks, then 3000mg daily for 1 month. •Glycine 1000mg for sediment control; •Enzymedica PURIFY to dissolve lesions. Use •*Uva Ursi* tea, •*Una da Gato* caps; •*Nettles* extract or •*horsetail-nettles* tea to reduce prostate swelling rapidly. •Echinacea/goldenseal extract drops 4x daily; •Garlic caps 8 daily, or •Pau d'arco tea 3 cups daily; •mixed carotenes 100,000IU. •GABA relieves frequent urination and fights infection. •Vitamin E 800IU daily.

3—**Soothe the pain with EFAs:** •Evening Primrose oil 4000mg daily; •Udo's PERFECTED OIL BLEND; •Barleans lignan-rich flax oil 3x daily; •Crystal Star ANTI-FLAM™ caps, 4 at a time as needed. —**For prostatitis:** •Quercetin 1000mg daily with Bromelain 1500mg daily (helps stop pain). A *saw palmetto/pygeum* formula, like •Solaray PROSTA-GEUM, with •Barleans lignan-rich flax oil 3x daily; •zinc 100mg daily, •vitamin E 800IU daily with selenium 200mcg or •Eidon SELENIUM liquid.

4—**Flavonoids deter cancer-causing hormones:** •Grapeseed PCOs 300mg daily; •Bilberry extract 2x daily, or •vitamin C 5000mg with bioflavonoids daily.

Can't find a recommended product? Call the 800 number listed in Product Resources for the store nearest you.

Rheumatic Fever

Severe Systemic Inflammation, Roseola

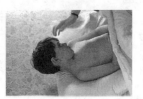

Rheumatic fever is a serious inflammatory condition following a strep infection. It normally affects small children between 3 and 12 years old. Full blown rheumatic fever affects the heart or brain; arthritis-like pain and stiffness often settles in the joints. A prolapse of the mitral valve, an abnormality of a gate within the heart may also be related to RF. Rheumatic fever can be prevented if the strep virus is killed within 10 to 12 days of infection, before it overwhelms the body's immune defenses. Once the disease has been contracted, recurrence is common. Treatment must be maintained for months, even years to prevent rheumatic heart disease. Natural treatment focuses on rebuilding immune response. *Roseola*, often called scarlet fever, is a similar child's infectious disease accompanied by high fever, nausea and a skin rash. **What are the signs?** An initial moderate fever, followed by chronic extreme weakness. There is often a skin rash, poor circulation, shortness of breath and a long term sore throat. The most common symptom of full-blown RF is arthritis. Roseola symptoms include a high fever for 3 or 4 days, usually with convulsions, and a rash covering chest, arms and tummy. **What causes RF?** Inflammation of the main circulatory system makes holes in the heart ventricles, especially in children. Allergic reaction may be present, often accompanied by acute viral disease, exposure to harmful chemicals, environmental pollutants, or radiation. *See Infections page 473.*

Diet and Lifestyle Support Therapy

Nutritional therapy plan:

1—Adhere to a fresh juice and liquid diet for the first bedridden stages of healing to reduce body work and strain.

2—Take potassium broth or essence, (page 291), and apple/alfalfa sprout juice daily during the acute period.

3—Take Red Star nutritional yeast or miso broths, or miso soup with snipped sea greens daily for B vitamins and strength. Add Amazake RICE DRINK for healing protein.

4—Then eat fresh and mildly cooked foods, including plenty of seafoods and vegetable protein from whole grains, tofu, sprouts, etc. Eat only small meals. Drink bottled water.

5—Avoid all sugars, salty, refined foods during healing. Keep fats low. No fried foods, caffeine or carbonated drinks during healing.

—**Use superfoods to rebuild immunity:** • Crystal Star RESTORE YOUR STRENGTH™ for iodine, potassium and broad spectrum nutrient support. (Excellent results.)
• Sun Wellness CHLORELLA 1 pkt. daily.
• Wakunaga KYO-GREEN drink.
• Esteem GREEN HARVEST drink.
• AloeLife ALOE GOLD drink.

—**Bodywork:**
•Bed rest is a key. Treatment may take months, or even years.
•Yoga and mild muscle-toning exercises, and/or massage therapy during confinement (which can last for several weeks) will prevent loss and atrophy of body strength.
•Take a catnip enema once a week to remove infection and reduce fever.
•Do not use aspirin as an anti-inflammatory. Notify your dentist of rheumatic heart disorder if having an extraction or anesthesia for any reason.
•Apply wintergreen oil compresses to chest.
•Use a tea tree oil rub on sore joints.

Herbal, Superfood and Supplement Therapy

Interceptive therapy plan: Choose 2 to 3 recommendations.

1—**Overcome infection:** •Crystal Star ANTI-BIO™ caps 4 daily for a month; •Garlic tabs 6 daily; •Lane Labs BENEFIN shark cartilage caps 2 daily as an antiviral; •Colloidal silver as directed; •Beta carotene 50-100,000IU daily. —**Homeopathic treatment is very effective in the initial phase.** See a homeopathic physician. Homeopathy may be used even of chemical medications are being taken. Reduce doses for kids.

2—**Reduce inflammation:** •Nutricology ENZOCAINE (very effective herbs, anti-arthritis nutrients, MSM and proteolytic enzymes); •Evening primrose oil caps 4 daily; •*dandelion* extract; *elderberry* tea 2 cups daily; or •Herbs, Etc. ECHINACEA TRIPLE SOURCE.

3—**Ease arthritis symptoms:** •Crystal Star DR. ENZYME™ with protease and bromelain; or •ANTI-FLAM™caps for pain and stiffness; •America's Finest BOSWELLIN & CURCUMINOIDS; •MSM 400-800mg daily, or methionine 250mg 2x daily; •High potency royal jelly 2 tsp. daily. Take •wintergreen leaf/white willow tea internally.

4—**Normalize cardiopulmonary activity:** •CoQ$_{10}$ 60mg 2x daily; •Crystal Star HEART PROTECTOR™ formulas, or •HAWTHORN extract drops in water; or •Heart Foods HAWTHORN PLUS to normalize circulation.

5—**Strengthen against recurrence:** •Crystal Star FEEL GREAT NOW™ caps (an energy tonic rich in ginseng and ginseng-like herbs); •Immudyne MACROFORCE caps with beta glucan; Effective antioxidants include: •MICROHYDRIN PLUS royalbodycare.com; •Vitamin E 4-800IU daily; •PCOs from grapeseed or white pine 50mg 3x daily; •Germanium 30mg 3x daily; •Solaray B$_{12}$ 2000mcg daily during healing. •Rainforest Remedies STRONG RESISTANCE.

6—**Flush the glands, especially the lymph system:** •Ascorbate vitamin C crystals with bioflavonoids, ¼ tsp. every hour in juice, or until stool turns soupy during acute periods, then reduce dosage to 3-5000mg daily.

7—**Probiotics replace friendly flora after long antibiotic courses:** •UAS DDS-JUNIOR with FOS or •Nutricology SYMBIOTICS powder ¼ tsp. in water 4x daily. •Enzymatic Therapy THYMU-PLEX caps for immune stimulation.

Can't find a recommended product? Call the 800 number listed in Product Resources for the store nearest you.

Schizophrenia

Psychosis, Mental Illness, Tardive Dyskinesia

Schizophrenia is a psychosis with severely disordered perception, characterized by hallucinations, delusions, extreme paranoia, and scattered, random thoughts. Personal relationships are abnormal, daily work is almost impossible. The schizophrenic usually withdraws emotionally and socially. Anti-psychotic (*neuroleptic*) drugs may do more harm than good. *Tardive dyskinesia* is a bizarre side effect disorder caused *exclusively* by anti-psychotic drugs, with symptoms similar to the psychosis - social withdrawal, a slow, shuffling gait, lethargy, grimaces and outbursts. Over 70% of patients taking antipsychotic drugs develop this grim disorder which almost totally isolates them socially. Natural therapies have been successful treating schizophrenia and reversing TD. For example, magnetic waves to certain brain areas show promise for reducing hearing voices in the head. **First signs?** Long lasting depression, lethargy, violent emotional swings, detachment from reality. **Schizophrenia develops from both genetic and environmental factors:** blood sugar imbalances from too many junk foods and sugars, severe gluten, dairy or chemical allergies, prescription or pleasure drug abuse, thyroid imbalance, even a gene fluke in the nicotine receptor. *See* Hypoglycemia Diet *suggestions page 463 for more information.*

Diet and Lifestyle Support Therapy

Nutritional therapy plan: *Improving body chemistry is a key.*

1—A hypoglycemia diet has been very successful in controlling schizophrenia.

2—Start with a short 3-day juice cleansing diet to normalize blood composition (pg. 203). Minimize fruit juices if hypoglycemia is involved. Try •Crystal Star RESTORE YOUR STRENGTH™ or Nutricology PRO GREENS, both with brain nourishing EFAs.

3—Then, eat largely fresh foods for the remainder of the week. Eat niacin-rich foods like broccoli, carrots, potatoes and corn.

4—Gradually add vegetable proteins (try •Garden of Life GOATEIN protein drink), gluten-free grains (like brown rice, millet and amaranth), fish (like salmon, tuna, halibut), and sunflower seeds. Turkey is a calming tryptophan source. Add calming food supplements like •Lewis Labs LECITHIN or NUTRITIONAL YEAST or •Jarrow GENTLE FIBERS with flax seed meal, or •Barleans GREENS with flax seed oil for high antioxidants.

5—Eliminate all refined sugars, caffeine, red meats, food with additives and preserved foods. Especially eliminate arginine foods like peanut butter and nuts. They can be toxic to a schizophrenic's brain.

—Bodywork:

•Get some exercise every day. The oxygen will do wonders for your head.

•Research implicates a lack of sunlight and vitamin D during pregnancy to added risk of schizophrenia for the child. 15 minutes of exposure to morning sunlight and a vitamin D supplement (400IU) during pregnancy can prevent this devastating mental illness.

•Take ocean walks for sea minerals; or visit a mineral-rich spring or spa.

•Regular massage therapy and spinal adjustment have had some success.

—For tardive dyskinesia: The herb *rauwolfia serpentina* (an Ayurvedic anti-psychotic remedy), works almost as well as *reserpine*, the schizophrenia drug derived from it, without side effects like tardive dyskinesia. Try •Himalaya Herbal Products SERPINA with Evening Primrose oil 4000mg daily; •CoQ-10 200mg daily; •Niacin 500mg 3x daily (flush-free OK);

•Avoid all pleasure drugs, and as many prescription drugs as possible.

•Frankincense aromatherapy for brain oxygenation and depression relief.

Herbal, Superfood and Supplement Therapy

Interceptive therapy plan: Choose 2 to 3 recommendations. *Consult with your physician before discontinuing drug therapy or beginning an herbal program. Avoid yohimbe in any supplement - it may aggravate schizophrenia.*

1—**Enhance neurotransmitter activity:** •Crystal Star DEPRESS-EX™ caps 6-8 daily; •Pacific BioLogic RECOVERY AMERICA formulas (highly recommended); •NADH, 10mg in the morning; •EGG YOLK LECITHIN 3x daily; •Country Life PHOS. CHOLINE COMPLEX softgels; •Wakunaga NEURO-LOGIC as needed, or Phosphatidyl serine (PS) 100mg 3 daily for 3 months; •High potency royal jelly 50,000mg or more, 2 tsp. daily, or •Prince of Peace GINSENG-ROYAL JELLY vials (good activity). •Magnesium 800mg 2x daily.

2—**For better cerebral circulation:** •Ginkgo Biloba extract; •*Siberian eleuthero* extract; •Crystal Star MENTAL CLARITY™ caps - 1 daily; •zinc 50mg 2 daily. —**Niacin/vitamin C therapy:** 1-3000mg daily or use •Solaray CHROMIACIN daily. (A baby aspirin before taking removes niacin flush.) Take with •vitamin C powder with bioflavonoids, ¼ tsp. every 2 waking hours to bowel tolerance for the first month of healing.

3—**EFAs lift mood, nourish the brain:** •DHA 200mg, 2 daily; •Source Naturals FOCUS DHA, or •New Chapter SUPERCRITICAL DHA (recommended). •Evening Primrose oil 4000mg daily; •Health from the Sun TOTAL EFAs; •Udo's PERFECTED OIL BLEND. For ocean EFAs: •Crystal Star OCEAN MINERALS caps, •Biotec PACIFIC SEA PLASMA, or kelp tabs 8 daily.

4—**Nerve stability against depression, anxiety:** •Crystal Star RELAX CAPS™ (fast acting) and FEEL GREAT NOW™ caps for balance. •St. John's wort extract or New Chapter ST. JOHN'S SC27 extract softgels to combat depression; •Gotu kola to restore nerves; •*Valerian, scullcap, California poppy* or VALERIAN-WILD LETTUCE extract to calm.

5—**Balance body chemistry with amino acid therapy:** •Anabol Naturals AMINO BALANCE combats depression (highly recommended); Glutamine 1000mg 3x daily; •Tyrosine 1000mg 2x daily; •Glycine 1000mg 2x daily; •GABA 500mg 2x daily •Crystal Star ANTI-HST™ to balance body histamine levels; •Enzymatic Therapy THYROID-TYROSINE.

6—**B vitamins are key:** •Stress B-complex 150mg; extra B₆ 500mg and folic acid 800mcg daily. •Real Life Research TOTAL B; •Premier GERMANIUM w. DMG.

Can't find a recommended product? Call the 800 number listed in Product Resources for the store nearest you.

Sciatica

Neuritis of the Sciatic Nerve

Sciatica, neuritis of the sciatic nerve, runs from the lower back across the buttocks, into the leg, calf and foot. Sciatic pain is caused by compression of the sciatic nerve, characterized by sharp, radiating pain running down the buttocks and the back of the thighs. The inflammation is arthritic in nature - extremely sensitive to weather change and to the touch. Natural treatment focuses on removing the pressure on the nerve - via chiropractic or massage therapy treatments, and on restoring the health of the nerve. **Do you have sciatica?** You probably do if you have severe sometimes debilitating pain in the leg along the course of the sciatic nerve - felt at the back of the thigh, running down the inside of the leg. Most sufferers have lower back pain, muscle weakness and wasting, and reduced reflex activity. **What causes sciatica:** Sciatic nerve compression resulting from a ruptured disc or arthritis, an improper buttock injection, poor posture and muscle tone, poor bone and cartilage development, exhausted pituitary and adrenal glands. Wearing high heels too often and too long is a big factor for women…. especially if they are overweight. Men with flat feet who don't exercise regularly also complain of sciatic nerve pain. Protein and calcium depletion plays a role, especially if green vegetables are lacking in the diet. *See Back Pain page 331 and Neuritis/Neuralgia page 508 for more information.*

Diet and Lifestyle Support Therapy

Nutritional therapy plan:

1—A mineral rich diet is important: Take a potassium broth (pg. 291) every other day for a month to rebuild nerve health. Add iodine foods like sea greens, sea foods, shellfish.

2—Have a leafy green salad every day. Take a little white wine with dinner to relieve tension and nerve trauma. Drink bottled mineral water, 6-8 glasses daily.

3—Eat calcium and magnesium rich foods, like green vegetables, spinach, tofu, whole grains, molasses, nuts, seeds and sea greens (or try •Crystal Star RESTORE YOUR STRENGTH™ drink for electrolyte minerals from sea greens). Replenish nerve minerals with drinks like •Wakunaga KYO-GREEN one packet daily for nerve rebuilding or •Futurebiotics VITAL K, 3 tsp. daily, or •Alacer ELECTROMIX to replenish minerals (recommended).

4—Take a good natural protein drink, such as •Pure Form WHEY PROTEIN drink.

5—Avoid caffeine foods, refined sugars, especially chocolate.

—Lifestyle measures:

•Apply ice packs or wet heat to relieve pain. Hot epsom salts baths relax the nerve. •Apply alternating hot and cold, (finishing with cold), or hops/lobelia compresses to stimulate circulation.

•Gentle morning and evening stretches, and daily yoga exercises are effective.

—Effective topical nerve help applications:

•Capsaicin creme, or •Nature's Way CAYENNE PAIN RELIEVER ointment. •Baywood TOPICAL SUPER COOL RELIEF with boswellia and emu oil or America's Finest BOSWELLIN CREAM.

•*Cayenne/ginger* compress, or a cold compress of chamomile or lavender essential oils. •TIGER BALM or Chinese WHITE FLOWER oil

•B&T TRIFLORA analgesic gel

•St. John's wort oil (very effective)

•Mix wintergreen, cajeput, rosemary oils. Massage into area.

Herbal, Superfood and Supplement Therapy

Interceptive therapy plan: Choose a recommendation in each category.

1—**Relieve nerve spasms:** •GINKGO BILOBA extract for facial neuralgia; •Crystal Star STRESS OUT™ muscle relaxer drops or MUSCLE RELAXER™ caps for spasmodic pain; •DLPA 1000mg as needed for pain. •Homeopathic- Hylands Calms or Calms Forte tabs

2—**Help repair and restore nerves:** •Crystal Star RELAX CAPS™ as needed for rebuilding nerve sheath, 4 daily (good fast results from many sufferers); •Crystal Star OCEAN MINERALS™ caps 2 daily for nerve restoration. •BILBERRY extract for tissue-toning flavonoids, or •Ascorbate C or Ester C with bioflavonoids and rutin, 5000mg daily, to rebuild connective tissue. •Country Life LIGATEND as needed.

3—**Reduce nerve inflammation:** •Solaray Curcumin (turmeric extract) or •Crystal Star ANTI-FLAM™ caps 4 daily to take down inflammation; •*Devil's claw* extract drops in water 2x daily; •Lane Labs ADVACAL ULTRA caps with high magnesium, 4 daily; •Quercetin 1000mg; •Bromelain 1500mg daily or •Crystal Star DR. ENZYME™ with protease and bromelain (a specific). •Eidon POTASSIUM liquid; •Homeopathic Aranea Diadema - radiating pain, or •Mag. Phos. for spasmodic pain (good results), or •Hypericum if there is nerve injury.

4—**Thyroid therapy is important:** •Crystal Star OCEAN MINERALS caps; •New Chapter OCEAN HERBS 4 daily (good results or both).

5—**Effective herbal nerve tonics:** •*Lobelia* extract drops; •*Passionflower* or *scullcap* tea; •*valerian/wild lettuce* extract, a powerful nerve relaxant; •Hylands Nerve Tonic. •Niacin therapy: 500-1500mg daily to stimulate circulation.

6—**Essential fatty acids nourish nerves:** •*Evening Primrose* oil 4000mg daily; •Omega-3 oils like flax and fish oils daily. •Phosphatidyl Choline (PC55); •Nature's Plus EGG YOLK LECITHIN; •Vitamin E 400IU daily. •Nutricology PRO GREENS w. EFAs.

7—**Neural nutrients for long term restoration:** •Country Life sublingual B-12, 2500mcg daily; and •Stress B-complex 100mg with extra B$_6$ 250mg; •Anabol Naturals AMINO BALANCE; •Taurine 500mg daily; •*Black cohosh* extract drops.

Can't find a recommended product? Call the 800 number listed in Product Resources for the store nearest you.

Seasonal Affective Disorder

S.A.D., Winter Blues, Pineal Gland Imbalance

S.A.D. makes people sad. Wintertime means depression for 35 million Americans. S.A.D. manifests itself after the autumn equinox as sunlight hours lessen. Unusual appetite and low energy aspects of S.A.D. show our ancient ties to seasonal rhythms as they affect our behavior. Over 80% of people affected are women (experts think women produce less serotonin, a mood enhancing brain chemical, than men). Work productivity noticeably declines; relationships suffer. S.A.D. disorder is latitudinal - in Mexico, Florida and Texas, only 1.4% of the population suffers from S.A.D. In Canada, over 17% of the population suffer from acute S.A.D. In the Northeast U.S., up to 50% of people have noticeable winter mood shifts. **Do you have winter S.A.D.?** •Do you: oversleep or struggle to get out of bed, even if you get enough sleep? feel lethargic or have poor concentration during the day? suffer from eyestrain or headaches? feel overwhelmed by simple tasks? have unusually strong cravings for sweets or carbs? gain weight in the winter (up to 10-15 lbs.), even if your diet hasn't really changed? **What causes S.A.D.?** Not enough full spectrum light in winter months (the pineal gland doesn't get enough light to stop secreting melatonin), hormone and body rhythm imbalance. •feel more anxious, or low-energy? •Do short periods of sunlight noticeably lift your spirits? •Do you experience a "summer high" where you feel elated and full of energy?

Diet and Lifestyle Support Therapy

Nutritional therapy plan:

1—Conscious diet improvement is the key to reducing S.A.D. symptoms. A diet for hypoglycemia has been effective, low in fats and sugars. Make sure your diet is balanced, with natural foods, rich in complex carbohydrates, (to shift the distribution of amino acids in the blood). Add Rainbow Light HAWAIIAN SPIRULINA, with B-complex 100mg to balance sugar use.

2—Include B-vitamin and mineral-rich foods, like brown rice and fresh vegetables. Whole grains, legumes and soy products help control sugar cravings. Take Red Star NU-TRITIONAL YEAST, or Biostrath original LIQUID YEAST as a source of B vitamins and chromium.

3—Eat more vitamin D-rich foods: eggs, fish, seafoods and sea greens (2 tbsp. chopped dry sea greens or 6 pieces of sushi a week). Vegans may be at a higher risk since they don't eat serotonin-enhancing foods like poultry, dairy foods and eggs.

—Lifestyle measures:

•Light therapy is a widely accepted treatment for S.A.D., more effective than antidepressant drugs. Try to get 20 to 30 minutes of early morning sunshine to balance your serotonin levels. Otherwise, be aware that indoor or fluorescent light is not effective. Only full-spectrum light shuts off melatonin secretion to reduce S.A.D. symptoms. Exposure for 2 to 3 hours of light therapy offers up to 60% reduction in symptoms in 1 week.

•Though not approved by the FDA light boxes have shown definite effectiveness, if used from mid-fall until spring. Depression typically begins to lift a week after "photo-therapy" begins. Consider Environmental Lighting Concepts OTT-LITE (800-842-8848).

•Going south for 3 to 4 short winter vacations helps relieve symptoms and helps sufferers function more normally for up to 4 weeks after they return.

•Get an outdoor exercise walk every day, especially running, walking or jogging. Becoming active in winter sports like skiing, means you'll be less disturbed by winter.

•Get a small greenhouse; spend regular time in it during the winter. Light does wonders for your pineal gland. Plant oxygen does wonders for your head.

Herbal, Superfood and Supplement Therapy

Interceptive therapy plan: **Choose 2 or more recommendations.**

1—**Relieve depression:** •SAMe 400mg daily; •Crystal Star DEPRESS-EX caps with •*St. John's wort* extract and *Lemon Balm* tea through the winter; •New Chapter ST. JOHN'S SC27 softgels; •Gaia PHYTO PROZ SUPREME; •HAWTHORN extract., •MICROHYDRIN PLUS (available at royalbodycare.com) all elevate mood. •Lane Labs ADVACAL ULTRA; •Stress B-complex 100mg daily; •Natural Labs Deva Flower DEPRESSION-GLOOM.

2—**Neurotransmitter normalizers:** •Crystal Star RELAX CAPS™ or •*St. John's wort* extract. •*Gotu kola* helps restore nerves to overcome mental dullness. •Anabol Naturals AMINO BALANCE improve neurotransmission.

3—**Vitamin D is a key:** Take natural •vitamin D 400 to 1000IU daily all during the winter; or •American Biologics EMULSIFIED A & D 2x daily; or •Twin Labs ALLERGY D, or •Now Foods A & D 25,000/1,000IU.

4—**Stimulate the pineal/pituitary:** •Glutamine 200mg daily. Rub •*Rosemary* essential oil on temples, or take *rosemary* extract drops in wine; •Herbs America MACA MAGIC powder; •GINKGO BILOBA extract 3x daily; or •Metab. Resp. GINKGO BILOBA caps.

5—**Thyroid health is critical:** •Crystal Star IODINE, POTASSIUM, SILICA extract or •OCEAN MINERALS™ caps 2x daily, or •Nature's Path TRACE-MIN-LYTE with sea greens, or •Crystal Star RESTORE YOUR STRENGTH™ drink for electrolyte minerals, or •Kelp tabs 8 daily, with cayenne 3 daily; •Solaray ALFA JUICE caps, or •alfalfa tabs 10 daily; •Nutricology TG100 for hypothyroidism or Enzymatic Therapy •THYROID/TY-ROSINE COMPLEX; or •Tyrosine 500mg with L-lysine 500mg 2x daily.

6—**EFAs help normalize and nourish the brain:** •EVENING PRIMROSE oil 4 daily; •Nature's Secret ULTIMATE OIL; •Spectrum NORWEGIAN FISH OIL or Omega-3 flax oil 3x daily. •Royal jelly 2 tsp. daily, or •Prince of Peace GINSENG-ROYAL JELLY vials.

7—**Ginsengs help control sugar cravings:** •Crystal Star FEEL GREAT NOW™ caps; or Imperial Elixir GINSENG-ROYAL JELLY; Ginseng/gotu kola capsules. Take with •Chromium picolinate 200mcg to control sugar levels and normalize brain chemistry.

Can't find a recommended product? Call the 800 number listed in Product Resources for the store nearest you.

Sexuality

Lack of Normal Sexual Libido

Is it just us? We tend, today, to think we're the only culture beset with libido-lowering elements. The latest unhappy statistics for America show that 43% of women have some type of sexual dysfunction, and 52% of men between the ages of 40 and 70 have impotence problems. Certainly there is no question that our nutrient-poor, high fat diets, over-use of drugs and stimulants, and rushed, high-pressured lifestyles lead to low energy and lack of time for love. But the reality is that people in every era have felt the need for help in the sexual area. After all, this part of our lives is at the most basic, elemental center of our being. The recommendations presented on this page are revitalizers for sexual energy as well as effective natural treatments for the most common sexual problems affecting men and women today - impotence and low libido. Look to herbs first. Herbs have a centuries-old reputation for effectiveness in working with the body toward sexual health and enhancement. Bonus: New studies show that an active sex life can make you look up to seven years younger! *Note:* Check your prescription drugs; some have side effects of impaired sex drive.

Is your libido low? If you've lost your interest in sex, check out some of the natural answers to low libido.

—If you're a woman in menopause (see page 492) have you gained unusual weight (low thyroid and metabolism) or lost your normal energy (adrenal exhaustion)?
—If you're a man in andropause (see page 458) have erections become slow and difficult (atherosclerosis) or painful (prostate swelling, poor circulation)?
—Have you become dissatisfied with the path your life is taking? Are you depressed? Have you been under a lot of emotional stress for a long period of time?
—Do you feel unattractive or that you've lost your looks as you've aged? Has your diet deteriorated to fast foods on the run? Are you avoiding exercise every week?
—Is there unusual tension in your job? Is your personal relationship unhappy? Have you resorted to prescription (or pleasure) drugs to get through your day?
—Was your childhood marked by physical abuse or great trauma? (Sometimes the feelings don't surface for years.) Hypnotherapy may be effective for you.
—Do you have a serious illness that affects the nerves, like MS, Parkinson's or diabetes?

Some answers to individual sexuality and libido problems:

MEN: —*For low libido and impotence:* •Brazilian Catuaba 4000mg or •Muira Puama 4000mg (highly recommended), •Optimal Nutrients POTENT POTION; •Crystal Star MALE PERFORMANCE™ with saw palmetto has a long history of success for low libido in older men. Try •5-HTP 100mg an hour before sex; •Histidine 500m with B-6 and niacin •Life Enhancement PROSEXUAL PLUS. Despite the popularity of Viagra and Cialis, better sex through drugs may not be the best way to go. Natural therapies correct underlying causes of most impotence - poor circulation and atherosclerosis of the penile artery. Herbal fiber eliminates fatty build-up that contributes to impotence. Try •Jarrow GENTLE FIBERS (takes about 3 months). •Ginkgo Biloba helps impotence caused by atherosclerosis. In a recent study, ginkgo was more effective than drug injections. 50% of patients showed regained potency- compared to 20% using injections. •Yohimbe, 1000mg helps more rapid erections. (Do not take if you have high blood pressure, take high blood pressure drugs, or diet products containing *phenylpropanolamine*, or have heart, kidney or liver disorders.) •TRIBULUS TERRESTRIS, •Crystal Star LOVE MALE™ caps or Pure Essence Labs VIRILITY FOR MEN all improve male sexual response; •Arginine 3000mg daily boosts nitric oxide involved in the erection mechanism. Try acupuncture - a new study shows 20 out of 29 men overcame impotence after acupuncture. —**To prolong erections, reduce premature ejaculation:** for all men, *saw palmetto*, a tissue building steroid-like herb, reduces premature ejaculation. •Crystal Star PROSTATE PROTECTOR™caps reduces BPH-related discomfort; •*horsetail-nettles* tea helps reduce prostate swelling rapidly. •Crystal Star PROSTATE PROTECTOR™ roll-on is especially effective for younger men. .

WOMEN: —**Tonify your system:** •Crystal Star FEEL GREAT NOW™, 3 caps daily; —**Libido-enhancers:** •Crystal Star LOVE FEMALE™ caps; •Futurebiotics MAXATIVA for women; •Esteem WOMAN ALIVE caps; •*Dong Quai/Damiana* extract; •Herbs America MACA MAGIC and Pure Essence Labs LIBIDO FOR WOMEN (both highly recommended); •Prince of Peace RED GINSENG-ROYAL JELLY vials boost acetylcholine for sexual response; •Histidine 500mg with B-6 10cmg. —**Essential fatty acids** improve skin tone and lubricate both internally and externally: •EVENING PRIMROSE OIL 3000mg daily; •Herbal Products PACIFIC HEMP SUPREME 7 oil blend. —**For depression-related libido problems:** •*St. John's wort*, or 5-HTP to increase serotonin; •*Ginkgo Biloba* improves low libido caused by anti-depressant drugs. —**For vaginal dryness and painful intercourse:** For immediate relief: Apply natural •vitamin E oil, sesame seed oil, •aloe vera gel or •Moon Maid VITAL VULVA to vaginal opening. (Take vitamin E internally for long term relief - improves blood supply to the vaginal walls). Take •Crystal Star WOMEN'S DRYNESS™ extract to produce more membrane fluid; or Ayurvedic •Shatavari (Asparagus racemosus)- a primary sexual tonic for women with vaginal atrophy.

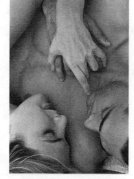

Can't find a recommended product? Call the 800 number listed in Product Resources for the store nearest you.

Sexuality

Diet and Lifestyle Support Therapy

Nutritional therapy: *Hormone-disrupting chemicals in produce, hormone-injected meats and dairy foods can wreak havoc on libido. Junk-y, chemicalized foods are part of a body not feeling "up to it." Avoid red meats; keep fats, salt and sugar low.*

—**For women:** 1) Soy foods offer a natural estrogenic effect. Cruciferous veggies help metabolize "bad" estrogens, release bloat. 2) Eat foods rich in EFA's: seafoods, sea greens, leafy greens, whole grains, nuts, and seeds. 3) Vitamin E foods mean more body moisture - soy foods, wheat germ, seeds, nuts, vegetable oils, and beta carotene foods like apricots, mangoes, carrots. 4) Boost adrenal energy with brown rice. 5) Eat magnesium-rich foods, like almonds, green salads, avocado, carrots, citrus fruits, lentils, salmon and flounder. 6) Celery stimulates the pituitary. 7) Seafoods boost an underactive thyroid for increased libido. 8) Chili peppers heighten arousal by setting pain sensors on alert.

—**For men:** A man's sex drive is dependent on testosterone and a good blood supply to the erectile tissue, factors that rely on good nutrition and exercise. 1) Eat zinc source foods: liver, oysters, nuts, seeds and legumes. 2) Dopamine (L-Dopa) is intimately associated with sex drive in men. One 16-oz. can of fava beans has almost a prescription dose! 3) Add mineral-rich foods like shellfish, greens and whole grains; EFA's from flaxseed and sea greens. 4) Eat fiber-rich foods like legumes, fruits and vegetables to avoid atherosclerosis of the penis. 5) Drink in moderation. Heavy drinking can lead to reduced erections. Two or three alcoholic drinks can delay orgasm in women or decreases its intensity. —**Lifestyle habits affect male sexual health:** •Extra weight means a smaller penis. Sexologists say a man loses ½ inch from his penis for every 15 pounds he gains. Extra weight causes a fat pad to creep over the shaft. •Long recreational drug use inhibits sperm production. •Heavy metal or radiation damages sperm/chromosome structure. •Sexually transmitted diseases scar the vas deferens obstructing sperm delivery to the penis; infertility results. •The cadmium in cigarettes interferes with use and absorption of zinc.

—**Bodywork for both:** Environmental estrogens in hormone-injected food animals, herbicides and pesticides affect male sperm counts and female hormone balance. Avoid hormone-injected meats and dairy foods, and herbicide-sprays (see page 459 for more). •Stimulate your sex drive reflexology point: Press the top of your foot with the fingers of one hand while pressing halfway between the anklebone and heel with the fingers of the other. Rotate your foot several times.
•Exercise can increase sex drive, especially exercise with your mate. Exercise like dancing, walking and swimming stimulates circulation to genitals, increases body oxygen. Research shows exercise is as effective as Viagra in men with heart problems who cannot use the drug.
•Try aromatherapy oils dotted on your sheets. Sex enhancing aromatherapy oils for men: cinnamon, sandalwood, lavender, patchouli, coriander, jasmine and cardamom. Sex enhancing oils for women: ylang, rose, clary sage, neroli and rosewood.

Herbal, Superfood and Supplement Therapy

Interceptive therapy for men: Choose 2 or more recommendations.
—*Ginseng and ginseng-like herbs are primary tonics for male virility:* •Velvet antler helps libido (and sports energy). •Yohimbe caps 750-1000mg stimulate testosterone (Do not take yohimbe if you take diet products with phenylpropanolamine, or have heart, kidney, liver disorders.) •Crystal Star LOVE MALE™ caps, or •MALE PERFORMANCE™ caps, recommended for long term help; •PROSTATE PROTECTOR™ roll-on for longer erections. —*EFA's boost seminal fluids:* Highest potency •royal jelly 60,000-120,000mg daily. •Ginkgo Biloba for erectile dysfunction. •Zinc 50mg 2x daily. —*For a stronger erection:* •Liquid niacin before intercourse; •Arginine 3000mg 45 minutes before sex for more penile blood flow (not if you have herpes). •Carnitine 1000mg 2x daily; •Life Enhancement PRO-SEXUAL PLUS. •Source Naturals TRIBULUS TERRESTRIS, or •Natural Balance COBRA, or •Pure Essence Labs VIRILITY FOR MEN, or •Muira puama caps. •*Mucuna pruriens* caps 1000mg, a natural source of L-dopa (not if taking antidepressant drugs). —*Effective superfoods for men:* •Unipro PERFECT PROTEIN; •Hsu's WILD AMERICAN GINSENG; •Trace Mineral Research CONCENTRACE for trace minerals.

Interceptive therapy for women: Choose 2 or more recommendations.
•Crystal Star LOVE FEMALE™ caps for 3 days before a special weekend. •Esteem WOMAN ALIVE; •Raintree Nutrition CLAVO HUASCA extract; •Yohimbe 500mg caps (see above for contra-indications.) or •Herbs America MACA MAGIC caps or extract (nice tingle). •Pure Essence Labs LIBIDO FOR WOMEN (highly recommended); •L-arginine 1500mg 45 minutes before sex to relax muscles and increase orgasm capacity (not if you have herpes); •Crystal Star WOMEN'S DRYNESS™, or •vitamin E, 800IU for vaginal fluids. •Moon Maid PRO-MENO cream, or Crystal Star PRO-EST BALANCE™ roll-on; •Paradise Herbs SENSUAL FIRE for women (recommended); •Pinnacle EXOTICA FOR WOMEN caps (good results). •Highest potency royal jelly 60,000-120,000mg daily.

For both men and women: Wild oats helps both sexes! 300mg of wild oats extract three days a week leads to dramatic increase in multiple orgasms for women! Results are very good for men in frequency of intercourse and orgasm. •Gaia Herbs WILD MILKY SEED OATS. •TRIBULUS TERRESTRIS works well for both (also indicated for diabetes help.) Increases female sex drive without the side effects of hormone drugs. In one study, ⅔ of women treated with tribulus report renewed sexual interest! Tribulus has a long history of reducing male impotence and may raise testosterone levels by activating luteinizing hormone (LH) in the pituitary gland. •Herbs America MACA MAGIC Express (highly recommended, helps build testosterone for both sexes); •2 *cayenne-ginger* caps for enhanced orgasm, or •Pinnacle HORNY GOAT WEED caps; •Kava is an intimacy aphrodisiac, best taken as extract drops in water. •Ashwagandha extract 3x a day for stress relief; mucous Niacin 100mg, 30 minutes before sex enhances sexual flush, mucous membrane tingling and orgasm intensity.

Can't find a recommended product? Call the 800 number listed in Product Resources for the store nearest you.

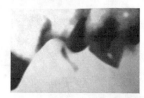

A New Look at Contraception, Fertility and STD Protection

Every method of contraception has risks, but the risk of contracting a sexually transmitted disease, and unwanted pregnancy are greater. Women especially, need to earnestly evaluate their lifestyles, sexual discipline and partner's attitudes to make a responsible choice. Unless you are in a long-term relationship, absolutely sure that your partner is monogamous, I believe you must take precautions against STD's. Be careful even if you know your partner is monogamous. Once a virus gets into your system, it never goes away. Sometimes people carry STD's from previous relationships and don't know it, or don't want to share the fact with a new partner. Don't forget that HIV and AIDS can kill you; herpes and HPV, (the virus that induces genital warts) are permanent. These STD's may become dormant, but they do not leave the body. STD's are especially dangerous to an unborn child because they can be transferred during birth. Even STD's that are not permanent cause a great deal of pain and can leave you permanently infertile.

—BARRIER METHODS: condom, diaphragm, cervical cap and vaginal sponge, are the most popular contraceptive devices. The latex (not lambskin) condom offers almost complete protection from STD's, but, failure rate from breakage, heat or wear is 15%. Use a back-up spermicide with a condom. Today, condom use has become less common, especially among teenagers, who have the greatest STD infection rates. The new female condoms, polyurethane ringed sheaths that fit over the cervix, can be inserted ahead of time, but they are clumsy and unromantic, hanging slightly outside the vagina. The female condom also has twice the failure rate of the male condom with an estimated 21 in 100 women becoming pregnant in the first year of use. They give the woman a choice if the man refuses to wear a condom, and they offer some protection against STD's. The diaphragm, fitted correctly, used with spermicide, without any tiny holes or cracks is an effective method of birth control, and provides some protection against STD's. Many sensitive women get bladder infections from the diaphragm rubbing against the urethra, and yeast infections from the spermicide. The cervical cap with spermicidal jelly creates a seal that prevents sperm penetration and inactivates sperm, is effective for 48 hours of birth control, but is not effective against STD's. The vaginal sponge, impregnated with spermicide, is effective for 24 hours. It is not a good choice for women who have had children, or for sensitive women who become irritated from a large dose of spermicide. It may become a cause of toxic shock syndrome when the women is unable to remove the sponge or when fragments remain. IUD's: have fallen from favor because of their many complications, increased risk of infertility, adverse health effects and high risk for STD's.

SPERMICIDES: creams, jellies, suppositories, foams, inserted in the vagina to kill or immobilize sperm. They have some ability to kill sexually-transmitted viruses, but should be used with a barrier method of contraception since they have up to 21% failure rate. Some tests show that Nonoxynol-9 contraceptive gel can put both men and women at more risk for STDs.

HORMONAL CONTRACEPTIVES: today's pills have much lower doses of hormones, but many women are still sensitive to the synthetic estrogen impact and wary of breast, cervical and uterine cancer risk. High blood pressure, migraine headaches, depression, water retention, thrush, gum inflammation, fibroid growth, weight gain, breast enlargement, low libido, and changes in skin pigment are still frequent side effects. The pill does not protect against STD's. Hormonal contraceptives are now available in skin patches and flexible rings you insert into the vagina. They are just as effective as the traditional pill, but come with similar side effects. The latest birth control pill (Seasonale) reduces a woman's period to just 4 times a year, highly desirable to many women. However, unless a woman has extenuating circumstances like chronic endometriosis which has not responded to natural therapies, I believe tampering with a woman's natural menstrual cycle may cause serious hormone disruption over the long term. Note: *St. John's wort* may decrease the effectiveness of the pill.

HORMONE IMPLANTS: (Norplant) surgically inserted into a woman's upper arm, releases tiny doses of hormone in the bloodstream. Side effects include irregular menstruation, intra-period spotting, headaches, depression. They are effective birth control for five years, but do not protect against STD's. They are painful and leave an unsightly scar when removed.

DEPO-PROVERA: (progestin) injections, used every 13 weeks, prevent egg release by the ovaries. The injections are highly effective against unwanted pregnancy, but I advise caution. Some women even report fibromyalgia that lasts months after Depo-Provera use is discontinued. —The "mini pill" is a progestin only birth control pill that can be used while breast-feeding. It has a high success rate, but must be used at the same time every day to be effective, making it inconvenient for the majority of users. Side effects like weight gain, irregular periods, breast soreness and nausea are common. The "mini pill" can also increase risk for ovarian cysts in susceptible women.

MORNING AFTER PILL: prevents ovulation to safeguard against pregnancy. Morning-after contraception can be used within three days of unprotected sex to prevent an unwanted pregnancy, but do not affect pregnancies that have already occurred. Nausea, dizziness and cramping are common side effects.

MALE BIRTH CONTROL: pills and injections are the newest hormone contraceptives. Male birth control uses testosterone to lower sperm counts in order to prevent pregnancy. Side effects include: infertility, low libido, impotence, depression and PMS like symptoms. The male birth control pill will not be available for another 5-10 years as studies evaluate its safety.

STERILIZATION: No sterilization form protects against STD's. Female sterilization: Tubal ligation means hormones, ovulation and menstruation continue as usual, but the egg disintegrates in the tubes and is absorbed by the bloodstream. Side effects are irregular bleeding, increased menstrual pain and excessively heavy periods, (a hysterectomy may be necessary to stop bleeding). Some women report bone loss, back pain, incontinence, loss of libido, hot flashes and night sweats. Male sterilization: Half a million American men undergo a vasectomy to become sterile every year. The tubes that carry the sperm to the penis are cut and tied. The man can continue to ejaculate semen without sperm. A vasectomy may raise risk of prostate cancer. Note: A no-scalpel vasectomy reduces body trauma and speeds recovery time. Ask your physician.

Can't find a recommended product? Call the 800 number listed in Product Resources for the store nearest you.

STD's - Sexually Transmitted Diseases

Chlamydia, Gonorrhea, Trichomonas, Vaginosis

STDs are a factor in every choice we make about our sexuality and reproductive lives. No decision about conception can be made without considering the STD quotient. STD's are more prevalent, more insidious, more dangerous than ever. Experts say 1 in 5 Americans has an *incurable* sexually transmitted infection; 15 million new infections occur each year. *Vaginosis*, a bacterial vaginal infection puts women at risk for serious pelvic inflammatory disease (PID), even for AIDS. Whether you believe our culture is paying for years of sexual freedom, or whether you believe STD's are the result of irresponsible behavior, they can't be ignored. Antibiotics are effective for bacterial sexually transmitted infections in early stages, less effective in advanced stages. Viral STD's can be minimized by medical treatment, but are incurable at this time. Natural therapies are a good choice at any stage, often producing dramatic results, reducing symptoms, cleansing infection, recharging immune response so the body is less vulnerable to repeat outbreaks. **Do you have an STD?** Symptoms usually appear 2 to 3 weeks after sexual contact. *Gonorrhea:* cloudy green or yellow discharge, painful urination, yeast infection, pelvic inflammation. *Syphilis:* First stage; rashy, flaky genital sores on the genitalia, fever, mouth sores, chronic sore throat. *Chlamydia:* thick discharge in some men and all women, urethritis; pelvic pain, sterility. *Trichomonas:* caused by a parasite, usually contracted via intercourse, severe itchiness, thin, foamy, yellowish discharge with a foul odor. *Vaginosis:* vaginal discharge; unpleasant odor.

Diet and Lifestyle Support Therapy

Nutritional therapy plan:

1—Follow a cleansing liquid diet for 3 days (pg. 172) during acute stages. Take one Potassium broth (pg. 291), one fresh carrot juice, one vegetable drink like Green Foods CARROT ESSENCE, Barleans GREENS, C'est Si Bon CHLORENERGY, or Wakunaga KYO-GREEN, or a simple apple/parsley juice to alkalize.

2—Continue with a cleansing fresh foods diet. Add several bunches of green grapes daily (an old remedy that works). Try Herbal Answers ALOE FORCE JUICE before meals.

3—Avoid starchy, fried and saturated fat foods. Avoid red meats, pasteurized dairy products, and caffeine during healing.

—**Bodywork:** *Call the National STD Hotline (800) 227-8922 for more info.*
•Strong doses of antibiotics are the usual medical treatment, but the most recent out-breaks (especially in teenagers) are showing resistance or non-response to these drugs.
•STD's like herpes and gonorrhea can be transmitted through oral sex. Experts advise using a condom during oral sex for protection. But beware: Nonoxynol-9 contraceptive gel can put both men and women at more risk for STD's.
•Overheating therapy is very effective in controlling virus replication. Even slight body temperature increases can lead to considerable reduction of infection. See page 225 in this book for effective technique.
•Smokers are 3 times more at risk than non-smokers for STD's. Smoking and a poor diet increase risk because they reduce immune defenses.
•Oral contraceptives potentiate the adverse effects of nicotine, and reduce levels of key nutrients like vitamins C, B-6, B-12, folic acid and zinc. Some oral contraceptives aggravate the formation of pre-cancerous lesions because of their imbalancing estrogen content.

—**For crabs** (pubic lice): wash pubic hair thoroughly; tweeze out die-hards; comb through a vinegar-water solution.

Herbal, Superfood and Supplement Therapy

Interceptive therapy plan: Choose 2 to 3 recommendations. *Note: Many STD's benefit from using GRAPEFRUIT SEED extract or SKIN SPRAY first.*

1—**For Gonorrhea:** *(800,000 new cases per year).* •Crystal Star ANTI-BIO™ caps or extract 6x daily, alternate with •Now OREGANO OIL soft gels. Add •Beta carotene 150,000IU daily; •Vitamin C crystals ½ tsp. every hour to bowel tolerance during acute phase; reduce to 5000mg daily for a month.

2—**For Chlamydia:** *(4 million new cases per year).* •Crystal Star DETOX BLOOD PURI-FIER™ caps with goldenseal -also open and apply to sores. •Or mix powders of *goldenseal, barberry, Oregon grape root and garlic* with vitamin A oil and apply directly to the cervix via an all-cotton tampon. •Premier Labs GERMANIUM 150mg; •CoQ$_{10}$ 60mg 4x daily; •American Health ACIDOPHILUS liquid; •Zinc 50mg 2x daily, (also mix in water and apply topically); •Vitamin E 400IU 2x daily; or •Am. Biologics or Schiff emulsified A & E; •Lane Labs BENE-FIN SHARK CARTILAGE 4 caps daily, or •East Park OLIVE LEAF extract caps as anti-viral agents.

3—**For Trichomonas:** *(3 million new cases per year- caused by a parasite).* •Crystal Star ANTI-BIO™ capsules for 2 months (alternate every 2 waking hours), with •Zinc 50mg 2x daily. •Bathe sores several times daily in a *goldenseal/myrrh* or *gentian* herb solution. •Use a TEA TREE oil vaginal suppository nightly. •Beta carotene 150,000IU daily; •Vitamin C crystals ½ tsp. every hour to bowel tolerance during acute phase; reduce to 5000mg daily for a month.

4—**For Syphilis:** *(up to 100,000 new cases per year!)* After antibiotics, use: •Crystal Star DETOX BLOOD PURIFER™ with goldenseal; •ECHINACEA, or •Herbs, Etc. ECHINACEA TRIPLE SOURCE, or *Sarsaparilla* extract for 4 months; •*Pau d' arco-Calendula* tea 3 cups daily, apply •*Calendula* ointment; •CoQ$_{10}$ 300mg daily; •Nuticology GERMANIUM 150mg (very effective); •MICROHYDRIN PLUS from royalbodycare.com.

5—**For Vaginosis:** •Vitamin E cream and 400IU internally daily; •B-complex 100mg daily.

Can't find a recommended product? Call the 800 number listed in Product Resources for the store nearest you.

STD's - Sexually Transmitted Diseases

Herpes 2 - Genital Herpes

Herpes Simplex 2 Virus is the most widespread of all STD's, affecting up to 100 million Americans - almost 1,000,000 new cases per year! A lifelong infection, it alternates between virulent and inactive stages, and can be transmitted by people who don't know they have herpes. More frightening: Up to 70% of cases are transmitted by people who don't know they have herpes. Men are more susceptible to recurrence than women, but women are more likely to be infected. Herpes can be transmitted from kissing, oral sex, intercourse, even skin discharges. Outbreaks are opportunistic.... they can be triggered by emotional anxiety, poor diet (especially excess arginine in the body), food allergies, too much drugs and alcohol, hormone imbalance related to the menstrual cycle, sunburn, fever, even a cold. Acyclovir, a drug widely used in herpes treatment, can cause side effects like nausea, vomiting, loss of appetite, and constipation or diarrhea. The natural therapies on this page are safe, gentle, and have been used successfully by a broad range people. **Do you have genital herpes?** The first herpes outbreak is usually the most potent, accompanied by swollen glands and fever, as the immune system rallies to fight the infection. Clusters of painful blisters appear on the groin, thighs and buttocks, accompanied by flu-like symptoms (headache, stiff neck, fever), and swelling of groin lymph glands. The genitals itch, the blisters swell and fester, shooting pains go through the thighs and legs. Blister's rupture in 1 to 3 days, then slowly heal in 3 to 5 days.

Diet and Lifestyle Support Therapy

Nutritional therapy plan:

1—Good nutrition for optimizing immune function is essential against herpes. A lysine-rich/arginine-poor diet has merit. Especially increase lysine-rich fresh fish. Arginine-containing foods aggravate herpes. Avoid them until blisters disappear: chocolate, peanuts, almonds, cashews, and walnuts; sunflower and sesame seeds, coconut. Reduce wheat, soy, lentils, oats, corn, rice, barley, tomatoes, squash. Avoid citrus during healing.

2—Have daily non-citrus fruit juices, a carrot/beet/cucumber juice or potassium broth (pg. 291). Other good healing drink choices: Herbal Answer's ALOE FORCE juice, Nutricology PROGREENS and Crystal Star ENERGY GREEN RENEWAL™ drink (both with detoxing nutrients from sea greens), Green Foods GREEN MAGMA and AloeLife FIBERMATE for internal cleansing

3—Then keep the diet consciously alkaline with miso soup, brown rice and vegetables often. Include broccoli, cabbage and brussels sprout regularly for indole 3 carbinole, a specific against herpes. Add cultured vegetable protein foods such as tofu and tempeh for healing and friendly G.I. bacteria.

4—Reduce dairy intake, especially hard cheeses, and red meat. Eliminate fried foods, nitrate-treated foods, and nightshade plants like tomatoes and eggplant.

—Bodywork:

• Apply ice packs to lesions for pain and inflammation relief. Ice may also be applied as a preventive measure when the sufferer feels a flare-up coming on.
• Get early morning sunlight on the sores every day for healing Vitamin D.
• Frequent hot baths provide overheating therapy to arrest the virus (pg. 183).
• During an outbreak don't touch the sores; wash hands if you do touch them. Don't touch your eyes if you have touched the sores. Apply a • wet black tea bag 5 minutes at a time for 4 days til lesion crusts over.
• Acupuncture helps herpes. Biofeedback, meditation and imagery help prevent outbreaks. Avoid immune-suppressing drugs, alcohol and tobacco.

Herbal, Superfood and Supplement Therapy

Interceptive therapy plan: Choose 2 to 3 recommendations.
Herbs have remarkable success against herpes- remitting symptoms, reducing outbreaks. Steroid drugs take over a long time for herpes weaken both the immune system and bone density.

1—**Control the viral infection:** Merix RELEEV® caps and topical solution (excellent results); • Olive leaf extract or • Nutricology PRO-LIVE olive leaf extract (very effective). Take • Lemon balm extract; apply lemon balm extract or tea directly to sores (remarkable anti-herpes activity), or • PSP Marketing VIRAMAX (good to shorten outbreaks and for prevention). Take • Crystal Star HERPEX caps, or • ANTI-BIO™ extract with antiviral support. • Pure Planet Red Marine Algae Plus, or • Vibrant Health GIGARTINA with red algae. • Indole 3 Carbinole helps inhibit HSV2. Consider I3C 600-800mg daily.

2—**Reduce inflamed outbreaks:** • Crystal Star HERPEX™ caps 4 daily with DR. ENZYME™ with protease and bromelain (highly recommended); take • Quercetin 1000mg with bromelain 1500mg (almost instant relief); and • Ester C powder ¼ tsp. every hour in water up to 10,000mg daily, or to bowel tolerance during an attack. Try • Source Naturals INFLAMA-REST tabs. Drink plenty of • peppermint tea (a specific against herpes). —**How lysine therapy works:** the HSV2 virus needs the amino acid arginine to replicate. Both lysine and arginine look similar to the virus. Lysine can essentially ambush the virus into taking it instead of arginine, blocking virus growth and keeping it from reactivating. Apply lysine cream frequently. Take lysine 500mg caps 6 daily until outbreaks clear.

3—**Heal the sores:** Take • Crystal Star ANTI-BIO™ caps 6 daily, and mix opened with aloe vera gel and apply. Apply • St. John's wort oil, • Crystal Star HERPEX™ LYSINE/LICORICE gel, or • ANTI-BIO™ gel with cat's claw, or • Nutribiotic GRAPEFRUIT SEED spray. Take • Diamond HERPANACINE caps 4 daily (excellent results); or • Echinacea extract 30 drops every 2 hrs, apply • echinacea powder to sores. —**Prevent future sores:** • Selenium 600mcg daily; • Premier Labs LITHIUM .5mg arrests viral replication (mix an opened capsule with water and apply to sores). • MICROHYDRIN PLUS available at royalbodycare.com.

536

STD's - Sexually Transmitted Diseases

Cervical Dysplasia, Condyloma, Venereal Warts (HPV)

Cervical dysplasia, precancerous cervical lesions is the newest sexually transmitted epidemic. It is silent, often unknown by the infected person. Venereal Warts (HPV), one of the most common STDs (up to 1 million new cases per year), infects ovaries, fallopian tubes, cervix, uterus, vaginal and anal areas. Infertility is a common result. Researchers suspect that two extremely contagious sexually transmitted viruses, *Human Papilloma Virus* (Condyloma warts), and *Herpes Simplex II* are involved, because these viruses also play a role in cervical cancer. Both conditions are the result of risky lifestyle habits and low immunity. Both can result in abnormal PAP smears (as can long use of some birth control pills because they deplete folic acid); both can possibly increase risk of anal cancer. Early age of first intercourse, multiple sexual partners, a fast food based, nutrient-poor diet and smoking are common risk factors. Natural therapies deal with the causes of genital warts and require strong commitment and significant lifestyle changes. **Common signs?** Heavy painful periods, bleeding between periods and pain during intercourse are first signs. Uncomfortable, itchy, unsightly warts in the genital or anal area are a clear sign. Other STD's like herpes, gonorrhea or a chronic yeast infection with heavy, pus-filled discharge are commonly involved. There is usually high fever during infection.

Diet and Lifestyle Support Therapy

Nutritional therapy plan:

1—Encourage strong immune response against dysplasia: Increase fresh fruits, vegetables (especially cruciferous veggies and leafy greens), and high fiber complex carbohydrates as protective factors. Add high folic acid foods like lima beans, whole wheat and nutritional yeast like Red Star NUTRITIONAL YEAST. Add vegetable juices (especially carrot) like Green Foods CARROT ESSENCE, and/or green drinks like Solgar EARTH SOURCE GREENS & MORE, or C'est Si Bon CHLORENERGY, 2 pkts. daily for immune support. Use AloeLife ALOE GOLD drink to help deter the virus . Also •Steep 4 garlic cloves in 4-oz. of aloe vera juice and apply 2x daily.

2—Add 2 tbsp. chopped sea greens daily for ocean carotenes; or try Crystal Star RE-STORE YOUR STRENGTH™ drink. Add cold water fish like salmon for omega-3 oils. Add leafy greens for folacin. Eat cultured foods to normalize intestinal flora. If there are mouth sores, treat as for thrush. (see page 362), or chew Enzymatic Therapy DGL tablets.

3—Reduce dietary fat, especially from animal foods. Reduce caffeine and hard liquor. Avoid foods that aggravate herpes-type infections like sugary junk foods and fried foods. Red meats and poultry may have been contaminated with estrogens or other hormones.

—Lifestyle measures:

•High risk lifestyle factors must be eliminated for permanent improvement and prevention of further invasive lesions. Eliminate smoking, excess alcohol, oral contraceptives and multiple sexual partners. Use a barrier contraceptive to prevent new contact with HPV or HVS II. Recurrence often occurs after standard surgery alone.
•Avoid surgery by using vaginal packs, Nutribiotic GRAPEFRUIT SEED extract, Body Essentials SILICA GEL, or chlorella powder paste, placed against the cervix draws out toxins and sloughs abnormal cells. Abstain from sexual intercourse during vag pack treatment. (See page 193 for a pack to make yourself.)
•Alternating hot and cold hydrotherapy promotes healing activity to the pelvic area.
•Well in Hand WART WONDER is a good choice for topical relief of viral warts. *Call 888-550-7774 for more information.*

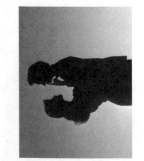

Herbal, Superfood and Supplement Therapy

Interceptive therapy plan: Choose 2 to 3 recommendations.

1—**Control the infection:** •*Usnea* extract helps deal with the virus; for 1 month, give your body an ascorbic acid flush with ¼ tsp. vitamin C powder with bioflav. every 2 hours until the stool turns soupy. Then take • vitamin C 5000mg daily with bioflavonoids for a month. Use •Crystal Star DR. ENZYME™ with protease and bromelain or •Quercetin 1000mg with bromelain 1500mg daily to reduce inflammation.

2—**Detoxify blood and liver:** Crystal Star •DETOX BLOOD PURIFIER™ caps for one month as a blood cleanser, followed by •FIBER & HERBS COLON CLEANSE™ to rid the colon of re-infection (very effective). Drink 1 cup daily •*burdock* or *dandelion root* tea, and take •MILK THISTLE SEED extract for 2 months. —**Flush lymph glands:** Echinacea extract, or cayenne caps daily; •Crystal Star ANTI-BIO™ caps 6 daily.

3—**For venereal warts:** Take dilute •oregano oil, 6 drops daily (1 part oregano oil to 4 parts olive oil); apply •East Park OLIVE LEAF extract cream. Make up •*Goldenseal/chaparral* vaginal suppositories (powders mixed with vitamin A oil)- extremely helpful for women with venereal warts or dysplasia, rendering many disease-free. Take •Crystal Star ANTI-BIO capsules 4 daily, with *elder-boneset-ginger-cayenne* tea to raise body temperature during acute stages; one week off, one week on until improvement (good results). —**Topicals:** Earth's Bounty O₂ SPRAY daily for a month, then rest a month; resume if needed. If improvement in the first month, body's defense forces will have taken over.

4—**For cervical dysplasia:** Take • B-complex with extra 800mcg folic acid and sublingual B-12, 2500mcg; a •vitamin C flush (see above); •vitamin A up to 100,000IU for a month (not if pregnant), or •beta-carotene 200,000IU, or PHYCOTENE MICROCLUSTERS from sea veggies, at royalbodycare.com. Take •Crystal Star CALCIUM-MAGNESIUM SOURCE™ caps or •*black cohosh* or *vitex* extract to prevent pre-cancerous lesions from becoming cancerous.•Nature's Way DIM-PLUS 400mg daily helps eliminate precancerous cells. •Sea greens 2 tbsp. daily or Green Foods ION KELP tabs for thyroid support.

5—**Antioxidants are keys:** •Grapeseed OPCs 300mg daily; •Nutricology germanium 150mg and N-acetyl cysteine 1000mg; •Vitamin E 800IU with selenium 400mcg daily.

Can't find a recommended product? Call the 800 number listed in Product Resources for the store nearest you.

Shingles

Herpes Zoster, Hives, Angioderma

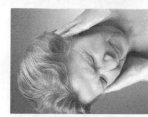

The CDC says up to 1 million Americans over age 50 are diagnosed with shingles every year! Shingles are the eruption of an acute nervous system infection caused by the **Herpes Zoster** virus (the same that causes chicken pox). Infectious, herpes-type blisters appear on the body torso. Flu-like symptoms, fever, headache and upset stomach accompany. Scarring, numbness and skin discoloration often result. You may be prone to shingles if you had chicken pox as a child; one in ten people who had chicken pox as children develop shingles later in life. The most common cause of shingles is a reaction to certain medications, usually multiple medications, especially antibiotics like penicillin). HCl depletion which leads to chronic constipation, then to acidosis is common. *Hives* are the same type of itchy blisters, but are caused by an allergic, histamine-type reaction to a chemical, like over-chlorinated drinking water, or to food, like dairy products, shellfish, wheat, MSG, or food additives. Like herpes, stress, adrenal and/or liver exhaustion, and lowered immunity also trigger outbreaks. **Do you have shingles signs?** Preliminary symptoms include chills, fever and an anxious feeling before very painful, swollen, red skin blisters develop. Pain radiates along one or several nerves preceding outbreaks; attacks last from 2 days to 2 weeks, leaving very irritated nerves, fever, chills and weakness after blisters are gone. *See Herpes page 377 and 535 for more information.*

Diet and Lifestyle Support Therapy

Nutritional therapy plan: *Note: Corticosteroid drugs are frequently prescribed for shingles. Corticosteroid drugs taken over a long period of time for shingles, weaken the immune system, allowing future attacks. Acetaminophen pain killers like Tylenol, can aggravate the blisters.*

1—Go on a short 3 day cleansing diet to eliminate acid wastes and alkalize the blood (pg. 203). Take a carrot-beet-cucumber juice, and a cranberry or carrot juice each day. Take an apple juice or celery juice each night.

2—Then, eat only fresh foods for 1-2 weeks, (fresh food enzymes reduce neuralgia recurring outbreaks). Add Jarrow GENTLE FIBERS to relieve constipation.

3—Alkalize and add B vitamins with miso soup, brown rice, vegetables, nutritional yeast and leafy greens. Have cultured foods like yogurt and kefir for friendly G.I. flora • Add Red Star Nutritional Yeast or Bio-Strath original LIQUID YEAST.

4—Avoid acid-forming foods: red meats, cheese, salty foods, eggs, caffeine, fried foods, and sodas. Avoid refined foods, sugars, aspirin, tetracyclines, and meats that may contain nitrates, nitrites and antibiotics. Avoid arginine-forming foods (see page 535).

5—Eliminate allergen foods - those with preservatives, flavorings, additives, colorings.

6—Effective drinks to help normalize, reduce itching and pain: •Herbal Answers ALOE FORCE aloe juice, •Green Foods CARROT ESSENCE.

—**Effective topical applications for pain:**

•Merix SHING-RELEEV antiviral spray. (Great feedback on this product!)

•Ice compresses, or Flax seed compresses. Epsom salt baths or oatmeal baths or compresses to neutralize acids.

•CAPSAICIN cream or Nature's Way CAYENNE PAIN RELIEVING OINTMENT, or *Cayenne-Ginger* compresses.

•Get early morning sunlight on the body for healing vitamin D.

•Relaxation and tension control techniques are effective. Stress creates an acid body condition, and erodes protective nerve sheathing. Acupuncture and Tai chi can relieve even the most stubborn cases of shingles.

Herbal, Superfood and Supplement Therapy

Interceptive therapy plan: Choose 2 to 3 recommendations.

1—Control eruptions: •Crystal Star ANTI-HST™ caps 4 to 6 daily to help produce normalizing antihistamines and open air passages. Add •HERPEX™ capsules, 2 caps 3x daily to calm itchy blistering. •Merix Health Products RELEEV to inhibit viral replication (good results); •PSP Marketing VIRAMAX or •Source Naturals RED MARINE ALGAE interfere with herpes virus (excellent results from both) —**Vitamin C controls eruptions:** Take Ester C powder with bioflavs., ¼ tsp. every hour in water up to 10,000mg or bowel to erance during an attack; reduce to 5000mg daily until blisters heal.

2—Reduce inflammation, relieve pain: Crystal Star DR. ENZYME™ with protease and bromelain (rapid action), or •Quercetin 1000mg with bromelain 1500. •Emulsified A & D 50,000/1,000IU 2x daily, with •Vit. E 400IU and selenium 200mcg 2x daily. •Apply E oil directly. •New Chapter ST. JOHN'S SC27 as an anti-inflammatory. •*Cayenne* caps 2 daily relieve pain, or •DLPA 750mg for pain. •Enzymatic Therapy HERPILYN caps. Apply •Crystal Star HERPEX™ lysine/licorice skin gel. **Homeopathics:** •B & T CALIFLORA gel. •B&T SSSTING STOP gel. •Biochemics PAIN RELIEF eucalyptus lotion.

3—Heal the blisters: •Diamond HERPANACINE caps 4 to 6 daily; or take MSM with MICROHYDRIN available at royalbodycare.com (notable results). Take •Lysine 1000mg internally, and apply LYSINE cream to blisters. Apply •Lemon Balm cream or lemon balm extract directly; or •calendula ointment; or •BioForce ECHINACEA cream; •Aloe Answers ALOE FORCE skin gel, or an •aloe vera/goldenseal solution.

4—Control viral lesion spread: Apply •Vibrant Health RMA (Red Marie Algae) *Gigartina* ointment for viral lesions; or spray lesions with •Earth's Bounty O₂ SPRAY several times daily. Take •East Park OLIVE LEAF extract caps with •Echinacea extract to flush lymph glands and •Omega-3 flax oil 3 tsp. daily.

5—Rebuild nerves: •Crystal Star RELAX CAPS™ as needed; •Stress B-complex 200mg with extra B₆ and B₁₂ 2000mcg sublingual; •*Scullcap* extract; •*St. John's wort* extract; •*Red clover/nettles* tea; •Reishi mushroom extract or •Planetary REISHI MUSHROOM SUPREME; •Magnesium 800mg 2x daily.

Can't find a recommended product? Call the 800 number listed in Product Resources for the store nearest you.

Shock and Trauma Control

Do you know what to do in an emergency?

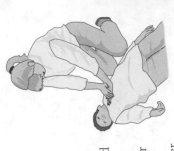

Shock is the condition that develops when blood flow drops below the levels needed to maintain vital body functions. Obviously, shock and trauma can happen during serious injuries when a great deal of blood and body fluids are lost. But it can also occur during severe infections, allergic reactions (anaphylactic shock), and nervous system malfunction (as in a severe reaction to a poisonous spider or snake bite). Major burns, heat prostration, a severe accident, a serious head injury or bone break, or bad fall.... every significant injury is accompanied by some degree of shock, because the autonomic nervous system responds to the trauma of injury by altering blood flow. It is usually wise to treat any severely injured person for shock in addition to treating them for the injury. If there is lots of bleeding, severe burns, or a head wound, treatment for shock should be very high priority.

Do you recognize shock? Here are the common signs:

1) Victim is weak, restless and unresponsive, with irregular deep breathing. 2) Victim's skin is cold, pale and damp to the touch, eye pupils are dilated. 3) Victim has a rapid weak heartbeat, possibly a heart attack or stroke sometimes with nausea. 4) Alertness and consciousness are low. Breathing is shallow.

Get medical care immediately! The following emergency measures are beneficial until medical help arrives:

Have the person lie down with legs elevated slightly above the head. Don't bend the legs. Loosen clothing. Protect the person from extremes of warmth and cold. If there is a chance of serious or life-threatening injury, do not move the person. Give small sips of fluids only if fully conscious - no solid food.

Know CPR. Cardiopulmonary resuscitation (CPR) is an important emergency procedure if a person's heart or breathing has stopped. CPR is essential in order to avoid brain damage, which usually begins in 4 to 6 minutes after cardiopulmonary arrest.

1. Be sure victim is truly unconscious. If shouting or shaking does not wake him or her, call immediately for help. Give precise directions and telephone number.
2. Lay the victim flat on the back on a straight, firm surface. If you have to roll the person over, roll him or her towards you with one of your hands supporting the neck as you turn.
3. Open the airway so the tongue is not blocking it. If you feel the person may have a neck injury, use your fingers to move the tongue out of the airway. If not, use the following procedure. Place one of your palms across the forehead, and using your other hand, lift the chin up and forward. At the same time, gently push down the forehead. This head and chin-tilt movement lifts the chin but does not fully close the mouth. As the jaw is tilted, the tongue will move out of the airway. Remove any dentures if present.
4. Check to see if the victim is breathing. Opening the airway may be all that is needed. If no signs of breathing are detected, move the tongue out of the airway again.
5. Begin mouth-to-mouth resuscitation. Remove your hand from the forehead and pinch the victim's nostrils together. Take a deep breath and place your open mouth over the victim's mouth. Exhale completely into the victim's mouth. Take your mouth away, inhale quickly, and repeat four times.
6. Check pulse on the side of the neck. You should feel the pulse of the carotid artery here. Move your fingers around if you don't feel it at once, and keep trying for 10 to 15 seconds.

If there is no pulse, begin chest compression to maintain circulation until medical help arrives.

- Kneel next to the victim's chest, midway between the shoulder and waist. Find the tip of the breastbone, and place your hands one over the other, palms down on this point.
- Shift your weight forward, and with your elbows locked, bear down on the victim's chest, compressing it 1½ to 2 inches.
- Compress the chest for half a second, then relax for a half second. Repeat. Count "1 and 2 and 3 and 4 and 5." Each time you reach 5 you should have done 5 compressions.
- After 15 compressions, take your hands off the chest and place them on the neck and forehead as before. Pinch the nostrils and administer 2 strong breaths into the victim's mouth.
- Do 15 more chest compressions. After 4 cycles of chest compressions and mouth-to-mouth breathing, check again for pulse and breathing.
- If neither pulse nor breathing have returned, resume until medical help arrives, or the victim revives, or you can no longer continue. Don't give up too soon!

Emergency herbals may be able to help.

—Deva Flowers FIRST AID remedy, or Nelson Bach RESCUE REMEDY; 2-4 drops on the tongue every 5 minutes until breathing normalizes.
—Dilute cayenne extract or powder in water (1-3 tsp., or 2-4 capsules); give with an eyedropper on the back of the tongue if necessary every 10 minutes to restore normal heart rate.
—Consciousness-reviving herbs such as strong incense, camphor, bay oil or musk can be used under the victim's nose as aromatherapy for revival.
—GINKGO BILOBA extract - a few drops in water, given on the tongue helps with stroke and allergic reactions such as dizziness, loss of balance, memory loss or ringing in the ears.
—Arnica Montana drops are usually the first homeopathic remedy to give for injury; every half hour to 1 hour on the tongue.
—Bromelain 500mg, or Quercetin with bromelain control body trauma; act like aspirin, anti-inflammatory without stomach upset. Open 1-2 capsules in water and give in small sips.
—Hops/valerian tincture, or Crystal Star STRESS OUT™ extract; 5-6 drops in water. Give in small sips every 10-15 minutes for calmness.

Thanks and credit to EVERYBODY'S GUIDE TO HOMEOPATHIC MEDICINES for this section. It is a needed family reference.

Can't find a recommended product? Call the 800 number listed in Product Resources for the store nearest you.

Sinus Infections

Sinusitis

For 40 million Americans, a chronic sinus infection is a daily energy drain. A sinus infection can be serious, spreading to the eyes and threatening vision. Although rare, a severe sinus infection can even spread to the brain and be life threatening! The sinuses are thin, air-filled chambers in the cartilage around the nose, sides of the forehead, the eye sockets and in the cheekbones. When sinus openings are obstructed, infected pus collects in these pockets causing pain and swelling. **Sinusitis** is an inflammation of the sinus mucous membranes. Chronic sinusitis may be a fungal infection and aggravate one by driving the infection deeper into sinus cavities. Natural healing methods revolve around relieving inflammation and cause of the clogging. **Do you have sinusitis?** Is breathing difficult, your head mucous-clogged and achy? Do you have pain behind the eyes, throbbing facial pain with a runny nose and inflamed nasal passages? Is there post-nasal drip with greenish discharge coughed up, loss of smell and taste, indigestion from mucous overload, and bad breath from low grade infection? Do you get frequent sore throat, earaches and toothaches? **What causes sinusitis?** A fungal, viral or bacterial infection, often triggered by an allergy (even from overusing nose drops with *benzalkonium chloride* preserver in the drops). Beware of: a diet with a lot of mucous-forming foods (dairy products and sugars), too many salty and fried foods, lack of green vegetables and lack of exercise.

Diet and Lifestyle Support Therapy

Nutritional therapy plan: *See my book COOKING FOR HEALTHY HEALING for a complete diet for respiratory health.*

1—Go on a 3 day mucous cleansing liquid diet. (pg. 202). Take a glass of lemon juice and water, or Herbal Answers ALOE FORCE juice each morning to thin mucous secretions. Add fresh carrot juice the 1st day. Add a pineapple/papaya juice, or dilute pineapple juice the 2nd day. Add a glass of apple juice the 3rd day.

2—Take an onion/garlic syrup each day. Or try this *Intensive Horseradish Decongestant:* soak fresh grated horseradish root in lemon juice. Add pinches of garlic, and ginger if desired. Take a spoonful and hang over a sink to expel lots of mucous all at once.

3—Then, eat only fresh foods for the rest of the week to cleanse encrusted mucous deposits. Drink 8 glasses of healthy liquids, including broths, herb teas and water to relieve congestion. (Add •Pure Planet CHLORELLA powder to boost immunity.)

4—Add lots of garlic, onions and mustard to your diet. Slowly add whole grains, vegetable protein, and cultured foods like Rejuvenative Foods VEGI-DELITE to your own tolerance. Avoid heavy starches, red meats, dairy foods, caffeine, refined sugars for 3 months.

—Bodywork:
- Take a hot sauna for 20 minutes daily during acute phase.
- Mix several drops of tea tree oil in a vaporizer. Use at night for clear morning sinuses.
- Apply hot compresses to sinus area for best results. Alternate with cold compresses for best results.
- Apply TIGER BALM or Chinese WHITE FLOWER OIL to sinus area.

—Acupressure points: (Acupuncture is also effective for chronic sinusitis.) 1) Massage under the big toes for 1 minute. 2) Squeeze ends of each finger and thumb hard for 20 seconds. 3) Press your thumb and index finger gently on the top of your nose on either side for 5 seconds. Repeat 3 times.

—For nasal polyps from sinus infection: Make a water solution of *goldenseal*, *echinacea* and *myrrh* powders - snuff up the nose to thoroughly rinse nasal sinuses.

Herbal, Superfood and Supplement Therapy

Interceptive therapy plan: Choose 2 to 3 recommendations.

1—**Address the infection:** •Planetary 3 SPICES SINUS COMPLEX. Use with Crystal Star ANTI-BIO™ caps, or •Pure Essence Labs ALLER FREE with enzymes to fight allergic response. •XLEAR Nasal Wash with Xylitol (highly recommended) or •Nutribiotic GRAPEFRUIT SEED extract diluted, as an antibiotic nasal rinse. •Osha root or Goldenrod tea, and Nutricology PRO-LIVE olive leaf extract tabs are gentle anti-virals.

2—**Relieve congestion:** •Vitamin C therapy: Use Ester C powder with bioflavonoids, 1/4 tsp. every hour to bowel tolerance during acute phase. And dissolve vitamin C crystals in water and drip into nose with eye-dropper. •*Ephedra* extract 15 drops 4x daily; •*Ephedra* tea (see contraindications pg. 70); •*Lobelia* extract drops in water; Zand DECONGEST HERBAL; •Gaia Herbs EYEBRIGHT-BAYBERRY; •Nature's Path NASAL-LYTE.

3—**Reduce inflammation:** •Crystal Star DR. ENZYME™ with protease and bromelain; •Quercetin 1000mg with bromelain 1500mg daily or •Source Naturals ACTIVATED QUERCETIN. •Propolis tincture drops or high potency royal jelly 2 tsp. daily.

4—**Cleanse sinus passages:** *Fenugreek/thyme* tea or *nettles* tea, or use *calendula* tea as a nasal wash. •Crystal Star ZINC SOURCE™ drops in water as a nasal rinse. —**Salt water sinus cleanse:** dissolve 1/4 tsp. sea salt to 1 cup warm water. Close one nostril, inhale enough solution through other nostril to be able to spit it out of mouth. Repeat daily one month. •Steam face and head with *eucalyptus/mullein*, or a *chamomile* steam.

5—**Long term relief:** •Lifespan Nutrition SNEEZE-EZE nasal spray forms an invisible, gel like mucus lining in the nasal tract, that acts as a filter for sinus irritants (outstanding immediate results); •Astragalus extract drops; •*Usnea* extract; garlic caps 6 daily; •CoQ$_{10}$ 200mg daily Add 2x daily each: •N-acetyl-cysteine (NAC) 500mg, and •Beta carotene 50,000IU. Add •zinc picolinate 50mg, or •zinc lozenges, or •Source Naturals OPTI-ZINC. •B-complex 100mg with pantothenic acid 500mg, and B$_{12}$ 2000mcg sublingual daily. •Biotec CELLGUARD 6 daily in high risk seasons.

—Effective homeopathic remedies: •Boiron SINUSITIS tabs; •BioForce SINUS RELIEF drops; •*Euphorbium* nasal spray; •*Euphrasia* (good results); •*Kali bichromium*.

Can't find a recommended product? Call the 800 number listed in Product Resources for the store nearest you.

Skin

Health and Beauty

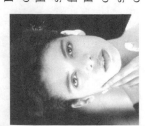

Beautiful skin is more than skin deep. The skin is the body's largest organ of both nourishment and elimination… the essence of renewable nature…it sloughs off old, dying cells every day for a new start. The skin's protective acid mantle inhibits the growth of disease-causing bacteria. Skin mirrors our emotional state and hormone balance, and is a sure sign of poor nutrition. (Allergies show up first on the skin.) On the other hand, relaxation, nourishment and improved nutrition show up quickly in skin beauty. **What causes skin problems?** Skin problems reflect a stressed lifestyle, a poor diet and lack of rest almost immediately. Avoid fast foods, fatty foods, caffeine and sugars. Keeping essential fatty acids and bioflavonoids high enhances skin texture, helps manage PMS and boosts liver function. Herbal nutrients are great for skin - packed with absorbable minerals, antioxidants, EFAs and bioflavonoids to cleanse, hydrate, heal, alkalize, and balance. Watch out for hormone disrupting chemicals in topical creams for bodybuilding and enhanced sexual performance. A recent article in Pediatrics documents significant signs of puberty in a 2 year old boy who had frequent contact with his father's skin and exercise equipment after application of a testosterone cream. Sores, spots, cracks, oiliness or dryness, scaling, itching, chapping, redness and rashes mean unbalanced skin and protective acid mantle. *See the following pages for more.*

Diet and Lifestyle Support Therapy

Nutritional therapy plan:

1—Great skin starts with a good diet: for dry skin, eat potassium-rich foods: leafy greens, bell peppers, bananas, broccoli, sesame and sunflower seeds, fish and sea greens.
2—Eat cultured foods: yogurt, tofu and kefir. Apply •Yogurt to balance skin pH.
3—Eat vitamin C, E, carotene-rich foods: fresh fruit, vegetable and fruit juices, celery, cucumbers, seafoods and fresh greens (or try •Barleans GREENS with EFAs).
4—Healthy skin contains 50 to 75% water. Drink 6 glasses of water every day. Try •Penta Water for purity. Drink watermelon juice when it is available - rich in natural silica to keep the system flushed and alkaline. Try Herbal Answers HERBAL ALOE FORCE juice and Jarrow GENTLE FIBERS for inside out activity. Use •Crystal Star GREEN TEA CLEANSER™ each morning to detox from environmental pollutants.
5—Eliminate red meats, fried, fatty and fast foods. Reduce caffeine, dairy foods, salty, sugary foods. They show up on your skin.

—Kitchen cosmetics:

•Make an AHA wrinkle treatment with a mix of egg whites, honey and red wine. Smooth on; leave on 20 minutes. Rinse off.
•Make a plant facial for moisture and tone: mix in your hand, 1 tsp. kelp granules and 1 tablespoon aloe vera gel. Apply to face and neck. Leave on 10 minutes, rinse.
•My own nourishing make-up remover: Mix in a dark bottle, avocado, almond, kukui nut, and sesame oils - makes your skin feel great.

—Bodywork:

•Use a balancing mask once a week. Smooth on a blend of aloe vera gel and vitamin E oil.
•Swirl 3TBS honey in bath water for silky skin. Apply body lotion after your shower before you dry off for the most moisture to your skin.
•Get 20 minutes of early morning sunlight on the skin for Vitamin D.

—Exfoliate for glowing skin: •Masada DEAD SEA SALTS. •Loofa sponge, ayate cloth, dry skin brush; •Rub with cucumber or papaya skins; •Rub with a honey/almond/oatmeal scrub; •Mychelle INCREDIBLE PUMPKIN PEEL and FRUIT FIESTA PEEL (a staff favorite).

Herbal, Superfood and Supplement Therapy

Interceptive therapy plan: Choose 2 to 3 recommendations.

1—Essential fatty acids are critical: Eat •chia, sesame, sunflower seeds; take •Evening primrose oil 4000mg daily; apply •Sesame seed, jojoba, or Kukui nut oil, (nourish while cleaning off make-up); •Yoanna ALOE PEARL or PANTHENOL COLLAGEN cream (recommended); •Nutricology SKIN GLOW Hyaluronic Acid softgels; Vitamin A & D 25,000/1,000. •Lane Labs SKIN PERFECT moisturizing cream (great under make-up).

2—Skin detox cleansers and pH balancers: •Aubrey BLUE-GREEN ALGAE cleanser. •Crystal Star HOT SEAWEED BATH™. •Zia SEA TONIC with aloe. •Dreamous BIOPATHIC SERUM and PURIFYING EARTH masque, •Lane Labs SKIN SMOOTHING BAR and SKIN REJUVENATOR CREAM -great results! —**Environmental pollutant cleansers:** • Planetary YELLOW DOCK SKIN CLEANSE; •Herbs Etc. DERMATONIC; •*Dandelion* caps 4 daily, or drink 2 cups of roasted *dandelion* tea daily. •Alpha Lipoic acid 300-600mg daily enhances antioxidant effectiveness. •Nutricology GERMANIUM 150mg. •*Suma* root capsules 4 daily. •Biotec AGELESS BEAUTY 6 daily, •Vitamin E with selenium 400IU; •ginkgo biloba extract (photo-protective).

3—Smoothing/hydrators for skin: • Source Naturals SKIN ETERNAL SERUM (ester C, Lipoic acid, DMAE); •Maitake Products AQUAMELLA (excellent for hydration); • Eidon SILICA; •Mychelle PERFECT C SERUM or •Yoanna OXYGEN FIRMING C complex (DMAE, Beta Glucan, Ester C); •American Health HYALURONIC ACID cream (for smoother skin); • MSM, 1000mg daily for soft skin. Pat on •Lavender for puffiness; •Rose hips tea-lemon juice blend to tighten; •Chamomile tea to tone; •Rose oil to hydrate.

4—For oily, shiny skin: •Mychelle FRUIT ENZYME CLEANSER; •Lavender essential oil; •Zia OIL CONTROL extract; • Rachel Perry CALENDULA CUCUMBER oil-free moisturizer. •a green clay mask. • Prince of Peace GINSENG-ROYAL JELLY vials.

5—Total skin support: •Diamond HERPANACINE 2 daily; •Crystal Star BEAUTIFUL SKIN™ tea - internally and externally (pat on problem spots); •Ester C with bioflavs., 3000mg daily; •Lane Labs TOKI, collagen replacement drink (boosts collagen 114%); •Yoanna VITAMIN E oil (highly nourishing); •Derma-E PYCNOGENOL MOISTURIZER inhibits collagen deterioration. • Noni of Beverly Hills PROTEIN CONDITIONER.

Can't find a recommended product? Call the 800 number listed in Product Resources for the store nearest you.

Skin

Dry, Wrinkled Skin, Brown Age Spots and Liver Spots

Skin aging is due to: 1) skin cells overloaded with toxins (free radical damage caused by smog and pollutants, too much tobacco, fried foods, caffeine, and alcohol); 2) poor circulation preventing oxygen delivery (broken capillaries, weak vein walls, atherosclerosis); 3) dehydration (too much sun exposure, especially with a thinned ozone layer, sometimes a result of estrogen depletion or imbalance from birth control pills); 4) shrunken skin tissues from lack of fatty acids and muscle tone, stress, poor diet, poor digestion of fats, liver malfunction and exhaustion.

Age spots, brown mottled spots on the hands, neck and face, are an external sign of waste accumulation, especially in the liver, (shows up as sallow skin), and of free radical damage in skin cells. Lipofuscin is the age-related skin pigment that oxidizes to actually appear as brown age spots. **Wrinkled, rough skin** texture is a sign of poor dermal collagen health. When collagen becomes hard from free radical attacks on skin cell membranes, it crosslinks with neighboring collagen fibers. Skin can't hold moisture or maintain elasticity, so it collapses on itself, forming a fish net below the surface of the skin, seen as wrinkles, dry skin and sagging skin. *See the following pages for more information on other skin problems.*

Diet and Lifestyle Support Therapy

Nutritional therapy plan:

1—Age spots and a yellowish, old skin look are signs that the liver is throwing off metabolic wastes through the skin. Go on a short liver detox cleansing diet (pg. 199) to cleanse accumulated toxins. Then drink carrot/beet/cucumber juice or Herbal Answers ALOE FORCE juice once a week for the next month to keep the liver clean.

2—Your diet is your most powerful weapon against wrinkles: lots of vegetable proteins from whole grains, seafoods (salmon is especially beneficial), sprouts and soy foods; mineral-rich foods, like leafy greens onions, cruciferous vegetables and molasses; pure water; and foods rich in carotenes (critical for collagen) like carrots, canteloupe, berries, greens, sea greens, broccoli. Keep constipation at bay with Jarrow GENTLE FIBERS.

3—Drink 8 glasses of water, like PENTA bottled water, or healthy liquids like Alacer EMERGEN-C for minerals and vitamin C. Include a glass of lemon juice and water; apply lemon juice to age spots. Take a high B skin food mix 2 tbsp. daily in juice: lecithin granules, wheat germ, Red Star Nutritional Yeast, molasses.

4—Refined sugars are as bad for your skin as too much sun. Avoid red meats, and caffeine containing foods. They dry out your skin. Avoid rancid nuts and oils.

—Lifestyle measures:

•Massage therapy releases toxins from lymph glands and tones facial muscles.
•Anti-wrinkle food facials: 1) rub the insides of fresh papaya skins on the face; 2) pat on a mix of whipped egg white and cream. Let dry; rinse off. 3) apply a yogurt mask to help reduce age spots and freckles. 4) For velvety skin, mix 1 tsp. kelp granules in a small bowl with 1 tbsp. aloe vera gel. Apply to face and neck. Leave on 10 minutes, rinse.
•Cigarette tar and nicotine deprive skin of oxygen, causing shriveling, wrinkling.
•Use sunscreen regularly. Sunscreens prevent age spots from darkening.

—For facial rejuvenation: Get plenty of fresh air; exercise 3x a week.

•For crepey eyelids, squeeze eyes closed, count to 12; then relax with eyes shut. Repeat 5 times daily. Change visible in 2 weeks.

Herbal, Superfood and Supplement Therapy

Interceptive therapy plan: Choose 2 to 3 recommendations.

1—**For age spots:** •Yoanna ALOE PEARL cream lightens discoloration; •Ginkgo Biloba extract to prevent lipofuscin build-up; •Anabol Naturals AMINO BALANCE is a specific; •Arginine blocks enzyme glycosylation 2000mg daily. •Reviva BROWN SPOT REMOVER~ 2% hydroquinone cream helps block melanin production of spots; •Crystal Star ADRENAL ENERGY BOOST™ caps with •LIVER CLEANSE FLUSHING™ tea for freckling. Apply •Lane Labs SUN SPOT ES. Results in about 3 weeks.

2—**For wrinkles:** • Lane Labs TOKI, collagen replacement drink (significant improvement in age spots, wrinkles). • Yoanna OXYGEN FIRMING C COMPLEX (Lipoic acid, vitamin C and DMAE, an antioxidant membrane stabilizer); •American Health HYALURONIC ACID cream (reduces fine lines); •Crystal Star DR. ENZYME™ to reduce inflammation linked to skin wrinkling; •Alpha lipoic acid 200mg daily, or Derma-E ALPHA LIPOIC moisturizer a skin antioxidant. Apply *chamomile* tea or •Mychelle SUPREME POLYPETIDE cream; •CoQ-10, 300mg daily, or •Avalon CoQ-10 WRINKLE DEFENSE cream; apply •Zia ULTIMATE MOISTURE or HERBAL MOISTURE gel for redness. •Grape seed extract caps 200mg; Lines around lips? •Baywood LIP MAXIMIZER (recommended).

3—**Combat sun aging with EFAs:** sea greens rehydrate skin, hold moisture. •Eat 2 tbsp. dry, snipped sea greens over rice, soup or salad, or 6 pieces of sushi a day, (noticeable in 3 to 4 weeks). •Evening primrose oil caps 4 daily; •Mychelle "THE PERFECT" C SERUM and DEEP REPAIR CREAM (even for serious sun damage). •Steam face with a mix of EFA herbs: *chamomile, eucalyptus, rosemary, nettles.*

4—**Renew skin elasticity:** Estrogen-collagen helps. •Crystal Star EST-AID™ caps 4 daily; •CC Pollen ROYAL JELLY cream; •Yoanna ELASTIN COLLAGEN LOTION; •Immudyne REJUVENATING SERUM (with beta glucan); •Premier One ROYAL JELLY 2 tsp. daily, or •Derma E RECOVERY COMPLEX. •MSM, 1000mg for soft elasticity.

5—**Alternatives to AHAs:** better skin tone and texture, less wrinkles, brown spots. •Yoanna ALOE CHAMOMILE EXFOLIATOR (excellent); Zia SEAWEED LIFT SERUM, • Earth Science Beta Ginseng AHAs; •Noni of Beverly Hills PROTEIN CONDITIONER.

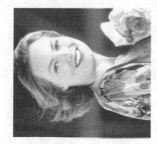

Can't find a recommended product? Call the 800 number listed in Product Resources for the store nearest you.

Skin, Cellulite

Fatty Deposits Showing through the Skin

Cellulite is a combination of fat, water and trapped wastes beneath the skin - usually on otherwise thin women. When circulation and elimination processes become impaired, connective tissue loses its strength. Unmetabolized fats and wastes become trapped in pockets just beneath the skin instead of being expelled through normal means. Over time, the waste materials harden and form the puckering skin effect we know as cellulite. Because it is unattached material, dieting and exercise alone can't dislodge cellulite. An effective program for cellulite release should be in four parts: 1) Stimulate elimination functions; 2) Increase circulation and metabolism; 3) Control excess fluid and waste retention; 4) Re-establish connective tissue elasticity. **Do you have cellulite?** It looks like lumpy, rippled skin around thighs, hips and love handles. When regular fat is squeezed, the skin appears smooth - cellulitic skin will ripple like an orange peel, or have the texture of cottage cheese. Cellulite is also characterized by heaviness in the legs, soreness and tenderness when tissue is massaged. **Why do you get it?** Sometimes its a family trait, more often its linked to poor nutrition resulting in liver exhaustion, excess estrogen build up, and poor fat metabolism. Inadequate exercise, poor elimination and insufficient water intake increase trapped wastes and toxins. Other causes? Crash dieting with rapid regain of weight increases cellulite formation. Smoking impedes both circulation and metabolism. Don't get too much sun. UV rays contribute to cellulite. *See WEIGHT LOSS, pages 564-569 or my book Cooking For Healthy Healing for more.*

Diet and Lifestyle Support Therapy

Nutritional therapy plan: *A good diet helps empty fat cells and carry off wastes.*

1—Add daily flushers to free trapped toxins: pineapple (bromelain), apples and berries (pectin fiber) and citrus (vitamin C). Carrot/beet/cucumber juice cleans the liver so it can metabolize fats better. Drink 6 to 8 glasses of water, juices and green tea every day. Graze - eat smaller, more frequent meals, instead of 2 to 3 large ones to keep fat burning.

2—Fruits and juices each morning. Two fresh or steamed vegetables at every other meal. A fresh salad and brown rice once a day. A liver cleanse works wonders. See pg. 199.—**The cellulite blacklist:** •All fried, fatty dairy foods; •High caffeine, carbonated sodas, hard liquor; •Red meats; •Extra salty foods (use herbal seasoning instead).

3—Balance estrogen: add cruciferous veggies like broccoli to keep excess estrogen flushed. Have Omega-rich fish and seafood twice a week. Have 2 tbsp. snipped dried sea greens 3 or 4 times a week in a soup, salad or rice; or 6 pcs. sushi daily.

—**Bodywork:**

•Use a dry skin brush or loofa to stimulate lymph glands. A seaweed bath afterward releases trapped toxins. A spa body wrap is a rapid fluid and inch-loss treatment. Get a massage treatment at the spa to release even more trapped fats.

•**10-minute daily cellulite exercises work.** They keep a slim subcutaneous fat layer, increase circulation, maintain underlying tissue integrity. Do them all each day for 10 minutes. 1) Standing arm swings 50 count both arms. 2) 100 tummy sucks. 3) 100 torso twists. 4) Wall pushups with each arm and both arms. 5) Standing leg circles, 50 each leg. 6) Weight lifting that focuses on the lower body helps develop the muscles in the hips and thighs. 7) Deep breathing moves out lymph congestion that shows as cellulite (one reason why yoga and pilates are so effective).

—**Rub-on cellulite-fighting essential oils:** •Antioxidant oils *rosemary* and *thyme.* •*Peppermint* oil increases metabolism. •*Juniper* stimulates circulation. •Apply Earth's Bounty O₂ SPRAY to fatty areas. (In some cases, the fat globules release by coming out through the skin in little white bumps.)

Herbal, Superfood and Supplement Therapy

Interceptive therapy plan: Choose 2 to 4 recommendations.

1—**Release trapped fats and shrink cellulite cells:** •Crystal Star HOT SEAWEED BATH™ stimulate circulation and potentiate lipolysis. •Crystal Star CELLULITE BODY-SHAPER™ roll-on gel with CELLULITE RELEASE™ caps (recommended, also helps balance hormones). •Health from the Sun LEAN FOR LESS program; •Biotec AGELESS BEAUTY tabs dissolve, flush rancid fats. •Nomie of Beverly Hills AHA SKIN CLEANSER.

2—**Help the liver to metabolize fats instead of storing them:** •Crystal Star LIVER CLEANSE FLUSHING™ tea; •*Milk Thistle Seed* or *Artichoke* leaf extract for liver congestion; •Anabol Naturals AMINO BALANCE caps; •Gaia MILK THISTLE-YELLOW DOCK extract; •Bromelain 1500mg daily to break down proteins and help metabolize fats.

3—**Raise metabolism to burn cellulite:** •Crystal Star THERMO THINNER™ caps with •Crystal Star THYROID META-MAX™ caps, or •Co-enzyme A Technology BODY IMAGE for thermogenesis; •Ginkgo Biloba extract 200mg daily.

4—**Essential fatty acids speed fat digestion, improve skin texture:** •Health from the Sun CLA 700mg (great for stubborn cellulite in the thigh area); Evening primrose oil 3000mg daily; •Borage oil caps 1000mg 2x daily (also reduces swelling).

5—**Repair/tighten connective tissue to free trapped wastes:** •Weleda BIRCH CELLULITE OIL to improve skin texture (highly recommended); Crystal Star IODINE, POTASSIUM, SILICA extract for collagen support; •Jarrow BIOSIL; •Body Essentials SILICA GEL internally, 1 tbsp. in 3-oz. liquid, externally on problem areas; •Solaray CENTELLA VEIN caps. •Bilberry or grape seed extract caps 200mg daily.

6—**Do thigh creams work?** Some of them do. Choose one with AHA's, herbal antioxidants and theophyllisilane for better skin tone. •Body Innovations CELLULITE ERASER body spray firms the skin, reducing the look of cellulite for five hours. •Or, make your own thigh cream with a blend of ¼ cup each jojoba and kukui nut oil. Add 5 drops *each* essential oils: juniper oil, grapefruit, rosemary and clary sage. Rub into affected skin areas 2x daily to help release water retention and increase circulation.

Can't find a recommended product? Call the 800 number listed in Product Resources for the store nearest you.

Skin, Damaged

Scars, Sunburn, Stretch Marks

Every blistering sunburn you get doubles your risk of skin cancer. Even on a cloudy day, 80% of the sun's harmful UV rays come through. **Sun damage** is cumulative, so moderation is the key. Sunlight helps you avoid breast and prostate cancer (a lack of protective vitamin D provided by sunlight may be involved). People who get almost no sun are at *higher* risk for melanoma than those who get moderate early morning sun. Practice good sun sense. Don't fry now and pay later. **High Risk Factors:** 1) Beware tanning beds. They have actually been implicated in accelerated skin aging, cataracts, immune system disorders. (Try Tyrosine 1000mg daily as an activator instead.) 2) Your adult skin will reflect frequent sunburns as a child. 3) Double your protection if you have light-colored eyes and hair, and fair or freckled skin; 4) Watch out if you've been on immune-suppressing, or photosensitive drugs - antibiotics, diuretics, hypoglycemia drugs, soaps w. *hexachlorophene,* and *Phenergan* in creams. Check labels. 5) Protect more if you've moved from a northern climate to the south, or from a high altitude to a flat land, or if you work all day outdoors. **Is your skin damaged?** It probably is if you have slow healing skin wounds, with continuing redness, roughness, irregular weals. Sunburn dehydrates skin, loss of elasticity is a sign, along with heat-exposure signs like throbbing headache, high blood pressure and a racing pulse. *Stretch marks* come with post-pregnancy stretching or serious weight-loss, and with the wide ranging nutrient deficiencies that accompany both circumstances. *See page 55 for facial surgery scar healing.*

Diet and Lifestyle Support Therapy

Nutritional therapy plan:

1—Have a veggie drink 3x a week during healing. Try •Nutricology PRO-GREENS with EFAs, or •Fit for You, International MIRACLE GREENS with high sea greens. Make a healing skin mix: nutritional yeast, wheat germ, lecithin granules; take 2 tbsp. daily with any meal.

2—Eat a high vegetable protein diet for faster healing. Include whole grains, sprouts, tofu, a protein drink every morning, like Garden of Life GOATEIN with colostrum for skin, or All One Multiple Vitamin and Mineral drink with rice protein.

3—Drink 6-8 glasses of mineral water daily to rehydrate from within. Try Penta water for 6 glasses, AloeLife ALOE GOLD juice for 2 glasses (noticeable results).

4—For scars and sun damaged skin, try Lane Labs TOKI collagen replacement drink every day (outstanding results, even for old scars). Eat avocados for skin elasticity.

•**For sunburns:** apply yogurt, black tea, oatmeal compresses or vinegar to burned areas. Apply grated apple to burned eyelids for fast relief. —Electrolyte drinks for skin fluid replacement: Effervescent C-2 packets daily, like Alacer EMERGEN-C, or Potassium broth (pg. 291). No alcoholic beverages - they dehydrate.

•**For stretch marks:** Massage aloe vera gel mixed with Yoanna VITAMIN E oil, or AHA's on stomach. Earth Mama Angel Baby STRETCH OIL for pregnancy stretch marks.

•**For scars:** Massage scar well with •Mtn. Ocean MOTHER'S BLEND oil, or sesame oil, kukui nut or wheat germ oil to bring up healthy circulation, skin tone. Add drops of lavender or frankincense essential oil to accelerate results. •Aloe vera or calendula gel.

—Sun sense skin burn prevention:

•Minimize exposure to mid-day sun. •Wear sunglasses with 100% UV filters. •Use a sunscreen with SPF 15 or more. I like Mychelle SUN SHIELD SPF 30. •Wear lip balm with sunscreen. •Drink plenty of water before, after and during exposure to replenish and moisturize your skin from within.

•For sun damage, take a cool bath immediately (no soap, no hot water); apply cold compresses to really burned areas. After burn subsides, try Mychelle INCREDIBLE PUMPKIN PEEL to heal damaged tissues (good results).

Herbal, Superfood and Supplement Therapy

Interceptive therapy plan: Choose 2 to 3 recommendations.

1—For scars: •Transformation PUREZYME (excellent results); •Home Health SCAR-GO. •Earth's Bounty O₂ SPRAY. •Crystal Star SCAR REDUCER™ gel or New Chapter TAMANU oil to break down scar material. •GOTU KOLA extract caps 4 daily; apply •fresh pineapple to scar and take Bromelain 1500mg daily, or •Crystal Star DR. ENZYME™ with protease and bromelain for 3 months. •Homeopathic *Thiosinaminum.* Apply •Pure Essence Labs FEM CREME for 3 months. •Derma E SCAR GEL. To heal sun damaged skin, Lane Labs SUNSPOT ES (outstanding results for raised, red, scaly spots). **—Healing minerals:** •Crystal Star OCEAN MINERALS™ •Nature's Path TRACE-LYTE with sea greens; •GERMANIUM 150mg for 2 months. Silicon treatment takes 3-4 months: •Eidon SILICA liquid or Alta Health SILICA. Apply •Body Essentials SILICA gel.

2—Boost skin EFAs: •Herbal Answers ALOE FORCE skin gel; •Evening Primrose Oil 4000mg daily; •Omega Nutrition ESSENTIAL BALANCE, 2 daily. •Prince of Peace GINSENG-ROYAL JELLY vials. Apply •shea butter cream or Tamanu oil.

3—Sunburn protection: •Alpha lipoic acid 400-600mg daily shields from oxidative damage. If your tissues are loaded with carotene A, vitamin C, E and B complex, your skin stands much less chance of damage by the sun. •Zinc 50mg daily and apply zinc oxide cream. •B-complex 100mg daily with extra PABA caps 1000mg and PABA cream. •For a natural looking tan without the skin damage, try Europharma SOLAIRE caps. —**Herbal sunburn remedies:** •Sea buckthorn oil (also heals radiation burns); •CamoCare CHAMOMILE ointment; •Jason WITCH VERA gel speeds healing; •Beehive Botanicals PROPOLIS & HONEY; or •apply a wheat germ oil, A & D oil, comfrey leaf and honey poultice (stretch marks, too). •CC Pollen PROPOLIS SKIN CREAM •AHA's reduce sun wrinkling, like Noni of Beverly Hills PROTEIN CONDITIONER.

—Antioxidants protect skin: COQ-10 200mg; •PCO's 100mg daily and apply •Derma-E PYCNOGENOL MOISTURIZER or Yoanna OXYGEN FIRMING COMPLEX; •Vitamin C therapy, up to 5000mg during healing; pat a C solution on burned areas. •Take MSM to repair sun-damaged skin.

Can't find a recommended product? Call the 800 number listed in Product Resources for the store nearest you.

543

Skin Infections

Dermatitis, Inflamed Itches and Rashes, Ulcerations

What does your skin rash mean? Our skin is the mirror of our lifestyle. Deep body imbalances often reveal themselves in skin problems.

Many skin problems start with internal toxicity, allergies, hormone imbalance and poor digestion. Stress and a poor diet clearly aggravate and contribute to skin disorders. Beyond these general conditions, the underlying reasons for unhealthy skin reflect our lives..... 1) DIET: essential fatty acid depletion, too many dairy foods, over-processed and chemicalized foods. 2) STRESS: emotional unhappiness, work-related anxiety. 3) DRUGS: Recreational or prescription reaction, detergents and household products. 4) SYSTEM OVERLOADS: especially liver exhaustion, adrenal malfunctions, nervous system, and bowel sluggishness. Investigate your symptoms before you attempt treatment to get best results. The following symptom list is designed to point you in the right direction in determining what a skin rash may mean.

Eczema is an increasingly common but aggravating skin condition related to food allergies (particularly eggs, soy foods, wheat and milk), essential fatty acid depletion, low hydrochloric acid in the stomach causing poor digestion, leaky gut syndrome and emotional stress.

Dermatitis is an inflamed skin condition with itch and rash that can stem from a wide variety of causes..... a systemic reaction to an allergen..... or to emotional stress, or to a severe deficiency of essential fatty acids. Atopic dermatitis is a severe type of eczema usually caused by allergies to chemicals, plants, clothing, topical medications, or jewelry metals. The systemic nature of these conditions means that they can and do spread, and can become quite severe. However, both conditions are usually temporary and can often be reversed by eliminating the offending allergen, improving digestion and boosting EFA intake.

Signs that you may have eczema or dermatitis:

- Inflamed, angry red, dry thickened skin patches (frequently on the cheeks, ankles or wrists)
- Crusting, tiny, oozing blisters on the skin; itching, weeping skin
- Thickened, lumpy skin; scaling and bumps on the skin
- Tingling, unpleasant skin prickling

See FUNGAL SKIN INFECTIONS page 420 and ECZEMA AND PSORIASIS, page 403–404, for more information.

Psoriasis is a troublesome, mysterious chronic skin disorder, affecting 6.4 million Americans. Psoriasis is characterized by an abnormal growth of skin cells. Normal skin cells mature within about a month, but a psoriatic skin cell takes only three to six days. A recent study links psoriasis to immune system malfunction. It isn't contagious, with effects ranging from mild to significant, but each year, about 400 people die from complications due to severe psoriasis. (In extreme cases, large areas of skin are lost, leaving the body susceptible to serious infections.) Natural therapies focus on stress reduction and anti-inflammatories for relief. In clinical studies, supplementation with omega-3 fatty acids has produced good results.

Signs that you may have psoriasis: See ECZEMA AND PSORIASIS SKIN INFECTIONS page 403–404 for more information.

- Inflamed skin lesions with white scales (usually on the scalp, knees, elbows, hands and feet)
- Intense skin sloughing (severe erythrodemic psoriasis)
- Joint inflammation with arthritic pain (10% of people with psoriasis have psoriatic arthritis)
- Pitting of the nails can be a sign of psoriasis

Rosacea is a skin disorder related to adult acne occurring mainly in middle-aged people of Celtic descent. There is no known cure for acne rosacea. Doctors treat it in much the same way as other forms of acne, with oral and topical antibiotics. Eliminating food triggers, particularly spicy foods and alcohol, and avoiding excessive emotional stress, sun, and environmental pollutants is key to control of rosacea breakouts.

Signs that you may have rosacea: See PAGE 546 for more information.

- Flushing and redness of the cheeks, chin, nose, and forehead
- Acne-like bumps and pimples
- Dilated blood vessels on the face
- A red, bumpy nose; bloodshot eyes or gritty feeling in eyes
- Small, hard bumps on both eyelids

Can't find a recommended product? Call the 800 number listed in Product Resources for the store nearest you.

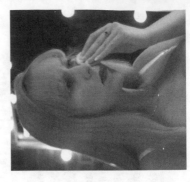

Skin Infections

Diet and Lifestyle Support Therapy

Nutritional therapy plan:

1—Rashes are often symptoms of food allergies - avoid common allergens like milk and wheat products, eggs, red meats (that usually have nitrates), fast foods, sugary foods, fried foods, chocolate, shellfish, peanut butter.

2—Go on a short 3 day juice cleanse (page 208) to clear acid waste from the system. Try Crystal Star GREEN TEA CLEANSER™ to neutralize acids if the condition is chronic.

3—Then eat a diet with plenty of leafy greens and other mineral-rich foods, like seafoods and sea vegetables to rebuild healthy tissue and good adrenal function.

4—Reduce both fats and calories. Use olive oil, flax or sesame oil, or grapeseed oil for EFAs.

5—Eat cultured foods like yogurt or kefir frequently, or try Solgar WHEY TO GO protein drink, or Jarrow GENTLE FIBERS drink for healthy G.I. flora.

6—Make a skin mix of ¼ cup each: toasted wheat germ, molasses and nutritional yeast; take 2 tbsp. daily. Or try WHEAT GERM ESSENCE for liver support.

—For ulcerations: Keep the diet simple. Add more fresh fruits and vegetables. Add protein sources for faster healing: whole grains, soy foods, seafoods and cultured foods. Include carotene-rich foods from yellow-orange vegetables and sea vegetables, or Green Foods CARROT ESSENCE. Include vitamin C-rich foods for collagen and tissue health. Include silicon-rich foods from vegetables, whole grains and seafoods to build connective skin tissue. Take a skin healing mix of 1 tsp. each, wheat germ oil and nutritional yeast in aloe vera juice 2x daily. Drink 6-8 glasses of bottled water or healthy juices and herbal teas (Crystal Star DR. VITALITY™ tea is a specific for skin) to keep acid wastes flushed. Avoid saturated and trans fats, sugars and caffeine-containing foods.

Lifestyle measures:

• Get early morning sunlight on the skin every day possible for healing vitamin D.
• Take an oatmeal bath for itchy skin.
• Avoid detergents on the skin. Use mild castile soap. Avoid perfumed cosmetics.

Effective skin healers:

• Calendula gel for ulcerations, or • B & T CALIFLORA gel for open ulcerations.
• Body Essentials SILICA GEL
• PCO's 100mg daily and apply Derma-E PYCNOGENOL MOISTURIZER
• Dreamous BIOPATHIC SERUM
• Herbal Answers ALOE FORCE SKIN GEL
• Earth's Bounty O₂ SPRAY (usually a noticeable change in 3 weeks)
• Tea tree oil if fungus is the cause
• Aubrey Organics ANTI-ITCH HERBAL REMEDY
• Beehive Botanicals DERMA CREAM

Herbal, Superfood and Supplement Therapy

Interceptive therapy plan: Choose 2 or 3 recommendations.

1—Control infection: •Crystal Star ANTI-BIO™ gel as needed, and • ANTI-BIO™ caps 6 daily. •Diamond HERPANACINE (works well in stubborn cases); •Nutribiotic GRAPEFRUIT SEED extract, or mix 4 drops in 5-oz. water and apply directly, or use the gel (good results in about 4 days); *St. John's wort* oil, or •Nature's Apothecary HERBAL FIRST AID oil; •Nutricology GERMANIUM 150mg; •GINKGO BILOBA extract 4x daily. •Allergy Research OREGANO OIL as directed; Vitamin C 5000mg daily to deter eruptions. •Crystal Star

2—Form new smooth skin: •Flora VEGE-SIL for healthy new growth. •Crystal Star OCEAN MINERALS drops, or •Jarrow BIOSIL for collagen formation. •MSM, 1000mg daily or •Eidon SULFUR liquid to smooth; •Vitamin C therapy: ascorbate C powder; mix with water to a solution. Apply to area, and take 1 tsp. every hour for collagen-connective tissue growth. •Stress B-complex 100mg 2x daily with extra Biotin 600mcg.

3—For inflamed skin and eruptions: Crystal Star ANTI-HST™ capsules, 4-6 daily to relieve a histamine weal-type rash. Very effective. Homeopathic *Urtica urens,* or *Natrum muriaticum.*
•*Burdock* tea 3x daily; make a paste of •vitamin C powder and aloe vera juice and apply.
•Place cold wet *chamomile* tea bags on inflamed area or a compress of cold *chamomile* tea; •mix 3 drops of *lavender* essential oil in 4 tbsp. aloe vera gel and apply. •devil's claw extract; •Crystal Star •BEAUTIFUL SKIN™ capsules, 4 daily with DR. ENZYME™ with protease and bromelain 3 daily. Make, drink and apply an herbal itch tea: *dandelion root, burdock root, echinacea root, kelp, yellow dock root, chamomile.* •Quercetin 1000mg daily with bromelain 1500mg daily; •Zinc 50mg. 2x daily.

4—Essential fatty acids for smooth skin: •Evening primrose oil 4 daily; •Barleans lignan rich omega-3 flax oil 3 daily; •Nature's Secret ULTIMATE OIL •Apply wheat germ oil; •Suma caps 3-4 daily. •Udo's PERFECTED OIL BLEND.

5—Effective skin healing applications: •Aloe vera gel mixed with *goldenseal* powder.
•Crystal Star BEAUTIFUL SKIN TEA™ - apply to neutralize acids coming out on the skin;
apply •HEALTHY SKIN™ gel to a minor rash (sometimes overnight results). •Apply A, D & E oil, take emulsified A & D oil caps; •Prime Pharm. PRIMADERM cream.

6—For pH balance: •UAS DDS-PLUS with FOS; •Trimedica ALKAMAX; •Pancreatin 1300mg.

—For ulcerations: Hot •*comfrey* compresses, •tea tree oil, •propolis tincture, a •green clay poultice. Apply frequently a •paste of aloe vera gel and *goldenseal* powder and a few drops of *tea tree* oil. Take •Crystal Star DR.ENZYME™ with protease and bromelain or Bromelain 1500mg; •Barleans lignan-rich Omega-3 flax oil 3x daily. Take •Crystal Star BEAUTIFUL SKIN™ caps and apply Crystal Star ANTI-BIO™ gel if there is infection. Make a healing tea: •Steep *burdock* and *dandelion root* and *echinacea* EXTRACT; take 3 cups daily. •Herbal Answers ALOE FORCE SKIN GEL, and •Flora VEGE-SIL for connective tissue regrowth.

Can't find a recommended product? Call the 800 number listed in Product Resources for the store nearest you.

Therapy for other Skin Problems

Rosacea, Vitiligo, Strawberries, Hard Bumps

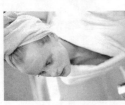

Your skin heals from the inside out. Don't forget the importance of diet and nutrition to skin regeneration.

WHITE HARD BUMPS on UPPER ARMS and CHEST: —**Effective natural therapies:** Apply mix of crushed garlic and honey to bumps; Take •Vitamin A 25,000IU 2 daily, •zinc picolinate 50mg daily. •Ester C 550mg with bioflavonoids 3 daily; *butternut* bark capsules (good results), or •Crystal Star FIBER & HERBS caps with butternut. (*Butternut tea* internally and externally also produces good results for skin bumps, a colon problem.) Dab with pineapple juice and take •bromelain 1500mg daily. Take •EFAs: Evening Primrose oil 3000mg. Health from the Sun CLA. Dry skin brush areas morning and night until skin is pink. Try a natural body scrub like MASADA MINERAL HERB SPA body glow, or take hot seaweed bath for skin oxygen, slough off dead cells and speed cell renewal.

VITILIGO (*leukoderma*): A progressive immune system disorder causing skin depigmentation when the body stops making melanin. Some victims are helped when the condition is treated as if it were radiation poisoning for 6 to 9 months (see page 53). Steroid drug treatments offer some repigmentation, but higher risk of skin cancer. —**Effective natural therapies:** The newest treatment: •phenylalanine 1000mg one hour before exposure to UV light, •high dose vitamin C 3-5grams daily, • sublingual B-12 10,000mcg daily, and •folic acid 800mcg daily. Good reports from •PABA 1000mg with 2 tbsp. molasses daily as an iron source, HCl 600mg daily, •pantothenic acid 1000mg; •magnesium 1500mg daily; •Solaray TURMERIC capsules 4 daily; •Flora VEGE-SIL tabs, or •Crystal Star IODINE, POTASSIUM, SILICA drops, •astragalus caps and •sea greens to stimulate the thyroid. •Evening Primrose oil caps 6 daily; •KHELLA is the herb of choice in Europe (available here from Herb Pharm); and • Ginkgo Biloba extract. •Calendula gel is a good topical.

SCLERODERMA: A runaway healing process where the body inexplicably begins, then continues to produce too much collagen and connective tissue, replacing normal cell structure. This causes scar tissue to build up on skin, lungs and circulatory organs. It begins with discolored skin, followed by lesions, swelling and horrible pain. —**Effective natural therapies:** Drink fresh carrot and mixed vegetable juice at least three times a week. Take a protein drink like •Nutricology PRO-GREENS with EFAs every day. Add aloe vera gel and avocado oil to your bath water. Take •MSM, 1000mg daily for soft, pliable skin. Take •gotu kola (*centella asiatica*) caps 4 daily and •PABA 1000mg daily for significant skin softening. Apply •calendula gel to lesions and take •Crystal Star DR.ENZYME™ with protease and bromelain, or Bromelain 1500mg daily to reduce swelling. Get regular exercise to increase perspiration, stimulate metabolism, and rid the body of carbon dioxide build-up. Stop smoking. Add antioxidants: •CoQ₁₀ 300mg daily, •beta carotene 150,000IU daily, •2 tbsp. sea greens (any kind) daily to resmoisturize, •vitamin C with bioflavonoids, 5000mg daily, •glutathione 50mg daily, •PCO's from grapeseed or white pine 50mg 4x daily, •B₆ 250mg daily, and• zinc 30mg daily.

STRAWBERRIES, EXCESS PIGMENTATION: —**Effective natural therapies:** Reduce too high copper levels by adding more zinc and iron-rich foods. Reduce clogging waste with a gentle herbal laxative like Planetary TRIPHALA INTERNAL CLEANSER. Apply •B&T CALIFLORA ointment, take •pantothenic acid 1000mg, B₆ 500mg and alpha lipoic acid 600mg. Check for zinc deficiency with Ethical Nutrients ZINC STATUS (also is a supplement).

ROSACEA: Redness of the central face, small red bumps and enlarged blood vessels on face, neck and chest. Rosacea triggers: tomatoes, red spices, chocolate, meat marinades, hot drinks, citrus fruits, vinegar, red wine and red meats. May be caused by a parasite, "*human demodex*." —**Effective natural therapies:** •Stay well hydrated. Drink plenty of quality water (like PENTA bottled water) and eat plenty of fresh fruits and vegetables. Avoid excess alcohol and smoking which contribute to dehydration. Take •Crystal Star RED SKIN RELIEF™ caps with herbal anti-inflammatories (excellent results), along with Dr. Diamond HERPANACINE capsules (long term balance). Add plenty of •EFAs to your diet - EVENING PRIMROSE oil 4000mg daily, or Health from the Sun TOTAL EFA, or add Omega-3 rich flax or perilla oil in your salad dressings. Add •B complex vitamins 100mg daily and •vitamin E 400IU with selenium 200mcg. Add •sea greens to your diet 2 tbsp. daily, or take •Crystal Star IODINE, POTASSIUM, SILICA drops for thyroid stimulation and minerals, or •OCEAN MINERALS™ with sea greens. Apply •Dreamous BIOPATHIC SERUM (great results); or GRAPEFRUIT SEED extract. For inflammation relief, spray on soothing Mychelle FRUIT ENZYME MIST and apply CAPILLARY CALMING SERUM 2-3x daily (fast results). Yoanna CUCUMBER PEARL MOISTURIZER nourishes and reduces redness; Mix •2 tsp. turmeric powder and 6 tsp. coriander powder with enough milk to make a paste. Apply and leave on 10 minutes when you see a breakout. Or use •Zia 10-minute CRANBERRY PEEL or wash with Mychelle CRANBERRY CLEANSER (a specific for rosacea). Drink •Crystal Star BEAUTIFUL SKIN™ tea and pat on face with cotton balls. •Saw Palmetto is a specific for Rosacea. Drink •*echinacea-pau d'arco* tea 3 cups daily to flush fats from the blood stream. Add probiotics like •American Health ACIDOPHILUS liquid (dairy-free) or UAS - DDS PLUS, and B-12, up to 5000mcg daily. Consider enzymes and supplemental HCl 600mg daily, to optimize digestion of fats. After outbreaks, consider Anabol Naturals AMINO BALANCE to speed skin healing (recommended). Consider Yoanna MINERAL MAKEUP, good coverage for sensitive, rosacea-prone skin. *Contact the National Rosacea Society (888) 662-5874 for more info.*

Can't find a recommended product? Call the 800 number listed in Product Resources for the store nearest you.

Smoking

Second-Hand Smoke, Smokeless Tobacco

Wow! Look at these numbers! Each cigarette takes 8 minutes off your life; a pack a day takes 1 month off your life each year; 2 packs a day, takes 12-15 years off your life. Cigarettes have over 4000 known poisons, any of which can kill a grown man. One drop of pure nicotinic acid can kill a grown man. Still, one in six Americans smoke cigarettes. Depending on the age that you quit, your life expectancy can increase from 2-5 years. Secondhand or passive smoke, (the third leading cause of preventable death in the U.S.), and chewing tobacco are just as dangerous, especially for women. Passive smoke reduces fertility, successful pregnancies, and normal birth weight babies. It increases the instance of cervical, uterine and lung cancer (in pets who are exposed, too), heart disease and osteoporosis. Don't be discouraged. Quitting is hard work, but it gets easier every day, as the body loses dependence on nicotine. New trials on a nicotine vaccine are currently underway in Belgium. If successful, the new vaccine, TA-NIC, will offer smokers another tool to break them of this life-threatening addiction.

Is your disease risk on the rise from smoking? Are you getting chronic bronchitis and allergies? Do you have a constant hacking cough? Is your breathing getting noticeably more difficult? Do you come up tired and short of breath with almost any physical exertion? Do you have CCPD (emphysema)? Is your breathing dry? Do you think you have lung cancer or other degenerative lung disease like T.B? Do you have smoking-related problems? Adrenal exhaustion; poor circulation affecting vision; high blood pressure; premature aging; hair loss and wrinkled, dehydrated skin with poor color and elasticity (smoke decreases blood flow to the skin); stomach ulcers; osteoporosis; severe gum disease; low immunity. The cost of smoking-related illness is over 50 billion dollars today in medical bills alone. *See POISONING, HEAVY METAL page 523 in this book for more information.*

Are you trying to quit smoking?

I hope so. Every 72 seconds someone dies from smoking. Here's the best motivational chart I've ever seen to illustrate the benefits for your body and your life once you really quit. *Sources: The American Cancer Society and Centers for Disease Control.*

What happens after you quit smoking?

Within 20 minutes of smoking, your body begins a series of changes that continues for years. You lose all benefits by smoking just one cigarette a day says the American Cancer Society.

20 MINUTES:
- Blood pressure drops to normal
- Pulse rate drops to normal
- Temperature of hands and feet normalizes

8 HOURS
- Carbon monoxide level in blood drops to normal
- Oxygen level in blood increases to normal

24 HOURS
- Chance of heart attack decreases

48 HOURS
- Nerve endings start regrowing
- Ability to smell and taste is enhanced

2 WEEKS TO 3 MONTHS
- Circulation improves
- Walking becomes easier
- Lung function increases up to 30%

1 to 9 MONTHS
- Coughing, sinus congestion, fatigue, and short-ness of breath decrease
- Cilia regrow in lungs, allowing lungs to handle mucous, keep clean and reduce infection.
- Body's overall energy rises

1 YEAR
- Coronary disease risk is half that of a smoker

5 YEARS
- Lung cancer death rate for average former pack a day smoker decreases by almost half
- Stroke risk is reduced to that of a nonsmoker five to 15 years after quitting
- Risk of cancer of the mouth, throat, and esophagus is half that of a smoker's

10 YEARS
- Lung cancer death rate similar to a nonsmoker
- Precancerous cells are replaced
- Risk of cancer of the mouth, throat, esophagus, bladder, kidney, cervix, pancreas decreases

15 YEARS
- Risk of coronary disease same as a nonsmoker

Can't find a recommended product? Call the 800 number listed in Product Resources for the store nearest you.

Smoking

Diet and Lifestyle Support Therapy

Nutritional therapy plan:

1—There must be a lifestyle and diet change for permanent success against smoking. Start with a 3 day liquid cleansing diet- fresh fruit and vegetable juices and miso soup to neutralize and clear the blood of nicotinic acid and to fortify blood sugar. Include lots of vegetable proteins. Add magnesium-rich foods like dark leafy veggies, whole grains, sea seafoods, sea vegetables and legumes.

2—Follow with a fresh foods only diet for 3 days. Have carrot juice, plenty of carrots and celery, leafy green salads and lots of citrus fruits to promote body alkalinity. (pH 7 and above readings show less desire for tobacco.) —Green drinks like •Pure Planet CHLORELLA and •Nutricology PRO-GREENS + EFA's help neutralize nicotine toxicity.

3—Avoid junk foods and sugar that aggravate cravings. Avoid oxalic acid-forming foods like chocolate and cooked spinach or rutabaga that bind up magnesium in the body.

4—Take a cup of green tea or Crystal Star GREEN TEA CLEANSER™ or a squeezed lemon in water daily to reduce carcinogens. Add •New Chapter GINGER WONDER syrup—1 tbsp. in 8-oz. water 2x daily to boost circulation. *Consider a Chemical-Pollutant Cleanse (pg. 178) about 2 months after quitting smoking to help release cigarette toxins.*

—Bodywork:

•Do deep breathing exercises and aerobic exercise for more body oxygen whenever you feel the urge for tobacco until the desire decreases, in about 4 minutes.

•To help curb craving for chewing tobacco, chew licorice root sticks or cloves.... helps your breath, too.

•Acupuncture treatments along with anti-smoking counseling can help even long time smokers quit.

Info you may not know about smoking:

—If your parents smoke, you may inherit an addiction even before birth. Fetuses absorb nicotine, CO_2 and tar in the womb (some even pull away from the uterine wall). Passive smoke is almost as bad. The family of a heavy smoker has lung damage and lung cancer risk equal to smoking 1 to 10 cigarettes a day!

—Smokers are prone to heartburn and ulcers. Smoking inhibits a protective bicarbonate secretion in the small intestine that neutralizes acid. Cigars are even worse than cigarettes.

—Smoking reduces the size of a man's erection. All muscles (not just the penis) grow slower and need longer recovery time if you smoke.

—Smoking gives your face wrinkles because it constricts blood vessels, depriving your tissues of oxygen as well as vitamin A, B, C and D, thus harming connective tissue. Nicotine depletes elastin stores that make your skin soft and pliable.

Herbal, Superfood and Supplement Therapy

Interceptive therapy plan: Choose 2 to 3 recommendations.

1—**Control the cravings:** Take •*Lobelia* tea or •*oats/scullcap* tea, 2 cups throughout the day in sips to keep tissues flooded with agents that discourage the taste for nicotine. (Add 1 pinch ginger, or •New Chapter GINGER WONDER syrup for best results.) •Homeopathic Natra-Bio NICO-RX kit (works); •Herbs, Etc. SMOKE FREE softgels; or •Gaia NICOTINE RELIEF liquid phytocaps help; •Red Earth Herbal Drops NICO-FREE extract.

•Make a nicotine addiction-fighting tea to lessen desire, strengthen adrenals, and cleanse lungs. Steep one part each: Oatstraw and seed, lobelia seed and leaf, black pepper, licorice root, calamus root, sassafras. Sip slowly throughout the day for at least 2 weeks.

2—**Flush nicotine out of the lymph system and lungs:** •*Echinacea*, very effective lymph flusher; •*Ephedra* tea, *Fenugreek* seed tea, or •Herbs Etc. LUNG TONIC softgels to cleanse lungs.

3—**Help neutralize cancer-causing compounds:** Solaray TURMERIC caps 6 daily.

—**For nico-toxicity take daily:** N-acetyl-cysteine 1000mg, 2 Glutamine 1000mg, 4 Vitamin C 1000mg, 4 Evening primrose oil, 20 Sun Wellness CHLORELLA tabs.

4—**Calm the nerves:** •Crystal Star RELAX CAPS™ 6 daily (highly recommended); •WITHDRAWAL SUPPORT™ for addiction caps to calm tension; •Magnesium 800mg daily; •Stress B-complex 100mg daily; •VALERIAN/WILD LETTUCE drops in water.

5—**Protect against heart and artery problems with EFA's:** Smoking is a big contributor to high blood pressure because smoke narrows arteries. Nicotine revs up heartbeat. When the body calls for more oxygen-laden blood, the arteries can't deliver it. Slow suicide. •Spectrum NORWEGIAN FISH OIL or •Barleans high-lignan flax oil caps, 3 daily; •Biotec PACIFIC SEA PLASMA sea greens 6 daily; •Natures Path TRACE-MIN- LYTE with sea greens. •Taurine 1500mg daily.

6—**Ginseng helps normalize and control cravings:** •*Ginseng-licorice* extract also helps blood sugar balance; •Crystal Star FEEL GREAT NOW™ caps help rebuild nerves; •Imperial Elixir AMERICAN GINSENG. •Prince of Peace American Ginseng-Bee Pollen-Royal Jelly vials help circulation, sugar cravings and energy.

7—**Guard against secondary smoke:** •Royal Bodycare MICROHYDRIN PLUS; •New Chapter SMOKE SHIELD (good results in clinical trials); •Glutathione 50mg daily; •Ascorbate vitamin C powder + bioflavonoids, ½ tsp. in water each hour to bowel tolerance during withdrawal stage, then reduce to 5000mg daily; •PCO's 100mg daily.

8—**Antioxidants are lung protectors against tobacco:** •Premier Labs GERMANIUM 150mg; •Twin Labs LYCOPENE 10mg for lungs; •CoQ 10, 300mg daily (recommended); •Niacin therapy: 500-1000mg daily, with •Beta-carotene 200,000IU daily.

Can't find a recommended product? Call the 800 number listed in Product Resources for the store nearest you.

Snake Bite

Poisonous Spider Bites, Scorpions

Get emergency medical help immediately! Time is critical. Use the methods below only until this help arrives. There is anti-venin for snake bites today, but it is often snake-specific and carries the risk of anaphylactic shock. Buy a snake bite kit before you go on any trip where you can't reach medical help in a reasonable time. Know what poisonous snakes live your area. If you're not sure, treat it as if it is poisonous – the black widow and the brown recluse. There is anti-venin for black widows, but none for brown recluse spiders. 2 spiders in the U.S. are highly poisonous - the black widow and the brown recluse. There is anti-venin for black widows, but none for brown recluse spiders. Shock, convulsions may occur. **Were you bitten by a poisonous snake or spider?** *Snake bite:* slow, upward spreading red lines as poison moves toward the heart; swelling, sometimes severe pain and nausea; sweating, rapid heartbeat, dizziness, weakness, difficulty breathing, labored breathing, headache, swollen face, fever, chills, profuse sweating and shock. *Black widow bite:* severe chest and abdominal pain, sometimes fainting. *Brown recluse bite:* within a few days to a week after bite, a small raised blister forms. Then an ulcer that lasts for weeks, even months. There is general weakness, nausea, hive breakouts and kidney problems. *California scorpions* (from areas other than around the Colorado River) are not dangerous unless you are allergic. *Texas/Southwest scorpions* are poisonous and dangerous to pets and people. Get medical help.

Diet and Lifestyle Support Therapy

Nutritional therapy plan:

1—For snake bite: wash bite with soap and water. •Do not pour alcohol on a bite. It is useless and may speed up the venom spread. Ice packs or compresses are no good either for snake bite because they may damage tissue. Native American healers applied a tobacco and saliva poultice to a bite.

2—Give the victim only small sips of water. No alcoholic drinks. The poison will spread through the body faster.

3—Plant onions and garlic to keep snakes away. Eating daily onions before going into snake country may be protective against the poison of some bites.

4—Green drinks can help to detoxify and restore normal body composition after bite has been treated and crisis has passed. Try aloe vera juice first; then Crystal Star RESTORE YOUR STRENGTH™ for iodine/potassium therapy. C'est Si Bon CHLORENERGY 2 packets daily for chlorella, or Nutricology PRO-GREENS with flax EFAs.

—Bodywork:

•Take precautions if you are going on a camping trip, tropical hike, or working around snake havens like sheds and outbuildings. Wear heavy boots and leggings that fangs can't penetrate.

•Keep victim still and calm. Immobilize the bite area and keep it lower than the heart. Until medical help arrives, put a constricting band 2 to 4" above the bite. Don't cut off circulation. Move band up if swelling reaches the band.

•If you can't get to medical help within 15 minutes, and swelling is rapid and pain severe, make a small cut with a sharp knife up and down, not across, through each fang mark. Use suction by mouth or a suction cup for at least 30 minutes, repeatedly. Spit out blood. Rinse mouth immediately.

•A Springlife POLARIZER, if used immediately may reduce swelling and adverse reactions.

Herbal, Superfood and Supplement Therapy

Interceptive therapy plan: Choose 1 or 2 recommendations.

A) In a life-threatening situation, where the victim may go into cardiac arrest, *cayenne* may save the victim's life. •Cayenne, 2 capsules or 8-10 drops of cayenne extract in warm water, as a shock preventive can help strengthen the victim's heart. Seek medical help.

B) In a life-threatening situation, where the victim may go into shock or convulsions, massive doses of vitamin C may save the victim's life. Use •Calcium ascorbate vitamin C powder, ¼ tsp. in water every 15 minutes as a detoxifier during acute reaction phase. Seek medical help.

C) Use •Echinacea extract drops under the tongue or in water in either case to flush poisons from the lymph glands. Use echinacea pulp as a poultice after the bite has been lanced and poison drained.

1—**Reduce swelling:** Take •Crystal Star ANTI-HST™ caps to help calm a histamine swelling reaction. Take •*yellow dock* tea with *echinacea* extract drops every hour until swelling goes down. Apply •Black cohosh tea or open an •Enzymedica PURIFY (protease) capsule and apply as an antidote to venom, as well as take in water.

—**Effective compresses to reduce swelling:** •*Plantain*; •*Rue*; •Fresh comfrey leaf; •*Slippery elm*.

2—**After the bite crisis has passed, and AFTER poison is out of the body:** Use •Golden Pride ORAL CHELATION therapy with EDTA. •Metabolic Response Modifiers CARDIOCHELATE or •alpha lipoic acid 600mg to detoxify the system. Use •Niacin therapy: up to 500mg daily, to dilate and tone blood vessels.

3—**Heal skin from the bite:** •*Aloe/comfrey* salve or *Aloe vera* gel; •*Comfrey* tea; •*Calendula* gel; •Chinese WHITE FLOWER OIL; •Vitamin E 400IU, take internally; prick capsule and apply locally; •Vitamin A & D 25,000IU, take internally; prick capsule and apply locally.

Can't find a recommended product? Call the 800 number listed in Product Resources for the store nearest you.

Spinal Meningitis
Encephalitis

Meningitis is an infectious, viral disease that causes inflammation of nerves, spine and brain tissue. It is characterized by deficient blood supply to these areas and thus deprives the brain of oxygen. Children are especially at risk for permanent brain damage or paralysis. Coma or death may ensue if prompt treatment is not undertaken. Medical treatment has been successful for meningitis if received early. Unfortunately the *meningoccocus* microbe is becoming resistant to antibiotics. *Encephalitis* is a rarer form of the infection, with many of the same symptoms. *Acute bacterial meningitis* can be rapidly fatal, especially for infants or the elderly. Get emergency help right away for acute symptoms. Be aware that the new popular pain killing drug, Vioxx, has been linked to rare but serious cases of non-bacterial meningitis. **Do you have early signs of meningitis?** Many signs look like other illness. Oxygen deprivation means lethargy, slow thought and movement. There may be chronic cold symptoms - a sore throat, stiff neck, nausea and fever, severe headaches and light sensitivity, as well as a dark red skin rash. (Infants also have a bulging soft spot on the skull.) Emergency symptoms include stupor, coma (change in temperature and sleep patterns may precede a coma), and convulsions with acute inflammation of the brain and spinal cord. **What causes meningitis?** A wide array of viruses, possibly insect-borne. Dehydration, heavy metal or chemical poisoning are often involved.

Diet and Lifestyle Support Therapy

Nutritional therapy: *Nutritional therapies increase healing rate substantially.*

1—There must be diet and lifestyle upgrade for permanent improvement.

2—During healing, a 24 hour liquid diet (pg. 173) should be used one day a week to keep the body flushed and alkaline.

3—The diet should be 50-75% fresh foods and vegetable juices, with fresh carrot juice or •Green Foods CARROT ESSENCE drink, and a potassium broth (pg. 291) or veggie drink like •Crystal Star RESTORE YOUR STRENGTH™, or for kids, •Omega Nutrition ESSENTIAL BALANCE JR.2 twice a week.

4—Add cultured foods, like yogurt and kefir, for friendly G.I. flora establishment.

5—Drink only healthy liquids, 8 glasses daily; take 1 to 2 electrolyte drinks daily, like Natures Path TRACE LYTE, or •Alacer EMERGEN-C and ELECTROMIX (highly recommended). Other effective drinks: •C'est Si Bon CHLORENERGY, and •Nutricology PROGREENS w. flax oil EFAs.

6—Reduce mucous-forming foods, like dairy foods, red meats, caffeine-containing and refined foods. No sugar, fried, or junk foods at all.

—**Bodywork:** *Steroid drugs over a long period of time for meningitis weaken both bone structure and immunity.*

•Immerse back of the head in warm epsom salts solution several times daily to draw out inflammation.

•Alternate hot and cold packs on the neck and back of the head to stimulate circulation to the area.

•Use catnip enemas to reduce fever, during acute phase and to clear body quickly of infection.

•Avoid aluminum cookware, deodorants, and other alum containing products.

•Get some fresh air and early morning sunshine every day.

•Get plenty of rest during healing.

Herbal, Superfood and Supplement Therapy

Interceptive therapy: Choose 2 to 3 recommendations.

1—**Reduce infection and help overcome the virus:** •Crystal Star ANTI-BIO™ extract with anti-viral support to control infection. •ECHINACEA extract 3 to 4x daily to help flush lymph glands and fight infection. •Ester C powder with bioflavonoids, ¼ tsp. •Vitamin C powder with bioflavonoids, ¼ tsp. •Vitamin A & D 10,000IU/400IU for children as soon as rash appears. —**For encephalitis:** •Homeopathic *Belladonna* 200c, and •Alacer EMERGEN-C electrolyte replacement. •ROYAL JELLY or Long Life IMPERIAL TONIC (Royal Jelly + EPO), or •Prince of Peace GINSENG-ROYAL JELLY vials. •Germanium 150mg, in divided doses. •Enzymatic Therapy VIRAPLEX 4 daily to address the virus.

2—**Reduce inflammation:** •Crystal Star DR. ENZYME™ with protease and bromelain, or •Quercetin 1000mg with bromelain 1500mg with meals, or •Nature's Plus QUERCETIN with Vitamin C and bromelain. •Enzymedica PURIFY; •Fresh comfrey leaf tea 5 cups daily. •Crystal Star ANTI-FLAM™ caps 2-4 at a time.

3—**EFA's help normalize brain and nerve health:** •Health from the Sun TOTAL EFA; Evening Primrose oil or •Nature's Secret ULTIMATE OIL caps 4 daily; •High omega-3 flax oil 3 tsp. daily; •Kelp tabs 6-8 daily. —**For nerve support:** •Gotu Kola caps 4 daily; •*Scullcap* tea daily; •Herbs Etc. NERVINE TONIC; •Lobelia drops in water (OK for kids).

4—**Enhance immune response with antioxidants:** •Enzymatic Therapy THYMUPLEX caps; •KYOLIC Aged Garlic Extract 6 to 8 capsules daily; •Nutricology THYMUS ORGANIC GLANDULAR; •Royal Bodycare MICROHYDRIN PLUS; •PCO's from grapeseed or white pine 50mg 3x daily; •Solgar OCEANIC carotene 50,000IU; •Chondroitin up to 1200mg for degeneration. •Zinc lozenges 1 to 2 daily.

5—**Nourish brain tissue and increase blood flow to the brain:** •Phosphatidyl choline (Twin Lab PC 55); •B Complex 50mg, with extra B₆ 100mg, and •Solaray B₁₂ 2000mcg daily. •Anabol Naturals AMINO BALANCE for tissue repair. •Golden Pride FORMULA ONE oral chelation with EDTA; •Niacin therapy: 100-500mg daily. (If a child, use no flush niacin; if adult, use a baby aspirin first to avoid niacin flush.)

Can't find a recommended product? Call the 800 number listed in Product Resources for the store nearest you.

Sports Injuries

Torn Ligaments, Sprains, Muscle Pain, Tendonitis

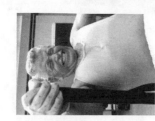

A *strain* or *pulled muscle* is any damage to the tendon that anchors the muscle. A *sprain* is caused by a twisting motion that tears the ligaments that bind up the joints. It takes much longer to heal than a strain. *Tendonitis* is the painful inflammation of a tendon, usually resulting from a strain, and developing as a dull, dragging sensation after exercise. You can help yourself prevent sports injures. Start your workout slowly; warm your body up at least 2 degrees before you start pushing yourself; end your workout with a cool down period to prevent lactic acid build-up. Experts agree: The first three days after an injury are the most critical for rapid healing. Acupuncture and acupressure, massage therapy and shiatsu all help. **Do you suffer from a sports injury?** Most common are muscle pulls, wrenched knees, twisted ankles, sprained wrists, shin splints, tennis elbows and torn ligaments. Arthritis-like, painful joints and nerve endings dominate with tendon inflammation, shooting ankle, foot and knee pains. Cramping and soreness follow muscle exertion with limited range of motion and leg cramps at night. **What puts you most at risk for injury?** Conditions like minerals deficiencies - especially calcium and magnesium; a poor diet, low in green vegetables and whole grains, high in fried foods, fats and sugars; poor circulation. *See ATHLETES' NEEDS page 254 and MUSCLE CRAMPS page 502 for more information.*

Diet and Lifestyle Support Therapy

Nutritional therapy plan:

1—A good diet helps you avoid injuries. During healing eat about 50% fresh foods. Add vegetable proteins for faster healing. Muscles need complex carbs from green foods to heal. Add a green drink like •Green Kamut JUST BARLEY, •Crystal Star ENERGY GREEN RENEWAL™, •Green Foods MAGMA PLUS™, or •Nutricology PRO-GREENS with EFA's.

2—Eat chromium-rich foods - lobster, low fat cheeses, nutritional yeast.

3—Eat silicon-rich foods - rice, oats, green grasses and leafy greens.

4—Drink electrolyte replacements: Knudsens RECHARGE, Nature's Path TRACE LYTE, Alacer ELECTRO-MIX powder (highly recommended). Drink extra water and fluids.

5—Eat magnesium-rich foods - whole grains, nuts, beans, squashes for muscles.

6—Eat high vitamin C/bioflavonoid foods - a drink of lemon juice/honey/water at night, grapefruit or pineapple juice each morning. Add •New Chapter GINGER WONDER SYRUP to reduce swelling. Or try •Jarrow GENTLE FIBERS with bioflavs.

7—Avoid foods like red meats, sugars, caffeine, carbonated drinks during healing.

8—Antioxidant bars have a place in injury prevention, especially as a source of MCT's.

Check out your natural food store for healthy ones.

—Bodywork:

•Elevate the injured area; apply ice packs immediately. Leave on for 30 minutes. Remove for 15 minutes. Repeat process for 3 hours to decrease internal bleeding from injured vessels. Wrap sprains with an ACE bandage (over the ice if necessary) to limit swelling. Apply alternating hot and cold packs the next day for circulation, to take down swelling and relax cramps. Elevate legs and slap them hard with open palms to stimulate circulation. •Massage affected areas frequently. Add a few drops of peppermint oil and lavender to reduce pain and muscle stress.

—Healing applications for injuries:

•BHI TRAUMEEL (highly recommended). •Nature's Way CAYENNE PAIN RELIEVING ointment. •DMSO liquid roll-on.

Herbal, Superfood and Supplement Therapy

Interceptive therapy plan: Choose 2 to 3 recommendations.

1—Reduce trauma; reconstruct cartilage: •Glucosamine 1500mg-Chondroitin 1200mg (alternative to NSAIDS drugs); •Crystal Star MUSCLE RELAXER™ or •STRESS OUT™ extract for pain (very fast acting). •Flora VEGE-SIL caps for collagen regrowth.

2—Reduce inflammation, swelling: •St. John's Wort oil; •New Chapter ZYFLAMEND, COX-2 Inhibitor; •Nature's Answer SEACENTIALS GOLD for lactic acid build-up; •Peppermint oil (rapid action); •Country Life LIGATEND (recommended).

3—Enzyme therapy heals soft tissue: •Crystal Star DR. ENZYME™ with protease and bromelain; •Enzymedica PURIFY protease; ginger extract (New Chapter DAILY GINGER) a protease component. •quercetin 1000mg and bromelain 1500mg (Nature's Plus); •Biotec CELL GUARD, 6 daily; *Boswellia serrata* 1200mg.

4—Speed recovery: •Creatine 1000mg for muscles and joint injuries; •New Chapter ZYFLAMEND (highly recommended); •Esteem SUPER PRO with DMG. •Chromium picolinate 200mcg daily; •Vitamin C crystals with bioflavs, ½ tsp. in water, or •Alacer EMERGEN-C every hour for collagen and connective tissue healing.

—Healing topicals: •Earth's Bounty O₂ spray; •TIGER BALM analgesic rub; •Tea tree oil; •Miracle of Aloe MIRACLE FOOT REPAIR for cracked feet. •Hot salt pack: Heat 1 lb. salt in a heavy pan. Pour in a heavy cotton sock, about ¾ full. Place on painful area for 30 minutes. (Remarkable). •Wakunaga GLUCOSAMINE SOOTHING cream for joints. •Nature's Apothecary HERBAL FIRST AID oil.

5—For muscle pulls, leg cramps: •Arnica Montana; •Biochemics PAIN RELIEF lotion; •Magnesium 800mg daily or Flora MAGNESIUM liquid; •Stress-B-complex 100mg daily with extra B-6 250mg. •*Kava kava* relaxes muscles; •Siberian eleuthero extract for lactic acid build-up. •Ho-shou-wu for ligament, nerve healing.

6—Homeopathic sports remedies: •Arnica for dislocations, sprains, bruises; •Bryonia alba for red, swollen joints; •Ruta Graveolens for pulled tendons; •Hypericum for damaged nerves; •Rhus Tox. for swelling; Boiron Sportenine for tendonitis; •Silicea for torn ligaments; •Bellis Perennis for repetitive strains; •Hylands Arnicaid.

Can't find a recommended product? Call the 800 number listed in Product Resources for the store nearest you.

Strep Throat

Sore Throat, Swollen Glands, Laryngitis, Hoarseness

Here are the differences between **strep throat** and *sore throat irritation* from a cold: Onset of strep throat is rapid; a cold is slow. Throat is very sore with strep throat, not so sore with a cold. You have a fever and aches with strep throat; mild achiness with a cold. You have swollen, tender lymph nodes with strep throat; not with a cold. There are usually complications with strep throat, like streptococcal pneumonia or middle ear infections; sinusitis with a cold. Antibiotics work for strep throat, not usually for a cold. *Hoarseness,* the result of inflammation of the vocal chords, is typically the result of a virus, or extensive yelling. *Laryngitis,* raspy, breathy voice, is often due to voice fatigue from a cold. **Do you have strep throat?** Putting the signs together…. look for a sore, aching, inflamed, throat and tonsils. Talking is difficult…. most people can't speak above a whisper because of swollen throat tissues. A simple medical test confirms diagnosis. **What causes strep throat?** A viral or strep infection (if chronic, it may be mononucleosis), recurring tonsillitis (even in adults), the beginnings of a cold or flu. Strep infection is far more common among smokers, for those under stress (adrenal exhaustion), and for people who eat a lot of clogging dairy foods that form harboring mucous. *See Colds & Flu, and Viral, Staph and Bacterial Infection pages for more information.*

Diet and Lifestyle Support Therapy

Nutritional therapy plan:

1—Go on a 24 hr. liquid cleansing diet (pg. 173), or a 3 day mucous cleansing diet (pg. 202). Soak 1 chopped garlic bulb and 1 small chopped onion in 1 pt. honey and water overnight; take 1 tsp. every hour. Take grapefruit or cranberry juice throughout the day.

2—Take lemon juice and honey in hot water with a pinch of cayenne pepper each morning, and a potassium broth (pg. 291) daily. Eat plenty of leafy greens. Eat plenty of plain yogurt. Take Red Star NUTRITIONAL YEAST or miso broth at night before retiring. Cook with a piece of astragalus bark for extra immune support.

3—To keep strep throat away, avoid dairy foods, sugary, fried and fatty foods. Add AloeLife ALOE GOLD juice, or Crystal Star DR. VITALITY™ green and white tea to your morning regimen.

—**Effective gargles remove excess phlegm:** (about every ½ hr.): 1) Lemon juice and brandy; 2) black tea; 3) liquid chlorophyll ½ tsp. in water with pinches of cayenne; 4) lemon juice and sea salt in water. 5) cider vinegar and honey in water every hour until relief. 6) *Goldenseal/myrrh* solution or *Myrrh* tincture, ½ tsp. in water. Or try •New Chapter GINGER WONDER syrup - use as a gargle.

—**Throat applications:** 1) Hot ginger compresses. 2) Eucalyptus steams. 3) Color therapy glasses: wear blue. 4) Hot parsley compresses on the throat. 5) Drip black walnut extract in throat. 6) *White oak bark tea.*

—**For laryngitis and hoarseness:** 1) Apply *ginger/cayenne* compresses to throat. 2) Spray *ginseng-licorice* extract in throat. 3) Take a steamy mineral or epsom salts bath. 4) Hum a little, don't whisper to reduce swelling.

—**Bodywork:**
• Take hot 20 minute saunas daily.
• Stick tongue out as far as it will go. Hold for 30 seconds. Release and relax. Repeat 3 times to increase blood supply to the area.
• Take a catnip enema to cleanse infection from a strep throat.

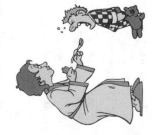

Herbal, Superfood and Supplement Therapy

Interceptive therapy plan: Choose 2 to 3 recommendations.

1—**Control the infection:** •Crystal Star ANTI-BIO™ extract every hour, and •ECHINACEA extract to flush lymph glands for at least 7 days. •Add *elder-boneset-ginger-cayenne* tea to help induce a cleansing sweat; •Immudyne MACROFORCE with beta glucan for an immune boost; •Enzymatic Therapy ESPERITOX chewables and VIRAPLEX caps as directed. •Merix C & F caps for swollen glands (good results); •Lane Labs BENE-FIN SHARK CARTILAGE caps as directed. •Nutribiotic GRAPEFRUIT SEED extract in water, or capsules for infection. •Colloidal silver drops as needed for a week, or •Eidon IMMUNE SUPPORT liquid; •Garlic capsules 8 daily or •Wakunaga AGED GARLIC EXTRACT. •Pure Essence Labs FLORALIVE or American Health ACIDOPHILUS liquid.

2—**Reduce inflammation:** •Crystal Star DR. ENZYME™ with protease and bromelain; •Alacer EMERGEN-C every few hours (very good results). Hold in the mouth as long as possible and take •Vitamin C chewable 500mg every hour during acute stages.

—**For chronic low-grade strep infection:** •Crystal Star ZINC SOURCE™ throat rescue drops (apply directly on throat); take •Enzymatic Therapy THYMU-PLEX caps with vitamin C 5000mg daily, and •Lysine 500mg; add •Zinc lozenges as needed.

3—**Soothe the throat tissues:** •*Ginseng-licorice* extract in water as needed (good results), or •*thyme* tea as needed; •Hylands SORE THROAT and C PLUS tabs; •*Chamomile* tea; •Bladderwrack gargle to help coat irritated throat membranes.

—**Good lozenges:** •Herbon Naturals ECHINACEA THROAT DROPS; •Zand HERBAL INSURE lozenges; •Zinc gluconate or •propolis lozenges every 2 hours as needed; •Olbas lozenges; •Thayers ROSE HIPS AND C, or •Wild cherry lozenges.

4—**Remove congestion:** •Crystal Star D-CONGEST™ fast relief spray; •Zand DE-CONGEST HERBAL; •Yogi BREATHE DEEP tea; Salt-sage gargle: make 2 cups sage leaf tea; strain, and add 1 tsp. sea salt.

—**For laryngitis and hoarseness:** •Licorice root; •Alacer EMERGEN-C. •Beehive Botanical PROPOLIS throat spray; •Gargle tea tree oil, 3 drops in water.

Can't find a recommended product? Call the 800 number listed in Product Resources for the store nearest you.

Stress

Tension, Nerves, Anxiety, Low Energy

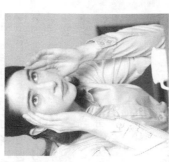

Are you stressed out? Is your energy at all-time low? Over 20 million Americans suffer from health problems linked to chronic stress. New statistics show that up to 95 percent of visits to health care professionals are stress-related. Everyone is affected by varying degrees of stress.... people who work in polluted atmospheres, people at control desks with machines or instruments demanding continual attention, people who travel coast to coast constantly, people with mundane, boring jobs, etc. At best, stress causes useless fatigue; at worst, it is dangerous to health. Profound stress, such as that caused by job loss or the loss of a loved one takes a serious physical toll. Medical experts agree. The more "stressed out" you become, the more vulnerable you are to colds, flu, ulcers, allergies, even heart attacks and high blood pressure. Stress especially drains our energy, targeting organs like the adrenal glands and wiping out their stores. Long term stress invariably leads to severe fatigue from adrenal exhaustion, and regularly results in depression. Stress shows up in how you look, too. Blemishes may appear around the chin; nails become brittle and peel, hair is dull and lifeless. Stress can even make your hair fall out!

Not all stress is bad. It can be a motivating factor in our lives. The human body is designed to handle stressful situations, even to thrive on some of them. You can never avoid all stress, but you can maintain a high degree of health to handle and survive stress well.

What puts you at greatest risk for serious stress? Emotional problems, job pressure and money worries appear at the top of most stress lists, coupled with lack of rest, and aggravated by the overuse of drugs, tobacco, caffeine or alcohol, our most common stress "relievers." Physical stress triggers? Allergies, hypoglycemia, mineral depletion, environmental pollutants, all leading to adrenal dysfunction figure in.

What's your stress level? **There are four levels of stress symptoms:**

1) losing interest in everything, eye-corner sagging, forehead creasing, becoming short-tempered, bored, nervous;

2) tiredness, anger, insomnia, paranoia, sadness;

3) chronic head and neck aches, high blood pressure, upset stomach, looking older;

4) skin disorders, kidney malfunction, frequent infections, heart disease, nervous breakdown, unexplained weight gain around the waist and stomach.

Do something about your stress. **Deep breathing relieves and rejuvenates:**

Deep breathing activates relaxation centers in the brain, reducing overall body stress and increasing creative mental energy. When you're tense, your breathing is shallow. When you're emotionally distressed, your oxygen levels decrease. When you're angry or fearful, your breathing rate increases (normal breathing is about 16 times per minute). When body fluid and congestion build up, immunity suffers because breathing affects the circulation of lymph. Breathing is controlled by two sets of nerves — the involuntary (autonomic) nervous system, and the voluntary nervous system. Breathing enhances the autonomic nervous system and many of its involuntary functions.

Use your breathing as a stress release meditation:

1: Shift your focus away from your racing mind and stressed emotions. There is a basic connection between your breath and your state of mind. Sit quietly and focus on your breath.

2: Consciously take slow, deep, and regular breaths... your mind will become more calm.

3: Recall a pleasant past experience. Feel appreciation about the good things and people you have in your life. Shifting your focus to positive feelings helps neutralize the stress.

Breath and Body Stretch:

1: Stand tall and raise your hands above your head. Stretch your arms and fingers as if you are reaching for the sky — pretend you are trying to climb up with your hands and arms. As you reach, inhale deeply through your nostrils while rising on your toes.

2: Exhale slowly, and gradually return to the starting position, with your arms hanging loosely at your side. Repeat this at least 5 times. This is a great warm-up to a brisk walk.

Filling a Balloon:

1: Breathe in through the nose and imagine that the in-coming breath is filling a balloon in your belly, then continues up your torso and fills your entire upper body with air.

2: After you are completely filled up with air, exhale, let go and feel the balloon emptying. Do a few of these deep breaths. Relaxation is just a breath away.

Can't find a recommended product? Call the 800 number listed in Product Resources for the store nearest you.

Stress

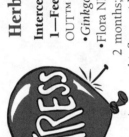

Diet and Lifestyle Support Therapy

Nutritional therapy plan: *Good nutrition is a good answer to stress.*

1—As stress increases, protein needs increase. Protein and mineral-rich foods are the best choice. Vegetable proteins from whole grains, sea greens, sea and soy foods, eggs and sprouts offer notable results.

2—Have fresh carrot juice and fresh fish or seafood at least once a week. Add magnesium-rich foods from green vegetables and whole grains. Add more potassium-rich foods like potatoes, salmon, bananas, seafood and avocados to your diet. Potassium helps reduce stress-related high blood pressure, and regulates blood sugar. Intake should be about 3 to 5 grams daily. Cut down on high sodium foods which dehydrate the body.

3—Eat B vitamin-rich foods like brown rice and other whole grains. Avoid trans fats from fried foods, red meats and highly processed foods for adrenal health. These foods are high in chemicals that overburden the body's elimination systems. Add bee pollen and royal jelly for body-balancing B's; •CC Pollen DYNAMIC TRIO or •Prince of Peace GINSENG-ROYAL JELLY vials.

4—Reduce caffeine intake. Drink green tea or Crystal Star DR. VITALITY™ green and white blend each morning instead for energy and antioxidants.

5—Take a glass of wine before dinner. No liquids with meals. Drink bottled water.

6—Make an anti-stress mix of brewer's yeast, toasted wheat germ, sunflower seeds, molasses, flax oil; take 2 tbsp. daily in food. Take miso soup before bed to relax.

7—Feed your adrenals with foods like sea greens, like Crystal Star RESTORE YOUR STRENGTH™ drink and green drinks, like Esteem GREEN HARVEST.

—Watchwords:

• You have to unwind before you can unleash. Work addiction is the health hazard of our time. Take a break to….. strengthen family and friendship ties; celebrate your life's rituals; build a good diet, adequate rest and exercise into your life; develop creative pastimes (not computer games); delegate at least some responsibilities; live for today.

• Take a rest and relaxation period every day. Listen to soft music. Meditate. Do 3 minutes of neck rolls.

• Have a good laugh every day.

—Stress reduction / relaxation techniques:

• Massage therapy once a month, especially cranial sacral therapy (highly recommended). Hypnotherapy, aromatherapy, and shiatsu have all shown effective results against stress.

• Quiet your mind with deep, rhythmic deep breathing exercises every day.

• Get regular exercise for tissue oxygen. Walk your dog.

• Don't smoke. Nicotine constricts the blood vessels, causing increased stress.

• Go on a short vacation. Take a long weekend. It will do wonders for your head.

Herbal, Superfood and Supplement Therapy

Interceptive therapy plan: Choose 2 to 3 recommendations.

1—Feed your nerves: •Crystal Star RELAX CAPS™ - nerve repair, or •STRESS OUT™ extract as needed; •*Gotu kola* or *Ginseng/gotu kola* caps - nerve support; •*Ginkgo Biloba* extract - a feeling of well-being. •Herbs Etc. NERVINE TONIC; •Flora NERVE GUARD drops; Country Life sublingual B-12, 2500mcg daily for 2 months; •5-HTP 50-100mg daily before bed for 2 months. •Vitamin C with bioflavonoids, 3000mg daily. •B complex 150mg with extra B-6 250mg daily. •Stress B Complex 100mg 2-3x daily, with extra B-6 250mg and pantothenic acid 1500mg; •Niacinamide for valium-like activity.

2—Feed your adrenals: •Crystal Star ADRENAL ENERGY BOOST™ caps; •*Licorice* root extract, or •*Ginseng/Licorice* drops; or •Planetary SCHIZANDRA ADRENAL support; •Country Life RELAXER tabs for fast relief •Nutricology PRO-GREENS with EFAs.

3—Amino acids boost your brain energy: •SAMe 400mg daily (important in synthesizing brain chemicals); •Glutamine 1000mg daily; •Country Life MOOD FACTORS capsules, or •Anabol Naturals AMINO BALANCE; Tyrosine 500mg; •DLPA 1000mg as needed; •GABA 1000mg mimics valium without sedation.

4—Stabilizing minerals: •Crystal Star STRESS ARREST™ tea or •CALCIUM MAGNESIUM SOURCE™ caps. •Magnesium 1200mg daily, or •Lane Labs ADVACAL ULTRA with high magnesium. •Nature's Path TRACE-LYTE with sea greens for electrolytes.

5—Fight depression with essential fatty acids: •New Chapter SUPERCRITICAL DHA; •Evening Primrose oil 2000mg 2x daily; Barleans high lignan omega-3 flax oil 2 tbsp. daily; or •Udo's PEFECTED OIL BLEND; •Phosphatidylserine 200-300mg daily to help the brain manage stress.

6—Adaptogens strengthen resistance to stress: •*Siberian eleuthero* extract, *rhodiola rosea* (excellent results), astragalus or schizandra extracts have fast results; or try •Crystal Star FEEL GREAT NOW™ with Siberian eleuthero, jiaogulan, bee pollen, Fo Ti; •Una da gato to increase immune response for 2 months. •Homeopathic *Nux Vomica* tabs, excellent for stress-related indigestion and diarrhea.

7—Calm your mind: •Bach RESCUE REMEDY drops; •Liddell FEELING OVERWHELMED homeopathic drops; •Prime Advantage VITAL STRESSX (recommended). •Rub St. John's wort oil on the temples. •*Kava Kava* extract or •Herb Pharm PHARMA-KAVA drops; •Pure Essence 4 WAY STRESS SUPPORT.

8—Fight fatigue with antioxidants: •CoQ10, 100mg 4x daily, and •Alpha Lipoic Acid 600mg daily, increase ATP chemical energy. •Royal Bodycare MICROHYDRIN PLUS; •NADH 5 to 10mg if you're tired all the time. •Ascorbate vitamin C with bioflavonoids, 500mg every 4 hours during acute periods, or take •Alacer EMERGEN-C; •Premiere Labs GERMANIUM with DMG.

Can't find a recommended product? Call the 800 number listed in Product Resources for the store nearest you.

Taste and Smell Loss

Deviated Septum

Do you have trouble smelling odors or tasting foods? Around 6 million Americans suffer from taste and smell loss. It's a desensitization problem, perhaps becoming bigger than might appear at first glance.... affecting our weight, and our ability to tell what foods are good for us (an ancient, innate sense). Affecting all ages, causes extend from a deviated septum, to a temporary response to common drugs people take for colds and flu, to damaged nerve endings from arthritis or osteoporosis. Other than surgery for a deviated septum, modern medicine has not tackled the problem, largely because of its amorphous, tangential nature. (The food industry, however is well aware of its importance and has intensified the smell and taste of many products artificially to deal with it (which may unintentionally, desensitize even more). Natural healing methods focus on overcoming nutritional deficiencies first in order to deal with the root causes. Aromatherapy is gaining importance for taste and smell problems because what we call "taste" (as much as 90%) is actually smell. In most cases, if total atrophy has not developed, at least partial taste and smell can be restored. **Besides mechanical reasons, like atrophied nerve ending and a deviated septum, what reduces our taste and smell?** Zinc depletion, today a result of too many antibiotics, causing zinc excretion. Gland imbalances, especially thyroid depletion. A chronic low grade throat and sinus infection with post-nasal drip. A common side effect of chemotherapy, some high blood pressure medicines, some over-the-counter cold medicines, and certain diuretic drugs.

Diet and Lifestyle Support Therapy

Nutritional therapy plan:

1—A mineral-rich, low fat, low salt diet is a key. Keep your diet free of mucous-clogging foods, like heavy starches, red meats and dairy foods.

2—Add plenty of fresh, crunchy, high texture foods like celery and apples. Have a fresh green salad every day. Have green tea every morning, or Crystal Star DR. VITALITY™ green and white tea blend, to clear mucous clogs.

3—Eat zinc-rich foods: seafoods and fish, and sea greens snipped over your salads, rice, pizza, soups. Or add Pure Planet 100% PURE SPIRULINA (spirulina is one of the most highly absorbable zinc sources in the natural world).

4—Boost minerals and B-vitamins: Have some brown rice, miso soup, whole grains and green leafy vegetables, and sea greens every day for at least 3 months. Try Crystal Star RESTORE YOUR STRENGTH™ drink with sea veggies, or Nutricology PRO-GREENS with EFAs for at least 3 months.

5—Make sure the diet is low in salt and refined sugars. Use herbal salt-free seasonings.

6—**Think green!** For people who may have become desensitized by chemicalized foods, chlorophyll can help re-establish taste and smell pathways. Add Liquid chlorophyll, 1 tsp. before meals in water. Green drinks like C'est Si Bon CHLORENERGY or Green Kamut JUST BARLEY can sometimes do wonders. Use them for at least 3 months to see results. Other green drinks to try Crystal Star ENERGY GREEN RENEWAL™ caps; •Nature's Secret ULTIMATE GREEN; •Pines MIGHTY GREENS caps; •Solaray ALFAJUICE caps.

—Bodywork:

•Use a catnip or chlorophyll enema to cleanse clogging mucous.
•Regular exercise with deep diaphragmatic breathing to keep passages clear (see page 250).

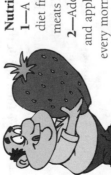

Herbal, Superfood and Supplement Therapy

Interceptive therapy plan: Choose 2 to 3 recommendations.

1—**Boost minerals to enhance your sense of smell:** •Magnesium 1200mg daily; •Zinc up to 100mg daily. Most people with sensory, especially taste, loss have a zinc depletion. Check for deficiency with Ethical Nutrients ZINC STATUS liquid (also as a supplement); •Crystal Star OCEAN MINERALS™ caps 4 daily, for natural foundation minerals; •Flora CALCIUM-MAGNESIUM-ZINC liquid; •*Fenugreek tea*, a specific 2 cups daily.

2—**Boost your circulation:** •GINKGO BILOBA extract 4x daily, a primary sensory aid. Add •Country Life sublingual B-12, 2500mg daily (acts on taste), with B-complex 100mg daily, and extra B_6 100mg and flush-free niacin 100mg for best results. •*Cayenne* caps or *ginger-cayenne* caps; •*Rosemary* aromatherapy applied on the temples; •*Gotu kola* caps 6 daily for better nerve ending activity (makes a noticeable difference).

3—**Enhance your thyroid activity:** Add •sea veggies, 2 tbsp. chopped dry, daily over soup, salad or rice (or 6 pieces of sushi a day); •Crystal Star IODINE, POTASSIUM, SILICA drops; •Solgar OCEANIC BETA CAROTENE up to 100,000IU daily, or •PHYCOTENE MICROCLUSTERS mixed carotenes available from Royal Bodycare. •Take Kelp tabs 8 daily for 3 months or Green Foods IONKELP tabs; •New Chapter OCEAN HERBS, or •Nature's Path TRACE-LYTE with sea greens, 2 daily; or •Arise & Shine LIQUID ORGANIC SEA MINERALS; •Ester C 550mg with bioflavonoids 4-6 daily.

4—**Boost your neurotransmitters:** •phosphatidylcholine 3000mg, •GABA 1000mg or Choline 600mg. (If your choline levels are low, try Huperzine A 50mg to allow levels to rise.) •Take ¼ tsp. each: Glutamine powder and Glycine powder; or Glutamine 1000mg 2 daily, •Evening primrose oil 2-4 daily.

5—**Herbal adaptogens like ginseng help normalize body systems:** •Imperial Elixir Siberian eleuthero and royal jelly capsules 3-4 daily; or •Siberian eleuthero extract capsules 2 daily; or •Crystal Star FEEL GREAT NOW™ with several ginsengs. •Prince of Peace GINSENG-ROYAL JELLY vials. •Beehive Botanicals PROPOLIS & HERB spray under the tongue 3-4x daily (works well, very convenient).

Can't find a recommended product? Call the 800 number listed in Product Resources for the store nearest you.

Teething

Children's Tooth and Mouth Pain

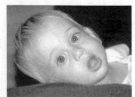

Although it may seem like an ailment to every parent who soothes a fussy child on numerous sleepless nights, teething is a natural process of the first baby teeth breaking through the gums. Normally beginning around the seventh or eighth month, a baby will add another tooth about every month, until the complete set of 20 teeth comes in - usually around thirty months. Pain from teething can be minimized with natural methods. Gentle herbs have been used for centuries to help children over this rough growing patch in their lives. (Teething is also a natural reminder to Moms that it's time to wean the child from breast feeding.) Many of the same remedies apply for wisdom teeth breakthrough in later years (see page 389).

Is your child teething? Check for sore, inflamed gums where teeth are pushing through the skin. There's often slight fever and infection in the process. The child will whimper or cry from irritability and the discomfort, and usually has trouble sleeping. Most babies drool more than usual, so they have red, chapped cheeks and chin from it. The child will want to chew or suck on anything and everything to relieve the inflammation. Watch out for any periodic diarrhea, skin rashes, runny nose and loss of appetite which might indicate infection beyond just teething. *See also Children's special section page 224-236.*

Diet and Lifestyle Support Therapy

Nutritional therapy plan:

1—Include vitamin A-rich vegetables, vitamin D-rich eggs, fish and sea greens and high bioflavonoid foods in the child's diet.

2—Feed plenty of chilled foods; fresh fruits, yogurt, etc. to relieve discomfort. Give a dilute solution of Jarrow GENTLE FIBERS drink several times a week to balance gastric upset.

3—Give lots of cool water daily. Can mix with aloe vera juice. Apply •aloe vera gel to gums as needed.

—**Chilled food chews:**

Cold, hard cookies or bagels or Earth's Best TEETHING BISCUITS.
Let child chew on chunks of frozen banana or cold raw carrot sticks.
Give a teething ring that has been kept in the fridge.

—**Effective food applications on gums:**

•Try New Chapter GINGER WONDER syrup. Put a few drops in juice and rub on gums with a cotton swab (very effective).

•Massage child's gums lightly with a little honey or propolis, like Beehive Botanical PROPOLIS & HERB SPRAY, recommended.

•Make a weak tea tree oil solution with water, and rub on gums for swelling or infection.

•Garlic oil rub if there is infection.

•Sea salt and honey mix.

•Dilute wine or brandy if there is swelling.

—**Bodywork:**

•Let the child play in the sun for 15 to 20 minutes every morning for full-spectrum vitamins - especially sunlight vitamin D.

Herbal, Superfood and Supplement Therapy

Interceptive therapy plan: Choose 2 to 3 recommendations.

1—**Reduce infection and inflammation:** Make a weak •goldenseal and honey solution with water. Give with an eye dropper on back of the tongue. Rub on gums as an anti-infective; •Myrrh extract drops; or •Bilberry extract, or •Gaia Herbs BILBERRY alcohol free extract, an anti-inflammatory; •Ascorbate vitamin C powder with bioflavonoids - a weak solution in water. Give internally and apply to gums every few hours. •UAS DDS-JUNIOR with FOS (open up capsule and swab teeth, gums and throat).

—**Effective rub-ons:** •Noveya BABY TEETHING GEL; •Herbs for Kids GUM-OMILE OIL or *Licorice root* extract; or let the child chew on natural licorice sticks. •*Lobelia* extract or •Peppermint oil - use only a drop or two of these extracts or oil; blend the oils with a few drops of flax oil to dilute; blend the extracts with a little water. •Clove oil is especially good (for cutting wisdom teeth, too); •Soak yarrow flowers in bran and water for 3 days. Strain and rub on gums.

2—**Soothe pain naturally:** Make weak teas of any of the following herbs: give internally and pat on with a soft cloth. •*Slippery elm*; •*Chamomile*; •*Raspberry*; •*Catnip*; •*Peppermint*; •*Fennel seed*.

3—**Give minerals for stronger teeth:** •Mezotrace CHEWABLE MINERAL complex. (Break in half or dissolve in juice.)

4—**Homeopathic remedies are a good, fast-working choice:** •Hylands TEETHING tabs and gel; •Boiron Camilia gel; •Calcarea carbonica; •Chamomilla; •Hyland's Calc.-Phos. tabs (dissolve in juice); rub •Plantago Majus tincture on tender gums.

Can't find a recommended product? Call the 800 number listed in Product Resources for the store nearest you.

Tinnitus

Ringing in the Ears, Meniere's Syndrome, Inner Ear Malfunction, Vertigo

Over 50 million Americans suffer from tinnitus... 80% of people with hearing problems have it. *Tinnitus* means "ringing in the ears." It starts as a low ringing, like the humming of a transformer, eventually becomes permanent and robs you of sleep every night. *Meniere's syndrome* is a recurring, progressive set of symptoms that include ringing and pressure in the ears with some hearing loss and dizziness. *Vertigo* is a result of equilibrium (inner ear) disturbance with the sensation of moving around, or of having objects move around you. It occurs when your brain and central nervous system get conflicting messages from the body sensors that maintain balance - ears, eyes and skin pressure receptors (the feeling you get on a boat in choppy waters). Vertigo starts with ear pain, ringing, pressure, a feeling of unsteady, lightheadedness upon standing quickly, sometimes hearing loss. **What causes tinnitus?** Chronic ear infection or wax build-up, unrelenting loud noise or music, ear bone softening (possible prelude to osteoporosis), too much aspirin, and TMJ disorder are all implicated. **How about vertigo?** Poor circulation, blood pressure imbalance, lack of brain oxygen or brain tumors, chemical allergies, neurological disease, hypoglycemia, B vitamin deficiency, drug reaction to antihistamines, steroids, antidepressants, anti-seizure drugs, cephalosporin antibiotics, pain killers or the artificial sweetener, aspartame. *See TMJ page 389 and MOTION SICKNESS page 400 for more.*

Diet and Lifestyle Support Therapy

Nutritional therapy plan: Natural therapies have been successful.

1—Attain ideal body weight for better body balance. The diet should be low in saturated fats and cholesterol, high in vegetable proteins and B vitamin foods - brown rice, broccoli, tofu, seafoods, and sprouts. Boost circulation with New Chapter GINGER WONDER syrup- 1 tbsp. in 8-oz. water 2x daily, or Aloe Falls ALOE juice with ginger.

2—Have a potassium broth (pg. 291) or a green drink like Pure Planet CHLORELLA, Wakunaga KYO-GREEN with EFAs, or Crystal Star ENERGY GREEN RENEWAL™ drink once a week.

3—Make a mix of Red Star NUTRITIONAL YEAST and toasted wheat germ (or 2 tsp. wheat germ oil and BioStrath YEAST ELIXIR), take 1 tbsp. daily on a fresh salad.

4—Eliminate common allergy foods: wheat, corn, dairy foods, sprayed foods like oranges and lettuce. Avoid salty, fried foods, chemical-containing foods. You'll notice a difference. Avoid caffeine, especially full-strength coffee, sodas, colas and chocolate. They may affect your calcium balance. Surprise, a little wine daily seems to help.

—Bodywork:

•A series of cranial treatments from a good massage therapist have notable results for TMJ (and therefore tinnitus) sufferers. Chiropractic adjustment, acupuncture and shiatsu massage show improvement for both tinnitus and vertigo. **—Acupressure point:** •Pinch between the eyebrows 3x for 10 seconds each time during an attack. •Press top of the wrist line for 15 seconds at a time.

•You can mask tinnitus ringing with white noise or soothing sounds from a machine at night. The machines are widely available today.

•Stress management techniques, like meditation, hypnosis, biofeedback, yoga help.

•Reduce or avoid aspirin. Avoid alcohol, marijuana, methamphetamines, cocaine, hallucinogens, and balance-changing drugs.

•Heat your feet to move blood away from your ears.

Herbal, Superfood and Supplement Therapy

Interceptive therapy plan: Choose 2 to 3 recommendations.

1—Relieve ringing: 1) *Boost circulation, clear blocks:* Proven good results program: •Dr. Bob Martin's HEARALL caps, •Clear Products CLEAR TINNITUS, •*Cayenne-ginger* caps for circulation, •*Ginkgo Biloba* extract 4x daily (improvement usually in 2 months). •*Ginger* caps 4 daily for 3 months; •CoQ-10, 300mg daily for 3 months, or •VINPOCETINE 30mg 2x daily; (good results); •Histidine caps 1000mg daily. *Bilberry* extract; •Niacin therapy 250mg 3x daily. 2) *Boost calcium:* •Crystal Star CALCIUM MAGNESIUM SOURCE™ caps or •1500mg calcium with magnesium and zinc daily. 3) *Clear low grade ear infection:* •Crystal Star ANTI-BIO™ caps (6) or extract 3x daily.

2—Help repair nerves: •Crystal Star RELAX CAPS™ for nerve rebuilding, to restore mental equilibrium; •*Black cohosh* extract drops 3x daily. •Premier GERMANIUM with DMG daily (excellent). •Ligustrum caps. •Amla C or Ester C with bioflavonoids and rutin, up to 5000mg daily. •Herbs, Etc. DEEP SLEEP softgels for interrupted sleep.

3—Reduce your cholesterol and triglyceride levels: •Crystal Star CHO-LO FIBER TONE™ caps, 3 daily for 2 months; •Maitake Products REISHI capsules; •Red yeast rice.

4—Relieve pain, congestion: •Crystal Star ANTI-HST™ caps up to 6 daily; •*Lobelia* extract drops in water; or •*Mullein/Lobelia* tea. •Crystal Star EAR DEFENSE™ extract (good results). •Metabolic Response Modifiers CARDIO-CHELATE with EDTA, MSM. •Douglas Labs GLUTATHIONE PLUS with NAC drains congesting fluid; •Lane Labs Palm Vitee Tocotrienols. •Fluid elimination tea: *uva ursi, parsley leaf, red clover, fennel seed, flax seed.*

5—Boost B-vitamins: Especially B-12. •Now sublingual B-12, 2500mcg daily; B-complex 100mg with extra B-6 100mg. Bee products are a specific: •Prince of Peace GINSENG-ROYAL JELLY vials; •Beehive Botanicals ROYAL JELLY/GINSENG capsules; •Montana Big Sky ROYAL JELLY 2 tsp. daily; •Ginseng/royal jelly and honey in water as a daily drink.

6—Silica helps strengthen vascular walls: •Crystal Star IODINE, POTASSIUM, SILICA SOURCE extract, or •*Horsetail/oatstraw* tea or •Eyebright tea or •Flora VEGE-SIL caps daily. •Add sea greens to your diet, 2 tbsp. dried, snipped, daily (any kind).

Can't find a recommended product? Call the 800 number listed in Product Resources for the store nearest you.

Tonsillitis

Tonsil Lymph Inflammation

The tonsils are part of the lymphatic gland tissue on either side of the entrance to the throat. They strain and process poisons from the body. (Removal of these glands reduces your ability to respond to pathogens taken in by mouth.) **Tonsillitis** is tonsil inflammation, usually caused by *streptococcal* organisms. While tonsillitis itself may not be serious, it always indicates a deeper immune response let-down, and can lead to serious problems, like rheumatic fever and nephritis. Scar tissue accumulates with every tonsillitis attack. If your tonsils do need conventional medical attention, ask about today's partial laser operation that just trims the tonsils with a carbon-dioxide laser. It's an inexpensive, out-patient procedure that leaves you with a minor sore throat instead of a major trauma, and leaves some tonsil-straining ability of the body intact. **Do you have tonsillitis?** Painful, tender, swollen tonsils and lymph glands on either side of the jaw with difficulty swallowing are the main sign. Flu signs like fever and chills; aches and pains in the back and extremities; vomiting sometimes accompany. There's bad breath because of the infection, congested ears and hearing difficulty because of the swollen glands. Poor diet (not enough green vegetables, too many starches and sugars) aggravates this type of sporadic infection. An allergy to dairy foods or wheat may be involved. *See STREP THROAT page 507 for more information.*

Diet and Lifestyle Support Therapy

Nutritional therapy plan:

1—Go on a 24 hr. (pg. 173) or 3 day liquid cleansing diet (pg. 172) to clear out body toxins. Take a potassium broth (pg. 291) once a day. Have an onion/garlic broth each day. Then eat only fresh foods for the rest of the week during an attack. Get plenty of vegetable protein for healing. Take New Chapter GINGER WONDER syrup- 1 tbsp. in 8-oz. water 2x daily, during these cleanses to reduce inflammation.

2—Have lemon juice and water each morning, or Herbal Answers ALOE FORCE JUICE with plenty of other high vitamin C juices throughout the day, like orange, pineapple, and grapefruit juice.

3—Avoid sugars, dairy products especially, and all fast foods until condition clears.

4—Drink 6-8 glasses of bottled water daily to keep the body flushed.

Amazingly, tonsillitis is regularly reported as part of the destructive behavior that characterizes learning disorders like ADD. Tests show that the swelling and inflammation of the tonsils cause sleep apnea. Removing the tonsils in these cases has markedly lessened the tonsils cause sleep apnea. Removing the tonsils in these cases has markedly lessened behavior problems because the sleep apnea is cured.

—Bodywork:
•Take a garlic or catnip enema during an attack to clear body poisons.
•Chill the throat with a towel wrapped around crushed ice.
•Hot mineral salts baths frequently.
•Get plenty of bed rest during acute stage.

—Gargles to reduce throat inflammation:
•Warm salt water gargles 3x daily.
•Thyme tea as a gargle.
•Slippery elm tea to soothe.
•Liquid chlorophyll 1 tsp. in water.
•Goldenseal/myrrh solution in water as a gargle

Herbal, Superfood and Supplement Therapy

Interceptive therapy plan: Choose 3 or more recommendations.

1—**Control the infection:** •Crystal Star ANTI-BIO™ caps 4-6 daily, or •*usnea* extract drops to flush lymph glands and clear infection. •Garlic oil; or swab •Black walnut extract directly on throat. •Use Herbs, Etc. PHYTOCILLIN, and spray throat with •Nutribiotic GRAPEFRUIT SEED extract as a gargle as directed, for anti-infective activity. •Nature's Plus CHEWABLE ACEROLA C 500mg with bioflavonoids, 1-2 every hour during acute stages (especially if there is constipation which there often is if a dairy allergy is involved).

2—**Soothe throat pain and swelling:** •Enzymatic Therapy ESBERITOX chewables is a specific (fast results); •Crystal Star ANTI-FLAM™ caps to take down inflammation; •Crystal Star DR. ENZYME™ with protease and bromelain caps for pain relief (good results). •Echinacea extract or cleavers tea as lymphatics to clear lymph tissue. •*Licorice* root or •*ginseng/licorice* extract. •Nature's Path THROAT-LYTE; •Solaray pantothenic acid 1500mg with B₆ 250mg to take down swelling. •Quercetin 500mg with •bromelain 500mg to relieve inflammation.

3—**Help clear sinus and throat congestion:** •Crystal Star ZINC SOURCE™ throat rescue drops as a soothing throat coat. •Gargle a weak *tea tree* oil solution in water every 2-3 hours to counter inflammation. •*Mullein* or •*lobelia* tea as a throat compress; •Zinc gluconate throat lozenges as needed. •Propolis lozenges or tincture as needed. •Herbon Naturals ECHINACEA THROAT DROPS.

4—**Enhance immune response:** •Beehive Botanical PROPOLIS SPRAY. •Prince of Peace GINSENG-ROYAL JELLY vials for EFA's. •Nutricology PRO GREENS with EFA's. •*Lobelia* drops if there is high fever. •Enzymatic Therapy VIRAPLEX caps 4 daily; or THYMULUS extract. •Solaray ALFAJUICE caps. •Nutramedix IMMUN-X for long term support.

—Note: Investigate raw glandular extracts; they offer biochemical nutritional support for stress and fatigue affecting glands. They can improve gland health dramatically by delivering cell-specific and gland specific factors.

Can't find a recommended product? Call the 800 number listed in Product Resources for the store nearest you.

Tumors

Malignant Tumors, Brain Tumors

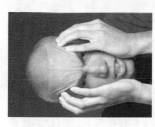

Malignant tumors should be addressed quickly to control spreading to other tissues. *Brain tumors* should especially be acted upon immediately, because both malignant and benign tumors can cause irreversible neurological damage. Brain tumors are likely to return if not completely excised. Immune enhancement is the key in natural treatment. A whole foods diet and natural supplementation program has been successful in both reducing and in some cases, completely eliminating tumors. **Do you think you might have a tumor?** Have you noticed growing, changing lumps and nodules, often inflamed, weeping, and painful, sometimes with adhesions to other tissue. Brain tumor signs include: chronic headaches, personality changes, unexplained vomiting, weakness and lethargy, double vision, unusual muscle coordination and intellectual deterioration, sometimes seizures and stupor. **What causes tumors?** Experts are commenting on environmental, heavy metal or radiation poisoning conditions. Some point to X-rays and low grade radiation tests, like mammograms, causing protective iodine depletion and thyroid malfunction. Viral infections like Epstein-Barr, herpes simplex and Kaposi's sarcoma may play a role. Nutritionists and holistic doctors, say high level of exposure to excitotoxins (food additives which can cause brain toxicity) like fluoride, MSG, and aspartame may be to blame. *See CANCER pages 345-357 for more information.*

Diet and Lifestyle Support Therapy

Nutritional therapy plan:

1—Go on a short mucous cleansing liquid diet (pg. 202). Then, for 1 month, have one each of the following juices daily: 1) Cranberry/pineapple juice; 2) Potassium broth (pg. 291) or one Herbal Answers ALOE FORCE JUICE drink; 3) A veggie drink like Sun Wellness CHLORELLA drink, Crystal Star ENERGY GREEN RENEWAL™ for iodine, potassium and green therapy, Green Foods GREEN MAGMA or Fit for You, Intl. MIRACLE GREENS with sea greens, esp. for hormone driven tumors.

2—Add whole grains, high fiber foods and steamed vegetables during the 4th week. Eat primarily fresh foods, especially sprouts, for the next month.

3—Add high sulphur foods: Garlic, onion and cruciferous vegetables or Wakunaga AGED GARLIC EXTRACT capsules and AloeLife ALOE VERA juice with herbs.

4—Avoid heavy starches, high sugar foods, and all fried foods. Keep the system clean and the liver functioning well with a diet high in greens, low in dairy foods and fats.

5—Drink only distilled bottled water - 6-8 glasses daily to quickly clear toxic wastes.

There has been an enormous increase in numbers of brain tumors reported in the last decade. Can aspartame (Nutrasweet) play a role in brain tumors? Studies from its own labs show that aspartame produced a high incidence of brain tumors at all concentrations examined, and was the reason that the FDA first rejected aspartame for human consumption. The more aspartame consumed, the more likely tumors would develop. In fact, brain tumors rates have increased by 10% since this substance was added to our food supply. Coincidence? Maybe not.

While experts still dispute the findings, evidence shows that, over time, a breakdown product of aspartame, DKP (*diketopiperizine*), may be causing the tumors. There also appears to be some proof that aspartame further breaks down into formaldehyde and that a high intake of MSG (*monosodium glutamate*) from foods may increase aspartame's toxicity to brain cells. Soft drink companies now date their colas. Heating aspartame also speeds up the DKP breakdown. Using in hot beverages or for cooking is especially hazardous.

Herbal, Superfood and Supplement Therapy

Interceptive therapy plans: Choose 2 or 3 recommendations.

1—Reduce tumor size and growth: •Lane Labs NOXYLANE 4 (clinically shown to triple natural killer cell activity); •Dr. Rath's VITACOR PLUS (helps stop replication of cancer cells to deter metastasis); Carnivora Research, Inc. •CARNIVORA® Immune Enhancer caps; •Nutricology MODIFIED CITRUS PECTIN to reduce tumor spread. •Enzymedica PURIFY or •Crystal Star DR. ENZYME™, or Quercetin 1000mg with bromelain 1500mg for enzyme therapy; •Vitamin K 100mcg inhibits growth; •Add COQ-10 300mg daily; and vitamin E 400IU + selenium 200mcg. Take •Nutricology GERMANIUM 150mg, and apply a •germanium-water solution. •PHYCOTENE MICROCLUSTERS available at Royal Bodycare (proven), or •beta carotene 200,000IU. •Apply •Crystal Star ANTI-BIO™ gel with una da gato; Take •pycnogenol PCO's 300mg daily; •Natural Balance creatine 3000-5000mg daily (for a short time); •Natural Energy Plus CAISSE'S tea.

2—Iodine therapy is important: •Crystal Star IODINE, POTASSIUM, SILICA SOURCE extract, or •OCEAN MINERALS™ caps 4 daily; or •Kelp tabs 10 daily; •Vitamin E 800IU with selenium 200mcg; or •New Chapter OCEAN HERBS with sea greens.

3—EFA's - important balancing nutrients: •EVENING PRIMROSE OIL 6 daily; •Nature's Secret ULTIMATE OIL especially for radiation/chemical caused tumors. Add •Lane Labs BENEFIN shark cartilage. •Also open a shark cartilage capsule and mix with ¼ tsp. vitamin C crystals; or •MSM 1000mg daily. Results usually in 3 to 4 weeks.

4—Certain herbs can reduce tumors: •Dr. Christopher's BLACK DRAWING OINT-MENT (very strong, use on external tumors). •Reishi, shiitake, or maitake mushroom caps, 6 daily, or Grifron PRO-MAITAKE D-Fraction extract; •Planetary PAU D'ARCO DEEP CLEANSER for internal use, or •*Pau darco/butternut bark* tea for natural quercetin (also apply pau d' arco extract and echinacea extract drops mixed into aloe vera gel). Use •Calendula gel, or make an •escharotic ointment through which tumor cells can exit: equal parts *garlic*, *goldenseal*, *zinc* powders mixed in calendula ointment. Apply daily for 4 weeks. Commercial product is •HERBAL VEIL 8 by Viable Herbal Solutions. •Chaparral and una da gato are good in a tumor-reducing poultice, plus take 4 capsules daily.

Can't find a recommended product? Call the 800 number listed in Product Resources for the store nearest you.

Varicose Veins

Spider Veins, Peripheral Vascular Problems

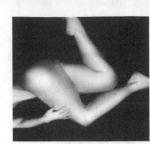

Peripheral vascular problems like varicose veins are more than a cosmetic nuisance. They're a result of leaky valves and they can be painful, cause unusual fatigue, heaviness and cramping, leg and ankle swelling. *Varicose veins* develop when a defect in the vein wall dilates the vein and damages vein valves (sometimes even dangerous clots in veins). When vein valves don't function well, blood pressure increases resulting in bulging. *Spider (thread) veins* are thin, red, unsightly lines on the face, upper arms and thighs. Women are affected four times as frequently as men. Vein fragility increases with age due to loss of tissue tone, and weakening of vein walls. **Do you have varicose veins?** Check for distended, swollen, painful leg veins, a heavy, tight, tired feeling in the legs, sometimes with numbness and tingling. **Spider veins?** Look for thin red lines and muscle cramping. **What causes unsightly veins?** Look to your diet first... Is it low in fiber? Too high in red meat, fried foods and dairy foods? Is your diet nutrition-poor? (lack of vitamin E, C, and A, and essential fatty acids means weakness of vascular walls due to weak connective tissue). Are you constipated a lot? Or overweight? (puts straining pressure on the veins). Is your posture poor? Have long periods of standing, heavy lifting or sitting? (affects vein circulation) See Circulation page 373.

Vasculitis is an inflammation of the veins.

Diet and Lifestyle Support Therapy

Nutritional therapy plan:

1—Keep weight down to relieve heaviness on the legs. Go on a 24 hour (pg. 173) liquid diet to clear circulation. Eat fresh foods for the rest of the week - plenty of green salads and juices. Add a glass of cider vinegar and honey each morning. (Add 1 tsp. New Chapter GINGER WONDER SYRUP to boost circulation.) Cider vinegar compresses help.

2—Then follow a vegetarian, high fiber diet for the rest of the month. Varicose veins are rarely seen in parts of the world where people eat high fiber diets. Boost your fiber with fresh fruits and vegetables, and whole grains. Include seafoods, beans, whole grains, brown rice, steamed veggies. Add •Jarrow GENTLE FIBERS drink for venous integrity (very good results). Take an epsom salts bath once a week.

3—Have a high vitamin C juice every day, like pineapple, carrot, citrus fruit, or a veggie drink like Barleans GREENS or Futurebiotics VITAL K.

4—Eat foods with high PCO's, like cherries, berries, currants and grapes.

5—Reduce dairy foods, fried foods, prepared meats, red meats and saturated fats of all kinds. Avoid salty, sugary and caffeine foods.

—Bodywork exercises: *Sitting for long periods of time is the worst for varicose veins. Take short, frequent breaks in your work schedule. Sit with a stool to prop your feet on.* •Walk every day; swim as much as possible, for the best leg exercises. Walk in the ocean whenever possible for strengthening sea minerals. Walk in the early morning dewy grass. •Elevate legs when possible. Avoid standing for long periods. Go barefoot, or wear flat sandals. Do not use knee high hosiery. The elastic band at the top impedes circulation. •Massage feet and legs every morning and night with diluted myrrh oil. •Use alternating hot and cold hydrotherapy (pg. 185) daily.

—For broken capillaries: Take HCl 600mg daily. Apply white oak bark compresses, and take 8 white oak caps daily.

Herbal, Superfood and Supplement Therapy

Interceptive therapy plan: Choose 2 to 3 recommendations. *Note: Sclerotherapy injections for spider veins can produce good results but are usually not covered by insurance. Use vitamin E oil after the procedure to speed healing.*

1—**Strengthen vascular fragility, stimulate circulation:** A highly effective 3-month program–noticeable improvement in 2 months: •Crystal Star VARI-VEIN™ caps (with horse chestnut and grape seed PCOs) with •Evening Primrose Oil 3000mg, or •Natural Balance GREAT LEGS caps, and apply Derma-e CLEAR VEIN CREME (recommended). •GINKGO BILOBA extract caps 3 daily; •Gotu kola caps 4 daily for spider veins; or •Solaray CENTELLA VEIN capsules to maintain connective tissue. •Planetary HAWTHORN HEART tabs. •Reviva VITAMIN P DAY CREAM for venous tone. •Lane Labs TOKI collagen replacement drink helps reduce varicose veins and spider veins (highly recommended).

2—**Boost flavonoids for vein tone:** •Horse Chestnut cream; •Quercetin 1000mg with Bromelain 1500mg daily, or •Nature's Plus BROMELAIN 1500mg daily, or •Solaray QBC caps 2 daily. •BILBERRY extract 4x daily or •PCOs from grapeseed, 300mg daily for 2 months; •Derma E CLEAR VEIN CREAM with alpha lipoic acid (good results). •Vitamin C crystals with bioflavs and rutin, ½ tsp. every 4 hours to bowel tolerance daily for 1 month, for connective tissue, collagen formation, or •Pure Planet AMLA C PLUS.

3—**Reduce pain and heaviness:** •Crystal Star MUSCLE RELAXER™ 4 daily (very effective through the day if you sit a lot); •Apply Earth's Bounty O₂ SPRAY to the legs and feet. Homeopathic remedies: •BioForce VenaForce gel and tablets; •B&T CALIFLORA gel; or •Hamamelis for swelling. —**Effective leg compresses:** Apply •Witch hazel compresses 2x daily; or •Calendula compresses morning and evening; or •Ginger compresses and take 4 capsules ginger daily. Use •Butcher's broom tea and compresses for circulation increase.

4—**Reduce inflammation:** •Crystal Star DR. ENZYME™ with protease and bromelain thelps break down fibrin; •Apply aloe vera gel. Elevate legs while application soaks in. •Take vitamin E 400IU with •Zinc 30mg daily, and apply a mix of ¼ tsp. vitamin E oil and 2 tbsp. liquid lecithin. (Feet and legs tingle and feel hot as if thawing out). Take •Capsicum caps 4 daily; or •Capsicum-Ginger root caps, 6 daily; •Vitamin K cream for spider veins daily and vitamin K cream for spider veins.

Can't find a recommended product? Call the 800 number listed in Product Resources for the store nearest you.

Vaginal Yeast Infections

Leukorrhea, Bacterial Vaginosis (BV), Vulvitis

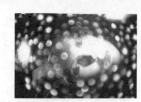

Thirty million women a year get them. **Trichomonas**: caused by a parasite, contracted via intercourse. **Leukorrhea**: a yeasty infection when normal vaginal acidity is disrupted. **Bacterial Vaginosis (gardnerella)**: thrives when vaginal pH is disturbed. **Vulvitis**: a vulva inflammation caused by allergic irritation, bacterial or fungal infection. Natural therapies can address most vaginal yeast infections, but long-term cure is not likely unless diet and lifestyle changes are made. *Note:* Douching excessively with commercial brands loaded with perfumes and additives, can lead to problems. Commercial douches disrupt normal vaginal balance, wash out "friendly" bacteria that help protect against infections like candida and BV (*bacterial vaginosis*). Try herbal douches instead for a limited time. **Do you have a vaginal infection:** *Yeast infection:* smells like bread or beer, sometimes fishy. *Leukorrhea:* itchy, inflamed vaginal tissues, a foul, yeasty discharge; sex is painful. *Trichomonas:* severe itch, foamy, yellow discharge with foul odor. *Bacterial Vaginosis:* a foul, fishy odor, white discharge, moderate itchiness. *Vulvitis:* itching, redness, swelling, with fluid-filled blisters. **Causes?** Long exposure to antibiotics weakens immune response, imbalances hormones. Spermicidal cream Nonoxynol-9, aggravates cystitis and Candida infections, and can kill friendly lactobacilli that protect the vagina against micro-organisms. *See SEXUALLY TRANSMITTED DISEASES and CANDIDA ALBICANS healing suggestions for more information.*

Diet and Lifestyle Support Therapy

Nutritional therapy plan:

1—Keep the diet primarily fresh during healing. Have a large green salad with alfalfa sprouts every day. Keep meals light without heavy starches, fatty foods, sugars, or dairy foods. Avoid red meats, hard liquor, sugar and caffeine while clearing.

2—Eat cultured foods - yogurt or kefir (8-oz daily can improve a yeast-triggered infection by as much as 70%), especially if you have been taking antibiotics.

3—Normalize body chemistry: drink 3-4 glasses unsweetened cranberry juice daily.

4—Schiff GARLIC/ONION caps 6 daily (with watermelon seed tea if also bladder infection).

5—Use green drinks both orally and as douches, like Chlorophyll liquid 1 tsp. to 1 qt. water, or Barleans GREENS, or Wakunaga KYO-GREEN drink.

—**Effective douches:** •Cider vinegar- 2 tbsp. to 1 qt. water; add a pinch cayenne or 2TBS green clay if desired. •Diluted mineral water, or a plain yogurt and mineral water douche. •Baking soda 2 tsp./honey 1 tsp./1 qt. water.

—**Bodywork:** Be kind to your mate. Many infections bounce back and forth between partners. Treat your sexual partner with a penis soak. Avoid sex during an infection, or use barrier protection. Birth control pills have been implicated in some infections.

•**Effective vaginal douches:** Add 1-oz. herbs to 1-qt. water. Steep 30 min., strain. Calendula - esp. for candida infections; Tea tree oil drops; Witch hazel bark/leaf or chaparral leaf; Sage leaf or white oak bark in white vinegar; 3% H_2O_2, 1 tbsp. in 1 qt. water.

•**Vaginal packs or suppositories to rebalance vaginal pH:** Apply on a tampon, or mix with cocoa butter and simply insert. Try dilute tea tree oil; Home Health ROSE WATER KIT; Acidophilus powder or capsules, or alternate Boric acid with acidophilus; Dolisos homeopathic Yeast Clear; Crystal Star FUNGEX™ gel, or coconut oil for vulvitis.

•**For BV and trichomonas:** Drink cranberry juice, insert tea tree oil or garlic suppositories for 14 days (change 3x daily), alternate salt water and vinegar douches for a week, and take vitamins B-complex and C daily.

Herbal, Superfood and Supplement Therapy

Interceptive therapy plan: Choose 2 to 3 recommendations.

1—Normalize vaginal biochemistry: •Crystal Star WOMAN'S BEST FRIEND™ caps 6 daily, with •Natren GY-NA-TREN for 4 days for a mild infection. Use with •UAS DDS-PLUS with FOS for more severe problems. Add •Crystal Star ANTI-BIO™ caps 6 daily or an *Oregon grape root-goldenseal root* compound to boost activity. Drink •*Pau d' arco* tea 3 cups daily; •*Garlic* 8 caps daily; or •*Black walnut hulls* extract 2x daily (also effective in a douche). Recurrent infections— •Pure Essence Labs CANDEX with enzyme support; •Nutricology PROLIVE (olive leaf extract); •American Biologics DIOXYCHLOR, or Enzymedica PURIFY. —**Phyto-estrogen herbs help body-balancing against yeast infections:** •Crystal Star EST-AID™ caps, or Esteem TOTAL WOMAN.

2—Vitamin therapy effective for vaginal yeast infections: •Zinc 50mg daily is primary (usually results in 3 weeks for trichomonas even if drugs have not been effective). •Beta carotene 100,000IU daily, or Vitamin A 25,000IU suppositories (not if pregnant). •Vitamin E 400IU 2x daily. •Vitamin C (ascorbic acid) crystals, ½ tsp. every 2 hours during healing, up to 5000mg daily. A weak water solution may also be used as a douche. •B complex 100mg daily, with extra B_6 100mg. •Vitamin K 100mcg 3x daily.

3—Vaginal herbal suppositories: •Mix powders of *cramesbill, goldenseal, echinacea root, white oak bark, raspberry* with cocoa butter to bind. Roll into suppositories and chill. Insert at night. Seal with a napkin or tampon. Especially for chronic vaginitis - more than a yeast infection. •*Garlic-goldenseal* powders mixed with a little yogurt and smeared on a tampon. •Nutribiotic GRAPEFRUIT SEED concentrate 20 drops in 1 gal. water. May also use orally as directed (very effective). •Use vitamin A: prick an oil capsule and smear on a tampon, or simply insert the capsule into vagina twice daily (it will dissolve).

4—Probiotics are critical: •UAS DDS-PLUS with FOS or Pure Essence FLORALIVE or other acidophilus - ½ tsp. or contents of 5 capsules in 1 tbsp. yogurt. Douche in the morning with ¼ tsp. acidophilus in water. Take ¼ tsp. in water orally, or 6 capsules daily.

Can't find a recommended product? Call the 800 number listed in Product Resources for the store nearest you.

Warts
Moles, Skin Tags

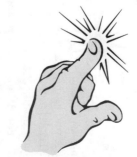

Warts are single or clustered, soft, irregular skin growths found on the hands, feet, arms and face, ranging in size from a pinhead to a small bean. They also occur on the throat or voice box and affect the speaking voice tone. Usually caused by a virus, they are contagious and will spread if picked, bitten, or nicked in shaving. **Moles** are discolored growths elevated above the skin surface, and may appear because of a liver or lung condition. They are harmless unless continually irritated. **Skin tags** (*acrochordons*) are small outgrowths of skin tissue connected to a soft stalk. They usually appear after age 45 or 50, and can be bent easily (unlike a tumor lump). They can be removed with a scalpel or scissors, burned off, or frozen off with liquid nitrogen, a quick, painless procedure from a dermatologist. **What is that skin bump?** Warts are flat or raised nodules on the skin surface, with a rough, pitted discolored surface, sometimes causing pain and discomfort when rubbed or chafed; if virally caused, warts are often contagious. Moles are generally smooth and rounded. General causes focus on a viral infection, or Vitamin A and mineral depletion, usually from widespread use of antibiotics and vaccinations that depress normal immunity. *See GENITAL WARTS page 534 and CYSTS, WENS & LIPOMAS page 385 for more information.*

Diet and Lifestyle Support Therapy

Nutritional therapy plan:

1—Add vitamin A rich foods to the diet, like yellow and green fruits and vegetables, eggs, and cold water fish.

2—Add sulphur-containing foods, like asparagus, garlic and onion family foods, fresh figs, citrus fruits and eggs.

3—Include high vitamin C foods with bioflavonoids, like citrus fruits and broccoli.

4—Add yogurt and other cultured foods to the diet. Take a vegetable drink like Aloe-Life ALOE GOLD drink, Jarrow GENTLE FIBERS drink or Crystal Star ENERGY GREEN RENEWAL™ drink with sea vegetables, every day for a month.

—Effective food applications:

• Use very soft brown-black bananas. Place a small section of peel (inside down) on the wart. Cover with a bandage and leave on 24 hours. Repeat until wart is gone.

• Apply a mixture of lemon juice, sea salt, onion juice and vitamin E oil.

• Papaya skins or pineapple slices; or •Raw potato.

—Bodywork:

• Hypnosis therapy has been successful in controlling warts and moles.

• Some skin therapists use an electric current passed through a wart to make it shrink.

• Rough up the wart with the smooth side of an emery board. Make a blend of essential oil of thuja and castor oil (equal parts). Apply 1 or 2 drops to wart twice daily. Wart or mole will slowly shrink and slough off. Do not squeeze or pick. Or, paint on Gaia Herbs CELANDINE tincture 2-3x daily. Warts disappear within weeks (good activity).

• Soak warts in hot water first. Then apply:
—Castor oil (very effective) or Calendula ointment, or B&T CALI-FLORA ointment.
—Herbal Answers ALOE FORCE gel.
—Lysine cream applications, and take lysine capsules 500mg 3-4x daily.

• For moles: Dilute frankincense with castor oil and apply. Or, mix one to two drops frankincense oil in tea tree oil and apply.

Herbal, Superfood and Supplement Therapy

Interceptive therapy plan: Choose 2 or 3 recommendations.

1—**Address the infection:** •Crystal Star ANTI-BIO™ caps 6 daily or *usnea* extract if there is inflammation or bacterial infection. Apply •Crystal Star ANTI-BIO™ gel. Or apply •*tea tree* oil or *oregano* oil to wart, or •Allergy Research Oregano Oil religiously for 1-2 months, 3-4 times daily. Wonderful results. Apply Nutribiotic GRAPEFRUIT SEED extract full strength, or SKIN SPRAY 2 to 3x daily. •Crystal Star DR. ENZYME™ with protease and bromelain for inflammation relief.

2—**High dose vitamin therapy can help:** The high dosages recommended here should be used for no longer than 2-3 months at a time. •Zinc 75mg daily. •Emulsified A 100,000-150,000IU or •PHYCOTENE MICROCLUSTERS available at royalbodycare. com, as an anti-infective. (Nothing seems to happen for 1 to 2 months, then growths may disappear in a week or so, all at once.) •B-complex up to 200mg daily, with extra B₆ 250mg daily. •Vitamin C crystals with bioflavonoids; take internally, ½ tsp. in water every 4 hours daily. Apply locally to affected area. Also important for immunity against warts.

3—**Boost immune response:** •Immudyne MACROFORCE with beta glucan; or •Eidon IMMUNE SUPPORT liquid. •Flora VEGE-SIL 4 daily. •N-acetyl cysteine (NAC) 2000mg daily. MICROHYDRIN PLUS from Royal Bodycare (fights viral and bacterial infections).

4—**Applications for warts and moles:** Well in Hand WART WONDER- especially for childhood warts (highly recommended). •Put several drops of *lomatium* extract and several drops of castor oil on a bandaid and apply. Open and apply contents of a •MAI-TAKE MUSHROOM capsule daily. •For a mole, wart or skin tag, use a bloodroot paste mixed with castor oil, takes about 30 days. •Apply a paste of garlic cloves directly and cover with a plastic strip. Use vitamin E oil on surrounding skin so it doesn't burn; also take Vitamin E 800IU daily. Usually takes a week for the wart to fall off. For wart and moles caused by a virus: (not HPV-caused warts). •Rough up a viral wart with the smooth side of an emery board and apply a drop of 3% H₂O₂ to kill the virus. For plantar warts: soak foot in the hottest water you can stand about 30 minutes daily for a month. Apply Earth's Bounty O₂ SPRAY or H₂O₂ 3% solution.

Can't find a recommended product? Call the 800 number listed in Product Resources for the store nearest you.

Water Retention

Bloating, Edema

Water retention, where too much fluid accumulates in body tissues and cavities, is more often a problem of NOT ENOUGH WATER - a condition of body imbalance. If we don't get sufficient water, fluid levels go out of balance, and the body begins to retain more water in an effort to compensate. Kidney, liver, blood pressure, circulation, pre-menstrual and pregnancy problems are all associated with water retention. **Why do we hold on to too much fluid?** Serious weight control dieting can take away foods that previously provided water. You may have a diet imbalance... too much salt, red meat or MSG, not enough protein, potassium and B complex vitamins. Medical diuretics, alcoholic drinks, oral contraceptives and steroid drugs can dehydrate (sometimes accompanied by a kidney or bladder infection). Persistent edema is linked to kidney, liver, bladder and circulatory problems. You may just not be drinking enough healthy fluids. A natural program should concentrate on balancing body chemistry rather than simply releasing water. **Are you retaining water?** You probably are if your hands, feet, ankles look and feel swollen, if your tummy feels bulgy (your clothes are too tight). If you head feels achy and your clothes fit fine one day and too tight the next, bloating is probably related to PMS or menopausal hormonal changes (especially excess estrogen). Climate changes, allergy reactions, constipation and lack of exercise all play a role. *See PMS page 515 for more information about pre-period edema.*

Diet and Lifestyle Support Therapy

Nutritional therapy plan:

1—Reduce salt and salty foods intake.

2—Eat largely fresh foods for 3-5 days to increase your body's food water content without density.

3—Have a leafy green salad every day with plenty of kale or dandelion greens, cucumbers, parsley, alfalfa sprouts and celery. Green drinks, like Barleans GREENS, Green Foods GREEN MAGMA can provide both needed minerals and body acid/alkaline balance.

4—Eat potassium-rich foods like broccoli, seafoods and sea greens for fluid balance. Both Futurebiotics VITAL K 2-4 tsp. daily, and Crystal Star RESTORE YOUR STRENGTH™ drink are nutritious choices for potassium.

5—Avoid starchy, sugary, foods. Reduce meats, wheat products, dried foods and dairy foods that demand more water to dissolve.

6—Drink at least 6-8 glasses of bottled water daily for free flowing functions, waste removal, and appetite suppression. Caffeine drinks are diuretic, but should be avoided by women with pre-period edema.

7—Take electrolyte drinks daily like Alacer ELECTROMIX or Knudsen's RECHARGE, or Nature's Path TRACE-LYTE liquid electrolytes to quickly balance body fluids.

—Bodywork:

• Be careful of overusing chemical/medical diuretics. They can cause potassium and mineral loss, and eventually muscle weakness and fatigue.

• Take hot 20 minute saunas often. Or try •Crystal Star POUNDS OFF™ bath as a strong diaphoretic for sweating once a week.

• Exercise every day to keep circulation and body metabolism free-flowing.

• Elevate head and shoulders for sleeping.

• Weleda BIRCH CELLULITE OIL for better skin texture and tone.

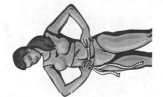

Herbal, Superfood and Supplement Therapy

If taking prescription diuretics, be sure to include potassium in your daily diet.

Interceptive therapy plan: Choose 2 to 3 recommendations.

1—Non-depleting, natural fluid balancers: •Crystal Star BLOAT RELEASE™ tea promotes better elimination and calorie burning; •TINKLE CAPS™, 4-6 daily, and/or •TINKLE™ tea (great for pre-period edema); •*Dandelion* leaf tea or •*Cornsilk/dandelion* tea, 3 cups daily; or •*Juniper/parsley/uva ursi* tea or *uva ursi* extract drops in water. •Ascorbic acid therapy: Vitamin C crystals with bioflavonoids and rutin, ½ tsp. in water or juice every 2-3 hours until relief. Then 3-5000mg daily for prevention. •Flora VEGE-SIL as natural diuretic; •Richardson Labs CHROMA SLIM (men).

2—Enhance adrenal activity to regulate salt and water balance: •Crystal Star ADRENAL ENERGY BOOST™ caps 2-4 daily; •Arise & Shine LIQUID ORGANIC SEA MINERALS; or •Nature's Path TRACE-MIN-LYTE with sea greens for mineral balance - very important if you have low adrenal function with water retention

3—Tone and strengthen genito-urinary tissue: •BILBERRY or HAWTHORN extract as needed daily for tissue tone and to increase circulation. Nature's Apothecary KIDNEY SUPPORT or Herbs, Etc. KIDNEY TONIC. •Transformation EXCELLZYME (a kidney antioxidant).

4—Enhance liver function: •Crystal Star CELLULITE RELEASE™ caps 3-4 daily for 1-3 months (highly recommended). •Enzymatic Therapy KIDNEY/LIVER COMPLEX. •B Complex 100mg daily with extra B₆ 250mg 2x daily.

5—Achieve hormone balance to achieve fluid balance: •[FE]MALE HARMONY™ caps and tea produce good results. Or •Ester[...] COMFORT caps. •ECHINACEA extract, 10 drops in 2 cups d[...] lymph glands and balance hormones. •Solaray ALFAJUIC[...] balance and as a detoxifier.

6—Proteolytic enzymes help lead to body balance with Protease & Bromelain to reduce bloat and body c[...] tion; Bromelain 1500mg daily for a month, or •Enzy[...]

Can't find a recommended product? Call the 800 number listed in Product Resources for the store nearest you[...]

Weight Loss

Weight Control, Excess Fat Retention

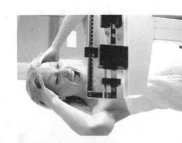

The latest statistics are shocking. One out of every two Americans is overweight! This doesn't count kids who are rapidly becoming an entire overweight g... Right now, two-thirds of Americans are trying to lose weight. Amazingly, of those, only 20% are actually reducing their calories or exercising. Next to smo... obesity is the second leading preventable cause of death in the United States, contributing to an excess of 300,000 deaths each year. The natural recommendations presented on the following pages can be used successfully for a wide variety of men and women struggling with their weight. Notes: Yo-yo dieting increases the risk of gallstones. For the best results, start slowly on your weight loss program and stick with it. The five keys to an effective weight control diet: low fat, high fiber, regular exercise, stress control, lots of water. *See the following pages and* SKIN, CELLULITE CONTROL *page 541 for more.*

The Seven Most Common Weight Loss Challenges

There are almost as many different weight loss problems as there are people who have them. I've identified seven of the most common and developed comprehensive programs to address them. Each plan has years of observed success behind it. Once you make the decision to be a thin person, analyze what your weight loss challenge really is. Identify your most prominent weight control problem, especially if there seems to be more than one. As improvement is realized in the primary area, secondary problems are often overcome in the process.

1. Lazy Metabolism and Thyroid Imbalance: Is your metabolism sluggish?

• Are you often weak and tired? (especially in the morning) Are you unusually depressed and anxious for no great reason?
• Do you get frequent digestive disturbances like heartburn and indigestion?
• Do you have breast fibroids? Are you over 50 and experiencing unusual hair loss?

Weight gain after 40 or after menopause usually means lowered thyroid and metabolic activity. Huge studies reveal that 1 in 10 women over 65 have early stages of hypothyroidism! Boosting metabolism and supporting your thyroid is easy. Add sea vegetables to your diet like kelp, dulse, arame and nori, rich in natural iodine, as a mainstay. Or take sea greens in capsules or extracts, like •Crystal Star OCEAN MINERALS™ caps. Herbal formulas show good results for weight problems caused by low thyroid activity. Try •Crystal Star THYROID META MAX™ caps or Gaia Herbs THYROID SUPPORT phytocaps. Add thermogenic spices like cinnamon, cayenne, mustard and ginger to speed up your fat burning process. Try dipping raw veggies in mustard throughout the day. One tsp. of mustard can increase metabolism 25% for up to 3 hours! Add ice to your drinks to boost calorie burning.... up to 25 more calories per drink! Avoid breads and pastries; if you have any tendency to wheat or gluten allergies you'll bloat when you eat them.

2. Overeating Fat, Sugar and Calories: Empty calories like junk food are the downfall of dieters.

• Do you binge on junk foods, especially fatty and sugary foods, about every ten days? Do you have second and third helpings at a meal but still feel hungry?
• Do you eat all your calories at one meal and then try to eat nothing for the rest of the day when you're dieting? (Most people can't do it.)

Overeating is a big reason why it's so hard for people to lose weight, especially men. From a young age, men are encouraged to take second, even third helpings as a sign of manliness or approval for the cook. Women are hit hardest by food cravings during their periods, at the onset of menopause and when they're depressed. We all tend to overeat when we're under stress or tired.... circumstances under which many of us eat today. Our lifestyles don't help. 45% of every food dollar is spent eating out and restaurant portions are bigger than ever. Control portions so you don't overeat. Reduce fats to 20% of your food intake. Don't replace fats with fat substitutes like Olestra. Smell food first before you eat, take your time eating. An herbal appetite suppressant with *St. John's wort* can help against cravings for fatty foods. Hypericin, a St. John's wort constituent, makes the user feel full, much as the drug fenfluramine does, but without the risks. •Crystal Star WILL POWER™ caps with hoodia reduce appetite surges and overeating binges; •Trimedica SLIM SWEET for sugar cravers weight loss; •Nature's Secret CRAVE LESS; or •Source Naturals DIET-PHEN. Enzyme therapy improves fat metabolism: •Transformation LIPOZYME.

3. Sugar Craving and Blood Sugar Imbalances: Sugary foods raise insulin levels too much, your body's signal to make fat, bad for weight loss.

• Are you moody, easily frustrated with a tendency towards crying spells? Do you get very, very tired especially after sugar binges?
• Do you have a wired feeling that is only relieved by eating sweets?

Can't find a recommended product? Call the 800 number listed in Product Resources for the store nearest you.

Dieters who drastically lower their fats often replace them with empty carbohydrates like sugar and starches trying to make up for the missing taste. Increase healthy essential fatty acids (EFAs) from seafood, sea greens, flax seed oil to reduce sweets craving. Try •Health from the Sun CLA 3000mg daily. Consider •Crystal Star ENERGY GREEN RENEWAL™ drink mix for protein stabilization. Target excess sugar in the blood with herbs for weight loss. •Crystal Star SUGAR CONTROL™ formulas, or Planetary TRIPHALA GARCINIA program for high or low blood sugar reactions. Try •Crystal Star DETOX FAT and SUGAR RELEASE™ caps if you eat too much of these foods. Banaba shows good weight loss results for some type 2 diabetes patients. Use acupressure for sugar willpower. Pinch the bud of cartilage directly above your ear canal for 1 minute to short-circuit nerve impulses that cause cravings.

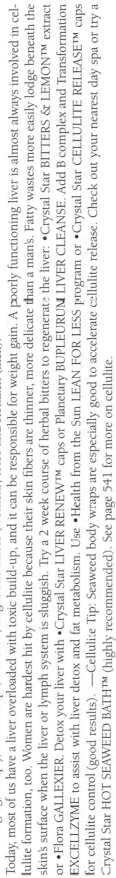
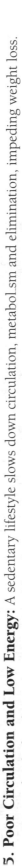

4. Liver Malfunction and Cellulite Formation:
Liver malfunction is directly related to sugar and fat metabolism as a cause of weight gain.

- Have you experienced extreme, unrelenting fatigue or unusual depression and sadness lately for no reason?
- Have you gained weight but your diet hasn't changed? (Your liver metabolizes fats.) Are you experiencing food and chemical sensitivities?
- Has your digestion noticeably worsened? (worsens after fatty meals); with chronic constipation and heartburn?
- Bulging, dimply, skin on hips, buttocks, thighs and knees (women); torso and stomach (men)?

Today, most of us have a liver overloaded with toxic build-up, and it can be responsible for weight gain. A poorly functioning liver is almost always involved in cellulite formation, too. Women are hardest hit by cellulite because their skin fibers are thinner, more delicate than a man's. Fatty wastes more easily lodge beneath the skin's surface when the liver or lymph system is sluggish. Try a 2 week course of herbal bitters to regenerate the liver: •Crystal Star BITTERS & LEMON™ extract or •Flora GALLEXIER. Detox your liver with •Crystal Star LIVER RENEW™ caps or Planetary BUPLEURUM LIVER CLEANSE. Add B complex and Transformation EXCELLZYME to assist with liver detox and fat metabolism. Use •Health from the Sun LEAN FOR LESS program or •Crystal Star CELLULITE RELEASE™ caps for cellulite control (good results). —Cellulite Tip: Seaweed body wraps are especially good to accelerate cellulite release. Check out your nearest day spa or try a Crystal Star HOT SEAWEED BATH™ (highly recommended). See page 541 for more on cellulite.

5. Poor Circulation and Low Energy:
A sedentary lifestyle slows down circulation, metabolism and elimination, impeding weight loss.

- Do your hands, feet, face and ears become cold easily?
- Has your memory gotten noticeably worse? Do you have ringing in your ears?

For some dieters, initial weight loss is rapid, but then a plateau is reached and further weight loss becomes difficult because restricted food intake slows down metabolism, reduces energy and affects circulation. Boost circulation with •Crystal Star HEARTSEASE CIRCU-CLEANSE™ tea or Natural Balance GREAT LEGS caps (excellent results), Crystal Star FEEL GREAT NOW™ caps or •Futurebiotics CIRCUPLEX. Ginkgo biloba extract is a specific. Add •CoQ₁₀, ~ 200mg daily for antioxidant enzyme activity. Mineral electrolytes turn body energy circuits back on: •Nature's Path TRACE-LYTE. Dry brush your skin before showers to speed up your circulation and improve daily energy (great for cellulite, too).

6. Poor Elimination that keeps you congested (and overweight):
An astounding 30 million of us have chronic constipation, a major factor in weight control.

- Are your bowel movements infrequent? Do you get frequent bad breath, body odor or coated tongue?

If your colon is sluggish, your body hangs on to toxins and wastes that would normally be removed via elimination channels. This waste material build-up slows down all systems and your weight loss program. Take 2 tbsp. of aloe vera juice in the morning for effective relief. Consider an herbal formula like •Crystal Star FIBER & HERBS COLON CLEANSE™ caps, Zand CLEANSING LAXATIVE tabs or •Planetary TRIPHALA INTERNAL CLEANSER. Use massage therapy on your lower back (near the kidneys) to relieve colon congestion. If you get backaches when you're constipated, your transverse colon is probably blocked by impacted wastes. A light massage work can help to break up congestion and release accumulated material.

7. High Stress-Cortisol:
It's not what you're eating, it's what's eating you! Research shows high stress boosts the hormone cortisol which increases appetite and cravings for sugary, high carb foods that the body stores as tummy fat. Menopausal women who overeat when they're unhappy are especially affected because they already have more deep abdominal fat stores.

- Do you have a tummy bulge or thick waist that doesn't go away even with exercise and diet improvements?
- Are you under chronic stress or feeling overwhelmed on a near daily basis? Are you tired in the daytime and sleepless at night?

If you're stuck on a weight loss plateau because of high stress, relaxation techniques and herbal appetite suppressants can offer dramatic benefits. Fight stress-related appetite surges with brain balancing herbs like St. John's wort and Rhodiola (excellent results). Crystal Star TUMMY BULGE CONTROL™ capsules combine these herbs and thermogenic herbs like garcinia cambogia for fat burning. Add mood stabilizing minerals like •Crystal Star CALCIUM MAGNESIUM SOURCE™ caps or Lane Labs ADVACAL ULTRA. "Good" fats help your body burn bad fats. •Health from the Sun CLA 3000mg daily or Evening Primrose Oil 3000mg daily. Deep breathing exercises really help because they move lymphatic wastes. See page 250.

Can't find a recommended product? Call the 800 number listed in Product Resources for the store nearest you.

Weight Control For Kids

Today's children are becoming an overweight generation....one in five school children are overweight. America's adults are paying more attention to their diets, but statistics show that U.S. kids are the fattest they've ever been. Obesity is the most prevalent but preventable nutritional disease of the kids in the U.S. Until the 1960's, weight control wasn't much of a problem for kids. But the fifties ushered in the fast food era - refined, chemicalized foods that changed people's metabolism and cell structure. As the fifties kids became parents, they passed on immune defense depletions and digestion problems to their kids - now the parents of the overweight, undernourished kids of today. In fact, the incidence of childhood obesity has doubled in just the past two decades! It's only the beginning. T.V. food advertising especially targets kids who are eating an ever widening array of chemical-laced, genetically altered foods, and junky foods with too much fat, salt, sugar and calories. Some kids eat out of a box most of the time!

U.S. schools have dropped the ball for children's health, offering kids more fatty, nutrient-starved meals and less physical exercise. The telecommunications age has brought kids computers, T.V.'s, and video games - but less active playtime, exercise and outdoor play than any previous generation. P.E. classes in U.S. schools, most sports and many extra-curricular activities have been dropped, and our kids are paying the price. Most kids attend only 1 or 2 physical education classes a week. Forty percent of boys 6-12 can't even touch their toes; American girls actually run *slower* today than they did 10 years ago. P.E. teachers have been reassigned to other classes in over three-quarters of U.S. schools. Today's kids watch up to 28 hours of TV a week. By the time U.S. kids reach their senior high school year, they've spent over 3 years of their lives watching TV. Even more alarming, heart disease is now traceable to early childhood. U.S. doctors are discovering that many American teens (even some 3 year olds) already have fatty deposits on their coronary arteries. And, type 2 diabetes is increasingly being diagnosed in overweight kids. Today's kids rely on junk foods. Children are rewarded with food for good behavior or denied food for punishment from an early age. As they grow older, kids tend to continue that cycle by rewarding themselves with salty, sugary, fatty snacks, soft drinks, and depression and rejection by peers. Getting weight problems under control at an early age is critical for later health. If a child's extra weight hangs on through teenage years, there's a 77% likelihood they will be overweight as adults. But, crash diets aren't the answer. Changing the focus to health, to having a fit body instead of a thin body can make all the difference in managing weight. Kids need mineral-rich building foods, fiber-rich energy foods, and protein-rich growth foods.

I recommend a light detox to start a good weight control program for an overweight child, who usually has a "toxic overload" from too many chemical-laced foods. A gentle detox normalizes body chemistry. My JUNK FOOD DETOX FOR KIDS is a 3 day diet. Avoid all highly processed, junky foods, red meats and dairy foods, except yogurt during this detox.

—**On rising:** give citrus juice with 1 teaspoon of acidophilus liquid, or a glass of lemon juice and water with honey or maple syrup.

—**Breakfast:** offer fresh fruits, such as apples, pineapple, papaya or oranges. Add vanilla yogurt or rice milk if desired.

—**Mid-morning:** give fresh carrot juice. Add ¼ tsp. ascorbate vitamin C or Ester C crystals to neutralize body toxins.

—**Lunch:** give fresh raw crunchy veggies with a yogurt dip; or a fresh veggie salad with lemon/oil or yogurt dressing.

—**Mid-afternoon:** offer a refreshing herb tea, such as licorice or peppermint tea with honey.

—**Dinner:** give a fresh salad, with avocados, carrots, kiwi, romaine and other high vitamin A foods; and/or a cup of miso soup or other clear broth soup.

—**Before bed:** offer a relaxing herb tea, like chamomile tea. Add ¼ tsp. vitamin C or Ester C crystals; or a cup of MISO broth for strength.

Once the light detox is over, begin a healthy diet. Breakfast is a key for weight loss for kids. A high fiber breakfast cuts a child's calories by up to 200 calories a day and holds appetite until lunchtime. Add fresh plant, enzyme-rich foods to the child's diet. Many of today's diets don't work because they rely on microwaved foods - a process that kills the enzymes. Enzyme dead foods create a nutritional gap for our kids (some experts say we would die if all we ate was micro-waved foods). For some children, this also means weight gain and constipation, a major problem for kids that eat a lot of dairy foods like milk, cheese and ice cream. 20% of Caucasian children and 80% of black children don't produce lactase, the enzyme necessary to digest milk. **#1 GREEN DRINK FOR KIDS:** Make it easy in a juicer. Use any fresh veggies that your child likes most. Include green leafy vegetables like spinach, sunflower greens and lettuces. I find that kids like baby veggies. Consider baby bok choy, baby carrots and sprouts. Don't forget sweet tasting veggies like cucumbers, celery and tomatoes. **#2 ENERGIZING FRUIT SMOOTHIE:** Use fresh fruit, not canned or frozen. Blend 1 banana and 1 orange with apple juice. Add half a papaya or one-quarter of a fresh pineapple.

Two enzyme rich juice recipes that even the pickiest of kids will ask for again and again.

If you don't have a juicer, give your child a good plant enzyme supplement to keep his metabolism going strong, like •Transformation's powdered DIGESTZYME, a quality product I've worked with. Check out my small library series book WEIGHT LOSS & CELLULITE CONTROL for a complete kid's weight loss diet and more tips. It has passed many tests for foods overweight and "couch potato" kids will eat. It focuses on good nutrition, so your child will have less craving for junk foods.

Can't find a recommended product? Call the 800 number listed in Product Resources for the store nearest you.

Weight Control After 40... It Isn't Easy

Everybody faces a disconcerting body thickening and a slow rise in weight in their 40's and 50's.... even people who have always been slim, who have a good diet, and who regularly exercise. Body fat typically doubles between the ages of 20 and 50. Both men and women go through a change of life in middle years that affects body shape. For women, a major calorie-burning process grinds to a halt after menopause, because her menstrual cycle consumes extra calories. Metabolism rises in the last two weeks of a menstrual cycle accounts for up to 20,000 calories per year, calories that start to add up when menstruation ceases! Women also develop more deep abdominal fat (but less fat around their hips and thighs) as estrogen levels drop with menopause. A woman needs to work a little harder to lose extra fat later in life. but once her body adjusts to its new hormone levels, weight gain stabilizes, and in many cases, falls back to premenopausal levels. Lower testosterone levels in andropausal men mean a decrease in muscle mass and increase in fat storage. By cutting back on fat and adding more fiber, most men can avoid middle-age spread. —**Add calcium (and magnesium) to your weight loss program after 40!** Large studies reveal a new diet fact. People over 40 on weight control diets lose weight if they have enough calcium but struggle to lose weight if their calcium is low. Magnesium works with calcium on a weight control diet because serotonin (a natural appetite suppressant) needs magnesium and Vitamin B₆ to activate. Herbal calcium formulas like Crystal Star CALCIUM MAGNESIUM SOURCE™ caps or Flora CALCIUM liquid have high absorbability and natural calcium-magnesium balance; for regular calcium sources, take at least 1600mg a day with 800mg magnesium or take Lane Labs ADVACAL ULTRA FAST RELEASE (excellent results). —**For weight loss after 40:** 1) Improve body chemistry at the hormone level; 2) Re-establish better metabolic rates.

#1 LOVE YOUR LIVER. The liver is your body's chemical plant responsible for fat metabolism. It is intricately involved with hormone functions, so it is the prime target to optimize for weight loss after 40. Weight gain and energy loss signal a liver that has enlarged through overwork, alcohol exhaustion and congestion. A good calorie-burning herbal formula with ginseng works extremely well. I have used •Crystal Star's THERMO THINNER™ caps along with CELLULITE RELEASE™ caps with success. •Gaia Herbs GINSENG SUPREME is a good choice; or add liver tonics: fresh vegetable juices, dandelion greens, milk thistle seed extract (accelerates liver regeneration by a factor of four). •Planetary BUPLEURUM LIVER CLEANSE; or •Herbs Etc. LIVER TONIC; or a liver tea: 4-oz hawthorn berries, 2-oz. red sage, and 1-oz. cardamom seeds. Steep 24 hours in 2 qts. water. Add maple syrup. Take 2 cups daily.

#2 CONSCIOUSLY EAT LESS. As metabolism slows, you don't need to fuel it up as much, because your body doesn't use up nutrients like it once did. If you eat like you did in your 20's and 30's, your body will store too much, mostly as fat. New research shows that moderate food intake may extend lifespan as much as ten years! —**Make sure you are eating a low fat diet.** Even with all the fat-conscious foods on the market today, Americans still consume one-third of their calories as fat. Your fat intake should be about 20% for weight control, 15% or less for weight loss. But remember: no-fat is not good for weight loss. Your body goes into a survival mode if you eliminate all fat, shedding its highly active lean muscle tissue to reduce your body's need for food. When lean muscle tissue decreases, fat burning slows or stops. —**Portion control is the cornerstone of weight control.** Eat smaller meals every 3 hours to keep your appetite hole from gnawing, and your metabolic rate high. Small meals virtually prevent carbohydrates and proteins from being converted into fat. Try an herbal control supplement to help. •Transformation LIPOZYME caps with active enzymes keep food from depositing as fat storage. —**Control hunger with safe herbal appetite suppressants.** Serotonin is the brain chemical linked to mood and appetite. Serotonin balancers like St. John's wort, 5-HTP, and evening primrose oil help stabilize mood and reduce food cravings. •Crystal Star TUMMY BULGE™ caps can help. Or take a green drink with herbs like barley grass, spirulina, sea greens and alfalfa such as •Crystal Star's ENERGY GREEN RENEWAL™ in mid-afternoon to decrease craving for high-calorie foods. —**Control cravings:** The herb gymnema sylvestre helps control sugar cravings, binding with sugar receptors in the mouth, causing sugary foods to lose their appealing sweet flavor, an effect that can last for up to 2 hours. Seven different clinical studies show garcinia cambogia or HCA (hydroxycitric acid) reduces food intake an amazing 46%. Try •Gaia DIET SLIM, or Crystal Star SUGAR CONTROL formulas to reduce blood sugar reactions that contribute to cravings and weight gain.

#3 RAISE YOUR METABOLISM. A higher metabolic rate means you burn more fat, lose weight easier, and maintain ideal body weight more comfortably. •Crystal Star THYROID META MAX™ caps and guggul 3000mg a day can help. —**Don't skip meals....** especially breakfast. Breakfast is the worst meal to skip if you want to raise metabolism. It sends a temporary fasting signal to the brain that food is going to be scarce. So stress hormones increase, and the body begins shedding lean muscle tissue in order to decrease its need for food. By the time you eat again, your pancreas is so sensitized to a lack of food, that it sharply increases blood insulin levels, your body's signal to make fat. Eat early in the day, when metabolism is at its best with hours of activity ahead to burn fats for weight loss. Reduce both sugars and fats - they slow metabolism. Fats have twice the calories, gram for gram, as protein and complex carbohydrates. Fats use only 2% of their calories before the fat storage process begins. Protein and carbohydrates burn almost 25% of their calories before storing them as fat. Limit alcohol consumption, even wine, to two glasses or less a day. With 7 calories per gram, alcohol sugars shift metabolism in favor of fat depositing. —**Eat fat-burning foods.** Fresh fruits and vegetables (full of enzymes), raise metabolism. Have an 8-oz glass of green tea and fruits for breakfast or between meals (if taken with or after meals, the fructose is likely to be converted to fat by the liver). Sea greens work especially well for women to recharge metabolism and thyroid action. Sea greens are also a rich source of vitamins D and K which help balance estrogen and DHEA.

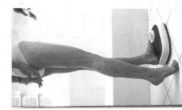

Can't find a recommended product? Call the 800 number listed in Product Resources for the store nearest you.

Try toasted nori, arame, dulse and sea palm, to recharge metabolism after menopause. Add 2 tablespoons chopped and dried to any salad, soup, rice dish or omelet for an active dose. Or add 6 pieces of sushi daily. —**Re-activate your fat-burning systems with herbs.** Herbs like *panax ginseng* and *Siberian eleuthero, suma, gotu kola,* and *licorice root* normalize body homeostasis; *ginkgo biloba* and *hawthorn* boost circulation; *bee pollen, alfalfa,* and phytohormone-containing herbs like *sarsaparilla* and *black cohosh* support the liver; spices and sea greens like *cayenne, ginger, kelp* and *spirulina* help the thyroid govern metabolism. •Crystal Star THYROID META-MAX™ caps greatly enhance fat burning. —**To increase lean muscle tissue as well as improve fat burning:** An herbal fat burner with coleus forskohlii before meals offers a thyroid-metabolic boost and longer calorie burning. —L-Phenylalanine (LPA), suppresses appetite, boosts energy, reduces food craving. (Avoid phenylalanine if taking anti-depressant medication, have high blood pressure, or are pregnant.) —L-Tyrosine is a thyroid precursor and reduces appetite. —L-Carnitine suppresses appetite, accelerates fat metabolism and helps control sugar levels. Amino acids combined in a formula like •AMINO BALANCE by Anabol Naturals work extremely well. —**Drink at least six 8-oz glasses water daily,** even if you're not thirsty. Water may be the most important catalyst for increased fat burning, because it increases the liver's main functions of detoxification and metabolism to process more fats. Water naturally suppresses appetite, helps maintain a high metabolic rate, promotes good digestion, regular bowel movements, and actually reduces fat deposits. Don't worry about fluid retention. High water intake actually lessens bloating, because it flushes out sodium and toxins. Studies show that *decreasing* water intake *increases* fat deposits. Expert dieters drink 8 glasses of water a day. They know each pound of fat burned releases 22 ounces of water which is flushed away along with fat breakdown. PENTA bottled water tastes great and rehydrates fast.

#4 EXERCISE FOR SURE. Strive for regular exercise. It's the key to permanent, painless weight control. Regular exercise extends life-span and cuts the risk of heart attack in half! But, recent statistics from the National Institutes of Health find that 58% of adult Americans get no or little exercise. No diet will work without exercise; with it, almost every diet will. Exercise before a meal raises blood sugar levels, increases metabolism and decreases appetite, often for hours afterward. Even with just a slight change in eating habits, you can still lose weight with a brisk hour's walk. Aerobic exercise, combined with a low fat, low calorie, fresh foods diet is particularly good for women. One study shows that overweight women who cut their calories and add an aerobic exercise program significantly reduce their PMS problems like mood swings and poor concentration. They have lower blood levels of monoamine oxidase (an enzyme linked to PMS).....and they lose an average of 36 pounds. Good exercise for women with the little tummy bulge that appears at menopause? Do hard tummy sucks to the count of 100 each morning. It works! —**Get out in the sun.** The sun receives a lot of criticism today, but sunlight is a natural serotonin trigger. In moderation, it increases metabolism and food digestion. One of the best choices is to eat outdoors. Sunlight can produce metabolic effects in the body similar to that of physical training.

Thermogenesis is critical to weight loss after 40. Thermogenesis is about fat burning. About 75% of the calories you eat work to keep you alive and support your resting metabolic rate. The rest are stored as white fat, or burned up by brown adipose tissue, (BAT), your fat-burning factory. The more active your brown fat is, the better your thermogenesis and the easier it is to maintain a desirable weight. Dieters who rely solely on restricting their calorie intake usually end up disappointed, because extreme calorie restriction lowers the rate of thermogenesis. Your body actually burns less fat than it did before you started dieting. People who yo-yo on and off low calorie diets have even more problems. When a yo-yo dieter begins to increase calorie intake after dieting, their metabolic rate does not return to pre-diet levels, so they store more calories as fat than they did before they started!

Middle-aged spread means too little thermogenesis after you eat. Everybody increases metabolism after eating, but the amounts of calorie burning vary widely. Lean people experience a 40% increase after a meal. Overweight people may have only an increase of 10%. Obesity occurs primarily when brown fat isn't working properly, only a little thermogenesis takes place, and the body deals with the excess calories by storing them as fat. Starting in our early 40's, a genetic timer shuts down the thermogenic mechanism. Turning this timer back on is the secret to re-activating thermogenesis and a more youthful metabolism. Here's how brown fat works to stimulate thermogenesis: A protein, called uncoupling protein, breaks down, or uncouples, the train of biochemical events that the cells use to turn calories into energy. Brown fat cells continue to convert calories into heat as long as they are stimulated, and as long as there is white fat for them to work on. Brown fat activity is self-perpetuating, automatically producing more brown fat cells, resulting in substantially more excess calories being burned off as heat through thermogenesis.

Research into the genetics of obesity shows that some people are born without enough brown fat. People who eat lightly but still can't lose weight, gain more weight at middle age because their small amount of brown fat is reduced even more. Thermogenic herbs like *Green tea, sida cordifolia, Siberian eleuthero, guarana* and *capsicum* can reactivate brown fat in middle age. •Thermogenic herbs boost blood flow to lean muscle tissue so it works faster and longer. •Thermogenic herbs help you eat less with less effort. •The longer you take thermogenic herbs, the more effective they become, because they help your body burn enough calories to make a difference. Crystal Star THIN AFTER 40™ caps contain liver support herbs, appetite control herbs, thermogenic herbs and metabolism boosters. If you put on pounds from fats and starches, add Transformation DIGESTZYME.

Weight loss is not easy in today's lifestyle. Reaching your ideal weight is a victory. Keeping it requires vigilance.

Can't find a recommended product? Call the 800 number listed in Product Resources for the store nearest you.

Weight Loss

Diet and Lifestyle Support Therapy

Nutrition diet watchwords: *Have 2 high fiber apples every day!*

1—The importance of cutting back on saturated fat cannot be overstated. Saturated fats are hard for the liver to metabolize. Focus on healthy fats from seafood, sea greens, nuts and seeds which curb cravings by initiating a satiety response. Fat isn't all bad. It's your body's chief energy source. Most overweight people have too high blood sugar and too low fat levels. This causes constant hunger; the delicate balance between fat storage and fat utilization is upset; your ability to use fat for energy decreases. Eating fast, fried, or junk foods aggravates this imbalance. You wind up with empty calories and more cravings. Fat becomes non-moving energy; fat cells become fat storage depots. But don't replace fats with fat substitutes like Olestra. Eating a one ounce portion of olestra potato chips on a daily basis reduces blood carotene levels by 50%! Fake fats fool your tastebuds, not your stomach. In one study, people who replaced 20% of their fat with fake fats were still hungry at the end of the day and ate twice as much food as normal!

2—Water can get you over diet plateaus. Dehydration slows resting metabolic rate (RMR) and can cause waste products like ketones to build up. Drink juices in the morning to wash out waste products. Don't eat carbs at night, you'll bloat in the morning.

3—A little caffeine after a meal raises thermogenesis (calorie burning) and boosts metabolic rate. Consider Crystal Star DR. VITALITY™ tea or caps. Use fat burning spices like *ginger, cinnamon, garlic, mustard and cayenne.*

—Bodywork:

•Daily exercise releases fat from cells. A brisk walk burns calories and cuts cravings. An outdoor walk in winter raises low serotonin levels. Exercise early in the day raises metabolism as much as 25%! Exercising before breakfast helps the body dip into its fat stores for quick energy and curbs the munchies all day. Even if eating habits just slightly change, you can still lose weight with a brisk hour's walk or 15 minutes of aerobic exercise.

•One pound of fat represents 3500 calories. A 3 mile walk burns up 250 calories. In about 2 weeks you'll lose a pound of real extra fat. That's 3 pounds a month and 30 pounds a year without changing your diet. It's easy to see how cutting down even moderately on fatty, sugary foods in combination with exercise can provide the look and body tone you want. Exercise promotes an afterburn effect, raising metabolic rate from 1.00 to 1.05-1.15 per minute up to 24 hours afterwards. Calories are burned at an even faster rate after exercise.

•Weight training increases lean muscle mass, replacing fat-marbled muscle with lean muscle. Muscle tissue burns calories; the more lean muscle you have, the more calories you can burn… important as aging decreases muscle mass. Exercise before a meal raises blood sugar levels and decreases appetite, often for several hours afterward. Deep breathing exercises increase metabolic rate and reduce stress. See pg. 250.

Herbal, Superfood and Supplement Therapy

Interceptive therapy plan: Choose 2 or more recommendations.

1—**Stimulate BAT (brown adipose tissue) thermogenesis:** •Evening Primrose oil 3000mg daily or Health from the Sun SUNPOWER CLA caps; •L-carnitine, up to 4000mg daily; •Arginine/ornithine 1000mg at bedtime. •Crystal Star THERMO THINNER caps (women); •Gaia DIET SLIM; •Source Naturals DIET PHEN with *hoodia extract* capsules; •Esteem TRIM & FIRM AM & PM; •Diamond Herpanacine DIAMOND TRIM. •Nature's Secret ULTIMATE WEIGHT LOSS; •Health from the Sun LEAN FOR LESS program.

—**Deficiencies can lead to food binges:** •B-complex with extra B-6 200mg (boosts serotonin and metabolizes carbohydrates); lack of minerals can lead to sugar craving: •Crystal Star OCEAN MINERALS™ or •Eidon ZINC liquid.

2—**Raise serotonin to control food cravings:** Crystal Star TUMMY BULGE™ with *St. John's wort,* a serotonin stimulant or WILLPOWER™ caps with *hoodia,* an appetite suppressant. •phenylalanine 500mg before meals (unless sensitive to phenylalanine): Try •chromium picolinate 400mcg; •L-glutamine 2000mg or •gymnema sylvestre for sugar cravings. •Spirulina and bee pollen for energy proteins and blood sugar balance. •Rainbow Light GARCINIA MAX DIET SYSTEM. •NADH 5mg in the morning for an energy lift and to help drop those last five pounds. •*Ginkgo biloba* extract 2-3x a day to help reduce stress linked to weight gain around the middle (not if you are taking Warfarin).

—**Superfoods help block appetite:** •Wakunaga HARVEST BLEND; •Crystal Star ENERGY GREEN RENEWAL™ (men); •Metabolic Response Modifiers WHEY PUMPED; •Esteem Products GREEN HARVEST; •All One MULTIPLE with green plant base.

3—**Natural fat blockers:** Crystal Star DETOX FAT & SUGAR RELEASE™ for a quick cleanse. Then, fat digesting enzymes, like •Transformation LYPOZYME; or garcinia cambogia in formulas like •Planetary TRIPHALA GARCINIA. Pyruvate aids in transforming blood sugar into energy; •Twin Lab PYRUVATE FUEL. Chitosan reduces dietary fat and cholesterol absorption; Natural Balance FAT MAGNET. (Gastrointestinal problems may result from excess use of pyruvate or chitosan.)

4—**Good fats help burn bad fats:** •CLA (conjugated linoleic acid) 3000mg daily (excellent results); •Barleans omega-3 flax oil or Udo's PERFECTED OIL BLEND for binging; •Richardson Labs CHROMA-SLIM lipotropic-carnitine formula.

5—**Boost metabolism:** Jump start weight loss with calcium, about 1600mg daily or Lane Labs ADVACAL ULTRA FAST RELEASE. •Genesis Today 4 WEIGHT CONTROL to help regulate thyroid or •Enzymatic Therapy THYROID/TYROSINE caps. For compulsive eating, tyrosine 1000mg with zinc 30mg daily. •Ayurvedic guggulsterone, like Solaray GUGGUL caps; •Crystal Star THYROID META MAX caps; or •Now Foods 7-KETO LEAN; •CoQ-10 (200mg daily turns fat into energy); •Bromelain 1500mg 3x daily for maximum metabolism (works amazingly well).

Can't find a recommended product? Call the 800 number listed in Product Resources for the store nearest you.

Look It Up!

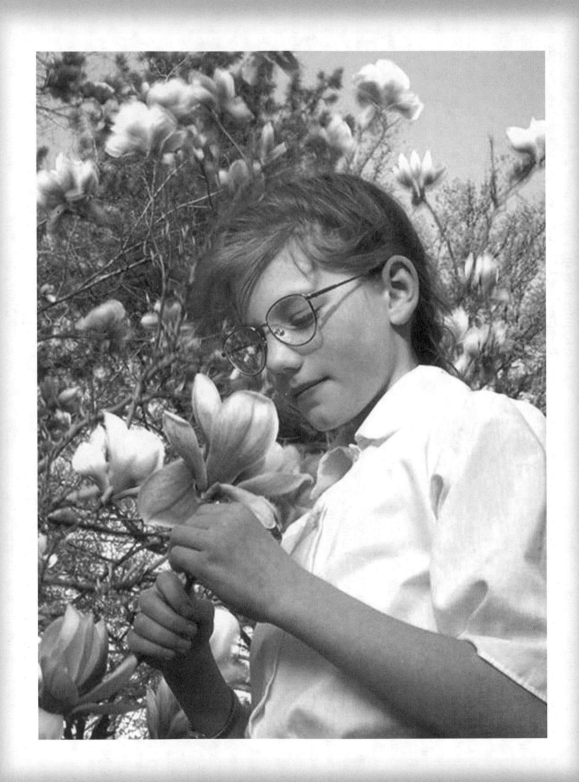

Your Natural Healing Arsenal
All you need to know about the help you need to get

This invaluable section is an encyclopedia-style reference that details the storehouse of alternative health care options available to Americans today. While covering all aspects of natural healing, the real value of this chapter lies in the information about effective alternative remedies, products, and healing techniques that consumers can access for themselves.

Look for general listings like Amino Acids, Antioxidants, B-vitamins or Raw Glandulars; check out the specifics of a special nutrient or herb, like DIM (*diindolyl-methane*), CoQ-10 or jiaogulan; look up important alternative healing procedures like anti-neoplaston therapy; get a clear understanding of current terms in the news like phyto-chemicals.

I've included a wealth of information from the latest worldwide research and testing, empirical observation, and alternative specialist and practitioner recommendations.

The survey is structured in easy-to-use alphabetical order—by name of substance, product, remedy or procedure. More than 350 entries are available in this exhaustive survey.

Just Look It Up!

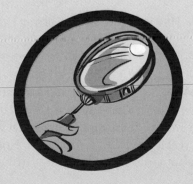

The Alternative Health Care Arsenal

Look It Up!

The alternative arsenal is an updated, exhaustive survey of the health care options available to Americans today. The value of this section lies in its quick reference data on effective alternative remedies, products and healing procedures that consumers can access for themselves. Information from worldwide studies, empirical observation, as well as natural healers and practitioners is included. The survey is structured in alphabetical order as an easy-reference guide. Access it by name of substance, product, remedy or procedure.

ACEROLA: derived from the ripe fruit of the cherry-like *Malpighia Glabra*, acerola is a rich source of vitamin C and bioflavonoids. Used as an antioxidant and for its ascorbic acid content.

• **ACIDOPHILUS CULTURE COMPLEX:** like *lactobacillus, bulgaricus, and bifida bacterium,* are beneficial bacteria that synthesize nutrients in the intestinal tract, counteract pathogenic micro-organisms like *candida albicans* and *E. coli,* and maintain a healthy intestinal environment. Acidophilus cultures also help auto-immune diseases that involve colon toxicity, like rheumatoid arthritis and chronic fatigue syndrome. Treats herpes simplex I and II, acne, mouth ulcers, even high cholesterol. Helps slow cancer growth, too. Use for digestion and for friendly flora restoration after protracted drug use.

• **ACONITE:** a homeopathic remedy for children's earaches. Helps the body deal with the trauma of sudden fright or shock. See HOMEOPATHIC REMEDIES on page 15.

• **ACUPUNCTURE AND ACUPRESSURE:** see ALTERNATIVE HEALING TECHNIQUES, pp. 33-35.

• **AGAR:** derived from *Gelidiella Acerosa*, a sea algae. Agar increases peristaltic action and relieves constipation. Agar can bond with heavy metals and radioactive toxins in the body, and help eliminate them.

• **ALANINE:** a non-essential amino acid which helps maintain blood glucose levels, particularly as an energy storage source for the liver and muscles. See also Amino Acids.

• **ALGAE, GREEN & BLUE-GREEN:** *phyto-plankton.* See GREEN SUPERFOODS, pg 100.

• **ALLYLIC SULFIDES:** organic sulphur compounds found in garlic and onions. Allylic sulfides act as powerful antioxidant compounds that inhibit bacterial and viral growth including staphylococcus, streptococcus and salmonella, and provide cardiovascular protection. They also lower cholesterol levels, decrease blood clotting, and as with all sulphur compounds, help skin tone and texture.

• **ALOE VERA,** *Aloe Barbadensis:* See HEALING POWERHOUSES OF THE DESERT, pg. 162.

• **ALPHA CAROTENE:** see Carotenoids.

• **ALPHA HYDROXY ACIDS (AHA'S):** naturally occurring substances found in foods like apples, grapes, citrus fruit, sugar cane and sour milk, as well as in the body. AHAs work by dissolving the glue-like lipids holding cells together, penetrating deep into the skin to loosen clingy bonds that clog and roughen skin. When top layers of skin are loosened and released they reveal a smoother complexion. Not all AHAs work the same. Glycolic acid from sugar cane acts fastest and deepest, but is also one of the most irritating.

Lactic acid from sour milk is often the AHA of choice because it doesn't penetrate as deeply so it's not as irritating. Tartaric acid from grapes, malic acid from apples, citric acid from citrus, and new synthetics, work only on or near the skin surface. They take longer to show improvement, but do not sting or redden the skin. Products advertised with high AHA's don't necessarily work better — only faster. The real difference is in the pH level of the product. Quicker results can be achieved from a product lower on the pH scale (2.5pH) than a product higher on the pH scale (4.5pH). Products between 3pH and 4.5pH have more moisturizing effects.

• **ALPHA-LINOLENIC ACID (LNA):** See FATS & OILS, page 134.

• **ALPHA LIPOIC ACID:** (alpha lipoic acid or thioctic acid) is a unique, "universal" antioxidant, both lipid and water soluble, able to quench free radicals in both fat and water mediums. It is among the most powerful liver detoxifiers ever discovered. Lipoic acid is a potent promoter of glutathione and an important co-factor in energy metabolism, especially in stress conditions. It also increases the effectiveness of other antioxidants, like vitamins C and E, showing great promise for heart disease (especially stroke recovery and atherosclerosis), diabetes (approved in Europe for diabetic retinopathy), neuro-degenerative diseases, such as Parkinson's and Alzheimer's, inflammatory diseases like arthritis and irritable bowel syndromes, HIV and AIDS, cataracts, heavy-metal toxicity and detoxification support. Helps with appetite control in a natural weight loss program. Note: Take with meals to prolong its delivery and to prevent a hypoglycemic response.

• **ALPHA TOCOPHEROL (vitamin E):** found in wheat germ, nut and seed oils, eggs, organ meats, oats and olives, vitamin E boosts fertility, improves circulation, promotes longevity, prevents blood clots, strengthens capillary walls, helps our bodies use vitamin A, maintains cell membrane health, and contributes to healthy skin and hair. Alpha tocopherol is an antioxidant proven in preventing heart disease, and protecting healthy cells from free radical destruction.

• **AMLA BERRY,** (Indian gooseberry) *Emblica Officinalis:* is one of the richest natural sources of bioflavonoids and vitamin C; each amla fruit contains up to 700mg of vitamin C. It is a natural ascorbate, synergistically enhanced by both bioflavonoids and polyphenols. Amla is revered for its anti-aging, immune enhancing properties. It has been used since ancient times for anemia, asthma, bleeding gums, diabetes, colds, chronic lung disease, hyperlipidemia, hypertension, yeast infections, scurvy and cancer. Studies show that amla protects against chromosome damage from heavy metal exposure.

• **AMINO ACIDS:** the 29 known building blocks of protein in the body — absolutely necessary to life, growth and healing. Protein is composed of, and depends upon the right supply of amino acids, from which over 1600 basic proteins are formed, comprising more than 75% of your body's solid weight of structural, muscle and blood protein cells. Amino acids are an important part of body fluids, antibodies that fight infection, and hormone-enzyme systems responsible for growth, maintenance and repair of our bodies throughout our lives. Amino acids are energy sources with a vital role in brain function, acting as neurotransmitters for the central nervous system. They are critical to rapid healing, and good acid-alkaline balance.

The liver produces about 80% of the amino acids it needs; the remaining 20% must be obtained from our foods. But poor diet, unhealthy habits and environmental pollutants mean that the "essential amino acids" (those we need but our bodies can't produce), may not be sufficient to produce the "non-essentials" (those formed by our metabolism). We can correct this situation by increasing intake of protein foods or supplementation (a food-source, pre-digested supplement may be used more quickly than dietary amino acids).

Specific amino acids produce specific pharmacological effects in the body, and can be used to target specific healing goals. Amino acids work well with other natural healers, like herbs, minerals and antioxidants.

The main amino acids are *Alanine, Arginine, Aspartic Acid, Branch Chain Aminos, Carnitine, Cysteine, Cystine, GABA, Glutamic Acid, Glutamine, Glutathione, Glycine, Di-methyl-glycine, Histidine, Inosine, Lysine, Methionine, Ornithine, Phenylalanine, Taurine, Threonine, Tryptophan, Tyrosine.* SEE REFERENCE BY NAME IN THIS CHAPTER.

<u>Tips for taking amino acids effectively</u>:
1: Take amino acids with extra water or other liquid for optimum absorption by the body.
2: If using a single free form amino acid, take a full spectrum amino acid compound sometime during the same day for increased absorption and results.
3: Free form aminos compete for uptake; take free forms separately from each other for best results.
4: Take single free form amino acids with their nutrient co-factors for best metabolic uptake.
5: Take free form amino acids, except those for brain stimulation, before meals.

Note: Amino acid names may be preceded by the letters "D," "L," or "DL." The prefixes are needed because many biological compounds exist in nature in two identical forms, except that they are mirror images of each other (like your right and left hands). In most cases, only one form is active in the body. "D" stands for dextro (right), "L" stands for levo (left). Sometimes the "D" form is active — D-glucose or D-alpha-tocopherol, sometimes the "L" form is active — L-carnitine or L-lysine, sometimes the "DL" form is active — DL-Phenylalanine. Only the active form is usually available for sale, so even if the initial isn't stated, the product is the active form.

• **AMINOPHYLLINE:** a theophylline-type extract of tea, is a primary ingredient in some spot reducing creams. How aminophylline works: fat cells are covered with switches called beta-receptors. When the body needs energy, beta-receptors release a substance that activates fat for fuel. But, long term storage cells, that reside in a woman's thighs and upper arms and on a man's belly, have only a few beta-receptors, so they hang on to their fat stores. Prolonging fat release in these cells can result in one to two inches of fat loss from fat depots. Aminophylline keeps fat releasing activated to prolong the mechanism of fat loss.

• **ANDROGRAPHIS:** a bitter herb native to India and Southern Asia, andrographis is credited for stopping the virulent Indian flu epidemic in 1919. A recent 1999 study shows good results for reducing cold symptom severity, too. One practitioner reports 70 to 80% effectiveness in reducing severe flu symptoms when andrographis is taken in the first 24 hours of onset. Andrographis has anti-inflammatory and antibiotic action, and works especially well in combination with vitamin C, bioflavonoids and echinacea.

• **ANDRO** (*Androstenedione*): a steroid hormone and a metabolite of DHEA, is naturally made in male and female gonads and the adrenal glands. A testosterone precursor, Andro is one step away from testosterone. Testosterone is a major player in development of male sex organs, muscles, body hair and in maintaining strength and energy. Serum levels of testosterone start rising about 15 minutes after oral administration of Andro, and stay elevated for up to 3 hours. Andro became a popular sports supplement in 1998 when baseball superstar, Mark McGwire revealed that he was taking it. Andro comes from Scotch pine tree pollen.

Is Andro safe? It's clearly a powerful hormone stimulant, not to be taken casually. We know very little about its long-term effects on health and hormone balance. In some men, Andro boosts testosterone levels too much, too fast, causing too much testosterone production, leading to aggressive behavior and acne.

…A study in the June 1999 JAMA finds that Andro may not always increase blood levels of testosterone, but may actually convert into estrogen. This especially concerns men, Andro's target market. Excess estrogen in males can increase risk for pancreatic cancer and heart disease. It also can cause side effects like enlarged breasts or water retention! In women, Andro may cause facial whiskers, chest hair growth or voice deepening.

<u>New information shows more serious concerns</u>.....
—After long-term Andro use, your body may perceive abnormal amounts of the hormone and may shut down natural testosterone production as happens with melatonin, another steroid hormone.
—Teens should be especially warned — abnormally high testosterone levels in kids can stunt growth and cause permanent heart and liver damage.
—Don't take Andro if you have prostate enlargement or cancers of the breast, prostate or testes.
—Avoid Andro if you have acne, liver disease, heavy menstruation or Cushing's syndrome.

• **ANTHOCYANIDINS:** flavonoids found in red wine, grape juice and grapes, blackberries, cherries, cranberry, blueberries (the richest food source), raspberries, bilberries, white pine and hawthorn herb. Anthocyanidins strengthen connective tissue like skin, tendons, ligaments and bone matrix. A very good choice for athletes who experience excessive free radical damage to connective tissue. (See OPC's for more.)

• **ANTI-NEOPLASTON THERAPY:** a relatively new cancer treatment developed by Dr. Stanislaw Burzynski. Antineoplastons consist of small peptides, components of protein, and peptide metabolites that are given orally or intravenously. They work by entering the cell and altering specific functions of the genes; some activate the tumor suppressor genes that prevent cancer, while others turn off the oncogenes that force the cancer cell to divide uncontrollably. Antineoplastons cause cancerous cells to either revert to normal or die without dividing. Burzynski first isolated the natural compounds from blood and urine in the early 1970's. He now synthesizes them at his own FDA regulated pharmaceutical lab. For complete information write to P.O. Box 1770, Pacific Palisades, CA 90272.

• **ANTIOXIDANTS:** Increasing evidence shows that people live more vigorous, less-diseased lives when antioxidants are a part of their nutritional program. This is especially true if a person shows signs of premature aging, reduced immune response, allergies, or is regularly exposed to environmental pollutants. Antioxidants unite with oxygen, protecting cells, and other body constituents like enzymes from being destroyed or altered by oxidation. Antioxidant mechanisms are selective, acting against undesirable oxygen reactions but not desirable oxygen actions. Although oxygen is vital to our body functions, either too much or too little oxygen creates toxic by-products called free radicals. These highly reactive substances can damage cell structures, impair immunity, even alter DNA codes — resulting in degenerative disease and premature aging. Free radical attacks are the forerunners of heart attacks, cancer, and opportunistic diseases such as HIV infection, candidiasis or chronic fatigue syndrome. Antioxidants "scavenge" or quench free radical fires, neutralize their damage and render them harmless. A poor diet, inadequate exercise, illness and long term emotional stress result in a reduction of the body's system antioxidants. See also Free Radicals, page 592.

Antioxidants you can use for protective health care and healing:
—**Alfalfa:** is rich in chlorophyll, which helps heal damaged tissue and promotes growth of new tissue. It is one of the oldest fatigue remedies known.

—**Barley Grass:** 3 times more potent than vitamin C, 2-0-GIV (2-O-glycosylisovitexin) derived from barley grass neutralizes free radicals linked to cell malignancies. Commercial barley grass products offer a therapeutic dose of 2-O-GIV.

—**Pycnogenol:** an antioxidant bioflavonoid extract of pine bark. 50 times stronger than vitamin E, 20 times stronger than vitamin C, pycnogenol crosses the blood-brain barrier to directly protect brain cells.

—**CoQ-10:** an essential catalyst co-enzyme for cellular energy in the body. Supplementation provides wide ranging therapeutic benefits. See ENZYMES & ENZYME THERAPY, pg. 19 for complete information.

—**Germanium:** A potent antioxidant mineral (*germanium sesquioxide*), that detoxifies, blocks free radicals and increases production of natural killer cells. An interferon stimulus for immunity and healing.

—**Ginkgo Biloba:** combats aging effects, especially boosting memory acuity and circulation. Helps protect cells against free radical damage. Reduces blood cell clumping leading to congestive heart disease.

—**Glutathione Peroxidase:** an antioxidant enzyme that scavenges and neutralizes free radicals by turning them into stable oxygen and H_2O_2, then into oxygen and water. See ENZYME THERAPY, pg.19.

—**SOD, Superoxide Dismutase:** an antioxidant enzyme that works with catalase to scavenge and neutralize free radicals. See ENZYMES & ENZYME THERAPY, pg.19.

—**Astragalus:** an herbal immune stimulant and body tonic that enhances adrenal function. Vasodilating properties lower blood pressure, increase metabolism and improve circulation.

—**Methionine:** a free radical deactivator; a lipotropic that keeps fats from accumulating in the liver and arteries. Protective against chemical allergic reactions.

—**Licorice:** offers immune-enhancing properties that increase the overall number of lymphocytes, and the activity of killer T-cells. It is antiviral and antibacterial, with powerful antioxidant properties. Tests indicate it may also have cancer-inhibiting properties.

—**Cysteine:** an antioxidant amino acid that works with vitamins C, E, and selenium to protect against radiation toxicity, cancer carcinogens, and free radical damage to skin and arteries. Stimulates immune white cell activity. Aids in the body's uptake of iron. Note: Take vitamin C in a 3:1 ratio to cysteine for best results.

—**Egg lipids, egg yolk lecithin:** a powerful source of choline and phosphatides. Used in treating AIDS and immune-deficient disease. Refrigerate; take immediately upon mixing with water to retain potency.

—**L-Glutathione:** an antioxidant amino acid that works with cysteine and glutamine to balance blood sugar; neutralizes radiation, inhibits free radicals; detoxes blood of chemotherapy, X-rays and liver toxins.

—**Wheat Germ Oil:** a wheat berry extract; rich in B vitamins, proteins, vitamin E, and iron. One tablespoon provides the antioxidant equivalent of an oxygen tent for 30 minutes.

—**Octacosanol:** a wheat germ derivative; often used by athletes to boost energy and increase oxygen use during exercise.

—**GLA, Gamma Linoleic Acid:** from evening primrose oil, black currant oil and borage seed oil. A source of cell energy, electrical insulation for nerves, a precursor of prostaglandins which regulate hormones.

—**Shiitake Mushrooms:** stimulates interferon for stronger immune function. Used in Oriental medicine to prevent high blood pressure and heart disease, and to reduce cholesterol.

—**Reishi Mushrooms** (*Ganoderma*): adapatogens that increase vitality, enhance immunity and prolong a healthy life. Helps reduce the side effects of chemotherapy for cancer.

—**Tyrosine:** an amino acid formed from phenylalanine — a GH stimulant that helps build the body's store of adrenal and thyroid hormones. A source of quick energy, especially for the brain.

—**Di-Methyl-Glycine** (DMG or B_{15}): an energy stimulant, used by athletes for endurance and stamina. Sublingual forms are most absorbable. For best results, take before sustained exercise. Note: Too much DMG disrupts the metabolic chain and causes fatigue. The proper dose produces energy; overdoses do not.

Some foods are also rich in antioxidants:

—**Selenium:** a component of glutathione; protects the body from free radical and heavy metal damage. Food sources: bran, brewer's yeast, broccoli, cabbage, celery, corn, cucumbers, garlic, mushrooms, onions, wheat germ and whole grains.

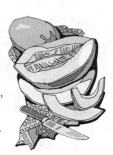

—**Vitamin E:** a fat soluble antioxidant and immune stimulant whose activity is increased by selenium. Neutralizes free radicals against aging; an effective anticoagulant and vasodilator against blood clots and heart disease. Food sources: almonds, soy, walnuts, apricots, corn, safflower oil, peanut butter, wheat germ.

—**Beta-carotene:** a vitamin A precursor, converting to vitamin A in the liver as needed. A powerful anti-infective and antioxidant for immune health, protection against pollutants, early aging and allergy control. Food sources: yellow and orange fruits and vegetables, and sea greens.

—**Vitamin C:** a primary preventer of free radical damage. Boosts immune strength, protects against infections; safeguards against radiation, heavy metal toxicity, environmental pollutants and early aging. Essential in forming new collagen tissue, supports adrenal and iron insufficiency, especially when you're under stress. Food sources: broccoli, lemons, grapefruit, bell peppers, kale, kiwi, oranges, potatoes, strawberries.

Note: Take vitamins A, C, E, selenium and beta carotene together for the most cancer-fighting potential.

• **ANTI-CARCINOGENS:** anticarcinogens are substances that prevent or delay tumor formation and development. Some herbs and foods have anti-carcinogenic properties: *panax ginseng, soy foods, garlic, echinacea root, goldenseal, licorice, black cohosh, wild yam, sarsaparilla root, maitake mushroom, reishi mushroom, shiitake mushroom, and cruciferous vegetables like broccoli and cabbage.*

• **ANTI-PARASITIC NUTRIENTS:** parasites are extremely common and persistent around the globe. Parasites have adapted and become stronger in order to survive, developing defenses against drugs designed to kill them. In fact, most drugs commonly used to treat parasites not only lose effectiveness against new parasite strains, but also cause a number of unpleasant side effects in the host. Herbal remedies, however, have been successfully used for centuries as living medicines against parasites, with few side effects. Natural antiparasitic herbs include *black walnut hulls, garlic, pumpkin seed, gentian root, wormwood, butternut bark, fennel seed, cascara sagrada, mugwort, slippery elm and false unicorn rt.*

• **ARGININE:** a semi-essential amino acid, augments growth hormone and regulates the thymus for immune health. For athletes and body builders, arginine increases muscle tone while curbing appetite and metabolizing fat for weight loss. Helps lower blood serum fats, and detoxifies excess ammonia. Promotes wound and skin healing, blocks tumor formation and increases sperm motility. Boosts nitric oxide (NO) production, optimizing both circulation and sexual function in men *and* women. Herpes virus and schizophrenia can be checked by "starving" them of arginine foods like nuts, peanut butter or cheese. Take with cranberry or apple juice for best results.

• **ARNICA:** a homeopathic remedy for pain relief and to speed healing, especially from sports injuries, like sprains, strains and bruises. May be used topically or internally. See HOMEOPATHIC REMEDIES pp. 12-18.

• **AROMATHERAPY:** see ALTERNATIVE HEALING CHOICES, pp. 42-48.

• **ARROWROOT:** powdered cassava herb, used as a thickener for sauces. Arrowroot works without the digestive, elimination and vitamin loss cornstarch can cause.

• **ARSENICUM ALBUM:** a homeopathic remedy for food poisoning accompanied by diarrhea; for allergic symptoms such as a runny nose; for asthma and colds. See HOMEOPATHIC REMEDIES pp. 12-18.

• **ARTICHOKE LEAF EXTRACT:** A liver protector and gentle diuretic, artichoke leaf extract increases bile flow and may help decrease hepatitis risk. Lowers "bad" LDL cholesterol and blood pressure by increasing cholesterol excretion and decreasing cholesterol synthesis in the liver. A proven remedy for indigestion and heartburn (improves digestion of fats and intestinal movement). Cautioned for people with gallstones.

• **ASPARTAME:** FDA has received more complaints about adverse reactions to aspartame than any other food ingredient in the agency's history. See SUGAR & SWEETENERS IN A HEALING DIET, pp. 145-153.

• **ASPARTIC ACID:** a non-essential amino acid, abundant in sugar cane and beets; used mainly as a sweetener. A precursor of threonine, it is a neurotransmitter made with ATP that increases your resistance to fatigue. Clinically used to counteract depression and in drugs to protect the liver.

• **ASTRAGALUS:** a prime immune enhancing herb, it is a strong antiviral agent, working to produce extra interferon in the body. Astragalus counteracts immune-suppressing effects of cancer drugs and radiation. Vasodilating properties help significantly lower blood pressure, reduce fluid retention, improve circulation. Research shows that astragalus is an anti-clotting agent in preventing coronary heart disease. Nourishes exhausted adrenals to combat fatigue. Effective in normalizing the nervous system and hormone balance.

BARLEY GRASS: See GREEN SUPERFOODS, page 100.

• **BEE POLLEN:** collected by bees from male seed flowers, mixed with bee secretions, then formed into granules. A highly bio-active, tonic nutrient rightly known as a superfood. Complete, balanced nutrients — vitamins, minerals, proteins, fats, enzyme precursors, and all essential amino acids.

Bee pollen is a full-spectrum rejuvenative food, especially beneficial for the extra nutritional and energy needs of athletes and those recovering from illness. A pollen / spore antidote during allergy season, bee pollen relieves respiratory symptoms like bronchitis, sinusitis and colds. Like royal jelly, pollen helps balance the endocrine system, with specific benefits for menstrual and prostate problems. Enzymes in bee pollen normalize chronic colitis and constipation-diarrhea syndromes. Research shows that pollen delays early aging effects increasing both mental and physical capability. Two teaspoons daily is a usual dose. Use only unsprayed pollen for therapy.

• **BEE PROPOLIS:** collected by bees from the resin under tree bark, propolis is the first line of defense against beehive infections. A strong, natural antibiotic and antifungal, in humans, propolis stimulates the thymus gland to enhance resistance to infection. Like all bee products, it is also a powerful anti-viral, effective against pneumonia and similar viral infections. Propolis is rich in bioflavonoids and amino acids, is a good source of trace minerals and high in B vitamins, C, E and beta-carotene.

—**Propolis has a wide range of healing uses:** it treats stomach and intestinal ulcers, speeds healing of broken bones and aids new cell growth. It is part of almost every natural treatment for gum, mouth and throat disorders. Research on propolis and serum blood fats confirms its value for lowering high blood pressure, reducing arteriosclerosis and lessening risk of coronary disease. Tests show healing effects on some skin cancers and melanomas. Propolis tincture may be applied to help warts, herpes lesions or other sores, mixed with liquids and taken internally, chewed as lozenges for mouth and gum healing. Dosage is 300mg daily.

• **BENTONITE:** a natural clay used for internal cleansing and externally as a poultice or mask.

• **BELLADONNA:** See Homeopathic Remedies, pp. 12-18 for sudden fever or sunstroke; for childhood fevers, stomach spasms or restless sleep.

• **BETA CAROTENE:** a vitamin A precursor, converting to vitamin A in the liver as needed. A powerful anti-infective and antioxidant for immune response, protection against environmental pollutants, the aging process, and allergy control. Supplements protect against respiratory diseases and infections. Beta carotene helps prevent lung cancer, and in developing anti-tumor immunity. Food sources: green leafy vegetables, green pepper, carrots and other orange vegetables, dandelion greens and sea vegetables. See Vitamins.

• **BETA-1, 3-D-GLUCAN:** a complex polysaccharide derived from baker's yeast. Other food sources: maitake, royal agaricus and reishi mushrooms, barley and oats. Beta glucan activates immunity by attaching to immune macrophages that engulf and render invading pathogens harmless. Speeds healing from wounds and reduces inflammation. Has anti-tumor activity for cancer protection. Especially promising as a preventive for colds, flu, and serious infections like sepsis and pneumonia. New reports find beta glucan also speeds recovery from sinusitis and bronchitis. A new winner in anti-aging skin care, studies show, used topically, beta glucan reduces wrinkles, improves skin texture and tone, renews skin elasticity, and fights skin dehydration. An injectable form shows promise against skin melanomas.

• **B COMPLEX VITAMINS:** B complex vitamins are essential to almost every aspect of body function, including metabolism of carbohydrates, fats, amino acids and energy production. B Complex vitamins work together. While the separate B vitamins can and do work for specific problems or deficiencies, they should be taken as a whole for broad-spectrum activity. See Vitamins.

• **BIOFEEDBACK:** see Alternative Healing Techniques, page 23.

• **BIOFLAVONOIDS:** part of the vitamin C complex, bioflavonoids prevent arteries from hardening, and enhance blood vessel, capillary and vein strength. They protect connective tissue integrity, and control bruising, internal bleeding and mouth herpes. Bioflavs lower cholesterol and stimulate bile production. They are antimicrobial against infections and inflammation. A major study shows that bioflavonoids, when combined with enzymes and vitamin C, perform as well as anti-inflammatory drug prescriptions in reducing swelling. They retard cataract formation, and guard against diabetic retinopathy. The body does not produce its own bioflavonoids; they must be obtained regularly from the diet. The strongest supplementary form is quercetin. Food sources include: blueberries, cherries, turmeric, ginger, alfalfa, the white part under the skin of citrus fruits and certain herbs like hawthorn and juniper berries. See Vitamins.

• **BIOTIN:** a B Complex member, needed for metabolizing amino acids and essential fatty acids, and for forming immune anti-bodies. Biotin helps your body use folacin, B_{12} and pantothenic acid. Naturally made from yeast, biotin supplements show good results in controlling hair loss, dermatitis, eczema, dandruff and seborrhea. It improves glucose tolerance in diabetics and shows enhanced immune response for Candida Albicans and CFIDS. If you take long term antibiotics, take extra biotin. Food sources: poultry, raspberries, grapefruit, tomatoes, tuna, nutritional yeast, salmon, eggs, organ meats, legumes and nuts. See Vitamins.

• **BITTERS:** herbs or substances with a bitter taste that promote the secretion of bile and hydrochloric acid. Bitters tone the muscles of the digestive tract, and improve nutrient absorption and waste elimination. They also enhance immune response, increasing levels of antibodies and improving gut resistance to infections. Beneficial for inflammatory bowel disease, chronic constipation, liver problems, lethargy and low energy. Best used in liquid preparations before meals. Examples of herbal bitters include: *gentian, lemon peel, goldenseal, dandelion, senna, angelica and Oregon grape.*

• **BORON:** a mineral which enhances the use of calcium, magnesium, phosphorus and vitamin D in bone formation and structure. Stimulates estrogen production to protect against the onset of osteoporosis. A significant nutritional deterrent to bone loss for athletes. Food sources: most vegetables, fruits and nuts.

• **BOSWELLIA:** *Boswellia glabra, Boswellia serrata* - an anti-inflammatory in Ayurvedic healing. Boswellia suppresses the proliferating tissue of inflamed areas and also prevents breakdown of connective tissue. Boswellia is highly effective for rheumatoid arthritis, osteoarthritis, low back pain, myositis and fibrocystitis.

• **BOVINE TRACHEAL CARTILAGE:** BTC is used to treat cancer, arthritis, rheumatism, acute and chronic skin allergies, and to accelerate the healing of wounds. BTC is a biological response modifier which activates and increases the ability of macrophages (white blood cells) to destroy bacteria and viruses. Paradoxically, BTC is a normalizer, stimulating the immune system to resist cancer and viruses, but suppressing it in rheumatoid diseases. Standard dosage of BTC is 9 grams daily.

• **BRANCH CHAIN AMINO ACIDS:** Leucine, Isoleucine, Valine (BCAAs) are essential amino acids called the stress amino acids; they must be taken together in balanced proportion. Easily converted into ATP, critical to energy and muscle metabolism, they aid hemoglobin formation, help stabilize blood sugar and lower elevated blood sugar levels. BCAAs show excellent results in tissue repair from athletic stress, rebuilding the body from anorexia deficiencies, and in liver restoration after surgical trauma.

• **BREWER'S YEAST:** See NUTRITIONAL YEAST and PROTEINS AND A HEALING DIET, pp. 98-99.

• **BROMELAIN:** an enzyme derived from pineapple stems, it is widely used to relieve painful menstruation and to treat all kinds of arthritis. Bromelain inhibits blood-platelet aggregation (clotting) without causing excess bleeding. It is an effective anti-inflammatory sports medicine to reduce bruising, relieve pain and swelling, and promote wound healing. It may be used externally as a paste applied to stings, to deactivate the protein molecules of insect venom. I highly recommend bromelain before and after surgery of all kinds to accelerate healing and reduce pain.

Typically, it is taken with meals, or 30 minutes before or 90 minutes after a meal to help treat sports injuries. See also ENZYMES & ENZYME THERAPY, pg.19.

• **BRYONIA:** a homeopathic remedy for the swelling and inflammation of arthritis when the symptoms are worse with movement and better with cold. Also for flu infections. See HOMEOPATHIC REMEDIES, page 12-18.

• **BUCKWHEAT:** (known as kasha when roasted) a non-wheat grain, OKAY for candida diets.

• **BURDOCK:** a hormone-balancer and strong liver purifier, burdock is a significant anti-inflammatory, antibacterial, antifungal and antitumor herb. A specific for blood cleansing, detoxification, immune enhancing combinations, it has special value for skin, arthritic and gland problems.

CALCIUM: the body's most abundant mineral, every cell needs calcium to survive. Calcium is necessary for synthesis of vitamin B_{12} and uses vitamin D for absorption. It works with phosphorus to build teeth and bones, with magnesium for cardiovascular health and skeletal strength. It helps blood clot, lowers blood pressure, prevents muscle cramping, maintains nerve health, deters colon cancer and osteoporosis, controls anxiety and depression, and insures quality sleep. Aluminum-based antacids, aspirin, cortisone, chemotherapy agents, calcium channel blockers and some antibiotics interfere with calcium absorption. Antibiotics, steroid drugs, heavy caffeine intake and smoking increase calcium needs. New reports reveal calcium may help prevent colon cancer by suppressing the growth of colon polyps. Calcium citrate has the current best record of absorbability.
Calcium may be more important for weight control than ever realized. Five different studies reveal that women with the lowest calcium levels weigh the most. High levels of calcium increase fat burning while low levels increase fat storage. And, a high calcium diet helps satisfy nutritional needs, reducing the food cravings that are the downfall of dieters. Note: The body leaches calcium from the bones if stores are in short supply. Good food sources: dark leafy greens, dairy foods, sea greens like nori, tofu, molasses and shellfish. Good herbal sources: lamb's quarters (1500mg per oz.), nettles, watercress, chamomile, valerian, pau d' arco bark. A high quality liquid herbal calcium preparation wih these herbs is highly bioavailable and works extremely well.
—**Calcium glucarate:** A natural compound of alfalfa sprouts, apples, grapefruit and broccoli. Best known as a cancer preventive, calcium glucarate (*D-Glucarate* is a derivative of calcium glucarate) stimulates glucuronidation, a body cleansing process that helps detoxify carcinogens. Used primarily against breast cancer; high doses, 10g per day given to women at high risk showed improvement without unpleasant side effects. Currently being tested as a possible prostate cancer preventive and for lung cancer. Found to lower cholesterol in animal tests.

• **CALCAREA FLUOR:** a homeopathic cell salt used to treat weak blood vessels, as found in hemorrhoids, varicose veins, hardened arteries and glands. See HOMEOPATHIC CELL SALTS, pp. 17-18.

• **CALCAREA PHOS:** a homeopathic cell salt used to strengthen bones and build blood cells. Deficiency results in anemia, emaciation, poor digestion and slow growth. See HOMEOPATHIC CELL SALTS, pp. 17-18.

• **CALCAREA SULPH:** calcium sulphate found in bile; promotes continual blood cleansing. When deficient, toxic build-up occurs in the form of skin disorders, respiratory clog, boils and ulcerations, and slow healing. Commonly used as a homeopathic cell salt. See HOMEOPATHIC CELL SALTS, pp. 17-18.

• **CAMPHOR:** Gum and bark are used therapeutically for a wide range of conditions. Camphor bark is best known for its key inclusion in an ancient Tibetan formula (Padma 28) designed to help promote healthy circulation. Within this complex formula, camphor relieves pain and reduces nerve sensitivity. Padma 28 is beneficial for Multiple Sclerosis, chronic viral hepatitis, PAO (peripheral artery occlusion) and intermittent claudication. The Padma 28 formula is available through Pacific BioLogic, now called Adaptrin. *Call 800-869-8783 for more info.*
—**Camphor Oil:** a mild antiseptic from the *cinnamonium camphora* tree, is used in skin preparations.

• **CANOLA OIL:** See Fats & Oils, pg. 130-131.

• **CANTHANXANTHIN:** see Carotenoids.

• **CAPRYLIC ACID:** a short-chain fatty acid long known for its antifungal action. Effective against all candida species, caprylic acid helps restore and maintain a healthy yeast balance. Caprylic acid is not absorbed in the stomach, making it an excellent choice for candida of the gut. Occurs naturally as a fatty acid in sweat, in cow's and goat's milk, and in palm and coconut oil.

• **CAPSICUM (cayenne):** Capsicum helps block production of "substance P" in the body, linked to the pain response. It reduces joint and muscular pain, and boosts circulation to the affected area (works on the central system), offering a cardiovascular lift by increasing circulation. Used topically, it is a superior pain reliever for arthritis, diabetic neuralgia, postherpetic neuralgia and fibromyalgia. *Note: may cause a mild burning sensation which normally disappears after a few applications.* Taken internally, cayenne is a wonderful tonic for the cardiovascular and digestive systems. *Capsicum* boosts calorie burning for weight loss, especially when combined with caffeine herbs or *ephedra*. Enhances the performance of other herbs in a formula.

• **CANTHARIS:** a homeopathic remedy for bladder infections and genito-urinary tract problems, especially if there is burning and urgency. Also good for burns. See Homeopathic Remedies, pp. 12-18.

• **CAROB POWDER:** a sweet powder with 45% natural sugars, made from the seed pods of a Mediterranean tree. It has a flavor similar to chocolate, but contains less fat and no caffeine.

• **CAROTENOIDS:** a major class of antioxidant nutrients used today to combat everything from infections and eye diseases to cancer. More than 600 have been identified; only a small handful have been studied extensively. While each carotenoid reviewed here is a proven health remedy by itself, a combination of carotenoids offers the most protection.
—**Alpha Carotene:** a vitamin A precursor. High food sources: carrots, pumpkin, and other red/orange and yellow fruits and veggies. Although alpha carotene has lower vitamin A activity than beta carotene, it is 38% stronger as an antioxidant and 10% more protective against skin, liver and lung cancer in animal tests.
—**Astaxanthin:** responsible for the pink pigment in the flesh of crustaceans, salmon, scallops, and some microalgae. Astaxanthin has 10 times the antioxidant activity as beta carotene, and 100 to 500 times the antioxidant capability of vitamin E. Boosts immune response; protects against Macular Degeneration. Able to cross the blood brain barrier, making it promising for Alzheimer's, Parkinson's, and ALS treatment.
—**Beta Carotene:** the most well know carotene, beta carotene is a vitamin A precursor, converting to vitamin A in the liver as needed. Food sources: spirulina, green leafy vegetables, green pepper, carrots and other orange vegetables, dandelion greens and sea greens. A powerful anti-infective and antioxidant for immune response, anti-tumor immunity protection, early aging and allergy control. Effective protection against environmental pollutants, respiratory diseases and infections. Helps prevent lung cancer.
—**Canthaxanthin:** an antioxidant carotenoid that improves immune response. Food sources: mushrooms, trout, crustaceans, like crab and mussels. Decreases skin cancer risk; inhibits other cancer cell growth.
—**Cryptoxanthin:** a vitamin A precursor. May reduce risk of cervical dysplasia. Food sources: corn, oranges and paprika, and other red/orange and yellow fruits and veggies.
—**Lutein and Zeaxanthin:** potent antioxidant carotenoids not converted to vitamin A (like beta-carotene). Of all carotenoids, lutein and zeaxanthin most support the eyes. They make up the yellow retinal pigment that specifically protects the macula. A Harvard study reports that people eating the most lutein and zeaxanthin foods are most likely to have healthy retinas and maculae. A new study shows high lutein diets also protect against colon cancer. Food sources: spinach, kale, most fruits and vegetables.

—Lycopene: a powerful antioxidant that gives many foods their reddish color, lycopene requires some fat to be absorbed in the body. A promising food medicine against cancer. Men who eat a high lycopene diet cut their risk for prostate cancer by 40%! The International Journal of Cancer reveals that lycopene also protects against cancers of the mouth, pharynx, esophagus, stomach, colon and rectum. A University of Illinois report shows that women with high lycopene levels have a 5 times lower risk for developing cervical cancer. A high lycopene diet may even cut heart attack risk in half! Food sources: tomatoes and in smaller quantities, watermelon, guava and pink grapefruit.

• **CARNITINE:** a vitamin-like amino acid, synthesized in the liver and kidney, and found principally in meat (hence the name carnitine). Carnitine's primary function is to facilitate fat metabolism by transporting long chain fatty-acid molecules into the mitochondria of cells where they are "burned" to produce energy (carnitine clearly increases the use of fat for energy). L-Carnitine enzymatically connects to the fatty acids, enabling them to cross the mitochondria membrane for fat breakdown. Although there are two forms, the D and L-isomers (mirror images of each other) only L-Carnitine is biologically effective. Signs of low carnitine include: fatigue, weight gain, high cholesterol and triglycerides, and weakened heart function.

Carnitine is very effective in speeding fat oxidation for weight loss. Further, high protein weight-loss diets cause ketosis, accumulation of fat waste ketones in the blood. Uncontrolled, ketosis in this type of weight-loss diet or in diabetes can be life-threatening. Carnitine prevents ketone build up.... a good idea if you are on the "zone" protein diet. Carnitine reduces ischemic heart disease by preventing fatty build-up. Its role in fat use helps prostaglandin metabolism and improves abnormal cholesterol-triglyceride levels. Good for sports enthusiasts to prevent muscle damage and delay lactate burn. May help patients with kidney failure who undergo dialysis, and people taking the cancer drug cisplatin or the chemotherapy drug ifosfamide, all of which deplete carnitine in the body. A specific for male infertility (increases sperm count and motility.)

—Acetyl-L-carnitine (ALC): is gaining a reputation as a nootropic (a brain nutrient) which can reduce age-related mental decline. ALC specifically increases alertness and attention span, improves learning and memory, and boosts eye-hand coordination.

• **CATECHIN:** the most abundant plant polyphenol, available in grapes, pomegranates, raspberries, huckleberries, strawberries and green tea. Catechin breaks up free radical cell chains of fats, prevents DNA damage, helps block carcinogens, and protects against digestive and respiratory infections. Green tea catechins show excellent antioxidant effects on fatty foods. Antioxidant properties of green tea catechins are 30 times more powerful than vitamin E and 50 times more potent than vitamin C.

• **CAT'S CLAW,** *(Una de Gato, uncaria tomentosa):* a rainforest botanical with a wide spectrum of therapeutic uses. It contains an immune stimulating oxindole alkaloid, isopteropodine that enhances the phagocyte (eater) ability of white blood cells and macrophages. A standardized compound with isolated active carboxyl-alkyl-esters has been found to also enhance the DNA repair process and lymphocyte function. Cat's claw helps cleanse the intestinal tract and heal numerous intestinal disorders, such as ulcers, Crohn's disease, diverticulitis, leaky bowel syndrome and colitis. Rich in antioxidant polyphenols and several plant steroids like beta-sitosterol, cat's claw is effective for cardiovascular health and hormone imbalances like prostate swelling and PMS. Other conditions that benefit from cat's claw include: arthritis, rheumatism, cancer, allergies, candidiasis, genital herpes, herpes zoster, HIV, bladder infections and environmental toxin poisoning.

• **CHAMOMILLA:** a homeopathic remedy for calming fussy children when they are crying because of pain, especially for teething pain. An aid in drug withdrawal. See HOMEOPATHIC REMEDIES, pp. 12-18.

• **CHARCOAL, ACTIVATED:** a natural agent that relieves gas and diarrhea. An antidote for almost all poisons. ***Note: For any case of poisoning, phone the Poison Control Center in your state.

• **CHITOSAN:** derived from a component in the exoskeletons of shellfish, chitosan is a natural product that reduces absorption of dietary fats and cholesterol in the intestines. Chitosan is an indigestible fiber that attaches to fat in the stomach before it is metabolized, then carries the fat (and cholesterol) through normal body channels to be eliminated instead of absorbed. A 1994 report showed that test subjects lost 8% of body weight in four weeks with chitosan. Note: Chitosan can interfere with the absorption of some minerals and fat-soluble vitamins..... gastrointestinal problems may result.

• **CHLORELLA:** See GREEN SUPERFOODS, page 100.

• **CHLORINE:** naturally-occurring chlorine stimulates the liver, bile and smooth joint-tendon operation. An electrolyte, it helps maintain acid/alkaline balance. Good food sources: seafoods, sea greens and salt.

• **CHOLINE:** a lipotropic, B complex family member, choline works with inositol to emulsify fats. A brain nutrient and neurotransmitter that aids memory and learning, and helps retard Alzheimer's disease and neurological disorders. It is a good part of any program to overcome alcoholism, liver and kidney disorders. Research shows success in cancer control. Helps dizziness, lowers cholesterol and supports liver function.

• **CHONDROITIN SULFATE A (CSA):** an anti-inflammatory agent from bovine cartilage. Use both topically and internally for problems like arthritic symptoms, circulatory and orthopedic therapy. Effective for cardiovascular disease. *Note: CSA may thin the blood. Avoid if taking other blood thinning drugs. CSA is contraindicated in prostate cancer.*

• **CHROMIUM:** an essential trace mineral needed for glucose tolerance and sugar regulation. Chromium deficiency means high cholesterol, heart trouble, diabetes or hypoglycemia, poor carbohydrate and fat metabolism, and premature aging. Chromium supplements can reduce blood cholesterol levels, increase HDL cholesterol levels, and diminish atherosclerosis. Most effective as a biologically active form of GTF (chromium, niacin and glutathione), it helps control diabetes through insulin potentiation. For athletes, chromium is a safe way to convert body fat to muscle. For dieters, chromium curbs appetite as it raises metabolism. Good food sources: nutritional yeast, clams, honey, whole grains, liver, corn oil, grapes, raisins.
　　—Chromium picolinate: an exceptionally bio-active source of chromium, it is a combination of chromium and picolinic acid, a substance secreted by the liver and kidneys. Picolinic acid is the body's best mineral transporter, combining with elements like iron, zinc and chromium to move them efficiently into the cells. Chromium helps weight control by sensitizing the body to insulin (fatty excess body weight tends to impair insulin sensitivity, making it harder to lose weight). Chromium picolinate helps build muscles without steroid side effects, promotes healthy growth in children, speeds wound healing and decreases proneness to arterial plaque accumulation. 200mcg of chromium picolinate seems to be the best dose.

• **CLA (conjugated linoleic acid):** an essential fatty acid, CLA converts the most energy from the least amount of food making it popular among athletes for nutrient-energy conversion, increasing muscle mass and burning fat. CLA studies were the first to show that fats can help you lose fat for weight loss. CLA especially inhibits body storage of saturated fat by increasing the use of fat reserves for energy. As other fatty acids, CLA has powerful antioxidants for immunity and shows remarkable results in lowering cholesterol.

• **COBALAMIN:** See Vitamin B_{12}. Cyanocobalamin may be made from sugar beets, molasses or whey.

• **COBALT:** an integral component mineral of vitamin B_{12} synthesis. Aids in hemoglobin formation. Good food sources: green leafy vegetables and liver.

• **COCONUT OIL:** See FATS AND OILS, pp. 130-131.

• **Co-ENZYME-A:** a metabolic enzyme critical to both aerobic and anaerobic energy metabolism. For example, co-enzyme-A is essential to the aerobic tricarboxylic acid cycle (the ATP, or Krebs cycle) which produces most of your body's energy, and helps release energy anaerobically from blood glycogen. Coenzyme-A is critical to fatty acid metabolism, too which helps your body maintain cholesterol and triglyceride levels. Co-enzyme-A deficiency means fatty acids cannot be converted into energy. Coenzyme-A starts the manufacture of acetylcholine in the brain and steroid hormones in the adrenal glands. Coenzyme-A activates white blood cells for immune response, contributes to hemoglobin formation and helps the body repair damaged RNA and DNA. Coenzyme-A helps make important components of connective tissue, like chondroitin sulfate and hyaluronic acid to keep joints flexible.

—**Pantethine:** a water soluble component of co-enzyme A derived from panthothenic acid. Although pantethine has been used in Japan for the past 30 years, in the U.S. we are just beginning to learn about its value. Research shows pantethine helps lower total cholesterol, LDL "bad" cholesterol, and triglycerides while increasing HDL "good" cholesterol that helps protect against heart disease. It's a good natural choice for diabetes and cholesterol management.

• **Co-ENZYME Q-10:** a vital enzyme catalyst in the creation of cell energy, Co-Q_{10} is synthesized in the liver. The body's ability to assimilate Co-Q_{10} declines with age; Co-Q_{10} supplementation has a long history of effectiveness in immune enhancement, raising cardiac strength against angina, promoting natural weight loss, inhibiting aging and overcoming gum disease (often when nothing else works). Co-Q_{10} is crucial in preventing and treating congestive heart and artery diseases. CoQ_{10} helps the heart muscle work stronger and more effectively. Studies show that quality of life improves for people with congestive heart failure, cardiomyopathy and mitral valve prolapse who take CoQ_{10} supplements. CoQ_{10} can reduce high blood pressure without other medication. Recent research showing effective doses of 300mg for breast and prostate cancer protection and treatment is extremely encouraging. Low levels of CoQ_{10} are also found in women with cervical and breast cancer; new treatment strategies should consider incorporating CoQ_{10} therapy. Food sources: dark green vegetables, alfalfa and barley grass, rice bran, wheat germ, beans, nuts, fish and eggs. Consider supplementing with Co-Q_{10} if you are taking drugs to lower cholesterol because these drugs can deplete Co-Q_{10}. Co-Q_{10} works synergistically in combination with vitamin E.

• **COLEUS FORSKOHLII:** an Ayurvedic herbal medicinal used for allergic conditions such as asthma and eczema. Forskolin in coleus forskohlii boosts the enzyme adenylate cyclase involved in smooth muscle relaxation, particularly helpful in relaxing bronchial muscles in asthmatics. Some research shows Coleus and Green Tea work together to modify the way adrenaline burns fat.... a boon to weight control. New studies also point to coleus in the treatment of psoriasis. Coleus seems to normalize out-of-whack cell division in psoriasis to reduce symptoms. Used frequently in extracts, coleus can be used alone or in conjunction with drug treatments.

• **COLLAGEN:** the most abundant protein of the body, is responsible for maintaining the integrity of vein walls, tendons, ligaments and cartilage. Collagen is similar to elastin and is the chief constituent in connective tissue. Connective tissue is dependant on nutrients from blood, so a healthy circulatory system aids in healthy skin, ligaments and tendons. (This is why smoking, a blood vessel constrictor, is so detrimental to connective tissue.) Exercise, a healthy diet and herbs like *ginkgo biloba, cayenne* and *garlic* help keep circulation healthy. *Horsetail herb*, high in silica, is an important trace mineral for connective tissue. Vitamin C complex, especially with OPC flavonoids, supports collagen growth and structure, and prevents collagen destruction. OPCs have the unique ability to reinforce the natural cross-linking of the collagen matrix of connective tissue.

• **COLLOIDAL MINERALS:** mineral preparations containing tiny mineral particles held in suspension in water by each particles' minute electrical charge. Proponents say colloidal minerals most closely resemble the way plants convert minerals pulled from the soil. Because of their tiny size, colloidal minerals may be better absorbed than other types of mineral preparations.

—**Colloidal Silver:** pure metallic ionic silver. Probably the most universal natural antibiotic substance, colloidal silver is not produced by a chemical process. It is tasteless, nonaddictive and nontoxic. Many forms of bacteria, viruses and fungi utilize a specific enzyme for their metabolism. Colloidal silver acts as a catalyst to disable the enzyme. It has proven toxic to most fungi, bacteria (including anthrax), parasites, and many viruses. Importantly, the bacteria, fungi and viruses do not seem to develop an immunity to silver as they do to chemical antibiotic agents. Cautions: Not for pregnant or nursing women. Not for long-term use because of depletion of friendly bacteria and, in very rare cases, a permanent blue-gray discoloration of the skin.

• **COLOSTRUM:** a mammary secretion in Mother's milk. It is rich in natural immune agents, *Immunoglobins IgG, IgA and IgM, Cytokines, Interferon, Nucleotides, Gamma Interferon, Orotic Acid, Lactobacillus bifidus acidophilus,* enzymes and vitamin A, E and B-12. It also contains lactoferrin and growth-enhancing factors. It triggers over 50 immune and growth processes in newborns. Colostrum supplements are obtained from bovine colostrum, with a higher concentration of IGF-1 (insulin growth factor 1) but a chemical structure virtually identical to that of humans. Studies using bovine colostrum show significant fitness improvements in stamina, muscle tone and growth, and shortened recovery time for athletes. It appears to increase bone density and returns elasticity to the skin. In adults, colostrum supplements help regulate immune response and inhibit the growth of a wide array of harmful pathogens. *Note: Choose a product from pasture-fed cows that are free of pesticides, antibiotics and hormones.*

• **COPPER:** a mineral that helps control inflammatory arthritis-bursitis symptoms. Aids in iron absorption, protein metabolism, bone formation and blood clotting. Helps prevent hair from losing its color. SOD (*superoxide dismutase*) is a copper-containing enzyme that protects against free radical damage. Copper deficiencies can be caused by mega-dose zinc therapy, or too much refined sugar. Deficiencies result in high cholesterol, anemia, heart arrhythmias and nervousness. Excess copper can result in mental depression.

• **CORDYCEPS MUSHROOM** *Cordyceps sinensis:* a mushroom-fungus used in traditional Chinese medicine as a tonic and energizer. Research suggests that cordyceps enhances immunity, increasing both T-cells and natural killer cell activity. Accelerates spleen regeneration, increases SOD (superoxide dismutase) activity, enhances oxygen uptake to the heart and brain, exhibits testosterone-like effects, improves libido and sperm count, and is effective in reducing uterine fibroid tumors (a specific against ovarian tumors). Increases life-span in animal lymphoma. A wonderful tool for recuperation from surgery, debility, fatigue, anemia or illness. Cordyceps took the spotlight in 1993 when a group of Chinese runners, previously considered mediocre, took a cordyceps-based tonic formula and broke nine world records!

• **COX-2- INHIBITORS** (Herbal): The COX-2 enzyme received a lot of media attention for its role in inflammatory diseases like arthritis and fibromyalgia. New research in the Journal of Clinical Investigation reveals COX-2 is also involved in the cancer cascade. Medical professionals are using COX-2 Inhibiting drugs to reduce tumor growth and increase the effectiveness of radiation treatments. But, COX-2 inhibitor drugs come with their own set of serious problems, like gastrointestinal bleeding. Herbal COX-2 inhibitors like *ginger, saw palmetto, rosemary, turmeric and green tea* may be better choices.

• **CREATINE** *(methyl guanidine-acetic acid):* is made naturally in the human liver, as creatine phosphate. Creatine is also found in red meat and fish. Creatine monohydrate supplements, with more weight of material than any other form, are popular with athletes today who want to gain weight and muscle mass, and increase their stamina. While research shows that using creatine along with an exercise program does increase lean body mass and muscle strength faster, creatine supplementation may cause an electrolyte imbalance. Creatine draws on water from other parts of the body. When using, drink lots of water.

• **CURCUMIN:** a constituent of *curcuma longa*, curcumin is a *turmeric* extract, the yellow spice used in curry. Curcumin is anti-inflammatory, it relieves arthritic symptoms, inhibits platelet aggregation; its fibrinolytic activity controls excess buildup of fibrin in blood vessels which can lead to blood clots. Curcumin increases bile secretion and protects against blood cholesterol rise from eating fatty foods. It is a powerful, oil-soluble antioxidant which can fight viruses. Curcumin inhibits tumor necrosis factor (TNF), a cytokine that increases HIV replication in T-cells. Numerous studies show the anti-tumor effect of *turmeric* and curcumin.

• **CYSTEINE:** a semi-essential antioxidant amino acid that works with vitamins C, E and selenium to protect against radiation, cancer carcinogens and free radical damage to skin and arteries. Stimulates immune white cell activity. Helps heal burns and surgery wounds, and renders toxic chemicals in the body harmless. Taken with evening primrose oil, cysteine protects the brain from alcohol and tobacco effects (highly effective in preventing hangover). Used for hair loss, psoriasis, dental plaque prevention and skin dermatitis. Relieves bronchial asthma by breaking down mucous plugs. *Note: Take vitamin C in a 3:1 ratio to cysteine for best results.*

　　—**N-acetyl-cysteine, NAC:** an antioxidant amino acid, a more stable, bio-available form of L-cysteine, converted in the body to glutathione, a prime immune T-cell enhancer (especially for people with HIV who have low glutathione). NAC detoxifies from alcohol, heavy metals, X-rays and radiation damage, treats viral diseases, protects the liver, and breaks up pulmonary-bronchial mucus. Reduces cold and flu symptoms. *Note: NAC is a powerful chelator of zinc and copper, capable of removing enough of these minerals from the body to produce deficiencies unless supplies are adequate.*

• **CYSTINE:** a semi-essential amino acid, cystine is the oxidized form of cysteine, and like it, promotes white blood cell activity, and heals burns and wounds. The main constituent of hair, essential to formation of skin. Cystine can sometimes be harmful to the kidneys, and should generally not be used clinically.

DEAD SEA SALTS: obtained from the Dead Sea in Israel, are composed of potassium, chlorine, sodium, calcium and magnesium salts, and sulfur and bromine compounds. Used in detoxifying baths.

• **DHA** *(docosahexaenoic acid):* the most predominant EFA in our brain tissue. Low levels of DHA are linked to mental problems like depression, memory loss, attention deficit/hyperactivity disorders, hostility, Alzheimer's disease, and senility. Studies show that DHA even protects against Alzheimer's and promotes clearer thinking. DHA can lower blood fats, and normalize high cholesterol and triglyceride levels. An 18-year study published in the journal Pediatrics reveals that breast-fed infants have academic advantage! The determining factor for this effect seems to be the high content of DHA in breast milk! Food sources include sea foods, sea plants and eggs.

• **DHEA,** *(dehydro-epiandro-sterone):* an abundant hormone produced from cholesterol by the adrenals, with smaller amounts made by female ovaries - part of an important cascade that ends in the making of estrogen and/or testosterone. DHEA helps maintain muscle and skin tone, and bone health. It stimulates immune defenses and T-cells to fight infections, and interferes with immune suppressive over-reactions (like lupus or rheumatoid arthritis) that attack the body. Research shows that HIV progression can be predicted by monitoring DHEA levels. (Full-blown AIDS does not develop until adrenal output of DHEA drops.)

　　…DHEA is effective therapy for menopause symptoms much the same as estrogen replacement, and for post-menopausal women with osteoporosis who are low in DHEA. Pre-menopausal women who have low levels of DHEA may develop breast cancer. Breast cancer risk associated with estrogen replacement therapy (ERT) is apparently reduced when DHEA is used, and may even be prevented by DHEA's immune support. (Animal studies show that mice susceptible to breast cancer do not develop it when treated with DHEA.)

　　…DHEA is of enormous interest as an anti-aging substance because it helps lower cholesterol, and promotes of energy and libido. Several studies show that DHEA does act as a kind of youth drug, because the older subjects who took it had more energy and muscle tone and better heart health. Yet, hormone activity is highly individual, so hormone test results are often inconclusive or contradictory. For example, a study shows that men with high DHEA levels have half the heart disease as those with low levels. But, women in the study with high DHEA have a <u>higher</u> risk of heart disease. Follow-up studies were even more contradictory, and didn't bear out long term DHEA benefits.

...DHEA has few side effects, but if you take too much, it suppresses your body's ability to make its own. People who get good results may have to take it for the rest of their lives to continue the results. Adult acne is a common side effect, as is excess face and body hair. DHEA dose falls between 5-15mg for women and 10-30mg for men. Most physicians today give it in combination with estrogen, progesterone and testosterone.

...DHEA supplements are synthesized from wild yam sterols. Unable to unravel all the actions of this complex plant, researchers currently disregard the idea that wild yam acts as a precursor to DHEA. But the fact that wild yam is used to manufacture both synthetic DHEA and synthesized progesterone shows that it works well for women's hormone problems that involve progesterone.

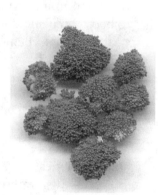

• **DIM** (*di-indolylmethane*): a plant indole found in cruciferous veggies like broccoli, cabbage, and cauliflower. DIM is the most biologically active cruciferous indole known. (Indole-3-carbinole must be converted into DIM to become active in the body.) —DIM might be called Nature's prescription for hormone harmony because of its role in natural hormone balancing therapy; it increases good estrogen metabolites, 2-hydroxy estrogens with antioxidant properties protect the brain and heart. DIM has a long history of safe use by both adults and children. As a fat soluble nutrient, DIM is best taken with a light meal along with healthy fats like those from seafood, or a flax oil dressing on a green salad. Dosage: 100-200mg for hormone balance, 200-400mg for men's health, 400mg for weight loss and cervical health. Try Nature's Way DIM Plus.

A few good things DIM can do for you....

...**Helps fight hormone-driven cancers.** Structurally similar to estrogen, DIM increases the chances of estrogen to be broken down into "good" estrogen metabolites which promote cell apoptosis (programmed cell death), helping to eliminate precancerous cells. Excess estrogen from unmetabolized estradiol,"bad" estrogen, is involved in women's problems like breast cancer and PMS, even low libido in men. Research studies show DIM successfully treats chemically-induced breast cancer in lab animals. New tests show DIM may play a role in natural prostate and uterine cancer protection, too.

...**Reports find DIM reduces PMS symptoms** like breast pain and moodiness, improves endometriosis and may even help reverse cervical dysplasia.

...**Promotes weight loss.** Proper estrogen metabolism means more efficient energy metabolism and faster weight loss, especially when used in conjunction with regular exercise....and especially in burning stored fat to help menopausal women lose weight.

...**Boosts male vitality and sports performance.** DIM enhances the activity of testosterone making it helpful for andropausal men and athletes seeking better performance and increased muscle growth.

...**DIM may improve safety of superhormones like DHEA and HRT drugs** by metabolizing excess estrogen resulting from supplementation or drug therapy. *Note: DIM's interaction with oral contraceptives is unknown at this time. Experts advise caution until studies have been done.*

...**New reports suggest DIM helps fight H. pylori infection** involved in stomach ulcers and cancers.

• **D-LIMONENE:** a nutraceutical in the rinds and seeds of citrus fruits and spices like caraway, dill and bergamot, D-limonene helps protects against cancer by accelerating liver detoxification. It also inhibits cancer of the stomach, lungs, and breasts. Phase 1 testing on the anti-cancer action of D-Limonene on humans with pancreatic and colorectal cancer is underway at the Charing Cross Hospital in London. Used as a natural solvent and disinfectant in environmentally-friendly household and industrial cleaning supplies.

• **DLPA, DL-PHENYLALANINE:** a safe, effective pain reliever and anti-depressant amino acid with an endorphin effect for arthritis, and lower back and cerebro-spinal pain. Increases mental alertness, and improves the symptoms of Parkinson's disease. Normal therapeutic dose is 500-750mg. Contra-indications: avoid DLPA if you have high blood pressure, are pregnant, or diabetic. See Amino Acids for more.

• **DMAE:** a naturally occurring nutrient that stimulates the production of choline. Choline is a building block of acetylcholine, a neurotransmitter involved in memory and learning. DMAE's mild stimulant feeling has also been found to elevate mood. DMAE is the precise salt of a substance called Deaner (DMAE p-acetamidobenzoate). In Europe, deaner is used for schizophrenia, phobias, low spirits and problems with learning and concentration. The FDA removed deaner from US citizens in 1983 because it was judged that although deaner was quite safe, the drug was not effective for hyperactivity in children, its only approved use.

• **DNA,** *deoxyribonucleic acid:* the substance in cell nuclei that genetically codes amino acids and determines the life form into which a cell develops. Derived from fish sperm, commercial DNA is used as a skin revitalizer to boost circulation and oxygen uptake. Repeated exposure to radiation causes DNA breakdown. Drastic medical treatments like chemotherapy help destroy cancers but also tend to alter normal cell DNA.

EDTA, *ethylenediamine tetra-acetic acid:* used in chelation therapy to remove toxic, clogging minerals from the circulatory system—particularly those that impair membrane function and contribute to free radical damage. EDTA puts these minerals into solution where they can be excreted by the kidneys.

• **EGG OIL:** fat-soluble emollients and emulsifiers extracted from eggs. Offers protection against dehydration and has lubricating, anti-friction properties when rubbed on the skin.
   —**Egg replacer** a cholesterol free, vegetarian combination of starches and leavening used to give the qualities of eggs in baking.

• **ELASTIN:** a protein and chief constituent in connective tissue, similar to collagen. Collagen and elastin give the skin its strength and elasticity. Elastin is also found in the artery walls. The skin is made up of 79% collagen, 11% lipids, 7% mucopolysaccharides, 2% elastin, and 1% carbohydrates. Elastin is used as an emollient in cosmetics to prevent water loss. *Horsetail herb*, high in silica, is an important trace mineral for connective tissue. Vitamins A (and-or beta-carotene), B, C, and D are essential for connective tissue health. Smoking harms connective tissue because it constricts the blood vessels.

• **ELECTROLYTES:** the ionized salts in blood, tissue fluids and cells, that transport electrical operating energy through the body. Electrolyte salts include sodium, potassium and chlorine. They are essential to cell function and body pH balance, but are easily lost through perspiration, so regular replacement is necessary from drinking electrolytic fluids. When electrolytes are low, we tire easily. When they are adequate, we have more energy. Electrolyte drinks are especially beneficial for athletes and those doing hard physical work.

• **EMOLLIENTS:** an agent that softens and smooths the skin, reduces roughness, cracking and skin irritation, and retards fine wrinkle lines - coating the skin with a film to retard evaporation of water. Some emollients, like glycerine and hyaluronic acid actually attract water to the skin. Seaweeds are some of Nature's best emollients.

• **ENERGIZERS and STIMULANTS, NATURAL:** natural energizers and stimulants help create a sense of well-being and self-confidence, relieving fatigue and drowsiness. In battling fatigue, natural energizers have great advantages over chemically processed stimulants. They have more broad-based activity so that they don't exhaust the body. They work better for individual needs; at correct dosage, supporting rather than depleting. The downside to stimulants (even some natural ones), is tolerance, dependency, nervousness, loss of focus, or after-effect headaches. Increasing a stimulant's strength can increase the toxicity and-or dependency potential. Taken too often, even natural stimulants can drive a body to exhaustion. Avoid stimulants, even natural ones, during pregnancy. The tiny body of the fetus cannot handle the systemic excitation.

…Specific remedies for fatigue are classified under central nervous system stimulants, metabolic enhancers, and adaptogens. The following list takes a quick look at natural stimulants and what they do. See individual nutrient entries for more information about their properties, activity and benefits.

—Central Nervous System (CNS) Stimulants: act by affecting the cerebral cortex and the medulla of the brain. Most contain either natural caffeine, naturally-occurring ephedrine, or certain free-form amino acids. CNS stimulators promote alertness, energy, and more rapid, clearer flow of thought. They also act as respiratory stimulants. Most central nervous system stimulants should be used for short-term energy needs. Long term use can result in a net loss of energy to the system.

Examples of food and herb source central nervous system stimulants:

Coffee and caffeine: America's most popular stimulant. See CAFFEINE, page 122.

Guaraña: a rich, natural source of rainforest guaranine, for long, slow endurance energy without coffee's heated hydrocarbons that pose health problems.

Glutamine: converts readily into 6-carbon glucose - an excellent brain nutrient and energy source. Improves memory recall, sustained concentration and alertness. Improves mental performance in cases of retardation, senility and schizophrenia. Increases libido and helps overcome impotence. See Amino Acids.

Kola Nut: a natural caffeine source without heated hydrocarbons. Allays hunger; combats fatigue.

L-Phenylalanine: a tyrosine precursor that works on the central nervous system with vitamin B-6 as an antidepressant and mood elevator. Successful in treating manic, post-amphetamine and schizophrenic depression. Aids in learning and memory retention. A thyroid stimulant that helps curb the appetite by increasing the body's production of cholecystokinin (CCK). See Amino Acids.

Tyrosine: builds adrenaline and thyroid stores. Rapidly metabolized as an antioxidant in the body; effective as a quick energy source for the brain. Safe therapy for depression, hypertension, in controlling drug abuse and aiding drug withdrawal. Increases libido. A growth hormone stimulant. See Amino Acids.

Yerba Maté: a South American herbal that naturally lifts fatigue and provides broad range nutrition to body cells. Rich in vitamins A, E, C and B (especially pantothenic acid), with measurable amounts of chlorophyll, calcium, potassium, iron and magnesium. Protects against stress effects. Helps open respiratory passages and overcome allergy symptoms. Yerba maté is a catalyst that increases the effects of other herbs.

Ephedra: a CNS stimulant that contains the biochemicals ephedrine and pseudoephedrine. Acts as an energy tonic to restore body vitality. A natural bronchodilator and decongestant for respiratory problems. Used in many weight loss formulas for its ability to increase thermogenesis. Ephedra is also a cardiac stimulant and should be used with caution by anyone with high blood pressure. See also *Ephedra*.

Ginkgo Biloba: a primary brain and mental energy stimulant. Increases both peripheral and cerebral circulation through vasodilation. A good stimulant choice for older people who suffer from poor memory and other aging-related CNS problems. Causes an increase in acetylcholine levels to better transmit body electrical impulses. Best results are achieved from the extract. See *Ginkgo Biloba*.

Damiana: a mild aphrodisiac, synergistic with other energy herbs in stimulating libido. A specific in a combination to treat frigidity in women and impotence in men. Also a mild anti-depressant tonic.

Yohimbe: A strong aphrodisiac herb affecting both male impotence and female frigidity. Stimulates the sympathetic nervous system for more rapid penile erections. *Note: Avoid if there is high blood pressure or heart arrythmia.*

—Metabolic Enhancers: improve the performance of biochemical pathways by providing energizing catalysts and co-factors that do not stress or deplete the body. Examples of metabolic enhancers include co-enzyme factors like B vitamins, fat mobilizers like L-carnitine, electron transporters like CoQ-10, lactic acid limiters like inosine and gamma oryzonal (GO), and tissue oxygenators like *Di-Methyl-Glycine* (B_{15}).

Examples of food and herb source metabolic stimulants:

Ginger: a warming circulatory stimulant and cleansing herb, useful in all formulas where circulation to the extremities is needed, such as arthritis. Ginger helps in lung-chest clearing combinations, in digestive stimulants and stomach alkalizers for clearing gas, in promoting menstrual regularity and cramping relief, and for all kinds of nausea, motion sickness and morning sickness. It may be used directly on the skin as a compress to stimulate venous circulation. Other uses include: catalytic action in nervine and sedative formulas, as a gargle and sore throat syrup, as a diaphoretic to remove wastes, and to stimulate kidney activity.

Capsicum: increases thermogenesis for weight loss, especially when used with xanthine herbs like guarana or kola nut. A circulatory system catalyst that enhances cardiovascular function and improves the performance of other herbs in a formula.

Bee Pollen: an energizing, nutritive "superfood." See Bee Pollen and Royal Jelly, pp. 162-164.

Royal Jelly: supplies key nutrients for energy, mental alertness and a general feeling of well-being. Enhances immunity and deep cellular health. One of the world's richest sources of pantothenic acid to combat stress, fatigue and insomnia. See Bee Pollen and Royal Jelly, pp. 162-164.

Green Tea: rich in flavonoids with antioxidant and anti-allergen activity. A beneficial fasting tea, providing energy support and clearer thinking during cleansing. Contains polyphenols (not tannins as commonly believed) that act as antioxidants, yet do not interfere with iron or protein absorption. Like other plant antioxidants, such as beta carotene and vitamin C, green tea antioxidants work at the molecular level, combatting free radical damage to protect against degenerative diseases. See Tea, page 125.

Lipoic Acid: a unique antioxidant, able to quench free radicals in both fat and water mediums. A potent promoter of glutathione and an important co-factor in energy metabolism. See Alpha lipoic acid, page 573.

Rosemary: an antioxidant herb, and strong brain and memory stimulant. A circulatory toning agent, and effective nervine for stress, tension and depression.

CoQ-10: an essential catalyst co-enzyme for cellular energy in the body. Supplementation provides wide ranging therapeutic benefits. See ENZYMES & ENZYME THERAPY, pg.19.

DMG: *Di-Methyl-Glycine,* B-15: a powerful antioxidant and energy stimulant. DMG is a highly reputed energizer and stimulant whose effects are attributed to its conversion to glycine. See Amino Acids.

—Adaptogens: herbal regulator tonics that help the body handle stress, build strength and maintain vitality. They are more for longterm revitalization than immediate energy — rich sources of strengthening nutrients like germanium, and steroid-like compounds that provide concentrated body support. These increase the body's overall immune function in a broad spectrum way rather than specific action. They promote recovery from illness and may be used synergistically with other tonic herbs to restore and normalize.

Examples of adaptogen herbs:

Panax Ginseng: is the most broad spectrum of all adaptogenic herbs; it includes Oriental red and white, and American Ginseng. Ginseng stimulates both long and short term energy, especially brain and memory centers. Ginseng has measurable amounts of germanium, helps to lower cholesterol and regulate sugar use in the body, promotes regeneration from stress and fatigue, and rebuilds strength. Panax is rich in phytohormones, thought to be responsible for its long tradition as an aphrodisiac, for both men and women's problems. Studies show that ginseng may be a source of phytotestosterone for men, and may be a protective factor for breast cancer in women because of its phytoestrogen content. Ginseng benefits are cumulative in the body. Taking panax for several months is more effective than short term doses. See *Ginseng, Panax.*

Siberian Eleuthero: a long-term energy tonic for the adrenal glands and circulatory health.

Schizandra: synergistic with eleuthero against stress, weight gain and fatigue. Supports sugar regulation, and liver function and strength. Helps correct skin problems through better digestion of fatty foods.

Gotu Kola: a brain and nervous restorative, especially effective as a toner after illness or surgery.

Astragalus: a superior tonic and strong immune enhancing herb. Provides therapeutic support for recovery from illness or surgery, especially from chemotherapy and radiation. Nourishes exhausted adrenals to combat fatigue. Helps normalize nervous, hormonal and immune systems. See *Astragalus.*

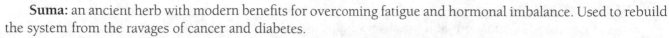

Suma: an ancient herb with modern benefits for overcoming fatigue and hormonal imbalance. Used to rebuild the system from the ravages of cancer and diabetes.

Fo-Ti, *(Ho-Shou-Wu):* a flavonoid-rich herb; a cardiovascular strengthener for longevity.

Reishi: an adaptogen mushroom for deep immune support, anti-cancer and antioxidant protection, liver regeneration and blood sugar regulation. Excellent for recovery from illness. See *Reishi Mushroom.*

Germanium, *(organic sesquioxide):* a potent adaptogen that detoxifies, blocks free radicals and increases killer cell production. An interferon stimulus for immune strength and healing. See *Germanium.*

Burdock: a hormone balancer with antibacterial, antifungal and antitumor properties. A specific in all blood cleansing and detoxification combinations; an important anti-inflammatory and anti-infective.

• **ENFLEURAGE:** the time-consuming, expensive technique of making essential oils from delicate flowers, such as roses and orange blossoms that cannot be steam distilled. Glass trays are lined with fat and scattered with fresh flowers. The next day the flowers are removed from the fat and replaced with fresh ones. The cycle is repeated for 4 to 5 weeks. The lard is then scraped from the trays and mixed with alcohol. When the alcohol is removed by distillation, a highly scented essential oil, or "absolute," is left behind.

• **ENZYMES:** see Enzymes & Enzyme Therapy, page 19.

• **EPHEDRA,** *Ma Huang:* used in Traditional Chinese Medicine for more than 5,000 years, cultivated for its healing properties longer than any other medicinal plant, few herbs are as misunderstood today. A wonderful bronchodilator for colds, coughs, flu, fever, headache, edema, asthma, sinus congestion and aching joints. Some uses for ma huang are approved by the FDA in over-the-counter (OTC) drugs, but Western manufacturers also use it for energy and diet products which are not FDA approved. Concerns over potency and safety, especially its isolated alkaloids have prompted a nationwide ban at this writing (2006). Ma huang contains a total of 0.5 to 2.5 percent of ephedra alkaloids, with ephedrine comprising between 30 and 90% of those alkaloids. Ephedrine is a potent isolate; it produces effects similar to adrenaline, raising blood pressure. In <u>large</u> doses, ephedrine causes nervousness, insomnia, dizziness, palpitations and skin flushing. *Note: The whole ephedra plant, which most knowledgeable herbalists use instead of the isolate, is generally safe when combined with other herbs, as an anti-asthmatic, bronchodilator, and peripheral vasoconstrictor. See pg. 70 for info on contraindications.*

• **ESCIN:** a saponin occurring in the seeds of the horse chestnut tree, *Aesculus hippocastanum.* Used externally to reduce swelling and increase skin tissue tone, increasing circulation and encouraging flexibility.

• **ESSENTIAL FATTY ACIDS:** includes linoleic, linolenic and arachidonic acids, necessary for cell membrane function, balanced prostaglandin production and metabolic processes. Food sources: seafoods, dark green vegetables, sesame and pumpkin seeds, flax seed, evening primrose oil, borage seed, hemp oil and black currant seed oil. See "Fats & Oils," page 130, and CLA, DHA and GLA listings for more.

• **ESSIAC:** an herbal tea formula of the Ojibway (Chippewa) Indians, made famous by Rene Caisse for treating cancer, newly rediscovered and popular today. The name "Essiac" is an anagram of her last name "Caisse." Her formula consists of *sheep sorrel, burdock root, turkey rhubarb* and *slippery elm bark.*

• **ESTROGEN:** natural estrogens are conjugated hormones, including estradiol, estrone and estriol, thought to be formed through the adrenals and the pituitary, especially after menopause.

—*Estradiol:* produced by the ovaries, with estrogenic properties; taken orally, converted to estrone.

—*Estrone:* an estrogen produced by the ovaries and by conversion of estradiol; linked to breast cancer.

—*Estriol:* believed to be a "good" estrogen (non-cancer-facilitating). Phytoestrogens (plant estrogens) are thought to be close in chemical makeup to human estriol.

FERRUM PHOS: a homeopathic cell salt used to treat colds and flu, inflammation and nausea. A remedy for first stage inflammations and infective wounds. See HOMEOPATHIC CELL SALTS, pp. 17-18.

• **FLAX SEED OIL:** see ESSENTIAL FATTY ACIDS & OMEGA-3 OILS, page 134-135.

• **FLUORIDE:** new research shows that fluoride is more poisonous than lead, only slightly less poisonous than arsenic. The difference between calcium fluoride (naturally occurring) and other forms is the higher availability of free fluoride ions in sodium-fluoride, and in fluoride from hydrofluosilicic acid. Fluoride is linked to cancer, Alzheimer's, poor child brain development, nervous system health, and fluorosis (fluoride poisoning of cells that form tooth enamel). Where calcium fluoride occurs naturally in the water, people age before their time, suffer from bone disease, tooth disorders, and premature atherosclerosis. Disastrous effects are more apparent in elderly populations, in people with low calcium-magnesium or vitamin C levels and people with cardiovascular and kidney disease. Postmenopausal women in fluoridated areas have more risk of fractures. As little as 0.7 parts per million fluoride in the water has been associated with skeletal fluorosis.

Fluoride depresses thyroid activity, and may be at least partly responsible for the surge in hypothyroidism in the U.S. Yet, <u>mandatory</u> water fluoridation continues to be pushed for its supposed dental benefits... even though new large-scale studies now show no difference in decay rates of permanent teeth in fluoridated and non-fluoridated areas. In fact, the studies reveal the rates of cavities actually decline when cities stop adding fluoride to their water. I recommend European bottled waters like Evian and Perrier as good fluoride-free choices, as well as artesian well water - the Cadillac of natural waters.

• **FOLIC ACID**, *Folacin:* a B vitamin that plays an important role in the synthesis of DNA, enzyme production and blood formation. Essential for division and growth of new cells, it is a good choice during pregnancy (400mcg daily) to guard against spina bifida and neural tube defects. It prevents anemia, helps control leukemia and pernicious anemia, is effective against alcoholism, even some precancerous lesions. It is critical in overcoming immune depression following chemotherapy with MTX. Folic acid reduces high homocysteine levels, which thicken the blood and facilitate the conversion of LDL (bad cholesterol) into free radical particles. New estimates are that 1 in 5 cardiac cases can be attributed to high homocysteine levels. A high intake of folic acid and B_6 lowers heart disease risk 45% for women by keeping homocysteine levels in check (February 1998 JAMA). Aluminum antacids, oral contraceptives, some HRT drugs, alcohol, long-term antibiotics and anti-inflammatory drugs increase need for folic acid. Food sources: leafy greens, organ meats, peas, nutritional yeast, broccoli, fruits, soy foods, chicken, brown rice, eggs and whole grains.

• **FOS** *(fructo-oligosaccharides):* food constituents in artichokes, onions, garlic and asparagus which nourishes friendly intestinal bifidobacteria in the digestive tract while reducing harmful bacteria. One gram a day boosts bifidobacteria five-fold. FOS produces B-vitamins (including B-12) and improves the liver's ability to detoxify system poisons. Prevents traveler's diarrhea, helps babies digest milk (reducing fecal odor) and fights harmful bacteria like *E. coli.* Promotes healthy peristalsis and bowel regularity.

• **FREE RADICALS:** stress related, unstable fragments of molecules produced from oxygen and fats in cells, which clutter up an unhealthy body. Your body takes 10,000 free radical hits a day just in normal, everyday living! Your immune system sometimes creates free radicals to neutralize certain viruses and bacteria. However, in today's world, over-exposure to environmental pollutants, pesticides, food additives and chemicals, UV rays from ozone depletion, smoke, drugs and fast food can cause excessive free radical production. Free radicals result when high energy chemical oxidation reactions in the body get out of control. An excess of free radicals affect the immune system so that it destroys its own tissue structure.

However, as with most activities in nature, the body produces the necessary substances to deactivate free radicals, antioxidants (in this case the antioxidant enzymes superoxide dismutase, catalase, and glutathione).

Still, if your body antioxidant levels are low, your health may be in real trouble. Free radicals that go unchecked by antioxidants are very dangerous- they can reprogram your DNA, degrade collagen and cause premature aging, immune breakdown and inflammatory reactions. Free radicals may be the missing link to many diseases, including atherosclerosis, Alzheimer's disease and immune compromised diseases like Fibromyalgia and Chronic Fatigue Syndrome. Cell damage, partially responsible for the effects of aging, is involved in cancer, triggers some forms of heart disease and is an integral part of eye diseases like cataracts and macular degeneration.

Specific antioxidant depleters are:
   —Infections from viruses, bacteria, or parasites.
   —Trauma from surgery, injury, inflammation, and wound healing.
   —Burns, and exposure to excessive heat or cold.
   —Smoking or passive exposure to cigarette smoke. Excessive alcohol and/or addictive drug intake.
   —Exposure to toxic chemicals, pesticide residues, fluoride, nitrites, nitrates, etc.
   —Exposure to radiation, including excessive UV rays from sunlight.
   —Cytotoxic drugs, such as the anticancer drug Adriamycin.
   —Oxidant drugs that steal electrons, such as acetaminophen (Tylenol).
   —Dietary lack of antioxidant-rich foods.

Some foods make free radicals more likely to occur. Polyunsaturated fats, in sunflower, corn and soy oils, and junk foods can lead to excessive free radical production. A low-fat diet reduces the damage of oxidation by free radicals. Iron and copper, okay in small quantities, increase free radical production in large amounts.

Antioxidants are free radical scavengers, neutralizing free radicals by donating one of their own electrons before free radical production gets out of control. Remarkably, antioxidants do NOT become free radicals themselves; they have the ability to remain stable in the unpaired form. However, our polluted environment means it is doubtful that our bodies receive enough antioxidants in our food to meet our needs. Supplements like zinc, carotenes and B vitamins work synergistically with antioxidants. Vitamins C and E, and the protein glutathione act as anti-oxidants themselves. Super antioxidant OPCs, *oligomeric proanthocyanidin complexes*, from grape seed extract or pine bark (trade name Pycnogenol), are 50 times stronger than vitamin E and 20 times stronger than vitamin C. They're available over-the-counter to supercharge your antioxidant defenses. Herbs like *garlic, ginkgo biloba, rosemary* and *ginsengs* are also rich in powerful antioxidants to use for healing.

• **FRUCTOSE:** a simple fruit sugar found in honey, in fruit and other parts of plants. Much sweeter than sucrose (cane sugar), *crystalline fructose* available commercially is usually made from corn starch and has a low glycemic index. See Sweeteners in a Healing Diet, page 147.

GABA, *Gamma-Aminobutyric Acid:* a non-essential amino acid useful in treating brain and nerve dysfunctions, like anxiety, depression, nerves, high blood pressure, insomnia, schizophrenia, Parkinson's and Alzheimer's diseases, and ADD in children. GABA is a natural tranquilizer, improves libido, and along with glutamine and tyrosine, helps overcome alcohol and drug abuse. Used with niacinamide, it is a relaxant.

• **GAMMA ORYZANOL (GO):** a substance extracted from rice bran oil, used as a medicine in Japan since 1962. A mild anti-inflammatory that also relieves anxiety, GO acts on the hypothalamus and pituitary gland. Many bodybuilders believe it increases growth hormone levels, but animal studies show it actually inhibits growth hormone secretion as well as prolactin, luteinizing hormone and thyroid-stimulating hormone. Studies show gamma oryzanol reduces menopausal hot flashes, and lowers cholesterol and triglyceride levels. Used successfully in the treatment of Irritable Bowel Syndrome (I.B.S.), gastritis and peptic ulcers.

• **GARLIC:** a therapeutic food with antibiotic, antifungal, antiparasitic and antiviral activity. Used extensively for disease prevention; internally against infection of all kinds; externally for eye, ear, nose and throat infections; and due to its thiamine content, to prevent mosquito and insect bites. Garlic has measurable amounts of germanium, an antioxidant for endurance and wound healing.

- **GELSEMIUM:** a homeopathic remedy for chronic lethargy. See Homeopathic Remedies, page 15.

- **GENISTEIN:** a phytohormone constituent of soy. See Soy Foods in a Healing Diet, page 109.

- **GERMANIUM,** *(organic sesquioxide):* an antioxidant mineral and interferon stimulus for immune strength. An anticancer agent activating macrophages and increasing production of killer cells in the body, especially if a tumor has metastasized. Facilitates oxygen uptake, detoxifies and blocks free radicals. Effective for viral, bacterial and fungal infections, osteoporosis, arthritis, heart, blood pressure and respiratory conditions. Studies show success with leukemia, HIV, and cancers of the brain, lung, pancreas and lymph system. Good sources: chlorella, garlic, tuna, oysters, green tea, reishi mushroom, aloe vera, ginseng, leafy greens.

- **GINGER:** an aromatic, spicy herb. Both fresh and dried ginger root have therapeutic properties for digestion, hypertension, headaches and other problems. Ginger is the world's greatest herbal inhibitor of 5-LO enzyme, a chemical cousin of COX-2 and the only food source for prostate cancer cells. Without this food source, prostate cancer cells die in only 1 to 2 hours.... so it's an especially good choice for prostate cancer protection. It's easy to have fresh ginger on hand. Peel fresh roots, chop in the blender, put in a plastic bag and freeze. Ginger thaws in less than 10 minutes, ready for use.

- **GINKGO BILOBA:** the leaf extract of an ancient Chinese tree, used therapeutically to combat the effects of aging. It improves circulation throughout the body, sends more blood and oxygen to the brain for better memory and mental alertness, and protects the brain against mental disorders. Ginkgo is effective for vertigo, dizziness and ringing in the ears. A potent antioxidant, it protects cells against free radical damage and reduces blood cell clumping which can lead to congestive heart disease. Helps return elasticity to cholesterol-hardened blood vessels. Reduces inflammation in the lungs leading to asthmatic attack. New research shows that ginkgo increases vascular strength and helps reverse impotence caused by penile atherosclerosis. In one study, ginkgo was 30% more effective than drug injections with 50% of patients showing regained potency.

- **GINSENG, PANAX:** the most effective adaptogen of all tonic herbs, *Panax ginseng*, and its American brother, *Panax Quinquefolium* are intensely studied today by science. Scientific research is incredibly expensive, so the wealth of testing on ginseng shows its importance in the minds of researchers everywhere. *Fortunately, even as scientific work goes on, we can buy and use this safe remedy during its testing, something impossible with drugs. Taking ginseng for several months to a year is far more effective than short term doses.*

A small sampling of modern scientific validation of the benefits of this ancient healing plant:
1) Ginseng aids treatment for cardiovascular disorders, including heart attack and heart disease. In clinical trials on patients with high blood pressure, ginseng tea helped produce a steady, consistent reduction in blood pressure (average drop, 23 in the blood pressure of patients with a systolic pressure above 140.)
2) Ginseng may inhibit growth and formation of liver cancer cells, one of the most difficult cancers to overcome. Tests show that ginseng stimulates protein synthesis and converts cancer cell characteristics functionally and morphologically to those of normal liver cells, a process induced in the cells by a *single ginsenoside!*
3) Ginseng polysaccharides protect against alcohol induced gastric ulcers. It's a good preventive medicine choice for anyone regularly drinking hard liquor with a damaged stomach lining.
4) Ginseng benefits hormone balance for both men and women, an explanation for its long reputation as an aphrodisiac. Amazingly, it works with the needs and qualities of the opposite male and female systems.
For men, ginseng has a long tradition as a reproductive restorative. While ginseng won't make a man a SUPERMAN, it may be the only herb to clinically test as a source of plant testosterone. Ginseng seems to increase sperm count and seminal vesicle weight, supports key adrenal and prostate functions. Like Viagra, ginseng enhances nitric oxide (NO) synthesis which regulates muscle tone of blood vessels that control flow to the penis. This effect and mild testosterone action, link ginseng to stronger erections for impotent men. Antioxidants help cardiovascular performance not only for sexual energy, but for sports and workouts... important for a man's outlook.

For women, ginseng helps normalize hormones, notably those that guard against breast cancer, endometriosis, and hormone driven problems. Ginseng has an estrogen-like effect due to the chemical similarity of ginsenosides and female steroidal hormones. It exerts an estrogen effect on the vaginal mucosa, to prevent thinning of vaginal walls after menopause, and menopause discomfort during intercourse. It affects a woman's mental energy through hypothalamus stimulation.... a factor in turning a woman's attention to love-making. Ginseng also has distinct, antioxidant cardiovascular benefits for women.

5) Ginseng has an insulin-like effect on sugar regulation, stimulating sugar removal.

6) Ginseng shows therapeutic activity against recurrent, severe viral infections and syndromes, like HIV and other immune deficient diseases, according to recent Russian studies.

7) Ginseng has powerful, intercellular antioxidants, particularly helpful for anti-aging capabilities, neutralizing free radicals and enhancing immunity.

8) Ginseng stimulates RNA synthesis in bone marrow cells, and has anti-toxic effects against radiation, heavy metals, and airborne pollutants.

9) Ginseng stimulates many parts of the immune system, including phagocyte action, antibody response and natural killer cell activity. It modifies cytokine production, strengthens the immune properties of cellular connective tissue, enhances interleukin and balances red and white blood cell count.

10) Ginseng plays a role in normalizing skin cancer cells and protects against aging skin and early wrinkling. This may be a boon to all the world as the ozone layer thins, exposing all of us to harmful UV rays.

11) Ginseng offers longterm mental and psychological benefits. European ginseng research with the elderly show clear improvement for mental outlook in depression, optimistic spirits and insomnia.

12) Ginseng assists memory, concentration, alertness and improved learning ability. It is currently being tested for Alzheimer's disease, and I myself have seen evidence that ginseng helps in Alzheimer's cases.

13) Ginseng is the quintessential herb for stress — the very thing people need to handle the growing pressure in their lives today. Stress is anything that lessens vitality, and it's the single greatest factor in the development of health problems. Beyond its specific abilities, ginseng superbly helps us to deal with stress.

• **GLA,** *Gamma Linoleic Acid:* obtained from evening primrose oil, black currant, and borage seed oil. A source of energy for the cells, electrical insulation for nerve fibers, a precursor of prostaglandins which regulate hormone and metabolic functions. Therapeutic use is wide ranging — from control of PMS and menopause symptoms, to help in nerve transmission for M.S. and muscular dystrophy.

• **GLANDULAR EXTRACTS, RAW:** Gland therapy, minute amounts of raw animal glandulars that support and normalize a particular organ or gland, is now seen as valid and safe. It's based on the premise that "like cells help like cells," and that glandular substance communicates biochemically with our bodies through micro-nutrients and polypeptides. For serious, organ debilitating diseases, like cancer, gland cell therapy augments the body's own gland substance so that it can better heal itself. Predigested gland tissue provides many benefits of whole fresh glands. Freeze-dried, de-fatted, dehydrated concentrates are also effective. Highest quality preservation is essential, since heat or salt precipitation render the glands useless. Every gland works with a particular amino acid, so a combination of a raw glandular and a harmonizing amino acid provides the human gland with more ability to produce its hormone secretions.

The most essential glandulars:
—**Raw Adrenal:** stimulates and nourishes exhausted adrenals. Reduces inflammation and increases endurance without synthetic steroids. Helps protect against chronic fatigue syndrome and candida albicans by normalizing metabolism. Increases resistance to allergy reactions and infections associated with poor adrenal function. Helps control hypoglycemic and diabetic reactions, and menopause imbalance symptoms.
—**Raw Brain:** improves brain chemistry, helping prevent memory loss, chronic mental fatigue and senility onset. Encourages better nerve stability and restful sleep. Beneficial support during alcoholism recovery.

—**Raw Female Complex,** (including ovary, pituitary, uterus): restores hormonal balance, especially between estrogen and progesterone. Helps regulate the menstrual cycle and stimulates delayed or absent menstruation. Normalizes PMS symptoms and controls cramping. Indicated for low libido and infertility.

—**Raw Heart:** improves heart muscle activity and reduces low density lipoproteins in the blood.

—**Raw Kidney:** aids in normalization of waste filtering function and kidney-urinary disorders. Helps normalize blood pressure, body fluid and acid-alkaline balance.

—**Raw Liver:** helps restore the liver after abuse, disease and exhaustion. Improves metabolic activity and filtering of wastes and toxins like alcohol and chemicals. Aids fat metabolism. Increases healthy bile flow and glucose regulation. Raw liver is effective for jaundice, hepatitis, toxemia and alcoholism.

—**Raw Lung:** supports the lungs against asthma, emphysema, congestion, bronchitis and pneumonia.

—**Raw Male Complex,** (contains raw orchic, pituitary, and prostate), re-establishes hormonal balance of testosterone-progesterone-estrogen. Helps normalize functions of diseased or damaged male organs. Supports male body growth and fat distribution, improves sperm count, virility, and chances of fertilization.

—**Raw Mammary:** helps heal breast-nipple inflammation. Controls profuse menstruation, period pain, and normalizes too-frequent cycles, especially at onset of menopause. Supports scant milk during lactation.

—**Raw Orchic:** helps increase male sexual strength and potency by stimulating testosterone production and sperm count. Raw orchic can bring noticeable improvement in male athletic performance.

—**Raw Ovary:** normalizes estrogen-progesterone balance. Helps correct endometrial misplacement and overgrowth, PMS symptoms and cramping. Supports hormone production slow down during menopause.

—**Raw Pancreas:** the pancreas is a triple function gland producing pancreatin for digestion, and insulin and glucagon for glucose metabolism and balanced blood glucose levels. Raw pancreas supports enzyme secretions for fat metabolism, hormone balance, food assimilation, and intestinal immune response.

—**Raw Pituitary:** the "master gland," stimulates overall body growth through electrolyte metabolism in the ovaries, testes, adrenals and skin. Plays a major role in reproduction, estrogen secretion, blood sugar metabolism, kidney function, skin pigmentation, water retention and bowel movements. Helps overcome hypoglycemia and infertility. Effective for athletes in controlling body stress, sugar balance and fatigue.

—**Raw Spleen:** aids in the building and storage of red blood cells to promote strength and tissue oxygenation. Filters harmful substances from the bloodstream and enhances immune function by increasing white blood cell activity. Increases absorption of calcium and iron.

—**Raw Thymus:** stimulates and strengthens immune response against foreign organisms and toxins. Raw thymus helps activate T-cells in the spleen, lymph nodes and bone marrow. Minimizes aging symptoms as the thymus gland shrinks with age. Use with zinc to help regenerate thymic tissue.

—**Raw Thyroid:** supports energy production, helps regulate metabolism and circulation, and controls obesity and sluggishness caused by low thyroid. Helps mental alertness, hair, skin and reproductive-sexual problems. Works synergistically with tyrosine and natural iodine. *Note: use a thyroxin-free compound.*

—**Raw Uterus:** helps menses dysfunctions like amenorrhea, habitual miscarriage, infertility and irregular periods. Helps prevent inflammation and infection of the cervical canal and vagina. Aids in calcium use for bone and muscle. Improves tissue growth and repair. Helps overcome birth control side effects.

• **GLUCOSAMINE SULFATE:** a proteoglycan, or amino sugar that promotes tissue elasticity and cushioning. Glucosamine stimulates manufacture of glycosaminoglycans, important cartilage components that help the body repair damaged or eroded cartilage. Glucosamine stimulates proper joint function and joint repair. Glucosamine sulfate is the form used because sulfur takes part in forming cartilage. Supplements are derived from chitin (exoskeleton of shrimp, lobsters or crabs).

• **GLUTAMIC ACID:** a non-essential amino acid, important for nerve health and metabolism of sugars and fats. Over 50% of the brain's amino acid composition is represented by glutamic acid and its derivatives. It is a prime brain fuel because it transports potassium across the blood-brain barrier. Helps correct mental and nerve disorders, like epilepsy, muscular dystrophy, mental retardation and severe insulin reactions.

• **GLUTAMINE:** a non-essential amino acid that converts readily into 6-carbon glucose, a prime brain nutrient and energy source. Supplements rapidly improve memory retention, recall, concentration and alertness. Glutamine helps mental performance in cases of retardation, senility, epileptic seizure and schizophrenia. It reduces alcohol and sugar cravings, protects against alcohol toxicity, and controls hypoglycemia.

• **GLUTATHIONE:** a non-essential amino acid that works with cysteine and glutamine as a glucose tolerance factor and anti-oxidant; neutralizes radiation toxicity, inhibits free radicals, helps white blood cells kill bacteria. Protects vitamins C and E from oxidation and enhances their effectiveness. Works with vitamin E to break down fat and protect against stroke and cataract formation. Binds to carcinogens, allowing them to be eliminated through the urine or bile. A prime immune booster that detoxifies your liver from heavy metal pollutants, cigarette toxins, alcohol and drug (especially PCP) overload, and from the effects of chemotherapy and radiation. Stimulates prostaglandin metabolism. Glutathione levels drop as you age. The amino acid N-acetylcysteine (NAC), is converted in the body to glutathione and is the best choice for absorption. Food sources: watermelon, asparagus, avocados, oranges, peaches. Dosage: 300-600 mg daily.

• **GLYCERINE, VEGETABLE:** a naturally-occurring substance, metabolized in the body like a carbohydrate, not a fat or oil, today extracted from coconut, and used in natural cosmetics as a smoothing agent.

• **GLYCINE:** a non-essential amino acid which releases growth hormone when taken in large doses. Converts to creatine to retard nerve and muscle degeneration, so therapeutically effective for myasthenia gravis, gout and muscular dystrophy. A key to regulating hypoglycemic sugar drop, (take upon rising).
  —**Di-Methyl-Glycine, DMG,** once known as B-15, is a powerful antioxidant and energizer. Used successfully to improve Down Syndrome and mental retardation, and to curb craving in alcohol addiction. DMG's highly reputed energy effects can be attributed to its conversion to glycine. Successfully used as a control for epileptic seizures, with notable therapeutic results for atherosclerosis, rheumatic fever, rheumatism, emphysema and liver cirrhosis. For best results, take sublingually before exercise. Note: Too much DMG disrupts the metabolic chain and causes fatigue. The proper dose produces energy, overdoses do not.

• **GLYCONUTRITIONALS:** supplemental carbohydrate saccharides that help improve overall health. Glycoproteins, present on the surface of every cell with a nucleus, require at least eight different carbohydrate saccharides for molecular communication. By improving the communication, experts believe glyconutritionals boost immune defenses against harmful bacteria and viruses, reduce inflammation, and accelerate toxin removal from cells. Specific disease states that may benefit from glyconutritional supplements: chronic fatigue syndrome, rheumatoid arthritis, lupus, fibromyalgia, quadriplegia, candida, cancer, and asthma.

• **GRAPEFRUIT SEED EXTRACT:** a natural antibiotic, for bacterial, viral and fungal infections; works against yeast infections like candida albicans and vaginal infections, moderate parasitic infestations, dysentery, traveler's diarrhea, infected cuts, gingivitis, strep throat, staph infections, ringworm, ear infections, nail fungus, dandruff and warts. Add 10-20 drops to water to sanitize counter tops, and bathrooms. For germ-killing action against tartar and gingivitis, add 3-4 drops grapefruit seed extract solution to water pic reservoirs.

• **GREEN TEA:** See Black, Green and White Teas and Their Healing Benefits, page 126.

• **GUAR GUM:** an herbal product that provides soluble digestive fiber and absorbs undesirable intestinal substances. Used therapeutically to lower cholesterol and to flatten the diabetic sugar curve.

• **GUM GUGGUL:** an Indian gum resin herb from the mukul myrrh tree, it is used as a natural alternative to drugs for reducing cholesterol. In Ayurvedic healing, it is used for rheumatism, nervous diseases, tuberculosis, urinary disorders and skin diseases. Guggulipid, an extract of guggul, is credited with the ability to lower both cholesterol and triglyceride levels because it increases the liver's metabolism of LDL cholesterol. Guggulipid prevents the formation of atherosclerosis and helps regress pre-existing atherosclerotic plaques. It also helps inhibit platelet aggregation, promotes fibrinolysis, and may prevent development of a stroke or embolism. Natural healers use it as a successful treatment for acne.

• **GYMNEMA SYLVESTRE:** See Sugar & Sweeteners in a Healing Diet, pp. 145-153.

HDLs and LDLs *(High and Low Density Lipoproteins):* water-soluble, protein-covered bundles, synthesized in the liver and intestinal tract, that transport cholesterol through the bloodstream. Bad cholesterol (LDL) carries cholesterol through the bloodstream for cell-building needs, but leaves excess behind on artery walls and in tissues. Good cholesterol (HDL) helps prevent narrowing of the artery walls by removing excess cholesterol and transporting it to the liver for excretion as bile.

• **H_2O_2, HYDROGEN PEROXIDE, Food Grade:** Controversy has surrounded the use of food grade hydrogen peroxide for therapeutic, anti-infective and antifungal health care. Our experience with this source of nascent oxygen has been successful in many areas, but a great deal of that success is predicated on the method and dosage with which H_2O_2 is used. Medicinal directions are very specific as to dosage and ailment. Read the bottle label carefully before embarking on a program that includes H_2O_2. Food grade H_2O_2 is available in two refrigerated forms: hydrogen dioxide (hydrogen peroxide), mainly for external use, or magnesium dioxide (magnesium peroxide). You can purchase OXY-TECH food grade hydrogen peroxide by calling 800-833-3256, or at your health food store. It contains less oxygen but is much more palatable and more stable.

Both compounds form a stable substance we know as oxygen. The 3% dilute solution may be used internally for asthma, emphysema, arthritis, candida albicans, and degenerative conditions like chronic fatigue syndromes and HIV infections. Other applications for a 3% solution include fungal infections, as a douche for vaginal infections, and as an enema solution for detox cleansing. It may be used as a mouthwash, skin spray, or on the skin to replace the skin's acid mantle that has been removed by soap.

Oxygen baths are valuable detoxifying agents, and noticeably increase body energy. About 1 cup H_2O_2 per bath produces significant effect for 3 to 7 days. Oxygen baths are stimulating rather than relaxing. Therapeutic benefits include body pH balance, reduction of skin cancers, clearing of asthma and lung congestion, arthritis and rheumatism relief, and conditions where increased body oxygen can prevent and control disease. Add ½ cup sea salt and ½ cup baking soda for extra benefits.

Some common guidelines: *See page 186 for how to use H_2O_2 safely.*

…H_2O_2 is not for health maintenance use. It should be taken only if there is a specific need. Once improvement is noticed, discontinue using H_2O_2. If you need to take H_2O_2 for more than 12 days orally or more than 60 days externally, contact a holistic physician for a custom protocol.

…Like many antibiotics, H_2O_2 also kills friendly bacterial culture in the digestive tract. When taking H_2O_2 orally, replace the intestinal flora (acidophilus, bifidus, and bulgaricus) by eating cultured foods, or take a supplement culture 2 hours after taking H_2O_2. If you experience nausea or bloating, discontinue use.

…Do not use H_2O_2 if you have had a heart or liver transplant.

• **HERBAL WRAPS:** the best European and American spas use herbal wraps as restorative body-conditioners. Wraps are good body cleansers that alkalize and release body wastes quickly. They should be used in conjunction with a short cleansing program and 6-8 glasses of water a day to flush out loosened fats and toxins. Seaweed wraps have taken America and Europe by storm as a "lean and clean" method for relieving bloating, cellulite and toning skin tissue. Enzyme wraps are an important part of every spa program in Japan to replace and rebalance important minerals, enhance metabolism and alkalize body chemistry.

• **HISTIDINE:** a semi-essential amino acid in adults, essential in infants. Abundant in hemoglobin and a key to the production of both red and white blood cells. Histamine is formed from histidine, a precursor to good immune response, for effective defense against colds, respiratory infections, and countering allergic reactions. It has strong vasodilating and hypotensive properties for cardio-circulatory diseases, anemia and cataracts. Synthesizes glutamic acid, aids copper transport through joints, and removes heavy metals from the tissues, making it successful in treating arthritis. Histidine raises libido in both sexes. See Amino Acids.

• **HOMEOSTATIC SOIL ORGANISMS (HSO's):** beneficial bacteria naturally present in the Earth's soil that protect plants from disease and help them digest nutrients. Supplemental HSO's help you: flush waste matter lodged in the intestines, improve nutrient absorption, and produce lactoferrin—a potent natural immune stimulant. Some manufacturers claim HSO's are more effective than traditional probiotic products because they can withstand heat, cold, chlorine, fluorene, ascorbic acid, stomach acids, even pH changes.

• **HOMOCYSTEINE:** an amino acid by-product of protein metabolism. New research implicates high homocysteine levels in heart disease, stroke and senility. Eating foods rich in vitamins B6, B12 and folic acid like beans, garlic, sea veggies, fish, nutritional yeast, brown rice and green foods helps to lower homocysteine levels in the blood. For more, see my 4 point program to help lower homocysteine levels on pg. 440.

• **HORNY GOAT WEED** (also known as *Epimedium* or Yin Yang Huo): A traditional Chinese aphrodisiac, horny goat weed was the food for "yin yang," a mythical animal that could achieve sexual climax up to one hundred times days. Today horny goat weed is considered one of the best sexual tonics for men and women. Its testosterone-like effects show success for boosting erectile function in men, relieve women's menopausal complaints, support kidney health and allay fatigue for both sexes.

• **HUPERZINE A:** the active alkaloid extracted, then standardized, from *Huperzia serrata*, a rare Chinese club moss. Huperzine A is a potent blocker of the enzyme acetylcholinesterase (AChE) that helps break down acetylcholine, the neurotransmitter essential for memory and brain function. The inhibition of AChE helps enhance thinking, concentration and memory. Alan Kozikowski, Ph.D., the scientist who first synthesized Huperzine A extract, says the product is effective for decreasing deterioration of brain cells by increasing the brain's levels of acetylcholine and other neurotransmitters. It appears to be effective for Alzheimer's disease.

• **HGH, Human Growth Hormone** (*also called somatotrophin*) is produced by the pituitary gland. HGH promotes the growth of bone and regulates height, stimulates the breakdown of body fat to produce energy, and the synthesis of collagen for cartilage, tendons and ligaments. HGH helps increase muscle mass, hence its promise for the sports community and anti-aging. HGH supplements today are synthetic, made from bacterial suspension with a methionine amino-acid terminal. Side effects of synthetic HGH include carpal tunnel syndrome, aching joints, increased risk of diabetes and severe fluid retention. Animal studies on HGH show shorter life spans, not longer. Amino acids and vitamins that stimulate natural release of the body's own HGH: glutamine 500mg daily with a niacin boost for more effects; also arginine, lysine, ornithine and glycine. *Homeopathic* microdoses of growth hormone retain the anti-aging benefits without its drawbacks.

• **HYALURONIC ACID (HA):** the newest rage in anti-aging therapies, hyaluronic acid is a naturally occurring mucopolysaccharide that helps the skin, eyes, joints and muscles retain youthful moisture. HA attracts water to help lubricate and regulate moisture in the tissues and movable parts of the body. It's a prime component of synovial fluid, which helps facilitate nutrient transport into the cells and the removal of metabolic waste. HA is used therapeutically to increase joint mobility in arthritis and other connective tissue disorders, to promote clear, healthy eyes, and as a superior anti-aging treatment for the skin. I have seen particular good results with HA for dramatically improving skin texture and glow, while decreasing some of the fine lines and wrinkles.

- **HYDROLYZE:** Hydrolysis, decomposing a compound into a simpler compound by water occurs during digestion — proteins in the stomach react with water and enzymes to form peptones and amino acids.
  —*Hydrolyzed animal elastin:* hydrolyzed animal connective tissue in emollients and creams.
  —*Hydrolyzed vegetable protein:* hydrolysate (liquefaction) of vegetable protein.
  —*Hydrolyzed milk protein:* moisturizer made of protein extracted from milk.

- **HYPERTHERMIA, CLINICAL:** see OVERHEATING THERAPY, page 182.

- **HYPNOTHERAPY:** see ALTERNATIVE HEALTH CHOICES, page 41.

- **HYPOALLERGENIC:** a term for cosmetics meaning less likely to cause an allergic reaction. Hypoallergenic cosmetics are made without the use of common allergens that most frequently cause allergic reactions. However, some people may still be sensitive to these products.

IGNATIA: a homeopathic female remedy to relax emotional hypertension; especially during times of great grief or loss. See HOMEOPATHIC REMEDIES, page 15.

- **INDIUM:** the 7th rarest trace mineral widely touted today as a "silver bullet" for anti-aging. Indium is not readily available from foods, and only recently tested as a nutritional supplement. Tests show indium can produce 90-694% higher gland mineral uptake, 333% increase in chromium, a possible increase in pituitary, thyroid and endocrine hormones, enhanced calcium uptake against osteoporosis, a 36% reduction in mouse cancers and 42% reduction of mouse tumors. Indium is especially effective in balancing hormones and nourishing glands. Anecdotal reports reveal indium may be able to reduce graying hair or baldness, improve sight, and fight serious illness like cancer and AIDS. Try Indium from Green Nutrition Brokerage at 209-339-9775. Use only as directed. Large amounts may cause vomiting or headaches.

- **INDOLE 3-CARBINOL:** an indole (plant glucosinolate) found in cruciferous veggies like broccoli, brussels sprouts and cauliflower. Indole 3 carbinol stimulates natural phase 2 enzymes that eliminate carcinogens before they bind to DNA and cause cancer. Research finds that indole 3 carbinol reduces pain and muscle weakness in 50% of fibromyalgia patients. The commercial product (I3C) is regularly used with success for warts on the larynx and genitalia. Powerful medicine for today's women who are bombarded daily with estrogen mimics from the environment and commercial food supply, like DIM, indole 3 carbinol stimulates estrogen metabolism to control excess estrogen. Reduces breast cancer risk and symptoms of estrogen dominance like weight gain, heavy menstruation and fibrocystic breasts.

- **INOSINE:** a non-essential amino acid that stimulates ATP energy; helps provide muscle endurance as the body's glycogen reserves run out. Take on an empty stomach with an electrolyte drink before exercise.

- **INOSITOL:** part of the B-complex family, a sugar-like crystalline substance found in the liver, kidney and heart muscle, and in most plants. Deficiency is related to loss of hair, eye defects and growth retardation.

- **IODINE:** a mineral which exerts antibiotic-like action and also prevents toxicity from radiation. A key component of good thyroid function and proper metabolism, necessary for skin, hair and nail health, and for wound healing. White blood cells absorb iodine from the blood and use it to enhance their pathogen killing capacity. Iodine also prevents mucous buildup. Iodine deficiency results in goiter, hypothyroidism, cretinism, confused thinking and menstrual difficulties. Good food sources: seafoods and sea vegetables.

- **IP-6** *(Inositol Hexaphosphate),* a natural compound of rice bran and other plants, research shows IP-6 helps prevent tumor formation and shrinks existing tumors by normalizing cell growth. IP-6 has seen good results in both animal and human cancers. Documented tests show IP-6 enhances natural killer cell activity, is a natural iron chelator, and has potent antioxidant activity.

• **IPRIFLAVONE:** a semi-synthetic isoflavonoid, ipriflavone, like other isoflavonoids has a chemical structure resembling estrogen. The estrogen-like effect helps reduce bone loss, giving ipriflavone the reputation of a "new bone builder." Studies suggest that ipriflavone and its metabolites protect bones by inhibiting bone resorption (bone-degrading osteoclast activity). Ipriflavone also may activate bone-building cells called osteoblasts. Three separate Italian studies show that 200mg of ipriflavone 3 times a day reduces postmenopausal bone loss. Another test shows ipriflavone may <u>reduce</u> the number of white blood cells — important for disease protection. Contra-indications: May interact with prescription drugs like theophylline, caffeine, Coumadin, tolbutamide and phenytoin. Ask your pharmacist. Use with caution if you have kidney disease.

• **IRON:** a mineral that combines with proteins and copper to produce hemoglobin; carries oxygen through the body. Iron deficiency means fatigue, dry hair, mental impairment, muscle weakness and anemia. Iron strengthens immunity, helps wound healing, and is important for women using contraceptive drugs and during pregnancy. It keeps hair color young, eyes bright, the body strong. However, free un-bound iron is a strong pro-oxidant, and can be toxic at abnormally high levels. Iron overload is linked to some cancers, heart disease, diabetes, arthritis and gland malfunction. Using herb or food source iron supplements avoids the problem. Food sources: molasses, cherries, prunes, leafy greens, poultry, liver, legumes, peas, eggs, fish and whole grains. Vitamin C-rich foods like tomatoes, citrus and vinegar greatly enhance iron absorption. Herbal sources: *alfalfa, bilberry, burdock, catnip, yellow dock root, watercress, dulse, sarsaparilla and nettles.*

• **ISOPRENOIDS:** fat soluble antioxidants that neutralize free radicals by anchoring themselves to fatty membranes, grabbing free radicals attached to the membranes and passing them to other antioxidants. CoQ-10 and vitamin E are isoprenoid antioxidants.

JIAOGULAN: China's immortality herb, jiaogulan is gaining notoriety in the West as a worthy adaptogen, comparable to ginseng. Jiaogulan actually contains three to four times as many saponins as panax ginseng. Jiaogulan is a natural antibacterial and antiinflammatory, and a proven remedy to help lower high cholesterol and blood pressure. Improves fat metabolism, soothes the nervous system, enhances strength and endurance, and can help facilitate weight loss by inhibiting the body's tendency to store sugars as fat.

• **JOJOBA OIL:** oil extracted from the bean-like seeds of the desert shrub, Simondsia Chinensis. A liquid used as a lubricant and a substitute for sperm oil, carnauba wax and beeswax. Mexican and American Indians have long used the jojoba bean wax as a hair conditioner and skin lubricant.

KALI MUR: potassium chloride, a homeopathic remedy for inflammatory arthritis. Deficiency results in glandular swelling, skin scaling, and excess mucous discharge. See HOMEOPATHIC CELL SALTS, pp. 17-18.

• **KALI PHOS:** potassium phosphate; a body deficiency is characterized by intense body odor. A homeopathic remedy to treat mental problems such as depression. See HOMEOPATHIC CELL SALTS, pp. 17-18.

• **KALI SULPH:** potassium sulphate, a homeopathic cell salt that oxygenates the skin. Deficiency causes tongue deposits, and slimy nasal, eye, ear and mouth secretions. See HOMEOPATHIC CELL SALTS, pp. 17-18.

• **KEFIR:** a cultured milk product, it comes plain or fruit-flavored, and may be taken as a liquid or used like yogurt or sour cream. Kefir provides friendly intestinal flora. Use the plain flavor, cup for cup as a replacement for whole milk, buttermilk or half and half; fruit flavors may be used in sweet baked dishes.
   —**Kefir Cheese:** a good cultured replacement for sour cream or cream cheese in dips and other recipes, kefir cheese is low in fat and calories, and has a slightly tangy-rich flavor that really enhances snack foods. Use it cup for cup in place of sour cream, cottage cheese, cream cheese or ricotta.

• **KOMBUCHA MUSHROOM:** actually a colony of yeast and bacteria, proponents of kombucha claim that it is a panacea for almost any disease. Used for weight loss because it contains caffeine, kombucha helps both liver and gallbladder activity. Advocated for bronchitis, asthma and muscle aches. One study shows the tea contains a strong antibacterial, effective against antibiotic-resistant strains of *staphylococcus*.

A mixture of black tea and sugar is brewed to which a Kombucha "mother" (starter) is added. The B vitamin-rich environment allows the bacteria to convert to a digestive "tea" vinegar, rich in amino acids and enzymes. To use kombucha tea, start with 2-oz. a day; do not exceed 8-oz. a day. People with uric acid problems or gout should limit use, since the active yeasts contain significant amounts of nucleic acid which increases uric acid in the blood. Diabetic use is controversial because kombucha contains 3-4% simple sugars. *Note: If mold is floating on the surface, or the mushroom falls apart when handled, discard tea entirely.*

• **KUZU:** a powdered thickening root for Japanese dishes and macrobiotic diets. Superior for imparting a shine and sparkle to stir-fried foods and clear sauces. A dairy alternative in cooking.

LACHESIS: a homeopathic remedy for PMS symptoms that improve once menstrual flow begins. For menopausal hot flashes. See Homeopathic Remedies, page 15.

• **LACTASE:** an enzyme normally produced in the small intestine, lactase supplements can be taken before or with meals that include dairy to aid in digestion. When there is insufficient lactase, unabsorbed lactose (milk sugar) migrates to the colon, where it ferments causing gastrointestinal problems.

• **LACTIC ACID:** a by-product of the metabolism of glucose and glycogen, present in blood and muscle tissue. Also present in sour milk, beer, sauerkraut, pickles, and other foods made by bacterial fermentation. Used in cosmetics to exfoliate skin.

• **LACTOBACILLUS:** there are several types of *lactobacilli*, including *L. acidophilus, L. bifidus, L. caucassus, and L. bulgaricus*, all beneficial bacteria that synthesize intestinal tract nutrients, counteract pathogenic microorganisms and maintain intestinal health. Lactobacillus organisms are readily destroyed by noxious chemicals and drugs, particularly chlorine and antibiotics. In fact, a single long course of antibiotics can destroy most bowel flora, leading to the overgrowth of yeasty pathogenic organisms, like *candida albicans*, which are resistant to antibiotics. Even eating antibiotic-laced meats and dairy products leads to an insidious decline in the number of Lactobacillus organisms within the human body. Skin disorders, chronic candidiasis, irritable bowel syndrome and other intestinal disorders, hepatitis, lupus and heart disease are all associated with a Lactobacillus deficiency. Top food sources: yogurt, kefir, miso, tempeh and uncooked sauerkraut.

• **LACTOFERRIN:** a protein isolated from colostrum (the first milk produced after giving birth) which blocks cancer angiogenesis and boosts immune response. There have even been reports of liver cancer going into remission after treatment with lactoferrin. Especially useful for people whose bodies are weakened and susceptible to infection from chemotherapy. Caution: Lactoferrin is contraindicated during pregnancy as high levels of lactoferrin may cause rejection of the fetus. Also contraindicated for leukemia or prostatitis. Lactoferrin's ability to stimulate white blood cell activity may aggravate these disorders.

• **LAETRILE (B-17):** a nutrient substance derived from apricot seeds discovered in 1950. Contains cyanide, benzaldehyde and glucose, and can be toxic at high doses. Even though it has had some success in cancer treatment, laetrile treatment has been banned in the U.S. because of potential toxicity.

• **LANOLIN:** also known as wool fat or wool wax, is a product of the oil glands of sheep. Chemically, a wax instead of a fat, lanolin is a natural emulsifier that absorbs and holds water to the skin.

• **LECITHIN:** a phospholipid (fat-like substance) produced in the liver, and present in some foods, lecithin consists mostly of phosphatidyl choline, so it's a source of phosphatidyl choline for the brain and nerves. High concentrations of lecithin appear in heart cells and around the brain, spinal cord and nerve sheathing. Choline is recognized as the direct precursor of acetylcholine, the neurotransmitter essential for memory. Acetylcholine deficiency is associated with Alzheimer's disease and senile conditions that involve memory and neurological abnormalities. Lecithin supplements significantly increase choline levels.

Today's lecithin comes from high phosphatide soy or eggs, is low in fat and cholesterol and helps thicken recipes without using dairy products. To use in recipes: substitute for ⅓ the oil. Add two teaspoons daily to almost any food to increase phosphatides, choline, inositol, potassium and linoleic acid. Lecithin is a natural emulsifier, breaking down fat particles, an action essential to control of cholesterol and triglyceride levels. Lecithin lowers dangerous LDL cholesterol, and elevates healthier HDL particles.

• **LEDUM:** a homeopathic remedy for bruises. May be used following arnica treatment to fade the bruise after it becomes black and blue. See HOMEOPATHIC REMEDIES, page 15.

• **LEMON,** *Citrus Limon:* rich in vitamin C and potassium, a traditional tonic for increasing salivary and gastric secretions, currently used to dissolve gallstones, and now showing promising anticancer properties.

• **LINOLEIC ACID:** See FATS & OILS, pp. 130-139.

• **LION'S MANE MUSHROOM,** *Hericium erinaceus:* named for its beautiful cascading tendrils, lion's mane is gaining popularity in the America for its ability to boost brain health. New studies reveal lion's mane may actually stimulate the growth of neurons, possibly inhibiting brain dysfunction caused by Alzheimer's disease, senility, stress or traumatic injury. In addition, lion's mane is a specific for constipation and indigestion, helps lower blood pressure and cholesterol, and is a good nervous system tonic.

• **LITHIUM:** an earth's crust trace mineral used clinically as *lithium arginate.* Successful in treating manic-depressive disorders, ADD in children, epilepsy, alcoholism, drug withdrawal and migraine headaches. Research shows it helps in malignant lymphatic growths, arteriosclerosis and chronic hepatitis. Overdoses may cause palpitations and headaches. Good food sources: mineral water, whole grains and seeds.

• **LUTEIN:** a carotenoid nutrient like alpha-carotene, beta-carotene, cryptoxanthin, lycopene and zeaxanthin. Carotenoids are found in spinach, kale and many fruits and vegetables. Lutein is not converted to vitamin A like beta-carotene, but does serve as a potent antioxidant. Of all the carotenoids, lutein and zeaxanthin lend the most support to the eyes. Lutein and zeaxanthin make up the yellow retinal pigment and appear to specifically protect the macula. A Harvard study reports that people eating the most lutein and zeaxanthin foods are most likely to have healthy retinas and maculae.

• **LYCOPENE:** see above, and Carotenoids.

• **LYCOPODIUM:** a homeopathic remedy that helps to increase personal confidence. Also favored by estheticians to soothe irritated complexions and as an antiseptic. See HOMEOPATHIC REMEDIES, page 15.

• **LYSINE:** an essential amino acid; a primary treatment for the herpes virus. May be used topically or internally. Add high lysine foods, like corn, poultry and avocados to your diet if you have recurrent herpes breakouts. Helps rebuild muscle and repair tissue after injury or surgery. Important for calcium uptake for bone growth, and in cases of osteoporosis, reduces calcium loss in the urine. Helps the formation of collagen, hormones and enzymes. Supplements are effective for Parkinson's disease, Alzheimer's and hypothyroidism.

MSM *(methylsulfonylmethane):* a dietary sulfur, MSM contains 34% sulfur important for body elements like hormones, enzymes, antibodies, antioxidants, in tissues and body proteins. Four major amino acids, methionine, cysteine, cystine, and taurine depend heavily on sulfur. MSM contributes to healthy hair and nails, skin softness, and encourages repair of damaged skin by stimulating the production of collagen. It increases blood circulation and maintains acid-alkaline balance. It boosts both natural detoxification and immune functions by helping the body produce immunoglobulins (antibodies). MSM is often used for muscle and joint pain stopping pain impulses before they reach the brain. It relieves constipation, and helps heal burns and scars. The supplement is derived from a naturally produced form of DMSO (dimethyl sulfoxide).

• **MACA:** A Rainforest herb with libido enhancing activity. For men, maca works to restore lost energy and recharge sexual performance. For women, maca's high iodine stimulates the thyroid, often imbalanced in low libido. Recent sexuality tests with animals have been quite dramatic. Maca extracts were fed to mice; none to control mice. Control mice had sex 13 times in 3 hours... the high potency maca mice had sex 67 times in 3 hours! For menopausal women, maca appears to boost the pituitary gland, increasing hormone production in the ovaries, often resulting in multiple orgasms. Some research shows maca increases estrogen levels after menopause or hysterectomy by as much as 70%! Used traditionally in high altitudes by Peruvian's as a fertility aid. New studies confirm this effect for animals living at high altitudes.

• **MAGNESIUM:** a critical mineral for osteoporosis and skeletal structure, necessary for good nerve and muscle function, healthy blood vessels, balanced blood pressure and athletic endurance. Important for tooth formation, heart and kidney health, and restful sleep. Counteracts stress, irregular heartbeat, emotional instability and depression. Calms hyperactive children. Supplements help alcoholism, diabetes and asthma. Deficiency means muscle spasms, cramps, stomach upsets, sometimes fibromyalgia. Magnesium is readily absorbed from dark leafy greens, seafood, whole grains, dairy foods, nuts, legumes, poultry and hot spices.

• **MAGNESIUM PHOS:** a homeopathic remedy for abdominal cramping or spasmodic back pain; particularly for menstrual cramps. See HOMEOPATHIC REMEDIES, page 15.

• **MAGNETS:** Static-magnetic-field-therapy, used for centuries, is currently undergoing a surge of new research for its pain relieving potential. Scientific studies show magnets increase blood and oxygen circulation, aid nutrient flow through the blood, balance endocrine glands and body pH, speed up proper calcium deposition, help heal nerve tissue and bones, and stimulate enzyme activity. Although the answers aren't in for the reasons magnets relieve pain, study after study is showing that magnets do work.

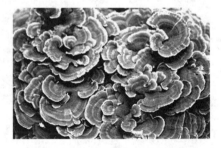

• **MAITAKE MUSHROOM,** *Grifola frondosa:* a rich source of beta 1,3 and 1,6 glucans that boost immunity against hormone-driven cancers. NCI testing reveals that maitake extract can actually prevent HIV from destroying the "helper" T-cells of the immune system. Scientists from NCI consider maitake as powerful as the drug AZT, but without the toxic side effects. Maitake helps reduce blood pressure and cholesterol levels, and lower blood sugar levels in non-insulin dependent diabetics. May also help CFS, diabetes, hepatitis, pneumonia, HBP, HIV-related infections, and arthritis. D-fraction compound from maitake is now FDA approved for phase 2 clinical trials against advanced breast and prostate cancer. Research from New York Medical College shows D-fraction inhibits tumor growth by up to 95% and induces cell apoptosis (cell death) of prostate cancer cells.

• **MANGANESE:** a mineral that nourishes brain and nerve centers to eliminate fatigue, nerves and low back pain, and aids in sugar and fat metabolism. SOD (*superoxide dismutase*), a powerful free radical quenching enzyme, is solely dependent on manganese for its immune enhancing activity. Manganese boosts calcium in nourishing bones, and reduces epileptic seizures. Deficiencies result in poor hair and nail growth (white spots on nails), hearing loss, blood pressure imbalances, impotence, latent diabetes, and poor muscle coordination. Tranquilizer drugs deplete manganese. Manganese supplements protect nerves from adverse effects of tranquilizers. Food sources: blueberries, ginger, rice, eggs, green vegetables, legumes, nuts and bananas.

• **MANNOSE:** A naturally-occurring simple sugar which can successfully treat up to 90% of urinary tract infections. D-mannose sticks to the offending *E. coli* bacteria which tend to adhere to the urinary wall, allowing it to be rinsed away through normal urination. Also helps treat kidney infections caused by *E. coli*. An excellent UTI preventive taken before intercourse or for people who are prone. Food sources: cranberry, pineapple. Available in supplements. Adult dosage: ½ tsp. every 3-4 hours. Children: ¼ tsp. every 3-4 hours.

• **MANUKA OIL:** Derived from the Manuka tree, indigenous to New Zealand, manuka oil is 20-30 times stronger than *tea tree oil* against gram postive bacteria. Helpful for a wide range of skin problems including acne, ezcema, psoriasis and minor cuts, manuka reduces foot and body odor by wiping out offending bacteria, even effective against athlete's foot and head lice! Good for pet skin problems and fleas, too.

• **MELATONIN:** an antioxidant hormone secreted cyclically by the pineal gland to keep us in sync with the rhythms of the day and the seasons. Melatonin helps us recover from the effects of jet lag faster.
   —**Protective functions give melatonin an anti-aging reputation:** 1: Helps protect the body from free radical damage. 2: Reduced immune function is an aging factor, as the thymus shrinks reducing our ability to generate T-cells. Melatonin slightly reverses thymus shrinkage, enabling it to produce more infection-fighting T-cells, and enhances immune antibody production. 3: Studies show that a nightly melatonin supplement boosts the performance during sleep of immune systems compromised by age, drugs or stress.
   Do you know?.....
   —Breast and perhaps prostate cancer, hormone driven cancers, may indicate a deficiency of melatonin.
   —Melatonin dampens estrogen release. High melatonin levels can even temporarily shut down the reproductive system (the theory basis for a new contraceptive combining high dose melatonin with progestin).
   —Melatonin decreases the size of the prostate gland (a melatonin deficiency allows it to grow). This is good news for older males with enlarged prostate. But melatonin supplements can greatly decrease sex drive and actually shrink gonads — certainly an unwanted effect.
   —Melatonin may be indicated in low-tryptophan diseases, like anorexia, hypertension, manic depression, Cushing's disease, schizophrenia, and psoriasis, because tryptophan is the raw material for melatonin.
   —If you supplement melatonin longterm, the body tends to shut down its own melatonin production.
   —Melatonin is not recommended for people under 40 except short-term, or for a specific purpose, like a sleep disorder or jet lag. If you don't have a sleep disorder, melatonin may actually disrupt sleep patterns.
   —High levels of melatonin can be found in delayed puberty, narcolepsy, obesity, and spina bifida.
   —Beta blockers suppress melatonin. Serotonin stimulants, like 5-HTP or chlorpromazine (an antipsychotic), raise melatonin levels.
   Consider carefully longterm melatonin supplements. Hormones are incredibly delicate substances with long-ranging effects we don't fully understand. I believe taking a hormone contraceptive drug that eventually shuts down the reproductive system is asking for trouble. If you decide to take melatonin as a protective measure against breast or prostate cancer, a small protective dose...about .1 to .3 mg at night, gives your body a chance to use the supplement yet still make its own hormone. You can always resume if needed. Herbal immune protectives that don't carry the hormone risk of melatonin, are *panax ginseng, ginkgo biloba or garlic.*

• **METHIONINE:** an essential amino acid; an antioxidant and free radical deactivator. A major source of organic sulphur for healthy liver activity, lymph and immune health. Protective against chemical allergic reactions. An effective "lipotropic" that keeps fats from accumulating in the liver and arteries, thus keeping high blood pressure and serum cholesterol under control. Effective against toxemia during pregnancy. An important part of treatment for rheumatic fever. Supports healthy skin and nails, and prevents hair loss.

• **MGN-3:** a natural weapon against cancer, MGN-3 is made by combining one of Japan's top cancer treatments—an extract from shiitake mushroom—and an antiviral extract from the outer shell of rice bran. In one study, cancer patients' natural killer cells were able to kill 27 times more cancer cells after just two months of treatment with MGN-3. Animal research shows MGN-3 may help all types of cancer, and reduce the toxic side effects of chemo and radiation. A highly contested and debatable 2004 court ruling against the manufacturer for improper marketing has unfortunately made MGN-3 unavailable to the American public. Looking for effective substitutes? Consider Lane Labs Noxylane 4, Maitake Products Maitake D-Fraction, or American Biosciences Imm-Power.

• **MINERALS and TRACE MINERALS:** the building blocks of life, minerals are nature's most basic nutrients, the bonding agents between you and food. Minerals are especially necessary for people in active sports, because you must have minerals to run. Minerals comprise only 4% of your body weight, but they are keys to major areas of your health. Minerals keep your body pH balanced — alkaline instead of acid. They are essential to bone formation and bone health. They regulate the osmosis of cellular fluids, nerve electrical activity and most metabolic functions. They transport oxygen, govern heart rhythm, help you sleep, and keep you emotionally balanced. Trace minerals are only .01% of body weight, but even deficiencies in these micro-nutrients can cause severe depression, PMS and other menstrual disorders, hyperactivity in children, blood sugar disorders, nervous stress, high blood pressure, premature aging, memory loss and poor healing.

…Minerals are important. Hardly any of us get enough. Your body doesn't synthesize minerals; they must be regularly obtained from your food.... in turn they allow your body to absorb the nutrients it takes in. Minerals from plants and herbs are higher quality and more absorbable than from meat sources. Today's diet of chemicalized foods inhibits mineral absorption. High stress lifestyles that rely on tobacco, alcohol, steroids and antibiotics contribute to mineral depletion. USDA research finds that men who consume five cans of cola a day for three months absorb less calcium, increasing risk for bone deterioration and injuries or breaks! Many minerals are no longer even sufficiently present in our fruits and vegetables, leached from the soil by chemicals and pesticide sprays used in commercial farming. Plant minerals from earth and sea herbs are one of the most reliable ways to get mineral benefits. Herbal minerals are whole foods that your body easily uses.

…Minerals can really give your body a boost. Eat organically grown produce whenever possible, and take a good herb or food-source mineral supplement.

• **MODIFIED CITRUS PECTIN (MCP):** MCP, a water soluble fiber derived from citrus fruits which seems to block cancer metastasis by acting as a decoy for lectins (cancer cell surface proteins). Cancer cell lectins seek out the sugar, galactose, in cells. MCP also contains galactose so when lectin meets MCP, it attaches to the pectin (like it would a regular cell) rendering the cancer cell incapable of spreading anywhere else in the body. In animal tests, MCP blocks prostate cancer metastasis. Results are also good in vitro (in cell lines) for human melanoma, and cancers of the colon and breast.

• **MOLYBDENUM:** a metabolic mineral, necessary in mobilizing enzymes. New research shows benefits for esophageal cancers and sulfite-induced cancer. Molybdenum amounts are dependent on good soil content. Good food sources: whole grains, brown rice, brewer's yeast and mineral water.

• **MUCOPOLYSACCHARIDES:** See polysaccharides and Aloe Vera plant, page 162.

• **MUSHROOMS:** Mushrooms are far more than tasty foods. They are powerful medicine used to combat everything from heart disease and cancer to AIDS. Specific mushrooms have a tonifying effect, strengthening the endocrine and immune systems, and improving liver health and mental acuity. See listings for *shiitake, reishi, poria cocos, lion's mane, agaricus, maitake and cordyceps* for more.

NADH *(nicotinamide adenine dinucleotide):* a potent antioxidant coenzyme derived from vitamin B3, involved in the synthesis of ATP *(adenosine triphosphate),* which enhances cellular energy in the brain and body. NADH actually donate free electrons to CoQ10, allowing it to function longer. Brain and muscle cells contain the highest amounts of NADH. Although NADH is in every living animal and plant cell, the first supplement was derived from yeast in 1993 (the finished product is yeast free), by George Birkmayer, M.D., Ph.D. NADH has a "metabolic burst" step that leads to the destruction of a cytotoxic invader and heightens immune response. It also repairs DNA, boosts two brain neurotransmitters, dopamine and norepinephrine and has anti-aging potential. NADH studies promise hope for Alzheimer's and Parkinson's disease, chronic fatigue syndrome and depression. Recommended dosage for energy enhancement is 2.5 to 5mg daily. Rare side effects include: nausea, nervousness, insomnia, and decreased appetite.

• **NATRUM MUR,** *sodium chloride:* regulates moisture within cells. Deficiency causes fatigue, chills, salt craving, bloating, profuse sweating, tearing, salivation and watery stools. HOMEOPATHIC CELL SALTS, pp. 17-18.

• **NATRUM PHOS,** *sodium phosphate:* regulates pH balance. Imbalance is indicated by a coated tongue, itchy skin, sour stomach, loss of appetite, diarrhea and flatulence. See HOMEOPATHIC CELL SALTS, pp. 17-18.

• **NATRUM SULPH,** *sodium sulphate:* imbalance produces tissue edema, dry skin with watery eruptions, poor bile and pancreas activity, headaches and gouty symptoms. See HOMEOPATHIC CELL SALTS, pp. 17-18.

• **NEXRUTINE:** a patent-pending extract of *Phellodendron* tree used as a natural pain reliever for arthritis or pain from over exertion. Selectively inhibits the COX-2 enzyme involved in inflammation. Note: Use with caution if there is impaired kidney function, high blood pressure or heart disease.

• **NEEM OIL,** *Azadirachta Indica:* a tropical tree related to mahogany, used medicinally for centuries, now rediscovered by alternative healers. Recent science validates the traditional uses of neem, including skin care, treatment of bacterial and viral infections, and immune system enhancement. Historically, a twig from the neem branch was used as a natural toothbrush to help prevent and treat periodontal disease in India. Today, neem oil is regularly included as a purifier and antimicrobial in natural toothpastes. Numerous studies show neem to be versatile, effective against skin and dental disease, fungi, viruses, bacteria and parasites, fever, allergies, inflammation, ulcers, tuberculosis, cardiovascular problems; it's even used as a spermicide. Used in shampoos or rinses, neem oil is an insecticide against fleas and ticks, and head lice in people.

• **NONI** *(Morinda Citrifolia):* also known as *nonu,* is a traditional Hawaiian medicinal herb, used by Polynesian islanders as a primary medicine for more than 1,500 years. It's highly effective for degenerative diseases like type II diabetes, high blood pressure and heart disease, and for arthritis, digestive disorders, colds, flu, sinus infections, headaches, menstrual problems, skin disorders and more. Noni has anti-tumor activity, anti-inflammatory effects, cell repair and regeneration effects and stimulates immune response. It is a notable pain reliever, especially for carpal tunnel syndrome, tennis elbow and sciatica. Research shows antibacterial properties against *M. pyrogenes, Ps. aeruginosa,* even *E. coli.* Try Matrix NONI caps or liquid. Noni contains vitamins, minerals, trace elements, enzymes and co-enzymes, plant sterols, antioxidants and bioflavonoids. Many believe the synergistic effect of all these nutrients is what gives it its powerful punch. Look for a freeze-dried whole fruit product for best results.

• **NUTRITIONAL YEAST:** a supplement and condiment with a distinct but pleasant aroma and taste. Formerly called brewer's yeast made from by-products of the beer brewing process, today's nutritional yeast is made from a carbohydrate sugar of molasses, and tastes and smells much better. For healing, nutritional yeast sold in capsules or in the bulk food section of the health food store is the best choice. Nutritional yeast is not the same as candida albicans yeast. It is one of the best sources of B-complex, high in minerals, protein, all the essential amino acids, and nucleic acid—vital for proper cell development. Improves skin problems like acne because it helps the liver break down fats. A good source of glutathione which boosts immune response and cleansing. Its chromium triggers insulin action—good for persons suffering from diabetes. Neutralizes bowel irritation, soothes inflammation and restores normal bowel movements. One of the best immune-enhancing supplements in food form - just 1 to 2 tsp. in a protein drink offer a daily energy lift.

• **NUX VOMICA:** a homeopathic remedy for gastrointestinal problems. A prime remedy for hangover, recovering alcoholics, drug addiction and migraine prevention. See HOMEOPATHIC REMEDIES, page 15.

OCTACOSANOL: a wheat germ derivative, used to counteract fatigue and increase oxygen use during exercise and athletic performance. Antioxidant properties help for muscular dystrophy and M.S.

• **OLIVE LEAF EXTRACT:** a potent herbal antibacterial, antiviral, antifungal, antiparasite and antioxidant. It stimulates the immune system by phagocyte production, restores energy and boosts stamina. Olive leaf's powerful punch comes from its *oleuropein* and oleuropein's hydrolysis. *Oleuropein* is a member of the iridoid group, a uniquely structured chemical class in which one member has the capability to transfer into another group, a biogenetic characteristic which gives *oleuropein* its antimicrobial power. Clinical research and experience show that olive leaf extract has a wide range of successes against viral, bacterial, fungal, and protozoan infections, particularly for treatment of herpes I and II, human herpes virus 6 and 7, HIV-AIDS, colds and flu, meningitis, Epstein-Barr virus, encephalitis, shingles, chronic fatigue, hepatitis B, pneumonia, tuberculosis, gonorrhea, malaria, severe diarrhea, blood poisoning, and dental, ear, urinary tract and surgical infections. Lab tests done by Upjohn Co. find that olive leaf extract kills 56 pathogens. Tests from East Park Research finds that olive leaf extract treats as many as 120 illnesses.

• **OMEGA-3 and OMEGA-6 FATTY ACIDS:** See FATS & OILS, pp. 130-131.

• **OREGANO OIL:** rich in polyphenolic flavonoids, two of which, carvacrol and thymol are potent antiseptics. (Note: Both oregano and thyme contain the active ingredients carvacrol and thymol. Carvacrol is the predominant polyphenol in oregano; thymol the predominant in thyme.) Oregano oil contains over 50 compounds with antimicrobial actions that inhibit candida yeast, bacteria, viruses and parasites. Oregano oil is also a powerful antioxidant. Oregano oil is particularly effective against chronic candida infections. Animal research from Turkey reveals that oregano oil slows down development of diabetes-related health complications. A good traveler's choice to protect from parasitic infestation and foreign bacteria. Can be applied topically to fight fungal nail infections.
Note: Direct contact with oregano essential oil can cause mild burns — avoid irritation by mixing with olive oil. Oregano oil is used externally or internally (capsule or diluted extract). Extract dosage: 4 drops 3x daily or as directed.

• **OREGON GRAPE CREAM** (*Mahonia aquifolium*)*:* has direct action on the skin when applied topically. Tests show it's over 80% effective in relieving psoriasis, eczema, dermatitis, dandruff, acne and dry scaly skin. Alkaloids extracted from the root and bark have strong anti-microbial and anti-fungal properties, and are potent antioxidants which neutralize skin damaging free radicals, reduce inflammation, and inhibit abnormal skin cell growth (as in psoriasis). Once used extensively by early American physicians, Oregon grape was replaced by cortisone creams. Today, it is again popular. An Oregon grape cream called PRIMADERM is by Prime Pharmaceutical Corp.

• **ORNITHINE:** a non-essential amino acid that works with arginine and carnitine to metabolize excess body fat; with the pituitary gland to promote growth hormone, muscle development, tissue repair, and endurance. Aids fat metabolism through the liver; builds immune strength; helps scavenge free radicals.

• **OPCs,** *Oligomeric Proanthocyanidin Complexes:* a class of bioflavonoids composed of polyphenols. Generally extracted either from grape seeds or white pine bark, these potent antioxidants destroy free radicals, activity widely accepted in slowing the aging process and enhancing immune response. Free radicals also weaken cell membranes, cause inflammation, genetic mutations, and contribute to major health problems like cancer and cardiovascular disease. Increasing evidence shows that people live less-diseased lives when OPCs are a part of their nutritional program. This is especially true for premature aging, immune deficiency, allergies or exposure to environmental pollutants. A side benefit of proanthocyanidin activity is the inhibition of histamine production, which allows the body to better defend against LDL-cholesterol.

Vitamin C activity is vastly increased with all OPCs, especially strengthening collagen in blood vessels, and increasing capillary resiliency. German studies show OPCs have a unique ability to bind to collagen structures and to inhibit collagen destruction. Blood vessel strength is enhanced by as much as 140% after OPC supplementation. Capillaries become more elastic, circulation noticeably improves. Easy bruising and varicose vein tendency lessens. New tests on grape seed extract indicate that its properties were the primary anti-carcinogen in the world famous "grape cure" against cancer widely used in the early part of this century.

—**Pycnogenol:** a trade name for pine bark OPCs, pycnogenol is a highly active bioflavonoid. It helps resist inflammation and free radical damage to blood vessels and skin. It strengthens the entire arterial system. Pycnogenol is used in Europe as an "oral cosmetic," because it stimulates collagen-rich connective tissue against atherosclerosis and helps joint flexibility. It is used against diabetic retinopathy, varicose veins and hemorrhoids. It is one of the few dietary antioxidants that crosses the blood-brain barrier to directly protect brain cells.

—**Grape seed extract:** highly bio-available proanthocyanidin bioflavonoids....a prime antioxidant. Studies show OPCs from grape seed extract scavenge free radicals 50% more effectively than vitamin E, and 20% more effectively than vitamin C. Vitamin E scavenges harmful free radicals in fatty environments of the body; vitamin C scavenges free radicals in the watery environments. Grape seed extract scavenges free radicals in both environments, and does so more efficiently.

…OPCs from herbs in particular do more than protect, they also help repair, and more:
—potent free radical scavengers, with tumor inhibiting properties.
—an arteriosclerosis antidote, strengthening capillary/vein structure.
—reduces vein fragility to help prevent bruising, varicose veins, restless legs and lower leg blood volume.
—anti-allergy properties, protective against early histamine production.
—specifically aids vascular fragility associated with diabetic retinopathy.
—improves skin elasticity, enhances circulation, fights inflammation and improves joint flexibility.
—helps PMS symptoms.

• **OSCILLOCOCCINUM:** a homeopathic remedy for flu. See HOMEOPATHIC REMEDIES, pg.15.

• **OVERHEATING THERAPY** (*Hyperthermia*): See page 182. *Note: simple overheating therapy may be used in the home. It stimulates the body's immune mechanism without the stress of fever-inducing drugs.*

• **OYSTER MUSHROOM:** *Pleurotus ostreatus:* A nutritious edible mushroom with anti-tumor activity. Contains 8 essential amino acids, B-complex, high protein, EFA's, and minerals (esp. iron for anemia). In animal studies, oyster mushrooms inhibited breast tumors 89.7%! Animal research reveals oyster mushrooms help lower cholesterol levels. In the Czech republic, an extract of oyster mushrooms is regularly recommended for high cholesterol prevention in people. Used in TCM for joint and muscle relaxation.

• **OXALIC ACID:** a component of chard, spinach and beet greens that binds to calcium and iron in the body, thus preventing their absorption. To reduce oxalic acid in these foods, lightly steam or stir fry them until they turn bright green and slightly tender. Or, consider a Japanese variety of spinach called "Toyo" which contains less oxalic acid than regular spinach. It also works well in liver cleansing juices.

PABA, *Para-Aminobenzoic Acid:* a B Complex family member and component of folic acid, PABA has sunscreening properties, is effective against sun and other burns, and is used in treating vitiligo, (depigmentation of the skin). Successful with molasses, pantothenic and folic acid in restoring lost hair color. New research shows success against skin cancers caused by UV radiation (lack of ozone-layer protection). Good food sources: nutritional yeast, eggs, molasses and wheat germ. See Vitamins.

• **PANTOTHENIC ACID:** See vitamin B-5. Page 621.

• **pH:** the scale used to measure acidity and alkalinity. pH is hydrogen, or "H" ion concentration of a solution. "p" stands for the power factor of the H ion. pH of a solution is measured on a scale of 14. A neutral solution, neither acidic nor alkaline, such as water, has a pH of 7. Acid is less than 7; alkaline is more than 7.

• **PHENYLALANINE:** an essential amino acid; a tyrosine precursor that works with vitamin B-6 on the central nervous system as an anti-depressant and mood elevator. Successful in treating manic, post-amphetamine, and schizophrenic-type depression (check for allergies first). Aids in learning and memory retention. Relieves menstrual, arthritic and migraine pain. A thyroid stimulant that helps curb the appetite by increasing the body's production of CCK.

Contra-indications: phenylketonurics (people with elevated natural phenylalanine levels) should avoid aspartame sweeteners. Pregnant women and those with blood pressure imbalance, skin carcinomas, and diabetes should avoid phenylalanine. Tumors and cancerous melanoma growths have been slowed by reducing dietary intake of tyrosine and phenylalanine. Avoid if blurred vision occurs when using.

• **PHOSPHORUS:** the second most abundant body mineral. Necessary for skeletal structure, brain oxygenation and cell reproduction. Increases muscle performance; decreases muscle fatigue. Excess antacids deplete phosphorus. Good food sources: eggs, fish, organ meats, dairy foods, legumes, nuts and poultry.

• **PHOSPHATIDYL CHOLINE:** a natural lecithin factor, phosphatidyl choline is an essential component of cell membranes, maintaining membrane fluidity and playing a critical role in all membrane-dependent metabolic processes. Well known as a liver protector, phosphatidyl choline's emulsifying action controls cholesterol and triglyceride levels; often used to increase absorption of fat-soluble vitamins and herbs.

• **PHOSPHATIDYL SERINE, (PS):** a brain cell nutrient that rapidly absorbs and readily crosses the blood-brain barrier. PS helps activate and regulate proteins that play major roles in nerve cell functions and nerve impulses. Studies show that PS helps maintain or improve cognitive ability — memory and learning, especially for Alzheimer's victims. PS effectively helps individuals maintain mental fitness, with benefits persisting even for weeks after PS is stopped. Common foods have insignificant amounts of PS, and the body produces only limited amounts. Concentrated PS was once available only as a bovine-derived product with potential safety problems. A new concentrated, safe-source PS is derived from soybeans.

—**Phospholipids:** ingredients in lecithin which aid in the conversion of food into cell nutrients. Certain phospholipids boost mental performance, guard against high cholesterol or improve nutrient bioavailability. See entries for Phosphatidylcholine and Phosphatidyl Serine, above.

• **PHYTOCHEMICALS:** the natural constituents in plants that have specific pharmacologic action. Also known as neutraceuticals, the actions of phytochemicals are predictable in much the same way as pharmaceuticals, but they are foods. To use phytochemicals best, ingest the plant source in its whole form.

—**Anticarcinogens:** phytochemicals that prevent or delay tumor formation. Some herbs and foods with known anticarcinogens include: *ginseng,* some soy products, *garlic, echinacea, goldenseal, licorice, black cohosh, wild yam, sarsaparilla, maitake* mushroom and cruciferous vegetables.

—**Phytohormones:** many plants contain substances with hormonal actions. Plant hormone phyto-chemicals are quite similar to human hormones and capable of binding to hormone receptor sites in the human body. Unlike synthetic hormones, plant hormones show little or no adverse side effects. Some herbs with phytohormone activity: *soy, licorice, wild yam, sarsaparilla root, dong quai, damiana and black cohosh.*

—**Phytoestrogen:** plant estrogenic hormones remarkably similar to human estrogen hormones. Especially important in hormone-driven cancers, phytoestrogens bind to estrogen receptor sites in the body without the negative side effects of synthetic estrogens or even excess body estrogens. Recent studies show phytoestrogens inhibit the proliferation of both estrogen-receptor positive and negative breast tumor cells. Some herbs with phytoestrogenic activity: *dong quai, panax ginseng, licorice, fennel, alfalfa and red clover.*

——**Phytoprogesterone:** plant progesterone hormones similar to human progesterone. Biochemically, progesterone provides the material from which all other steroid hormones (like cortisone, testosterone, estrogen and salt-regulating aldosterone) can be made. Its simple molecular structure allows it to balance either an excess or deficiency of other hormones. An estrogen precurser, its tremendous increase during pregnancy serves to stabilize the hormone adjustment and growth of mother and child. This is especially visible in uterine and heart muscle tissue, the intestines and bladder. Less visibly, progesterone normalizes gland processes for both men and women. Deficient progesterone often means hypoglycemia, accompanied by obesity. Some plants with progesterone-like activity: *sarsaparilla, licorice root and wild yam.* Natural progesterone, synthesized from diosgenin in wild yam, can increase progesterone levels when used topically in hormone boosting creams. Whole herbs with progesterone-like activity have more subtle, balancing activity, but are also extremely helpful for women's problems.

——**Phyto-testosterone:** plant testosterone similar to the androgen or male hormone found in both men and women. Accelerates tissue growth, stimulates blood flow, balances secondary sexual characteristics. Testosterone is essential for normal sexual behavior and male erections. Few people realize that testosterone influences sex drive in both sexes. The body's production of testosterone decreases and in some cases, changes its structure with age. Ginseng is the only herb tested so far to stimulate testosterone production in the body.

• **PHYTOSOMES:** a new form of botanical technology, the phytosome process enhances and intensifies the power of certain herbal compounds. A phytosome is created by binding flavonoid molecules from herbs to molecules of phosphatidyl choline from lecithin. The union becomes a new molecule better used by the body. Phytosomes can deliver liposomes from plants directly into the body, providing extra phosphatidyl choline and magnifying the power of an herbal compound in its absorption through the skin.

• **PODOPHYLLUM:** a homeopathic remedy that helps diarrhea. See HOMEOPATHIC REMEDIES, page 15.

• **POLYSACCHARIDES:** long chains of simple sugars, plant polysaccharides have long been used in healing, particularly in stimulating the immune system. Aloe, green tea, echinacea, astragalus and maitake mushroom contain large amounts of polysaccharides.

——**Mucopolysaccharides:** polysaccharides that form chemical bonds with water. An important constituent of connective tissue, supporting and binding together the cells to form tissues, and the tissues to form organs. Mucopolysaccharides, especially in the form of Chondroitin Sulphate A (CSA), are beneficial for prevention and reversal of coronary heart disease. CSA is also anti-inflammatory, antiallergenic, and antistress. It is used successfully in treating osteoporosis and in accelerating recovery from bone fractures.

• **PORIA COCOS MUSHROOM,** *Sclerotium Poriae coco:* Strengthens the spleen; regulates excess fluid buildup; purifies body fluids; and prevents build-up of toxins. Recent animal tests show poria cocos may help prevent gastric ulcers by reducing gastric secretions and acidity, and may protect the liver from chemical-induced damage. Used in TCM formulas as a Qi tonic to help balance the effect of other Qi tonic herbs that may dry the system or cause palpitations or dizziness.

• **POTASSIUM:** an electrolyte mineral in body fluids, potassium balances the acid-alkaline system, transmits electrical signals between cells and nerves, and enhances muscle performance. It works with sodium to regulate the body's water balance, and protects the heart against hypertension and stroke (people taking high blood pressure medication are vulnerable to potassium deficiency). Potassium helps oxygenate the brain for clear thinking and controls allergy reactions. Stress, hypoglycemia, diarrhea, acute anxiety or depression generally deplete potassium stores. A vegetable potassium broth (page 291) is one of the best natural healing tools for cleansing and restoring body energy. Good food sources: fresh fruits, especially kiwis and bananas, potatoes, sea greens, poultry and fish, dairy foods, legumes, seeds, whole grains, and spices like *coriander, cumin, basil, parsley, ginger, hot peppers, dill, tarragon, paprika and turmeric.*

• **PREGNENOLONE:** called "preg," pregnenolone is a steroid hormone naturally made from cholesterol, the precursor hormone to DHEA on one of its pathways, and to progesterone on a different pathway. Supplements are lab produced by extracting diosgenin from wild yams, then converting it into pregnenolone through chemical processes. Like DHEA, preg produces a feeling of well-being and increases energy. At higher doses, it enhances visual and auditory perception, especially in men. May cause insomnia or shallow sleep, irritability, and anxiety at higher doses. At doses over 25mg a day, preg may cause headaches.

• **PROBIOTICS:** (meaning "for life") dietary supplements consisting of beneficial microorganisms. Friendly bacteria have a profound influence on our health. Most health professionals recommend a blend of varying species of lactobacillus and bifidophilus. The intestine is home to hundreds of species of microorganisms, both friendly and unfriendly, and competition for survival is fierce. When friendly microorganisms are plentiful and flourishing, they inhibit the growth of pathogenic organisms, boost the immune system, manufacture important vitamins (vitamin K and B vitamins - including B12), improve digestion, combat vaginal yeast infections, maintain the body's vital chemical and hormone balance and keep our bodies clean and protected from toxins. Food sources: yogurt, fermented soy foods, raw sauerkraut, vinegars, kefir products.

• **PROSTAGLANDINS:** a vital group of hormone-like substances derived from essential fatty acids (EFA's) that regulate body functions electrically. EFA's control reproduction and fertility, inflammation, immunity and communication between cells. Prostaglandins supplement and balance the body's essential fatty acid supply. Maintaining the proper prostaglandin balance is a key to health. An excess of prostaglandin E2 caused by a diet overloaded in saturated fats can increase your risk of heart attack and stroke. Fortunately high levels of prostaglandin E1 and E3 from diets high in Omega 3 fatty acids and Gamma Linolenic Acid (GLA) are protective against this reaction-- improving circulation, relaxing blood vessels and lowering blood pressure. Foods like ocean fish, seafoods, olive and flax oil, safflower or sunflower oils, sesame seeds, pumpkin seeds, pine nuts, and herbs like evening primrose are good choices for prostaglandin balance. Conversely, excess saturated fats and Omega 6 fatty acids in the body, especially from fatty animal foods, and large amounts of vegetable oils, imbalance prostaglandin production and proper hormone flow, leading to inflammation and the degenerative disease cascade.

• **PROTEASE:** Plant enzyme proteases are powerful therapeutic agents. Natural medicine uses protease to break up and assist the body in removing undesirable proteins in the blood- a major cause of chronic illness. Taken with food, protease helps digest protein; taken between meals, protease is a potent antioxidant, blood purifier and immune stimulant; taken on an empty stomach, protease goes directly to the bloodstream, reaching most body tissues rapidly for healing action.

Protease stimulates immune phagocytosis- the engulfing of pathogens by immune "eater" cells. Especially helpful for people with autoimmune disorders like Chronic Fatigue Syndrome (CFIDS), arthritis or fibromyalgia, or acute infections. Helps dissolve the fibrin coating on cancer cells, allowing the body's defenses to function better. Accelerates healing of breast and uterine fibroids, and tumors by breaking down fibrous tissue. Works well to reduce internal scarring caused by radiation therapy. Helps dissolve sebaceous gland cysts - 3 caps on an empty stomach between meals is a protective dose. Note: Not for use during pregnancy; if you have a stomach ulcer; before surgery; or if you're using anti-coagulant drugs or have a blood-clotting disorder.

• **PSYLLIUM HUSKS:** a lubricating, mucilaginous, fibrous herb with cleansing, laxative properties. A "colon broom" for constipation; effective for diverticulitis; a lubricant for ulcerous intestinal tract tissue.

• **PULSATILLA:** homeopathic remedy for child allergies or infections. HOMEOPATHIC REMEDIES, page 15.

• **PYRIDOXINE:** see vitamin B-6.

• **PYRUVATE:** Pyruvic acid is a natural element in the human body, an energy by-product of the metabolism of a sugar or starch. Today's popular attention to pyruvate is for its potential as a weight loss and fat loss enhancer. Tests show pyruvate supplements elevate the body's resting metabolic rate and enhance lean muscle mass. Researcher Ronald Stanko, M.D. of University of Pittsburgh Medical School found pyruvate supplements increase weight loss by 37% and fat loss by 48%. Other studies find pyruvate boosts endurance, reduces fatigue and increases energy levels. As a potent antioxidant, it inhibits free radicals, lowers bad LDL cholesterol, and is heart-healthy because it helps the heart pump more blood with less oxygen use.

QUERCETIN: a powerful bioflavonoid cousin of rutin, quercetin is isolated from blue-green algae. Its primary therapeutic use today is in controlling allergy and asthma reactions, since it suppresses the release and production of the two inflammatory agents that cause asthma and allergy symptoms — histamines and leukotrienes. Take quercetin with bromelain for best bioavailability and synergistic anti-inflammatory activity. Quercetin is also being tested with good results as an anti-viral against herpes, polio and respiratory viruses. A potential natural reverse transcriptase inhibitor for HIV-AIDS.

• **QUINOA:** an ancient Inca supergrain, essentially gluten-free, with complete protein from amino acids, and complex carbohydrates. Flavorful and light, use like like rice or millet

REFLEXOLOGY: see YOUR ALTERNATIVE HEALTH CARE CHOICES, page 31.

• **REISHI MUSHROOM,** *Ganoderma lucidum:* known as the "elixir of immortality," reishi is a rare mushroom from the Orient, now cultivated in America. Reishi, or *ganoderma*, increases vitality, enhances immunity and brain function, and prolongs a healthy life. It is a therapeutic antioxidant used for a wide range of serious conditions —anti-tumor, anti-HIV and anti-hepatitis activity. It reduces the side effects of chemotherapy and radiation, and accelerates recovery from these treatments. Research shows success against chronic fatigue syndrome and chronic bronchitis (antibacterial and antiviral). Reishi helps regenerate the liver, lowers cholesterol and triglycerides, reduces coronary risk and high blood pressure, and eases allergy symptoms. It is also a superior nervous system tonic for people affected by chronic stress or severe emotional upsets.

• **RESVERATROL:** a natural polyphenol found in grapes and in high amounts in red wine, resveratrol may help prevent cancer. Clinically, it causes leukemia cancer cells to change back to non-cancerous cells. Resveratrol has antioxidant and anticoagulant properties which protect the heart. Contains mild plant estrogens that protect a woman's heart when she goes through menopause. A glass of resveratrol-rich red wine with dinner benefits heart protection, and eases digestion and reduces stress. *Note: Has mild estrogenic effects that may aggravate hormone-dependent tumors, or add to high estrogen stores in women already using HRT drugs.*

• **RETIN-A:** a vitamin A derivative for treating acne, fine lines and hyperpigmentation, Retin-A is available through prescription in five strengths in cream, gel or liquid form. Retin-A works by decreasing the cohesiveness of skin cells, causing the skin to peel. Because it is a skin irritant, other irritants (like extreme weather, wind, cosmetics, or soaps) can cause severe irritation. Many people are sensitive to Retin-A. *Note: Alpha Hydroxy Acids (AHAs) are an alternative, but should be used cautiously.* See Alpha Hydroxy Acids.

• **RIBOSE:** a simple sugar found naturally in all body cells; a vital part of the metabolic process for ATP energy, the number one fuel used by cells. Maintaining an adequate level of ATP is necessary for peak energy to the heart and muscles. The best candidates for ribose are people with cardiovascular disease, or athletes who experience diminished heart and skeletal muscle nucleotides following high-intensity exercise. Athletes who experience anoxia (muscles using oxygen faster than the bloodstream can supply it), enhance their energy recovery with ribose. Ischemia, a heart condition of poor blood flow which causes a lack of sufficient oxygen to reach the cells decreases ATP levels by 50 percent or more. Ribose studies show that the heart is able to recover 85 percent of its ATP levels within 24 hours.

• **RHUS TOX:** a poison ivy derivative; used homeopathically for pain and stiffness in the joints and ligaments when the pain is worse with cold, damp weather. See HOMEOPATHIC REMEDIES, page 15.

• **RIBOFLAVIN:** see vitamin B-2.

• **ROYAL AGARICUS MUSHROOM,** *Agaricus blazei Murill:* highly popular in Japan, *royal agaricus* is most prized as an immune booster. Like maitake, *royal agaricus* is a rich source of beta 1, 3 and 1,6 glucans. New in vitro studies reveal *agaricus* increases immune cells and the effectiveness of natural killer cells' ability to fight cancer. Activates interferon for potent anti-viral action. Helpful for hepatitis A, B, C.

• **ROYAL JELLY:** the milk-like secretion from the head glands of the queen bee's nurse-workers, RJ is a powerhouse of B vitamins, calcium, iron, potassium and silicon. It has enzyme precursors, a sex hormone and all eight essential amino acids. In fact, it contains every nutrient necessary to support life. It is a natural antibiotic, stimulates immune response, supplies key nutrients for energy and mental alertness, promotes cell longevity, and is effective for wide ranging health benefits. RJ is one of the world's richest sources of pantothenic acid, known to combat stress, fatigue and insomnia, and is a necessary nutrient for healthy skin and hair. It has been found effective for gland and hormone imbalances that reflect in menstrual and prostate problems. The highest quality royal jelly products are preserved in their whole, raw, "alive" state, which promotes ready absorption by the body. As little as one drop of pure extract of fresh royal jelly can deliver an adequate daily supply.

SALICYLIC ACID: occurs naturally in wintergreen leaves, sweet birch, and white willow. Synthetically prepared, it is used in making aspirin, and as a preservative in cosmetics. It is antipyretic (anti-itch) and antiseptic. In medicine, it is used as an antimicrobial at 2 to 20% concentration in ointments, powders, and plasters. It can be absorbed by the skin, but large amounts may cause abdominal pain and hyperventilation.

• **SAMBUCUS NIGRA,** *(Black Elderberry):* has been used in herbal medicine since the days of Hippocrates. Dr. Madeleine Mumcuoglu, Ph.D., Pharm, has found that elderberry extracts successfully and consistently defeat the flu virus, accelerating flu recovery by two to four days compared with a placebo. Viruses have tiny protein spikes with H and N antigens. The H antigen of the virus binds to healthy cell receptors and punctures the cells walls - thus enabling it to reproduce. Active substances in black elderberry disarm the virus's tiny protein spikes of the H antigen, preventing the virus from reproducing itself, thus stopping the virus infection. Besides key antiviral components, elderberry contains high anthocyanin (antioxidant) content.

• **SAMe,** *(S-Adenosyl Methionine):* prescribed for two decades in 14 countries, SAMe is now in the US market. SAMe is normally produced in the brain from the amino acid methionine. It becomes an active methionine in the body when the amino acid L-methionine combines with ATP (primary energy molecule). The supplement form of SAMe is made by first producing the amino acid L-methionine by a micro-fermentation process, then artificially zapping it with ATP. SAMe is an important methyl donor in a process called methylation, important to the biochemical pathway of cellular DNA. Methylation affects everything from fetal development to brain function. Neurotransmitters such as L-dopa, dopamine and related hormones are the products of methylation reactions.

...SAMe is useful for:

—**Depression:** Widely prescribed in Italy, clinical studies show that SAMe is an effective natural antidepressant. Synthesis of SAMe is impaired in depressed patients. Supplementing with SAMe results in increased levels of serotonin and dopamine, and improved binding of neurotransmitters to receptor sites. SAMe has a quicker onset of action and is better tolerated than tricyclic antidepressants.

—**Osteoarthritis pain:** SAMe relieves the pain of osteoarthritis by aiding chemical processes that control pain and inflammation. The U.S. Arthritis Foundation states that SAMe "provides pain relief."

—**Liver disease:** Studies show that SAMe helps cirrhosis, hepatitis, cholestasis (bile ducts blockage), and may prevent liver damage caused by some drugs. Alcohol harms the liver partly by depleting SAMe.

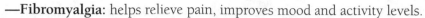

—**Fibromyalgia:** helps relieve pain, improves mood and activity levels.

—**Migraine headaches:** provides pain relief.

—**Alzheimer's disease:** studies show its neurotransmitter improvement enhances memory centers.

Common dose: 200 to 400mg, with higher therapeutic doses. SAMe is extremely safe, but people with bipolar (manic) depression should consult a physician. Include a B vitamin complex when taking SAMe. When a SAMe molecule loses its methyl group, it breaks down to become homocysteine. Homocysteine is toxic to cells if it builds up. Vitamin B-6, B-12 and folic acid beneficially convert homocysteine into the antioxidant glutathione.

• **SANGRE DE GRADO:** a sap taken from Croton trees, used for hundreds of years by those living in the Amazon basin rainforests, not only for topical treatments, but also diluted, as a remedy for gastrointestinal complaints, ulcers and diarrhea. Used externally for insect bites and also to stop hemorrhaging. The sap is amazingly effective in healing cuts and wounds. The newest studies reveal Sangre de Grado helps form crust at the site of the wound, regenerate skin, and form new collagen. Peruvian herbalists use Sangre de Grado internally for vaginal infections, ulcers (mouth, stomach, intestines), fractures, hemorrhoids and bone fractures. Modern research points to Sangre de Grado as one of the most potent herbal antivirals available. It is currently undergoing FDA Phase 2 and Phase 3 clinical trials for viral respiratory infections (used orally) and for herpes (topically). Research shows Sangre de Grado is 30 times more effective than penicillin or chloramphenicol against bacteria. It even fights deadly *E. Coli* bacteria.

• **SAUNA HEAT THERAPY:** a sauna is excellent overheating therapy. A long sauna not only induces a healing, cleansing fever, but also causes profuse therapeutic sweating to remove toxic substances. (In overheating therapy, your skin acts as a "third kidney" to eliminate body wastes through perspiration.) Professional saunas are available in every health club and gym as part of the membership, and the new home-installed models are not only adequate but reasonable in price. For optimum skin cleansing and restoration, take a sauna once or twice a week.

…**Some of the health benefits of a dry sauna:** 1: speeds up metabolism; 2: inhibits the replication of pathogenic organisms; 3: stimulates activity of all vital organs and glands; 4: supports the body's immune system and accelerates its healing functions; 5: dramatically increases detoxifying capacity of the skin; 6: a proven jump-start technique for a weight loss program, especially for sugar cravers.

Note: Although induced fever is a natural, constructive means of biological healing, advice from an expert practitioner is recommended. A heart and general vitality check is advisable. Some seriously ill people lose their ability to perspire; this should be known before using overheating therapy. See page 183 for more about saunas.

• **SEA GREENS:** including *arame, bladderwrack, dulse, hijiki, kelp, kombu, nori, sea palm, and wakame* are foods with superior nutritional content. They are rich sources of proteins, carbohydrates, antioxidants, minerals and vitamins, especially healing carotenes. They are good body alkalizers, and can be used in place of salt or other seasonings. Sea vegetables are the mainstay of iodine therapy for wide ranging health needs. See ABOUT SEA GREENS & IODINE THERAPY, pg. 156 for more information on their healing properties.

• **SELENIUM:** a component of glutathione and powerful antioxidant, selenium protects the body from free radical damage and heavy metal toxins. An anticancer substance and immune stimulant, it works with vitamin E to prevent cholesterol build-up, protect against heart and degenerative disease and enhance skin elasticity. Used in China with impressive results against an *Ebola*-like hemorrhagic fever outbreak. (Researchers saw a 37% mortality rate in the selenium treated patients, the disease normally has a 100% mortality rate.) Deficiency results in aging skin, liver damage, hypothyroidism and sometimes in digestive tract cancer. The most effective supplement is organic seleno-methionine. Very high doses of selenium (over 900mcg) can be toxic. Between 50-200mcg is a safe daily dose to consider. Food sources: nutritional yeast, sesame seeds, garlic, tuna, sea greens, wheat germ, oysters, fish, organ meats, vegetables, nuts and mushrooms.

• **SEPIA:** a homeopathic remedy for treating herpes, eczema and hair loss. See HOMEOPATHY, page 15.

• **SEROTONIN:** a neurotransmitter with widespread and often profound implications, serotonin has a number of functions in the central nervous system, blood vessels and intestines. It plays a role in sleep, mood, depression, appetite, memory, learning, body temperature, sexual behavior, cardiovascular function, muscle contraction, and endocrine regulation. Serotonin is also a precursor to the neurohormone, melatonin, well known for its role in reducing sleep disorders and jet lag. New research shows imbalanced serotonin in the brain can lead to food binges (especially on sugary foods and carbohydrates), depression, obsessive compulsive disorder, aggressive behavior and multiple addictions. About 2% of all serotonin is located in the brain.

• **SHARK CARTILAGE:** contains a biologically active protein that strongly inhibits development of new blood vessel networks (angiogenesis). Angiogenesis is a primary cause of rheumatoid arthritis and cancer tumor growth. Other conditions dependent on angiogenesis blood supply may be corrected somewhat by shark cartilage: eye diseases like diabetic retinopathy, macular degeneration and glaucoma; lupus erythematosus; inflammatory bowel diseases like Crohn's disease; scleroderma; yeast diseases like candida enteritis; cancers like Kaposi's sarcoma and solid tumors; skin disorders such as eczema and psoriasis.
Note: Because of its efficient inhibition on the formation of new capillary networks, there are some contraindications: a pregnant woman should not supplement with shark cartilage because she wants capillary growth for her fetus. If you have heart disease or peripheral vascular disease, avoid shark cartilage since new capillaries are desirable. Shark cartilage is unsuitable if you suffer from liver dysfunction or disabling kidney disease. Large amounts of shark cartilage can cause gastric upset — take smaller dosages throughout the day. Daily dosage: between 20 and 90 gm daily; the course of therapy often runs from six to nine months.

• **SHIITAKE MUSHROOM,** *Lentinus edodes:* usually sold dry, shiitake is a tonic mushroom useful for system weakness, and immune defense. At least two different extracts, *LEM*, an extract from immature shiitake's, and *Lentinan*, an extract from the mushroom fruit body, act as immune system stimulators and antiviral activators. Shiitake mushrooms stimulate immmune macrophages and NK (natural killer) cells to act rapidly and aggressively against invading pathogens and increase antibody production and interferon for better disease resistance. Animal tests reveal shiitake offers more powerful protection against influenza A than the anti-viral drug, amantadine. A compound in shiitake, called *eritadenine*, lowers serum cholesterol by as much as 45 percent. Also shows healing results against hypertension, cataracts, anemia, allergies and immune compromised diseases like Chronic Fatigue, candida, encephalitis, cancer and retro viruses like HIV. Shiitake may even assist the body in making antibodies to Hepatitis B. Use shiitake a few each time; a little goes a long way. *Note: In large amounts, may cause diarrhea or skin rash. Consult with your physician if you are taking blood thinners, shiitake has mild anti-clotting properties.*

• **SILICA,** *silicon dioxide:* a chemical compound of silicon and oxygen, silica comprises a large percent of the earth's crust and mantle, rocks and sand. Quartz consists solely of silica. There is some confusion between silica and silicon, both available in health food stores. Silicon is the elemental silicon mineral that is found in man, animals and plants. Silica is generally silicon dioxide, the most abundant silicon compound.
Silica gel, derived from quartz crystals, contains hydrogen, oxygen and silicon, one form of which is used to absorb moisture in containers for certain foods and in the bottles of our supplements. Some silica supplements are water-soluble extracts of the herb horsetail. Others are derived from purified algae. In addition to its benefits for healthy hair, skin and nails, and for calcium absorption in bone formation, silica/silicon maintains flexible arteries and plays a significant role in cardiovascular health. Beneficial food sources: grain husks (particularly barley, oats, millet, wheat), seeds, green leafy vegetables, red beets, asparagus, Jerusalem artichokes, parsley, bell peppers, sunflower seeds and horsetail herb.
—**Silicon:** a mineral necessary for collagen synthesis, and responsible for connective tissue growth and health. Regenerates body infrastructure (silicon supplements may help bone recalcification), including skeleton, tendons, ligaments, cartilage, connective tissue, skin, hair and nails. Silicon counteracts the effects of aluminum on the body,

and is important in the prevention of Alzheimer's disease, osteoporosis and arteriosclerosis. Silicon levels decrease with age and are needed in larger amounts by the elderly. Food sources: whole grains, horsetail herb, well water, bottled mineral water and fresh vegetables.

—**Silicea,** *(silica):* a homeopathic cell salt essential to health of bones, joints, skin and glands. Deficiency produces respiratory system catarrh, pus discharges from the skin, slow wound healing and offensive body odor. Very successful in the homeopathic treatment of boils, pimples and abscesses, for hair and nail health, blood cleansing, and rebuilding the body after illness or injury. See HOMEOPATHIC CELL SALTS, pp. 17-18.

• **SODIUM:** an electrolyte mineral that helps regulate kidney and body fluid function. Involved with high blood pressure only when calcium and phosphorous are deficient in the body. Works as an anti-dehydrating agent. Beneficial food sources include: celery, seafoods, sea vegetables, cheese, dairy products.

• **SORBITOL:** a humectant that gives a velvety feel to skin. Used as a replacement for glycerin in emulsions, ointments, mouthwashes, toothpastes, and cosmetics. Used in foods as a sugar substitute. First found in the ripe berries of the mountain ash, it also occurs in other berries, cherries, plums, pears, apples, seaweed and algae. Medicinally used to reduce excess body water and for intravenous feeding. If ingested in excess, it can cause diarrhea and gastrointestinal disturbances.

• **SOY:** see SOY FOODS & THERAPEUTIC BENEFITS, page 109.

• **SPIRULINA:** a blue-green algae that the Aztecs and Mayans relied on as a primary food and health maintenance source. Used widely today for body cleansing, as a high quality nutrient source and its newly discovered cancer protective qualities. See GREEN SUPERFOODS, page 100 for more information.

• **STEVIA REBAUDIANA,** *(sweet herb):* see SUGAR & SWEETENERS IN A HEALING DIET, pp. 145-153.

• **STEROLS & STEROLINS:** plant constituents including beta sitosterol and beta sitosterolin that resemble animal fat cholesterol, but have different biological activity. Plant sterols enhance immune response in three important ways: They increase immune T-cell division; they enhance T-cells' secretion of lymphokines involved in cellular immunity, and they boost the activity of cytotoxic cells (key to fighting pathogens). New research reveals plant sterol therapy can improve or eliminate a wide variety of disorders including: Chronic Fatigue Syndrome (CFIDS), hepatitis C, prostatitis, cervical cancer, rheumatoid arthritis, HIV and allergies. A good choice to help normalize cholesterol levels, and reduce adrenal stress. Abundant in all plants, raw nuts and seeds, and shellfish. Largely derived from pine in commercial supplements.

• **SULFORAPHANE:** a sulphur compound in cruciferous vegetables, mustard, horseradish and broccoli sprouts. Sulforaphane activates phase 2 enzymes (like indole 3 carbinol) that detoxify cancer-causing substances from the body. Sulforaphane helps delay onset of cancer, and inhibits size and number of tumors. Reduces breast cancer occurrence by up to 60% in lab animals. Colon cancer risk can be cut in half by eating 2-lbs. of sulforaphane-rich broccoli a week. The newest research reveals sulforaphane can also kill *H. pylori*, a bacteria responsible for some stomach ulcers and stomach cancers. Broccoli sprouts are sweet tasting and contain 30 to 50 times more sulforaphane than broccoli itself. *Note:* broccoli seeds are often heavily treated with fungicides and pesticides, so organic broccoli sprouts are the best choice.

• **SULPHUR:** the "beauty mineral" for smooth skin, glossy hair, hard nails and collagen synthesis. It is critical to protein absorption. Good food sources: eggs, fish, onions, garlic, hot peppers and mustard.

• **SUPER OXIDE DISMUTASE (SOD):** an enzyme, SOD prevents damage caused by the toxic oxygen molecule known as superoxide. Manganese and zinc especially, stimulate production of SOD. Many experts do not believe that antioxidant enzyme levels in cells can be increased by taking antioxidant enzymes like SOD orally. In fact, human tests with SOD don't appear to increase the levels of SOD in the blood or tissues. See Antioxidants.

TAURINE: a non-essential amino acid, taurine is a potent anti-seizure nutrient. A neurotransmitter that helps control hyperactivity, nervous system imbalance after drug or alcohol abuse, and epilepsy. Normalizes irregular heartbeat, helps prevent circulatory and heart disorders, hypoglycemia, hypothyroidism, water retention and hypertension. Taurine is the most abundant amino acid in the retina and is important for proper eye functioning. Taurine may even play a role in preventing cataract development. Lowers cholesterol levels. Found in high concentrations in bile, mother's milk, shark and abalone. Supplementation is necessary for therapy.

• **TESTOSTERONE:** the key male hormone, although it's a part of women's sexuality, too. Male energy, strength, muscle growth and sexuality are largely dependent on an adequate supply of testosterone. While a man's hormone fluctuations are less dramatic than a woman's, testosterone levels start to decline around age 40, falling up to 10% each decade. Low energy, impotence and prostate problems are three of the main problems men complain about as they experience these hormonal changes. As a result, natural testosterone boosters like panax ginseng, super hormone supplements like Andro, and even testosterone drugs are in high demand to help keep an older man feeling and performing at his best.

• **THIAMINE:** see Vitamin B-1.

• **THREONINE:** an essential amino acid that works with glycine to aid in overcoming depression, and neurologic dysfunctions such as genetic spastic disorders and M.S. Works with aspartic acid and methionine as a lipotropic to prevent fatty build-up in the liver. Helps to control epileptic seizures. An immune stimulant and thymus enhancer. Important for the formation of collagen, elastin and enamel.

• **THUYA:** a homeopathic remedy for warts and sinusitis. See Homeopathic Remedies, page 15.

• **TRANSFER FACTORS:** molecular messengers of the immune system (specifically immune T-lymphocytes) which confer immunity to a pathogen. Naturally present in human blood, but extracted from cow's colostrum in supplement form. Very promising as part of a natural healing arsenal to fight viral, bacterial, fungal and parasitical illness. May one day treat even serious diseases like antibiotic-resistant "supergerms," cancer, malaria and AIDS.

• **TREMELLA MUSHROOM,** *Tremella fuciformis:* legend says that Concubine Yang, thought to be the most beautiful woman in Chinese history, used tremella as her beauty secret. Tremella is very rich in dietary fibers and vitamin D. Used therapeutically for asthma, cardiovascular health and as a tonic for degenerative disease. Boosts red cell production and protects against radiation poisoning.

• **TRIPHALA:** the most widely used cleansing formula in Ayurveda composed of harada fruit (*Terminalia chebula*), amla fruit (*Embilica officinalis*) and Behada fruit (*Terminalia belerica*). Less likely to cause laxative dependence than other formulas, gentle enough for anyone to use. Astringent properties tonify the colon and promote natural detoxification. Often noted for its ability to treat psychosomatic conditions affecting the digestive tract.

• **TRYPTOPHAN:** an essential amino acid; a precursor of the neurotransmitter serotonin that regulates mood and metabolism. Tryptophan is a non-addictive tranquilizer for restful sleep. Dilates blood vessels to decrease aggressive behavior, migraine headaches, and schizophrenia. Counteracts compulsive overeating, smoking and alcoholism. An effective anti-depressant, it raises low blood sugar, and reduces seizures in petit mal epilepsy. Produces nicotinic acid (natural niacin) now being tested to counteract the effects of nicotine from cigarettes.
    —**5-HTP** (*L-5-Hydroxytryptophan*): 5-HTP is the step between tryptophan and serotonin, so it plays an important role in the serotonin story. Tryptophan helps synthesize serotonin in our bodies; once tryptophan is

taken up into a nerve cell, it is converted into 5-HTP with the help of the enzyme *tryptophan hydroxylase*. The 5-HTP is then converted to serotonin. The supplement 5-HTP is extracted from *Griffonia* seed to boost serotonin. Many researchers consider 5-HTP to be the safest tryptophan alternative available, and successful studies using 5-HTP show that it alleviates serotonin-deficiency by elevating brain serotonin.

• **TURKEY TAIL MUSHROOM,** *Coriolus versicolor:* studies on turkey tail have been going on since the 1970's in Japan. Its constituents PSP and PSK are well known for their powerful immunomodulating action. Like most medicinal mushrooms, turkey tail has anti-cancer activity, improving survival rates and recovery from chemo and radiation therapies. Used in TCM to clear dampness and phlegm.

• **TYROSINE:** a semi-essential amino acid and growth hormone stimulant formed from phenylalanine, tyrosine helps to build the body's natural store of adrenaline and thyroid hormones. It rapidly metabolizes as an antioxidant throughout the body, and is effective as a source of quick energy, especially for the brain. It converts to the amino acid L-Dopa, making it a safe therapy for depression, hypertension, and Parkinson's disease, helps control drug abuse and aids drug withdrawal. It helps reduce appetite and body fat in a weight loss diet. For some, it increases libido and sex drive. It produces melanin for skin and hair pigment making it helpful for those with vitiligo and prematurely grey hair. *Note: Tumors, cancerous melanomas and manic depression are slowed through dietary reduction of tyrosine and phenylalanine.*

UMEBOSHI PLUMS: pickled Japanese apricots with alkalizing, bacteria killing properties; part of a macrobiotic diet.

• **UREA,** *carbamide:* used in yeast food and wine production, also to "brown" baked goods like pretzels. Commercial urea consists of colorless or white odorless crystals that have a cool, salty taste. Widely used as an antiseptic in antiperspirants and deodorants, mouthwashes, shampoos, lotions and similar products.

VANADIUM: a mineral cofactor for several enzymes. Deficiency is linked to heart disease, poor reproductive ability and infant mortality. Recent studies have found that vanadium improves sugar metabolism for non-insulin dependent diabetics. But high levels of vanadium can be toxic; elevated vanadium levels are linked to manic depressive illness. I only recommend taking vanadium in small dosages. 1mg doses of vanadium within a broad spectrum multi-vitamin and mineral formula is a safe choice for a blood sugar stabilizing program. Good food sources: whole grains, fish, olives, radishes, vegetables.

• **VINEGAR:** brown rice, balsamic, apple cider, herb, raspberry, ume plum — vinegars have been used for 5000 years as healthful flavor enhancers and food preservers. As condiments, like relishes or dressings, they help digest heavy foods and high protein meals. The most nutritious vinegars are not overly filtered, and still contain the "mother" mixture of beneficial bacteria and enzymes in the bottle. They look slightly cloudy.

• **VINPOCETINE:** a derivative of *vincamine*, an extract of periwinkle, used in Hungary for senility and blood vessel disorders for 25 years. Vinpocetine is a memory enhancer that improves cerebral blood flow, brain cell ATP and utilization of oxygen and glucose. Guards against stroke, memory impairment, motor disorders, inner ear imbalance and hearing loss. Improves vision in 70% of subjects tested. Preliminary research finds vinpocetine may relieve urinary incontinence. *Note: rare occurrences of dry mouth and heart palpitations.* Dosage: One 10mg capsule 1 to 3x daily. Available through Olympia Nutrition 1-888-366-9909.

• **VITAMINS:** organic micro-nutrients that act like spark plugs in the body, keeping it "tuned up" and functioning normally. You can't live on vitamins; they are not pep pills, substitutes for food, or components of body structure. They stimulate, but do not act as, nutritional fuel. They are catalysts, often working as co-enzymes at the cell level, regulating metabolic processes through enzyme activity, to convert proteins and carbohydrates to tissue and energy. Most vitamins cannot be synthesized by the body, and must be supplied by food or supplement. Excess amounts are excreted in the urine, or stored by the body until needed.

Even with their minute size and amounts in the body, vitamins are absolutely necessary for growth, vitality, resistance to disease, and healthy aging. It is impossible to sustain life without them. A growing number of studies show that even small to modest vitamin deficiencies can endanger the whole body.... especially your immune response. Unfortunately, it takes weeks or months for signs of most vitamin deficiencies to appear because the body only slowly uses its supply. Even when your body is "running on empty" in a certain vitamin, problems may be hard to pinpoint, because the cells usually continue to function with decreasing efficiency until they receive proper nourishment or suffer irreversible damage.

Vitamin therapy does not produce results overnight. Regenerative changes in biochemistry may require as much time to rebuild as they did to decline. Vitamins fill nutritional gaps at your body's deepest levels and need to be taken for a long time for real effectiveness in preventing diseases. However, vitamin test results so far indicate that longterm benefits of vitamin therapy are worthwhile. In most cases, a program of moderate amounts over a longer period of time brings about better body balance and more permanent results.

Today, poor dietary habits, over-processed foods, and agri-business practices lead most health professionals to believe that supplements are needed for adequate nutrition. Even as basic as the RDA recommendations are, not one dietary survey shows that Americans consume anywhere near RDA amounts in their normal diets. One large USDA survey of the daily food intake of 21,500 people over a three day period showed that not a single person got 100% of the RDA nutrients. Only 3% ate the recommended number of servings from the four food groups. Only 12% got the RDA for protein, calcium, iron, magnesium, zinc or vitamins A, C, B_6, B_{12}, B_2, and B_1. The study concluded that trying to change long-held dietary habits and ignoring vitamin supplements left much of the American population at nutritional risk.

People most affected by vitamin deficiencies include:
1: Women with excessive menstrual bleeding who may need iron supplements.
2: Pregnant or nursing women who may need extra iron, calcium and folic acid.
3: The elderly, many of whom don't even get two-thirds of the RDA for calcium, iron, vitamin A or C. (*Note: Seniors take more than 50% of all drug prescriptions in the U.S. 90 out of the 100 most prescribed drugs interfere with nutrient metabolism, so it's a sad fact that many older people don't absorb even very much of the nutrition that they do eat.*)
4: Everyone on medications that interfere with nutrient absorption, digestion or metabolism.
5: People on weight loss diets with extremely low calorie intake.
6: People at risk for heart and circulatory blockages, and those at risk for osteoporosis.
7: People who have recently had surgery, or suffer from serious injuries, wounds or burns.
8: People with periodontal disease or malabsorption problems.
9: Vegetarians, who may not receive enough calcium, iron, zinc or vitamin B_{12}.
10: People who live in communities where municipal water supplies are fluoridated.

Vitamins help us go beyond average health to optimal health. Here's what vitamins do for you:
—**VITAMIN A:** is a fat soluble vitamin, requiring fats, minerals (especially zinc) and enzymes for absorption. Available in both plants and animals, plants contain the beta carotene form while animal sources contain retinol. Vitamin A counteracts night blindness, weak eyesight, and strengthens the optical system. Supplementation lowers risk of many types of cancer. Retinoids inhibit malignant transformation, and reverse pre-malignant changes in tissue. Vitamin A is particularly effective against lung cancer. It is also an anti-infective that builds immune resistance. It helps develop strong bone cells, a major factor in the health of skin, hair, teeth and gums. Deficiency results in eye dryness and the inability to tear, night blindness, rough, itchy skin, poor bone growth, weak tooth enamel, chronic diarrhea and frequent respiratory infections. Vitamin A is critical to adrenal and steroid hormone synthesis, and is a key to preventing early aging. Good food sources: fish liver oils, seafood, sea greens, dairy foods, yellow fruits and vegetables, dark leafy greens, yams, sweet potatoes, liver, watermelon and canteloupe, and eggs. *Note: Avoid high doses of Vitamin A during pregnancy.*

—**VITAMIN B-1,** *(Thiamine)*: known as the "morale vitamin" because it enhances nerves and mental attitude. Promotes proper growth in children, aids carbohydrate utilization for energy and supports the nervous system. Enhances immune response. Helps control motion sickness. Wards off mosquitos and stinging insects. Pregnancy, lactation, diuretics and oral contraceptives require extra thiamine. Smoking, heavy metal pollutants, excess sugar, junk foods, stress and alcohol all deplete thiamine. Deficiency results in insomnia, fatigue, confusion, poor memory and poor muscle coordination. Food source thiamine is sensitive to heat and chlorine. Avoid washing or cooking thiamine-rich foods in chlorinated water if you suspect you are thiamine deficient. A high sugar diet or too much alcohol also increases your thiamine needs. Good food sources: asparagus, brewer's yeast, brown rice, beans, nuts, seeds, wheat germ, organ meats and soy foods.

—**VITAMIN B-2,** *(Riboflavin)*: commonly deficient in the U.S. diet. Necessary for energy production, and for fat and carbohydrate metabolism. Helps prevent cataracts and corneal ulcers, and generally benefits vision. Promotes healthy skin, especially in cases of psoriasis. Helps protect against drug toxicity and environmental chemicals. Pregnancy and lactation, excess dairy and red meat consumption, prolonged stress, sulfa drugs, diuretics and oral contraceptives all require extra riboflavin. Deficiency is associated with alcohol abuse, anemia, hypothyroidism, diabetes, ulcers, cataracts and congenital heart disease. Good food sources: almonds, nutritional yeast, broccoli, green leafy veggies, eggs, mushrooms, yogurt, organ meats and caviar.

—**VITAMIN B-3,** *(Niacin)*: a vitamin involved with energy production, sex hormone synthesis and good digestion, boosting production of hydrochloric acid in the stomach. Niacin improves joint function, strength and endurance in people with osteoarthritis. Niacin can significantly lower cholesterol. A new study reveals niacin combined with chromium can lower cholesterol as much as 30%! Niacin promotes healthy skin and nerves, relieves diarrhea and digestive problems, migraines and vertigo. Depletion results in dermatitis, headaches, gum disease, sometimes high blood pressure and schizophrenic behavior. However, because niacin can rapidly open up and stimulate circulation, (a niacin skin flush is evidence of this), it can act quickly to reverse deficiency disorders. Niacin works with chromium to regulate blood sugar for diabetes and hypoglycemia. To boost energy, look for products containing B3's active coenzyme, NADH (nicotinamide adenine dinucleotide). Food sources: almonds, avocados, nutritional yeast, fish, legumes, bananas, whole grains, cheese, eggs and sesame seeds.

—**VITAMIN B-5,** *(Pantothenic Acid)*: an antioxidant vitamin vital to proper adrenal activity, pantothenic acid is a precursor to cortisone production and an aid to natural steroid synthesis. It is important in preventing arthritis and high cholesterol. It fights infection by building antibodies, and defends against stress, fatigue and nerve disorders. It is a key to overcoming postoperative shock and drug side effects after surgery. Pantothenic acid inhibits hair color loss. Deficiency results in anemia, fatigue and muscle cramping. Individuals suffering from constant psychological stress have a heightened need for B$_5$. Good food sources include: nutritional yeast, brown rice, poultry, yams, organ meats, egg yolks, soy products and royal jelly.

—**VITAMIN B-6,** *(Pyridoxine)*: a key vitamin in red blood cell regeneration, and protein metabolism, and carbohydrate use. A primary immune stimulant with particular effectiveness against liver cancer. Supplementation inhibits histamine release in treating allergies and asthma. Supports all aspects of nerve health including neuropsychiatric disorders, epilepsy and carpal tunnel syndrome. Works as a natural diuretic, especially in premenstrual edema. Controls acne, promotes beautiful skin, relieves morning sickness and is an anti-aging factor. Protects against environmental pollutants, smoking and stress. Oral contraceptives, *thiazide* diuretics, penicillin and alcohol deplete B-6. Deficiency results in anemia, depression, lethargy, nervousness, water retention and skin lesions. Food sources: bananas, nutritional yeast, buckwheat, organ meats, fish, avocados, legumes, poultry, nuts, rice bran, brown rice, wheat bran, sunflower seeds and soy foods.

—**VITAMIN B-12,** *(Cyano Cobalamin)*: an anti-inflammatory analgesic that works with calcium for absorption. Critical to DNA synthesis and red blood cell formation; involved in all immune responses. A specific for sulfite-induced asthma. Research shows some success in cancer management, especially in tumor growth. Energizes, relieves depression, hangover and poor concentration. Supplied largely from animal foods, B-12 may be deficient for vegetarians, and a deficiency can take five or more years to appear after body stores are depleted. Deficiency results in anemia, nerve degeneration, dizziness, heart palpitations and excess weight loss. Long use of cholesterol drugs, oral contraceptives, anti-inflammatory and anti-convulsant drugs deplete B-12. Food sources: cheese, poultry, sea greens, yogurt, eggs, organ meats, nutritional yeast and fish.

—**VITAMIN C,** *(Ascorbic Acid):* a primary factor in immune strength and health. Protects against cancer, viral and bacterial infections, heart disease, arthritis and allergies. It is a strong antioxidant against free radical damage. Safeguards against radiation poisoning, heavy metal toxicity, environmental pollutants and early aging. Accelerates healing after surgery, increases infection resistance, and is essential to formation of new collagen tissue. Vitamin C controls alcohol craving, lowers cholesterol, and is a key factor in treating diabetes, high blood pressure, male infertility, and in suppressing the HIV virus. Supports adrenal and iron insufficiency, especially when the body is under stress. Relieves withdrawal symptoms from addictive drugs, tranquilizers and alcohol. Aspirin, oral contraceptives, smoking and tetracycline inhibit vitamin C absorption and deplete C levels. Deficiency results in easy bruising, receding gums, slow healing, fatigue and rough skin.

In spite of these clear benefits, vitamin C has been the subject of controversy for the last few years. Much of the concern started in 1998 when a group of British scientists published a study stating that vitamin C could actually cause cell damage by promoting free radical cascades. Critics at the Linus Pauling Institute immediately declared that the study was flawed and that its conclusions were unwarranted. They stated that the study focused too narrowly on a biological marker that has not been proven as a good indicator of cell damage. Still, we know that oxidized vitamin C does have pro-oxidant and anti-oxidant activity, and that's why you get better best results by combining vitamin C with other antioxidants. Other antioxidants freely give their own electrons to Vitamin C to neutralize this reaction. Antioxidants like Vitamin E, N-Acetyl-Cysteine, and green tea have been found to neutralize any free radical reaction caused by vitamin C alone and also boosts its antioxidant activity.

—**Ester C™,** a metabolite form of vitamin C, is biochemically the same as naturally metabolized C in the body. Both fat and water soluble, and non-acid, Ester C is absorbed twice as fast into the bloodstream and excreted twice as slowly as ordinary vitamin C. Good food sources: citrus fruits, green peppers, papaya, tomatoes, kiwi, potatoes, greens, cauliflower and broccoli.

—**VITAMIN D:** a critical fat soluble vitamin, D works with vitamin A to utilize calcium and phosphorus in building bones and teeth. Although we call it a vitamin, D is really a hormone produced in the skin from sunlight. Cholesterol compounds in the skin convert to a vitamin D precursor when exposed to UV radiation. Twenty minutes a day of early morning sunshine make a real difference to your body's vitamin D stores, especially if you are at risk for osteoporosis. Vitamin D helps in all eye problems including spots, conjunctivitis and glaucoma. Helps protect against colon cancer. Deficiency results in nearsightedness, psoriasis, soft teeth, muscle cramps and tics, slow healing, insomnia, nosebleeds, fast heartbeat and arthritis. Good food sources: cod liver oil, yogurt, cheese, butter, herring, halibut, salmon, tuna, eggs and liver.

—**VITAMIN E:** a fat soluble antioxidant and important immune stimulating vitamin. An effective anticoagulant and vasodilator against blood clots and heart disease. Retards cellular and mental aging, alleviates fatigue and provides tissue oxygen to accelerate healing of wounds and burns. Works with selenium against the effects of aging and cancer by neutralizing free radicals. Beneficial for chronic, so-called incurable diseases like arthritis, lupus, Parkinson's disease and MS. Improves skin tone and texture; helps control alopecia and dandruff. Synergistic with CoQ10. Deficiency results in muscle and nerve degeneration, anemia, skin pigmentation. Good food sources: almonds, leafy vegetables, seafoods and sea greens, spirulina, soy, wheat germ, palm oil, wheat germ oil and organ meats. Still, it is hard to obtain enough vitamin E from foods to help prevent disease. When purchasing supplements, look for natural vitamin E, d-alpha tocopherol (Tocopherol is another term for vitamin E and its related compounds), which is far more bioavailable than synthetic forms. In one study, it took 300mg of synthetic vitamin E to reach the blood levels achieved by 100mg of natural vitamin E! In addition, research from Oregon State University shows that synthetic vitamin E is excreted by the body 3 times faster than the natural form.

—**Tocotrienols:** compounds related to vitamin E tocopherols, tocotrienols lower cholesterol, with potent antioxidant and anti-cancer properties. Studies show tocotrienols are more effective than tocopherols in decreasing both total and LDL cholesterol levels. Although tocotrienols and tocopherols both offer significant protection against damage to the arterial wall - tocotrienols have a stronger lipid lowering effect. Vitamin E supplements containing natural mixed tocopherols, including the tocotrienols, offer the best choice.

—**VITAMIN K:** a fat soluble vitamin necessary for blood clotting and may be taken as a guard against too-easy bleeding. Vitamin K is easy to get from the normal diet and is stored in the body. Deficiency occurs from poor nutrient absorption, from conditions like celiac disease, intestinal worms or chronic colitis. Antibiotic overload contributes to many cases of vitamin K deficiency because these drugs deplete and destroy friendly intestinal flora. Vitamin K reduces excessive menstruation, helps heal broken blood vessels in the eye, aids in arresting bone loss and post-menopausal brittle bones. Vitamin K is an integral part of liver function and is a good source of help for cirrhosis and jaundice of the liver. Good food sources: seafoods, sea greens, dark leafy vegetables, liver, molasses, eggs, oats, crucifers and sprouts.

WATERMELON SEED: a diuretic used in herbal teas to flush out bacteria from UTI's and reduce urinary stone accumulations. High in amino acids citrulline and arginine, watermelon seed increases synthesis of urea in the liver, accounting for its diuretic action. A gentle body cleanser for skin conditions like hives. Used in TCM for constipation.

• **WHEAT GERM, WHEAT GERM OIL:** wheat germ is the embryo of the wheat berry, rich in B vitamins, protein and iron. It goes rancid quickly, buy in nitrogen-flushed packaging. Wheat germ oil is a vitamin E source and body oxygenator, an excellent cosmetic oil for the skin, adding highly absorbable EFA's that noticeably help skin texture. One tablespoon provides the antioxidant equivalent of an oxygen tent for 30 minutes.

• **WHEAT GRASS:** See GREEN SUPERFOODS, page 100.

XYLITOL: a low glycemic, low calorie sweetener made from birchwood chips or plums, xylitol is safe for hypoglycemics and diabetics used in small amounts. Xylitol is one of the few sweeteners that can actually help strengthen your teeth and prevent cavities. Xylitol helps reduce cavities by neutralizing mouth acids, and enhances tooth remineralization. A potent anti-infective, xylitol is a specific for ear infections, sinusitis, the common cold and flu. Xylitol works especially well in a nasal spray to help wash away irritants linked to allergies and asthma. *Note: Taken in large amounts, xylitol may cause diarrhea.*

ZEAXANTHIN: See Carotenoids.

• **ZINC:** a mineral that acts as a co-factor of SOD to protect against free radical damage, is essential to the formation of insulin, immune strength, gland, sexual and reproductive health. Helps prevent birth defects, enhances sensory perception, accelerates healing. Zinc is a brain food that helps control mental disorders and promotes mental alertness. Stress depletes zinc, impairing immune response and the ability to heal. People who get little sleep, work a 16-hour day (or more than one job), or those recovering from injury need to increase zinc levels in their diet. The picolinate form is highly absorbable. Food sources: crab, herring, liver, lobster, oysters, turkey, poppy, sunflower, pumpkin and caraway seeds, nutritional yeast, eggs, mushrooms and wheat germ.

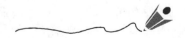

Product Resources

Where you can get what we recommend.....

The following list is for your convenience and assistance in obtaining further information about the products I recommend in HEALTHY HEALING. The list is unsolicited by the companies named. Each company has a solid history of testing and corroborative data that is invaluable to me and my staff, as well as empirical confirmation by the stores that carry these products who have shared their experiences with us. We hear from thousands of readers about the products they have used. I consider their information with every edition of HEALTHY HEALING. I realize there are many other fine companies and products who are not listed here, but you can rely on the companies below for their high quality products and good results.

- Alacer Corp., 19631 Pauling, Foothill Ranch, CA 92610, 800-854-0249
- All One, 719 East Haley St., Santa Barbara, CA 93103, 800-235-5727
- Aloe Life International, P.O. Box 710759, Santee, CA 92072, 800-414-2563
- Always Young, 827 Route 82, Suite 281, Hopewell Junction, NY 12533 800-252-8572
- American Health, 2100 Smithtown Avenue, Ronkonkoma, NY 11779, 800-445-7137
- Anabol Naturals, 1550 Mansfield Street, Santa Cruz, CA 95062, 800-426-2265
- Arise & Shine, P.O. Box 400, Medford, OR 97501, 800-688-2444
- Ark Naturals Products for Pets, 6166 Taylor Rd. #105, Naples, FL 34109, 800-926-5100
- Barleans Organic Oils, 4936 Lake Terrell Rd., Ferndale, WA 98248, 800-445-3529
- Baywood Intl., 14950 N. 83rd Pl., Ste.1, Scottsdale, AZ 85260, 800-481-7169
- Beehive Botanicals, Route 8, Box 8257, Hayward, WI 54843, 800-233-4483
- BHI (Heel Inc.) P.O. Box 11280, Albuquerque, NM 87192, 800-621-7644
- Biostrath, 75 Commerce Drive, Hauppauge, NY, 11788-3943, 800-439-2324
- Body Ecology, 218 Laredo Drive, Decatur, GA 30030, 800-511-2660
- Bodyonics (Pinnacle), 140 Lauman Lane, Hicksville, NY 11801, 800-899-2749
- Boericke & Tafel Inc.,(B & T) 2381 Circadian Way, Santa Rosa, CA 95407, 707-571-8202
- Bragg/Live Food Products, Inc., 7340 Hollister Ave., Santa Barbara, CA 93102, 805-968-1028
- Cat's Paw 1-800-CATSPAW (228-7729)
- CC Pollen Co., 3627 East Indian School Rd., Suite 209, Phoenix, AZ 85018-5126, 800-875-0096
- C'est Si Bon, 1308 Sartori Ave. Suite 205, Torrance, CA 90501, 888-700-0801
- Champion Nutrition, 2615 Stanwell Dr., Concord, CA 94520, 800-225-4831
- Clear Products, 4320 Vandever Ave Suite A, San Diego, CA 92120, 888-257-2532
- Coenzyme-A Technologies Inc., 12512 Beverly Park Road B1, Lynnwood, WA 98037, 425-438-8586
- Country Life, 180 Vanderbilt Motor Pkwy, Hauppauge NY, 11788, 800-645-5768
- Crystal Star Herbs, 121-B Calle Del Oaks, Del Rey Oaks, CA 93940, 800-736-6015
- Dancing Paws, 2832 Walnut Avenue, Suite B, Tustin, CA 92780, 888-644-7297
- Designing Health, 28410 Witherspoon Parkway, Valencia, CA 91355, 800-774 -7387
- Diamond/Herpanacine Ass, 145 Willow Grove Ave. #1 Dept. #WP 5, Glenside, PA 19038, 888-467-4200
- Dreamous, 2720 Monterey Ave. Suite 401, Torrance, CA 90503, 800-251-7543
- Dr. Goodpet, P.O. Box 4547, Inglewood, CA 90309, 800-222-9932
- Dr Rath's Vitamins, 1260 Memorex Drive, Suite 200, Santa Clara, CA 95050, 800-624-2442
- EAS, 555 Corporate Circle, Golden, CO 80401, 800-923-4300
- Earth Mama Angel Baby, 9866 SE Empire Court, Clackamas, OR 97015, 503-607-0607
- East Park Research, Inc., 2709 Horseshoe Drive, Las Vegas, NV 89120, 800-345-8367

- Eidon Mineral Products,12330 Stowe Drive, Poway, CA 92060, 800-700-1169
- Enzymatic Therapy, 825 Challenger Drive, Green Bay, WI 54311, 800-783-2286
- Enzymedica, 752 Tamiami Trail, Port Charlotte, FL 33954, 888-918-1118
- Earth's Bounty/Matrix Health Products, 1101 N.E. 144th St. #109, Vancouver, WA 98685, 800-736-5609
- Esteem Products Ltd.,1800 136th Pl. NE Suite 5, Bellevue, WA 98005, 800-954-5515
- Ethical Nutrients/Unipro, 971 Calle Negocio, San Clemente, CA 92673, 800-668-8743
- Fit for You, Intl., 971 S Bundy Dr., Brentwood CA 90049-5828, 800-521-5867
- Flint River Ranch, 1243 Columbia Avenue B-6, Riverside, CA 92507-2123, 888-722-4589
- Flora, Inc., 805 East Badger Road, P.O. Box 73, Lynden, WA 98264, 800-446-2110, (Info.) 604-451-8232
- Futurebiotics, 70 Commerce Drive, Hauppauge, NY 11788, 800-645-1721
- Gaia Herbs, Inc., 108 Island Ford Road, Brevard, NC 28712, 888-917-8269
- Golden Pride, 1501 Northpoint Pkwy., Suite 100, West Palm Beach, FL 33407, 561-640-5700
- Green Foods Corp., 320 North Graves Ave., Oxnard, CA 93030 800-777-4430
- Grifron/Maitake Products, Inc., 1 Madison St. Bldg. F, East Rutherford, NJ 07073, 800-747-7418
- Halo Purely For Pets, Inc. 3438 East Lake Road #14, Palm Harbor, FL 34685, 800-426-4256
- Health from the Sun/Arkopharma, P.O. Box 179, Newport, NH 03773, 800-447-2229
- Herbal Answers, Inc., P.O. Box 1110, Saratoga Springs, New York 12866, 888-256-3367
- Herbal Magic, Inc., P.O. Box 70, Forest Knolls, CA 94933, 800-684-3722
- Herbal Products & Development, P.O. Box 1084, Aptos, CA 95001, 831-688-4200
- HerbaSway Laboratories, 101 North Plains Industrial Road, Wallingford, CT 06492, 800-672-7322
- Herbs Etc.,1340 Rufina Circle, Santa Fe, NM 87507, 888-433-1212
- Home Health, 2100 Smithtown Avenue, Ronkonkoma, NY 11779, 800-445-7137
- Immudyne, 7453 Empire Drive, Suite 300, Florence, Kentucky 41042, 888-246-6839
- Isagenix International, 2225 S. Price Road, Chandler, AZ, 85248, 877-877-8111
- Imperial Elixir, P.O. Box 970, Simi Valley, CA 93062, 800-284-2598
- Jagulana Herbal Products, Inc., P.O. Box 45, Badger, CA 93603, 888-465-3686
- Jarrow Formulas, 1824 South Robertson Blvd., Los Angeles, CA 90035, 800-726-0886
- Jason Natural/Earth's Best, 4600 Sleepytime Dr., Boulder, CO 80301, 800-434-4246
- Lane Labs, 25 Commerce Drive, Allendale, NJ 07401, 800-526-3005
- Lane Labs TOKI, 1-888-AGELESS, Please mention code #6404
- Liddell Laboratories, 1036 Country Club Drive, Moraga, CA 94556, 800-460-7733
- MagiaBella, 5742 West Harold Gatty Drive, Salt Lake City, Utah 84116, 800-871-9954
- MagneLyfe/Encore Technology, Inc., 115 W 29th Street Ste 1100-B, New York, NY 10001, 877-624-6353
- Maine Coast Sea Vegetables, 3 Georges Pond Road, Franklin, Maine 04634, 207-565-2907
- Maitake Products, Inc., 1 Madison St. Bldg. F, East Rutherford, NJ 07073, 800-747-7418
- Mendocino Sea Vegetable Co., P.O. Box 1265, Mendocino, CA 95460, 707-937-2050
- Merix Health Care Products, 18 E. Dundee Rd. #3-204, Barrington, IL 60010, 847-277-1111
- Metabolic Response Modifiers, 236 Calle Pintoresco, San Clemente, CA 92672, 800-948-6296
- Mezotrace Corporation, 415 Wellington St., Winnemucca, NV 89445, 800-843-9989
- Moon Maid Botanicals, 535 Tall Poplar Road, Cosby, TN 37722, 877-253-7853
- Motherlove Herbal Co., P.O. Box 101, Laporte, CO 80535, 970-493-2892
- MRI (Medical Research Institute), 444 De Haro St. Suite 209, San Francisco CA 94107, 888-448-4246
- Mychelle Dermaceuticals, Box 1, Frisco, CO 80443, 800-447-2076
- Natren Inc., 3105 Willow Ln., Westlake Village, CA 91361, 866-462-8736
- Natural Animal Health Products, Inc., 7000 U.S. 1 North, St. Augustine, FL 32095, 800-274-7387
- Natural Balance, 3130 N. Commerce Ct., Castle Rock, CO 80104-8002, 303-688-6633
- Natural Energy Plus, 4630 N. Paseo De Los Cerritos, Tucson, AZ 85745, 888-633-9233
- Natural Labs Corporation (Deva Flowers), P.O. Box 20037, Sedona, AZ 86341-0037, 800-233-0810
- Nature's Answer, 75 Commerce Drive, Hauppauge, NY, 11788-3943, 800-439-2324
- Nature's Apothecary/NOW Foods, 395 S. Glen Ellyn Rd., Bloomingdale, IL 60108, 888-669-3663

- Nature's Path Supplements, PO Box 7862, North Port, FL 34286, 800-326-5772
- Nature's Secret/Irwin Naturals, 5310 Beethoven St., Los Angeles, CA 90066, 800-297-3273
- Nature's Way, 1375 N. Mountain Springs Parkway, Springville, UT 84663, 800-962-8873
- Nelson Bach, Wilmington Technology Park, 100 Research Dr., Wilmington, MA 01887, 800-319-9151
- New Chapter, 90 Technology Dr., Brattleboro, VT 05301, 800-543-7279
- No-Miss Nail Care, 6401 E. Rogers Circle Suite 14, Boca Raton, FL 33487, 800-283-1963
- Nonie of Beverly Hills, Inc., 812 Seward St., Hollywood, CA 90038, 888-666-4324
- NOW, 395 S. Glen Ellyn Rd., Bloomingdale, IL 60108, 888-669-3663
- NutriCology /Allergy Research Group, 2300 North Loop Rd., Alameda, CA 94507, 800-545-9960
- Oshadhi, 1340 G Industrial Ave., Petaluma, CA 94952, 888-674-2344
- Pacific BioLogic, P.O. Box 520, Clayton, CA 94517-0520, 800-869-8783
- Penta Water, 2091 Rutherford Rd., Carlsbad, CA 92008, 800-531-5088
- PetGuard, P.O. Box 668, Green Cove Springs, Florida 32043, 877-PETGUARD
- Pines International, Inc., 1992 East 1400 Road, Lawrence, KS 66044, 800-697-4637
- Planetary Formulas, P.O. Box 533, Soquel, CA 95073, 800-606-6226
- Prince of Peace, 3536 Arden Road, Hayward, CA 94545, 800-732-2328
- PSP Marketing, 23241 Areco Ct., Laguna Nigel, CA 92677, 866-777-5050
- Pure Essence Laboratories, Inc., P.O. Box 95397, Las Vegas, NV 89193, 888-254-8000
- Pure Form, 3240 West Desert Inn Rd., Las Vegas, NV 89103, 888-363-9817
- Pure Planet, 1542 Seabright Ave., Long Beach, CA 90813, 562-951-1124
- Quantum, Inc., 754 Washington St., Eugene, OR 97401, 800-448-1448
- Rainbow Light, 125 McPherson St., Santa Cruz, CA 95060, 800-571-4701
- Rainforest Remedies, Box 325, Twin Lakes, WI 53181, 800-824-6396
- Real Life Research, Inc., 14631 Best Ave., Norwalk, CA 90650, 800-423-8837
- Rejuvenative Foods, P.O. Box 8464, Santa Cruz, CA 95061, 800-805-7957
- Royal Bodycare, 2301 Crown Court, Irving, TX 75038, 972-893-4002
- Solaray, Inc., 1400 Kearns Boulevard, Park City, UT 84060, 800-669-8877
- Source Naturals Inc., 19 Janis Way, Scotts Valley, CA 95066, 800-815-2333
- Spectrum Naturals, 5341 Old Redwood Hwy., Suite 400, Petaluma, CA 94954, 707-778-8900
- Springlife Inc., 4630 N. Paseo De Los Cerritos, Tucson, AZ 85745, 888-633-9233
- Starwest Botanicals, 11253 Trade Center Drive, Rancho Cordova, CA 95742, 800-800-4372
- Sun Wellness (Sun Chlorella), 3305 Kashiwa Street, Torrance, CA 90505, 800-829-2828
- Superior Trading, 835 Washington Street, San Francisco, CA 94108, 415-495-7988
- Tender Care Int. TUSHIES, 3925 North Hastings Way, Eau Claire, WI 54703, 800-344-6379
- Transformation Enzyme Corporation, 2900 Wilcrest, Suite 220, Houston, TX 77042, 800-777-1474
- Trimedica International, Inc., 1895 South Los Feliz Drive, Tempe, AZ 85281-6023, 800-800-8849
- UAS Laboratories, 9953 Valleyview Rd., Eden Prairie, MN 55344, 800-422-3371
- Vibrant Health, 403 Ashley Falls Road, Canaan, CT 06018, 800-242-1835
- Vitamin Research Products, 4610 Arrowhead Drive, Carson City, NV 89706, 800-877-2447
- Wakunaga of America / Kyolic, 23501 Madero, Mission Viejo, CA 92691, 800-421-2998 / 800-825-7888
- Wellements, 3925 E. Watkins St. Suite 200, Phoenix, AZ 85034, 800-255-2690
- Well in Hand, 5164 Waterlick Rd., Forest, VA 24551, 888-550-7774
- Wyndmere Naturals, Inc., 5417 Opportunity Court, Minnetonka, MN 55343, 800-207-8538
- Yoanna Skin Care, P.O. Box 610072, Redwood City, CA 94061, 800-366-4617
- Y.S. Royal Jelly and Organic Bee Farm, 2774 N. 4351 Rd., Sheridan, IL 60551, 800-654-4593
- Zand Herbal Formulas, 1441 West Smith Road, Ferndale, WA 98248, 800-232-4005
- Zia Natural Skincare, 4600 Sleepytime Drive, Boulder, CO 80301, 800-334-7546

Bibliography

Your Health Care Choices Today

Blate, Michael. "Headaches & Backaches." Healthy and Natural Journal. 1994.

Bowles, Willa Vae. "Enzymes for Energy." Total Health. 1993.

Cichoke, Anthony J., D.C. Enzymes & Enzyme Therapy. 1994.

Cichoke, Anthony J., D.C. "Enzyme Therapy." Let's Live. 1993.

Cichoke, Anthony J., D.C. The Complete Book of Enzyme Therapy. Avery Publishing Group. 1999.

Cohen, Kenneth S. "What Is Qigong?" Qigong Healing. www.qigonghealing.com/html/qigong.html

Drexler, Madeline. "Body & Soul." The Natural Way. April/May 1995.

"Evidence Prayer Can Heal." FOXnews.com. June 13, 2000.

Gates, Donna. The Body Ecology Diet. 1993.

Godfrey-June, Jean. "Reflexology: The Body's Mini-health Map." The Natural Way. June/July 1995.

Gregory, Scott J. A Holistic Protocol for The Immune System. 1995.

Grimm, Ellen. "Increase Your Energy with Self-Massage." Natural Health. 1994.

Higley, Connie & Alan. Reference Guide to Essential Oils. Abundant Health. 1998.

"Hypnosis, Meditation and Survival.Newton, B.W. original study: "The Use of Hypnosis in the Treatment of Cancer Patients." American Journal of Clinical Hypnosis 25 (2-3): 104-13 (1982-83).

International Institute of Reflexology. Petersburg, FL.

Krizmanic, Judy. "The Best of Both Worlds." Vegetarian Times. 1995.

Kunz, Kevin & Barbara. "Understanding the Science and Art of Reflexology." Alternative & Complementary Therapies. April/May 1995.

Liberman, Jacob, O.D., Ph.D. Light, Medicine of the Future. 1991.

Liu, Qinshang. "The Art of Qigong." Healthy & Natural, Volume 7, Issue 5.

Liu, Qinshang. "Qi and Qigong." Healthy & Natural, Volume 7, Issue 3.

McClennan, Sam (with Tom Monte). Integrative Acupressure. New York: A Perigee Book. 1998.

"Meditation Decreases Blood Pressure." Alternative Therapies, Vol. 5, No. 6. Nov. 1999.

"Meditation Speeds Healing." Natural Health. March 1999.

Mowrey, Daniel B., Ph.D. The Scientific Validation of Herbal Medicine. Cormorant Books. 1986.

Mowrey, Daniel, Ph.D. Next Generation Herbal Medicine. 1990.

Myss, Caroline, Ph.D. & C. Norman Shealy, M.D., Ph.D. The Creation of Health. 1993.

Newmark, Gretchen Rose, R.D. "Meditation is Something To Think About." Let's Live. Sept. 1994.

"Prevention: The Best Approach To Health." Vegetarian Times. Aug. 1997. Study: The American Journal of Managed Care, Jan. 1997.

Price, Shirley. Practical Aromatherapy: How to Use Essential Oils to Restore Vitality. Thorsons Publishers Limited. 1987.

Robbins, John. Diet For A New America. 1987.

Ruch, Meredith Gould. "Feeling Down?" Natural Health. 1993.

Schneider, J. "Report from Reflexologists: A Look at What People Do." Reflexions, Vol. 6, No. 1. 1985.

Springer, Shelley Cypher, M.D., MBA and Dorothy J. Eicher, M.D. "Effect of a Prayer Circle on a Moribund Premature Infant." Alternative Therapies, Vol. 5, No. 2. March 1999.

Steefel, Lorraine, R.N., M.A. "Use of Acupuncture for Detoxification." Alternative & Complementary Therapies. 1995.

Tisserand, Robert. Aromatherapy to Heal and Tend the Body. 1988.

Valnet, Jean, M.D. The Practice of Aromatherapy. Healing Arts Press. 1990.

Weiss, Rick. "Medicine's Latest Miracle: Acupuncture." The Natural Way. 1995.

Whitaker, Julian. 199 Health Secrets. 1993.

Zamarra, J.W., et al. "Usefulness of the transcendental meditation program in the treatment of patients with coronary artery disease." Am J Cardio, Vol. 77. 1996. pp. 867-70.

Herbal Healing

Abernathy, Sarah. "Herb-Nutrient-Drug Interactions: Facts You Need To Know." Healthy Healing. 2003.

Abernathy, Sarah. "Iatrogenic Disease." Healthy Healing. 2003.

American Herbal Products Association. Botanical Safety Handbook CRC Press. 1997.

Arnold, Kathryn. "Rainforest Medicine." Delicious! 1994.

Baar, Karen. The Real Options in Healthcare. 1995.

Chen, Ze-lin, M.D. & Mei-fang Chen, M.D. Comprehensive Guide to Chinese Herbal Medicine. 1992.

Colbin, Annemarie. Food and Healing. 1986.

Duke, James A., Ph.D. The Green Pharmacy. Rodale Press. 1996.

Fillius, Thomas J., et al. "Chief Two Moons Meridas: Indian Miracle Man?" HerbClip-ABC. 1995.

Frawley, David, M.D. "Ayurveda, the Science of Life." Let's Live. 1993.

Hultkrantz, Ake. Shamanic Healing & Ritual Drama. 1992.

Laux, Marcus. Cures from the Rainforest Pharmacy. 1995.

Marshall, Lisa Anne. "The Roots of Western And Herbal Medicine."Natural Foods Merchandiser. 1994.

Mehl-Madrona, Lewis E., M.D., Ph.D. "Coyote Medicine Heals Body and Spirit." Let's Live. Sept. 1999.

Mendelsohn, Robert & Michael J. Balick. "More Drugs Await Discovery in Rainforests."ABC. 1995.

Murray, Michael, N.D. & Joseph Pizzorno, N.D. Encyclopedia of Natural Medicine. Prima Publishing. 1998.

Page, Linda, N.D., Ph.D. Reduce Stress-Boost Energy. Healthy Healing. 1999.

Reid, Daniel. Chinese Herbal Medicine. Boston: Shambhala. 1993.

Schwontkowski, Donna. Herbal Treasures from the Amazon. 1995.

Treadway, Linda, Ph.D. & Scott Ph.D. Ayurveda & Immortality Berkeley: Celestial Arts. 1986.

Weil, Andrew, M.D. Spontaneous Healing. New York: Alfred A. Knopf Pub. 1995.

Werbach, Melvyn R., M.D. Nutritional Influences On Illness: A Sourcebook Of Clinical Research. 1988.

Wolfson, Evelyn. From the Earth To Beyond the Sky: Native American Medicine. 1993.

Yen-Hsu, Hong. How to Treat Yourself with Chinese Herbs. 1993.

Zucker, Martin. "Women's Health - Ayurveda Offers Ancient Solutions for Modern Times." Let's Live. 1995.

The Alternative Health Care Arsenal

"Cooked vs. Raw." Natural Health. 1999.

"Don't Give Yourself an Ulcer—Eat Broccoli," CNN.com, May 28, 2002.

Greenwood-Robinson, Maggie, Ph.D. "Artichokes For What Ails You." Let's Live. April 2001.

Haas, Elson, M.D. Staying Healthy with Nutrition. Berkeley: Celestial Arts. 1992.

Howard Loomis, D.C. "Indigestion: Why HCL, Antacids, and Pancreatin Are Not The Answer." American Chirop. April 1988.

Kirschman, G.J. and John D. Nutrition Almanac, 4th ed. 1996.

LaValle, James. "Nexrutine: A Breakthrough in Natural Pain Management." Total Health, Vol. 23, No. 4.

London, Cathleen, M.D. "Pantethine: A Critical Player in a Heart-Healthy Lifestyle." Total Health, Vol. 23, No. 4.

Mandile, Maria. "Vinpocetine." Natural Health. Jan/Feb 2002.

Maranan, Julia Tolliver. "NADH." Natural Health. Sept. 2001.

Murray, Michael T., N.D. Encyclopedia of Nutritional Supplements. 1996.

Murray, Michael T., N.D. "Introducing Coleus Forskholii." The Doctor's Prescription for Healthy Living, Vol. 3, No. 2.

"Mushroom Wisdom." Maitake Products Inc. 2002.

Page, Linda, N.D., Ph.D. How To Be Your Own Herbal Pharmacist. Healthy Healing. 1997.

Vanderhaeghe, Lorna. "Nature's Super Stars." Total Health, Vol. 22, No. 4.

Zeligs, Michael A., M.D. & A. Scott Connelly, M.D. All About DIM. Avery Pub. 2000.

Foods for Your Healing Diet

Althoff, Susanne. "The Truth about Coffee." Natural Health. April 2000.

"Americans Do Not Drink Enough Water." www.altmedicine.com 6/12/00.

"Antibiotics: Just Say No." Vegetarian Times. April 2002.

"Antitumor Properties of Chlorella." HerbalGram, No. 20. Spring 1989.

Antonios, F.T. & MacGregor, G.A. Deleterious effects of salt intake other than effects on blood pressure. Clin Exp Pharmacol Physiol., Volume 22. 1995. 180-184.

"A World Of News." Organic: A Way To Grow. Spring 2002.

Berdanier, Carolyn D. CRC Desk Reference For Nutrition. CRC Press. 1998.

Carper, Jean. The Food Pharmacy. Bantam Books. 1988.

Carper, Jean. Food-Your Miracle Medicine. Harper Collins. 1993.

Chua, Val. "Top of the Tea." Asia One Food & Entertaining. Dec. 20, 2001.

"Could Eating Tofu Speed Brain Decline?" CBS HealthWatch. April 3, 2000.

Dieg, et al. "Inhibition of herpes virus replication by marine algae extracts." Anitimicrb. Ag. Chemother, Vol. 6. 1974. pp.524-525.

"Digestive Health." Whole Foods. Dec. 1999.

"Drinking Green Tea May Help you Lose Weight." WebMD. March, 22, 2000.

Duke, James, Ph.D. The Green Pharmacy. Rodale Press. 1997.

"Eggs Might Not Be So Bad After All." WebMD Health. 2001.

Ehresmann, et al. "Antiviral Substances from California Marine Algae." J. Phycol., Vol. 13. pp. 37-40. 1979.

Elkins, Rita, M.H. "Barley Grass- Always Greener." Let's Live. April 2000.

Elmore, Vicki L. "Speaking Out Against GMO's- Genetically Modified Organisms." Healthy & Natural Journal, Vol. 7, Issue 1.

Ensminger, Konlande, & Robson. The Concise Encyclopedia of Foods & Nutrition. CRC Press. 1995.

Erickson, Kim. "Seaweed." Herbs for Health. Sept./Oct. 2001.

Garrison, R. & Somer, E. Nutrition Desk Reference. Keats. 1995.

Gittleman, Anne Louise, N.D., M.S., C.N.S. "Get Your Healthy Fats the Easy Way." Herbs for Health. Nov/Dec. 2001.

Gonzales et al. "Polysaccharides as antiviral agents: antiviral activity of carrageenan." Antimicrobial Agents and Chemotherapy, Vol. 3. 1987. pp. 1388-1393.

"Green Foods Versus Pesticides." Healthy & Natural, Vol. 7, Iss. 1.

Gursche, Siegfried. "Healing With Herbal Juices." Alive, No. 134.

Hausman, Patricia & Judith Benn Hurley. The Healing Foods. Rodale Press. 1989.

Healthwell daily news: "Essential Fatty Acids May Slow or Reverse the Progression of Huntington's Disease." June 8, 2002.

"Heart Attack Victims Should Drink Tea." BBC News. May 7, 2002.

Hobbs, Christopher, L.Ac. Medicinal Mushrooms: An Exploration of Tradition, Healing & Culture. Botanica Press. 1996.

Hobbs, Christopher, LAc., A.H.G. "White Tea: A New Brew." Let's Live. January 2002.

Holloway, William Jr. & Herb Joiner-Bey, N.D. Water: The Foundation of Youth, Health and Beauty. Impakt Health. 2002.

"Hopkins Health Watch: Drinking Milk Doesn't Do A Body Good: Another Risk Factor For Ovarian Cancer." The John R. Lee, M.D. Medical Letter. Aug. 1999.

"How Good Is Soy?" Cnn.com. June 26, 2001.

"In Praise of Coffee." Health & Healing, Vol. 10, No. 9.

Jacobi, Dana. "Soya, oh Boya! A Whole New World of Taste." Better Nutrition. May 1998.

Ji B-T, Chow, et al. "Green tea consumption and the risk of pancre-atic & colorectal cancers." Int J Cancer, Vol. 70. 1997. p. 255-8.

Joiner-Bey, Herb, N.D. "Athlete Alert! The Winning Edge: Optimal Cell Hydration." 1999.

Kaylor, Mark, Ph.D. " Amazing Mushrooms: Reishi, Maitake & Lion's Mane." Health Prdts Business. Jan. 2002.

Khalsa, Karta Purkh Singh, C.N., A.H.G. "Overcome Sugar Addiction." Herbs for Health. Jan./Feb. 2002.

Khalsa, Siri. "Barley Grass, Wheat Grass, and Alfalfa: The Green Grasses." Nutrition News. 2000.

Khalsa, Siri. "Big Fat Lies." Nutrition News. 2001.

Khalsa, Siri. "Mushrooms: Magic, Myth and Medicine." Nutrition News. 1998.

Khalsa, Siri. " The Two Sides Of Soy." Nutrition News. 2000.

Kincaid-Smith, P. & Alderman, M. "Universal recommendations for sodium intake should be avoided." MJA, Vol. 170. 1999. pp. 174-175.

Kliger, Craig. "Diet Nutrition," WebMD. Jan. 2001.

Laird, Harrison. "Soy Comparable to Some Diabetes Drugs." WebMD Inc. 2002.

Landau, Meryl Davids. "Top 10 Natural Remedies." Natural Health.

"Low Salt Diets Could Be Hazardous To Your Health, U.S. doctors warned on Friday." CNN.com. March 13, 1998.

Luke, J. Fluoride Deposition in the Aged Pineal Gland. Caries Research, Vol. 35. 1999. pp. 125-128.

Madison, Deborah. Vegetarian Cooking For Everyone. Broadway Books. 1997.

Mercola, Joseph, Ph.D. "The Potential Dangers of Sucralose." Optimal Wellness Center. www.mercola.com.

Moll, L., et al. Vegetarian Times Complete Cookbook Macmillan.1995.

"More Bitter Truth About Artificial Sweeteners." seasilver.threadnet.com/Preventorium/artifici-2.htm.

Moss, Ralph, Ph.D. Chlorella Shows Promise As Anti-Cancer Supplement Sept. 1994.

Mowrey, Daniel, Ph.D. "Cordyceps: Energy Blast from China." Physical. Oct. 1998.

Murray, Michael T., N.D. Encyclopedia of Nutritional Supplements.1996.

Nachatelo, Melissa. "How Drugs Are Polluting Our Water." Natural Health. Sept. 2001.

Onstad, Dianne. Whole Foods Companion. Chelsea Green. 1996.

"Organic: What's in a Word." CBS Healthwatch. 12/21/00.

"The Organic Report." March 2001.

Osborne, Sally. "Does Soy Have A Dark Side?" Natural Health March 1999.

"Research Shows Milk May Cause Constipation in Some Children." CNN.com. Oct. 15, 1998.

Robbins, John. "It's in the Water." The Connection. March 2000.

Robbins, John. The Food Revolution. Conari Press. 2001.

Runestad, Todd. "GMOs Down on the Pharm." Nutrition Science News. May 2000.

Scheer, James. "Royal Jelly: Hiveful of Healing." Better Nutrition for Today's Living. Dec. 1994.

"Spirulina." Nutrition News. 1998.

"Study: Caffeine may protect the brain from Parkinson's." CNN. com May 23, 2000.

"Study Reports Spirulina Boosts Immune System." Health Products Business. Feb. 2001.

"Tempeh." Natural Health. March 1999.

Tenneson, Michael. "Water." Health. June 2000.

"The Big Lie: Fluoridation helps the poor." IFIN, No. 583. June 24, 2002.

"The Many Health Benefits of Vinegar." Julian Whitaker's Health & Healing. May 1997.

"Tofu Is A Superfood For the 90s." Let's Live. June 1995.

Turner, Lisa. "Energy in a Glass: Green Foods." Let's Live. 1997.

"White House Opposes Biotech Labels." BIO 2002 Conference AP news. www.healthy.net.

Williams, David, M.D. "Alternatives: Health Technology Report." Vol. 9, No. 11.

Williams, David G., M.D. "Humans as Toxic Waste Dumps." Alternatives for a Health-Conscious Individual, Volume 9, No. 12

"Wine, Women, and Greens." Health. May 2000.

www.kushiinstitute.org.

www.macrobiotics.org.

www.nrdc.org/water/drinking/nbw.asp.

www.rejuvenative.com.

www.xlear.com.

Zhou, James, Ph.D. "Luohan: The Magic Fruit." Herbal Wisdom. March 1, 2000.

A Basic Guide to Detoxification

Airola, Paavo, Ph.D. How To Get Well. 1974.

Anderson, Richard, N.D., N.M.D. Cleanse & Purify Thyself. 1994.

Baker, Elizabeth & Dr. Elton. The Uncook Book - Raw Food Adventures to a New Health High. 1983.

Barrettt, Jennifer. "Yoga Basics." Vegetarian Times. Jan. 2002.

Benninger, Jon. "Detox." Energy Times. July 1994.

Blauer, Stephen. Rejuvenation. 1980.

Cassata, Carla. "How To Balance Body Chemistry." Let's Live. March 1995.

Duncan, Lindsey, C.N. "Internal Detoxification." Healthy & Natural Journal. October 1994.

Easterling, John. "Rainforest Bio-Energetics."Healthy & Natural Journal. October 1994.

Gates, Donna. The Body Ecology Diet. 1996.

Goldberg, Burton. Alternative Medicine: The Definitive Guide. 1993.

Haas, Elson M, M.D. The Detox Diet. Berkeley: Celestial Arts. 1996.

Harrison, Lewis. 30 - Day Body Purification: How To Cleanse Your Inner Body & Experience the Joys of Toxin-Free Health. 1995.

Hobbs, Christopher. "Herbs For Health - Losing Addictions Naturally." Let's Live. April 1993.

Hobbs, Christopher."Tonics, Bitters, Digestion, and Elimination." Let's Live. August 1990.

Kennedy, David C., DDS. Letter & Paper (Addressing Fluoride's Relationship to Dental Fluorosis, Hip Fracture, Cancer, & Tooth Decay Costs Savings). June, 18, 1998

Jensen, Bernard, D.C. Tissue Cleansing Through Bowel Management. 1981.

Langer, Stephen, M.D. "Keeping Environmental Toxins At Bay." Better Nutrition For Today's Living. July 1993.

Larson, Joan Mathews, Ph.D. Seven Weeks To Sobriety. 1992.

Lewallen, Eleanor and John. Sea Vegetable Gourmet Cookbook & Wildcrafter's Guild. 1996.

Markowitz, Elysa. Living With Green Power: A Gourmet Collection of Living Food Recipes. 1997.

McCay, Julie. "What is Yoga?" Healthy & Natural Journal, Vol. 6, Issue 1.

Murray, Michael, N.D. & Joseph Pizzorno, N.D. Encyclopedia of Natural Medicine. Prima Publishing. 1998.

"Nutrients and Herbs for the Recovering Addict." Health World. July 1992.

Rafkin, Louise. "Yoga Keeps Many Feeling Young." CNN.com Aug. 17, 2000.

Rogers, Sherry A., M.D. "Doctors' Dialogue: Toxic Encephalopathy." Let's Live. March 1995.

Rosen, Kelli. "Yoga, Yoga Everywhere." Herbs for Health. May/June 2001.

Schaeffer, Rachel. "Calm Digestive Upset With Yoga." Natural Health. July 2002.

Schechter, Steven, N.D. Fighting Radiation & Chemical Pollutants with Foods, Herbs & Vitamins: Documented Natural Remedies that Boost Your Immunity & Detoxify. 1994.

Thomson, Bill. "Rejuvenate Yourself in Three Weeks." Natural Health. January 1993.

Walker, Norman, D.SC., Ph.D. Colon Health. 1979.

Walker, N.W. D. Sci. Raw Vegetable Juices. Jove Books. 1987. www.yogasite.com.

"Yoga: Healing the Body, Quieting the Mind." CNN.com. June 3, 1999.

Healing Programs for People with Special Needs

Abel, Robert, Jr., M.D. The DHA Story. Basic Health Pub. 2002.

Aesoph, Laurie, N.D. "When Should Parents Worry?" New Hope Communications. Sept. 1992.

Anderson, Nina and Howard Peiper, Ph.D. "Bad Scraps, Vegetarian Pets, and Ringworm." Healthy & Natural Jnal. V. 4, Issue 5.

Anderson, Nina and Howard Peiper, Ph.D. "Essential Fatty Acids Important To Pets." Healthy & Natural Journal. V. 4, Issue 6 .

"An E-asy Answer To Infertility Problems." Natural Foods Merchandiser. March 1998.

"Are germs killing your sperm?' Men's Health, March 1999.

"Ask the Experts." Natural Health. April 2000.

Barclay, Laurie, M.D. "Homeopathy a Good Alternative for Treating Ear Infections." WebMD. Feb 16. 2001.

Barela, Sharon. "The Secrets of Longevity." Veggie Life. 1997.

Batmanghelidj, F., M.D. Your Body's Many Cries for Water. 1996.

Bauman, Edward, Ph.D. Eating For Health: A Regenerative Five Food Group System. 1994.

Bennett, Michael L., PharmD. "Vanity Medicine with Human Growth Hormone." Nutrition Science News. Nov. 2000.

Borysenko, Joan & Miroslav. The Power of the Mind to Heal: Renewing Body, Mind & Spirit. 1994.

"Brain Function Harmed." Allergy Hotline. Nov. 1998.

"Breast Time for Baby." Vegetarian Times. July 1998.

Broadhurst, C. Leigh, Ph.D. "The Essential PUFA Guide for Dogs and Cats." Nutrition Science News. Oct. 2001.

Brown, Donald, N.D. Herbal Prescriptions for Better Health. 1995.

Burgstiner, Carson B., M.D. "You Are What You Eat." Health Counselor. 1991.

Burke, Edmund, Ph.D. "ACSM Conference Unveils Performance Enhancers." Nutrition Science News, Vol. 6, No. 9. Sept. 2001.

Burke, Edmund R., Ph.D. "What To Do When Exercise Is Through." Nutrition Science News. May 1999.

Bushkin, Gary, Ph.D., CNC and Estitta Bushkin, Ph.D, CNC. "Children's Health, Naturally." Health Prts Business. Oct. 2002.

Calechman, Steve. "Consumer Guide: Feel Younger Than You Are." Natural Health. April 2002.

"Cat's Claw." The Healthy Cell News. Fall/Winter 1997.

Challem, Jack. "Consumer Guide: Vitamins That Protect Against Aging." Natural Health. April 2002.

Chang, Helen. "Lactobacillus." The Natural Foods Merchandiser July 2002.

"Children's Dietary Needs Go Unmet." Nutrition Science News. February 1998.

"Cholesterol Kids Is Your Child at Risk?" Let's Live. March 1997.

Cichoke, Anthony J., M.D. The Complete Book of Enzyme Therapy. Avery Pub. 1999.

Colgan, Michael. M.D. Optimum Sports Nutrition. 1993.

Connelly AS, A. Effect of leucine metabolite beta-hydroxy-beta-methylbutyrate on muscle metabolism during resistance-exercise training. J Appl Physiol, Vol. 81. 1996. pp. 2095-2104.

"Consumer News: Natural Critter Care." E-Mag. May/June 1998.

"Creatine May Help People with Muscular Dystrophy and ALS." NNFA Today, Volume 13, No. 4. April 1999.

DeCava, Judith, C.C.N., L.N.C. "Exercise and Physical Health." ANMA 2000.

Denda, Margare E. & Phyllis S. Williams. The Natural Baby Food Cookbook. 1982.

"Deodorant For Your Pet." Life Enhancement. Sept. 1998.

DeNoon, Daniel. "Growth Hormone Linked to Cancer." WebMD. July 25, 2002.

"Does Sugar Make You Old Before Your Time?" Natural Health. Jan/Feb 1993.

Dossey, Larry, M.D. Healing Words. 1993.

"Drop the Pounds with Pooch." Letsliveonline.com. Oct 2002.

Dustman, Karen Dale. "Is Your Dog a Doctor?" Natural Health. Jan/Feb 1999.

"Expert: Aerobic Exercise Can Help Manage Glaucoma." FOXnews.com. June 5, 2000.

"Fat Cats and Big Dogs." Vegetarian Times. Jan 1999.

Fitzgerald, Frances. "Working On Muscles Without Bulking Up." Health Counselor, Vol. 9, No. 1.

Fontaine, Darryl & David Minard. Forever Young: How To Energize Your Body Naturally. 1993.

Fremerman, Sarah. "Shots in the Dark." Natural Health. Nov./Dec. 1999.

Gallia, Katherine. "How Schools Are Failing Our Kids." Natural Health. July 2002.

Goldstein, Martin, D.V.M. The Nature of Animal Healing. 1999.

"Good News on SIDS." Time. June 22, 1998.

"Growth Hormone Improves Symptoms in Crohn's Disease Patients."CNN.com. June 1, 2000.

"Health Bites." The Healthy Cell News. Spring/Summer 1997.

"Health Bulletin: The Weakest Drink." Men's Health. July 2002.

"Health News: Thanks for the Memories, Lecithin!" Natural Health. Sept/Oct 1995.

"Healthy Eating After 70." Health News. 1999.

Hobbs, Christopher. Ginkgo: Elixir of Youth. 1995.

Hobbs, Christopher. "Herbs For Fitness."Let's Live. 1991.

Hoffman, Jay M., M.D. Hunza: 15 Secrets of the World's Healthiest& Oldest Living People. 1979.

Howell, Edward, M.D. Enzyme Nutrition: The Food Enzyme Concept. 1985.

Huemer, Richard P., M.D. "The Facts of Lice." Let's Live. Sept. 1999.

"Improve Energy Fight Aging with Alpha Lipoic Acid." Herbs for Health. Sept./Oct. 1999.

"Inoculations May Be Rx For Disaster." The John R. Lee, M.D. Medical Letter. Nov. 1999.

"Intestinal Parasites." MotherNature.com.

"Is there a Limit to Human Life Expectancy?" Life Extension. Sept. 2002.

Jaret, Peter. "Alternative Medicine for Rover." WebMD.com.

Jones, Susan Smith. The Main Ingredients of Health & Happiness.1995.

Kervran, Louis, Ph.D. "Silica-Secret To Longevity." Flora Herbal Medicine Research Report, Vol. 1, No. 1. Winter 1998.

Khalsa, Siri. "Beat the Clock." Nutrition News. 1997.

Khalsa, Siri. "Cat's Claw: The Claw of the Jungle." Nutrition News. 1996.

Khalsa, Siri. "It's Time to Get Fit." Nutrition News. 2000.

Kidd, Parris M., Ph.D. Phosphatidylserine Offers Nutritional Support for brain function. Vitamin Retailer Magazine. Jan 1996.

Kidd, Randy, D.V.M. "Herbal First Aid for Pets." Herbs for Health. Nov./Dec. 2001.

Kidd, Randy, D.V.M. "Herbal Help for Ear Infections." Herbs for Health. May/June 2002.

Kidd, Randy, D.V.M. "Seven-step Herbal Health Program for Pets." Herbs for Health. Jan/Feb 2002.

King, Frank, Jr., Ph.D. "Homeopathic Answers for Vaccination." Healthy & Natural Journal, Vol. 6, Issue 4.

Krastek, Caroline. "Pet Power." Whole Foods. March 1998.

Kugler, Hans, Ph.D. "Interview." Nutrition & Healing. 1995.

"Lack of Sleep Alters Hormones, Metabolism." Doctor's Guide Oct. 22, 1999.

"Learn 2 Take a Pulse." Learn2.com.

Lee, John, M.D. "Getting Pregnant and Staying Pregnant." The John R. Lee M.D. Medical Letter. Sept. 1998.

Lee, John, M.D. "Kids and Nutrition." The John R. Lee, M.D. Medical Letter. June 2002.

"Let's Get Physical." Whole Foods. Feb. 1998.

Lewy AJ, et al. Melatonin treatment of winter depression: Pilot study. Psychiatry Res, Vol. 77. 1998. pp. 57-61.

Loehr, Dr. James E. & Dr. Jeffrey A. Migdow. Take A Deep Breath. 1986.

Maltin, Liza Jane. "High Protein Diets Cause Dehydration: Can Be Dangerous to even Most Physically Fit." WebMD. April 22, 2002.

Mars, Brigitte. " Herbs To Know About During Pregnancy." Let's Live. Feb. 1991.

"Massage Delivers Babies." Natural Health. Nov/Dec 1998.

"Melatonin Helps Break Valium Dependence." Nutrition Science News, Vol. 6, No. 3. March 2001.

Morantz, Alison. "Creatine." Natural Health. May/June 1998.

Morien, Krista. "Herbs in the News: Results Of Fertility Study Unfruitful." Herb Research Foundation, Vol.3, No 1.

"Mold Menacing Students Costing Millions." CNN.com. Nov. 25, 2002.

Murray, Michael T., N.D. "Evaluating Magnesium." American Journal of Natural Medicine. Dec. 1996.

Murray, Michael T., N.D. Healing Power of Herbs. 1992.

Murray, Michael T., N.D. The Complete Book of Juicing. 1992.

Murray, Michael T., N.D. The Healing Power of Foods. 1993.

"Mussels for Dogs." Letsliveonline.com. July 2000.

"Natural Response." Nutrition & Healing, Vol. 6, Iss. 4. April 1999.

"Nature's Medicine." Nutrition News, Vol. XX, No. 12. 1996.

"New Study Demonstrates that CordyMax® Cs-4 Enhances Endurance and Exercise Performance." http://www.pharmanex.com/eHealth/articles/Cordymax.shtml.

"Newsbites: Currying Flavor." Vegetarian Times. March 2002.

Nissen, S, et al. Natural Healing for Dogs & Cats. 1999.

"Nutrition Supplement: Vitamins, Minerals, and More." Herbs for Health. Sept/Oct. 1999.

Orey, Cal. "Top Dog- Good Nutrition for Healthy Pets." Let's Live. Nov. 1997.

Passwater, Richard A., Ph.D. The New Super Nutrition. 1991.

Peiper, Howard & Nina Anderson. Are You Poisoning Your Pets? 1995.

Peiper, Howard & Nina Anderson. Over 50 Looking 30! 1996.

"Pesticides Residues: Cause For Concern." Health News, April 15, 1999.

Peters, Bonnie. "Baby Massage Eases Colic." Healthy & Natural, Vol.7, Issue 4.

Phillips, Bill. Supplement Review. 1996.

"Phospatidylserine." Life Extension. Sept. 2002.

Pitcairn, Richard H., D.V.M., Ph.D. & Susan H. Pitcairn. Natural Health for Dogs & Cats. 1995.

Pizzorno, Lara, M.A., L.M.P. "Longevity." Delicious! May 1994.

Pizzorno, Lara, M.A., L.M.P. "Pregnancy: Grounds for a Caffeine Break." Delicious! May 1994.

"Pregnant? 2 Cans of Tuna Per Week OK." WebMD.com. July 31, 2002.

"President Bush Launches Healthier US Initiative." June 2002.

"Protect Against Brain Aging." Life Extension. Sept. 2002.

"Protection Against Dirty Air." Men's Health. Dec. 1998.

Province, MA, et al. The effect of exercise on falls in elderly patients. A preplanned meta-analysis of the FICSIT trials JAMA, Vol. 273. 1995. pp. 1341-7.

Rostler, Suzanne. "Type 2 Diabetes Epidemic in Children Coming." Yahoo! Daily News. September 13, 2000.

Samuels, Mike, M.D. & Nancy Samuels. The Well Adult. 1988.

"Selenium Supplements Can Reduce Cancer Rates, New Study Shows." Cornell University. Jan 7, 1999.

Shaw, Gina. "Couch-Potato Culture: Trading Convenience for Health." CBS HealthWatch. April 2000.

"Should Schools Report That Kids are Fat?" Natural Health. Aug. 2002.

Shuman, Jill M., M.S., R.D. "Healthful Aging." NFM's Nutrition Science News. April 1996.

Siegel, Bernie, M.D. How To Live Between Office Visits. 1993.

Silberman, Alex. "Forever Young?" Vegetarian Times. Feb. 2000.

"Sleep's healing properties." CNN.com. Aug. 25, 1999.

Smith, Ian, M.D. "Crazy for Creatine." Time. June 12, 2000.

Smith, Ian, M.D. "Hard Knocks." Time. Oct. 2, 2000.

Swift, Russell, D.V.M. "Dealing with Kidney Failure Holistically." www.pettribune.com.

"Tea for Two." Men's Health. Dec. 1998.

"The Natural Way to Take Care of Your Pet." Whole Foods. 1995.

"The Truth Behind the Headlines." Dr. Julian Whitaker's Health & Healing. March 2000.

Toews, Victoria Dolby, M.P.H. "Protect your Child from the Fat Epidemic." Letsliveonline.com. Feb 2002.

"True Life Story of the Effect of Aspartame on the Unborn Child." Leading Edge Research. 1996.

Tunella, Kim, C.D.C. "Enzymes...The Spark of Life." 1994.

"Vaccines Against Natural Processes." www.mercola.com/article/vaccines/against_natural_processes.html.

"Vaccine Refusal May Cause NY To Take Children." Healthkeepers Magazine. Spring Summer 2001.

Vierhile, Tom. "The 'Paw'ticulars of Natural Pet Food." Health Products Business. April 2002.

"Vitamin E in the Golden Years." Vegetarian Times. Oct. 1997.

"Vitamin E Prevents Muscle Damage After Weight Lifting." Quarterly Review of Natural Medicine Summer. 1998.

Walford, Roy L. "Calorie Restriction: Eat Less, Eat Better, Live Longer." Life Extension. Feb 1998.

"Walking reduces women's heart attack risk." CNN.com. 1999.

Weil, Andrew, M.D. "hGH: Forever Young." Herbs for Health. March/April 2000.

White, Linda, M.D. "Can You Take Herbs During Pregnancy?" Delicious! May 1997.

White, Linda B., M.D. & Sunny Mavor. Kids, Herbs & Health: A Parent's Guide to Natural Remedies. May 1999.

Wigmore, Ann. Recipes for Longer Life. 1978.

Williams, David, Ph.D. "Keep Your Cells Young for 100 Years or More." Alternatives for the Health-Conscious Individual. 2001.

"Workplace Chemicals Drop Sperm Count: Printers, Painters at Highest Risk." WebMD. Sept. 13, 2001.

www.arknaturals.com

www.dogshealth.com

Zand, Janet, LAc, OMD, et al. Smart Medicine For a Healthier Child. 1994.

Zucker, Martin. "Cholesterol Kids: Is Your Child at Risk?" Let's Live. March 1997.

Ailment Analysis & Health Programs

"ACAM Convention 2002." Life Extension. Feb. 2003.

"ADHD Options." Choices, Vol. 2, No. 3. May 2002.

Aesoph, Laurie, N.D. "Everything You Should Know about Sexually Transmitted Diseases." Delicious! March 1993.

Aesoph, Lauri, N.D. "Get Your Blood Flowing." letsliveonline.com, Nov. 2000.

Ahmed, Aftab J., Ph.D. "Osteoporosis: Diet, Acidity and Calcium." Total Health, Vol. 24, No. 2.

Almada, Anthony L., BSc, MSc. "OTC Fire Extinguishers: Natural Options for Arthritis." Health Products Business. April 2000.

"Alternative Approaches to Treating ADD." Let's Live. Sept. 1998.

Althoff, Susanne. "Getting Under Your Skin." Natural Health. Jan/Feb 2000.

"Aluminum and the risk of hip fractures." American Journal of Natural Medicine, Vol. 2, No. 3. April 1995.

"Alzheimer's Disease Could Triple by 2050." WebMD July 22, 2002.

American Journal of Obstetrics & Gynecology, Vol. 170, No.5, Pt 2. 1994. pp. 1543-9.

"Anemia Alert." First for Women. Sept. 29, 1997.

"Antioxidant May Improve Men's Fertility." Health Products Business. Nov. 2002.

Anton, Rein, M.D., Ph.D. "Reversing Heart Disease Through Oral Chelation." 1997.

"Are My Breasts Normal?" First for Women. June 17, 2002.

"Are You Using The Best Birth Control?" First For Women. March 4, 2002.

"Artichoke Extract: Triglyceride Buster." The Doctors' Prescription for Healthy Living, Vol. 3 No. 2.

Azmeh-Scanlan, Kathy. "Breathe Easy This Spring." Herbs for Health. March/April 2002.

"Bad News: Alpha Trouble." Time. March 20, 2000.

"Bad News: STD Update." Time. Dec. 18, 2000.

"Bad to the Bone." Health Sciences Institute e-Alert. April 30, 2003.

Balch, James, M.D. "Bone Up- But Don't Count on Calcium Alone." Prescriptions for Healthy Living, Issue 37.

Balch, James, M.D. & Phyllis Balch C.N.C. Prescription for Nutritional Healing. Penguin Putnam. 2000.

Benagh, Barbara. "Asthma Answers." Yoga Journal. July/August 2000.

Berkson, D. Lindsay. "Hormone Deception." Total Health, Vol. 24, No. 5.

"Body Battles HIV." The ANMA and AANC Journal. April 1995.

Bojic L., et al. Oxygenation in the Treatment of Macular Degeneration. Split, Yugoslavia: Split Naval Medical Institute. pp. 1-4.

Bouchez, Colette. "Some Breast Cancer Drugs May Body's Defense Against Recurrence." Health on the Net Foundation. April 17, 2003.

"Bowel Goes Wacky After Laparoscopic GERD Surgery." Joseph Mercola M.D. http://www.mercola.com.

Boyles, Salynn. "Anorexics' Survival Rate Normal." WebMD. March 13, 2003.

Broadhurst, C. Leigh, L, Ph.D. "PUFAs for Bone Growth and Repair." Nutrition Science News. March 2001.

"Brain Cells Regenerate." HealthKeepers Magazine. Spring-Summer 2001.

"Broccoli May thwart Herpes Virus." WebMD. Sept. 15, 2003.

Cancer Epidemiol Biomarkers Prev. "Chlorine in water linked to bladder, rectal cancers." AztecOne. Vol. 11, No. 8. 2002. pp. 713-8.

Cancer Facts & Figures 2003. American Cancer Society. 2003.

"Can Coffee Promote Osteoporosis?" Nutrition Science News. Sept. 2000.

"Chlorine May Start Heart Disease." PersonalMD.com. Journal of Clinical Investigation. 1996. p. 98.

"Cancer Prevention: Why Aren't We Trying." WebMD. March 10, 2003.

"CDC Reports Jump in Flu-related Deaths." CNN.com. Jan 7, 2003

Challem, Jack. "Gut Feelings and the Origin of Autism." letsliveonline.com. May 2001.

Challem, Jack. " How To Heal A Failing Heart." Letsliveonline.com, Aug. 2000.

Challem, Jack. "How to Use Vitamins and Minerals as Home Remedies." Natural Health. March/April 1994.

Challem, Jack. "St. John's Wort Works." Letsliveonline.com. March 2002.

Chang, Vivian. "On the Lookout for Hidden Lactose." Digestive Health & Nutrition. March/April 2002.

Christy, Martha M. Overcoming the Acid Crisis. Wishland. 2002.

"Cigarettes and Hair." Allure. Sept. 2003.

Circulation. Journal of the American College of Cardiology, Vol. 36, No. 1. 2000. pp. 102, 326-340, 380-385.

"CLA Combined with Cellulite Therapy Shows Dramatic Improvement." Life Extension. March 2003.

Clark, Carol. "Paying the price of AIDS." CNN.com. 2003.

"Clearing up the picture on laser eye surgery." CNN.com. February 26, 2003.

"Clinical Tip 30: Preventing Herpes Simplex with Selenium." Nutrition & Healing. Nov. 1998.

"Clinical Tip 66: Keep Your Gallbladder....Quit Eating Your Allergies." Nutrition & Healing. March 2000.

"Coffee May Cause Incontinence." Herbs for Health. Nov/Dec 2000.

Cumming RG and Klineberg RJ: Aluminum in antacids and cooking pots and the risk of hip fractures in elderly people. Ageing, Vol. 23. 1994. pp. 468-72.

"Daily Tooth Care Tips." Natural Health. May 2000.

Darlington, Joy. "Beating the Blood Sugar Blues." Vegetarian Times. April 2000.

"David Beats Goliath Again." Health Sciences Institute e-Alert, May 15, 2003.

"D! Briefs." Delicious! Jan. 1999.

DeCava, Judith, C.C.N., L.N.C. "Exercise and Physical Health." ANMA. 2000.

DeNoon, Daniel. "Deep Kiss Could Spread Cancer Virus." WebMD Medical News. Nov. 8, 2000.

DeNoon, Daniel. "Tai Chi Each Day Keeps Shingles Away." WebMD Medical News. Sept. 22, 2003.

"Diet Axes Jet Lag." The Natural Foods Merchandiser. Nov. 2002.

"Diet Deters Alzheimer's." letsliveonline.com. Oct. 2002. Study: JAMA, Vol. 287 2002. pp. 3223-3237, 3261-3263.

"Diet, Exercise Slow Prostate Cancer As Much As 30%." Daily University Science News. Sept. 11, 2001.

"Doctor on Call." First for Women. 11/23/98.

"Do You Have Hepatitis C?" Men's Health. March 1999.

"Do You Know What's Best For Your Back." Health. May 2000.

Drury, Kathyrn. "Lip Service." Vegetarian Times. Oct 2000.

DuBow, Wendy, Ph.D. "Good Night." Delicious Living. March 2003.

"Ease Anxiety with Shankhpushpi." Natural Health. Sept. 2002.

Elkins, Rita, M.H. "Fight Emphysema with Supplements." letsliveonline.com. Nov. 2002.

Elkins, Rita, M.H. "Foil the Flu." letsliveonline.com. Feb 2003.

"Endometriosis." Herbs for Health. July/August 2002.

"Exercise May Reduce Gallbladder Disease Risk." CNN.com. Sept. 8, 1999.

Fahey, Catherine. "Keep Your Adrenals Healthy." letsliveonline. Dec. 2001.

Faloon, William. "The Hidden Cancer Epidemic." Life Extension. Feb. 2003.

Faraji, M.H. & A.H. Haji Tarkhani. "Effect of sour tea (Hibiscus sabdariffa) on essential hypertension." Journal of Ethnopharmacology, Vol.7. 1999. pp. 231-236.

"Fatigue Brought to Its Knees." Health Products Business. June/July 2002.

"FDA Issues Vioxx Warning." CNN.com. March 25, 2002.

"Fibroid Help." Herbs For Health. May/June 2002.

"Fibroid Removal and Future Pregnancy." The John R. Lee, M.D. Medical Letter. Dec. 2002.

"Food Allergy & Crohn's Disease." Nutrition & Healing. April 1995.

"Food for Thought: The Role of Triglycerides." Science News Online. Sept. 21, 1996.

"For patients- What is a Pacemaker?" www.ccspace.com/PAT/patinf.html

"Fraction from Sangre de Grado Treats AIDS Related Diarrhea." HerbClip. May 30, 2000.

"From My Readers." The John R.Lee, M.D. Medical Letter. Feb. 2003.

Freundlich, Naomi. "A Vaccine Worse Than The Disease." Business Week. Oct.23, 2000.

"Gene Shows Who's 'Got Milk.'" CNN.com. Jan 13, 2002.

"Ginseng May Fight Bacterial Infection, Help Cystic Fibrosis Sufferers." CBS HealthWatch. May 25, 2001.

Gittleman, Ann Louise, M.S., CNS. Guess What Came to Dinner? Avery Pub. 2001.

Golin, Mark. "Morning Forecast: A 14 Point Health Checklist." Men's Health. July 1995.

Gorman, Christine. "Are Some People Immune to AIDS?" Time. March 1993.

Gormley, James. "Gutsy Moves." Health Products Business. Dec.2002.

Gottlieb, Bill (ed). Prevention Magazine Health Books. New Choices in Natural Healing: Over 1,800 of the Best Self-Help Remedies from the World of Alternative Medicine. 1995.

"Green Tea for Diabetes." Delicious Living. March 2003.

"Green Tea Protects Against Alcohol-induced Liver Injury." Life Extension. Sept. 2002.

"Growing evidence indicates that exercise cuts chance of breast cancer." CNN.com. March 13, 2000

Haas, Elson, M.D. The False Fat Diet. Ballantine Pub. 2000.

Haas, Elson, M.D. Staying Healthy With Nutrition. Celestial Arts Pub. 1992.

"Have Ageless Eyes." First For Women. 7/16/01.

"Headache hope." Vegetarian Times. Aug. 2002.

Head, Kathi, N.D. & Peter Chowka. "Avoid Kidney Stones with Good Nutrition." letsliveonline.com. March 2003.

Head, Kathi, N.D. "Coping with Diabetes Naturally." letsliveonline.com. Dec. 2002.

"Health Bulletin: A bad drug combination." Men's Health. Jan-Feb. 2002.

"Health Bulletin: Bake Away Back Pain." Men's Health. Oct. 2002.

"Health Bulletin: Depression can cloud more than your judgement." Men's Health. Nov. 1999.

"Health Bulletin: Heart Stopping Cell Phones." Men's Health. Nov. 1997.

"Health Bulletin: LDL on the Brain." Men's Health. Sept. 2002.

"HealthNews." Business Week. Nov. 19, 2001.

"Health officials: SARS could come back." CNN.com. Sept. 26, 2003.

"HealthWatch." Yoga Journal. 2001.

"Heart Disease Risk and Abdominal Fat." Life Extension. Nov. 2002.

"Helping the Brain Heal Itself." Let's Live. April 2000.

Hematol Oncol Clin North Am, Vol.14, No.2. April 2000. pp. 339- 53.

Herbal Research Publications. The Protocol Journal Of Botanical Medicine. 1995.

"Herb Mix Nixes Prostate Cancer in Lab." WebMD. Dec. 13, 2002.

Hobbs, Christopher, L.A.c. & Beth Baugh. "Get Over Your Hangover." letsliveonline.com. Dec. 2002.

Hobbs, Christopher, L.A.c. "Take the Ouch Out of Ear Infections." letsliveonline.com. Nov. 2002.

"Hopkins Health Watch: Electromagnetic Radiation and Miscarriage." The John R. Lee, M.D. Medical Letter. March 2003.

"Hopkins Health Watch: Iron Update." The John R. Lee, M.D. Medical Letter. June 2000.

"Hopkins Health Watch: Oh No, Not Another Cousin of Fosamax." The John R. Lee, M.D. Medical Letter. Dec. 1998.

"Hopkins Health Watch: Statin Lowers LDL but not Death Rate." The John R. Lee, M.D. Medical Letter. Jan. 2003.

"Hormone Replacement Therapy Poses Greatest Risk Of Heart Attack In First Year Of Use For Most Women." www.ahaf.org/whatsnew/H_HRT_Aug_2003.htm.

Horn, Clare. "Bad Breath Solutions." Natural Health. April 2000.

"Hot Tub Therapy May Help Diabetics." CNN.com. Sept. 16, 1999.

"How effective are latex condoms in preventing HIV?" www.cdc.gov/hiv/pubs/faq/faq23.htm.

Huemer, Richard, M.D. "Crohn's: Are Steroids To Blame." Let's Live. Jan 2000.

Hurd, Lyle. "The Gonzales-Isaacs Cancer Program." Total Health, Vol. 22, No. 4.

"Interview: A Promising New (yet old) Treatment for MS." The John R. Lee, M.D. Medical Letter. Dec. 1999.

"Ipriflavone: A Foundation For Healthy Bones." Total Health. 2002.

"I Tried Naet." Natural Health. August 2002.

"Is High Blood Pressure Inevitable." CNN.com. Feb. 27, 2002.

Jaffe, Harry. "New Coke." Men's Health. June 2002.

Jnadourek A, Vaishampayan JK, & Vazquez JA. Efficacy of melaleuca oral solution for the treatment of fluconazole refractory oral candidiasis in AIDS patients. AIDS, Vol. 12. 1998. pp. 1033-7.

Jones, Cindy, L.A., Ph.D. "Ginkgo for Arterial Disease." Herbs for Health. March/April 2002.

Johnson, Lois, M.D. "Help for Polycystic Ovary Syndrome." Herbs for Health. March/April 2001.

Kahn, Sherry. M.H.P. "The Hyperactivity Puzzle." letsliveonline.com. Aug. 2001.

Kane, Emily, N.D., L.A.c. "Clear Up Your UTI." Letsliveonline.com. July 2001.

Kane, Emily, N.D., L.A.c. "Toothaches and Gum Problems." Let's Live. July 1998.

Kane, Emily. N.D., L.A.c. "Turn Down TheVolume on Tinnitus." letsliveonline.com. Aug. 2002.

Karlson, Amy Elizabeth. "In Fine Form: How Posture Plays a Role in Your Health." Vegetarian Times. Oct. 2002.

Khalsa, Dharma Singh, M.D. & Malcolm Riley D.D.S. "Stress, Aging and the Brain." Total Health, Vol. 24, No. 3.

Khalsa, Karta Purkh Singh, C.D.N., A.H.G. "Butterbur: Nature's Newest Antihistamine." Let'sliveonline.com. Sept. 2002.

Khalsa, Karta Purkh Singh, C.D.N., R.H. "Fighting Fibromyalgia." Herbs for Health. May/June 2003.

Khalsa, Karta Purkh Singh. "Find Relief From Eczema." letsliveonline.com. March 2003.

Khalsa, Karta Purkh Singh, C.N., A.H.G. "Peruvian Sex Herb and More... Maca." Let's Live. Nov. 1999.

Khalsa, Siri. "Many Things Nobody Ever Told You About Menopause." Nutrition News. 2002.

Khalsa, Siri. "Windows to the Soul." Nutrition News. 1999.

Kidd, Parris, Ph.D. "Phosphatidylserine for Energy, Stress and Mood." Total Health. 2003.

"Kidney and Urological Diseases Statistics for the United States." National Kidney and Urological Diseases Information Clearing House. 1996.

"Kids at Risk for Asthma Epidemic." Healthy & Natural Journal, Vol. 7, Issue 4. Aug. 2000.

Kirchheimer, Sid. "In Vitro Linked to Rare Bladder Defects." WebMD. March 19, 2003.

Kirchheimer, Sid. "Is Acne Fed by the Western Diet." WebMD. Dec. 19, 2002.

Knittel, Linda. "Anti-Aging." letsliveonline.com. April 2003.

Koontz, Katy. "Use it or Lose it." Vegetarian Times. Aug. 2000.

La Puma, John, M.D., FACP. "Clinical Briefs: Writing Therapy to Reduce Asthma and RA Symptoms." Alternative Medicine Alert, Vol. 2, No. 6.

LeVan, Barry. "New Therapy For Irritable Bowel Syndrome." Life Extension. Nov. 2002.

Lohn, Martiga. "The Bowl Turn." Natural Health. April 1999.

"Long term vitamin C consumption lowers early-onset cataract incidence." Life Extension. May 2002.

"Low Cholesterol Can Be Too Low." Alternative Medicine. July 1999.

Lyn, Tan Ee. " SARS Virus Likely Came from Civet Cats." Netscape News. May 23, 2003.

"Macular Degeneration Linked to Infection." WebMD. April 24, 2003.

"Magnet Therapy May Quiet Voices in Schizophrenia." Archives of General Psychiatry, Vol. 60. 2003. pp. 49-56.

"Mammogram Guidelines Expanded." CNN.com. Feb. 21, 2002.

"Mammography Mix-Up." Vegetarian Times. July 1998.

"Many Gays with HIV Don't Know It." MSNBC news. June 8, 2002.

"Many Mammograms Have False-Positive Outcomes." FOXnews.com. Oct. 18, 2000.

Margulies, Paul, M.D., F.A.C.P., F.A.C.E. "Addison's Disease: The Facts You Need to Know." NADF. 1999.

Maranan, Julia. "Consumer Guide: Annual Women's Health Guide." Natural Health. Dec. 2002.

Mead, Paul S. et al. Food-Related Illness and Death in the United States. Centers for Disease Control and Prevention. Atlanta.

"Medical Updates: Coenzyme Q10 and Kidney Failure." Life Extension. Sept. 2002.

Medline (The Physician's National Medical Research Database). Physical Conditions Affected By A Deficiency Of The Metabolic Catalysts. Hawaii Medical Library, Inc.

"Melatonin Helps Break Valium Dependence." Nutrition Science News, Vol. 6, No. 3. March 2001.

Melatonin in Epilepsy: First Results of Replacement Therapy and First Clinical Results. Fautek J-D, Schmidt H, et al: Biol SignalsRecept, Vol. 8, No. 1. 1999. pp. 105-110.

Miller, Alan, N.D. "Healing Eczema From the Inside Out." Letsliveonline.com. Dec. 2002.

Morris, Lois B. "Mood News: Shots for Sadness." Allure. May 2003.

Morrison, Kara G. Screening and Education: Most people with STDs Never Show Symptoms and Annual Physical Exams Don'tTest For Them. Detroit News. Nov. 6, 2002.

Myers, Charles, M.D. "Natural Doesn't Always Mean Harmless: Arthritis Supplement Could Lead to the Spread of Prostate Cancer." Health Sciences Institute. July 2002.

Nachatelo, M. "Ease Your Asthma." Natural Health. Nov/Dec 2000.

"Natural Health Newswire: Cacium is the Best Hearing Aid." Let's Live. Dec. 1998.

"Nerve finding helps explain why emotional memories endure." CNN.com. Dec. 21, 1998.

"New Hope for Alzheimer's." Alternatives. March 2002.

"News and Notes: Massage your Gums." Natural Health. July 2002.

"Niacinamide Works." Alternatives. March 2002.

Nicksin, Carole. "The Heartbreak of Psoriasis." Vegetarian Times. April 2000.

"Nicotine Vaccine Tests Launched." September 10, 2001. http://news.bbc.co.uk/1/hi/health/1535852.stm.

"No Safe Haven." E-Magazine. Sept./Oct. 1998.

"Nutrition Bulletin." Men's Health. May 2002.

"Nutrition Bulletin: Shell Shocker." Men's Health. April 2002.

Panda S, Kar A. Ocimum sanctum leaf extract in the regulation of thyroid function in the male mouse. Pharmacol Research, Vol. 38. 1998. pp. 107-10.

"Patients Taking Cholesterol Drugs May Need Extra Co-enzyme Q." NFM's Nutrition Science News. March 1996.

Pizzorno, Lara. "Nature's Arsenal Against AIDS." Health & Nutrition Breakthroughs. March 1998.

"Playing Chicken." Time. March 9, 1998.

"Preliminary FoodNet Data on the Incidence of Food-borne Illnesses -- Selected Sites, United States, 2000. " CDC Food-Borne Diseases Active Surveillance Network (FoodNet).

"Preliminary FoodNet Data on the Incidence of Food-borne Illnesses -- Selected Sites, United States, 2001." CDC Foodborne Diseases Active Surveillance Network (FoodNet).

"Prevent Heat Exhaustion." First For Women. Aug. 18, 1997.

Quillin, Patrck, Ph.D., R.D., C.N.S. "Reversing Prostate Cancer." letsliveonline.com. Nov. 2002.

"Q & A." Life Extension. Dec. 2002.

Quillin, Patrick, Ph.D., R.D., C.N.S. "Nutritional Therapies For Colon Cancer." Letsliveonline.com. March 2002.

"Quit Smoking with Acupuncture." Natural Health. April 2003.

"Quiz: Are You Depressed?" Depression.com.

Randall, C. et al. Nettle sting of urtica dioica for joint pain- an exploratory study of this complementary therapy. Complement Ther Med, Vol. 7, No. 3. Sep. 1999. pp. 126-31.

Rea, William, M.D. "Could Chemical Overload be the Cause of Your illness." The John R. Lee, M.D. Medical Letter. Aug. 2000.

"Red Flag Raised Over 'Normal' Blood Pressure." CNN.com. May 14, 2003.

Reilly, Lee. "The Search for a Baldness cure." Vegetarian Times. May 1997.

"Research Roundup." Dr. Whitaker's Health & Healing. Oct. 2000.

Rodriguez-alfageme, C. et al. B cells malignantly transformed by Human Immunodeficiency Virus are polyclonal. Virology, 252. 1998. pp. 34-38.

Rountree, Robert, M.D. "7 Herbal Antibiotics." Letsliveonline.com. July 2001.

Rowland, Rhonda. "Scientists find stress linked to acne." CNN.com. May 15, 2002.

"SAMe Aids Arthritis Without Side Effects." Life Extension. Oct. 2002.

Sardi, Bill. "A New Look at Eye Health." Nutrition Science News. April 2001.

Schiavetta, Michael,."Stimulating Trends in Sexual Health." Health Products Business. June 2003.

Schulze, Richard. "Your Colon: The Root of all Health." Healthy & Natural Journal, Vol. 6, Issue 1.

"Scoop: Oil Change." Vegetarian Times. July 2002.

Segal, E. F. "Let the Eyes Have It." Vegetarian Times. Aug. 1998.

"Sex & Health: Bed Bugs that Really Bite." Men's Health. July/Aug. 1998.

Sheehan, Jan. "Taming TMJ." Delicious! Sept. 1999.

"Should Ritalin be Required for Hyperactive Kids?" Natural Health Magazine. Oct./Nov. 2001.

Siblerud RL, Motl J, & Kienholz E. Psychometric evidence that dental amalgam mercury may be an etiological factor in manic depression. J. Orthomolec Med, Vol. 13. 1998. pp. 31-40.

Sloan, Mark, N.D. "Mammograms: Prove To Be No Better Than Self-Exams." World Health News, Vol. 5, No. 3. Fall 2001.

"Smoking and Skin Cancer." Total Health. June 1993.

Soeken, KL. et al. Safety and efficacy of SAM-e for osteoarthritis. J. Fam Pract, Vol. 51, No. 5. 2002. pp. 425-43,

"Soothing Compounds." Herbs for Health. May/June 2002.

SPV-30 boxwood extract LEF book + U.S. study Int. J. Phytother. Phytopharmacol. 1998.

Stein, Diane. The Natural Remedy Book For Women. 1995.

"Stem Cells come through again." Alternatives. Jan. 2003.

"St. John's Wort May Stave Off Pink Elephants." Health Products Business. Feb. 1999.

Strauss, Edward, M.D, "Bone Density Scans The Test Women Don't Think About." Total Health, Vol. 24, No. 3.

"Stroke Deaths Expected to Double by 2032." WebMD. Feb 14, 2003.

"Study: Plant estrogen requires lower dose." Herbs for Health. March/April 1998.

Strum, Stephen M.D., FACP. "Understanding the Global Threat of SARS (Severe Acute Respiratory Syndrome)." Life Extension. June 2003.

"Study finds hay-fever medication worse than alcohol in impairing driver skills." CNN.com. March 6, 2000.

"Study: Head Injuries Early in Life May Lead to Alzheimer's Disease." CNN.com. Oct. 24, 2000.

"Study Outlines Faulty Mammogram Readings." CNN.com. Sept. 18, 2002.

Sullivan, Karin Horgan. "The Iron File." Vegetarian Times. July 1996.

"Summary of probable SARS cases with onset of illness from 1 November to 31 July 2003" (revised 26 Sept. 2003). WHO website.

"Super bugs pose bigger threat than SARS." WebMD April 30, 2003.

Suttman, U. et al. Weight gain and increased concentrations of receptor proteins for tumor necrosis factor after patients with symptommatic HIV infection received fortified nutrition support. J Am Diet Assoc, Vol. 96. 1996. pp. 565-69.

"Taurine Reverses Damage Done by Smoking and Protects Against Heart Disease." Life Extension. March 2003.

Teitelbaum, Jacob, M.D. "Say goodbye to Chronic Fatigue Syndrome and Fibromyalgia." Total Health, Volume 24, No. 4.

The $35.00 Blood Panel: A Guide For Patients.

"The Dangers of Cholesterol-Lowering Drugs." Dr. Julian Whitaker's Health & Healing. Sept. 1998.

"The Hidden Cancer Epidemic." Life Extension. Feb. 2003.

The Life Extension Foundation. Disease Prevention & Treatment.2000.

"The Lowdown on Aspartame." Dr. Whitaker's Health & Heaing, Vol. 12, No. 3. March 2000.

"The New Cholesterol Tests." American Health. Sept. 1999.

"The Role Of The Epstein-barr And Human Immunodeficiency Viruses In Aids Lymphoma." http://www.fccc.edu/research/reports/report98/astrin.html.

"The Truth About Cholesterol." First For Women. June 28, 1997.

"The Truth Behind the Headlines." Health & Healing. March 2000.

The Under-Over." Health Sciences Institute e-Alert. Feb. 6, 2003.

"The Watchful Eye." Herbs for Health. July/August 1999.

Thiel, Robert J., Ph.D., N.M.D. "Nutrition and Down Syndrome: Clinical Rationale and Results." ANMA. 1996.

"This is Your Brain on French Fries." Lipids, Vol. 29, No. 4. 1994. pp. 251-58. sln.fi.edu/brain/nutrition/fats/transfats.html.

Tillson, Rodney. "Straighten Up." Energy Times. March 2003.

Toews, Victoria, M.P.H. "Protect Your Child from the Fat Epidemic." letsliveonline.com. Feb. 2002.

"Too Many Bypasses." Men's Health. March 1998.

"Top Remedies to Prevent Prostate Problems." letsliveonline. com. June 2002.

Torsegno, M. & Zucchi, M. "Treatment of Mental Patients with a Preparation of the Total Alkaloids of Rauwolfia serpentina Benth." Minerva Med., Vol. 46. (Turin, Italy). Sept. 1955. pp. 604-607.

"Tracking the Hidden Epidemics: Trends in STDS in the United States." Centers for Disease Control and Prevention. 2000.

"Treat Allergies- Prevent Pain." First. April 2, 2001.

"Treating Sinusitis Naturally." Natural Health. April 2003.

Tse, Paul, A.H.C.M., C.E.T., C.T., R.Ac. The Detoxification, Immunostimulation and Healing Properties of Chlorella. World Convention of Traditional Medicine & Acupuncture. Singapore. March 18-19, 2000.

Tucker, Arthur, Ph.D. "Herbal Remedies for Warts." Herbs for Health. May-June 1999.

"Update on vitamin E for Patients with Tardive Dyskinesia." Quarterly Review of Natural Medicine. Winter 1998.

Vanderhaeghe, Lorna. "Alzheimer's and the Immune System." Total Health, Vol. 24, No. 4.

"Viagra Deaths Explained By New Understanding Of Platelet Clumping." University of Illinois at Chicago. Jan. 10, 2003.

"Vitamin A May Impede Retinitis Pigmentosa." Better Nutrition for Today's Living. Sept. 1993.

"Vitamin C for Gallbladder Health." Herbs for Health. July/August 2000.

Vogel, J. Phillip. "A New Era for SAMe." Life Extension. June 2003.

"Weight Loss Improves Incontinence." The John R. Lee, M.D. Medical Letter. Dec. 2002.

Weil, Andrew, M.D. "Ask Dr. Weil." Self-Healing. March 2000.

"Wheat grass and colitis." Life Extension from Scandinavian Journal of Gastroenterology, Vol.37, Iss 4. 2002. pp. 444-449.

"WHO: SARS in China 'linked to STD'" CNN.com. April 4, 2003.

"Why Are Migraines in Young Women on the Increase?" The John R. Lee M.D. Medical Letter. Feb. 2000.

Williams, David, M.D., "Sunlight, Son Bright." Alternatives. Oct. 2001.

Willard, Terry, Cl.H., Ph.D. "Shine Energizing Light on those Mid-Winter Blues." Healthy & Natural, Vol 7, Issue 1. Feb 2000.

"Women's Heart Disease, Heart Attacks, and Hormones." The John R. Lee, M.D. Medical Letter. Aug. 1998.

Wood, Sharon J. "Uncovering Lesser-Known Symptoms." Digestive Health & Nutrition. March/April 2002.

www.cdc.gov

www.apdaparkinson.org

www.cfids.org

www.copa.org/med/sperm.htm

www.epilepsyfoundation.org

www.globalchange.com/viagranews2.htm

www.healthrecovery.com/nicotine_addiction_relapse.html

www.heartprotect.com

www.jonkaiser.com

www.madsci.org/dtm/estro.html

www.pneumotox.com

www.sanavita.com/dermazinc/dandruff.html

www.seasonale.com

www.skfriends.com/is-vasectomy-risky.htm

www.thermography.net

"Your Health: Sunlight and Cataracts." Let's Live. Sept. 2000.

Zucker, Martin. "From Fatigued to Fabulous." letsliveonline.com. Feb 2003.

Zucker, Martin. "How to Treat your Feet Naturally." letsliveonline. com. Jan. 2002.

Zucker, Martin. "It's in Your Hands." Vegetarian Times. May 1998.

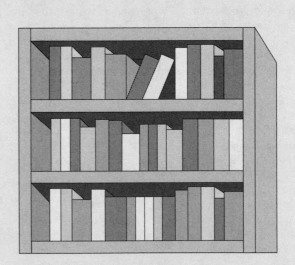

Index

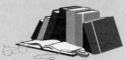

H

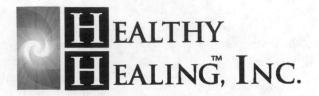

Healthy Healing, Inc.

HEALTHY HEALING - *Twelfth Edition, A Guide to Self Healing for Everyone* - by Linda Page, Ph.D. and Traditional Naturopath - An over 650-page alternative healing reference used by professors, students, health care professionals and private individuals. $32.95 - ISBN 1-884334-92-X   •New - Spiral bound version! $35.95 - ISBN - 1-884334-93-8

DIETS FOR HEALTHY HEALING - *Natural Solutions to America's 10 Biggest Health Problems* - by Linda Page, Ph.D. and Traditional Naturopath - Your primary guide to using food as your best medicine. 256 pages $18.95 - ISBN 1-884334-83-0 • New - eBook CD-ROM version! $18.95

DO YOU WANT TO HAVE A BABY? - *Natural Fertility Solutions and Pregnancy Care* - by Linda Page, Ph.D. and Traditional Naturopath, and Sarah Abernathy - Experience the journey of fertility, conception, pregnancy and birth, naturally! 176 pages $14.95 - ISBN 1-884334-39-3

HOW TO BE YOUR OWN HERBAL PHARMACIST - *Herbal Traditions, Expert Formulations* - by Linda Page, Ph.D. and Traditional Naturopath - A complete reference guide for herbal formulations and preparations. 256 pages $18.95 - ISBN 1-884334-78-4

DETOXIFICATION - *All You Need to Know to Recharge, Renew and Rejuvenate Your Body, Mind and Spirit!* - by Linda Page, Ph.D. and Traditional Naturopath - A complete encyclopedia-guide of detailed instructions for detoxification and cleansing. 264 pages $21.95 - ISBN 1-884334-54-7

PARTY LIGHTS - *Healthy Party Foods & Earthwise Entertaining* - Linda Page, Ph.D. and Traditional Naturopath, and Doug Vanderberg - A party reference book with over 70 parties and more than 500 original recipes you can prepare at home. 358 pages $19.95 - Sale! $9.95- ISBN 1-884334-53-9

THE BODY SMART SYSTEM - *The Complete Guide to Cleansing & Rejuvenation* - by Helene Silver - A complete 21 day regimen and guide that includes diet, relaxation techniques, massage and bath, exercise programs and recipes. 242 pages $19.95 - ISBN 1-884334-60-1

DVD-VIDEO "UNLEASHING THE HEALING POWER OF HERBS" - Linda Page presents information about herbs in this beautifully produced, educational, hour long video program. $19.95 - ISBN 1-884334-95-4

EXPANDED LIBRARY SERIES
by Linda Page, Ph.D. and Traditional Naturopath   ISBN - 1884334 -

14-8 **FATIGUE SYNDROMES 46 pages - Sale! $1.98**

64-4 **RENEWING FEMALE HEALTH 48 pages - Sale! $2.25**

90-3 **MENOPAUSE & OSTEOPOROSIS 64 pages - Sale! $2.98**

36-9 **CANCER 96 pages - Sale! $4.48**

15-6 **SEXUALITY 96 pages - Sale! $4.48**

66-0 **WEIGHT LOSS** & Cellulite Control **96 pages - Sale! $4.48**

67-9 **STRESS & ENERGY** Larger Format **96 pages - Sale! $4.98**

THE HEALTHY HEALING LIBRARY SERIES
by Linda Page, Ph.D. and Traditional Naturopath
32 pages, Sale! $1.75 each. ISBN - 1884334 -

13-X **REVEALING THE SECRETS OF ANTI-AGING**

47-4 **COLDS, FLU & YOU** - Building Optimum Immunity

34-2 **BOOSTING IMMUNITY WITH POWER PLANTS**

30-X **RENEWING MALE HEALTH & ENERGY**

(**Book availability and prices subject to change.**)

To Order:
**Healthy Healing, Inc. • 121-b Calle Del Oaks • Del Rey Oaks, CA 93940
Call: 1-800-736-6015 or fax: 1-800-260-4349
www.healthyhealing.com**   Code: HH12 8/06